THIRD EDITION

Hematopoietic Stem Cell Transplantation:
A Manual for Nursing Practice

Edited by
Kim Schmit-Pokorny, RN, MSN, OCN®, BMTCN®, and
Seth Eisenberg, RN, ADN, OCN®, BMTCN®

Oncology Nursing Society
Pittsburgh, Pennsylvania

ONS Publications Department

Publisher and Director of Publications: William A. Tony, BA, CQIA
Senior Editorial Manager: Lisa M. George, BA
Assistant Editorial Manager: Amy Nicoletti, BA, JD
Acquisitions Editor: John Zaphyr, BA, MEd
Staff Editor: Andrew Petyak, BA
Associate Staff Editor: Casey S. Kennedy, BA
Design and Production Administrator: Dany Sjoen
Editorial Assistant: Judy Holmes

Library of Congress Cataloging-in-Publication Data

Names: Schmit-Pokorny, Kim, editor. | Eisenberg, Seth, editor. | Oncology
  Nursing Society, issuing body.
Title: Hematopoietic stem cell transplantation : a manual for nursing
  practice / edited by Kim Schmit-Pokorny, Seth Eisenberg.
Other titles: Hematopoietic stem cell transplantation (Ezzone)
Description: Third edition. | Pittsburgh, Pennsylvania : Oncology Nursing
  Society, [2020] | Includes bibliographical references and index.
Identifiers: LCCN 2020007411 (print) | LCCN 2020007412 (ebook) | ISBN
  9781635930405 (paperback) | ISBN 9781635930412 (ebook)
Subjects: MESH: Hematopoietic Stem Cell Transplantation--nursing
Classification: LCC RD123.5 (print) | LCC RD123.5 (ebook) | NLM WH 380 |
  DDC 616.02/774--dc23
LC record available at https://lccn.loc.gov/2020007411
LC ebook record available at https://lccn.loc.gov/2020007412

Publisher's Note

This book is published by the Oncology Nursing Society (ONS). ONS neither represents nor guarantees that the practices described herein will, if followed, ensure safe and effective patient care. The recommendations contained in this book reflect ONS's judgment regarding the state of general knowledge and practice in the field as of the date of publication. The recommendations may not be appropriate for use in all circumstances. Those who use this book should make their own determinations regarding specific safe and appropriate patient care practices, taking into account the personnel, equipment, and practices available at the hospital or other facility at which they are located. The editors and publisher cannot be held responsible for any liability incurred as a consequence from the use or application of any of the contents of this book. Figures and tables are used as examples only. They are not meant to be all-inclusive, nor do they represent endorsement of any particular institution by ONS. Mention of specific products and opinions related to those products do not indicate or imply endorsement by ONS. Websites mentioned are provided for information only; the hosts are responsible for their own content and availability. Unless otherwise indicated, dollar amounts reflect U.S. dollars.

ONS publications are originally published in English. Publishers wishing to translate ONS publications must contact ONS about licensing arrangements. ONS publications cannot be translated without obtaining written permission from ONS. (Individual tables and figures that are reprinted or adapted require additional permission from the original source.) Because translations from English may not always be accurate or precise, ONS disclaims any responsibility for inaccuracies in words or meaning that may occur as a result of the translation. Readers relying on precise information should check the original English version.

Printed in the United States of America

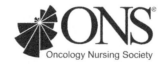

Innovation • Excellence • Advocacy

We dedicate this book to our patients and their families. We thank the authors of each chapter for their expertise and contributions to complete the third edition of *Hematopoietic Stem Cell Transplantation: A Manual for Nursing Practice*. We also appreciate the thoughtful comments from the field reviewers.

I thank my husband, Kevin, and children, Christopher and Megan, for their love and encouragement that supported me throughout this project. I also thank my colleagues at my work and across the country for their support and the work that they do for our patients.

—Kim Schmit-Pokorny

In addition, I thank Rosemary Ford for her unwavering passion for hematopoietic stem cell transplantation nursing practice and education, as well as for her invaluable guidance and mentorship.

—Seth Eisenberg

Contributors

Editors

Kim Schmit-Pokorny, RN, MSN, OCN®, BMTCN®
Manager, Blood and Marrow Transplant Program
Nebraska Medicine
Omaha, Nebraska
Chapter 5. Stem Cell Collection

Seth Eisenberg, RN, ADN, OCN®, BMTCN®
Professional Practice Coordinator, Infusion Services
Seattle Cancer Care Alliance
Seattle, Washington
Chapter 10. Hepatorenal and Bladder Complications

Authors

Jody B. Acheson, RN, DNP, MPH, OCN®, BMTCN®
Bone Marrow Transplant/Hematologic Malignancies Program Manager
St. Luke's Cancer Institute
Boise, Idaho
Chapter 4. Considerations in Program Development and Sites of Care

Shelley Burcat, MSN, RN, AOCNS®, CCCTM
Clinical Nurse Specialist
Philadelphia, Pennsylvania
Chapter 3. Current Research

Katherine Byar, MSN, APN, BC, BMTCN®
Nurse Practitioner
Nebraska Medicine
Omaha, Nebraska
Chapter 6. Transplant Treatment Course and Acute Complications

Suni Dawn Elgar, MPH, BSN, RN, OCN®
Associate Director of Clinical Operations, Apheresis, Blood and Marrow Transplant, Hematology, and Immunotherapy
Seattle Cancer Care Alliance
Seattle, Washington
Chapter 13. Relapse and Subsequent Malignancies

Kelly A. Hofstra, RN, BSN, OCN®, BMTCN®
Program Coordinator
St. Luke's Cancer Institute
Boise, Idaho
Chapter 4. Considerations in Program Development and Sites of Care

Keriann Kordas, MSN, APN
Advanced Practice Provider, Hematology/Oncology, Cellular Therapy
University of Chicago Medicine
Chicago, Illinois
Chapter 12. Neurologic Complications

Martha Lassiter, RN, MSN, AOCNS®, BMTCN®
Clinical Nurse Specialist
Division of Cellular Therapy and Hematologic Malignancies
Duke University Health System
Durham, North Carolina
Chapter 1. Overview of Hematopoiesis and Immunology

Theresa Latchford, RN, MS, BMTCN®, AOCNS®
Oncology Clinical Nurse Specialist
Stanford Health Care
Stanford, California
Chapter 16. Emerging Cellular Therapies: Chimeric Antigen Receptor T Cells

Rebecca Martin, BSN, RN, OCN®, BMTCN®
Staff Registered Nurse/Educator
Froedtert Hospital, Medical College of Wisconsin
Milwaukee, Wisconsin
Chapter 9. Gastrointestinal Complications

Sandra A. Mitchell, PhD, CRNP, AOCN®
Research Scientist, Outcomes Research Branch
Nurse Practitioner, Chronic Graft-Versus-Host Disease Clinic and Study Group
National Cancer Institute
Rockville, Maryland
Chapter 7. Acute and Chronic Graft-Versus-Host Disease

Joyce L. Neumann, PhD, APRN, AOCN®, BMTCN®
Program Director, Stem Cell Transplantation and Cellular Therapy
Adjuvant Ethicist, Section of Integrated Ethics
University of Texas MD Anderson Cancer Center
Houston, Texas
Chapter 15. Ethical Considerations

Kimberly A. Noonan, DNP, ANP-BC, AOCN®
Nurse Practitioner
Dana-Farber Cancer Institute
Boston, Massachusetts
Chapter 9. Gastrointestinal Complications

Rebecca Pape, MSN, APN, FNP-C
Advanced Practice Provider, Hematology/Oncology, Cellular Therapy
University of Chicago Medicine
Chicago, Illinois
Chapter 12. Neurologic Complications

Pamela D. Paplham, DNP, AOCNP®, FNP-BC, FAANP
Nurse Practitioner (BMT Survivorship)
Roswell Park Comprehensive Cancer Center
Buffalo, New York
Assistant Dean of MS/DNP Programs
Clinical Professor of Nursing
State University of New York at Buffalo
Buffalo, New York
Chapter 7. Acute and Chronic Graft-Versus-Host Disease

Lisa A. Pinner, RN, MSN, CNS, CPON®, BMTCN®
Clinical Nurse Specialist
Stanford Children's Hospital
Palo Alto, California
Chapter 14. Late Effects and Survivorship Care

Jean A. Ridgeway, DNP, MSN, APN, AOCN®
Advanced Practice Provider, Hematology/Oncology, Cellular Therapy
University of Chicago Medicine
Chicago, Illinois
Chapter 12. Neurologic Complications

Robin Rosselet, DNP, APRN-CNP, AOCN®
Director of Oncology Advanced Practice Providers
Assistant Professor, The Ohio State University College of Nursing
Arthur G. James Cancer Hospital and Solove Research Institute at
    The Ohio State University
Columbus, Ohio
Chapter 8. Hematologic Effects

Elaine Z. Stenstrup, MSN, APRN, ACNS-BC, AOCNS®, BMTCN®
Clinical Nurse Specialist, Oncology and Blood and Marrow Transplant
University of Minnesota Health
Minneapolis, Minnesota
Chapter 2. Basic Concepts of Transplantation

Jennifer M.L. Stephens, MA, PhD, RN, OCN®
Assistant Professor
Athabasca University
Athabasca, Alberta, Canada
Staff Nurse
Leukemia/Bone Marrow Transplant Program of British Columbia
Vancouver General Hospital
Vancouver, British Columbia, Canada
Chapter 11. Cardiopulmonary Complications

Kelli Thoele, PhD, RN, ACNS-BC, BMTCN®, OCN®
Clinical Nurse Specialist
Robert Wood Johnson Future of Nursing Scholar
Indiana University School of Nursing
Indianapolis, Indiana
Chapter 17. Professional Practice

D. Kathryn Tierney, RN, BMTCN®, PhD
Oncology Clinical Nurse Specialist
Blood and Marrow Transplantation
Stanford Health Care
Stanford, California
Clinical Assistant Professor, Division of Primary Care and Population
    Health
Stanford University School of Medicine
Stanford, California
Chapter 14. Late Effects and Survivorship Care; Chapter 16. Emerging Cellular Therapies: Chimeric Antigen Receptor T Cells

Mihkaila Maurine Wickline, MN, RN, AOCN®, BMTCN®
Nursing Supervisor, Long-Term Follow-Up
Seattle Cancer Care Alliance
Seattle, Washington
Chapter 13. Relapse and Subsequent Malignancies

Disclosures

Editors and authors of books and guidelines provided by the Oncology Nursing Society are expected to disclose to the readers any significant financial interest or other relationships with the manufacturer(s) of any commercial products.

A vested interest may be considered to exist if a contributor is affiliated with or has a financial interest in commercial organizations that may have a direct or indirect interest in the subject matter. A "financial interest" may include, but is not limited to, being a shareholder in the organization; being an employee of the commercial organization; serving on an organization's speakers bureau; or receiving research funding from the organization. An "affiliation" may be holding a position on an advisory board or some other role of benefit to the commercial organization. Vested interest statements appear in the front matter for each publication.

Contributors are expected to disclose any unlabeled or investigational use of products discussed in their content. This information is acknowledged solely for the information of the readers.

The contributors provided the following disclosure and vested interest information:

Kim Schmit-Pokorny, RN, MSN, OCN®, BMTCN®: Juno Therapeutics, Kite Pharma, Novartis, consultant or advisory role, honoraria

Seth Eisenberg, RN, ADN, OCN®, BMTCN®: B. Braun Medical, Genentech, ICU Medical, United States Pharmacopeia, consultant or advisory role; ICU Medical, honoraria

Katherine Byar, MSN, APN, BC, BMTCN®: Creative Educational Concepts, honoraria

Keriann Kordas, MSN, APN: Kite Pharma, consultant or advisory role; Merck, honoraria

Theresa Latchford, RN, MS, BMTCN®, AOCNS®: Kite Pharma, honoraria

Rebecca Martin, BSN, RN, OCN®, BMTCN®: Jazz Pharmaceuticals, honoraria

Kimberly A. Noonan, DNP, ANP-BC, AOCN®: Celgene, consultant or advisory role

Pamela D. Paplham, DNP, AOCNP®, FNP-BC, FAANP: American Society for Transplantation and Cellular Therapy, honoraria

D. Kathryn Tierney, RN, BMTCN®, PhD: American Society for Transplantation and Cellular Therapy, Oncology Nursing Society, honoraria

Licensing Opportunities

The Oncology Nursing Society (ONS) produces some of the most highly respected educational resources in the field of oncology nursing, including ONS's award-winning journals, books, online courses, evidence-based resources, core competencies, videos, and information available on the ONS website at www.ons.org. ONS welcomes opportunities to license reuse of these intellectual properties to other organizations. Licensing opportunities include the following:

- **Reprints**—Purchase high-quality reprints of ONS journal articles, book chapters, and other content directly from ONS, or obtain permission to produce your own reprints.
- **Translations**—Translate and then resell or share ONS resources internationally.
- **Integration**—Purchase a license to incorporate ONS's oncology-specific telephone triage protocols or other resources into your institution's EMR or EHR system.
- **Cobranding**—Display your company's logo on ONS resources for distribution to your organization's employees or customers.
- **Educational reuse**—Supplement your staff or student educational programs using ONS resources.
- **Customization**—Customize ONS intellectual property for inclusion in your own products or services.
- **Bulk purchases**—Buy ONS books and online courses in high quantities to receive great savings compared to regular pricing.

As you read through the pages of this book, think about whether any of these opportunities are the right fit for you as you consider reusing ONS content—and the contents of this book—for your organization.

Contact licensing@ons.org with your licensing questions or requests.

Contents

Preface

Hematopoietic stem cell transplantation (HSCT) has evolved into a treatment option for many types of diseases, and indications for HSCT continue to expand. The term *HSCT* will be used to identify transplantation throughout the book. The reader must read carefully to determine if the source of stem cells is autologous, syngeneic, or allogeneic; if the stem cells are collected from the bone marrow, peripheral blood, or umbilical cord blood; and if the preparative regimen is myeloablative or nonmyeloablative.

This publication was preceded by nursing manuals related to bone marrow (1994) and peripheral blood stem cell transplantation (1997) that were published by the Oncology Nursing Society (ONS). Many institutions used these books as guidelines for nursing practice and education. For many years, HSCT was seen as highly experimental treatment as pioneers in the field sought to improve outcomes and look for innovative ways to mitigate side effects. As a result of this research, standards have emerged for medicine and nursing practice, which ultimately paved the way for certification.

The first and second editions of *Hematopoietic Stem Cell Transplantation: A Manual for Nursing Practice* were published by ONS in 2004 and 2013, respectively. We thank the previous editor, Susan Ezzone, for her work as editor on both editions. In this edition, we want to continue to promote the expansion and dissemination of knowledge regarding HSCT for nurses working in the specialty and nurses caring for patients prior to and after transplantation. The specialty of HSCT and nursing practice continues to grow and evolve. As editors, we hope this publication will be a valuable educational resource for nurses caring for patients as they journey through the HSCT continuum.

CHAPTER 1

Overview of Hematopoiesis and Immunology

Martha Lassiter, RN, MSN, AOCNS®, BMTCN®

Introduction

Hematopoiesis and immunology provide the foundation for oncology principles and are the scientific basis of hematopoietic stem cell transplantation (HSCT). Hematopoiesis is one of the best understood stem cell–associated processes (Jankowski et al., 2018). It is a multistep process involving the interplay among hematopoietic stem cells (HSCs), the bone marrow microenvironment, cellular adhesion molecules (CAMs), chemokines, and cytokines. Cell renewal mechanisms are important because of senescence, utilization, and emigration (Wilson & Trumpp, 2006). Thus, the main objective of hematopoiesis is to maintain the peripheral blood with a constant level of different types of blood cells. Given that the specialized cells of the immune system develop from HSCs, immune function is partially dependent on hematopoiesis. The immune system is a configuration of cells and organs with specialized roles in defending against infection. Two types of immune responses exist: innate and acquired. *Innate* responses occur naturally and use phagocytic cells that release inflammatory mediators, as well as natural killer (NK) cells. *Acquired* responses involve antigen-specific B and T cells and are either humoral or cell mediated (Richards, Watanabe, Santos, Craxton, & Clark, 2008). Although immune function cells develop from HSCs, they must interact with primary and secondary immune system organs to complete their development and participate in immune interactions. Problems arise within the immune system as a result of overwhelming infection, inherited genetic mutations, acquired disorders, aging, and medications that interfere with normal immune function (Hunt, Walsh, Voegeli, & Roberts, 2010). In addition, malignancies and therapies affecting cells originating from HSCs also contribute to immune malfunction.

The purpose of this chapter is to provide an overview of hematopoiesis and immunology so that oncology nurses caring for HSCT recipients may gain and apply fundamental knowledge to clinical practice and educate patients and their caregivers throughout the transplant process.

Hematopoiesis and Immunology Across the Life Span

Aging is a common occurrence that affects all healthy cells, tissues, and organs, including the bone marrow; thus, age-related hematologic changes occur throughout the life cycle. Two types of marrow exist: red and yellow. Red marrow consists of HSCs and originates in flat and long bones. Yellow marrow consists of fat cells and resides in the hollow interior of the middle portion of long bones. At birth, all bone marrow is red, and as a person ages, the marrow converts to yellow (University of Western Australia School of Anatomy and Human Biology, 2009).

During early fetal development, hematopoiesis occurs in the liver and yolk sac. By the 20th week of gestation, the bone marrow begins to produce blood cells, and by the 30th week, the bone marrow has achieved a normal cellularity (Prabhakar, Ershler, & Long, 2009). As bones form prior to birth, the marrow cavities produce a network of epithelial cells called *bone marrow stroma*. Shortly before birth, HSCs fully populate the marrow cavities. During childhood, hematopoiesis occurs in the long bones. In the bone marrow, HSCs decline from 90% at birth to a level of approximately 50% by age 30 years. By adulthood, hematopoiesis occurs almost exclusively in the axial skeleton, pelvis, vertebrae, ribs, sternum, and skull. By age 70 years, the percentage of hematopoietic tissue occupying the marrow will have declined to 30% cellularity. Regardless of age, if bone marrow injury occurs, hematopoiesis can resume in the liver and spleen. This is referred to as *extramedullary hematopoiesis* (Prabhakar et al., 2009).

In immune function cells and organs, maturation processes occur. For example, the thymus gland plays a critical role in the immune system by initially developing and training T cells for adaptive immune function. The thymus gland develops and is most active from birth through puberty. However, during puberty, the thymus undergoes involution and anatomically reduces in size and is replaced with fatty tissue. Additionally, as a person matures, the bone marrow undergoes age-related changes. Previously, these age-related changes were thought to be due to increased adipogenesis and decreased osteogenesis. However, researchers have recently discovered that adipocytes support hematopoietic recovery through stem cell factor signaling (Sarkaria, Decker, & Ding, 2018). Thus, the decline in immune function with aging bone marrow may be due to vasculature changes as opposed to adipogenesis. The end result of marrow and thymic changes is still a decline in hematopoietic tissue and adaptive immunity (Prabhakar et al., 2009).

Hematopoietic Structure and Function

Hematopoietic Stem Cells

All blood cells arise from HSCs, which are primitive blood cells that reside within the bone marrow. The proportions of HSCs differ depending on the source. For example, in healthy individuals, at steady state, peripheral circulation of HSCs is 0.06%, whereas in the marrow, it is 1.1% (Körbling & Anderlini, 2001). However, HSCs spend a majority of time outside the cell cycle, quiescent, and are activated for the purpose of homeostasis or tissue repair (Prohaska & Weissman, 2009). Studies have demonstrated that approximately 5% of HSCs are active in cell cycling and regenerate every two to three months (Viale & Pelicci, 2009). When HSCs propagate, some of their daughter cells remain as HSCs, a process known as self-renewal, so that the consortium of HSCs is not depleted. Conversely, progenitor cells always commit to one of the other differentiation pathways that lead to the production of specific types of blood cells. Thus, progenitor cells cannot self-renew (Martinez-Agosto, Mikkola, Hartenstein, & Banerjee, 2007; Ueno, Itoh, Sugihara, Asano, & Takakura, 2009). In summary, HSCs belong to two cellular pools: one that is dormant, proliferates every few months, and maintains self-renewal potential and another that proliferates every 30 days and does not have self-renewal ability.

HSCs express numerous proteins on the surface of their cell membrane. These surface proteins serve as "markers" that identify the type and function of the cell. In addition, they provide molecular signaling patterns that allow cells to communicate with one another. The interaction of these markers with their respective receptors forms the basis of cell-to-cell interactions (Lataillade, Domenech, & Le Bousse-Kerdilès, 2004). Examples of the various markers HSCs express include CD34+, Thy-1lo (low expression of Thy-1, as opposed to high or absent expression), and c-kit. CD34 is the commonly recognized marker of HSCs and is used to separate them from other populations of leukocytes. As an HSC differentiates, it loses CD34, as well as other stem cell markers, and acquires the markers specific to its lineage. For example, T cells will acquire CD4 or CD8, and B cells will acquire surface immunoglobulins (Prohaska & Weissman, 2009).

The cluster of differentiation (CD) system is the nomenclature used to classify and analyze cell surface proteins present on leukocytes. Immunophenotyping, by use of flow cytometry, is a laboratory method commonly used to detect cell lineage, differentiation, and maturation. For accurate analysis, fresh blood or bone marrow is required. The tissue sample passes through a laser beam using fluorescent dyes and monoclonal antibodies (Taylor & Abdel-Wahab, 2018). Through immunophenotyping, the CD system aids in identifying the evolutionary stage of blood cells, dictates the next steps in cell maturation, serves as a regulatory signaler, and associates cells with certain immune functions and properties (Zola, Swart, Boumsell, & Mason, 2003;

Zola et al., 2005; Zola, Swart, Nicholson, & Voss, 2007). Additionally, immunophenotyping identifies whether the HSC is lineage positive or negative. For example, HSCs are CD34+; however, they can also be labeled *lineage negative*, indicating that the cell does not possess a surface marker specific to any mature blood cell.

Types of Progenitor Cells

The majority of cells produced by the hematopoietic system are derived from long-term HSCs (also known as LT-HSCs) that primarily reside in the bone marrow microenvironment. These HSCs have the capacity for self-renewal as previously described. However, a subset of long-term HSCs will differentiate into short-term HSCs (also known as ST-HSCs), which give rise to multipotent progenitors that enter the pathway of blood cell formation for the myeloid or lymphoid cell lineage.

The common myeloid progenitor gives rise to two types of progenitors: the granulocyte-monocyte progenitor and the megakaryocyte-erythrocyte progenitor. The granulocyte-monocyte progenitor produces the granulocyte lineages, which further generate neutrophils, basophils, and eosinophils; the monocyte-macrophage lineages; and the dendritic cell lineages (see Figure 1-1). The megakaryocyte-erythrocyte progenitor produces the erythroid-lineage cells and megakaryocytes (Prohaska & Weissman, 2009). From the short-term HSCs, the common lymphoid progenitor differentiates into the precursors of the B- and T-lymphocyte and NK lineages. Table 1-1 further describes the lineage, progenitor origin, type, and function of each blood cell.

Bone Marrow Microenvironment

All bone marrow consists of flexible, liquid tissue located in the hollow interior of bones. It is present within all bones of the skeletal system and is the primary location of hematopoiesis. Within the marrow exists a unique interplay among its structure, function, and regulation, all of which contribute to the formation of blood cells. Thus, the bone marrow microenvironment is important, and damage to it can cause failure of hematopoiesis. The interaction between HSCs and the bone marrow microenvironment regulates the biologic activities and trafficking of HSCs (Motabi & DiPersio, 2012).

In the bone marrow microenvironment, stromal cells provide and maintain the infrastructure in which HSCs reside. Stromal cells are a type of connective tissue found in the uterine mucosa, ovaries, prostate gland, bone marrow precursor cells, and the hematopoietic system. They are composed of fibroblasts, macrophages, adipocytes, osteoblasts, osteoclasts, and endothelial cells. Bone marrow stromal cells contribute to hematopoiesis by indirectly facilitating the movement of HSCs out of the bone marrow microenvironment and into peripheral circulation. The initiation, trafficking, and homing of HSCs involve complex cellular communication pathways with CAMs, cytokines, and chemokines (Lapid et al., 2012; Lataillade et al., 2004; Pelus,

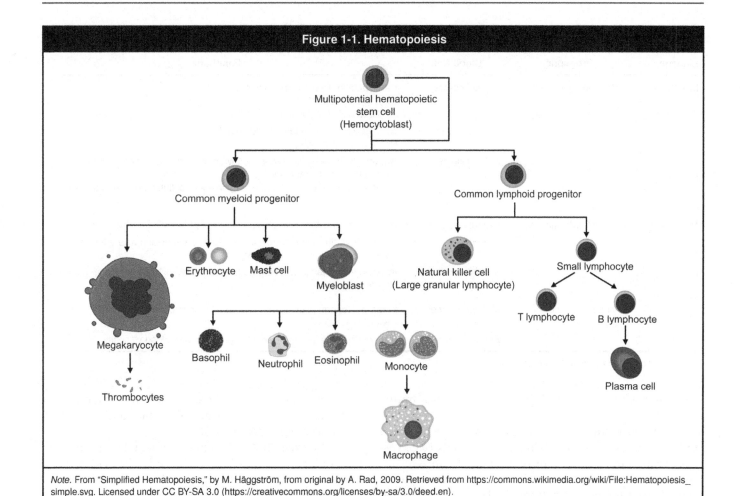

Figure 1-1. Hematopoiesis

Note. From "Simplified Hematopoiesis," by M. Häggström, from original by A. Rad, 2009. Retrieved from https://commons.wikimedia.org/wiki/File:Hematopoiesis_simple.svg. Licensed under CC BY-SA 3.0 (https://creativecommons.org/licenses/by-sa/3.0/deed.en).

2008). Knowledge of the bone marrow microenvironment has advanced over the past 10 years, with identification of more molecular and cellular players. Novel mechanisms of maintaining HSCs and other hematopoietic cells are sure to be discovered (Sarkaria et al., 2018).

Cellular Communications

CAMs are proteins located on the surface of all cells and are involved in directing cellular interactions. By binding their cell surface for cellular processes to occur, CAMs retain cells, mobilize and home cells from the blood into the marrow, and facilitate cell growth and differentiation, embryogenesis, inflammation, and immune cell transmigration (Agas, Marchetti, Douni, & Sabbieti, 2015). CAMs also are capable of transmitting information from the extracellular matrix into the cell (Lataillade et al., 2004; Schwarz & Bhandoola, 2006). Thus, target cells receive information from their environment through a class of proteins known as receptors, which also reside on the cell membrane surface. The four major types of CAMs are the immunoglobulin superfamily, integrins, cadherins, and selectins (Agas et al., 2015). In addition to CAMs, other mediators of the immune and hematopoietic response include cytokine and chemokine responses.

Cytokines are intracellular signaling proteins that have autocrine (i.e., same cell), paracrine (i.e., neighboring cell), and endocrine (i.e., distant tissue) functions (Liongue, Sertori, & Ward, 2016). Cytokines act by binding to a receptor on a target cell. Three broad classes of cytokines exist: lymphokines and monokines, which are produced by the immune system and control immune function, and growth factors, which control proliferation of blood cells (Liongue et al., 2016). Furthermore, cytokines assist in regulating the innate immune system (NK cells, macrophages, and neutrophils), adaptive immune system (T- and B-cell immune responses), inflammatory reactions, wound healing, cancer, and hematopoiesis (Cameron & Kelvin, 2003; Delves, Martin, Burton, & Roitt, 2017; Liongue et al., 2016).

A variety of cytokines stimulate HSCs to proliferate and differentiate. To induce proliferation and differentiation of the myeloid lineage, the cytokines interleukin (IL)-1, IL-3, IL-6, stem cell factor, erythropoietin, and granulocyte–colony-stimulating factor primarily stimulate HSCs. Other cytokines in the bone marrow microenvironment include interferons and tumor necrosis factors. IL-1, IL-6, stem cell factor, and *fms*-like tyrosine kinase-3 ligand induce proliferation and differentiation of the lymphoid lineage (Prohaska & Weissman, 2009). In addition to cytokines,

Table 1-1. Blood Cell Functions

Lineage	Progenitor	Blood Cell	Functions
Lymphoid	Common lymphoid	T lymphocytes	Participate in delayed-type hypersensitivity Directly kill infected cells Assist with B-cell function
		B lymphocytes	Synthesize and secrete immunoglobulins Become plasma cells
		Natural killers	Are able to kill selected tumor cells without having to be activated or immunized against a tumor cell Participate in early host defenses against intracellular organisms and viral infections
Myeloid	Granulocyte-monocyte	Granulocytes	Produce neutrophils, basophils, and eosinophils
		Monocytes	Migrate from the bone marrow into peripheral circulation where they enter tissues and mature into macrophages
		Dendritic cells	Involved in antigen processing and presentation to T cells of the immune system
	Megakaryocyte-erythrocyte	Megakaryocytes	Fragment to form platelets just before release into the circulation, assisting with coagulation
		Erythrocytes	Involved in tissue nourishment, oxygenation, and blood viscosity

Note. Based on information from Abbas et al., 2020.

chemokines play a role in HSC regulation and immune activity.

Belonging to the cytokine family, chemokines are small proteins produced by nonhematopoietic cells (e.g., gastrointestinal tract, ovaries, prostate gland, thymus, heart, spleen) and hematopoietic cells (e.g., platelets, stromal cells) (Lapidot & Petit, 2002; Lataillade et al., 2004). Chemokines guide the migration of cells that are attracted to them by following the signals of increasing chemokine concentrations toward its source. They play a part in wound healing, infection, and stem cell mobilization. For example, during an infection or anti-inflammatory response, leukocytes are stimulated to the site of infection or injury (Laing & Secombes, 2004; Lapidot & Petit, 2002). In stem cell mobilization, IV administration of chemokines, including IL-8, proteases, growth-regulated oncogene beta, and stromal cell–derived factor-1 alpha (SDF-1α), resulted in mobilization of hematopoietic progenitor cells (Lataillade et al., 2004; Pelus, 2008; Schwarz & Bhandoola, 2006). The main difference between chemokines and cytokines is that multiple chemokines may bind to a single receptor, whereas cytokines are activated by interactions with a unique and specific ligand (Lataillade et al., 2004).

Pathways of Hematopoietic Stem Cell Mobilization

Requirements for hematopoietic homeostasis and successful proliferation and differentiation of HSCs include a source of HSCs, cytokines, chemokines, and stromal cell interactions. Stromal cells express SDF-1α, a chemokine widely expressed on many tissues and secreted by bone marrow osteoblasts and endothelial cells. SDF-1α is involved in retaining progenitor cells within the bone marrow micro-environment as well as releasing HSCs and leukocytes from the marrow and into peripheral circulation (Pelus, 2008; Schwarz & Bhandoola, 2006).

For a given time in their development, HSCs express the chemokine receptor CXCR4. CXCR4 has been identified as important in the regulation of trafficking and homing of cells involved in hematopoiesis and the immune system (Lataillade et al., 2004). HSC retention within the bone marrow microenvironment occurs as a result of the SDF-1α gradient, CAMs, and the binding action of CXCR4. When a loss of attachment occurs between stromal cells, SDF-1α, and CXCR4, degradation of CAMs occurs, releasing HSCs into the peripheral circulation (Lataillade et al., 2004). This is commonly observed after chemotherapy or cytokine administration. For example, proliferation of HSCs following filgrastim administration occurs by the release of neutrophil-secreted proteases (i.e., elastase, cathepsin G, and matrix metalloproteinase-9 [MMP-9]), which cleave vascular cell adhesion molecule-1 (VCAM-1) and very late antigen-4 (VLA-4), which are CAMs expressed on stromal cells. The neutrophil-secreted proteases prevent the adhesion of HSCs to stromal cells via VLA-4, degrading VCAM-1. As a result, the HSC gets passed along toward the bone marrow sinus, where it will be exported out of the marrow and into circulation.

Within the past decade, newer pathways of HSC mobilization have been identified with the use of chemokine antagonists, such as plerixafor (Genzyme, 2019). Chemokine antagonists block the CXCR4 receptor on the HSC surface. When this occurs, HSCs are inhibited from binding to SDF-1α, allowing the release of HSCs into the peripheral circulation (Broxmeyer et al., 2005; Liles et al., 2003).

Immune Function: Cells and Responses

The bone marrow produces the basic cells of the immune system, which are derived from white blood cells (WBCs). Several different types of WBCs possess commonalities yet are distinct in form and function. A distinguishing morphologic feature of WBCs is the presence or absence of granules. *Granulocytes* (polymorphonuclear neutrophils) are identified by the presence of granules in cytoplasm when stained with specific dyes and viewed under light microscopy (Green & Wachsmann-Hogiu, 2015). These granules are membrane-bound enzymes that primarily aid in the digestion of foreign particles, a process known as *phagocytosis*. The three types of granulocytes are neutrophils, basophils, and eosinophils. *Agranulocytes* (mononuclear leukocytes) are characterized by the apparent absence of granules in their cytoplasm. These cells include monocytes, macrophages, and lymphocytes (Green & Wachsmann-Hogiu, 2015; Khanna-Gupta & Berliner, 2018; Tagliasacchi & Carboni, 1997; University of Western Australia School of Anatomy and Human Biology, 2009). Cells from the myeloid progenitors respond early and nonspecifically to infection, whereas lymphoid progenitors respond later and are dependent on the production of cytokines from antigen-presenting cells (APCs) (Gutcher & Becher, 2007). Myeloid-derived cells of the immune system include monocytes, macrophages, and granulocytes. Lymphocyte-derived cells of the immune system include T cells, B cells, and NK cells. Table 1-1 provides an overview of myeloid and lymphoid progenitors and their role in immune function.

Myeloid-Derived Immune Cells

Monocytes are produced from granulocyte-monocyte progenitor cells and mature in the bloodstream. Their functions include maintaining homeostasis, stimulating the differentiation of macrophages and dendritic cells, and responding to inflammation and infection (Dayyani et al., 2003; Swirski et al., 2009; Ziegler-Heitbrock, 2007). CD14 and CD16 are the most common surface markers expressed by monocytes (Dayyani et al., 2003; Ziegler-Heitbrock, 2007). Survival in circulation is short (8–72 hours); however, when they enter the tissues and become macrophages, their life span may extend up to two to three months (Khanna-Gupta & Berliner, 2018). Reserves of monocytes have been identified in murine spleen models and may further assist in the regulation of inflammation (Swirski et al., 2009). Monocytes present fragments of pathogens to T cells so that the pathogens may be recognized and destroyed, further eliciting an antibody response. When monocytes leave the bloodstream, they migrate to the tissues, where they continue to differentiate into types of macrophages or dendritic cells depending on the signals they receive from T and B lymphocytes (Ziegler-Heitbrock, 2007).

Macrophages express CD14 and CD45 and are commonly referred to as *scavengers* or APCs. Two types of tissue macrophages exist: (a) resident macrophages, which originate from either the bone marrow or the specific organ from which they arise (e.g., Kupffer cells [hepatic], alveolar macrophages [pulmonary], osteoclasts [bone], microglia [central nervous system]), and (b) exudative or elicited macrophages, which are derived from blood monocytes in response to infection or inflammation (Jankowski et al., 2018; Rao, 2018). Additionally, macrophages are involved in immune regulation and removal of apoptotic blood and tissue cells (Jankowski et al., 2018). Macrophages seize and engulf foreign materials and then present these antigens to the lymphoid-derived cells (T and B cells) of the immune system. Thus, macrophage activation is one of the first important steps in initiating immune response.

Dendritic cells, which originate from the myeloid lineage, are considered the most potent cells involved in antigen processing and presentation to B and T lymphocytes. They are extremely hard to isolate, which makes it challenging to study their specific functions. Dendritic cells circulate in the peripheral blood and tissues as immature cells. Once they encounter and capture a pathogen (e.g., virus, parasite, bacteria), cytokines are stimulated, and the dendritic cells navigate to the primary or secondary lymphoid organs where they mature. As a result, T- and B-cell activation occurs, which further initiates and shapes the innate immune response. Activated T lymphocytes then migrate to reach the injured tissue. After lymphocyte interaction, dendritic cells undergo apoptosis. Dendritic cells are present in tissues that are in contact with the external environment including the skin, the inner lining of the nose, the lungs, the stomach, and the intestines (Manches, Muniz, & Bhardwaj, 2018; Medzhitov, 2013).

Granulocytes are composed of three cell types: neutrophils, eosinophils, and basophils. Neutrophils are the first to arrive at the site of an infection or tissue damage and contribute to acute inflammatory response. As neutrophils roll along the vasculature, the cytokines G-CSF and granulocyte macrophage–colony-stimulating factor (GM-CSF) are released from macrophages. Myeloid precursors are stimulated to produce and release additional neutrophils into circulation, commonly referred to as *leukocytosis*. Neutrophils home into the site of infection and engulf the pathogen on contact, and cytokines send out warning signals. Eosinophils attack parasites and secrete leukotrienes, prostaglandins, and other cytokines (Wilson & Trumpp, 2006). Basophils possess receptors for immunoglobulin E; thus, when involved in allergic responses, inflammatory mediators such as histamine, prostaglandins, and serotonin are triggered (Wilson & Trumpp, 2006).

Lymphoid-Derived Immune Cells

After macrophages present APCs to the lymphocytes within the lymphoid tissue, antigen development specific for T- or B-cell activation and differentiation begins. T lymphocytes leave the lymphoid tissue and home into the disease site or release antibodies from activated B cells into the peripheral blood (Eberl, Colonna, Di Santo, & McKenzie,

2015). Thus, lymphoid progenitors are effectors and regulators of immune response. To generate T lymphocytes, lymphoid progenitors must leave the bone marrow, enter the bloodstream, and migrate to the thymus for maturation (Eberl et al., 2015; Schwarz & Bhandoola, 2006). Several subsets of T cells exist, each with a distinct function, including helper T cells (T_H cells), cytotoxic T cells (T_C cells), regulatory T cells (T_{reg} cells), memory T cells, and NK cells. Table 1-2 provides an overview of T-cell functions.

T_H cells initiate specific immunity, including maturation of B cells and activation of T_C cells and macrophages (Jiang & Chess, 2004; Krensky & Clayberger, 2005). T_H cells become activated when they are presented with peptide antigens by major histocompatibility complex (MHC) class II molecules that are expressed on the surface of APCs. Once activated, T_H cells divide rapidly and secrete cytokines that regulate or assist in activating immune response. Thus, T_H cells may be referred to as cytokine-secreting helper cells as well as CD4 T cells because they express the CD4 cell surface molecule (Gutcher & Becher, 2007; Jiang & Chess, 2004, Krensky & Clayberger, 2005).

T_C cells are involved in eradicating viral infections; however, studies demonstrate they also may play a role in autoimmunity and allogeneic organ rejection (Gutcher & Becher, 2007; Jiang & Chess, 2004; Krensky & Clayberger, 2005). T_C cells recognize their targets by binding to antigens associated with MHC class I molecules. These molecules are ubiquitous in the body and are responsible for lymphocyte recognition and antigen presentation. After binding to its target cell, the T_C cell inserts cytolytic proteins that contribute to DNA fragmentation and apoptosis. T_C cells are also known as CD8+ T cells because they express the CD8 protein on their surface (Eberl et al., 2015).

T_{reg} cells, formerly known as suppressor T cells, are a specialized population of T cells whose role is to suppress T cell–mediated immunity toward the end of an immune reaction and to suppress autoreactive T cells that escape maturation in the thymus. T_{reg} cells may have a crucial role in the generation and maintenance of immune tolerance. Two major classes of T_{reg} cells are those that arise from the thymus and those that differentiate from naïve T cells (i.e., mature T cells that have not been activated or encountered by an antigen) (Groux, 2001; Shevach, 2002). T_{reg} cells express CD4, CD8, and CD25. Interest in T_{reg} cells is occurring as a result of experimental murine models revealing the immunosuppressive potential of T_{reg} cells. Potential therapeutic benefits include the treatment of autoimmune diseases, chronic inflammatory diseases, and infectious diseases; cancer immunotherapy; and development of host transplantation tolerance, such as after allogeneic HSCT (Beyer & Schultze, 2006; Maloy & Powrie, 2001).

Upon the initial encounter during a bacterial or viral infection, exposure to a carcinogen, or previous vaccination, naïve T-cell proliferation occurs. Traditionally, memory T cells have been referred to as the "survivors" of effector cells, which then regress into a state of quiescence after the initial encounter (Sallusto & Lanzavecchia, 2001). Newer models of T-cell generation have demonstrated that the type, duration, amount of cytokine, and homing capabilities determine how memory T cells differentiate (Lanzavecchia & Sallusto, 2005). Two subtypes of memory T cells identified are central memory cells (TCMs) and effector memory cells (TEMs). TCMs home to the lymph nodes and have a low activation threshold. Upon restimulation in the lymph nodes, TCMs proliferate and differentiate into TEMs. TEMs home to the peripheral tissues, rapidly produce cytokines upon stimulation, and combat infection; however, they have limited proliferative capabilities. TCMs are involved in secondary immune responses and long-term protection, and TEMs are involved in immediate protection (Lanzavecchia & Sallusto, 2005). Memory cells may be CD4+ or CD8+, and both TEM and TCM cells express CD45RO+ (Liongue et al., 2016).

The chemokine receptor CCR7 controls homing to secondary lymph organs and has been identified in determining the difference between TEMs and TCMs. The CCR7− subset has characteristics that express receptors for migration to inflamed tissues and display effector functions; these are TEMs. TCMs express CCR7+ lymph homing receptors and lack immediate function; however, upon subsequent exposure, they differentiate and express CCR7− (Sallusto, Geginat, & Lanzavecchia, 2004; Sallusto, Lenig, Förster, Lipp, & Lanzavecchia, 1999).

NK cells are a subtype of T cells that are similar to killer T cells, directly killing tumors, such as melanomas and lymphomas, and virus-infected cells. The difference between

Table 1-2. T-Cell Functions

T-Cell Subsets	Functions
Helper T cells (T_H cells)	Initiate specific immunity Regulate and assist in activating immune response
Cytotoxic T cells (T_C cells)	Involved in eradicating viral infections May play a role in autoimmunity and organ rejection
Regulatory T cells (T_{reg} cells)	Suppress T-cell–mediated immunity May play a crucial role in immune tolerance
Memory T cells • Central memory cells (TCMs) • Effector memory cells (TEMs)	Suppress autoreactive T cells May play a role in immune tolerance Home to the lymph nodes and have low activation threshold (TCMs) Home to the peripheral tissues; combat infection but have limited proliferation capabilities (TEMs)
Natural killer cells	Directly kill tumors and virus-infected cells

Note. Based on information from Abbas et al., 2020.

NK cells and killer T cells is that NK cells destroy their targets without a prior "conference" in the lymphoid organs.

B-cell development occurs in the bone marrow and depends on adhesion interactions with stromal cells. The two main types of B cells are plasma cells and memory cells. Plasma cells are B cells that actively produce antibodies against antigens to which they have been exposed. Plasma cells secrete immunoglobulin (Ig), the antigen-specific antibodies. There are five known classes of immunoglobulin (IgG, IgA, IgM, IgE, and IgD), four subclasses of IgG, and two subclasses of IgA (Joshua, 2004). The primary actions of the classes of antibodies are listed in Table 1-3.

Table 1-3. Immunoglobulin Actions

Immunoglobulin	Actions
G	Major immunoglobulin in the blood Enters tissue spaces Coats microorganisms, speeding their destruction by other cells of the immune system
A	Guards the entrance to the body Concentrates in body fluids such as tears, saliva, and secretions of the respiratory and gastrointestinal tracts
M	Links together in the bloodstream to kill invaders
E	Participates in allergic reactions
D	Regulates cell activation on B-cell membranes

Note. Based on information from Abbas et al., 2020.

Antibodies are Y-shaped structures that contain two light chains and two heavy chains, known as the hypervariable region/antigen-binding region. The molecular configuration of the upper part of the "Y" varies to match a specific antigen. This portion is referred to as the fragment antigen-binding (Fab) region because of its antigen-binding capabilities. The molecular configuration of the bottom of the "Y" is the fragment crystallizable (Fc) region. The Fc region interacts with cell surface receptors and proteins of the complement system, stimulating antibodies to activate the immune system (Joshua, 2004).

APC function is mediated by the uptake of foreign antigens into the B cell followed by its processing and presentation on the cell surface with MHC class I (i.e., antigens found on the surface of all nucleated cells in the body) or MHC class II (i.e., antigens found on B cells and macrophages) proteins. Antibody production occurs after the Fab portion of the antibody is bound, leading to exposed Fc regions. These exposed regions activate the complement pathway, which then activates phagocytosis and macrophages (Joshua, 2004). This is a critical method of signaling other cells to engulf, kill, or remove a substance from the body. In addition to their role in humoral immunity, B lymphocytes are required for the initiation of T-cell responses (LeBien & Tedder, 2008). B-cell lineage surface markers have been identified, including CD19, CD20, CD21, CD22, CD23, CD24, CD40, CD72, CD79a, and CD79b (LeBien & Tedder, 2008). Plasma cells generally are short lived with a half-life of a few days. However, some plasma cells may survive for weeks within the bone marrow. Memory B cells are activated B cells that are specific to the antigen encountered during the primary immune response. These cells are long term and respond quickly, particularly following a second exposure to the same antigen (Kurosaki, Kometani, & Ise, 2015).

Organs of the Immune System

Organs of the immune system are involved in the production, maturation, and activity of immune cells. WBCs meet and interact with each other and with antigens in multiple organs. They are strategically located to intercept invaders and to allow immune cells to efficiently eliminate the invaders. In addition to the bone marrow, other organs of the immune system include nonencapsulated lymphoid organs such as the tonsils and adenoids in the upper respiratory tract, the liver, Peyer patches or small intestines, and the appendix (Belkaid & Harrison, 2017). The major organs that will be reviewed include the thymus, lymph nodes, and spleen.

The thymus gland is located in the anterior mediastinum. The thymus develops around the sixth week of gestation and begins to decline after birth at a rate of 3% per year until middle age; thereafter, thymic function declines by less than 1% annually throughout life (Jiménez, Ercilla, & Martínez, 2007; Prabhakar et al., 2009). Normally, immature thymocytes leave the bone marrow and migrate into the thymus gland. A process referred to as *thymic education* occurs, in which T cells that are beneficial to the immune system are spared while T cells that are not are eliminated. Mature T cells are then released into the bloodstream (Kurosaki et al., 2015).

Lymph nodes are small bean-shaped glands formed in clusters throughout the body. They are located in the neck, axilla, chest, pelvis, and inguinal regions, as well as in association with the blood vessels of the intestines, and are connected by lymphatic vessels. The two main types of lymph vessels are afferent and efferent. Afferent lymph vessels are found only in lymph nodes, and efferent lymph vessels are found in lymph nodes, the thymus, and the spleen. Immune cells and foreign particles enter the lymph nodes via the afferent lymph vessel. Each lymph node contains specialized compartments where immune cells congregate and encounter antigens. Thus, lymph nodes function as an immunologic filter. All lymphocytes exit lymph nodes through efferent lymph vessels. These lymph vessels and blood vessels provide immune transportation systems. Once in the bloodstream, lymphocytes are transported to tissues throughout the body. Lymphocytes are ubiquitous, patrolling for foreign antigens and gradually migrating back into the lymphatic system to begin the cycle again (Kurosaki et al., 2015).

The spleen, an encapsulated lymphoid organ located in the abdomen, is known for removing aging red blood cells, recycling iron, and eliciting an immune response for antibacterial and antifungal stimulation and immune reactivity. B cells become activated to produce antibodies in the spleen. The spleen is made up of T cells, B cells, macrophages, dendritic cells, NK cells, and red blood cells. Migratory macrophages and dendritic cells bring antigens to the spleen via the bloodstream. The spleen captures antigens from the blood that passes through it; thus, the spleen often is described as the immunologic filter for the blood. The white pulp of the spleen, known as the lymphoid region, is thought to participate in immune response when the macrophage or dendritic cells present the antigen to the appropriate B or T cell. Furthermore, the role of the spleen in protection from infections has been demonstrated in studies of splenectomized patients, as they cannot mount an immune response to certain infections and must therefore be on lifelong prophylactic antibiotics (Mebius & Kraal, 2005).

Genetic Basis of Hematopoietic Stem Cell Transplantation

Widespread use of high-resolution DNA-based typing has increased the accuracy and specificity of tissue typing. Studies have demonstrated that precise typing between the donor and recipient improves overall survival, reduces incidence of acute and chronic graft-versus-host disease (GVHD), and improves rates of engraftment (Bray et al., 2008; Morishima et al., 2002; Petersdorf et al., 2001).

MHC molecules control the immune response through recognition of self and nonself and serve as targets in transplant rejection. Therefore, they play an integral role in the immune system and autoimmunity. The gene in the MHC region that encodes antigen-processing polypeptides on the cell surface is known as the human leukocyte antigen (HLA). The HLA region is located on the short arm of chromosome 6 and is divided into three subgroups: class I (found on every cell in the body and presents antigens to T_C cells), class II (found on B cells, macrophages, and other APCs and presents antigens to T_H cells), and class III (involved in complement pathways and cytokines) (Petersdorf, 2016).

MHC molecules are anchored in the cell membrane where they display short peptides to T cells via T-cell receptors. HLAs are proteins located on the surface of WBCs and other tissues in the body (Petersdorf, 2016). If individuals are deemed to be HLA compatible, their tissues are immunologically compatible with one another (for HSCT purposes, the HLA-A, HLA-B, HLA-C, HLA-DRB1, and HLA-DQB1 antigens are the most important) (Bray et al., 2008).

Determination of the HLA alleles of an individual is called HLA typing. It is done to uniquely identify individuals and to facilitate and predict outcomes of cell, tissue, and organ transplantation. HLA typing traditionally has been performed by serologic methods, identifying HLA proteins expressed on WBCs. This testing is accomplished by mixing sera-containing antibodies with specific HLAs (Petersdorf, 2016). Production of antigen–antibody complexes is evidence that the specific HLA is produced by WBCs. This type of testing identifies the phenotype of the individual but not the genotype. Advances in molecular biology, using polymerase chain reaction–based methods, assist in detecting single nucleotide differences between two unique alleles of the same antigen (Petersdorf, 2016). Molecular testing permits more precise identification of the individual's HLA type. Some HLA alleles will appear serologically identical when they are not molecularly identical. Although some of these molecular variations in HLA alleles are not clinically significant, others can have important implications for outcomes in tissue transplantation, such as graft rejection and GVHD (Petersdorf, 2016).

Each nucleated human cell has two HLA haplotypes, one inherited from the mother and the other inherited from the father. Because parental haplotypes can segregate in different combinations, there is a 25% chance that any one sibling would be identical to the other. Aside from monozygotic twins, who share exactly the same HLA genotype, full siblings are most likely to share the same HLA haplotypes because they come from the same gene pool.

Some HLA alleles are very common in all populations, but some are rare in certain ethnic groups. Ethnic tendencies in HLA inheritance can make matching with an unrelated transplant donor difficult for members of ethnic minorities or people with mixed ethnic heritage (Bray et al., 2008). As a result, high-resolution matches are warranted.

In addition to HLA typing, peripheral blood HSC mobilization studies have demonstrated several factors related to the inability to mobilize sufficient numbers of HSCs to ensure rapid and durable engraftment. For patients or donors who unexpectedly fail to mobilize adequate HSCs, genetic factors are a potential culprit. Because interactions within the bone marrow microenvironment regulate HSC mobilization, the critical point in this process is the interaction between SDF-1α and stromal cells. Murine and human models have confirmed that if genetically deficient of SDF-1, or its receptor CXCR4, an individual will be unsuccessful in mobilizing HSCs (Benboubker et al., 2001). Prior exposure to alkylating or purine analog drugs, disease involvement in the bone marrow, and pelvic irradiation also may cause poor mobilization.

The gene for SDF-1α is located on chromosome 10q11.1 (Lewellis & Knaut, 2012). Studies have shown that autologous and allogeneic donors who possess this genotype mobilize a higher quantity of HSCs than patients without it, thus suggesting biologic relevance (Benboubker et al., 2001; Bogunia-Kubik, Gieryng, Dlubek, & Lange, 2009).

Post-Transplant Immune Reconstitution

After HSCT, bone marrow reconstitution consists of two distinct phases: numeric recovery of marrow cellular elements (i.e., WBCs, red blood cells, platelets) and functional recovery of cellular interactions (i.e., B cells, T cells, NK cells) (Guillaume, Rubinstein, & Symann, 1998; Storek et al., 2008). Depending on the source of stem cells, WBC engraftment occurs fairly promptly, usually within the first three to four weeks after transplantation. Despite prompt engraftment after transplant, recovery of humoral and cell-mediated immunity with full lymphocyte function takes much longer. This accounts for patient susceptibility to viral and opportunistic infections for several months after autologous transplantation and for many months to years after allogeneic transplantation.

Immune reconstitution is the recovery of antigen-specific T-cell function, production of cytokines, and cooperation with B lymphocytes in antibody production. Immune reconstitution may take months to years after cessation of therapy and may be affected by innate and adaptive/acquired immunity. Numerous factors can affect post-transplant immune reconstitution—for example, the type of HSCT (i.e., autologous vs. allogeneic, myeloablative vs. reduced intensity vs. T-cell depletion), source of stem cells (e.g., bone marrow, peripheral blood, umbilical cord blood), recipient age, malignancy and the treatment employed (e.g., chemotherapy, radiation), donor immunity, thymus function, histoincompatibility, immunosuppressive medications, donor age and sex, GVHD status, and presence of graft rejection (Bernstein, Boyd, & van den Brink, 2008; Jiménez et al., 2007). Strategies to enhance post-HSCT immune reconstitution are emerging and remain under clinical investigation. This has included inhibition of sex steroids (e.g., gonadotropin-releasing hormone agonist treatment), growth factor therapies (e.g., G-CSF, GM-CSF), cytokine therapies (e.g., IL-7), and cellular therapies (e.g., T-cell administration, adoptive transfer of NK cells to enhance malignancy/viral-specific immunity) (Bernstein et al., 2008; Zakrzewski, Holland, & van den Brink, 2007).

A potential sequela of immunosuppressive therapy is the development of opportunistic infections. Quantitative recovery of immunity does not always correlate with qualitative cellular function. Therefore, an important consideration for oncology nurses is to remember and educate others that normal laboratory parameters do not absolve the HSCT patient's risk of infection. In determining the patient's risk of infection, obtaining or having knowledge of the patient's history is crucial. In addition to a thorough history and physical examination, laboratory investigations to assess immune reconstitution have been examined and may assist in determining if prophylactic antimicrobials or IV immunoglobulin administration is warranted, as well as if immunosuppressive therapy can be tapered. Such tests include T-cell analysis by immunophenotyping (T-cell subsets), B-cell analysis (i.e., quantitative and IgG subclass analysis), NK-cell reconstitution, and dendritic cell and chimerism analysis. Additionally, disease-specific tests, as well as infection surveillance and detection strategies (such as blood cultures and polymerase chain reaction), can assist with identifying infection risk and the need for further evaluations and treatments.

Summary

A basic understanding of hematopoiesis and immunology provides the foundation for the therapy of HSCT. Dramatic advances in the field of genomics because of the Human Genome Project (International Human Genome Sequencing Consortium, 2004) are quickly increasing knowledge in these two areas. The field of HSCT is changing rapidly, with therapies becoming more effective and less toxic. Nurses and other healthcare professionals are being challenged to remain knowledgeable and to develop methods to effectively educate patients and families about the effects of these advances on therapy options, treatments, and outcomes.

The author would like to acknowledge Hollie Devine, RN, MSN, ANP-BC, AOCNP®, for her contribution to this chapter that remains unchanged from the previous edition of this book.

References

Abbas, A.K., Lichtman, A.H., & Pillai, S. (2020). *Basic immunology: Functions and disorders of the immune system* (6th ed.). Philadelphia, PA: Elsevier.

Agas, D., Marchetti, L., Douni, E., & Sabbieti, M.G. (2015). The unbearable lightness of bone marrow homeostasis. *Cytokine and Growth Factor Reviews, 26*, 347–359. https://doi.org/10.1016/j.cytogfr.2014.12.004

Belkaid, Y., & Harrison, O.J. (2017). Homeostatic immunity and the microbiota. *Immunity, 46*, 562–576. https://doi.org/10.1016/j.immuni.2017.04.008

Benboubker, L., Watier, H., Carion, A., Georget, M.-T., Desbois, I., Colombat, P., ... Domenech, J. (2001). Association between the *SDF1-3'A* allele and high levels of CD34+ progenitor cells mobilized into peripheral blood in humans. *British Journal of Haematology, 113*, 247–250. https://doi.org/10.1046/j.1365-2141.2001.02717.x

Bernstein, I.D., Boyd, R.L., & van den Brink, M.R.M. (2008). Clinical strategies to enhance posttransplant immune reconstitution. *Biology of Blood and Marrow Transplantation, 14*(Suppl. 1), 94–99. https://doi.org/10.1016/j.bbmt.2007.10.003

Beyer, M., & Schultze, J.L. (2006). Regulatory T cells in cancer. *Blood, 108*, 804–811. https://doi.org/10.1182/blood-2006-02-002774

Bogunia-Kubik, K., Gieryng, A., Dlubek, D., & Lange, A. (2009). The CXCL12-3'A allele is associated with a higher mobilization yield of CD34 progenitors to the peripheral blood of healthy donors for allogeneic transplantation. *Bone Marrow Transplantation, 44*, 273–278. https://doi.org/10.1038/bmt.2009.30

Bray, R.A., Hurley, C.K., Kamani, N.R., Woolfrey, A., Müller, C., Spellman, S., ... Confer, D.L. (2008). National Marrow Donor Program HLA matching guidelines for unrelated adult donor hematopoietic cell transplants. *Biology of Blood and Marrow Transplantation, 14*(Suppl. 9), 45–53. https://doi.org/10.1016/j.bbmt.2008.06.014

Broxmeyer, H.E., Orschell, C.M., Clapp, D.W., Hangoc, G., Cooper, S., Plett, P.A., ... Srour, E.F. (2005). Rapid mobilization of murine and human hematopoietic stem and progenitor cells with AMD3100, a CXCR4 antagonist. *Journal of Experimental Medicine, 201*, 1307–1318. https://doi.org/10.1084/jem.20041385

Cameron, M.J., & Kelvin, D.J. (2003). Cytokines and chemokines—Their receptors and their genes: An overview. In P. Santamaria (Ed.), *Advances in experimental medicine and biology: Vol. 520. Cytokines and chemokines in autoimmune disease* (pp. 8–32). Georgetown, TX: Landes Bioscience/Eurekah.com and Springer.

Dayyani, F., Belge, K.-U., Frankenberger, M., Mack, M., Berki, T., & Ziegler-Heitbrock, L. (2003). Mechanism of glucocorticoid-induced depletion of human CD14+CD16+ monocytes. *Journal of Leukocyte Biology, 74*, 33–39. https://doi.org/10.1189/jlb.1202612

Delves, P.J., Martin, S.J., Burton, D.R., & Roitt, I.M. (2017). *Roitt's essential immunology* (13th ed.). Hoboken, NJ: Wiley-Blackwell.

Eberl, G., Colonna, M., Di Santo, J.P., & McKenzie, A.N.J. (2015). Innate lymphoid cells: A new paradigm in immunology. *Science, 348*, aaa6566-1–aaa6566-8. https://doi.org/10.1126/science.aaa6566

Genzyme. (2019). *Mozobil® (plerixafor injection)* [Package insert]. Cambridge, MA: Author.

Green, R., & Wachsmann-Hogiu, S. (2015). Development, history, and future of automated cell counters. *Clinics in Laboratory Medicine, 35*, 1–10. https://doi.org/10.1016/j.cll.2014.11.003

Groux, H. (2001). An overview of regulatory T cells. *Microbes and Infection, 3*, 883–889. https://doi.org/10.1016/s1286-4579(01)01448-4

Guillaume, T., Rubinstein, D.B., & Symann, M. (1998). Immune reconstitution and immunotherapy after autologous hematopoietic stem cell transplantation. *Blood, 92*, 1471–1490. Retrieved from https://ashpublications.org/blood/article/92/5/1471/247373/Immune-Reconstitution-and-Immunotherapy-After

Gutcher, I., & Becher, B. (2007). APC-derived cytokines and T cell polarization in autoimmune inflammation. *Journal of Clinical Investigation, 117*, 1119–1127. https://doi.org/10.1172/jci31720

Hunt, K.J., Walsh, B.M., Voegeli, D., & Roberts, H.C. (2010). Inflammation in aging part 1: Physiological and immunological mechanisms. *Biological Research for Nursing, 11*, 245–252. https://doi.org/10.1177/1099800409352237

International Human Genome Sequencing Consortium. (2004). Finishing the euchromatic sequence of the human genome. *Nature, 431*, 931–945. https://doi.org/10.1038/nature03001

Jankowski, M., Dyszkiewicz-Konwińska, M., Magas, M., Skorupski, M., Gorecki, G., Bukowska, D., ... Kempisty, B. (2018). Haematopoiesis: "Living in the shadow" of stem cell differentiation. *Journal of Biological Regulators and Homeostatic Agents, 32*, 1–6.

Jiang, H., & Chess, L. (2004). An integrated view of suppressor T cell subsets in immunoregulation. *Journal of Clinical Investigation, 114*, 1198–1208. https://doi.org/10.1172/jci200423411

Jiménez, M., Ercilla, G., & Martínez, C. (2007). Immune reconstitution after allogeneic stem cell transplantation with reduced-intensity conditioning regimens. *Leukemia, 21*, 1628–1637. https://doi.org/10.1038/sj.leu.2404681

Joshua, D.E. (2004). Immunoglobulins. In J.S. Malpas, P.L. Bergsagel, R.A. Kyle, & K.C. Anderson (Eds.), *Myeloma: Biology and management* (3rd ed., pp. 3–20). Philadelphia, PA: Saunders.

Khanna-Gupta, A., & Berliner, N. (2018). Granulocytopoiesis and monocytopoiesis. In R. Hoffman, E.J. Benz Jr., L.E. Silberstein, H.E. Heslop, J.I. Weitz, J. Anastasi, ... S.A. Abutalib (Eds.), *Hematology: Basic principles and practice* (7th ed., pp. 321–333). Philadelphia, PA: Elsevier.

Körbling, M., & Anderlini, P. (2001). Peripheral blood stem cell versus bone marrow allotransplantation: Does the source of hematopoietic stem cells matter? *Blood, 98*, 2900–2908. https://doi.org/10.1182/blood.v98.10.2900

Krensky, A.M., & Clayberger, C. (2005). Granulysin: A novel host defense molecule. *American Journal of Transplantation, 5*, 1789–1792. https://doi.org/10.1111/j.1600-6143.2005.00970.x

Kurosaki, T., Kometani, K., & Ise, W. (2015). Memory B cells. *Nature Reviews Immunology, 15*, 149–159. https://doi.org/10.1038/nri3802

Laing, K.J., & Secombes, C.J. (2004). Chemokines. *Developmental and Comparative Immunology, 28*, 443–460. https://doi.org/10.1016/j.dci.2003.09.006

Lanzavecchia, A., & Sallusto, F. (2005). Understanding the generation and function of memory T cell subsets. *Current Opinion in Immunology, 17*, 326–332. https://doi.org/10.1016/j.coi.2005.04.010

Lapid, K., Glait-Santar, C., Gur-Cohen, S., Canaani, J., Kollet, O., & Lapidot, T. (2012, August). Egress and mobilization of hematopoietic stem and progenitor cells: A dynamic multi-facet process. In *StemBook*. https://doi.org/10.3824/stembook.1.39.1

Lapidot, T., & Petit, I. (2002). Current understanding of stem cell mobilization: The roles of chemokines, proteolytic enzymes, adhesion molecules, cytokines, and stromal cells. *Experimental Hematology, 30*, 973–981. https://doi.org/10.1016/s0301-472x(02)00883-4

Lataillade, J.-J., Domenech, J., & Le Bousse-Kerdilès, M.-C. (2004). Stromal cell-derived factor-1 (SDF-1)\CXCR4 couple plays multiple roles on haematopoietic progenitors at the border between the old cytokine and new chemokine worlds: Survival, cell cycling and trafficking. *European Cytokine Network, 15*, 177–188.

LeBien, T.W., & Tedder, T.D. (2008). B lymphocytes: How they develop and function. *Blood, 112*, 1570–1580. https://doi.org/10.1182/blood-2008-02-078071

Lewellis, S.W., & Knaut, H. (2012). Attractive guidance: How the chemokine SDF1/CXCL12 guides different cells to different locations. *Seminars in Cell and Developmental Biology, 23*, 333–340. https://doi.org/10.1016/j.semcdb.2012.03.009

Liles, W.C., Broxmeyer, H.E., Rodger, E., Wood, B., Hübel, K., Cooper, S., ... Dale, D.C. (2003). Mobilization of hematopoietic progenitor cells in healthy volunteers by AMD3100, a CXCR4 antagonist. *Blood, 102*, 2728–2730. https://doi.org/10.1182/blood-2003-02-0663

Liongue, C., Sertori, R., & Ward, A.C. (2016). Evolution of cytokine receptor signaling. *Journal of Immunology, 197*, 11–18. https://doi.org/10.4049/jimmunol.1600372

Maloy, K.J., & Powrie, F. (2001). Regulatory T cells in the control of immune pathology. *Nature Immunology, 2*, 816–822. https://doi.org/10.1038/ni0901-816

Manches, O., Muniz, L.R., & Bhardwaj, N. (2018). Dendritic cell biology. In R. Hoffman, E.J. Benz Jr., L.E. Silberstein, H.E. Heslop, J.I. Weitz, J. Anastasi, ... S.A. Abutalib (Eds.), *Hematology: Basic principles and practice* (7th ed., pp. 247–261). Philadelphia, PA: Elsevier.

Martinez-Agosto, J.A., Mikkola, H.K.A., Hartenstein, V., & Banerjee, U. (2007). The hematopoietic stem cell and its niche: A comparative view. *Genes and Development, 21*, 3044–3060. https://doi.org/10.1101/gad.1602607

Mebius, R.E., & Kraal, G. (2005). Structure and function of the spleen. *Nature Reviews Immunology, 5*, 606–616. https://doi.org/10.1038/nri1669

Medzhitov, R. (2013). Pattern recognition theory and the launch of modern innate immunity. *Journal of Immunology, 191*, 4473–4474. https://doi.org/10.4049/jimmunol.1302427

Morishima, Y., Sasazuki, T., Inoko, H., Juji, T., Akaza, T., Yamamoto, K., ... Kodera, Y. (2002). The clinical significance of human leukocyte antigen (HLA) allele compatibility in patients receiving a marrow transplant from serologically HLA-A, HLA-B, and HLA-DR matched unrelated donors. *Blood, 99*, 4200–4206. https://doi.org/10.1182/blood.v99.11.4200

Motabi, I.H., & DiPersio, J.F. (2012). Advances in stem cell mobilization. *Blood Reviews, 26*, 267–278. https://doi.org/10.1016/j.blre.2012.09.003

Pelus, L.M. (2008). Peripheral blood stem cell mobilization: New regimens, new cells, where do we stand. *Current Opinion in Hematology, 15*, 285–292. https://doi.org/10.1097/moh.0b013e328302f43a

Petersdorf, E. (2016). Histocompatibility. In S.J. Forman, R.S. Negrin, J.H. Antin, & F.R. Appelbaum (Eds.), *Thomas' hematopoietic cell transplantation: Stem cell transplantation* (5th ed., pp. 112–125). https://doi.org/10.1002/9781118416426.ch10

Petersdorf, E., Anasetti, C., Martin, P.J., Woolfrey, A., Smith, A., Mickelson, E., ... Hansen, J.A. (2001). Genomics of unrelated-donor hematopoietic cell transplantation. *Current Opinion in Immunology, 13*, 582–589. https://doi.org/10.1016/s0952-7915(00)00263-6

Prabhakar, M., Ershler, W.B., & Long, D.L. (2009). Bone marrow, thymus and blood: Changes across the lifespan. *Aging Health, 5*, 385–393. https://doi.org/10.2217/ahe.09.31

Prohaska, S., & Weissman, I.L. (2009). Biology of hematopoietic stem and progenitor cells. In F.R. Appelbaum, S.J. Forman, R.S. Negrin, & K.G. Blume (Eds.), *Thomas' hematopoietic cell transplantation: Stem cell transplantation* (4th ed., pp. 36–63). Hoboken, NJ: Wiley-Blackwell. https://doi.org/10.1002/9781444303537.ch5

Rao, D.S. (2018). Overview and compartmentalization of the immune system. In R. Hoffman, E.J. Benz Jr., L.E. Silberstein, H.E. Heslop, J.I. Weitz, J. Anastasi, ... S.A. Abutalib (Eds.), *Hematology: Basic principles and practice* (7th ed., pp. 199–209). Philadelphia, PA: Elsevier.

Richards, S., Watanabe, C., Santos, L., Craxton, A., & Clark, E.A. (2008). Regulation of B-cell entry into the cell cycle. *Immunological Reviews, 224,* 183–200. https://doi.org/10.1111/j.1600-065x.2008.00652.x

Sallusto, F., Geginat, J., & Lanzavecchia, A. (2004). Central memory and effector memory T cell subsets: Function, generation, and maintenance. *Annual Review of Immunology, 22,* 745–763. https://doi.org/10.1146/annurev.immunol.22.012703.104702

Sallusto, F., & Lanzavecchia, A. (2001). Exploring pathways for memory T cell generation. *Journal of Clinical Investigation, 108,* 805–806. https://doi.org/10.1172/jci14005

Sallusto, F., Lenig, D., Förster, R., Lipp, M., & Lanzavecchia, A. (1999). Two subsets of memory T lymphocytes with distinct homing potentials and effector functions. *Nature, 401,* 708–712. https://doi.org/10.1038/44385

Sarkaria, S.M., Decker, M., & Ding, L. (2018). Bone marrow microenvironment in normal and deranged hematopoiesis: Opportunities for regenerative medicine and therapies. *BioEssays, 40*(3), 1–14. https://doi.org/10.1002/bies.201700190

Schwarz, B.A., & Bhandoola, A. (2006). Trafficking from the bone marrow to the thymus: A prerequisite for thymopoiesis. *Immunological Reviews, 209,* 47–57. https://doi.org/10.1111/j.0105-2896.2006.00350.x

Shevach, E.M. (2002). CD4⁺CD25⁺ suppressor T cells: More questions than answers. *Nature Reviews Immunology, 2,* 389–400. https://doi.org/10.1038/nri821

Storek, J., Geddes, M., Khan, F., Huard, B., Helg, C., Chalandon, Y., ... Roosnek, E. (2008). Reconstitution of the immune system after hematopoietic stem cell transplantation in humans. *Seminars in Immunopathology, 30,* 425–437. https://doi.org/10.1007/s00281-008-0132-5

Swirski, F.K., Nahrendorf, M., Etzrodt, M., Wildgruber, M., Cortez-Retamozo, V., Panizzi, P., ... Pittet, M.J. (2009). Identification of splenic reservoir monocytes and their deployment to inflammatory sites. *Science, 325,* 612–616. https://doi.org/10.1126/science.1175202

Tagliasacchi, D., & Carboni, G. (1997, April). Let's observe the blood cells. *Fun Science Gallery.* Retrieved from http://www.funsci.com/fun3_en/blood/blood.htm

Taylor, J., & Abdel-Wahab, O. (2018). Stem cell model of hematologic diseases. In R. Hoffman, E.J. Benz Jr., L.E. Silberstein, H.E. Heslop, J.I. Weitz, J. Anastasi, ... S.A. Abutalib (Eds.), *Hematology: Basic principles and practice* (7th ed., pp. 111–119). Philadelphia, PA: Elsevier.

Ueno, M., Itoh, M., Sugihara, K., Asano, M., & Takakura, N. (2009). Both alleles of *PSF1* are required for maintenance of pool size of immature hematopoietic cells and acute bone marrow regeneration. *Blood, 113,* 555–562. https://doi.org/10.1182/blood-2008-01-136879

University of Western Australia School of Anatomy and Human Biology. (2009, June 8). Blue histology—Blood. Retrieved from http://www.lab.anhb.uwa.edu.au/mb140/corepages/blood/blood.htm

Viale, A., & Pelicci, P.G. (2009). Awaking stem cells from dormancy: Growing old and fighting cancer. *EMBO Molecular Medicine, 1,* 88–91. https://doi.org/10.1002/emmm.200900019

Wilson, A., & Trumpp, A. (2006). Bone-marrow haematopoietic-stem-cell niches. *Nature Reviews Immunology, 6,* 93–106. https://doi.org/10.1038/nri1779

Zakrzewski, J.L., Holland, A.M., & van den Brink, M.R.M. (2007). Adoptive precursor cell therapy to enhance immune reconstitution after hematopoietic stem cell transplantation. *Journal of Molecular Medicine, 85,* 837–843. https://doi.org/10.1007/s00109-007-0175-4

Ziegler-Heitbrock, L. (2007). The CD14+ CD16+ blood monocytes: Their role in infection and inflammation. *Journal of Leukocyte Biology, 81,* 584–592. https://doi.org/10.1189/jlb.0806510

Zola, H., Swart, B., Boumsell, L., & Mason, D.Y. (2003). Human leucocyte differentiation antigen nomenclature: Update on CD nomenclature. Report of IUIS/WHO Subcommittee. *Journal of Immunological Methods, 275,* 1–8. https://doi.org/10.1016/s0022-1759(03)00057-7

Zola, H., Swart, B., Nicholson, I., Aasted, B., Bensussan, A., Boumsell, L., ... Warren, H. (2005). CD molecules 2005: Human cell differentiation molecules. *Blood, 106,* 3123–3126. https://doi.org/10.1182/blood-2005-03-1338

Zola, H., Swart, B., Nicholson, I., & Voss, E. (2007). *Leukocyte and stromal cell molecules: The CD markers.* Hoboken, NJ: Wiley.

CHAPTER 2

Basic Concepts of Transplantation

Elaine Z. Stenstrup, MSN, APRN, ACNS-BC, AOCNS®, BMTCN®

Introduction

The area of hematopoietic stem cell transplantation (HSCT) has a long history and has grown immensely since its beginnings. The roots of bone marrow transplantation (BMT) can be traced back to 1949 when Leon Jacobson and his colleagues performed mouse experiments and discovered that mice could recover from lethal irradiation if their spleens were shielded (Salhotra & Nakamura, 2017). Lorenz, Uphoff, Reid, and Shelton demonstrated in 1951 that radiation protection could be provided with the infusion of syngeneic (identical twin) marrow. In 1955, Main and Prehn showed that mice protected with an allogeneic marrow infusion could permanently accept a skin graft from a marrow donor. By the mid-1950s, several laboratories had shown by cytogenetic markers that the radioprotective effect of BMT was the result of the replacement of the host's damaged hematopoietic system with healthy cells from a donor (Perumbeti & Sacher, 2018). In 1959, Dr. E. Donnall Thomas initiated the first attempt to treat leukemia using high-dose chemotherapy followed by syngeneic marrow transplantation (Salhotra & Nakamura, 2017). In early trials, transplantation using donors other than identical twins proved unsuccessful because of a lack of understanding of human leukocyte antigens (HLAs) and their importance to histocompatibility (Singh & McGuirk, 2016). By the mid-1960s, it had been discovered, in dogs, that successful allogeneic marrow transplantation could be achieved by matching at the major histocompatibility complex (Singh & McGuirk, 2016).

Many of the early transplants were unsuccessful because of only transient engraftment of cells and disease progression. The first successful allogeneic transplant for leukemia occurred in the late 1960s at the University of Minnesota. The donor was a matched sibling, and the recipient was an infant with an immune-deficiency disease (de la Morena & Gatti, 2011). The first unrelated allogeneic transplant was performed in 1973. Autologous marrow transplantation was first used successfully in patients with lymphoma in the late 1970s and became more widespread throughout the 1990s (D'Souza, Lee, Zhu, & Pasquini, 2017). Currently, HSCT is used in a variety of malignant, nonmalignant, and genetically determined diseases and is the only known cure for many malignant and nonmalignant diseases (see Table 2-1). Transplantation may

Table 2-1. Common Diseases Treated With Hematopoietic Stem Cell Transplantation

Type of Disease	Autologous Transplant	Allogeneic Transplant
Malignant		
Hematologic malignancies	Hodgkin lymphoma Multiple myeloma Non-Hodgkin lymphoma	Acute lymphoblastic leukemia Acute myeloid leukemia Chronic lymphocytic leukemia Chronic myeloid leukemia Hodgkin lymphoma Juvenile chronic myeloid leukemia Multiple myeloma Myelodysplastic syndromes Myelofibrosis Non-Hodgkin lymphoma
Solid tumors	Germ cell tumors Medulloblastoma Neuroblastoma	–
Nonmalignant		
Hematologic	Amyloidosis Autoimmune disorders	Chronic granulomatous disease Congenital neutropenia Diamond-Blackfan anemia Fanconi anemia Severe aplastic anemia Sickle cell disease Thalassemia
Immunodeficiency	–	Severe combined immunodeficiency disease Wiskott-Aldrich syndrome
Genetic	–	Adrenoleukodystrophy Epidermolysis bullosa Gaucher disease Hunter syndrome Hurler syndrome Metachromatic leukodystrophy
Miscellaneous	–	Glycogen storage diseases Langerhans cell histiocytosis Osteopetrosis

Note. Based on information from Perumbeti & Sacher, 2017; Salhotra & Nakamura, 2017.

be referred to by different terms, including BMT, HSCT, peripheral blood stem cell (PBSC) transplant, or umbilical cord transplant.

HSCT is the transplantation of hematopoietic stem cells, which can proliferate, repopulate the marrow spaces, and mature. Blood counts and immunity are reestablished and recover when the mature blood cells enter the bloodstream (de la Morena & Gatti, 2011). Historically, hematopoietic stem cells were collected from the bone marrow. Now physicians can select from three sources: bone marrow, peripheral blood, and umbilical cord blood (UCB) (de la Morena & Gatti, 2011). This cell source is now used more often than bone marrow in adults undergoing allogeneic transplantation (Gregory, 2017). Transplantation of UCB was successfully performed for the first time in 1988 to treat a child with Fanconi anemia. The patient received UCB from a sibling who was a perfect HLA match (Gluckman & Ruggeri, 2017). Since then, much has been learned about UCB and its role in transplantation. Multiple UCB banks have been established in the United States and Europe. With these and other advances, UCB transplant is a viable option for adult and pediatric HSCT (Gluckman & Ruggeri, 2017). Advantages and disadvantages for each type of cell source are explained later in this chapter.

The use of HSCT has increased for several reasons. It allows for the administration of dose-intensive systemic chemotherapy and radiation that would be lethal without transplantation. In addition, HSCT from an allogeneic donor has an additional antitumor effect (Perumbeti & Sacher, 2018). Several characteristics of hematopoietic stem cells make transplantation possible. The first is their ability to regenerate in the marrow. Each hematopoietic stem cell is pluripotent and able to self-replicate, proliferate, and develop into myeloid (red blood cells, platelets, neutrophils, and macrophages) or lymphoid (T and B lymphocytes) pathways. A small number of stem cells can replicate to repopulate a patient's entire hematopoietic system (Perumbeti & Sacher, 2018). The second characteristic is the cells' ability to find their way to the marrow following IV infusion, a process that is not yet clearly understood (Nuss, Barnes, Olson, & Skeen, 2011). The third important characteristic of hematopoietic stem cells is that they can be safely cryopreserved, allowing storage for future use (Perumbeti & Sacher, 2018).

Types of Hematopoietic Stem Cell Transplants

HSCT is categorized based on the origin of the cell source. Categories include autologous, allogeneic, and syngeneic (identical twin).

Autologous Transplantation

Autologous HSCT refers to the use of stem cells collected from a patient, or "self," to be reinfused or "transplanted" back into the patient at a later date. Autologous HSCT is performed following myeloablation or high-dose chemotherapy. Stem cells are collected and cryopreserved; they may be stored indefinitely until needed for reinfusion at the time of stem cell rescue. Autologous transplantation following myeloablative therapy is used in a variety of diseases, and the goal is to rescue the bone marrow after it has been destroyed by the previous lethal therapy. For some diseases, it is considered part of the initial treatment plan; for others, it is reserved for relapse or persistent disease states. Diseases treated with autologous transplantation include multiple myeloma, non-Hodgkin lymphoma, Hodgkin lymphoma, germ cell tumors, neuroblastoma, brain tumors, sarcomas, and recurrent Wilms tumors. Autologous transplantation has expanded to the treatment of autoimmune disorders, such as Crohn disease and juvenile rheumatoid arthritis. Clinical trials continue to evaluate the effectiveness of this treatment for other solid tumors, severe autoimmune disease, and some rheumatologic disorders (National Marrow Donor Program [NMDP], n.d.-c). Advantages of autologous transplant include ready access to stem cells, decreased incidence and severity of side effects, earlier engraftment, and no risk of graft-versus-host disease (GVHD) (Perumbeti & Sacher, 2018). However, the risk of potential tumor contamination in the infused cell product and the lack of the immunologic graft-versus-tumor effect may contribute to relapse (Perumbeti & Sacher, 2018).

Allogeneic Transplantation

Allogeneic HSCT uses a related or unrelated donor as the source of stem cells (see Table 2-2). It is the treatment of choice for patients with cancer who have diseased bone marrow or patients with genetic and immunologic diseases wherein their disease requires specific new genetic material or immune function (Perumbeti & Sacher, 2018; Salhotra & Nakamura, 2017; see Table 2-1). Standard allogeneic transplantation uses myeloablative chemotherapy followed by infusion of stem cells from a compatible donor. Appropriate donors are identified through HLA typing. HLA compatibility is a key factor in predicting transplant-related morbidity and mortality. Because the antigens are genetically acquired, siblings are more likely to have similar HLA-matched stem cells. However, because of the pairing and various combinations of HLA antigens in a family, a patient with one sibling has an approximately 25% chance of a match. For the average American family, a person has only a 30% chance of finding an HLA-matched family donor (Salhotra & Nakamura, 2017). If an HLA-compatible match is not found in the family, unrelated donors may be sought through bone marrow donor registries or umbilical cord blood registries, the largest of which is the NMDP (n.d.-g). A *haploidentical* transplant (type of allogeneic transplant typically using a parent, sibling, or child donor) may be considered if a suitable or fully matched donor cannot be found. The donor in this case is exactly half-matched (NMDP, n.d.-e). This expands the donor pool of immediate family members. Advantages to allogeneic HSCT

Table 2-2. Types of Allogeneic Hematopoietic Stem Cell Transplantation

Type of Transplant	Cell Source	Advantages	Disadvantages
Syngeneic	Identical twin	No need for immunosuppression	No graft-versus-tumor effect
Matched sibling/related	Human leukocyte antigen (HLA)-identical relative	No potential stem cell disease contamination Access to cells because donor is related	Only 25% of population has a sibling match Risk of graft-versus-host disease (GVHD)
Mismatched related	HLA-nonidentical relative	No potential stem cell disease contamination Increased number of potential donors	Increased risk of GVHD Increased risk of graft failure related to HLA disparity
Matched unrelated	HLA-identical unrelated donor	No potential stem cell disease contamination	Increased risk of GVHD Limited numbers of non-Caucasian donors Waiting period to identify donor
Mismatched unrelated	HLA-nonidentical unrelated donor	No potential stem cell disease contamination	Increased risk of GVHD High treatment-related mortality
Umbilical cord blood	Umbilical cord unit	Easy access to cell source	Limited number of cells Delayed time to engraftment Increased infection rates

Note. Based on information from Salhotra & Nakamura, 2017.

include not only replacement of diseased or damaged stem cells with healthy ones, but also the addition of a powerful immune reaction in which the newly transplanted immune cells may react against any residual disease—known as the *graft-versus-tumor effect* (Forman & Nakamura, 2011; Perumbeti & Sacher, 2018).

As a result of the immune modulation with allogeneic transplantation, patients are at risk for GVHD, a clinical syndrome that results when immunocompetent donor T lymphocytes recognize and attack minor HLA-related antigens in the recipient, or host, and trigger an immune reaction (Perumbeti & Sacher, 2018). GVHD can be acute or chronic (see Chapter 7). It generally is believed that patients undergoing allogeneic HSCT tend to have more complications. Toxicities related to transplant vary depending on conditioning regimen, donor type, level and length of immunosuppression, and organ status prior to transplantation (Majhail et al., 2015).

Syngeneic Transplantation

The term *syngeneic transplant* refers to an allogeneic transplant in which stem cells are collected from one identical twin and infused into the other twin following high-dose chemotherapy. The advantage of a syngeneic transplant is an exact match and better engraftment outcomes, as well as the low risk of GVHD. The disadvantage of this type of transplant is the lack of graft-versus-tumor effect.

Nonmyeloablative Hematopoietic Stem Cell Transplantation

Because of the potential dangers of allogeneic HSCT, it traditionally has been reserved for patients younger than 60 years without comorbidities. However, today more transplantations are being performed in older patients because of advances in the field (NMDP, n.d.-g). Evidence suggests that the dose-intensive chemotherapy previously thought to be the curative agent in allogeneic HSCT may not be solely responsible for patients' durable remissions. Rather, the powerful graft-versus-tumor effect may be concurrently responsible (Perumbeti & Sacher, 2018). Based on this theory, newer, potentially safer ways to perform these transplants have been developed.

Nonmyeloablative allogeneic HSCT, a treatment using standard doses of chemotherapy followed by infusions of donor stem cells, has been developed to take advantage of the graft-versus-tumor effect while providing an effective yet less toxic modality for performing allogeneic HSCT. Nonmyeloablative therapy is used as a milder conditioning regimen in treating patients who are ineligible for standard high-dose allogeneic HSCT and for salvaging patients after relapse from previous autologous HSCT. Results of published studies demonstrate that allogeneic HSCT following nonmyeloablative conditioning has significant activity in patients with chronic myeloid leukemia, acute myeloid leukemia, low-grade lymphoma, and mantle cell lymphoma (Salhotra & Nakamura, 2017). Ongoing research is also looking at effectiveness in other solid tumors.

Sources of Stem Cells

Stem cells may be collected from the bone marrow, PBSCs, or UCB. Each source has advantages and disadvantages.

Bone Marrow

Traditionally, bone marrow was the exclusive source of stem cells. When cells are collected or harvested from bone marrow, the donor is placed under general or epidural anesthesia in an operating room. Bone marrow is obtained by performing multiple needle aspirations of marrow from the posterior iliac crests. If an inadequate number of cells are harvested, the anterior iliac crests may be used (Perumbeti & Sacher, 2018). The bone marrow is mixed with anticoagulant and filtered to remove bone chips, fat cells, blood clots, and cellular debris. According to AABB et al. (2018), the filtered marrow contains "mature red cells, white cells, platelets, committed progenitors of all lineages, mast cells, fat cells, plasma cells, and pluripotent hematopoietic cells" (p. 3). If the donor and recipient are not ABO compatible, the red blood cells can be removed through red cell depletion from the collected marrow, thus avoiding the problem of red cell lysis after infusion of the marrow (Forman & Nakamura, 2011; Perumbeti & Sacher, 2018).

Advantages to bone marrow collection are that it can be completed in several hours and is generally well tolerated by donors; therefore, it may be performed as an outpatient procedure or require only a one-night stay. More significantly, bone marrow as a graft source may result in a decreased risk of GVHD, which may have a profound impact on the recipient's long-term outcome and quality of life (Perumbeti & Sacher, 2018). For diseases that do not require a graft-versus-tumor effect, such as aplastic anemia, sickle cell disease, or metabolic disorders, many consider it advantageous to use bone marrow. Disadvantages include the need for general or epidural anesthesia and the risk of infection, bleeding, and bone damage (Nuss et al., 2011; Perumbeti & Sacher, 2018).

Peripheral Blood Stem Cells

During the past 25 years, the use of PBSCs as a rescue following myeloablative therapy has increased significantly (Juric et al., 2016). PBSCs were initially only used for autologous transplants. However, in recent years, the collection of PBSCs from allogeneic donors has grown. Currently, 75% of adults receive allogeneic PBSCs during transplantation (Anasetti et al., 2012; Juric et al., 2016).

Stem cells are mobilized, or moved out of the bone marrow into the peripheral blood, with the use of filgrastim (granulocyte–colony-stimulating factor) with or without chemotherapy (Perumbeti & Sacher, 2018). Sargramostim (granulocyte macrophage–colony-stimulating factor), a granulocyte–colony-stimulating factor that also acts on macrophages, is rarely used in mobilization because of its effect on liver function tests, retention of fluid, and reactions with first doses (hypotension and hypoxia) (Perumbeti & Sacher, 2018). Typically, an allogeneic donor receives growth factors for four to six days, and as cells are mobilized into the bloodstream, they can then be collected from the peripheral blood by a process called *apheresis* (Devine, 2016; Nuss et al., 2011). If chemotherapy and growth factor is used to mobilize stem cells for autologous transplants, apheresis will be performed once recovery of peripheral blood counts has begun—usually approximately 17 days after the chemotherapy was administered (Devine, 2016).

Apheresis uses centrifugation to remove stem cells from the blood, with the remaining blood components remixed and returned to the donor. In autologous transplants, donors may receive mobilization chemotherapy followed by filgrastim or sargramostim. Once the autologous stem cells are obtained, they are mixed with an anticoagulant and DMSO (dimethyl sulfoxide) and cryopreserved. DMSO is a preservative used to protect the stem cells from ice crystals that can cause cell injury during cryopreservation. In the allogeneic setting, cells may be administered directly following apheresis or may be cryopreserved (AABB et al., 2018). The cells can be processed to remove ABO-incompatible red cells, ABO-incompatible plasma, or donor T lymphocytes if required (AABB et al., 2018). The number of cells with the stem cell marker (the CD34 antigen or CD34+) will determine whether enough stem cells were collected. Forman and Nakamura (2011) reported that to have an adequate number of cells for engraftment, a minimum of 2×10^6 CD34+ cells/kg body weight must be collected.

Some advantages of PBSC collection are that it can be performed as an outpatient procedure with no need for anesthesia, and it is generally tolerated well by donors of all ages. Most pediatric centers use a cutoff weight for safely apheresing allogeneic donors because of the potential exposure to blood products due to potential loss of red cells during apheresis relative to the smaller size of the donor. Another important advantage is that cells obtained from the blood are more mature and engraft earlier than cells obtained from bone marrow (Gregory, 2017). This quicker hematologic recovery time is favorable because it decreases length of neutropenia, use of antibiotics, length of thrombocytopenia, risk of bleeding, use of blood products, and organ toxicity, and it also causes fewer infections. All these lead to shorter hospital stays and lower costs.

An important consideration is to determine how the PBSCs will be collected. For autologous transplants, tunneled multilumen apheresis catheters are inserted into the patient for stem cell collection and may stay in place throughout the transplant process. Otherwise, a percutaneous nontunneled "dialysis" catheter can be placed in a central vein for the procedure. Peripheral IV access usually is used for allogeneic donors if good venous access is available and the donor can tolerate it for the duration of the apheresis procedure. Stem cell collection may take one to three or more apheresis procedures over several days, with each procedure lasting four to six hours (Forman & Nakamura, 2011; Gregory, 2017).

Umbilical Cord Blood Units

UCB has been a source of stem cells for transplantation for 15–20 years (Juric et al., 2016). It is a rich source of stem cells collected from the umbilical cord and placenta at the time of childbirth (AABB et al., 2018). This source can induce engraftment in some children and adults. Because the cells from UCB have not matured immunologically, they may be used in transplants in which a true HLA match cannot be obtained, such as when a matching sibling donor is unavailable or when no donor match is found in a transplant registry (Gluckman & Ruggeri, 2017; NMDP, n.d.-b). The UCB stem cells can be frozen and stored in a cord blood bank to be used in the registry for related or unrelated HSCT. Some mothers who are in childbearing years may choose to have another child to produce a related UCB source for a sick child.

Advantages of using UCB as a graft source include easy access to the UCB units, the speed with which a unit can be obtained once selected, and a simple collection procedure with no risk to the mother or child. Additional advantages over unrelated BMT are a lower risk of GVHD and rejection and decreased rate of virus transmission (Gluckman & Ruggeri, 2017). Disadvantages of UCB include the potential for passing genetic diseases to the recipient, a limited number of cells, slower engraftment (cells take time to mature), delayed post-transplant immune reconstitution, decreased graft-versus-tumor effect, and high costs of UCB units. It also is impossible to go back to the donor if additional cells are needed, and the risk of graft failure is greater (Perumbeti & Sacher, 2018). In UCB transplants, the cell dose is a more important determinant of outcome and survival than the cell source (Gluckman & Ruggeri, 2017; Nuss et al., 2011).

Be The Match (National Marrow Donor Program)

For the 70% of patients who do not have an HLA-compatible related donor, registries such as Be The Match (founded in 1986 as NMDP) provide potential unrelated donor options. With more than 19 million potential volunteer donors and 249,000 UCB units listed in its registry, it is the world's largest single database of unrelated marrow, UCB units, and stem cell donors. Be The Match offers a single point of access to finding unrelated marrow, blood stem cells, and UCB units. Through Be The Match, approximately 6,200 transplants are performed each year, under the mission to facilitate worldwide unrelated BMT and PBSC transplants. Since its inception, more than 92,000 transplants and cellular therapies have been facilitated (NMDP, n.d.-f).

Be The Match initiatives include supporting research (comprehensive database), empowering patients, educating medical professionals, and working to reduce the time needed for a donor search and the time between finding the donor and the transplant. Donor recruitment is a priority. Although Caucasians are well represented in registries, powerful initiatives are underway for targeted minority recruitment. Efforts are focused on African Americans, Native Americans and Alaska Natives, Asians and Pacific Islanders, and Hispanics and Latinos.

The initial step to finding an adult unrelated donor is to obtain the patient's HLA typing using the recommended molecular (DNA) testing methods. The search to find a donor may take several weeks to months, although searching cord blood banks can reveal blood units that are available immediately. A preliminary search is performed, which is a "single snapshot" of potential donors on the registry. It is a computerized search of all stem cell donors and UCB unit information contained in the registry that day. The preliminary search is free, and results usually are available within 24 hours. The search can be performed for any physician, by NMDP, or by an NMDP-approved transplant center. After the preliminary search is completed, patients and physicians receive information about unrelated donor transplantation from Be The Match (NMDP, n.d.-d).

If the decision is made to proceed with the transplant process, the patient must then be referred to a Be The Match–approved transplant center. A formal search is then initiated. Formal searches include further laboratory testing performed at the transplant center. This testing is done to confirm the initial HLA results as well as potential matches. Once a donor is identified and the typing is confirmed to be an appropriate match with the patient, the transplant center's physicians may request that the donor proceed to the workup phase. The donor will be contacted and educated about the donation process for the stem cell product requested (bone marrow or PBSCs). The potential donor will undergo a comprehensive physical evaluation, including blood work and any additional medical testing deemed necessary for safe procurement of the blood cell product (NMDP, n.d.-a, n.d.-d).

The goal of this evaluation is to protect the safety of the donor and the recipient. The potential transmission of communicable diseases from the donor to recipient is a serious concern. Therefore, laboratory testing includes complete blood count, electrolytes, and renal, hepatic, and endocrine testing. Infectious disease testing includes hepatitis B, hepatitis C, HIV, cytomegalovirus, herpes simplex virus, syphilis, and human T-lymphotropic virus, as well as other infectious disease testing the transplant center deems appropriate. The donor also will have blood and Rh typing, HLA testing, and pregnancy testing if applicable. A thorough physical examination and medical history, including travel, immunization, and transfusion histories, will be obtained (Perumbeti & Sacher, 2018).

Preparative Regimens

Many combinations of preparative regimens consisting of chemotherapy, immunotherapy, or radiation therapy are given before transplantation. The agents used in preparative regimens vary depending on the type of transplant (allogeneic vs. autologous), the disease being treated, and the desired effects of the HSCT. The goals of preparative regimens in traditional (myeloablative) allogeneic transplants include eradicating any malignant disease and suppressing the immune system to prevent graft rejection (Juric et al., 2016; Salhotra & Nakamura, 2017). In autologous transplants, immunosuppression is unnecessary because the host is the source of the new stem cells. Thus, the main goals are to eradicate disease and ablate the bone marrow. The goal of HSCT for treatment of nonmalignant diseases is to provide immunosuppression and bone marrow ablation to transplant a missing or defective gene (Juric et al., 2016; Perumbeti & Sacher, 2018). For additional information on preparative regimens, see Chapter 6.

Preparative regimens have evolved over time as more has been learned about various diseases and their responses to different drugs. Early BMTs used total body irradiation (TBI) alone for conditioning. TBI is the exposure of the entire body to gamma radiation. It is delivered in varying doses, usually to patients with lymphoid malignancies, and may be given as a single dose or in fractionated doses over three or four days (Juric et al., 2016). Although TBI can produce immunosuppression, bone marrow ablation, and some antitumor effects, it is not entirely effective in eradicating diseased marrow. Therefore, chemotherapy is added to optimize the conditioning regimen (Juric et al., 2016).

Preparative regimens vary depending on the disease, stem cell source, type of transplant, and goals of conditioning. Preparative regimens can be myeloablative, meaning the patient typically receives high-dose chemotherapy with or without radiation therapy, or nonmyeloablative, which are less-intensive regimens associated with decreased toxicity. Myeloablative preparative or conditioning regimens may last from two days to more than a week and are used to ablate the bone marrow by destroying diseased cells and killing or suppressing all other marrow cells, thus causing enough immunosuppression to enable donor cells to engraft (Juric et al., 2016; Perumbeti & Sacher, 2018). Nonmyeloablative regimens are less toxic because of reduced doses of chemotherapy and TBI and are used most often in older adult patients, patients with comorbid diseases, or patients who need the benefit of the associated graft-versus-tumor effect (Juric et al., 2016; Perumbeti & Sacher, 2018).

Choice of a preparative or conditioning regimen is largely based on the disease being treated and the goal of therapy. For hematologic and immunodeficiency diseases, high doses of chemotherapy, with or without TBI, will eradicate stem cells in the bone marrow to make space for engraftment of healthy allogeneic cells. The new donor cells will produce healthy white blood cells, red blood cells, and platelets and restore immunity (AABB et al., 2018). The goal of HSCT for hematologic malignancies is to administer high-dose chemotherapy to aggressively treat the disease, followed by reinfusion of stem cells to rescue the patient from the side effects of myeloablation. In genetic and metabolic disorders, chemotherapy is given to destroy abnormal cells in the bone marrow. Donor cells are infused and,

upon engraftment, produce adequate amounts of previously deficient enzymes, proteins, or genes, thus hopefully stopping disease progression and symptoms related to the disorder and possibly repairing disease damage (Perumbeti & Sacher, 2018).

The preparative regimen for nonmyeloablative allogeneic HSCT is different than that for traditional allogeneic HSCT because although the process is similar, the goals are different. Patients are conditioned with chemotherapy and/or radiation. The goal of this preparative regimen is not to eradicate the malignancy; rather, the intent is to provide adequate immunosuppression to achieve mixed chimerism initially and, ultimately, full donor chimeric engraftment of an allogeneic blood cell graft. *Chimerism* is the presence of donor hematopoietic cell lines in an allogeneic transplant recipient. This is evaluated by using genetic markers to confirm engraftment and to distinguish the donor from the recipient. The optimal conditioning regimen is yet to be determined. Regimens typically consist of highly immunosuppressive chemotherapy agents, such as purine analogs (e.g., fludarabine) or alkylating agents (e.g., busulfan, cyclophosphamide) in nonmyeloablative doses alone or in combination with immunosuppressive agents (e.g., antithymocyte globulin), monoclonal antibodies (e.g., alemtuzumab), or low-dose total nodal irradiation or TBI (200 cGy). The combination of chemotherapy, radiation, and immunotherapy is intended to suppress the recipient's immune system and allow engraftment of donor cells, as well as induce a graft-versus-tumor response (Salhotra & Nakamura, 2017).

Clinical Evaluation

Because many life-threatening complications are associated with HSCT, the decision to use this treatment is based on a thorough patient evaluation. Some variation exists among transplant centers in terms of eligibility requirements, diseases treated, and the pretransplant clinical evaluation. In an effort to standardize, as well as promote quality medical practices, the Foundation for the Accreditation of Cellular Therapy (FACT) was formed in 1996 by the American Society for Blood and Marrow Transplantation (now the American Society for Transplantation and Cellular Therapy) and the International Society for Cell and Gene Therapy (FACT & Joint Accreditation Committee–ISCT and EBMT [JACIE], 2018). FACT is a national voluntary inspection and accreditation program that encompasses all phases of hematopoietic cell collection, processing, and transplantation. It was developed to oversee and encourage standardization of quality practices in transplant centers. Centers that meet rigorous standards of quality medical care and laboratory practice are recognized with certificates of accreditation. FACT requirements for patient evaluation are listed in Figure 2-1.

General considerations for eligibility include determining that the patient has a chemotherapy-sensitive disease, adequate organ function, and no life-threatening viral exposures or comorbidities. Additionally, the patient's age, performance status, and ability to adhere to treatment instructions are considered. A clinical evaluation, including a complete health history documenting the history of the present illness, should be obtained. Information should include the disease and treatment course from diagnosis to the time of transplant. A general health history, including past medical and surgical history and family, social, and travel history, should be obtained, along with documentation of allergies, medications, and, if female, gynecologic history. A complete physical examination should be performed, including laboratory studies and diagnostics assessing vital organ function and infectious disease testing (FACT & JACIE, 2018).

In addition to the clinical assessment, a psychosocial assessment of the patient and family should be performed (Nuss et al., 2011). The patient should be evaluated for comprehension of the procedure, potential risks, side effects, and complications as well as the ability to adhere to treatment instructions. Psychosocial evaluation should include social and spiritual issues, psychological well-being, financial issues, and family concerns. Children should have neuropsychological testing performed to set a baseline for further assessments. Finally, consent must be obtained prior to HSCT. If the patient is a minor, a parent or guardian must consent; however, children younger than 18 years of age may sign an assent form.

Allogeneic transplant donors must undergo a thorough clinical evaluation and psychosocial assessment. They should have a complete medical history and physical examination to rule out genetic or infectious diseases and significant health problems that may pose a risk to either the patient or the donor during the collection of stem cells (see Figure 2-1). The stem cell donor evaluation is described in Chapter 5. Psychological intervention allows donors to express any fears they have regarding collection of stem cells or bone marrow and discuss ways to cope with those fears. Intervention should be provided to assist donors in processing feelings of guilt or anxiety related to the transplant recipient's outcome. The identity of an unrelated donor is typically kept confidential for at least one year. Some centers allow recipients to have anonymous contact with their donor during the first year via letters or cards; some allow direct contact one or more years after transplant if the donor and recipient consent; and some do not allow any contact (NMDP, n.d.-c). Informed consent is obtained prior to collection of PBSCs or donation of bone marrow.

Patient and Family Education

Transplantation is a very intense, complicated process that requires educational efforts throughout all phases of treatment. Nurses have an excellent opportunity to provide this education to patients, donors, and families or support people at each transplant phase. Education can be delivered using discussions, written materials, informational web-

Figure 2-1. Clinical Evaluation Requirements for Transplantation

Laboratory Evaluation
- Complete blood count with differential
- Chemistry profile
- Electrolytes, liver function tests, blood urea nitrogen/creatinine, prothrombin time/partial thromboplastin time, international normalized ratio
- Hepatitis B surface antigen[a,b]
- Hepatitis C antibody[a,b]
- HIV antibody[a,b]
- HIV1/2 antibody[a,b]
- Human T-cell leukemia virus 1[a,b]
- Rapid plasma reagin test[a,b]
- Cytomegalovirus immunoglobulin G, IgM[a,b]
- Herpes simplex virus immunoglobulin G
- ABO/Rh[a,b]
- Human leukocyte antigen typing for allogeneic transplants[b]
- Toxoplasmosis antibody
- Cocci serologies
- Varicella zoster virus immunoglobulin G
- Glomerular filtration rate/creatinine clearance
- Pregnancy test[a,b]

Organ Function Testing
- Multigated acquisition scan/echocardiogram
- Pulmonary function test
- 12-lead electrocardiogram
- Dental examination

Disease Evaluation
- Bone marrow aspirates and biopsies
- Lumbar puncture
- Computed tomography scans
- Magnetic resonance imaging
- Bone scan
- Positron-emission tomography scan
- Tumor markers
- 24-hour urine protein electrophoresis
- Immunoglobulins
- Urine catecholamines (vanillylmandelic acid/homovanillic acid)

[a] Required by Foundation for the Accreditation of Cellular Therapy
[b] Required for donor also

Note. Based on information from Foundation for the Accreditation of Cellular Therapy & Joint Accreditation Committee–ISCT and EBMT, 2018.

sites, and audiovisual aids if available. Barriers to learning should be identified and addressed.

Donors should be instructed regarding the diagnostic studies and laboratory tests required to evaluate their health status prior to donation of stem cells. Donors should have a thorough understanding of the collection process, the potential risks and complications, and the potential outcomes they may experience, along with the potential outcomes for the recipient of their donated cells. Donors also should know how to seek medical attention if they develop complications or have questions following collection.

Pretransplant education for patients and families should be individualized and ongoing, with continued evaluation of their comprehension and understanding of the process. Many patients have received other therapies prior to transplantation and may have previous experience with chemotherapy or radiation therapy and hospitalization. Many centers use printed (booklets or binders) or electronic educational materials related to each phase of transplant. Education should begin during the pretransplant time and may comprise the many roles involved with transplant: nurse, provider, pharmacist, social worker, and nutritionist. Assessment of a patient's prior experience with side effects may guide the nurse in providing appropriate pretransplant education. The nurse should discuss the route of administration, dosage, side effects, and administration of all medications, such as chemotherapy agents, anti-infectives, immunosuppressants, antiemetics, immunomodulators, analgesics, and growth factors. For patients undergoing autologous HSCT, information should be provided regarding the reinfusion and potential side effects and complications occurring during aplasia, including organ toxicity, infection, and bleeding. For patients undergoing allogeneic HSCT, education should include the risks, clinical presentation, and treatments for GVHD and hematopoietic growth factors. Additionally, the potential side effects of immunosuppressive medications, such as high risk of infection, hepatotoxicity, and nephrotoxicity, should be discussed.

Because of the level of caregiver burden for families and support people of patients undergoing HSCT, family structure and function should be assessed early in the transplant process. Many transplant centers require identification of a competent adult caregiver prior to initiation of transplantation, especially if most of the care will occur in the ambulatory setting, as in autologous or nonmyeloablative transplants. Efforts should include educating families on both the physical and psychosocial aspects of the process. Helping families to identify key support people and teaching them to delegate activities to maximize available resources are key elements in managing caregiver burden. Family members should be encouraged to express their fears and concerns regarding the possibility of death of the patient and their expectations and hope for a positive outcome. Patients and families need to be aware that transplantation may not be curative. Nurses, social workers, and psychosocial staff should address these issues and acknowledge changing roles within the family and their impact on the HSCT process. Whenever possible, families and support people should be encouraged to participate in groups and use other available support networks.

The education of a child undergoing transplantation requires special attention. Many pediatric transplant centers employ child life specialists who can assist with developing appropriate education. Educational efforts should be directed toward the child's developmental stage (Nuss et al., 2011). Although children may not understand everything, the healthcare team should attempt to help them understand why they are in the hospital, what is going to happen, how they may feel, and what they can do during the transplant process. Teaching should be conducted at appropriate times, and children should always be told what to expect prior to procedures or administration of medications. Children should be given the opportunity to ask questions and share their concerns. Parents may need help in addressing their children's questions or needs. Child life specialists, nurses, and other staff should be available to assist with education of children and families (Nuss et al., 2011).

Much of the basics of PBSC transplant and BMT can be applied to both adults and children. However, special considerations exist for children. Pediatric patients have unique growth and developmental needs. Children's ability to cope will depend on their developmental level, along with the trust and support they feel from the family and the transplant staff (Toruner & Altay, 2018). Children should have opportunities to have their emotional and developmental needs met. This could include enabling them to continue schoolwork, activities, play, and exercise, if possible. Peer interaction should be continued via computers, cell phones, and letters, if age appropriate. Social interaction with family, friends, and staff will be very important. Staff who are familiar with pediatric patients and their needs should be involved in the care of these patients when possible. Family involvement is crucial when a child is undergoing the transplant experience, and the entire family will need to be cared for and included.

Finally, discharge education is very important and should be initiated early to optimize planning and resources. Because of the high level of anxiety of patients and caregivers, information should be presented clearly and reinforced frequently during the hospital stay. Discharge instructions should be explained verbally by the nurse and reinforced by providing printed materials to take home. They should be realistic regarding life after transplant. Information provided should include the risk of infection, practices to prevent infection, physical activity expectations and restrictions, and medication administration. Patients and caregivers need information on how to meet daily nutritional requirements to combat fatigue. The possibility of GVHD and long-term complications of each organ system should be addressed. A follow-up plan should be outlined for patients and families (Khera et al., 2017).

Teaching at discharge should include family members and support people. Family roles may change throughout the transplant process as patients require changing levels of support. Family members should be instructed in ways to cope with the stress associated with this dynamic process (Khera et al., 2017). Everyday family life may be disrupted with frequent follow-up office visits in addition to the long-term effects of treatment (e.g., fatigue, GVHD). The family also may be dealing with financial issues, uncertainty about the future, fear of relapse, and fear of death (Khera et al., 2017). Recurrence anxiety is a predominant theme rarely addressed by the professional team because assessment of symptoms and recovery take priority. The family should be given time to discuss all these issues and express any concerns prior to discharge so that a follow-up plan can be cooperatively developed (Khera et al., 2017).

Summary

HSCT is a very complex process that continues to grow and develop. It is essential for nurses to maintain current knowledge of the basics so that they can continually improve the quality of care provided to patients and families. Treatment advances are occurring rapidly, and nurses have a tremendous opportunity to prepare and assist patients throughout the transplant process.

The author would like to acknowledge Dawn Niess, CNP, MS, RN, for her contribution to this chapter that remains unchanged from the previous edition of this book.

References

AABB, America's Blood Centers, American Red Cross, American Society for Apheresis, American Society for Blood and Marrow Transplantation, College of American Pathologists, … World Marrow Donor Association. (2018, October). *Circular of information for the use of cellular therapy products.* Retrieved from http://www.aabb.org/aabbcct/coi/Documents/CT-Circular-of-Information.pdf

Anasetti, C., Logan, B.R., Lee, S.J., Waller, E.K., Weisdorf, D.J., Wingard, J.R., … Confer, D.L. (2012). Peripheral-blood stem cells versus bone marrow from unrelated donors. *New England Journal of Medicine, 367,* 1487–1496. https://doi.org/10.1056/NEJMoa1203517

de la Morena, M.T., & Gatti, R.A. (2011). A history of bone marrow transplantation. *Hematology/Oncology Clinics of North America, 25,* 1–15. https://doi.org/10.1016/j.hoc.2010.11.001

Devine, H. (2016). Blood and marrow stem cell transplantation. In B.H. Gobel, S. Triest-Robertson, & W.H. Vogel (Eds.), *Advanced oncology nursing certification review and resource manual* (2nd ed., pp. 293–344). Pittsburgh, PA: Oncology Nursing Society.

D'Souza, A., Lee, S., Zhu, X., & Pasquini, M. (2017). Current use and trends in hematopoietic cell transplantation in the United States. *Biology of Blood and Marrow Transplantation, 23,* 1417–1421. https://doi.org/10.1016/j.bbmt.2017.05.035

Forman, S.J., & Nakamura, R. (2011). Hematopoietic cell transplantation. In R. Pazdur, L.D. Wagman, K.A. Camphausen, & W.J. Hoskins (Eds.), *Cancer management: A multidisciplinary approach: Medical, surgical, and radiation oncology* [Online ed.]. Retrieved from https://www.cancernetwork.com/cancer-management/hematopoietic-cell-transplantation

Foundation for the Accreditation of Cellular Therapy & Joint Accreditation Committee–ISCT and EBMT. (2018). *FACT-JACIE international standards for hematopoietic cellular therapy product collection, processing, and administration* (7th ed.). Retrieved from https://www.ebmt.org/sites/default/files/2018-06/FACT-JACIE%207th%20Edition%20Standards.pdf

Gluckman, E., & Ruggeri, A. (2017). Historical perspective and current trends of umbilical cord blood transplantation. In M. Horwitz & N. Chao (Eds.), *Cord blood transplantations. Advances and controversies in hematopoietic transplantation and cell therapy* (pp. 1–12). https://doi.org/10.1007/978-3-319-53628-6_1

Gregory, S.J. (2017). Hematopoietic stem cell transplantation. In J. Eggert (Ed.), *Cancer basics* (2nd ed., pp. 323–353). Pittsburgh, PA: Oncology Nursing Society.

Juric, M.K., Ghimire, S., Ogonek, J., Weissinger, E.M., Holler, E., van Rood, J.J., … Greinix, H.T. (2016). Milestones of hematopoietic stem cell transplantation—From first human studies to current developments. *Frontiers in Immunology, 7,* 470. https://doi.org/10.3389/fimmu.2016.00470

Khera, N., Martin, P., Edsall, K., Bonagura, A., Burns, L.J., Juckett, M., … Majhail, N.S. (2017). Patient-centered care coordination in hematopoietic cell transplantation. *Blood Advances, 1,* 1617–1627. https://doi.org/10.1182/bloodadvances.2017008789

Lorenz, E., Uphoff, D., Reid, T.R., & Shelton, E. (1951). Modification of irradiation injury in mice and guinea pigs by bone marrow injections. *Journal of the National Cancer Institute, 12,* 197–201. https://doi.org/10.1093/jnci/12.1.197

Main, J.M.M., & Prehn, R.T. (1955). Successful skin homografts after the administration of high dosage X radiation and homologous bone marrow. *Journal of the National Cancer Institute, 15,* 1023–1029. https://doi.org/10.1093/jnci/15.4.1023

Majhail, N.S., Farnia, S.H., Carpenter, P.A., Champlin, R.E., Crawford, S., Marks, D.I., … LeMaistre, C.F. (2015). Indications for autologous and allogeneic hematopoietic cell transplantation: Guidelines from the American Society for Blood and Marrow Transplantation. *Biology of Blood and Marrow Transplantation, 21,* 1863–1869. https://doi.org/10.1016/j.bbmt.2015.07.032

National Marrow Donor Program. (n.d.-a). Before you donate. Retrieved from https://bethematch.org/support-the-cause/donate-bone-marrow/donation-process/before-you-donate

National Marrow Donor Program. (n.d.-b). Cell sources. Retrieved from https://bethematchclinical.org/transplant-therapy-and-donor-matching/cell-sources

National Marrow Donor Program. (n.d.-c). Contacting your donor. Retrieved from https://bethematch.org/patients-and-families/life-after-transplant/contacting-your-donor

National Marrow Donor Program. (n.d.-d). Donor or cord blood unit search process. Retrieved from https://bethematchclinical.org/transplant-therapy-and-donor-matching/donor-or-cord-blood-search-process

National Marrow Donor Program. (n.d.-e). Haploidentical transplant. Retrieved from https://bethematch.org/patients-and-families/about-transplant/what-is-a-bone-marrow-transplant/haploidentical-transplant

National Marrow Donor Program. (n.d.-f). Our story. Retrieved from https://bethematch.org/about-us/our-story

National Marrow Donor Program. (n.d.-g). Patient eligibility for HCT. Retrieved from https://bethematchclinical.org/transplant-indications-and-outcomes/eligibility

Nuss, S., Barnes, Y., Fisher, V., Olson, E., & Skeens, M. (2011). Hematopoietic cell transplantation. In C. Baggott, D. Fochtman, G.V. Foley, & K.P. Kelly (Eds.), *Nursing care of children and adolescents with cancer and blood disorders* (4th ed., pp. 405–466). Glenview, IL: Association of Pediatric Hematology/Oncology Nurses.

Perumbeti, A., & Sacher, R.A. (2018, August 6). Hematopoietic stem cell transplantation. *Medscape.* Retrieved from https://emedicine.medscape.com/article/208954-overview#a14

Salhotra, A., & Nakamura, R. (2017). Overview of hematopoietic cell transplantation. In J.A. Cotliar (Ed.), *Atlas of graft-versus-host disease* (pp. 1–11). https://doi.org/10.1007/978-3-319-46952-2_1

Singh, A.K., & McGuirk, J.P. (2016). Allogeneic stem cell transplantation: A historical and scientific overview. *Cancer Research, 76,* 6445–6451. https://doi.org/10.1158/0008-5472.can-16-1311

Toruner, E.K., & Altay, N. (2018). New trends and recent care approaches in pediatric oncology nursing. *Asia-Pacific Journal of Oncology Nursing, 5,* 156–164. https://doi.org/10.4103/apjon.apjon_3_18

CHAPTER 3

Current Research

Shelley Burcat, MSN, RN, AOCNS®, CCCTM

Introduction

Research studies leading to wide application of hematopoietic stem cell transplantation (HSCT) began more than 50 years ago (Thomas, 1999). In 1977, a transplant team in Seattle reported on 100 patients with advanced acute leukemia who were prepared with cyclophosphamide and total body irradiation (TBI) and then given bone marrow from a human leukocyte antigen (HLA)-matched sibling. Seventeen of the patients were alive one to three years later (Thomas et al., 1977). The success of HSCT in even a few patients with advanced disease allowed researchers to consider treating patients earlier in the course of their disease (Thomas, 1999). Today, more than 90% of patients with early-stage hematologic malignancies and nonmalignant disorders can be cured if an optimal donor recipient combination is available (World Health Organization [WHO], n.d.). Currently, HSCT is performed in more than 500 centers in more than 50 countries, with approximately 50,000 HSCTs performed worldwide annually, and the number increases every year (D'Souza & Fretham, 2018; WHO, n.d.). In the United States, approximately 23,000 transplants are performed annually, and that number increases by 3% each year (Blood and Marrow Transplant Clinical Trials Network [BMT CTN], 2019). More recently, cord blood has been used as a stem cell source for patients without a donor, and more than 2,000 HSCTs are performed annually using cord blood (WHO, n.d.). Despite the advances made by the hundreds of teams performing HSCTs, obstacles remain (Wolff et al., 2011).

Ongoing clinical trials continue to define the role of HSCT in the treatment of many malignant and nonmalignant disease processes, including autoimmune diseases (ADs) and primary immunodeficiency diseases. This chapter will review the clinical trial process, current research, and future directions in HSCT.

Clinical Trials

Clinical trials are essential for the identification of effective therapies in modern medicine (Jones, Braz, McBride, Roberts, & Platts-Mills, 2016). The combination of earlier detection of most forms of cancer and the application of new treatments developed through clinical trials has improved the five-year survival rate from 1 in 3 four decades ago to 1 in 2 (Comis, Miller, Aldigé, Krebs, & Stoval, 2003). Nearly every new treatment, test, or intervention for cancer must be rigorously tested in clinical trials to be sure it is safe and effective before it can be used routinely in humans. In clinical trials, researchers test drugs, medical devices, and supportive care and other interventions in human volunteers, with the goal of improving all aspects of patient care (National Cancer Institute [NCI], n.d.). Clinical trials are used to find answers to different clinical questions, such as the following (NCI, n.d.): Can a new (or old) drug prevent cancer in people with higher risk of the disease? Can a drug or lifestyle change (e.g., exercise, diet) after treatment extend the lives of patients with cancer? Can a new drug or intervention improve quality of life?

Clinical trials are only conducted when there is a good reason to believe that a test or treatment may improve the care of patients. Before a clinical trial is opened to human participants, it must go through rigorous preclinical research. During preclinical research, scientists try to learn as much as they can about a compound, drug, or device. This may include animal studies. Once it is thought a drug or device may have clinical benefit, it is tested using human clinical trials. Clinical trials to test new cancer treatments involve a series of steps, called phases. If a new treatment is successful in one phase, it will proceed to further testing, using the next phase. Although clinical trials may be the only hope for finding a cure or symptom relief for a rare or terminal illness, patients are not enrolled in clinical trials to cure them. Table 3-1 describes the phases of clinical trials in detail. Types of clinical studies and trials are described in Tables 3-2 and 3-3.

Scientific Review Committee

The scientific review committee (SRC) conducts a peer review of local, national, and international research studies involving patients with cancer treated at its facility. NCI requires SRC review as part of cancer center designation. The SRC reviews all clinical intervention and nonintervention studies that involve cancer, cancer prevention, and survivorship. It is not responsible for reviewing studies that have undergone peer review by an NCI-accepted organization. The SRC also reviews all prospective studies

Table 3-1. Phases of Clinical Trials

Phase	Description
0	• First clinical trials performed using human participants • Aim to learn how a drug is processed in the body and how it affects the body • Very small dose of a drug given to approximately 10–15 people • Can help researchers decide if the new treatment should be tested in phase 1 trial • May also be referred to as pilot studies
1	• Help researchers identify the maximum tolerated dose for a new drug or new application for a drug • Study drug given to every person in the trial • Start with low doses given to a few patients, usually 3—referred to as a cohort • Dose increases with each cohort until side effects become too severe or the desired effect is achieved • May also collect information such as when and how often a drug should be taken and any side effects or problems • Usually enroll 15–30 people • May provide treatment benefit to participants, but primary goal is to determine safety • If a drug or treatment is found to be safe, progresses to phase 2 trial • 30% of drugs tested fail the phase 1 trial; 70% move to phase 2 trial • May be the only hope for finding a cure or symptom relief for a rare or terminal disease
2	• Conducted with larger numbers of patients to determine effectiveness of the potential treatment/drug in curing a disease or reducing symptoms • Include patients who have a certain type of cancer or disease • May also test new combinations of drugs • Usually enroll 30–120 patients • Participants assigned to either the study treatment or standard treatment • If drug is found likely to work and is as safe as the regular treatment, progresses to phase 3 trial

3	• Determine effectiveness of a drug or treatment for a specific disease
	• Compare a new drug or treatment to the current standard treatment
	• Assess side effects of each drug or treatment and determine which treatment works better
	• Patients are assigned to different groups or arms:
	  – Each group/arm receives a different treatment.
	  – Groups/arms are chosen using randomization.
	• Can enroll from 100 to several thousand people
	• Involve close observation of every participant
	• May be closed if side effects are too severe or one group has significantly better results
	• If a new treatment or drug is shown to be safe and effective, an application can be made for FDA approval:
	  – FDA reviews clinical trial results.
	  – Results that meet FDA standards are approved and the drug or treatment becomes available.

4	• Test treatments or drugs that have already received FDA approval • Test effectiveness, safety, and side effects over a long time • Help identify unknown or rare side effects • Include hundreds or thousands of patients • Can also be used to obtain FDA approval for a second indication

FDA—U.S. Food and Drug Administration

Note. Based on information from National Cancer Institute, 2016; National Comprehensive Cancer Network, n.d.; Statistics How To, 2016.

for tissue and/or body fluids with a scientific hypothesis that has not undergone a peer review, as well as studies that involve a cancer diagnosis regardless of whether the study's focus is cancer. The primary focus of the scientific review is for scientific merit, feasibility, and utilization of the cancer center's resources (Stanford Medicine, n.d.). The scientific review is completed prior to the institutional review board (IRB) review.

Institutional Review Board

All research that involves human participants should be reviewed by an IRB. Under U.S. Food and Drug Adminis-

tration (FDA) regulations, an IRB is an appropriately constituted committee designated to review and monitor biomedical and behavioral research involving human participants. The IRB comprises scientific experts and nonscientific members. It has the authority to approve, require modifications in (to secure approval), or disapprove research. The purpose of the IRB is to ensure appropriate steps are taken to protect the rights and welfare of humans participating in a research study. A goal of the IRB is to protect human participants from physical or psychological harm by reviewing research protocols and related materials. The protocol review assesses the ethics of the research and its methods, promotes fully informed and voluntary participation by prospective participants capable of making such choices (or, if that is not possible, informed permission given by a suitable proxy), and seeks to maximize the safety of participants (National Institute of Environmental Health Sciences, 2019; U.S. FDA, 2019).

National Cancer Institute National Clinical Trials Network

The Clinical Trials Cooperative Group Program, sponsored by NCI, is designed to promote and support clini-

Table 3-2. Types of Clinical Studies

Type of Study	Description
Case series and case reports	• Consist of collections of reports on the treatment of individual patients or a single patient • Have little to no statistical validity because they are reports of cases and no control groups are used to compare outcomes
Case-control studies	• Compare patients who have been diagnosed with a specific disorder to patients who do not have the disorder • Used to identify exposures that may have contributed to or may be associated with the condition • Frequently use medical records and patient recall for data collection • Are retrospective because they start with the outcome • Frequently less reliable than randomized controlled studies and cohort studies because showing a statistical relationship does not mean that one factor caused the other
Cohort studies	• Are observational studies • Follow groups or cohorts of patients who are receiving a treatment or have been exposed over time • Compare the group or cohort with similar groups that have not had the treatment or exposure being studied • Are not as reliable as randomized controlled studies, as the two groups may differ in ways other than the variable being studied
Retrospective cohorts (historical cohorts)	• Is an observational study used to estimate how often disease or life events happen in a certain population • Follow the same direction of inquiry as a cohort study: participants begin with the presence or absence of an exposure or risk factor and are followed until the outcome of interest is observed • Uses information that was collected in the past and kept in databases

Randomized controlled clinical trials	• Planned studies that introduce a treatment or exposure to study its effect on patients
	• Randomly assign patients to a treatment group or a control group:
	  – The treatment group receives the experimental treatment.
	  – The control group receives standard treatment or placebo.
	• May be blinded to reduce selection bias
	  – Blinded study: participants do not know which arm they are in
	  – Double-blinded study: neither researchers nor patients know which arm of the study participants are in
	• Must be an ethical reason for the trial to be conducted
	• Target a specific disease and have an event as a measure of the trial outcome
	• Allow for comparison between the intervention group and the control group
	• Can provide sound evidence of cause and effect

Systematic reviews	• Focus on a specific research question
	• Authors identify applicable studies on the topic being researched in the literature:
	  – Identify studies with sound methodology
	  – Review and combine studies using meta-analysis
	  – Summarize results according to predetermined criteria of the review question

Meta-analyses	• The use of statistical techniques to combine the data of several studies into one quantitative summary • Thoroughly examine a number of valid studies on a topic and mathematically combine the results, using statistical methodology to report the results as if it were one large study • Unable to determine statistical significance but can determine clinical significance—whether the difference is clinically meaningful or large
Quantitative vs. qualitative research	• Quantitative research uses statistics, whereas qualitative research does not use statistical methods. • If 50% of a group of patients chooses one treatment over another, that is quantitative research. • Asking why they chose one treatment over the other is qualitative research.
Qualitative research	• Allows researchers to better understand an event, organization, population, or culture using nonstatistical methods • Answers questions related to human responses to actual or potential health problems • Aims to describe, explore, and explain the health-related phenomena being studied

Note. Based on information from Cochrane Consumer Network, n.d.; Duke University Medical Center Library and Archives, 2019; Statistics How To, 2016; Uman, 2011.

Table 3-3. Types of Clinical Trials

Type	Description

Treatment	• A study that tests a new treatment (e.g., drugs, vaccines, surgical approaches, radiation treatments, or combination therapy)
	• Treatment studies for cancer patients who have been diagnosed with cancer.
	• Look to answer the following questions:
	  – What is the maximum tolerated dose?
	  – What are the optimal methods of administration?
	  – What are the side effects of the treatment?
	  – Does the treatment offer patients a durable response?
	  – Can the treatment stop the disease from metastasizing?
	  – Will the treatment offer the patient better quality of life (QOL) with fewer side effects?
	  – Will the treatment reduce relapse of the disease?

QOL, supportive care, and palliative care trials	• Studies to identify ways to improve the quality of life for patients with cancer
	• Look at ways to help patients deal with side effects from their disease and its treatment
	• QOL studies: may test drugs or activities to help patients and caregivers cope
	• QOL and supportive care studies look to answer the following questions:
	  – How are patients and their families affected by cancer and its treatment?
	  – What can be done to improve the comfort and QOL of patients with cancer?

Prevention	• Examine ways to prevent disease occurrence in individuals who have never had the disease or prevent recurrence of a disease
	• Are either action studies or agent studies:
	  – Action studies: explore whether the actions people take can prevent disease (e.g., exercise, diet)
	  – Agent studies: look at medications for prevention of illness; may be referred to as chemoprevention studies
	• Are performed to determine:
	  – How safe is a particular agent or activity for patients?
	  – Will this new approach prevent a disease?

Screening trials	• Test ways to diagnose disease earlier, prior to a patient developing symptoms
	• Will earlier diagnosis allow patients to respond to treatment and reduce the number of deaths attributed to the disease?
	• Harms with screening trials: overdiagnosis and false-positive findings
	• Are conducted to accomplish the following:
	  – Reduce deaths related to a disease by diagnosing the disease earlier
	  – Determine best tests for screening for a particular disease
	• Must ensure the benefit of the screening outweighs the harms

Note. Based on information from Heleno et al., 2013; National Cancer Institute, 2016.

cal trials of new cancer treatments, cancer control and prevention strategies, and quality-of-life issues during and after interventions, as well as cancer imaging trials that target therapy, surveillance, and biomarkers of therapeutic responses (NCI, 2007). This program has played a key role in developing new and improved cancer therapies. More than 25,000 patients and thousands of clinical investigators participate in the program's clinical trials annually. In recent years, however, many stakeholders have expressed concerns that the program is falling short of its potential to conduct the timely, large-scale, innovative clinical trials needed to improve patient care. New clinical trial designs are considering genetic aberrations found in multiple tumor types. Rather than testing a drug only in patients with the same tumor type, studies include all patients who have the same genetic abnormality (Wujcik, 2016). Actionable mutations, increased numbers of targeted drugs, and tumor sequencing developments have led to the need for new clinical trial designs (Wujcik, 2016). Four overarching goals were used to guide improvement efforts:

- Goal I. Improving the speed and efficiency of the design, launch, and conduct of clinical trials;
- Goal II. Making optimal use of scientific innovations;
- Goal III. Improving selection, prioritization, support, and completion of clinical trials;
- Goal IV. Fostering expanded participation of both patients and physicians. (Nass, Moses, & Mendelsohn, 2010, p. 11)

The nine former adult cooperative groups were consolidated into four adult groups in the National Clinical Trials Network, along with another large group that focuses solely on childhood cancers and a Canadian Collaborating Clinical Trials Network award (NCI, 2019; see Table 3-4). Several functions have been centralized to improve workflow, including the IRB, cancer trials support unit, imaging and radiation oncology core group, and common data management system central hosting (NCI, 2019).

Resources for Clinical Investigation in Blood and Marrow Transplantation

Despite the importance of clinical trials in setting a standard for care, only 3% of adult patients with cancer participate in clinical trials (Marshall, 2013; Sullivan, Muraro, & Tyndall, 2010). An analysis of cancer clinical trials for adults registered on ClinicalTrials.gov showed that 20% of trials never finish for reasons unrelated to how well the studied treatment or procedure works or its related side effects (Cancer.Net, 2019). Poor accrual is the most common reason for unfinished clinical trials (Cancer.Net, 2019). Many barriers for accrual to clinical trials have been identified. Physician barriers include the extra uncompensated time

Table 3-4. National Clinical Trials Network Cooperative Groups

Cooperative Group	Description
Alliance for Clinical Trials in Oncology	The Alliance for Clinical Trials in Oncology (n.d.) seeks to reduce the impact of cancer on people by uniting scientists and clinicians from many disciplines, who are committed to discovering, validating, and disseminating effective strategies for the prevention and treatment of cancer.
Canadian Cancer Trials Group (CCTG)	CCTG (n.d.) develops and conducts clinical trials to improve cancer prevention and treatment and ultimately reduce morbidity and mortality. It conducts trials in cancer therapy, supportive care, and prevention across Canada and internationally.
Children's Oncology Group (COG)	COG (n.d.) is the world's largest organization devoted to pediatric cancer research. COG and its predecessor organizations have been pivotal in transforming childhood cancer from a virtually incurable disease 50 years ago to one with a combined 5-year survival rate of 80% today.
ECOG-ACRIN Cancer Research Group	ECOG-ACRIN Cancer Research Group (n.d.) is dedicated to achieving research advances in cancer care and thereby reducing the burden of cancer and improving the quality of life and survival in patients with cancer. Research is organized into three scientific programs: Cancer Control and Outcomes, Therapeutic Studies, and Biomarker Sciences.
NRG Oncology	NRG Oncology (n.d.) joins the unique and complementary research areas of the National Surgical Adjuvant Breast and Bowel Project, the Radiation Therapy Oncology Group, and the Gynecologic Oncology Group.
SWOG Cancer Research Network	SWOG Cancer Research Network (n.d.) studies ways to improve the care patients with cancer receive and the quality of life for survivors once initial treatment ends—relieving pain, promoting physical and mental health, and creating better end-of-life care.

required to enroll participants, regulatory paperwork, and insurance overload. U.S. physician practices spend an estimated $23 billion to $31 billion on health plan interactions (Casalino et al., 2009; Sullivan et al., 2010). Health insurers may restrict protocol recruitment by denying or delaying coverage for treatment on a study (Sullivan et al., 2010). Patient barriers to enrollment in clinical trials include unavailability of appropriate trials, disqualification because of comorbidities, and concerns about transportation or insurance coverage (Sullivan et al., 2010).

The American Society for Transplantation and Cellular Therapy (ASTCT), formerly American Society for Blood and Marrow Transplantation (ASBMT), reviewed recent advances and problems in HSCT and identified priorities in basic and clinical research. The research areas are closely interrelated and of growing importance, as a greater number of higher-risk patients are receiving transplants. Each area has an interface between basic science and clinical practice. Research in each of these areas can have a direct and immediate clinical benefit (ASBMT, 2011). ASTCT has formed working groups to find solutions for its research priorities.

Barriers to clinical trials in HSCT include the rarity of the diseases studied, the low number of patients per center, and the different competing risk factors in the post-transplant setting (Appelbaum et al., 2015). An improvement that has resulted from the many continuing clinical trials is the use of transplantation in larger populations because of decreased toxicity (London, 2013).

BMT CTN was established in October 2001 as an NCI-funded initiative developed to conduct large, multi-institutional clinical trials to improve outcomes for patients undergoing HSCT (Center for International Blood and Marrow Transplant Research [CIBMTR], 2008). It was formed to address challenges faced by transplant teams and execute multicenter HSCT trials with broad national participation. It effectively fosters development of innovative and important concepts into well-designed trials that answer questions in the most efficient manner; supports timely implementation and completion of those trials; ensures protection of participants (both donors and recipients); provides high-quality data and adherence to regulatory requirements in an increasingly complex environment; and promotes timely publication of study results that advance the field of HSCT and affect patient care (BMT CTN, 2019). Since opening its first clinical trial in 2003, BMT CTN has enrolled more than 10,700 patients in clinical trials. It has launched 50 trials, including 4 trials from 2018–2019, and has completed accrual to 40 trials (BMT CTN, 2019). Among the four network-led protocols currently open, BMT CTN have achieved an overall accrual rate that is 86% of target projections (BMT CTN, 2019). Additional goals of BMT CTN include the development of consensus guidelines for diagnosing, monitoring, and grading important transplant-related endpoints, as well as the development and use of novel study designs to increase the efficiency and scientific validity of clinical trials in blood and marrow transplantation (CIBMTR, 2008). BMT CTN identified seven focus areas to frame its clinical agenda: expanding donor/graft sources, reducing regimen-related toxicity, improving graft-versus-host disease (GVHD) prevention and therapy, decreasing relapses, decreasing infections, improving late effects and quality of life, and increasing rare disease research (Appelbaum et al., 2015).

CIBMTR has been collecting health outcome data worldwide for more than 45 years. It has a database with information on more than 475,000 patients. The data are available to investigators with interest in treatments for cancer, marrow failure syndromes, and other life-threatening diseases (CIBMTR, 2017). CIBMTR research involves six major programs:

- **Clinical outcomes:** Fifteen scientific working groups use CIBMTR's research database to answer clinically important questions. Each committee focuses on a specific disease, use of HSCT, and complications of HSCT therapy.
- **Immunobiology:** CIBMTR maintains a repository of paired tissue samples (from donors and recipients, related and unrelated) used in studying the genetic, cellular, and immunologic factors that influence the outcomes of HSCT and cellular therapy.
- **Clinical trials:** BMT CTN conducts multicenter phase 2 and 3 trials focusing on HSCT issues, whereas the Resource for Clinical Investigation in Blood and Marrow Transplantation (RCI BMT) supports phase 1 and 2 trials and other prospective studies that bridge the gap between single-center and larger trials.
- **Health services:** CIBMTR conducts research in health disparities, health policy, and system capacity issues. Current studies focus on costs and cost-effectiveness, insurance coverage, individualized care plans, and informed consent.
- **Bioinformatics:** CIBMTR provides expertise in and conducts research on translational and operational bioinformatics.
- **Statistical methodology:** CIBMTR provides advice and statistical consultation for HSCT studies.

Recent endeavors include improving the HLA matching algorithm, analyzing next-generation sequencing typing data, and improving statistical methodology. The CIBMTR coordinating center provides advice and statistical consultation to researchers developing protocols for HSCT studies and investigates new statistical approaches and techniques for analyzing HSCT data (CIBMTR, 2017). In 2005, CIBMTR formed RCI BMT to provide statistical and data management services for smaller phase 1/2 clinical trials (Tomblyn & Drexler, 2008). Its goal is to bridge the gap between single-center pilot trials and larger phase 2/3 studies conducted by the BMT CTN (Tomblyn & Drexler, 2008). The RCI BMT coordinates and manages all aspects of the single-center pilot trials, including identification of up to 10 CIBMTR centers to participate in the trials to increase the rate of accrual (Tomblyn & Drexler, 2008).

Many advances in clinical oncology are the result of cooperative group trials, underscoring the importance of collaborative clinical trials to the medical community (Horwitz, Horowitz, DiFronzo, Kohn, & Heslop, 2011). Changing existing systems for conducting clinical trials will help to expedite clinical trials. Low accrual rates have a negative impact on clinical trials, often prolonging the duration of the trial, delaying the analysis of important results, or leading to early closure of important studies (Lara et al., 2001). Timely enrollment of patients into open clinical trials is critical to answering research questions while information is still relevant (CIBMTR, 2008). A current effort is underway to disseminate information about clinical trials to the public to increase participation. Figure 3-1 provides a list of websites that contain information on clinical trials.

Nurses are in an excellent position to educate patients about the existence and role of clinical trials. Nurses working with transplant recipients should be familiar with clinical trials, as many patients undergoing HSCT are involved in research studies. Nurses responsible for providing care for patients undergoing transplantation usually administer study medications and record patient responses. Many nurses are employed as study coordinators and data managers for clinical trials. Nurses usually are the members of the healthcare team who spend the most time with patients and their families and frequently are the ones patients and families turn to for interpretation of a doctor's explanation and information and support about treatment decisions.

Daly et al. (2017) looked at factors related to nurse engagement in discussion of clinical trials with patients. The purpose of the study was to obtain baseline data about nurses' knowledge, beliefs, attitudes, and barriers to engaging in such discussions with their patients. Despite recognition of the key role of nurses in educating and supporting patients considering a clinical trial, results of this survey suggested both knowledge and attitudinal barriers exist to fulfilling this responsibility (Daly et al., 2017).

Nurses can provide counsel, education, and emotional support for families who are making difficult treatment decisions based on their knowledge and experience in working with patients undergoing clinical trials. It is important for oncology nurses and nursing organizations to engage with all oncology care stakeholders in identifying the future needs of patients with cancer and the environment in which care will be delivered. Nurses must identify the roles necessary to ensure a workforce that is adequate in number and well trained to meet the challenges of care delivery (Wujcik, 2016). Currently, many resources exist for patients that explain and list available clinical trials. Examples are included in Figure 3-1.

National Marrow Donor Program/Be The Match formed a group of patients, caregivers, researchers, and other key stakeholders to set a patient-centered outcomes research (PCOR) agenda for the HSCT community. PCOR is used to help patients and caregivers make informed decisions about health care. To date, the clinical research enterprise has not routinely involved patients, caregivers, or other non-providers in the process of prioritizing, designing, and conducting research in HSCT. The PCOR working group held

Figure 3-1. Clinical Trial Resources

- **American Society for Transplantation and Cellular Therapy** (www.astct.org) is a national professional association that promotes advancement of the field of blood and bone marrow transplantation. Members are in both clinical practice and research.
- **Be The Match** (https://bethematchclinical.org; www.bethematch.org) is a site that provides information about bone marrow donation. It is operated by the National Marrow Donor Program and manages the largest, most diverse marrow registry in the world.
- **Blood and Marrow Transplant Clinical Trials Network** (https://web.emmes.com/study/bmt2) was established October 2001 to conduct large, multi-institutional clinical trials. The trials address important issues in hematopoietic stem cell transplantation, thereby furthering understanding of the best possible treatment approaches. Participating investigators collaborate to maintain continuity of operations, facilitate effective communication and cooperation among transplant centers and with collaborators at the National Institutes of Health, and offer trial participation to patients in all regions of the United States.
- **Bone Marrow and Cord Blood Donation and Transplantation** (https://bloodcell.transplant.hrsa.gov) is part of the Health Resources and Services Administration and gives access to information provided through the C.W. Bill Young Cell Transplantation Program. The program's purpose is to help patients who need a transplant from an unrelated marrow donor or cord blood unit through the following:
  - Providing information about bone marrow and umbilical cord blood transplantation to patients, families, healthcare professionals, and the general public
  - Providing an efficient electronic system for identifying matched marrow donors and cord blood units (single point of access)
  - Increasing the availability of unrelated marrow donors and cord blood units for transplantation
  - Collecting data and expanding research to improve patient outcomes
- **Cell Therapy Transplant Canada** (www.cttcanada.org) is a national, voluntary, interprofessional organization providing leadership and promoting excellence in patient care, research, and education in the field of hematopoietic stem cell transplant and cell therapy.
- **Center for International Blood and Marrow Transplant Research** (CIBMTR; www.cibmtr.org) collaborates with the global scientific community to advance hematopoietic stem cell transplantation and cellular therapy research worldwide. A combined research program of the National Marrow Donor Program and the Medical College of Wisconsin, CIBMTR facilitates research that has led to increased survival and an enriched quality of life for thousands of patients. It accomplishes prospective and observational research through scientific and statistical expertise, a large network of transplant centers, and a clinical database of more than 300,000 transplant recipients. CIBMTR does not make donor matches. Staff is available to answer questions about transplantation.
- The **Central Institutional Review Board** (CIRB; www.ncicirb.org) for the National Cancer Institute (NCI) is dedicated to protecting the rights and welfare of participants in cancer clinical trials. Institutions across the country rely on it to ensure clinical trials are reviewed efficiently and with the highest ethical and quality standards. It helps NCI accelerate scientific discovery and improve cancer prevention, treatment, and care.
- **ClinicalTrials.gov** (https://clinicaltrials.gov) is a registry of federally and privately supported clinical trials conducted in the United States and around the world. It provides information about a trial's purpose, who may participate, locations, and telephone numbers for details.
- **Clinical Trials Support Unit** (CTSU; www.ctsu.org/public/default.aspx) was launched by NCI in 1999 to streamline and harmonize support services for phase 3 Cooperative Group cancer clinical trials funded by NCI. The scope of CTSU has since expanded to include support of multiple NCI-funded networks and clinical trials of all phases and types, including cancer treatment, prevention and control, advanced imaging, and correlative science studies. CTSU collaborates with NCI and its funded organizations to develop and support operational processes and informatics solutions leading to cost-effective solutions that reduce administrative burden on clinical sites.
- **European Organisation for Research and Treatment of Cancer** (www.eortc.org) lists clinical trials available in Europe.
- **European Society for Blood and Marrow Transplantation** (EBMT; www.ebmt.org) is a nonprofit organization based in the Netherlands and established in 1974 to allow scientists and physicians involved in clinical bone marrow transplantation to share their experiences and develop cooperative studies. EBMT aims to promote all aspects associated with the transplantation of hematopoietic stem cells from all donor sources and types, including basic and clinical research, education, standardization, quality control, and accreditation for transplant procedures.
- **Jason Carter Clinical Trials Program** (www.jasoncarterclinicaltrialsprogram.org) helps patients find clinical trials. It also offers patient-friendly descriptions of trials for leukemia, lymphoma, and other blood cancers and disorders, as well as educational resources.
- The **Journal of Gene Medicine** (https://onlinelibrary.wiley.com/journal/15212254) clinical trial site allows users to search for trials by clinical phase and status (e.g., open, closed, under review), in addition to searching by country, investigator, disease, vector, and gene.
- The **Leukemia and Lymphoma Society** (www.lls.org/treatment/types-of-treatment/clinical-trials) has a Clinical Trial Support Center that provides personalized clinical trial navigation when appropriate. Clinical trial specialists will work one-on-one with patients throughout the entire clinical trial process. Clinical trial specialists are RNs with expertise in blood cancers.
- **National Cancer Institute** (www.cancer.gov) provides accurate information on cancer, including site-specific information, clinical trials, statistics, and research funding.
- **National Cancer Institute PDQ®** (Physician Data Query; www.cancer.gov/publications/pdq) is a comprehensive database that provides up-to-date cancer information for patients and families, healthcare professionals, and others interested in educating themselves about cancer.
- **National Marrow Donor Program** (https://bethematch.org) is funded by a federal contract with the American Red Cross, AABB, and Council of Community Blood Centers. It was created to improve the efficiency and effectiveness of donor searches to facilitate a larger number of unrelated bone marrow transplantations. It also provides information on and links to clinical trials.
- **OncoLink** (www.oncolink.org), by the Abramson Cancer Center of the University of Pennsylvania, provides clinical trial information and sources.
- The **Pediatric Blood and Marrow Transplant Consortium** (PBMTC; www.pbmtc.org) includes more than 100 pediatric bone marrow transplant centers in the United States, Canada, New Zealand, and Australia, with affiliated members in Europe, Asia, and South America. Its purpose is to engage in scientific and educational activities related to the use of hematopoietic stem cells in the treatment of diseases of children and adolescents. PBMTC is a core member of the National Institutes of Health–funded Blood and Marrow Transplant Clinical Trials Network and collaborates with the Children's Oncology Group and the American Society for Transplantation and Cellular Therapy.

(Continued on next page)

Figure 3-1. Clinical Trial Resources *(Continued)*

- The **Scleroderma: Cyclophosphamide or Transplantation** trial (www.sclerodermatrial.org) is a clinical research study designed for people with severe forms of scleroderma. It will compare the potential benefits of stem cell transplant and high-dose monthly cyclophosphamide in the treatment of scleroderma.
- **TrialCheck** (https://eviticlinicaltrials.com/Services) is an easy-to-search database of more than 300 cooperative group cancer clinical trials.
- **World Marrow Donor Association** (WMDA; https://wmda.info) is one of the founding members of the Worldwide Network for Blood and Marrow Transplantation (WBMT). WBMT is a nonprofit scientific organization that aims to promote excellence in stem cell transplantation, donation, and cellular therapy. It has an official relationship with the World Health Organization. The other three founding organizations of the WBMT are EBMT, CIBMTR, and the Asia-Pacific Blood and Marrow Transplantation Group. In 2017, WMDA took over the activities of Bone Marrow Donors Worldwide and the NetCord Foundation. Its work covers four areas: optimizing search, supporting global development, promoting donor care, and ensuring quality.

several symposia and identified six major areas of interest with priority research questions and recommendations (Burns et al., 2018):

- Patient, caregiver, and family education and support
- Emotional, cognitive, and social health
- Physical health and fatigue
- Sexual health and relationships
- Financial burden
- Models of survivorship care delivery

Using these six groups, the working group identified gaps in knowledge and priority recommendations for research (Burns et al., 2018). They found a lack of consistency in measures used and patient populations that made it difficult to compare outcomes across studies. The group recommended investigators incorporate uniform measures and homogenous patient groups in future research (Burns et al., 2018).

Patients need to work with physicians and take ownership of treatment decisions when receiving information about new treatment options, risk–benefit ratios, and outcomes. The DECIDES study (an exploratory cross-sectional qualitative study into decision making and expectations in autologous HSCT examined decision making in patients diagnosed with severe Crohn disease (Cooper, Blake, Lindsay, & Hawkey, 2017). Researchers examined the choice that patients with severe Crohn disease made related to treatment with autologous transplant versus no treatment. Therapeutic misconception and misestimating were influencing factors for many patients in their decision making and expected personal outcomes in relation to HSCT and participation in the Autologous Stem Cell Transplantation International Crohn's Disease (ASTIC) trial (Cooper et al., 2017). The researchers concluded that when patients are presented with newer treatment options, doctors should consider the potential "therapeutic misestimation" (Cooper et al., 2017, p. 1). Documenting a patient's goals of care at the beginning of treatment and revisiting those goals throughout the course of care will help to ensure continuous informed consent regarding treatment expectations, outcomes, and quality of life (Wujcik, 2016). Dr. Keith M. Sullivan, a professor of medicine in the Division of Cellular Therapy at Duke University Medical Center, advocates for patients with autoimmune disease to be referred to centers with experience in HSCT for autoimmune diseases. "It is shared decision making, but if the patient never hears about the option from an experienced transplant team, they can't make that informed decision," Sullivan said (as cited in Nierengarten, 2017, para. 18). The development of decision-making tools for future participants in clinical trials, such as HSCT, are recommended, especially if the research involves individual and sociocultural influencing factors on decision making (Cooper et al., 2017).

Nursing Research

HSCT is a rapidly growing field. Nurses caring for transplant recipients work in many settings, such as inpatient and outpatient transplant units, physician offices, research institutions, and home care. They are expected to have the knowledge needed to provide care for patients who are experiencing a wide range of transplant-related side effects, symptoms, and problems. These may be physical or psychosocial in nature and can involve the patient directly or a family member. As with most nursing specialties, HSCT nurses strive to base nursing interventions on evidence-based solutions. However, the conceptual foundation that currently guides HSCT nursing practice is stronger than the existing empirical or research base for practice (Haberman, 2007).

Bevans et al. (2009) conducted a survey to review HSCT nursing practice variations. Results from the study showed that practice variations existed from published guidelines. Nurses are in a position to take ownership of their practice and to define best practices to improve patient care during and after HSCT (Bevans et al., 2009). Many of the nursing interventions used in HSCT were based on research from other disciplines; however, more recently, nursing is developing evidence-based standards for practice. The body of nursing research in HSCT has been increasing, and many of the studies performed relate to performance improvement and the use of evidence-based practice (Wyant, 2018). Continued nursing research in the field of HSCT is needed.

Healthcare organizations are trying to bridge the gap between research and evidence-based practice to improve patient outcomes, further the quality of care, and reduce healthcare costs (Brant, 2015; Fisher, Cusack, Cox, Feigenbaum, & Wallen, 2016). The Health and Medicine Division of the National Academies of Sciences, Engineering, and Medicine (formerly the Institute of Medicine) set a goal of 90% of clinical decisions to be evidence based by 2020 and recognized the leadership of nursing to accomplish this (Brant, 2015; Shalala et al., 2011). In general, care provided by nurses often relies on tradition or intuitive processes as rationale for interventions (Fisher et al., 2016; Fliedner, 2002). Nursing interventions may be based on what a nurse has previously learned through formal education and practice, which results in variations in practice without a valid rationale (Fisher et al., 2016). Research is important to clinical nursing practice to improve healthcare quality. Although generating research-based evidence is crucial, findings must be implemented to have an impact on clinical practice (Pintz, Zhou, McLaughlin, Kelly, & Guzzetta, 2018; Titler, 2008). Currently, it can take 10–20 years for research to be translated into clinical practice (Agency for Healthcare Research and Quality, 2001; Pintz et al., 2018). Implementation of evidence-based practice remains low because the demands of patient care take precedence and conducting research in the clinical setting can prove challenging (Kleinpell, 2009). Research indicates that patients who receive care based on evidence from well-designed studies experience better care and better outcomes (Kleinpell, 2009). Cox, Arber, Gallagher, MacKenzie, and Ream (2017) conducted a study to establish priorities for oncology nursing research and suggested that patient and nurse involvement in the development of nursing research projects would make the research more relevant and beneficial for all parties involved. Several studies have examined the use of nursing research and barriers to use of research in cancer practice (Hagan, 2018; Hagan & Walden, 2017; Hendricks & Cope, 2017; Hweidi, Tawalbeh, Al-Hassan, Alayadeh, & Al-Smadi, 2017; O'Nan, 2011). The studies reported that dissemination of the findings through reading literature, attending educational offerings, and observing the practice of others was important. Barriers to use included a lack of time to read research and implement new ideas, as well as a lack of authority to change patient care. Other reasons cited were that the research is not generalizable to every practice setting, lack of support from physicians and other staff, and difficulty understanding research language and statistics. Hendricks and Cope (2017) conducted a study to look at barriers to research utilization and found a major barrier was a lack of knowledge of the research evidence presented. They suggested developing skills in the nursing staff to help them interpret research language and results.

When valid research findings are identified, implementing them into practice should be a priority. Policies, procedures, and standards should be revised to incorporate new findings into practice. Practice changes should be communicated to all healthcare workers involved in patient care, including physicians. Changes in practice can be piloted on selected units to work out the identified institutional problems, and then thorough educational in-servicing can be implemented as a practice change throughout the hospital.

Nursing management should encourage staff to join specialty organizations, obtain certification, attend conferences to maintain up-to-date knowledge of transplantation, and network with other healthcare workers involved in the care of HSCT recipients. Managers should support introduction of new nursing interventions based on valid research findings and encourage staff endeavors to implement new research findings when possible. Clinical staff should be encouraged to review current journals for new, relevant research findings. Staff should also be encouraged to question current nursing practices and look for gaps where there is a lack of research-based practice (Haberman, 2007). Identifying gaps in the literature and inconsistencies in HSCT practices is an important first step in designing evidence-based projects that can be used to standardize practice and link best practices to improved patient outcomes (Bevans et al., 2009).

Nursing research and evidence-based practice principles should be made understandable to frontline nursing staff (Steele-Moses, 2010). Nurses at the bedside are in the best position to identify problems for research. Bedside and research nurses must work together to identify and research areas of interest. Managers and advanced practice nurses are in a position to act as a bridge between nurses at the bedside and nurse researchers. Strategies to promote research in clinical practice include the use of journal clubs, formulation of a research committee, and identification of advanced practice nurses to champion research projects. Ways to showcase research projects and promote interest in research include nursing grand rounds, formal continuing education programs, and institutional newsletters (Kleinpell, 2009). Research should be kept in the forefront at all nursing gatherings within an institution (Steele-Moses, 2010).

Transplant nurses meetings were held during the ASTCT and CIBMTR Transplant Tandem Meetings since 1999. In 2019, these became the Transplantation and Cellular Therapy Meetings of ASTCT and CIBMTR, and the Transplant Nurses Meeting has continued as part of this combined meeting. The Transplant Nurses Special Interest Group (SIG) was established in 2010. Nurses originally were members of the Oncology Nursing Society (ONS) Blood and Marrow Stem Cell Transplant SIG and collaborated with ASBMT to plan and conduct the Transplant Nurses Meetings. Many of these nurses have become affiliate members of ASTCT. In 2010, the ASBMT board identified the need for nursing representation and involvement within the society and created the ASBMT Transplant Nurses SIG. The purpose of the SIG is to provide a forum for education, idea exchange, networking, promotion of transplant nursing, and dissemination of best practices within the field of blood and marrow transplantation (ASBMT, 2015). The ASTCT steering committee provides leadership for nurses within the organization and promotes nursing representation on organization committees. It also collaborates with ONS on various projects and represents ASTCT's interests on these projects (ASBMT, 2015).

The European Society for Blood and Marrow Transplantation (EBMT) Nurses Group has grown over the past two decades with the support of medical colleagues. Nurses have been taking a leading role in the holistic care of patients; HSCT nurses are involved in the decision-making process about treatment options for their patients, and they contribute to the enhancement of patients' quality of life (EBMT, n.d.). The Nurses Group has five committees dedicated to achieving the goals of EBMT:

- The Research Committee develops and promotes awareness of research projects. Examples of completed activities include management of related donors, including ethical issues; management of antithymocyte globulin administration; sexuality issues in HSCT recipients; risk of infectious complications in adults after HSCT depending on site of central venous catheter insertion; and role of nursing in skin care of patients with cutaneous chronic GVHD after allogeneic HSCT.
- The Communication and Networking Committee maintains the Nurses Group profile through communication channels including the website, newsletter, and social media platforms. It is committed to improving networking to develop educational activities for nurses and allied health professionals in hematology and HSCT.
- The Scientific Committee is a group of experienced nurses with specific interests in hematology and HSCT. They represent different specialties, from working as a nurse specialist, nurse coordinator, or nurse on a hospital ward, apheresis unit, outpatient clinic, or consultation unit. The committee is responsible for the nurse-oriented scientific program at the EBMT Annual Meeting.
- The Paediatric Committee was established in 2008 and is dedicated to improving the care of pediatric and adolescent hematology and HSCT patients.
- The Global Education Committee coordinates and organizes outreach meetings in cooperation with other nonprofit associations with the same mission and objectives. They coordinate and provide educational activities for nurses and allied health professionals within the field of hematology and HSCT.

The use of evidence-based practice contributes to high-quality patient care and better outcomes for patients (ASBMT, 2010; Pintz et al., 2018). It has been recognized by the healthcare community as the gold standard for the provision of safe, quality health care (Brant, 2015; Brown, Wickline, Ecoff, & Glaser, 2009). It is no longer considered acceptable to provide care based on ritualized practice, and organizations are working to ensure that nursing care delivery is based on the best evidence (Brown et al., 2009; Fisher et al., 2016). ONS is committed to developing knowledge through the research process and sharing that knowledge with nurses providing care to patients with cancer. Nurses can make a difference in nursing-sensitive patient outcomes through adoption of the ONS Putting Evidence Into Practice (PEP) resources (Doorenbos et al., 2008). ONS developed the PEP symptom interventions to provide nurses with the strongest evidence available. ONS is one of the leading nursing societies that focuses on identifying knowledge gaps, setting research priorities, and promoting evidence-based practice (Doorenbos et al., 2008).

Nurses should be able to locate, evaluate, and synthesize research findings (Theroux, 2010). Nurses are expected to participate in research activities by evaluating and interpreting research reports for applicability to nursing practice (Fain, 2017). Publication of research reports does not guarantee quality, value, or relative worth. Failing to adequately critique research reports may adversely affect outcomes of entire populations of patients (Fain, 2017).

Strategies to develop nursing infrastructures to complete valid and viable nursing research mirror those in the medical transplant community. Currently, most nursing studies involve single institutions with small patient samples. To develop meaningful research-based practice, nurses need to form cooperative groups consisting of researchers and clinicians representing the different areas of HSCT. These groups could develop research priorities that would be translated into multi-institutional trials. Performing multi-institutional trials increases the number of patient accruals, allows studies to be generalizable for more patients, and shortens the length of study time (Haberman, 2007). Recruitment of physicians and other healthcare team members in developing and conducting interprofessional research is another way for nurses to become involved in the research process. Because no single discipline is wholly responsible for the care of patients undergoing HSCT, it makes sense to perform research as a team. Including members from multiple disciplines allows studies to address the different interests identified by each of these disciplines. Interprofessional collaboration is important in the specialty of oncology. The complexity of new therapies and the associated side effect profiles benefit from a collaborative, interprofessional approach. HSCT recipients would benefit from interprofessional collaborations across the complexities of the care continuum (Knoop, Wujcik, & Wujcik, 2017). A small number of interprofessional research studies have been published (see Table 3-5), and it is hoped this trend will continue in the future.

Coleman et al. (2009) studied the effect of certification in oncology nursing on nursing-sensitive outcomes, surveying 93 nurses and 270 patients. Results showed that certified nurses scored higher than noncertified nurses on both the Nurses' Knowledge and Attitudes Survey Regarding Pain and the Nausea Management: Nurses' Knowledge and Attitudes Survey (Coleman et al., 2009). Employing certified nurses is necessary for an institution to achieve the American Nurses Credentialing Center's Magnet Recognition Program® award for excellence in nursing care (Shirey, 2005).

Gene Therapy

The use of hematopoietic stem cells (HSCs) has become a clinical standard to treat genetic diseases, but it

Table 3-5. Interprofessional Research in Hematopoietic Stem Cell Transplantation

Authors	Title	Study Design	Sample	Comments
Abad-Corpa et al., 2010	Effectiveness of the Implementation of an Evidence-Based Nursing Model Using Participatory Action Research in Oncohematology: Research Protocol	Prospective quasiexperimental design with 2 nonequivalent and nonconcurrent groups	40 nurses	Aims were to generate changes in nursing practice introducing an evidence-based clinical practice model through a participatory process and evaluate effectiveness of the changes in terms of nursing-sensitive outcomes.
Alaloul et al., 2016	Spirituality in Arab Muslim Hematopoietic Stem Cell Transplantation Survivors: A Qualitative Approach	Qualitative	63 HSCT survivors	Healthcare providers in the United States and other Western countries need to be aware of the unique religious and spiritual needs of Muslim cancer survivors to provide them with culturally sensitive care. More research on the spiritual needs of Muslim patients and survivors residing in Western countries is needed.
Appenfeller et al., 2018	Code BMT: A System for Seamless Patient Admission in an Outpatient BMT Program	Performance improvement	Unscheduled, after-hours admissions requiring a bed on the BMT unit	Maintaining a Code BMT practice requires frequent process improvements and ongoing education. The researchers found a successful Code BMT practice provides optimum care for a fragile patient population and a detailed plan of care for providers with many responsibilities. For programs initiating a similar process, non-BMT providers must acknowledge these patients require unique care. Regular meetings with nursing administration, physicians, and relevant support services are crucial. Education is also key to timely care. Training for nursing staff must include awareness of fever action plans and management of outpatient transplants. Patients and caregivers should be instructed on the reasons to call a BMT provider and the steps to take to receive appropriate care.
Assalone & McNinney, 2017	Dropping Knowledge, Not Patients: Reducing Falls on a Hematopoietic Stem Cell Transplant (HSCT) Unit	Performance improvement	13 patients	Oncology nurses play an important role in assessing patients' fall risks and educating on ways to prevent falls. To effectively prevent falls, all nurses and members of the interprofessional team should proactively educate patients and families on fall prevention.
Assalone & Wagner, 2018	Distress No More: The Effect of Early Intervention Palliative Care in Hematopoietic Stem Cell Transplant (HSCT)	Quantitative	11 patients total; 6 in control group and 5 in experimental group	Early palliative care consults help decrease patients' distress. HSCT nurses play a pivotal role in assessing distress level and facilitating prompt referrals, providing support and coping mechanisms.
Astarita et al., 2016	Experiences in Sexual Health Among Women After Hematopoietic Stem Cell Transplantation	Qualitative phenomenological	5 women	Implications for practice included designating time for pre- and post-HSCT education, improving current sexual health education provided by HSCT clinicians, engaging same-sex providers to discuss sexual health with patients, and increasing nurses' expertise in this area.
Baliousis et al., 2017	Perceptions of Hematopoietic Stem Cell Transplantation and Coping Predict Emotional Distress During the Acute Phase After Transplantation	Longitudinal, correlational	45 patients	Eliciting and discussing patients' negative perceptions of HSCT beforehand and supporting helpful coping may be important ways to reduce distress during HSCT.

(Continued on next page)

Authors	Title	Study Design	Sample	Comments
Barrell et al., 2012	Reduced-Intensity Conditioning Allogeneic Stem Cell Transplantation in Pediatric Patients and Subsequent Supportive Care	Retrospective medical record review	86 patients	For nurses to correctly educate patients and families and anticipate patients' needs, they need to have an understanding of the potential acute toxicities and supportive care in pediatric patients undergoing reduced-intensity conditioning versus myeloablative conditioning allogeneic HSCT.
Barrow et al., 2018	Central Line Associated Blood Stream Infection (CLABSI) Reduction in a Blood and Marrow Transplant Unit	Performance improvement	24-bed universal care unit	The interventions and methods used in this project can be universally applied to any inpatient oncology or BMT unit seeking to reduce CLABSI rates.
Bartel et al., 2017	Improving Oral Assessments and Implementing Preventative Low Level Laser Therapy in Hematopoietic Stem Cell Transplant Patients to Prevent Oral Mucositis	Performance improvement	–	Incorporating oral mucositis education during nursing orientation was suggested.
Bevans et al., 2010	An Individualized Dyadic Problem-Solving Education Intervention for Patients and Family Caregivers During Allogeneic Hematopoietic Stem Cell Transplantation: A Feasibility Study	Feasibility study; qualitative	34 adult dyads	Results suggested that dyads can participate in problem-solving education during HSCT and view it as beneficial. Participants identified the active process of solving problems as helpful.
Braga et al., 2015	Use of *Chamomilla Recutita* in the Prevention and Treatment of Oral Mucositis in Patients Undergoing Hematopoietic Stem Cell Transplantation: A Randomized, Controlled, Phase II Clinical Trial	Randomized, controlled, phase 2	40 patients	The results of this investigation will help nurses and other professionals in selecting the *C. recutita* dosage used to manage oral mucositis in patients undergoing HSCT.
Brassil et al., 2015	Exploring the Cancer Experiences of Young Adults in the Context of Stem Cell Transplantation	Qualitative	14 young adults	This study provides a foundation for addressing the psychosocial needs of young adults hospitalized for HSCT, paying particular attention to the development of specific interventions.
Brassil et al., 2014	Impact of an Incentive-Based Mobility Program, "Motivated and Moving," on Physiologic and Quality of Life Outcomes in a Stem Cell Transplant Population	Repeated measures design	83 participants	An incentive-based mobility program during hospitalization for HSCT has the potential to minimize fatigue and stabilize, if not improve, QOL.
Button, 2016	Prophylactic Treatment of Hepatic Veno-Occlusive Disease During Stem Cell Transplantation	Literature review	612 participants	Benefits are associated with administration of ursodeoxycholic acid in reducing the incidence of veno-occlusive disease and overall mortality in HSCT recipients.
Button et al., 2014	Exploring Palliative Care Provisions for Recipients of Allogeneic Hematopoietic Stem Cell Transplantation Who Relapsed	Retrospective chart review cohort study; cross-sectional survey	40 patients' charts; 14 advanced nurses	Palliative care should be integrated earlier. Nursing roles have the potential to address unmet needs for these patients.
Chan & Wang, 2018	Review Measurement Tools of Chronic Oral Graft-Versus-Host Disease	Performance improvement	–	Nurses should use the National Institutes of Health Oral Mucosal Score to screen for the incidence of chronic oral GVHD.

(Continued on next page)

Authors	Title	Study Design	Sample	Comments
Chiang & Hsiao, 2015	The Effect of Long-Term Follow-Up Clinic for Hematopoietic Cell Transplantation Survivors in Taiwan	Quantitative	110 HSCT survivors	Results indicated that long-term follow-up clinics provide early detection of HSCT survivors' symptoms and can prevent serious complications and maintain good QOL.
M.Z. Cohen et al., 2013	Understanding Health Literacy in Patients Receiving Hematopoietic Stem Cell Transplantation	Hermeneutic phenomenological approach	60 patients	Health literacy and communication concerns require a more nuanced approach to provide optimal patient-centered outcomes.
Coolbrandt & Grypdonck, 2010	Keeping Courage During Stem Cell Transplantation: A Qualitative Research	Qualitative	16 semistructured interviews with patients and 6 interviews with nurses	During HSCT, patients make many efforts to write a positive story and keep courage. These efforts involve more active strategies than the rather passive concept of hope suggests.
Cotter & Christianson, 2017	Preventing Pitfalls on the Road to Stem Cell Transplant: Development of an Early Psychosocial Screening Program	Qualitative	125 patients	Use of validated tools for screening helps to identify patient issues. Timing of screening and having solid processes for implementation and follow-through are essential.
Crable et al., 2018	Stem Cell Infusion: Guidelines and Practices	Literature review	–	Oncology nurses should understand the importance of proper hematopoietic progenitor cell handling and infusion, as well as be aware of possible side effects and toxicity management.
Cummings, 2017	Educating and Monitoring Nursing Staff Regarding the Care of Central Venous Access Devices (CVAD) in Stem Cell Transplant Patients	Performance improvement	Number of CLABSIs	Improved central venous access device best practices can reduce the number of CLABSIs in the BMT unit.
Dambrosio et al., 2018	Continuous Temperature Monitoring for Earlier Fever Detection in Neutropenic Patients: Patient's Acceptance and Comparison With Standard of Care	Comparative study	Data of 5,856 continuous hours were studied on 17 patients	The TempTraq® temperature skin patch, an FDA class II patch equipped with a small temperature sensor, was used to monitor body temperature in real time. Researchers compared standard-of-care intermittent temperature monitoring with a continuous temperature monitoring device on an inpatient HSCT unit. The patch data were successfully transmitted and displayed on the study tablet computer invariably. All patients were able to wear the patch through the hospital admission, and the majority reported it was comfortable to wear and were interested in wearing it during future admissions or at discharge.
Dandekar & Achrekar, 2016	Sleep Disturbance in Hospitalized Recipients of Hematopoietic Stem Cell Transplantation (HSCT)	Descriptive retrospective study	Patients undergoing HSCT	Planned nursing care should be initiated to ensure undisturbed sleep in patients undergoing HSCT.
Donofrio et al., 2017	Nurses Transition Post Stem Cell Transplant Care to the Home	Feasibility study	45 visits	RNs and advanced practice providers in this outpatient clinic established a workflow to care for patients after autologous HSCT in their home or home-like environment. The workflow supports interprofessional communication and teamwork by leveraging technology. The workflow enables safe, specialized, and holistic care to transplant recipients in the home environment.

(Continued on next page)

Authors	Title	Study Design	Sample	Comments
Eisenberg et al., 2013	Prevention of Dimethylsulfoxide-Related Nausea and Vomiting by Prophylactic Administration of Ondansetron for Patients Receiving Autologous Cryopreserved Peripheral Blood Stem Cells	Nonrandomized cohort using historical control	50 patients	Prophylactic administration of ondansetron had a positive effect on reducing nausea symptoms and episodes of vomiting during autologous stem cell infusions. These results prompted a change in clinical practice. More research is required to determine whether the inclusion of other antiemetic agents would provide even greater benefit.
Garbin et al., 2018	Serum Cyclosporine Levels: The Influence of the Time Interval Between Interrupting the Infusion and Obtaining the Samples: A Randomized Clinical Trial	Randomized clinical trial	32 adults	The results can help nurses choose how to collect blood samples through the central venous catheter, thus preventing patients from having a painful and stressful procedure such as peripheral venipuncture.
Gemmill et al., 2011	Informal Caregivers of Hematopoietic Cell Transplant Patients: A Review and Recommendations for Intervention and Research	Literature review	Studies published from 1980 to 2010 on informal caregivers of HSCT recipients	Beginning descriptive evidence provides the basis for interventions for informal caregivers of HSCT recipients. These interventions support caregiver QOL and role implementation depending on individual caregivers' resources and needs. Further evaluation and clinical research are needed.
Gibson et al., 2017	Nursing Operated Pulsed Xenon Ultraviolet-C Disinfection Robot Utilization and the Reduction of Hospital-Acquired *Clostridium Difficile* Infections (CDI) in Hematopoietic Stem Cell Transplant (HSCT) Patients	Performance improvement	HSCT unit at Honor Health in Arizona	Patient safety and infection prevention are the responsibility of all members of the healthcare team. The HSCT program successfully implemented an innovative program in which the nurses manage and operate the pulsed xenon ultraviolet C light machine to disinfect rooms, resulting in decreased hospital-acquired *Clostridium difficile* infections.
Granada et al., 2017	Isolation Coding System to Improve Ease of Identification of Infectious Organisms in Stem Cell Transplantation	Performance improvement	24-bed HSCT unit	Isolation dots facilitated quick, inexpensive identification of isolation type, thereby reinforcing appropriate personal protective equipment and precautions. In addition, the use of the colored dots allowed staff to recognize the infectious source while still protecting patients' privacy.
Hacker, 2017	Optimizing Health Through Exercise Following Hematopoietic Stem Cell Transplantation	Literature review	14 randomized clinical trials	Building teams with HSCT researchers and practitioners to develop pragmatic, effective interventions, such as clinic-based strength training, is vital for advancing science and clinical practice.
Hacker et al., 2017	Persistent Fatigue in Hematopoietic Stem Cell Transplantation Survivors	Quantitative	25 adult HSCT survivors with persistent fatigue and 25 matched healthy controls with occasional tiredness	This study provided preliminary support for the conceptualization of fatigue as existing on a continuum, with tiredness anchoring one end and exhaustion the other. Persistent fatigue experienced by HSCT survivors is more severe than the occasional tiredness of everyday life.

(Continued on next page)

Authors	Title	Study Design	Sample	Comments
Hacker et al., 2015	Sleep Patterns During Hospitalization Following Hematopoietic Stem Cell Transplantation	Secondary data analysis using a descriptive correlational design	40 patients	Attempts to streamline care during the night by not waking patients for routine care unless indicated by the patient's condition (as advocated by the American Academy of Nursing) and providing supportive care for symptoms (such as diarrhea) during the night may reduce the number of awakenings and possibly improve overall sleep quality.
Hacker et al., 2011	Strength Training Following Hematopoietic Stem Cell Transplantation	Pilot	19 participants	Preliminary evidence is provided for using strength training to enhance early recovery following HSCT. Elastic resistance bands are easy to use and relatively inexpensive.
Hsiao, 2015	The Quality Improvement of Long-Term Follow-Up Program in Hematopoietic Stem Cell Transplantation Recipient	Performance improvement	12 patients	This program can help prevent irreversible organ damage, improve survival, and increase QOL.
H.Y. Huang et al., 2015	The Trajectory and Associated Factors of Oral Mucositis of Patients Receiving Allogeneic Hematopoitic Stem-Cell Transplantation	Retrospective longitudinal study	50 patient charts	The findings contributed to the knowledge of the trajectory of oral mucositis and provided guidelines for setting the criteria for detecting patients at high risk for having oral mucositis in Taiwan.
Y.P. Huang et al., 2014	Experience of Nurses Caring for Child With Hematopoietic Stem Cell Transplantation in General Pediatric Ward	Descriptive phenomenological approach	12 nurses	Understanding and learning are gained from nurses who are able to seek meaning from HSCT through appreciating every caregiving effort and through valuing how their nursing role contributes to the quality of patients' care.
D.L. Kelly et al., 2015	Symptoms, Cytokines, and Quality of Life in Patients Diagnosed With Chronic Graft-Versus-Host Disease Following Allogeneic Hematopoietic Stem Cell Transplantation	Prospective, cross-sectional, cohort	24 adults with chronic GVHD	Better understanding of the interrelated symptoms of chronic GVHD and the biomarkers associated with these symptoms may lead to targeted symptom management interventions.
D.L. Kelly et al., 2018	Lifestyle Behaviors, Perceived Stress, and Inflammation of Individuals With Chronic Graft-Versus-Host Disease	Prospective observational study	24 adults (aged 18 years and older) with chronic GVHD	This study provided information about the role of lifestyle behaviors on inflammation and stress for nurses to offer anticipatory guidance to HSCT survivors regarding lifestyle choices that promote positive health outcomes.
Kemp et al., 2018	Implementation of a Bone Marrow Transplant Admission Checklist	Performance improvement	–	An admission checklist has many strengths to improve the admission process for BMT patients.
Kolke et al., 2019	Factors Influencing Patients' Intention to Perform Physical Activity During Hematopoietic Cell Transplantation	Longitudinal, descriptive design	54 patients	HSCT nurses have the opportunity, over an extended hospitalization, to assess physical and psychological symptoms. However, feasible interventions are needed to positively influence attitude and control toward physical activity in patients with a high symptom burden.

(Continued on next page)

Authors	Title	Study Design	Sample	Comments
Lawson et al., 2016	Effects of Making Art and Listening to Music on Symptoms Related to Blood and Marrow Transplantation	Randomized, 3-group, pre- and post-pilot design	39 adults	Art making and music listening are safe and desirable for patients undergoing BMT in an outpatient clinic. Nurses might consider partnering with therapists to offer these creative therapies as diversion during treatment.
Lawson et al., 2012	Effect of Art Making on Cancer-Related Symptoms of Blood and Marrow Transplantation Recipients	Pre- and post-test crossover design	20 patients	Individuals receiving BMT may benefit from participation in art-making interventions. Art making is easy to implement in a clinic setting and allows for positive interactions between nurses and patients.
Leung et al., 2012	Meaning in Bone Marrow Transplant Nurses' Work: Experiences Before and After a "Meaning-Centered" Intervention	Qualitative	14 nurses	Nurses can learn to be more responsive to patients' suffering beyond limits of cure. A minimal intervention, such as the meaning-centered intervention, supports BMT nurses in finding positive personal meaning and purpose in a highly stressful work culture.
Liu et al., 2016	Quality of Life After Hematopoietic Stem Cell Transplantation in Pediatric Survivors: Comparison With Healthy Controls and Risk Factors	Comparison study	43 pediatric transplant survivors and 43 age- and sex-matched healthy peers	The finding that children after transplant may achieve QOL similar to their healthy peers is important information as patients consider treatment options. For those sick children who cannot regularly attend school, their emotional and social functioning should be closely monitored.
Lu et al., 2016	Effects of Healing Touch and Relaxation Therapy on Adult Patients Undergoing Hematopoietic Stem Cell Transplant: A Feasibility Pilot Study	Feasibility pilot study	26 HSCT recipients; 13 who received healing touch daily and 13 who received relaxation therapy daily compared with retrospective clinical data of 20 patients who received HSCT	Reduction in length of stay could result in decreased cost. Second, mood and function improvements support QOL during HSCT.
Lucas et al., 2018	CAR-T Cell Education for ICU and BMT Nurses	Pre- and post-test	Oncology and intensive care unit staff	After 2 months of chimeric antigen receptor T-cell therapy education, nurses reported they had received adequate education to care for these patients.
Madden, Dockery, et al., 2018	Quality Improvement Initiative to Reduce *Clostridium Difficile* Infections in a Bone Marrow Transplant Unit	Quantitative	12-month pre- and postintervention on a tertiary BMT unit	Further research is warranted to determine the effectiveness of Bioquell hydrogen peroxide vapor decontamination on *Clostridium difficile* cross contamination between patients to improve outcomes for patients and reduce the risk of *C. difficile* infection.
Madden, Johnson, & Rudolph, 2018	Pre-Transplant Education Performed by a Designated Patient Educator: Can This Improve Knowledge, Behavior, Comprehension, and Satisfaction for Bone Marrow Transplant Patients?	Quantitative	BMT patients and their caregivers	Sustained and ongoing interprofessional involvement evaluating each aspect of educating patients and caregivers about the BMT process should continue to be a focus of transplant programs to improve outcomes and reduce costly readmissions for this specialty population.

(Continued on next page)

Authors	Title	Study Design	Sample	Comments
McNinney & Assalone, 2018	Can We Give You Some TIPS? Tailored Interventions for Patient Safety on a Hematopoietic Stem Cell Transplant (HSCT) Unit	Performance improvement	16-bed inpatient HSCT unit	To effectively prevent falls, nurses and the interprofessional team should proactively and consistently implement individualized patient interventions.
Morrison et al., 2018	Follow the Yellow Brick Road: Self-Management by Adolescents and Young Adults After a Stem Cell Transplant	Qualitative	17 adolescents and young adults (aged 13–25 years at transplant) and 13 caregivers (dyads)	Nurses play an instrumental role in adolescents' and young adults' self-management practices by providing information, education, and social support. Psychosocial issues were prominent in the self-management process and should be addressed in future research and interventions with adolescents and young adults and caregivers.
Nance & Santacroce, 2017	Blogging During Hematopoietic Stem Cell Transplant	Qualitative	Emerging adults (those aged 18–29 years) during protective isolation following HSCT	Including uncertainty in studies that use the psychoneuroimmunology paradigm should be considered when moving this line of investigation forward, given the finding that uncertainty played a central role for the emerging adults in this case study and the role of biopsychosocial mechanisms in mediating the effects of stress on health outcomes among emerging adults diagnosed with cancer.
O'Brien et al., 2018	Co-Design of a Hematopoietic Cell Transplant e-Learning Module for Patients on Fertility Preservation and Family Planning	Descriptive/qualitative	–	Six e-learning sections covered information on the basics of fertility, transplantation, fertility for men and women, family planning, financial considerations, legal and ethical considerations, and strategies for communicating with the healthcare team. HSCT recipients/caregivers and healthcare professionals served as reviewers.
Olausson et al., 2014	The Impact of Hyperglycemia on Hematopoietic Cell Transplantation Outcomes: An Integrative Review	Integrative review	12 empirical quantitative reports	Understanding the effects of hyperglycemia, as well as factors that place patients at risk for hyperglycemia, allows nurses to provide well-informed, proactive interventions aimed at glycemic control.
Otsuka et al., 2015	Search for Meaning of Hematopoietic Stem Cell Transplantation in Japanese Elderly	Qualitative	10 patients	This study suggested the necessity of nursing to enhance patients' wisdom and toughness in learning from their life experiences and support them in sharing their distress or increasing their motivation for life.
Rimkus & Trost, 2018	Tacrolimus Dosing: Can We Do It Better?	Prospective review; performance improvement	–	This project aimed to use data to better understand current practice, identify cost savings that could be achieved by reducing drug monitoring, and establish guidelines for a tacrolimus dosing program. The researchers planned to audit the process to evaluate GVHD rates.
Rodgers et al., 2013	Feasibility of a Symptom Management Intervention for Adolescents Recovering From a Hematopoietic Stem Cell Transplant	Quantitative, repeated measures design	16 patients	Healthcare providers need to continue to develop and evaluate innovative methods to educate adolescents on effective self-care strategies throughout HSCT recovery.

(Continued on next page)

Authors	Title	Study Design	Sample	Comments
Rodgers et al., 2014	Symptom Prevalence and Physiologic Biomarkers Among Adolescents Using a Mobile Phone Intervention Following Hematopoietic Stem Cell Transplantation	Repeated measures design	16 adolescents	Nurses should assess symptom frequency and distress to fully understand patients' symptom experiences. Nurses should monitor patients' weight and body mass index throughout HSCT recovery.
Rodgers et al., 2010	The Meaning of Adolescents' Eating Experiences During Bone Marrow Transplant Recovery	Phenomenological study	13 adolescents	Eating issues do not end when a BMT recipient is discharged from the hospital, and caregivers need to have a better understanding of the ongoing issues affecting adolescents throughout the recovery phase.
Rodriguez et al., 2017	A Nursing Led Implementation of a Homebound Stem Cell Transplant Program	Pilot	4 patients	Nurses effectively delivered care in the home while maintaining the same standards of quality and excellence as in the outpatient clinic.
Russell et al., 2011	Patients' Experiences of Appearance Changes Following Allogeneic Bone Marrow Transplantation	Qualitative	6 men and women	This study highlighted the need to identify and support those with long-term appearance changes.
Sabo et al., 2013	The Experience of Caring for a Spouse Undergoing Hematopoietic Stem Cell Transplantation: Opening Pandora's Box	Qualitative	4 men and 7 women	Nurses need to integrate regular psychosocial assessments of caregivers to recognize the early signs of distress and intervene to support and promote psychosocial health and well-being.
Sams et al., 2015	Community Respiratory Virus Infection in Hematopoietic Stem Cell Transplantation Recipients and Household Member Characteristics	Retrospective exploratory study	720 adults	As indicated by the potentially high number of days from transplantation to acquisition of community respiratory virus infection, education and continuing focus on prevention of infection should be reinforced throughout the lengthy transplantation period.
Sannes et al., 2018	Caregiver Sleep and Patient Neutrophil Engraftment in Allogeneic Hematopoietic Stem Cell Transplant: A Secondary Analysis	–	124 patients; 124 caregivers	Despite limitations in available patient data, findings appear to link caregiver well-being to patient outcomes. This underscores the interrelatedness of the patient–caregiver dyad in allogeneic HSCT. Potential may exist to improve patient outcome by focusing on caregiver well-being.
Sayre, 2015	Objective Measure of Strength in Fall Prevention for Patients Receiving Hematopoietic Stem Cell Transplant	Quantitative	45 patients	Routine measurement of hand grip strength may assist in identifying patients who are becoming weaker, thus leading to more targeted fall prevention intervention.
Schoulte et al., 2011	Influence of Coping Style on Symptom Interference Among Adult Recipients of Hematopoietic Stem Cell Transplantation	Qualitative, longitudinal; secondary analysis of data	105 adult patients	An intervention to teach alternate coping strategies should be implemented prior to treatment and tested for prevention of symptom-related life interference.
Siefker & Vogelsang, 2018	Nursing Interventions for the Patient Experiencing Mucositis	Quality improvement intervention	34 nurses	This quality improvement initiative was a successful addition to hospital nursing care and resulted in consistent treatment for patients experiencing mucositis. The nurses were more confident in assessing mucositis severity and using consistent interventions.

(Continued on next page)

Authors	Title	Study Design	Sample	Comments
Sinclair et al., 2016	Factors Associated With Post-Traumatic Growth, Quality of Life, and Spiritual Well-Being in Outpatients Undergoing Bone Marrow Transplantation: A Pilot Study	Pilot study; cross-sectional, descriptive, exploratory	100 patients	Findings suggested spirituality not only is important to patients undergoing BMT but also may be an integral to post-traumatic growth, QOL, and spiritual well-being.
Singh et al., 2017	Experiences of Women With Gestational Trophoblastic Neoplasia Treated With High-Dose Chemotherapy and Stem Cell Transplantation: A Qualitative Study	Qualitative	10 patients	Nurses need to develop services that effectively communicate the challenges of HSCT to patients and provide family-centered care and late effects and rehabilitation services.
Son et al., 2017	Adaptation of a Coping Intervention for Stem Cell Transplantation Patients and Caregivers	Qualitative	6–10 patients, caregivers, and dyads and 5–7 clinicians to review coping intervention, then additional 14–16 patients, caregivers, and dyads to further inform refinement	This intervention can facilitate coping with HSCT-related challenges and reduce distress and burden.
Sundaramurthi et al., 2017	Hematopoietic Stem Cell Transplantation Recipient and Caregiver Factors Affecting Length of Stay and Readmission	Secondary data analysis	136 total; 68 dyads	Educating patients and caregivers on infection prevention is critically important to reduce length of stay and 30-day readmission after HSCT.
Tierney et al., 2015	Sexuality, Menopausal Symptoms, and Quality of Life in Premenopausal Women in the First Year Following Hematopoietic Cell Transplantation	Prospective longitudinal study	63 women	Nurses and other healthcare providers working with HSCT recipients can provide anticipatory guidance on potential sexuality changes and menopausal symptoms to facilitate adaptation by reducing discordance between expectations and new realities.
Uggla et al., 2018	Music Therapy Effect Health Related Quality of Life in Children Undergoing HSCT; A Randomized Clinical Study	Randomized clinical study	38 children 0–17 years of age undergoing HSCT	The music therapy creative interaction is vital and provides children with a sense of control and facilitates emotional regulation. The combination of lower heart rate after intervention and higher health-related QOL at discharge may indicate that music therapy should be a complementary intervention and support for children during HSCT.
van der Lans et al., 2019	Five Phases of Recovery and Rehabilitation After Allogeneic Stem Cell Transplantation: A Qualitative Study	Qualitative	10 hemato-oncology patients were interviewed 1 year after transplant	Nurses can play an important role in achieving improvements in post-transplant care by tailoring care to individual needs of patients within distinct phases.
Velez et al., 2018	A Clinical Nurse's Role in Improving the Care of the BMT Recipient Receiving High Dose Chemotherapy	Performance improvement	Audits of 13 charts	BMT nurses must continue to update their knowledge and review standards and evidence-based guidelines to practice effectively. Assessing changes in practice and the impact on patient experience is critical to improving patient care.
Von Ah et al., 2016	The Caregiver's Role Across the Bone Marrow Transplantation Trajectory	Qualitative	15 family caregivers	A greater understanding of the adaptation of caregivers will lead to development of effective interventions for families going through BMT.

(Continued on next page)

Authors	Title	Study Design	Sample	Comments
Ward et al., 2017	Pilot Study of Parent Psycho-physiologic Outcomes in Pediatric Hematopoietic Stem Cell Transplantation	Pilot study	12 parent–child dyads	Routine psychological and physical health screening of parents of children undergoing HSCT is needed. Interprofessional psychosocial support services should be offered to parents at regular intervals during their child's HSCT.
Wheatley, 2018	Implementing and Evaluating a Nurse-Led Educational Intervention for Bone Marrow Transplant Patients in the Acute Care Setting	Performance improvement	–	A BMT basics class could provide a patient-centered approach to improving quality of care when implemented in addition to current evidence-based practice.
Williams et al., 2018	Symptom Monitoring and Burden in Autologous Stem Cell Transplantation for Multiple Myeloma	Randomized	204 patients	Patients receiving high-dose busulfan and melphalan experience more severe symptom burden than patients receiving high-dose melphalan during autologous HSCT. The benefit of longer time to progression of myeloma with the high-dose busulfan and melphalan regimen may offset the greater symptom burden. Nurses can provide symptom management for patients on more intense regimens, thus allowing them to achieve optimal treatment benefit.

BMT—bone marrow transplantation; CLABSI—central line–associated bloodstream infection; FDA—U.S. Food and Drug Administration; GVHD—graft-versus-host disease; HSCT—hematopoietic stem cell transplantation; QOL—quality of life

is limited by the availability of suitable matched donors and potential immunologic complications. Gene therapy using autologous HSCs is being evaluated for its ability to cure many of these diseases without the need for matched donors and risk of GVHD (Morgan, Gray, Lomova, & Kohn, 2017). Human gene therapy is the administration of genetic material to modify or manipulate the expression of a gene or to alter the biologic properties of living cells for therapeutic use (American Society of Gene and Cell Therapy, n.d.; Rein, Yang, & Chao, 2018). HSCT and gene therapy operate under the same premise: to introduce foreign DNA into patients with the goal of treating or curing disease (Rein et al., 2018). According to the American Society of Gene and Cell Therapy (n.d.), five therapeutic strategies are used in gene therapy:

- **Gene addition:** Gene addition involves insertion of a new copy of a gene into target cells to produce more of a protein. A modified virus such as adeno-associated virus is used to carry the gene into the cells. Therapies based on gene addition are being developed to treat many diseases, including adenosine deaminase–deficient severe combined immunodeficiency (SCID).
- **Gene correction:** Gene correction involves using gene editing technology (CRISPR/Cas9, TALEN, or zinc-finger nucleases) to remove repeated or faulty elements of a gene or to replace a damaged or dysfunctional region of DNA. The goal is to produce a protein that functions normally instead of in a way that contributes to disease.

Experimental work has used gene correction to extract HIV from the genome of affected laboratory mice.

- **Gene silencing:** Gene silencing is a process that prevents the production of a specific protein by targeting messenger RNA (mRNA; an intermediate required for protein expression from a gene) for degradation so that no protein is produced. Human and animal cells have single-stranded mRNA, whereas viruses have double-stranded RNA. Human and animal cells recognize double-stranded RNA as viral and destroy it. Gene silencing uses small sequences of RNA to bind unique sequences in the target mRNA and make it double stranded. This triggers destruction of the mRNA using the cellular machinery that destroys viral RNA. Gene silencing is used to treat diseases in which too much of a protein is produced. For example, too much tumor necrosis factor-alpha (TNF-α) often is observed in the afflicted joints of patients with rheumatoid arthritis. TNF-α is needed in small amounts in the rest of the body; gene silencing is used to reduce TNF-α levels only in the affected tissue.
- **Reprogramming:** Reprogramming involves adding one or more genes to cells of a specific type to change those cells' characteristics. This technique is powerful in tissue in which multiple cell types exist and the disease is caused by dysfunction in one type of cell. For example, type 1 diabetes mellitus (T1D) occurs because many of the insulin-producing islet cells of the pancreas are damaged. However, cells of the pancreas that

produce digestive enzymes are not damaged. Reprogramming these cells so that they can produce insulin would cure T1D.

- **Cell elimination:** Cell elimination strategies typically are used to destroy malignant tumor cells but also can be used to target overgrowth of benign tumor cells. Tumor cells can be eliminated by the introduction of suicide genes, which enter the tumor cells and release a prodrug that induces cell death. Viruses can be engineered to have an affinity for tumor cells. These oncotropic viruses carry therapeutic genes to increase toxicity to tumor cells, stimulate the immune system to attack the tumor, or inhibit the growth of blood vessels that supply the tumor with nutrients.

There are two basic ways to deliver gene and cellular therapies: vector and nonvector. A transmission vector is either delivered to the patient (in vivo transfer) or cells are harvested from a patient or donor, cultured ex vivo, and transferred back to the recipient (ex vivo transfer) (Rein et al., 2018).

Nonvector methods include electroporation, passive delivery, and ballistic delivery. Simple strands of naked DNA or RNA can be pushed into cells using high-voltage electroporation. This is a common technique in the laboratory. Naked DNA or RNA may also be taken up by target cells using a normal cellular process called endocytosis, after addition to the medium surrounding the cells. Finally, sheer mechanical force can be used to introduce genetic material with an instrument called a "gene gun."

Membrane-bound vesicles can also be used. Genetic material can be packaged into artificially created liposomes that are more easily taken up into the cells than naked DNA or RNA. Different types of liposomes are being developed to preferentially bind to specific tissues. Recent work has used a subtype of membrane vesicles that are endogenously produced and released by cells to carry small sequences of RNA into specific tissues.

Viral vectors for gene therapy are modified to use the ability of viruses to enter cells after disabling the capacity of the virus to divide. Different types of viruses have been engineered to function as therapy vectors. In the case of adeno-associated virus and retrovirus/lentivirus vectors, the genes of interest and control signals replace all or most of the essential viral genes in the vector so that the viral vector does not replicate. The integrating property of retroviruses allows the transmission of therapeutic information to all progeny of a transduced HSC (Morgan et al., 2017). For oncolytic viruses, such as adenovirus and herpes simplex virus, fewer viral genes are replaced and the virus is still able to replicate in a restricted number of cell types. Different types of viral vectors preferentially enter a subset of different tissues, express genes at different levels, and interact with the immune system differently.

Gene therapy can be combined with HSCT protocols. HSCs are collected from the patient or donor and then purified and expanded in vitro. The gene product is delivered to collected cells using one of the previously described methods. Cells that express the therapeutic gene are then readministered to the patient (American Society of Gene and Cell Therapy, n.d.).

Success in the treatment of X-linked SCID, adenosine deaminase–deficient SCID, and chronic granulomatous disease using gene therapy has been achieved, but this progress was tempered by serious adverse events linked to the genetic modification of HSCs (Cavazzana, 2014; Dunbar, 2007; Kohn, 2008). Researchers remain optimistic that gene therapy will become an effective treatment for several diseases. The spectrum ranges from the treatment of inherited or acquired genetic disorders to cancer, AIDS, cardiopathies, and autoimmune and neurologic diseases (Watts, Adair, & Kiem, 2011).

Obstacles to successful gene therapy include inadequacies of gene delivery systems with poor expression of recombinant genes and risk of insertional mutagenesis when using integrating vectors, which remains a safety concern (Morgan et al., 2017; Srivastava & Shaji, 2017). The requirements for successful gene transfer include the ability to insert the correct gene into the correct cell type and the cell's adequate expression of the inserted gene (Bordignon & Roncarolo, 2002; Nathwani, Davidoff, & Linch, 2004; Rein et al., 2018). Currently, HSCs, most commonly autologous, are the favorite target for human trials of gene therapy because stem cells carrying a therapeutic gene could be a lifelong source of the gene (Kirby, 1999; Kohn, 2008). Transfer of genes into the cell for gene or cellular therapies is done either in vivo or ex vivo (Rein et al., 2018).

HSCs are desirable targets for gene therapy for several reasons. They are easily accessible, able to replicate into all cell lineages, and can be removed from the body, modified ex vivo, and retransplanted with preservation of their function (Cavazzana, 2014; Fraser & Hoffman, 1995; Kirby, 1999; Kohn, 2008; Morgan et al., 2017; Rein et al., 2018). HSCs have been used successfully as a source of long-term repopulation of cells, so these cells should provide a lifelong source of amplified progeny expressing the introduced gene (Cavazzana, 2014; Cavazzana-Calvo, Bagnis, Mannoni, & Fischer, 1999; Civin, 2000; Schmitz et al., 1996). Progenitors of HSCs are involved in many human disorders (Havenga, Hoogerbrugge, Valerio, & van Es, 1997; Watts et al., 2011). Natural and laboratory viruses can gain entry and integrate into the DNA of early hematopoietic progenitor cells (Civin, 2000).

Stem cell transduction, or the ability to transfer the gene of interest to the stem cell while preserving the ability to self-renew and maintain multilineage potential, has remained a challenging problem for researchers (Becker, 2005; Cuaron & Gallucci, 1997; Kirby, 1999). HSCs constitute no more than 1 cell in 10,000 and perhaps as few as 1 in 100,000 (Kirby, 1999). The number of harvested HSCs represents only a small percentage of HSCs in the body, making it impossible to transduce most of the cells with the intended gene (Beutler, 1999). Stem cells resist transduction because they have trace receptors on the cell surface for vectors to interact with (Kirby, 1999). HSCs spend most of their time in a resting stage, making transduction efficiency low because they are not dividing. Attempts to induce the HSC to enter a dividing state with colony-stimulating factor, a combination of chemotherapy and growth factors, or novel agents have led to the loss of some of the properties of the stem cell. HSCs are abnormally incapable of engrafting when forced to cycle (Becker, 2005; Kirby, 1999; Romano, Micheli, Pacilio, & Giordano, 2000). Humans have evolved mechanisms for inactivating externally introduced fragments of DNA, which must be overcome for gene therapy to be successful (Becker, 2005).

The purification of HSCs for gene therapy relies mainly on mobilizing stem cells from the bone marrow into the peripheral circulation using an agent such as colony-stimulating factor or chemotherapy; cells are then selected. Using a positive-enrichment method requires the existence of cell surface markers that are potentially specific for stem cells. Gene therapy with HSCT consists of the replication of incompetent retroviral vectors that are modified to carry the gene of interest into pluripotent stem cells of the body. A commonly used strategy involves harvesting progenitor cells, incubating a portion of these cells with the transducing vector, and then reinfusing these cells back into the patient after a conditioning regimen designed to reduce the number of cancerous cells (Cuaron & Gallucci, 1997; Morgan et al., 2017; Rein et al., 2018).

The first reports of successful gene therapy were for the treatment of X-linked SCID. In this trial, 10 infants younger than one year of age received gene transfer into CD34+ cells using murine leukemia viruses (MLVs), a class of simple gammaretroviruses (gRVs). Peripheral mature T cells were detected in 10–12 weeks. T-cell counts reached normal levels in 8 of the 10 patients within three months of therapy and were still normal after five years (Cavazzana-Calvo, Lagresle, Hacein-Bey-Abina, & Fischer, 2005; Kohn, 2008; Morgan et al., 2017; Rein et al., 2018). However, 5 (of 10 total) boys who received the MLV gRV-modified CD34+ cells developed aggressive T-cell leukemias two to six years after the gene therapy, one of whom died (Dunbar, 2007; Morgan et al., 2017). The occurrence of T-cell acute lymphoblastic leukemia in patients receiving MLV gRVs was the result of the long-terminal repeat–driven gRV vector landing upstream of proto-oncogenes and ectopically activating their expression (Hacein-Bey-Abina et al., 2008; Howe et al., 2008; Kohlscheen, Bonig, & Modlich, 2017; Morgan et al., 2017). Since starting the use of gene-modified stem cells in 1999 for children with X-linked SCID, approximately 70 patients have been successfully treated (Cavazzana, 2014).

Thompson et al. (2018) reported on gene therapy in patients with transfusion-dependent beta-thalassemia (β-thalassemia). In two phase 1–2 trials, they treated 22 patients (aged 12–35 years) with transfusion-dependent β-thalassemia and transduced the cells ex vivo with Len-tiGlobin BB305 vector, which encodes adult hemoglobin (HbA) with a T87Q amino acid substitution (HbA^{T87Q}). Cells were reinfused after the patients received conditioning with busulfan. They monitored for adverse events, vector integration, and levels of replication-competent lentivirus. At a median of 26 months (range 15–42) after infusion of the gene-modified cells, all but one of the 13 patients who had a non β⁰/β⁰ genotype had stopped receiving red cell transfusions, the levels of HbA^{T87Q} ranged from 3.4 to 10 g/dl, and the levels of total hemoglobin ranged from 8.2 to 13.7 g/dl. Correction of biologic markers of dyserythropoiesis was achieved in evaluated patients with hemoglobin levels near normal ranges. In nine patients with β⁰/β⁰ genotype or two copies of the IVS1-110 mutation, the median annualized transfusion volume was decreased by 73%, and red cell transfusions were discontinued in three patients. Treatment-related adverse events were typical of those associated with autologous HSCT. No clonal dominance related to vector integration was observed. Results indicated the gene therapy with autologous CD34+ cells transduced with the BB305 vector reduced or eliminated the need for long-term red cell transfusions in 22 patients with severe β-thalassemia without serious adverse events (Thompson et al., 2018).

Gene therapy has been used to successfully correct genetic disorders for years. Recently, with the use of chimeric antigen receptor (CAR) T-cell therapy, researchers have applied gene therapy for the use of antitumor immunity (Wilkins, Keeler, & Flotte, 2017). CARs are engineered fusion proteins that incorporate antigen recognition for a specific tumor antigen target (Rein et al., 2018). These cells work most effectively against B-cell malignancies (Rein et al., 2018). CAR T-cell therapy is the first gene transfer therapy to receive commercial approval by FDA (June & Sadelain, 2018).

Nonmalignant Diseases Treated With Hematopoietic Stem Cell Transplantation

The use of HSCT has expanded to include many nonmalignant diseases, including genetic disorders, errors in metabolism, and autoimmune diseases. The first successful allogeneic HSCTs reported were for patients with primary immunodeficiencies (Sullivan, Parkman, & Walters, 2000). Currently, nonmalignant diseases account for 5% of HCT therapy. One-half to two-thirds of the procedures are performed for a broad range of inherited blood and immune system diseases in children (Appelbaum et al., 2015). Since 2004, through numerous early-phase observational or small randomized clinical trials, HSCT has proved to be a feasible tool for repairing diseases characterized by dysfunctional hematopoiesis and immunity (Appelbaum et al., 2015). Transplant-related morbidity and mortality remain a serious concern when considering HSCT for the treatment of nonmalignant diseases. These include regimen-related toxicities, fertility issues, GVHD, nonengraftment, and infection (Slatter et al., 2018; Steward, 2000; Sullivan et al., 1998). Advances in supportive care for patients with many genetic disorders, autoimmune diseases, and errors in metabolism now allow patients to experience good quality of life for many years after diagnosis (Steward, 2000). However, HSCT is the only curative therapy for patients with many primary immunodeficiencies and inherited metabolic diseases (Laberko & Gennery, 2018; Ochs & Petroni, 2018; Prasad & Kurtzberg, 2008; Sullivan et al., 1998). The risks versus benefits of HSCT for these patients are sometimes difficult to determine with current transplantation techniques.

Primary Immunodeficiency Diseases

Primary immunodeficiency diseases is a term used to describe a large number of disorders, with more than 300 genetically defined disorders identified (Laberko & Gennery, 2018; Ochs & Petroni, 2018). HSCT is curative for many immunodeficiency diseases and is the treatment of choice for patients with SCID (Hagin, Burroughs, & Torgerson, 2015; Laberko & Gennery, 2018; Ochs & Petroni, 2018; Sullivan et al., 2000). Patients with primary immunodeficiency benefit from early diagnosis and transplantation prior to developing serious infections, as active infection pretransplant adversely affects survival (Heimall et al., 2017). For all stem cell sources, successful outcomes are more likely when patients are still very young—preferably younger than six months (Dvorak & Cowan, 2008). The major factors when considering HSCT for immunodeficiency and immune dysregulation disorders include selecting a suitable donor to provide stem cells capable of successfully engrafting; curing the underlying disease and avoiding extensive reaction against the host (GVHD); selecting a conditioning regimen capable of opening sufficient space in the bone marrow to allow engraftment without creating severe life-threatening side effects; and selecting a post-transplant immunosuppressive regimen capable of preventing GVHD while allowing engraftment and expansion of donor cells (Hagin et al., 2015). Generally, the risks of graft rejection and GVHD are proportional to the degree of HLA mismatch between donor and recipient, and the risk of toxicity and death from infection is proportional to the intensity of the pretransplant conditioning regimen (Hagin et al., 2015). The European Society for Immunodeficiencies Inborn Errors Working Party is working to improve the outcome of transplant and gene therapy for severe congenital immunodeficiencies through enhanced interactions among HSCT centers, collaborative studies, education, development of guidelines, and creation of a registry of treatment results (European Society for Immunodeficiencies, n.d.).

The preferred choice of stem cells for patients with SCID is an HLA-identical sibling donor, in which case the overall survival exceeds 90% if the transplant is performed promptly (Dvorak & Cowan, 2008). When HLA-matched related donors are not available, three alternative sources

exist: a haplocompatible relative, an HLA-matched unrelated adult volunteer, or an unrelated banked umbilical cord blood unit (Cowan, Neven, Cavazanna-Calvo, Fischer, & Puck, 2008). Most of these patients are treated with T-cell-depleted haplocompatible stem cells (Sullivan et al., 2000). Overall three-year survival is 53%–79% in those receiving haplocompatible transplants, with significantly better success rates in more recent years and in more experienced centers (Dvorak & Cowan, 2008). Overall survival for patients undergoing HSCT from matched unrelated donors is 63%–67% (Dvorak & Cowan, 2008).

The use of reduced-toxicity conditioning is preferred in patients with primary immunodeficiency diseases, in whom there is no malignant disease to eradicate (Slatter et al., 2018). Preparative chemotherapy improved one-year post-HSCT median CD4 counts (p = 0.02) and freedom from IV immunoglobulin (p < 0.001) (Heimall et al., 2017). Stable mixed chimerism achieves cure for most patients, and many enter HSCT with chronic infection and end-organ comorbidities. In addition, many HSCT recipients are infants, who may be more susceptible to toxicity (Malär, Sjöö, Rentsch, Hassan, & Güngör, 2011; Slatter et al., 2018). Less toxic regimens may reduce early and late adverse effects, particularly effects on fertility (Lawitschka et al., 2015; Panasiuk et al., 2015; Slatter et al., 2018). Initial results from reduced-intensity HSCT suggest that specific conditioning regimens may be preferable in certain primary immunodeficiency diseases with severe comorbidities, with specific donor types and stem cell sources, and appear to enhance toxicity in children younger than one year old (Ritchie, Seymour, Roberts, Szer, & Grigg, 2001; Slatter et al., 2018; Straathof et al., 2009). The absence of conditioning therapy has been associated with graft failure in patients with T-cell-negative, B-cell-negative, NK-cell-positive SCID (an extreme form of SCID) and adenosine deaminase deficiency (Amrolia et al., 2000; Porta & Friedrich, 1998). Many patients have poor B-cell reconstitution requiring continued IV immunoglobulin administration (Amrolia et al., 2000; Buckley et al., 1999; Cowan et al., 2008; Sullivan et al., 2000).

Abd Hamid, Slatter, McKendrick, Pearce, and Gennery (2017) evaluated long-term clinical features, longitudinal immunoreconstitution, donor chimerism, and quality of life of patients with IL2RG/JAK3 SCID more than two years post-HSCT at their center. The difference between the groups was not statistically significant, but, given the small sample size, the observation is likely to be real. A biologic explanation may be that in conditioned patients, the thymic niche is consistently reseeded from bone marrow–derived stem cells leading to ongoing thymopoiesis, whereas for unconditioned recipients, initial seeding of the thymic niche at time of infusion is not generally followed by reseeding, as donor stem cell engraftment does not consistently occur in the bone marrow and thymic seeding may have a finite lifetime, eventually leading to thymic exhaustion. A subgroup analysis of patients in this trial showed that patients who discontinued immunoglobulin infusions appeared to have a normal health-related quality of life compared to normal controls, whereas those who remained on immunoglobulin had significantly worse results. The researchers concluded that in patients with IL2RG/JAK3 SCID, thymopoiesis is durable over time but is better in those who received conditioning. Low toxicity, myeloablative regimens achieve better donor stem cell engraftment, with few significant short-term toxicities, although long-term follow-up will be required to assess late effects. Freedom of immunoglobulin replacement leads to normal quality of life and is most associated with preparative chemotherapy (Abd Hamid et al., 2017).

Slatter et al. (2018) provide results of a follow-up study of treosulfan and fludarabine conditioning for HSCT in children with primary immunodeficiency. This study showed that the combination of treosulfan and fludarabine is suitable for pre-HSCT conditioning in patients with a diverse range of primary immunodeficiency diseases, regardless of age and with all types of donors and stem cell sources, providing a uniformly applicable conditioning strategy in primary immunodeficiency (Slatter et al., 2018).

Fox et al. (2018) reported a successful outcome following allogeneic HSCT in adults with primary immunodeficiency. Controversy exists regarding optimum timing and use of allogeneic HSCT in adults because of a lack of experience and previous poor outcomes. Based on the results, the researchers concluded that allogeneic HSCT is safe and effective in young adults and in patients with severe primary immunodeficiency and should be considered for patients who have an available donor (Fox et al., 2018).

Wiskott-Aldrich Syndrome

Wiskott-Aldrich syndrome management requires early diagnosis, supportive care, and HSCT (Thakkar et al., 2017). The only curative strategy is HSCT, and patients require pretransplant immunosuppression and ablation of host HSCs (Dvorak & Cowan, 2008; Sullivan et al., 2000). Matched sibling donor HSCT after myeloablative conditioning is the standard (Thakkar et al., 2017). Initially, the combination of cyclophosphamide and TBI had been used. However, TBI has been replaced by busulfan and cyclophosphamide to permit adequate immunosuppression and ablation of the abnormal recipient HSCs without the long-term toxicity of irradiation (Sullivan et al., 2000). Myeloablative strategies have been used for conditioning because of the concern for mixed donor chimerism (Ngwube et al., 2018). However, several reports of successful reduced-intensity conditioning with alternative donors exist in the literature (Thakkar et al., 2017).

An analysis of 170 patients reported to the International Bone Marrow Transplant Registry and National Marrow Donor Program demonstrated the five-year overall survival of patients transplanted from HLA-identical siblings was 87%. However, results from unrelated HSCT were significantly tied to age at transplant (Dvorak & Cowan, 2008; Fil-

ipovich et al., 2001; Sullivan et al., 2000). Haploidentical related donor transplant survival has been less successful, with an overall survival of 45%–52% (Dvorak & Cowan, 2008; Sullivan et al., 2000). Survival of unrelated donor recipients younger than five years old was 85%, whereas all 15 patients transplanted at age five years or older died (Dvorak & Cowan, 2008; Filipovich et al., 2001). Histocompatible or unrelated donor transplant in patients younger than five years old is the treatment of choice for Wiskott-Aldrich syndrome (Sullivan et al., 2000). HSCT from HLA-identical family members or matched unrelated donors, rather than the use of a haploidentical donor, is recommended (Griffith et al., 2009).

Ngwube et al. (2018) reported on a retrospective analysis of 12 children they transplanted for Wiskott-Aldrich syndrome. The long-term overall survival regardless of donor type remains excellent despite mixed chimerism.

Thakkar et al. (2017) reported on three successful reduced-intensity conditioning alternate donor HSCTs for Wiskott-Aldrich syndrome. They concluded that with newer conditioning regimens and GVHD prophylaxis, alternate donor HSCT can become a safe and effective treatment option.

Griffith et al. (2008) held a workshop and made recommendations for research into HSCT as a treatment for Wiskott-Aldrich syndrome, which includes a descriptive cross-sectional study of HSCT outcomes in North America and a long-term retrospective follow-up study of patients with Wiskott-Aldrich syndrome who have received HSCT. Collaborative studies by a consortium of institutions in North America are recommended to answer and achieve these goals (Griffith et al., 2008). Not all patients have a matched sibling donor, so there is a need to develop alternate donors through matched related donor, unrelated cord blood, and haploidentical donor HSCT programs (Thakkar et al., 2017).

Thalassemia Major

Allogeneic HSCT to replace the defective gene was initiated as curative therapy for thalassemia major in the 1980s (Lucarelli et al., 1990; Srivastava & Shaji, 2017). Since 1981, more than 4,000 patients worldwide have received HSCT for thalassemia major (Issaragrisil & Kunacheewa, 2016). HSCT remains the only curative option (Issaragrisil & Kunacheewa, 2016; Lucarelli & Gaziev, 2008; Srivastava & Shaji, 2017; Strocchio & Locatelli, 2018). Results using HLA-identical sibling donors are excellent, and all patients with thalassemia major who have an available HLA-identical sibling donor should be considered for HSCT at an early stage in the disease before development of significant iron overload–related complications (Issaragrisil & Kunacheewa, 2016; Peters, 2018; Saba & Flaig, 2002; Smiers, Krishnamurti, & Lucarelli, 2010; Strocchio & Locatelli, 2018). Lucarelli et al. (1998) performed analyses of transplantation results in patients younger than age 17 who had thalassemia, which resulted in the

Pesaro classification. The Pesaro classification has three classes of risk using the following criteria: degree of hepatomegaly greater than 2 cm, degree of portal fibrosis, and quality of chelation treatment given before transplantation. Patients with none of the adverse criteria constituted class 1, patients with one or various associations of two of the adverse criteria formed class 2, and those for whom all three criteria were adverse constituted class 3. Most patients older than age 16 have disease characteristics that place them in class 3, with very few in class 2. Patients categorized as class 3 have a higher incidence of graft failure than patients in class 1 or 2 (Smiers et al., 2010; Strocchio & Locatelli, 2018). All patients with an HLA-identical donor are assigned to protocols based on class at the time of transplantation, independent of age (Lucarelli et al., 1998).

The Pesaro classification system has been validated in children who received adequate medical care prior to HSCT. Limitations for the classification approach were seen when it was applied to patients who had inadequate pretransplant medical care, which is commonly seen in developing countries (Strocchio & Locatelli, 2018). Mathews et al. (2007) developed a risk evaluation based on patient age (younger or older than seven years of age) and liver size (more or less than 5 cm below the costal margin), which identifies a very high-risk subset within the Pesaro class 3 group. This observation has been confirmed by an analysis based on data reported to CIBMTR (Mathews et al., 2007; Sabloff et al., 2011; Strocchio & Locatelli, 2018). EBMT reported a retrospective review on 1,493 consecutive patients with thalassemia major who received HSCT between 2000 and 2010, and a significant threshold age of 14 for optimal results was identified (Baronciani et al., 2016; Strocchio & Locatelli, 2018).

Progress has been made in identification of conditioning regimens. Busulfan and cyclophosphamide have been the conditioning regimen of choice for patients undergoing HSCT for thalassemia major (Lucarelli et al., 1990; Strocchio & Locatelli, 2018). The regimen is associated with a high incidence of hepatic toxicity. To reduce the conditioning toxicity, other protocols have been developed replacing cyclophosphamide with fludarabine and thiotepa (Locatelli & Stefano, 2004; Strocchio & Locatelli, 2018) and using treosulfan as an alternative to busulfan, with encouraging results (Bernardo et al., 2012; Strocchio & Locatelli, 2018). The Pesaro group transplanted 22 children given a T-cell–depleted allograft from haploidentical relatives leading to a disease-free survival of 61% (Locatelli, Merli, & Strocchio, 2016; Sodani et al., 2010).

Researchers are exploring the option of haploidentical donors. Concern exists about the use of T-cell–depleted marrow because of the high risk of graft failure (Locatelli et al., 2016; Sodani et al., 2010). Anurathapan et al. (2016) recently reported the outcomes of 31 patients with thalassemia major who received T-cell-replete peripheral blood haploidentical HSCT. Two-year overall survival and event-free survival were 95% and 94%, respectively (Anurathapan et al., 2016; Locatelli et al., 2016).

Mixed chimerism is a common phenomenon after myeloablative transplantation for thalassemia. Approximately 10% of patients develop a condition of stable coexistence of donor and recipient stem cells, or persistent mixed chimerism, in the presence of a functional graft, suggesting that engraftment of a few donor cells might be sufficient for correction of disease phenotype in patients with thalassemia once donor host tolerance is established (Smiers et al., 2010; Srivastava & Shaji, 2017; Strocchio & Locatelli, 2018). A state of mixed chimerism can be classified as level 1 (less than 10%), level 2 (10%–25%), and level 3 (greater than 25%). Mixed chimerism has been reported during the post-HSCT period up to day 100, occurring in 30%–45% of patients (Srivastava & Shaji, 2017). A group of 335 patients had a 32.2% incidence of mixed chimerism. None of the 227 patients with complete chimerism rejected their grafts, and 35 of the 108 patients with mixed chimerism lost their graft, suggesting that mixed chimerism after HSCT for thalassemia is a risk factor for rejection (Smiers et al., 2010). The percentage of residual host hematopoietic cells after transplantation was predictive for graft rejection. Nearly all patients experiencing graft rejection had residual host hematopoietic cells exceeding 25% (Smiers et al., 2010). Based on studies conducted, the best time to transplant is in very young patients with HLA-identical siblings; however, current supportive therapy can provide good quality of life (Srivastava & Shaji, 2017; Strocchio & Locatelli, 2018; Sullivan et al., 2000).

The disease-free survival for related donor cord blood transplantation in patients with thalassemia is approaching 90%. The main complication is graft rejection, which may be reduced by increasing pretransplant immunosuppression (Pinto & Roberts, 2008). Patients receiving unrelated cord blood transplantation demonstrate higher rates of graft failure and delayed hematopoietic recovery because of inadequate cell dose in the graft (Strocchio & Locatelli, 2018; Strocchio et al., 2015). Ruggeri et al. (2011) described the outcomes from 35 patients with thalassemia treated with unrelated cord blood transplantation. Overall survival and disease-free survival estimates were 62% and 21%, respectively, with cumulative incidences of grade 2–4 acute GVHD and chronic GVHD of 23% and 16%, respectively. Primary graft failure was the main cause of treatment failure, occurring in 20 out of 35 patients with thalassemia major. A total nucleated cell dose greater than or equal to 5×10^7/kg was associated with better outcomes (Ruggeri et al., 2011; Strocchio & Locatelli, 2018). The major obstacles to unrelated cord blood transplantation are graft failure and delayed hematopoietic recovery. To overcome the risk of graft failure and delayed engraftment, current recommendations for cord blood transplantation in nonmalignant disorders suggest using units containing at least 3.5×10^7 total nucleated cells/kg of recipient body weight before cryopreservation and having fewer than two

HLA disparities (Gluckman, 2011; Strocchio & Locatelli, 2018). Strategies aimed at overcoming the cell dose limitation include cotransplantation of multiple units (Sideri et al., 2011; Strocchio & Locatelli, 2018) and cotransplantation of umbilical cord blood and either T-cell-depleted, HLA-identical CD34+ cells or mesenchymal stromal cells (Kim, Chung, Kim, Kim, & Oh, 2004; Kwon et al., 2014; Strocchio & Locatelli, 2018).

Sickle Cell Disease

Sickle cell disease (SCD) is an inherited genetic disorder associated with significant morbidity (Nickel & Kamani, 2018). Although substantial clinical advances have occurred in the treatment of SCD, which have improved conservative management, the only potential for cure is HSCT (Abboud, 2009; Bauer, Brendel, & Fitzhugh, 2017; Bhatia & Walters, 2008; Shenoy, 2013). Despite success with HSCT in SCD, it remains an underused treatment option. HSCT remains largely unacceptable to medical caregivers because offering a therapeutic option like HSCT that has a low, yet finite, risk of mortality in a condition generally not fatal in the short term presents a "dilemma of choice" (Nickel & Kamani, 2018; Platt & Guinan, 1996). Other barriers to successful HSCT in SCD include lack of a suitable donor; transplant-related morbidity, including infertility and GVHD; risk of mortality caused by the treatment; and immunologic graft rejection accompanied by disease recurrence (Bernaudin et al., 2007; Meier, Dioguardi, & Kamani, 2015; Walters, 2005).

Clinical trials using HSCT to treat SCD began in 1984 (Bauer et al., 2017; Bhatia & Walters, 2008; Hoppe & Walters, 2001; Johnson et al., 1984; Kassim & Sharma, 2017; Meier et al., 2015; Shenoy, 2007; Walters, 2015). EBMT and CIBMTR registries reported that 611 and 627 patients, respectively, have received HSCT for SCD as of 2013 (Gluckman, 2013; Meier et al., 2015; Walters, 2015). Overall survival at three years is greater than 90% for HSCT in children but only 62% in adults because of increased disease- and transplant-related mortality (Bhatia & Walters, 2008; Shenoy, 2007). This is especially true in the unrelated donor setting (Shenoy, 2007). Several studies have examined patient and healthcare provider attitudes related to HSCT for SCD (Chakrabarti & Bareford, 2007; van Besien et al., 2001; Vichinsky, Brugnara, Styles, & Wagner, 1998). The national collaborative group study found that 315 (6.5%) of 4,848 patients with SCD were younger than age 16 and met eligibility for the study. Of these patients, 239 had siblings, of whom 46% were not HLA typed because of parental refusal, physician concerns, lack of financial support, or other reasons. Eight percent of eligible patients were transplanted (Vichinsky et al., 1998).

Researchers van Besien et al. (2001) conducted a survey to determine the attitudes of adult patients and their healthcare providers regarding the risks and benefits of transplantation. The researchers wanted to determine an acceptable death rate of a curative treatment for adults with SCD. They surveyed 100 patients, 63 of whom were willing to accept some short-term risk of mortality in exchange for the certainty of cure. Fifteen patients were willing to accept more than 35% mortality risk. Results of the survey demonstrated adults with SCD are interested in a potentially curative treatment, even with a risk of treatment-related death. There is a lack of agreement between the recommendations of healthcare providers and the risk accepted by patients (van Besien et al., 2001).

Chakrabarti and Bareford (2007) surveyed 30 adult patients with SCD on their perception of reduced-intensity conditioning HSCT. Of the patients surveyed, 28 (93%) were aware of HSCT, but only 5 (16%) said it was discussed as a treatment option. Sixty-four percent of the patients surveyed would accept a risk of transplant-related mortality greater than 10%, and 30% of the patients were willing to accept a greater than 30% risk. However, 24 (80%) were unwilling to accept significant chronic GVHD in exchange for a cure, and 15 (50%) were not willing to accept infertility (Chakrabarti & Bareford, 2007).

Meier et al. (2015) replicated a study examining attitudes of parents and patients toward HSCT for SCD. They used a convenience sample of 69 parents of children with SCD and 18 adolescents with SCD, including 16 parent–adolescent dyads. Almost 44% of the participants reported having severe SCD based on clinical events. Nearly 21% reported moderate SCD, with 34.5% reporting mild clinical events of SCD. Seventy-two percent (64/89) of all respondents would be willing to accept a 5% or greater risk of mortality. Additionally, 56% of participants would accept a 10% or greater risk of mortality if the HSCT cured the SCD. Twenty-two percent of respondents were unwilling to accept any risk of mortality. Of those participants who were willing to accept 5% mortality, 75% would accept a 10% risk of GVHD. Overall, 56% of the participants were willing to accept the risk of infertility post-HSCT. However, more parents were willing to accept infertility risk compared to the adolescent patients surveyed. Results of this study suggest that, despite excellent outcomes following matched-sibling HSCT for patients with SCD, a number of parents and adolescents are unwilling to accept any risk of mortality or morbidity in exchange for a cure. However, a significant number of patients with SCD and parents of children with SCD are willing to accept risks of mortality and morbidity in exchange for a cure of SCD (Meier et al., 2015).

A lack of HLA-identical sibling donors remains an obstacle. It has been reported that 14% of patients with SCD will have a suitable HLA-identical sibling donor and 19% will have a very well matched unrelated marrow donor (Bolaños-Meade & Brodsky, 2009; Walters, 2015). The use of alternative donors and improving HLA typing methodology may allow appropriate donors to be identified, thus making this a treatment option available to more patients (Bhatia & Walters, 2008; Bolaños-Meade & Brodsky, 2009). Alternative sources of stem cells currently being evaluated include umbilical cord blood, matched unrelated donors, and haploidentical stem cells (Bolaños-Meade & Brodsky, 2009; Kassim & Sharma, 2017; Vichinsky et al., 1998; Walters, 2015).

The overwhelming majority of HSCTs for SCD are HLA-matched related donor transplants in children. Of the more than 1,200 transplants reported by EBMT and CIBMTR performed for SCD, approximately 75% were from matched sibling donors (Kassim & Sharma 2017; Meier et al., 2015). Patients without a matched related donor must rely on alternative donors to receive an HSCT. The use of unrelated cord blood transplantation has been reported. The National Heart, Lung, and Blood Institute BMT CTN trial of reduced-intensity conditioning cord blood transplantation in symptomatic patients with SCD was closed early to accrual secondary to increased graft rejection. Researchers have experienced success using reduced-intensity conditioning with haploidentical donor transplant for patients with hematologic malignancies and are developing protocols to expand this donor pool to patients with SCD (Bolaños-Meade & Brodsky, 2009; J. Filicko O'Hara, personal communication, April 20, 2010). Related donor cord blood transplantation for SCD has been reported with encouraging results. Eurocord reported a series of 44 patients with hemoglobinopathies transplanted with umbilical cord blood. The patients transplanted for SCD had 100% overall survival and 90% event-free survival. Nineteen evaluable patients with SCD had a five-year overall event-free survival rate of 94% ± 6% with a median follow-up of 32 months (Pinto & Roberts, 2008). Adamkiewicz et al. (2007) reported on seven children transplanted with unrelated umbilical cord blood. Three (43%) of the patients were cured. Four patients received myeloablative conditioning, three had sustained engraftment, and two developed grade 2–4 acute GVHD. One of the two died, and one developed extensive chronic GVHD.

HSCT for SCD in children has been reported with excellent results, with long-term disease-free survival of 82%–86% (Abboud, 2009). The majority of patients who have undergone HSCT for SCD have been younger than 16 years of age and have had multiple painful crises, recurrent episodes of acute chest syndrome, and occlusive stroke or evidence of end-organ dysfunction (Abboud, 2009).

Patients selected for transplant had preexisting complications of SCD, such as stroke, recurrent episodes of acute chest syndrome, or vaso-occlusive crises (Hoppe & Walters, 2001). Hsieh et al. (2009) reported on a trial using a nonmyeloablative regimen to treat patients with SCD. They concluded that nonmyeloablative HSCT using TBI with alemtuzumab and sirolimus will allow patients to achieve a stable, mixed donor–recipient chimerism and reverse the sickle cell phenotype (Hsieh et al., 2009).

Research efforts in HSCT for SCD need to target newer interventions directed at improving safety and efficacy of HSCT, minimizing areas of risk, and making a curative intervention available to more patients (Shenoy, 2013).

Autoimmune Diseases

HSCT trials were initiated in the late 1990s for treatment of ADs, including but not limited to systemic lupus erythematosus, multiple sclerosis, systemic sclerosis, and rheumatoid arthritis. Supported by random reports, HSCT has been evolving as a specific treatment for patients with ADs that have responded poorly or are refractory to conventional treatments (Farge et al., 2010; Hough, Snowden, & Wulffraat, 2005; Kelsey et al., 2016; Snowden et al., 2017; Snowden, Brooks, & Biggs, 1997; Swart et al., 2017). The goal is to eradicate autoreactive immune cells and regenerate a naïve, self-tolerant immune system (Sureda et al., 2015; Swart et al., 2017). More than 3,000 patients have been transplanted worldwide for ADs (Swart et al., 2017). EBMT reported that 1,951 patients from 1994 through 2015 with ADs have been treated with autologous HSCT and 105 patients have received allogeneic HSCT (Snowden et al., 2017). The rationale for autologous HSCT is that after the profound depletion of immune cells, including autoreactive T and B cells, a new and naïve immune system reconstituted from the stem cell graft will reestablish immune tolerance through the thymus (Swart et al., 2017). It remains unknown how HSCT rewires the out-of-control immune system (Swart et al., 2017). Clinical remissions in autoimmune disease after HSCT are the result of a true reconfiguration of the immune system instead of long-term immunosuppression (Swart et al., 2017).

Consensus conferences have been held in the United States and Europe to define the role of HSCT in ADs and develop strategies for conducting more meaningful trials. The two main objectives of the conferences were to show, through prospective randomized controlled trials (RCTs) whether autologous HSCT offered a durable and significantly improved quality of life for patients with severe ADs and to study immune reconstitution in patients with ADs to better understand the cellular and molecular mechanisms involved (Sullivan et al., 2010). The decision of the consensus conferences was to initially treat patients with ADs using autologous HSCT because of its lower morbidity and mortality (Sullivan et al., 1998, 2010; van Bekkum, 1999).

Adult patients with the underlying ADs should be considered for autologous HSCT when presenting with the following (Mancardi et al., 2015; Saccardi et al., 2012; Sureda et al., 2015; van Laar et al., 2014):
- Severe systemic sclerosis
  - Disease duration of less than five years since the onset of first non-Raynaud symptoms
  - Modified Rodnan skin score of 15 or higher
  - Respiratory with a diffusing capacity of the lung for carbon monoxide and/or forced vital capacity 80% of predicted
  - Evidence of interstitial lung disease on high-resolution computed tomography scan
  - Conduction or rhythm disturbance
  - Pericarditis

- Renal involvement
- Severe systemic sclerosis of less than two years
  - No major organ dysfunction as previously defined
  - Modified Rodnan skin score of at least 20
  - Acute-phase response
- Multiple sclerosis
  - Relapsing-remitting phase
  - High clinical and magnetic resonance imaging inflammatory activity
  - Rapid deterioration despite use of one or more lines of approved treatments
  - "Malignant" (Marburg) form
  - Secondary progressive disease, when some inflammatory activity is still evident
  - Clinical relapses or new T2 magnetic resonance imaging inflammatory activity still evident on two subsequent scans
  - Sustained and increased disability in the previous year, Expanded Disability Status Scale upper limit of 6.5, except for the malignant form (level II)
- Systemic lupus erythematosus
  - Early in disease course, with sustained or relapsed activity defined by British Isles Lupus Assessment Group category A
  - Creatinine clearance greater than 30 ml/min/m² on renal biopsy of less than 12 months
  - Evidence of WHO class III or IV glomerulonephritis
  - Neurologic, cardiovascular, pulmonary, vasculitis, or autoimmune cytopenias after at least six months of the best standard therapy
  - Use of mycophenolate mofetil or cyclophosphamide with or without anti-CD20
- Crohn disease
  - Refractory to immunosuppressive agents and anti-TNF-α monoclonal antibodies
  - Sustained endoscopic or computed tomography scan–proven activity
  - Extensive disease in which surgical resection would expose the patient to the risk of small bowel syndrome
  - Refractory colonic disease
  - Perianal lesions and refusal of coloproctectomy with a definitive stoma by the patient

Farge et al. (2010) reported an observational study analyzing all first autologous HSCTs for ADs reported to the EBMT registry from 1996 to 2007. Nine hundred patients with ADs underwent autologous HSCT. This observational study shows that autologous HSCT can induce sustained remissions for more than five years in patients with severe AD refractory to conventional therapy. The type of AD, rather than transplantation technique, was the most relevant determinant of outcome. Results improved with time and were associated with transplant center experience (Farge et al., 2010).

Allografting of stem cells from matched sibling donors is the most attractive model for treatment of AD because it is aimed at cure through replacement of a defective immune system with one derived from a healthy donor. However, the current risk of transplant-related toxicity in the allogeneic setting is a limit of the procedure, except for carefully and specifically selected patients entered into clinical trials (Griffith et al., 2005; Saccardi, Di Gioia, & Bosi, 2008). With experience in autologous HSCT, reduced-intensity conditioning regimens for hematologic malignancies, and better prevention and treatment of GVHD and infections, the safety profile of allogeneic transplant has improved, thereby making it possible to attempt investigational studies involving patients with life-threatening or severely disabling ADs (Daikeler et al., 2009; Griffith et al., 2005; Sullivan et al., 2010).

The National Institute of Allergy and Infectious Diseases and NCI held a workshop on the feasibility of allogeneic HSCT for ADs in 2005. At the workshop, researchers identified disease candidates, potential patient populations, specific limitations, and questions for allogeneic HSCT in ADs (Griffith et al., 2005). Patients identified as candidates for allogeneic HSCT are those who have the following disease characteristics:

- Aggressive course of disease with poor prognostic features
- Failure to respond to conventional therapy
- Failure to respond to high-dose immunosuppressive therapy and autologous HSCT
- High genetic load conveying disease susceptibility by criteria yet to be developed

Limitations and questions regarding allogeneic HSCT for AD identified by Griffith et al. (2005) included the following: What are the adverse events and safety in patients with significant organ dysfunction? Does allogeneic HSCT offer advantages over immunosuppression and autologous HSCT? Will relapses occur because sibling donors share too much genetic material with the patient?

Daikeler et al. (2009) performed a retrospective analysis of all patients reported to the EBMT data management system who had received an allogeneic HSCT for an AD. Thirty-five patients undergoing 38 allogeneic HSCTs for various hematologic and nonhematologic ADs were identified. Researchers were unable to identify any single factor that could predict outcomes (Daikeler et al., 2009).

More than 300,000 patients with multiple sclerosis are currently alive in the United States, but fewer than 50 transplants for multiple sclerosis are reported each year (Appelbaum et al., 2015). ASTCT recently released a position statement on autologous HSCT for multiple sclerosis. They consider it the standard of care for individuals with treatment-refractory relapsing disease with high risk of future disability (J.A. Cohen et al., 2019). This decision is based on recent studies indicating autologous HSCT is an efficacious and safe treatment for active relapsing forms of multiple sclerosis (J.A. Cohen et al., 2019).

The ASTIC (Autologous Stem-Cell Transplantation in Crohn's Disease) trial (Nottingham Digestive Diseases Centre, n.d.) evaluated the safety and tolerability of HSCT and the impact of this therapeutic approach on the clinical course of patients with Crohn disease (Allez et al., 2010; Snowden et al., 2018). Forty-five patients with active Crohn disease were randomized to HSC mobilization followed by high-dose immunoablation and autologous HSCT (n = 23) versus HSC mobilization only followed by best clinical practice (n = 22). After completion of the trial, 17 patients from the best clinical practice group went on to receive autologous HSCT. The trial failed to achieve its primary endpoint of sustained clinical remission off medication with no evidence of active disease on endoscopy or imaging (Lindsay et al., 2017; Snowden et al., 2018). Several important issues have been raised that affect interpretation of the benefit of HSCT in the ASTIC trial (Burt, Ruiz, & Kaiser, 2016; Hawkey, Lindsay, & Gribben, 2016; Lindsay et al., 2017). The predefined primary endpoint was the most stringent ever used for a clinical trial in Crohn disease. The data from this trial represent the largest report of patients with refractory Crohn disease undergoing autologous HSCT in terms of steroid-free clinical remission, enhanced quality of life, and mucosal healing. The large number of serious adverse events (76) suggests this treatment strategy should only be used in patients who are refractory to biologic therapies (Lindsay et al., 2017; Snowden et al., 2018).

Cooper et al. (2017) reported on the DECIDES study. The aim of this study was to explore factors influencing decision making and expectations of people considering or participating in the autologous HSCT trial. The conclusions were that decision making and expectations of this patient population in relation to autologous HSCT are a complex process influenced by participants' history of battling with their conditions, a frequent willingness to consider novel treatment options despite potential risks, and, in some cases, a raised level of expectation about the benefits of trial participation. When having discussions with patients who are considering novel treatments, potential therapeutic misestimation should be taken into account, enhancing shared decision making, informed consent, and communication with those deemed ineligible. The researchers concluded that future research should include longitudinal study designs taking greater account of the impact of individual, socioeconomic, cultural, and health service factors to capture outcomes for those receiving HSCT and for those ineligible for the trial (Cooper et al., 2017).

Crohn disease is the third most common indication for autologous HSCT in autoimmune disease, after multiple sclerosis and systemic sclerosis (Kelsey et al., 2016; Snowden et al., 2018). The EBMT registry contains 172 transplant registrations for Crohn disease as of 2017, with 164 for autologous HSCT (Snowden et al., 2018; unpublished data). In a joint initiative, the European Crohn's and Colitis Organisation and EBMT produced a state-of-the-art review of the rationale, evaluation, patient selection, stem cell mobilization and transplant procedures, and long-term follow-up (Snowden et al., 2018). The availability of new treatments for Crohn disease means that HSCT is not a suitable treatment method for most patients because of its greater toxicity, even though efficacy may be superior (Hawkey, 2017). It has been recommended that autologous HSCT should only be performed in experienced centers with expertise in both hematologic and gastroenterologic aspects of the procedure. Patients should be enrolled in clinical trials, and data registered centrally. Future developments should be coordinated at both national and international levels (Snowden et al., 2018).

Initial studies using autologous HSCT in the treatment of scleroderma had a high mortality rate because the transplants were mostly performed on patients with late-stage diffuse scleroderma with significant organ damage (Helbig et al., 2018). According to the Scleroderma Education Project (n.d.), as of December 2016, four autologous HSCT trials for treatment of scleroderma have been completed or are underway. Van Laar et al. (2014) reported on the Autologous Stem Cell Transplantation International Scleroderma (ASTIS) trial. The objective of the study was to compare the efficacy and safety of HSCT versus 12 successive monthly IV pulses of cyclophosphamide. Enrollment began in 2001 and ended in 2009. The investigators concluded that among patients with early diffuse cutaneous systemic sclerosis, HSCT was associated with increased treatment-related mortality in the first year after treatment. However, HSCT conferred a significant long-term event-free survival benefit (van Laar et al., 2014).

Sullivan et al. (2018) reported on myeloablative autologous HSCT for severe scleroderma. The researchers compared myeloablative CD34+ selected autologous HSCT with immunosuppression by means of 12 monthly infusions of cyclophosphamide in patients with scleroderma. The researchers found that myeloablative autologous HSCT achieved long-term benefits in patients with scleroderma, including improved event-free and overall survival, at a cost of increased expected toxicity (Sullivan et al., 2018).

Burt et al. (2011) reported on autologous nonmyeloablative HSCT compared with pulse cyclophosphamide once per month for systemic sclerosis (the ASSIST trial). They assessed the safety and efficacy of autologous HSCT in a phase 2 trial compared to standard of care, cyclophosphamide. Results of this study showed that nonmyeloablative autologous HSCT improved skin and pulmonary function in patients with systemic sclerosis for up to two years and was preferable to the current standard of care; however, longer follow-up is needed (Burt et al., 2011).

Burt (2019) is continuing this research with a randomized study of different nonmyeloablative conditioning regimens with HSC support in patients with scleroderma (ASSIST-IIb trial). The researchers propose to compare the ASSIST I conditioning regimen of cyclophosphamide and rabbit antithymocyte globulin to a less intense regimen of rabbit antithymocyte globulin, cyclophosphamide, and fludarabine. This study will determine if the lesser cardiotoxic regimen will be safer than and as effective as the standard regimen. They plan to randomize 160 participants.

Enrollment began September 2011, and the study is anticipated to be completed September 2021.

The Fred Hutchinson Cancer Research Center (2019) is conducting the STAT study (Scleroderma Treatment With Autologous Transplant). The primary objective is to evaluate the safety and potential efficacy of high-dose immunosuppressive therapy followed by autologous HSCT and maintenance therapy with mycophenolate mofetil in patients with systemic scleroderma by evaluating the effects on event-free survival at five years post-transplant.

The European League Against Rheumatism (EULAR) and EBMT have set forth transplant recommendations for systemic sclerosis. The most recent recommendations (Kowal-Bielecka et al., 2017) noted that, regarding HSCT, two RCTs showed improvement of skin involvement and stabilization of lung function in patients with systemic sclerosis and one large RCT reported improvement in event-free survival in patients with systemic sclerosis as compared with cyclophosphamide. HSCT should be considered for treatment of selected patients with rapidly progressive systemic sclerosis at risk for organ failure. In view of the high risk of side effects and early treatment-related mortality, careful patient selection and medical team experience are of key importance (Kowal-Bielecka et al., 2017). Dr. Sullivan stated, "Rheumatologists have two concerns: is this treatment approach safe, and are the improvements durable?" (as cited in Nierengarten, 2017, "Talking to Patients" section, para. 1). He advocated for rheumatologists to provide their patients with the information necessary to make an informed decision by referring them to a center with expertise in HSCT for scleroderma (Nierengarten, 2017).

Systematic long-term follow-up of patients is essential to trace the durability of remission and any associated late complications of the transplant procedure (Sullivan et al., 2000). However, single institutions cannot accrue enough patients to provide meaningful data. International multicenter trials should be undertaken to avoid duplication of effort and ensure a minimum amount of time is devoted to determining the role of this potentially lifesaving procedure (Burt et al., 2011; Tyndall & Gratwohl, 2000).

Members of the AD working party of EBMT consider HSCT "noncontributory to transplant patients with autoimmune disease outside the context of an approved, prospective RCT" (Sullivan et al., 2010, p. S52). Phase 1/2 trials are continuing in an effort to determine which ADs respond to transplant as well as the ideal timing of transplantation. Currently, randomized phase 3 trials are recruiting participants in the United States with systemic sclerosis, multiple sclerosis, and Crohn disease (Sullivan et al., 2010). The risk of transplant-related mortality within the first 100 days should be weighed against the risk of disease-related mortality, and careful selection and screening of patients before transplantation are essential (Swart et al., 2017). In all cases, safer but equally effective alternative treatments, including biologic therapies, should be considered first (Snowden et al., 2012; Swart et al., 2017). Toxic effects of HSCT arise from the selection of patients and conditioning regimen used, rather than the infused autologous HSCs. Nonmyeloablative autologous HSCTs produce fewer toxic events than myeloablative HSCTs. When possible, patients should be treated using a prospective clinical trial, ideally an RCT, or otherwise monitored in a prospective noninterventional study in a center accredited by an HSCT program. The "center effect" should be considered as well in the application of new technology to complex diseases. Effects causes by different centers or doctors can affect survival of patients undergoing HSCT for autoimmune diseases, which suggests a cautious approach (Atkins et al., 2016; Burt et al., 2011; Swart et al., 2017).

Autoimmune Type 1 Diabetes

T1D is one of the major ADs that affects children and young adults worldwide (D'Addio et al., 2014). T1D involves autoimmune destruction of beta cells, which leads to a lack of insulin production (Otonkoski, Gao, & Lundin, 2005; Voltarelli & Couri, 2009). To date, therapeutic approaches have not adequately addressed the problems of T1D, and no definitive cure currently exists (Mabed, 2011). Case reports reveal that T1D can be transmitted through allogeneic HSCT to a recipient (Voltarelli & Couri, 2009). Clinical studies suggested that moderate immunosuppression in patients with newly diagnosed T1D can prevent further loss of insulin production and can reduce insulin needs (Voltarelli et al., 2007). The successful use of HSCT for ADs led researchers to explore HSCT as treatment for T1D (Mabed, 2011).

Clinical trials examining the role of HSCT for T1D are continuing. Cantu Rodriguez and Gonzalez (2012), at the Hospital Universitario in Monterrey, Mexico, conducted a trial of HSCT in patients with T1D. The primary outcome measure was C-peptide levels before and after HSCT. The purpose of the study was to determine if nonmyeloablative autologous HSCT is able to induce prolonged and significant increases of C-peptide levels associated with absence or reduction of daily insulin dose. They concluded that autologous transplant is safe and may be a therapeutic intervention for early-onset T1D.

Carlsson, Schwarcz, Korsgren, and Le Blanc (2015) from Uppsala University Hospital in Uppsala, Sweden, conducted a trial on treatment of patients with new-onset T1D with mesenchymal stromal cells. The hypothesis was that the development of autoimmune diabetes may be halted at diagnosis by the immune modulatory properties of mesenchymal stromal cells. The researchers concluded that autologous mesenchymal stromal cell treatment in new-onset T1D constitutes a safe and promising strategy to intervene in disease progression and preserve beta cell function (Carlsson et al., 2015).

HIV

Autologous HSCT is now considered the standard of care for patients with HIV-related lymphomas who meet standard transplant criteria (Alvarnas, Zaia, & Forman, 2017). Trials of allogeneic HSCT as a primary treatment for HIV infection have failed to demonstrate benefit of this approach because of either recurrence of HIV infection or treatment-related death. However, investigators continue to evaluate HSCT-based therapies as a potential path toward cure of HIV infection itself (Alvarnas et al., 2017).

Outcomes from the BMT CTN 0803/AMC071 trial were compared with 151 non-HIV-infected, matched patients from the CIBMTR database. They found no significant differences between the groups for overall survival, progression-free survival, treatment-related mortality, risk of lymphoma progression, or time to engraftment (Alvarnas et al., 2016, 2017). The effectiveness of hematopoietic progenitor cell mobilization in patients with HIV also does not appear to differ from that in uninfected patients (Alvarnas et al., 2017; Re et al., 2013). Risk factors for mobilization failure in patients with HIV include CD4 T-cell count of less than 237/mm^3, a platelet count less than 160,000/mm^3, and mobilization with only granulocyte–colony-stimulating factor (Alvarnas et al., 2017).

Arslan et al. (2018) conducted a comprehensive systematic review of the literature for allogeneic HSCT, hematologic malignancies, and patients with HIV. They identified 49 patients who received HSCT for hematologic malignancy. The results indicated that clinical outcomes are not significantly different from patients without HIV (historical control). Reduced-intensity conditioning regimens portrayed a greater likelihood of survival compared to myeloablative regimens. They concluded that the improvements in supportive care, better donor availability, and novel conditioning regimens have led to the improvements in survival. In the current era of matched related donor, matched unrelated donor, cord blood transplantation, and haploidentical transplant, allogeneic HSCT remains a feasible therapy for hematologic malignancies in patients with HIV. The presence of HIV should not preclude these patients from potentially curative therapy, if indicated (Arslan et al., 2018; Kuritzkes, 2016; Mulanovich, Desai, & Popat, 2016).

The results of a review conducted by V. Gupta et al. (2009) demonstrated that because of improvements in supportive care, availability of reduced-intensity conditioning, and the ability to suppress HIV viral load with currently available medical care, allogeneic HSCT should be considered for HIV-positive patients with a hematologic malignancy (V. Gupta et al., 2009).

Since the discovery of HIV as the causative agent for AIDS in the 1980s, allogeneic cell therapy has been considered as a potential treatment option for infected patients (Hütter, 2016; Hužička, 1999). HIV invades predominantly bone marrow–derived cells carrying the CD4 receptor and a suitable chemokine receptor (commonly CCR5). In theory, effects from HSCT in hematologic malignancy would improve the course of HIV infection (Hütter, 2016). However, this approach has not eradicated HIV infection from patients.

Similar to the graft-versus-tumor effect, a donor-versus-HIV effect has been proposed (Hütter, 2016; Zaia & Forman, 2013). In practice, however, attempts to eradicate HIV by allogeneic HSCT have been unsuccessful. Prior to antiretroviral therapy, donor cells were infected by HIV rapidly after transplant. The introduction of antiretroviral therapy has had little impact on control of viral replication and elimination of viral reserve (Hütter, 2016; Kuritzkes, 2016). Cillo et al. (2013) performed a retrospective analysis of frozen specimens from patients on combination antiretroviral therapy who had no detectible HIV RNA in plasma. Specimens before and after autologous HSCT were studied with single-copy sensitive assay for HIV RNA and DNA as a surrogate measure of the HIV reservoir. Despite the absence of detectable HIV RNA in the plasma using conventional methods, 9 of the 10 patients were found to have detectable HIV DNA. The transplant recipients were likely "reinfected" with endogenous virus under cover of combination antiretroviral therapy. As a result of these data, researchers are focusing their efforts on modifying the infused T cells, making them resistant to HIV (Cillo et al., 2013; Zaia & Forman, 2013).

Two reports exist of patients with AIDS who experienced a "functional cure" of their HIV infection. The first is referred to in the literature as the "Berlin patient." This patient had been diagnosed with HIV-1 infection and was on antiretroviral therapy including tenofovir, emtricitabine, and efavirenz for four years prior to being diagnosed with acute myeloid leukemia. The patient received two HSCTs for acute myeloid leukemia using a myeloablative regimen. The donor chosen for this patient was an HLA-identical donor homozygous for the CCR5Δ32/Δ32 allele. After his second transplant from the same donor, the patient had a sustained remission of his acute myeloid leukemia and HIV-1 infection. At the time of the last follow-up, the patient had been off antiretroviral therapy for more than eight years without any evidence of his HIV-1 infection (Hütter et al., 2009; Kuritzkes, 2016). R.K. Gupta et al. (2019) recently reported a second patient to achieve HIV-1 remission after HSCT using a reduced-intensity conditioning regimen. The donor for this patient also had the CCR5Δ32/Δ32 allele. The researchers stated that 18 months may be too short of a time frame to call this a cure but would continue to follow and are optimistic (R.K. Gupta et al., 2019). Researchers plan to focus continued development strategies on preventing CCR5 expression (R.K. Gupta et al., 2019).

Allogeneic HSCT is not a generalizable treatment approach for healthy patients with HIV for use as a cure. However, for patients with hematologic malignancies who require HSCT for control of their disease, the priority should be to identify the best donor match to ensure success of the transplant and minimize GVHD risk. Identifying a CCR5-negative donor should be a secondary consideration (Kuritzkes, 2016).

Summary

Research in HSCT is continuing at a rapid pace with hundreds of transplant centers worldwide. Researchers are developing systems that will enable rapid translation of biologic science to clinical trials to make transplantation more available and safer. Nurses play an integral role in research to improve the HSCT process. They strive to provide safe, high-quality care for all patients while reducing and eliminating preventable harm (S. Kelly, 2010). Nurses are expected to improve and sustain quality outcomes for the care they provide, and nurses at the bedside are in the perfect position to improve quality of care with performance improvement (Dawson, 2019; S. Kelly, 2010).

Barriers to HSCT have been identified and criteria developed to overcome them and ensure the availability of HSCT for all individuals who could benefit. Clinical trials are ongoing to evaluate the psychosocial and physical aspects of HSCT, ensuring patients have optimal experiences before, during, and after transplant. As HSCT passes 50 years, many milestones have been achieved, and with continuing research, we can look forward to many more advances in the science.

References

Abad-Corpa, E., Meseguer-Liza, C., Martínez-Corbalán, J.T., Zárate-Riscal, L., Caravaca-Hernández, A., Paredes-Sidrach de Cardona, A., ... Cabrero-García, J. (2010). Effectiveness of the implementation of an evidence-based nursing model using participatory action research in oncohematology: Research protocol. *Journal of Advanced Nursing, 66*, 1845–1851. https://doi.org/10.1111/j.1365-2648.2010.05305.x

Abboud, M.R. (2009). Hematopoietic stem-cell transplantation for adults with sickle cell disease. *New England Journal of Medicine, 361*, 2380–2381. https://doi.org/10.1056/NEJMe0908574

Abd Hamid, I.J., Slatter, M.A., McKendrick, F., Pearce, M.S., & Gennery, A.R. (2017). Long-term outcome of hematopoietic stem cell transplantation for IL2RG/JAK3 SCID: A cohort report. *Blood, 129*, 2198–2201. https://doi.org/10.1182/blood-2016-11-748616

Adamkiewicz, T.V., Szabolcs, P., Haight, A., Baker, K.S., Staba, S., Kedar, A., ... Yeager, A.M. (2007). Unrelated cord blood transplantation in children with sickle cell disease: Review of four-center experience. *Pediatric Transplantation, 11*, 641–644. https://doi.org/10.1111/j.1399-3046.2007.00725.x

Agency for Healthcare Research and Quality. (2001). Translating Research Into Practice (TRIP)–II [Fact sheet]. Retrieved from https://archive.ahrq.gov/research/findings/factsheets/translating/tripfac/trip2fac.pdf

Alaloul, F., Schreiber, J.A., Al Nusairat, T., & Andrykowski, M.A. (2016). Spirituality in Arab Muslim hematopoietic stem cell transplantation survivors: A qualitative approach. *Cancer Nursing, 39*, E39–E46. https://doi.org/10.1097/NCC.0000000000000312

Allez, M., Karmiris, K., Louis, E., Van Assche, G., Ben-Horin, S., Klein, A., ... Chowers, Y. (2010). Report of the ECCO pathogenesis workshop on anti-TNF therapy failures in inflammatory bowel diseases: Definitions, frequency and pharmacological aspects. *Journal of Crohn's and Colitis, 4*, 355–366. https://doi.org/10.1016/j.crohns.2010.04.004

Alliance for Clinical Trials in Oncology. (n.d.). What we do. Retrieved from https://www.allianceforclinicaltrialsinoncology.org/main/public/standard.xhtml?path=%2FPublic%2FAbout

Alvarnas, J.C., Le Rademacher, J., Wang, Y., Little, R.F., Akpek, G., Ayala, E., ... Ambinder, R. (2016). Autologous hematopoietic cell transplantation for HIV-related lymphoma: Results of the BMT CTN 0803/AMC 071 trial. *Blood, 128*, 1050–1058. https://doi.org/10.1182/blood-2015-08-664706

Alvarnas, J.C., Zaia, J.A., & Forman, S.J. (2017). How I treat patients with HIV-related hematological malignancies using hematopoietic cell transplantation. *Blood, 130*, 1976–1984. https://doi.org/10.1182/blood-2017-04-551606

American Society for Blood and Marrow Transplantation. (2010, February). Evidence-based practice guidelines. In *BMT Tandem Meetings: Transplant Nursing Conference syllabus* (pp. 4–5). Arlington Heights, IL: Author.

American Society for Blood and Marrow Transplantation. (2011, October 20). Research priorities. Retrieved from http://asbmt.org/about/research-priorities

American Society for Blood and Marrow Transplantation. (2015). ASBMT Transplant Nursing Special Interest Group: Charter. Retrieved from https://higherlogicdownload.s3.amazonaws.com/ASBMT/43a1f41f-55cb-4c97-9e78-c03e867db505/UploadedImages/Transplant_Nursing_SIG_charter__2_.pdf

American Society of Gene and Cell Therapy. (n.d.). Gene and cell therapy FAQ's. Retrieved from https://www.asgct.org/education/more-resources/gene-and-cell-therapy-faqs

Amrolia, P., Gaspar, H.B., Hassan, A., Webb, D., Jones, A., Sturt, N., ... Veys, P. (2000). Nonmyeloablative stem cell transplantation for congenital immunodeficiencies. *Blood, 96*, 1239–1246. https://doi.org/10.1182/blood.V96.4.1239

Anurathapan, U., Hongeng, S., Pakakasama, S., Sirachainan, N., Songdej, D., Chuansumrit, A., ... Andersson, B.S. (2016). Hematopoietic stem cell transplantation for homozygous β-thalassemia and β-thalassemia/hemoglobin E patients from haploidentical donors. *Bone Marrow Transplantation, 51*, 813–818. https://doi.org/10.1038/bmt.2016.7

Appelbaum, F.R., Anasetti, C., Antin, J.H., Atkins, H., Davies, S., Devine, S., ... Horowitz, M.M. (2015). Blood and Marrow Transplant Clinical Trials Network State of the Science Symposium 2014. *Biology of Blood and Marrow Transplantation, 21*, 202–224. https://doi.org/10.1016/j.bbmt.2014.10.003

Appenfeller, A., Botterbush, J., Rimkus, C., & Fesler, M. (2018). Code BMT: A system for seamless patient admission in an outpatient BMT program. *Biology of Blood and Marrow Transplantation, 24*(Suppl. 3), S116. https://doi.org/10.1016/j.bbmt.2017.12.700

Arslan, S., Cummins, N.W., Rizza, S.A., Badley, A.D., Litzow, M.R., Navarro, W.H., & Hashmi, S.K. (2018). Outcomes and risks of allogeneic hematopoietic stem cell transplant for hematological malignancies in patients with HIV infection. *Blood, 24*(Suppl. 3), S340–S341. https://doi.org/10.1016/j.bbmt.2017.12.405

Assalone, D., & McNinney, T. (2017). Dropping knowledge, not patients: Reducing falls on a hematopoietic stem cell transplant (HSCT) unit [Poster abstract No. 12]. *Oncology Nursing Forum, 44*(2), 37. https://doi.org/10.1188/17.ONF.E88

Assalone, D., & Wagner, A. (2018). Distress no more: The effect of early intervention palliative care in hematopoietic stem cell transplant (HSCT) [Late-breaking abstract No. 17]. *Oncology Nursing Forum, 45*(2), 90. https://doi.org/10.1188/18.ONF.E34

Astarita, S., Caruso, L., Barron, A.M., & Rissmiller, P. (2016). Experiences in sexual health among women after hematopoietic stem cell transplantation. *Oncology Nursing Forum, 43*, 754–759. https://doi.org/10.1188/16.ONF.754-759

Atkins, H.L., Bowman, M., Allan, D., Anstee, G., Arnold, D.L., Bar-Or, A., ... Freedman, M.S. (2016). Immunoablation and autologous haemopoietic stem-cell transplantation for aggressive multiple sclerosis: A multicentre single-group phase 2 trial. *Lancet, 388*, 576–585. https://doi.org/10.1016/S0140-6736(16)30169-6

Baliousis, M., Rennoldson, M., Dawson, D.L., Mills, J., & das Nair, R. (2017). Perceptions of hematopoietic stem cell transplantation and coping predict emotional distress during the acute phase after transplantation. *Oncology Nursing Forum, 44*, 96–107. https://doi.org/10.1188/17.ONF.96-107

Baronciani, D., Angelucci, E., Potschger, U., Gaziev, J., Yesilipek, A., Zecca, M., ... Peters, C. (2016). Hemopoietic stem cell transplantation in thalassemia: A report from the European Society for Blood and Bone Marrow Transplantation Hemoglobinopathy Registry, 2000–2010. *Bone Marrow Transplantation 51*, 536–541. https://doi.org/10.1038/bmt.2015.293

Barrell, C., Dietzen, D., Jin, Z., Pinchefsky, S., Petrillo, K., & Satwani, P. (2012). Reduced-intensity conditioning allogeneic stem cell transplantation in pediatric patients and subsequent supportive care [Online exclusive]. *Oncology Nursing Forum, 39,* E451–E458. https://doi.org/10.1188/12.ONF.E451-E458

Barrow, C., Bellerive, C., Graham, S., & Shuey, K. (2018). Central line associated blood stream infection (CLABSI) reduction in a blood and marrow transplant unit [Poster abstract No. 22]. *Oncology Nursing Forum, 45*(2), 92–93. https://doi.org/10.1188/18.ONF.E34

Bartel, E., Layton, A., Hanchett, S., Quinn, A., & Rowe, C. (2017). Improving oral assessments and implementing preventative low level laser therapy in hematopoietic stem cell transplant patients to prevent oral mucositis [Poster abstract No. 67]. *Oncology Nursing Forum, 44*(2), 25. https://doi.org/10.1188/17.ONF.E88

Bauer, D.E., Brendel, C., & Fitzhugh, C.D. (2017). Curative approaches for sickle cell disease: A review of allogeneic and autologous strategies. *Blood Cells, Molecules, and Diseases, 67,* 155–168. https://doi.org/10.1016/j.bcmd.2017.08.014

Becker, P.S. (2005). The current status of gene therapy in autologous transplantation. *Acta Haematologica, 114,* 188–197. https://doi.org/10.1159/000088409

Bernardo, M.E., Piras, E., Vacca, A., Giorgiani, G., Zecca, M., Bertaina, A., … Locatelli, F. (2012). Allogeneic hematopoietic stem cell transplantation in thalassemia major: Results of a reduced-toxicity conditioning regimen based on the use of treosulfan. *Blood, 120,* 473–476. https://doi.org/10.1182/blood-2012-04-423822

Bernaudin, F., Socie, G., Kuentz, M., Chevret, S., Duval, M., Bertrand, Y., … Gluckman, E. (2007). Long-term results of related myeloablative stem-cell transplantation to cure sickle cell disease. *Blood, 110,* 2749–2756. https://doi.org/10.1182/blood-2007-03-079665

Beutler, E. (1999). Gene therapy. *Biology of Blood and Marrow Transplantation, 5,* 273–276. https://doi.org/10.1016/S1083-8791(99)70001-7

Bevans, M., Castro, K., Prince, P., Shelburne, N., Prachenko, O., Loscalzo, M., … Zabora, J. (2010). An individualized dyadic problem-solving education intervention for patients and family caregivers during allogeneic hematopoietic stem cell transplantation: A feasibility study. *Cancer Nursing, 33,* E24–E32. https://doi.org/10.1097/NCC.0b013e3181be5e6d

Bevans, M., Tierney, D.K., Bruch, C., Burgunder, M., Castro, K., Ford, R., … Schmit-Pokorny, K. (2009). Hematopoietic stem cell transplantation nursing: A practice variation study [Online exclusive]. *Oncology Nursing Forum, 36,* E317–E325. https://doi.org/10.1188/09.ONF.E317-E325

Bhatia, M., & Walters, M.C. (2008). Hematopoietic cell transplantation for thalassemia and sickle cell disease: Past, present and future. *Bone Marrow Transplantation, 41,* 109–117. https://doi.org/10.1038/sj.bmt.1705943

Blood and Marrow Transplant Clinical Trials Network. (2019). *Progress report May 2018–April 2019.* Retrieved from https://web.emmes.com/study/bmt2/Progress%20Reports.html

Bolaños-Meade, J., & Brodsky, R.A. (2009). Blood and marrow transplantation for sickle cell disease: Overcoming barriers to success. *Current Opinion in Oncology, 21,* 158–161. https://doi.org/10.1097/CCO.0b013e328324ba04

Bordignon, C., & Roncarolo, M.G. (2002). Therapeutic applications for hematopoietic stem cell gene transfer. *Nature Immunology, 3,* 318–321. https://doi.org/10.1038/ni0402-318

Braga, F.T., Santos, A.C., Bueno, P.C., Silveira, R.C., Santos, C.B., Bastos, J.K., & Carvalho, E.C. (2015). Use of *Chamomilla recutita* in the prevention and treatment of oral mucositis in patients undergoing hematopoietic stem cell transplantation: A randomized, controlled, phase II clinical trial. *Cancer Nursing, 38,* 322–329. https://doi.org/10.1097/NCC.0000000000000194

Brant, J.M. (2015). Bridging the research-to-practice gap: The role of the nurse scientist. *Seminars in Oncology Nursing, 31,* 298–305. https://doi.org/10.1016/j.soncn.2015.08.006

Brassil, K.J., Engebretson, J.C., Armstrong, T.S., Segovia, J.H., Worth, L.L., & Summers, B.L. (2015). Exploring the cancer experiences of young adults in the context of stem cell transplantation. *Cancer Nursing, 38,* 260–269. https://doi.org/10.1097/NCC.0000000000000200

Brassil, K.J., Szewczyk, N., Fellman, B., Neumann, J., Burgess, J., Urbauer, D., & LoBiondo-Wood, G. (2014). Impact of an incentive-based mobility program, "Motivated and Moving," on physiologic and quality of life outcomes in a stem cell transplant population. *Cancer Nursing, 37,* 345–354. https://doi.org/10.1097/NCC.0b013e3182a40db2

Brown, C.E., Wickline, M.A., Ecoff, L., & Glaser, D. (2009). Nursing practice, knowledge, attitudes and perceived barriers to evidence-based practice at an academic medical center. *Journal of Advanced Nursing, 65,* 371–381. https://doi.org/10.1111/j.1365-2648.2008.04878.x

Buckley, R.H., Schiff, S.E., Schiff, R.I., Markert, M.L., Williams, L.W., Roberts, J.L., … Ward, F.E. (1999). Hematopoietic stem-cell transplantation for the treatment of severe combined immunodeficiency. *New England Journal of Medicine, 340,* 508–516. https://doi.org/10.1056/NEJM199902183400703

Burns, L.J., Abbetti, B., Arnold, S.D., Bender, J., Doughtie, S., El-Jawahiri, A., … Denzen, E.M. (2018). Engaging patients in setting a patient-centered outcomes research agenda in hematopoietic cell transplantation. *Biology of Blood and Marrow Transplantation, 24,* 1111–1118. https://doi.org/10.1016/j.bbmt.2018.01.029

Burt, R. (2019, July 15). *Autologous stem cell systemic sclerosis immune suppression trial* (DIScl2011) (ClinicalTrials.gov Identifier: NCT01445821). Retrieved from https://clinicaltrials.gov/ct2/show/NCT01445821

Burt, R.K., Ruiz, M.A., & Kaiser, R.L., Jr. (2016). Stem cell transplantation for refractory Crohn disease. *JAMA, 315,* 2620. https://doi.org/10.1001/jama.2016.4030

Burt, R.K., Shah, S.J., Dill, K., Grant, T., Gheorghiade, M., Schroeder, J., … Barr, W. (2011). Autologous non-myeloablative haemopoietic stem-cell transplantation compared with pulse cyclophosphamide once a month for systemic sclerosis (ASSIST): An open-label, randomised phase 2 trial. *Lancet, 378,* 498–506. https://doi.org/10.1016/S0140-6736(11)60982-3

Button, E.B. (2016). Prophylactic treatment of hepatic veno-occlusive disease during stem cell transplantation. *Cancer Nursing, 39,* 335–336. https://doi.org/10.1097/NCC.0000000000000372

Button, E.B., Gavin, N.C., & Keogh, S.J. (2014). Exploring palliative care provision for recipients of allogeneic hematopoietic stem cell transplantation who relapsed. *Oncology Nursing Forum, 41,* 370–381. https://doi.org/10.1188/14.ONF.370-381

Canadian Cancer Trials Group. (n.d.). Who we are. Retrieved from https://www.ctg.queensu.ca/public/who-we-are

Cancer.Net. (2019, September). Phases of clinical trials. Retrieved from https://www.cancer.net/research-and-advocacy/clinical-trials/phases-clinical-trials

Cantu Rodriguez, O.G., & Gonzalez, J.E. (2012, December 10). *Hematopoietic stem cell transplantation in type 1 diabetes mellitus* (ClinicalTrials.gov Identifier: NCT01121029). Retrieved from https://clinicaltrials.gov/ct2/show/NCT01121029

Carlsson, P.-O., Schwarcz, E., Korsgren, O., & Le Blanc, K. (2015). Preserved β-cell function in type 1 diabetes by mesenchymal stromal cells. *Diabetes, 64,* 587–592. https://doi.org/10.2337/db14-0656

Casalino, L.P., Nicholson, S., Gans, D.N., Hammons, T., Morra, D., Karrison, T., & Levinson, W. (2009). What does it cost physician practices to interact with health insurance plans? *Health Affairs, 28*(Suppl. 1), w533–w543. https://doi.org/10.1377/hlthaff.28.4.w533

Cavazzana, M. (2014). Hematopoietic stem cell gene therapy: Progress on the clinical front. *Human Gene Therapy, 25,* 165–170. https://doi.org/10.1089/hum.2014.2504

Cavazzana-Calvo, M., Bagnis, C., Mannoni, P., & Fischer, A. (1999). Peripheral blood stem cell and gene therapy. *Best Practice and Research Clinical Haematology, 12,* 129–138. https://doi.org/10.1053/beha.1999.0012

Cavazzana-Calvo, M., Lagresle, C., Hacein-Bey-Abina, S., & Fischer, A. (2005). Gene therapy for severe combined immunodeficiency. *Annual Review of Medicine, 56,* 585–602. https://doi.org/10.1146/annurev.med.56.090203.104142

Center for International Blood and Marrow Transplant Research. (2008). The Blood and Marrow Transplant Clinical Trials Network. *CIBMTR Newsletter, 14*(2), 4–5. Retrieved from http://www.cibmtr.org/ReferenceCenter/Newsletters/Documents/Newsletter_Dec2008.pdf

Center for International Blood and Marrow Transplant Research. (2017). *2017 annual report.* Retrieved from https://www.cibmtr.org/About/AdminReports/Documents/2017%20CIBMTR%20Annual%20Report_web.pdf

Chakrabarti, S., & Bareford, D. (2007). A survey on patient perception of reduced-intensity transplantation in adults with sickle cell disease. *Bone Marrow Transplantation, 39,* 447–451. https://doi.org/10.1038/sj.bmt.1705622

Chan, Y.-T., & Wang, Y.-J. (2018). Review measurement tools of chronic oral graft-versus-host disease [Poster abstract No. 53]. *Oncology Nursing Forum, 45*(2), 109. https://doi.org/10.1188/18.ONF.E34

Chiang, M.K., & Hsiao, Y.M. (2015). The effect of long-term follow-up clinic for hematopoietic cell transplantation survivors in Taiwan [ICCN 2015 Abstract Book Manuscript Poster Abstract No. P-157]. *Cancer Nursing, 38*(Suppl. 4), S96. Retrieved from https://journals.lww.com/cancernursingonline/toc/2015/07001

Children's Oncology Group. (n.d.). About us. Retrieved from https://www.childrensoncologygroup.org/index.php/about-us

Cillo, A.R., Krishnan, A., Mitsuyasu, R.T., McMahon, D.K., Li, S., Rossi, J.J., ... Mellors, J.W. (2013). Plasma viremia and cellular HIV-1 DNA persist despite autologous hematopoietic stem cell transplantation for HIV-related lymphoma. *Journal of Acquired Immune Deficiency Syndrome, 63*, 438–441. https://doi.org/10.1097/QAI.0b013e31828e6163

Civin, C.I. (2000). Gene therapy in clinical applications: Overview: How do we translate gene therapy to clinical trials? *Stem Cells, 18*, 150–151. https://doi.org/10.1634/stemcells.18-2-150

Cochrane Consumer Network. (n.d.). What is a systematic review? Retrieved from https://consumers.cochrane.org/what-systematic-review

Cohen, J.A., Baldassari, L.E., Atkins, H.L., Bowen, J.D., Bredeson, C., Carpenter, P.A., ... Georges, G.E. (2019). Autologous hematopoietic cell transplantation for treatment-refractory relapsing multiple sclerosis: Position statement from the American Society for Blood and Marrow Transplantation. *Biology of Blood and Marrow Transplantation, 25*, 845–854. https://doi.org/10.1016/j.bbmt.2019.02.014

Cohen, M.Z., Jenkins, D., Holston, E.C., & Carlson, E.D. (2013). Understanding health literacy in patients receiving hematopoietic stem cell transplantation. *Oncology Nursing Forum, 40*, 508–515. https://doi.org/10.1188/13.ONF.508-515

Coleman, E.A., Coon, S.K., Lockhart, K., Kennedy, R.L., Montgomery, R., Copeland, N., ... Stewart, C. (2009). Effect of certification in oncology nursing on nursing-sensitive outcomes. *Clinical Journal of Oncology Nursing, 13*, 165–172. https://doi.org/10.1188/09.CJON.165-172

Comis, R.L., Miller, J.D., Aldigé, C.R., Krebs, L., & Stoval, E. (2003). Public attitudes toward participation in cancer clinical trials. *Journal of Clinical Oncology, 21*, 830–835. https://doi.org/10.1200/JCO.2003.02.105

Coolbrandt, A., & Grypdonck, M.H.F. (2010). Keeping courage during stem cell transplantation: A qualitative research. *European Journal of Oncology Nursing, 14*, 218–223. https://doi.org/10.1016/j.ejon.2010.01.001

Cooper, J., Blake, I., Lindsay, J.O., & Hawkey, C.J. (2017). Living with Crohn's disease: An exploratory cross-sectional qualitative study into decision-making and expectations in relation to autologous haematopoietic stem cell treatment (the DECIDES study). *BMJ Open, 7*, 1–13. https://doi.org/10.1136/bmjopen-2016-015201

Cotter, J., & Christianson, H. (2017). Preventing pitfalls on the road to stem cell transplant: Development of an early psychosocial screening program [Poster abstract No. 57]. *Oncology Nursing Forum, 44*(2), 53–54. https://doi.org/10.1188/17.ONF.E88

Cowan, M.J., Neven, B., Cavazanna-Calvo, M., Fischer, A., & Puck, J. (2008). Hematopoietic stem cell transplantation for severe combined immunodeficiency diseases. *Biology of Blood and Marrow Transplantation, 14*(Suppl. 1), 73–80. https://doi.org/10.1016/j.bbmt.2007.10.017

Cox, A., Arber, A., Gallagher, A., MacKenzie, M., & Ream, E. (2017). Establishing priorities for oncology nursing research: Nurse and patient collaboration. *Oncology Nursing Forum, 44*, 192–203. https://doi.org/10.1188/17.ONF.192-203

Crable, S., Scaramuzzo, L., & Brant, J. (2018). Stem cell infusion: Guidelines and practices [Poster abstract No. 68]. *Oncology Nursing Forum, 45*(2), 117. https://doi.org/10.1188/18.ONF.E34

Cuaron, L.J., & Gallucci, B. (1997). Gene therapy and blood cell transplantation. *Seminars in Oncology Nursing, 13*, 200–207. https://doi.org/10.1016/S0749-2081(97)80036-8

Cummings, A. (2017). Educating and monitoring nursing staff regarding the care of central venous access devices (CVAD) in stem cell transplant patients [Poster abstract No. 61]. *Oncology Nursing Forum, 44*(2), 55. https://doi.org/10.1188/17.ONF.E88

D'Addio, F., Valderrama-Vasquez, A., Ben Nasr, M., Franek, E., Zhu, D., Li, L., ... Fiorina, P. (2014). Autologous nonmyeloablative hematopoietic stem cell transplantation in new-onset type 1 diabetes: A multicenter analysis. *Diabetes, 63*, 3041–3046. https://doi.org/10.2337/db14-0295

Daikeler, T., Hügle, T., Farge, D., Andolina, M., Gualandi, F., Baldomero, H., ... Gratwohl, A. (2009). Allogeneic hematopoietic SCT for patients with autoimmune diseases. *Bone Marrow Transplantation, 44*, 27–33. https://doi.org/10.1038/bmt.2008.424

Daly, B., Meropol, N., Flocke, S., Fulton, S., Margevicius, S., & Schluchter, M. (2017). Factors related to nurse engagement in discussion of clinical trials with patients [Poster abstract No. 63]. *Oncology Nursing Forum, 44*(2), 56. https://doi.org/10.1188/17.ONF.E88

Dambrosio, N., Porter, M., de Lima, M., Bauer, E., Liedtke, D., Levitan, N., & Malek, E. (2018). Continuous temperature monitoring for earlier fever detection in neutropenic patients: Patient's acceptance and comparison with standard of care. *Biology of Blood and Marrow Transplantation, 24*(Suppl. 3), S108–S109. https://doi.org/10.1016/j.bbmt.2017.12.026

Dandekar, R., & Achrekar, M. (2016). Sleep disturbance in hospitalized recipients of hematopoietic stem cell transplantation (HSCT). *Cancer Nursing, 39*(Suppl. 6), S106.

Dawson, A. (2019). A practical guide to performance improvement: Beginning the process. *AORN Journal, 109*, 318–324. https://doi.org/10.1002/aorn.12614

Donofrio, L., Hambright, K., Kiss, C., Abboud, M., & Rodriguez, E. (2017). Nurses transition post stem cell transplant care to the home [Poster abstract No. 72]. *Oncology Nursing Forum, 44*(2), 59. https://doi.org/10.1188/17.ONF.E88

Doorenbos, A.Z., Berger, A.M., Brohard-Holbert, C., Eaton, L., Kozachik, S., LoBiondo-Wood, G., ... Varricchio, C. (2008). Oncology Nursing Society Putting Evidence Into Practice® resources: Where are we now and what is next? *Clinical Journal of Oncology Nursing, 12*, 965–970. https://doi.org/10.1188/08.CJON.965-970

D'Souza, A., & Fretham, C. (2018). Current uses and outcomes of hematopoietic stem cell transplantation (HCT): 2018 summary slides. Retrieved from https://www.cibmtr.org/ReferenceCenter/SlidesReports/SummarySlides/_layouts/15/WopiFrame.aspx?sourcedoc=/ReferenceCenter/SlidesReports/SummarySlides/Documents/2018%20Summary%20Slides%20-%20final%20-%20for%20web%20posting.pptx&action=default

Duke University Medical Center Library and Archives. (2019, November 22). EBP tutorial: Home. Retrieved from https://guides.mclibrary.duke.edu/ebptutorial

Dunbar, C.E. (2007). The yin and yang of stem cell gene therapy: Insights into hematopoiesis, leukemogenesis, and gene therapy safety. *American Society of Hematology Education Program Book, 2007*, 460–465. https://doi.org/10.1182/asheducation-2007.1.460

Dvorak, C.C., & Cowan, M.J. (2008). Hematopoietic stem cell transplantation for primary immunodeficiency disease. *Bone Marrow Transplantation, 41*, 119–126. https://doi.org/10.1038/sj.bmt.1705890

ECOG-ACRIN Cancer Research Group. (n.d.). About us. Retrieved from http://ecog-acrin.org/about-us

Eisenberg, S., Wickline, M., Linenberger, M., Gooley, T., & Holmberg, L. (2013). Prevention of dimethylsulfoxide-related nausea and vomiting by prophylactic administration of ondansetron for patients receiving autologous cryopreserved peripheral blood stem cells. *Oncology Nursing Forum, 40*, 285–292. https://doi.org/10.1188/13.ONF.285-292

European Society for Blood and Marrow Transplantation. (n.d.). Nurses Group—Who we are. Retrieved from https://www.ebmt.org/nursing/nurses-group-who-we-are

European Society for Immunodeficiencies. (n.d.). Inborn Errors Working Party (IEWP). Retrieved from https://esid.org/Working-Parties/Inborn-Errors-Working-Party-IEWP

Fain, J.A. (2017). *Reading, understanding, and applying nursing research* (5th ed.). Philadelphia, PA: F.A. Davis.

Farge, D., Labopin, M., Tyndall, A., Fassas, A., Mancardi, G.L., Van Laar, J., ... Saccardi, R. (2010). Autologous hematopoietic stem cell transplantation for autoimmune diseases: An observational study on 12 years' experience from the European Group for Blood and Marrow Transplantation Working Party on Autoimmune Diseases. *Haematologica, 95*, 284–292. https://doi.org/10.3324/haematol.2009.013458

Filipovich, A., Stone, J., Tomany, S., Ireland, M., Kollman, C., Pelz, C., ... Horowitz, M. (2001). Impact of donor type on outcome of bone marrow transplantation for Wiskott-Aldrich syndrome: Collaborative study of the International Bone Marrow Transplant Registry and the National Marrow Donor Program. *Blood, 97,* 1598–1603. https://doi.org/10.1182/blood.V97.6.1598

Fisher, C., Cusack, G., Cox, K., Feigenbaum, K., & Wallen, G.R. (2016). Developing competency to sustain evidence-based practice. *Journal of Nursing Administration, 46,* 581–585. https://doi.org/10.1097/NNA.0000000000000408

Fliedner, M.C. (2002). Research within the field of blood and marrow transplantation nursing: How can it contribute to higher quality of care? *International Journal of Hematology, 76*(Suppl. 2), 289–291. https://doi.org/10.1007/BF03165135

Fox, T.A., Chakraverty, R., Burns, S., Carpenter, B., Thomson, K., Lowe, D., … Morris, E. (2018). Successful outcome following allogeneic hematopoietic stem cell transplantation in adults with primary immunodeficiency. *Blood, 131,* 917–931. https://doi.org/10.1182/blood-2017-09-807487

Fraser, C.C., & Hoffman, R. (1995). Hematopoietic stem cell behavior: Potential implications for gene therapy. *Journal of Laboratory and Clinical Medicine, 125,* 692–702.

Fred Hutchinson Cancer Research Center. (2019, August 13). *Scleroderma treatment with autologous transplant (STAT) study* (ClinicalTrials.gov Identifier: NCT01413100). Retrieved from https://clinicaltrials.gov/ct2/show/NCT01413100

Garbin, L.M., Simões, B.P., Curcioli, A.C., & de Carvalho, E.C. (2018). Serum cyclosporine levels: The influence of the time interval between interrupting the infusion and obtaining the samples: A randomized clinical trial. *Cancer Nursing, 41,* E55–E61. https://doi.org/10.1097/NCC.0000000000000544

Gemmill, R., Cooke, L., Williams, A.C., & Grant, M. (2011). Informal caregivers of hematopoietic cell transplant patients: A review and recommendations for intervention and research. *Cancer Nursing, 34,* E13–E21. https://doi.org/10.1097/NCC.0b013e31820a592d

Gibson, D., Kendrick, S., McCreary, M., Davis, R., Szetela, A., & Costello, D. (2017). Nursing operated pulsed xenon ultraviolet-C disinfection robot utilization and the reduction of hospital-acquired *Clostridium difficile* infections (CDI) in hematopoietic stem cell transplant (HSCT) patients [Poster abstract No. 101]. *Oncology Nursing Forum, 44*(2), 69. https://doi.org/10.1188/17.ONF.E88

Gluckman, E. (2011). Milestones in umbilical cord blood transplantation. *Blood Reviews, 25,* 255–259. https://doi.org/10.1016/j.blre.2011.06.003

Gluckman, E. (2013). Allogeneic transplantation strategies including haploidentical transplantation in sickle cell disease. *American Society of Hematology Education Program Book, 2013,* 370–376. https://doi.org/10.1182/asheducation-2013.1.370

Granada, M.L.A., Estrella, J.M.E., & Ramirez, M.P.T. (2017). Isolation coding system to improve ease of identification of infectious organisms in stem cell transplantation [Poster abstract No. 106]. *Oncology Nursing Forum, 44*(2), 71. https://doi.org/10.1188/17.ONF.E88

Griffith, L.M., Cowan, M.J., Kohn, D.B., Notarangelo, L.D., Puck, J.M., Schultz, K.R., … Shearer, W.T. (2008). Allogeneic hematopoietic cell transplantation for primary immune deficiency diseases: Current status and critical needs. *Journal of Allergy and Clinical Immunology, 122,* 1087–1096. https://doi.org/10.1016/j.jaci.2008.09.045

Griffith, L.M., Cowan, M.J., Notarangelo, L.D., Puck, J.M., Buckley, R.H., Candotti, F., … Shearer, W.T. (2009). Improving cellular therapy for primary immune deficiency diseases: Recognition, diagnosis, and management. *Journal of Allergy and Clinical Immunology, 124,* 1152–1160.e12. https://doi.org/10.1016/j.jaci.2009.10.022

Griffith, L.M., Pavletic, S.Z., Tyndall, A., Bredeson, C.N., Bowen, J.D., Childs, R.W., … Nash, R.A. (2005). Feasibility of allogeneic hematopoietic stem cell transplantation for autoimmune disease: Position statement from a National Institute of Allergy and Infectious Diseases and National Cancer Institute–Sponsored International Workshop, Bethesda, MD, March 12 and 13, 2005. *Biology of Blood and Marrow Transplantation, 11,* 862–870. https://doi.org/10.1016/j.bbmt.2005.07.009

Gupta, R.K., Abdul-Jawad, S., McCoy, L.E., Mok, H.P., Peppa, D., Salgado, M., … Olavarria, E. (2019). HIV-1 remission following CCR5Δ32/Δ32 haematopoietic stem-cell transplantation. *Nature, 568,* 244–248. https://doi.org/10.1038/s41586-019-1027-4

Gupta, V., Tomblyn, M., Pedersen, T.L., Atkins, H.L., Battiwalla, M., Gress, R.E., … Keating, A. (2009). Allogeneic hematopoietic cell transplantation in human immunodeficiency virus-positive patients with hematologic disorders: A report from the Center for International Blood and Marrow Transplant Research. *Biology of Blood and Marrow Transplantation, 15,* 864–871. https://doi.org/10.1016/j.bbmt.2009.03.023

Haberman, M.R. (2007). Nursing research in blood cell and marrow transplantation. In S. Ezzone & K. Schmit-Pokorny (Eds.), *Blood and marrow stem cell transplantation: Principles, practice, and nursing insights* (3rd ed., pp. 479–490). Burlington, MA: Jones & Bartlett Learning.

Hacein-Bey-Abina, S., Garrigue, A., Wang, G.P., Soulier, J., Lim, A., Morillon, E., … Cavazzana-Calvo, M. (2008). Insertional oncogenesis in 4 patients after retrovirus-mediated gene therapy of SCID-X1. *Journal of Clinical Investigation, 118,* 3132–3142. https://doi.org/10.1172/JCI35700

Hacker, E.D. (2017). Optimizing health through exercise following hematopoietic stem cell transplantation [Poster abstract No. 109]. *Oncology Nursing Forum, 44*(2), 72. https://doi.org/10.1188/17.ONF.E88

Hacker, E.D., Fink, A., Peters, T., Park, C., Fantuzzi, G., & Rondelli, D. (2017). Persistent fatigue in hematopoietic stem cell transplantation survivors. *Cancer Nursing, 40,* 174–183. https://doi.org/10.1097/NCC.0000000000000405

Hacker, E.D., Kapella, M.C., Park, C., Ferrans, C.E., & Larson, J.L. (2015). Sleep patterns during hospitalization following hematopoietic stem cell transplantation. *Oncology Nursing Forum, 42,* 371–379. https://doi.org/10.1188/15.ONF.371-379

Hacker, E.D., Larson, J., Kujath, A., Peace, D., Rondelli, D., & Gaston, L. (2011). Strength training following hematopoietic stem cell transplantation. *Cancer Nursing, 34,* 238–249. https://doi.org/10.1097/NCC.0b013e3181fb3686

Hagan, J. (2018). Nurse satisfaction with opportunities to engage in research. *Western Journal of Nursing Research, 40,* 209–221. https://doi.org/10.1177/0193945916682472

Hagan, J., & Walden, M. (2017). Development and evaluation of the barriers to nurses' participation in research questionnaire at a large academic pediatric hospital. *Clinical Nursing Research, 26,* 157–175. https://doi.org/10.1177/1054773815609889

Hagin, D., Burroughs, L., & Torgerson, T.R. (2015). Hematopoietic stem cell transplant for immune deficiency and immune dysregulation disorders. *Immunology and Allergy Clinics of North America, 35,* 695–711. https://doi.org/10.1016/j.iac.2015.07.010

Havenga, M., Hoogerbrugge, P., Valerio, D., & van Es, H.H.G. (1997). Retroviral stem cell gene therapy. *Stem Cells, 15,* 162–179. https://doi.org/10.1002/stem.150162

Hawkey, C.J. (2017). Hematopoietic stem cell transplantation in Crohn's disease: State-of-the-art treatment. *Digestive Diseases, 35,* 107–114. https://doi.org/10.1159/000449090

Hawkey, C.J., Lindsay, J., & Gribben, J. (2016). Stem cell transplantation for refractory Crohn disease—Reply. *JAMA, 315,* 2620–2621. http://doi.org/10.1001/jama.2016.4033

Heimall, J., Logan, B., Cowan, M.J., Notarangelo, L.D., Griffith, L.M., Puck, J.M., … Dvorak, C.C. (2017). Immune reconstitution and survival of 100 SCID patients post-hematopoietic cell transplant: A PIDTC natural history. *Blood, 130,* 2718–2727. https://doi.org/10.1182/blood-2017-05-781849

Helbig, G., Widuchowska, M., Koclęga, A., Kopińska, A., Kopeć-Mędrek, M., Gaweł, W.B., … Markiewicz, M. (2018). Safety profile of autologous hematopoietic stem cell mobilization and transplantation in patients with systemic sclerosis. *Clinical Rheumatology, 37,* 1709–1714. https://doi.org/10.1007/s10067-017-3954-5

Heleno, B., Thomsen, M.F., Rodrigues, D.S., Jørgensen, K.J., & Brodersen, J. (2013). Quantification of harms in cancer screening trials: Literature review. *BMJ, 347,* f5334. https://doi.org/10.1136/bmj.f5334

Hendricks, J., & Cope, V. (2017). Research is not a 'scary' word: Registered nurses and the barriers to research utilisation. *Nordic Journal of Nursing Research, 37,* 44–50. https://doi.org/10.1177/2057158516679581

Hoppe, C.C., & Walters, M.C. (2001). Bone marrow transplantation in sickle cell anemia. *Current Opinion in Oncology, 13,* 85–90. https://doi.org/10.1097/00001622-200103000-00001

Horwitz, E.M., Horowitz, M.M., DiFronzo, N.L., Kohn, D.B., & Heslop, H.E. (2011). Guidance for developing phase II cell therapy trial proposals for consideration by the Blood and Marrow Transplant Clinical Trials Network. *Biology of Blood and Marrow Transplantation, 17*, 192–196. https://doi.org/10.1016/j.bbmt.2010.08.020

Hough, R.E., Snowden, J.A., & Wulffraat, N.M. (2005). Haemopoietic stem cell transplantation in autoimmune diseases: A European perspective. *British Journal of Haematology, 128*, 432–459. https://doi.org/10.1111/j.1365-2141.2004.05298.x

Howe, S.J., Mansour, M.R., Schwarzwaelder, K., Bartholomae, C., Hubank, M., Kempski, H., ... Thrasher, A.J. (2008). Insertional mutagenesis combined with acquired somatic mutations causes leukemogenesis following gene therapy of SCID-X1 patients. *Journal of Clinical Investigation, 118*, 3143–3150. https://doi.org/10.1172/JCI35798

Hsiao, Y. (2015). The quality improvement of long-term follow-up program in hematopoietic stem cell transplantation recipient [ICCN 2015 Abstract Book Manuscript Poster Abstract No. P-160]. *Cancer Nursing, 38*(Suppl. 4), S97. Retrieved from https://journals.lww.com/cancernursingonline/toc/2015/07001

Hsieh, M.M., Kang, E.M., Fitzhugh, C.D., Link, M.B., Bolan, C.D., Kurlander, R., ... Tisdale, J. (2009). Allogeneic hematopoietic stem-cell transplantation for sickle cell disease. *New England Journal of Medicine, 361*, 2309–2317. https://doi.org/10.1056/NEJMoa0904971

Huang, H.Y., Yang, C.I., & Chen, L.-M. (2015). The trajectory and associated factors of oral mucositis of patients receiving allogeneic hematopoitic stem-cell transplantation [ICCN 2015 Abstract Book Manuscript Poster Abstract No. P-109]. *Cancer Nursing, 38*(Suppl. 4), S83–S84. Retrieved from https://journals.lww.com/cancernursingonline/toc/2015/07001

Huang, Y.P., Kellett, U., Wang, S.Y., Chang, M.Y., & Chih, H.M. (2014). Experience of nurses caring for child with hematopoietic stem cell transplantation in general pediatric ward. *Cancer Nursing, 37*, E32–E39.

Hütter, G. (2016). HIV+ patients and HIV eradication—Allogeneic transplantation. *Expert Review of Hematology, 9*, 615–616. https://doi.org/10.1080/17474086.2016.1183478

Hütter, G., Nowak, D., Mossner, M., Ganepola, S., Müßig, A., Allers, K., ... Thiel, E. (2009). Long-term control of HIV by CCR5 delta32/delta32 stem-cell transplantation. *New England Journal of Medicine, 360*, 692–698. https://doi.org/10.1056/NEJMoa0802905

Hužička, I. (1999). Could bone marrow transplantation cure AIDS?: Review. *Medical Hypotheses, 52*, 247–257. https://doi.org/10.1054/mehy.1997.0638

Hweidi, I.M., Tawalbeh, L.I., Al-Hassan, M.A., Alayadeh, R.M., & Al-Smadi, A.M. (2017). Research use of nurses working in the critical care units: Barriers and facilitators. *Dimensions of Critical Care Nursing, 36*, 226–233. https://doi.org/10.1097/DCC.0000000000000255

Issaragrisil, S., & Kunacheewa, C. (2016). Matched sibling donor hematopoietic stem cell transplantation for thalassemia. *Current Opinion in Hematology, 23*, 508–514. https://doi.org/10.1097/MOH.0000000000000286

Johnson, F.L., Look, A.T., Gockerman, J., Ruggiero, M.R., Dalla-Pozza, L., & Billings, F.T., III. (1984). Bone-marrow transplantation in a patient with sickle-cell anemia. *New England Journal of Medicine, 311*, 780–783. https://doi.org/10.1056/NEJM198409203111207

Jones, C.W., Braz, V.A., McBride, S.M., Roberts, B.W., & Platts-Mills, T.F. (2016). Cross-sectional assessment of patient attitudes towards participation in clinical trials: Does making results publicly available matter? *BMJ Open, 6*, e013649. https://doi.org/10.1136/bmjopen-2016-013649

June, C.H., & Sadelain, M. (2018). Chimeric antigen receptor therapy. *New England Journal of Medicine, 379*, 64–73. https://doi.org/10.1056/NEJMra1706169

Kassim, A.A., & Sharma, D. (2017). Hematopoietic stem cell transplantation for sickle cell disease: The changing landscape. *Hematology/Oncology and Stem Cell Therapy, 10*, 259–266. https://doi.org/10.1016/j.hemonc.2017.05.008

Kelly, D.L., Lyon, D.E., Ameringer, S.A., & Elswick, R.K., Jr. (2015). Symptoms, cytokines, and quality of life in patients diagnosed with chronic graft-versus-host disease following allogeneic hematopoietic stem cell transplantation. *Oncology Nursing Forum, 42*, 265–275. https://doi.org/10.1188/15.ONF.265-275

Kelly, D.L., Lyon, D.E., Periera, D., Garvan, C., & Wingard, J. (2018). Lifestyle behaviors, perceived stress, and inflammation of individuals with chronic graft-versus-host disease. *Cancer Nursing, 41*, 11–22. https://doi.org/10.1097/NCC.0000000000000453

Kelly, S. (2010, September 11). Creating a self-sustaining professional culture of quality. *American Nurse Today*. Retrieved from https://www.americannursetoday.com/creating-a-self-sustaining-professional-culture-of-quality

Kelsey, P.J., Oliveira, M.-C., Badoglio, M., Sharrack, B., Farge, D., & Snowden, J.A. (2016). Haematopoietic stem cell transplantation in autoimmune diseases: From basic science to clinical practice. *Current Research in Translational Medicine, 54*, 71–82. https://doi.org/10.1016/j.retram.2016.03.003

Kemp, J., Chun, A., Wasmuth, K., Matula, M., Conover, L., & Campos, V. (2018). Implementation of a bone marrow transplant admission checklist [Poster abstract No. 130]. *Oncology Nursing Forum, 45*(2), 149. https://doi.org/10.1188/18.ONF.E34

Kim, D.-W., Chung, Y.-J., Kim, T.-G., Kim, Y.-L., & Oh, I.-H. (2004). Cotransplantation of third-party mesenchymal stromal cells can alleviate single-donor predominance and increase engraftment from double cord transplantation. *Blood, 103*, 1941–1948. https://doi.org/10.1182/blood-2003-05-1601

Kirby, S.L. (1999). Bone marrow: Target for gene transfer. *Hospital Practice, 34*(13), 59–63, 69–70, 73–74. https://doi.org/10.3810/hp.1999.12.176

Kleinpell, R.M. (2009). Promoting research in clinical practice: Strategies for implementing research initiatives. *Journal of Trauma Nursing, 16*, 114–119. https://doi.org/10.1097/JTN.0b013e3181ac9238

Knoop, T., Wujcik, D., & Wujcik, K. (2017). Emerging models of interprofessional collaboration in cancer care. *Seminars in Oncology Nursing, 33*, 459–463. https://doi.org/10.1016/j.soncn.2017.08.009

Kohlscheen, S., Bonig, H., & Modlich, U. (2017). Promises and challenges in hematopoietic stem cell gene therapy. *Human Gene Therapy, 28*, 782–799. https://doi.org/10.1089/hum.2017.141

Kohn, D.B. (2008). Gene therapy for childhood immunological diseases. *Bone Marrow Transplantation, 41*, 199–205. https://doi.org/10.1038/sj.bmt.1705895

Kolke, S.M., Kuhlenschmidt, M., Bauer, E., Anthony, M.K., Gittleman, H., Caimi, P.F., & Mazanec, S.R. (2019). Factors influencing patients' intention to perform physical activity during hematopoietic stem cell transplantation. *Oncology Nursing Forum, 46*, 746–756. https://doi.org/10.1188/19.ONF.746-756

Kowal-Bielecka, O., Fransen, J., Avouac, J., Becker, M., Kulak, A., Allanore, Y., ... Müller-Ladner, U. (2017). Update of EULAR recommendations for the treatment of systemic sclerosis. *Annals of the Rheumatic Diseases, 76*, 1327–1339. https://doi.org/10.1136/annrheumdis-2016-209909

Kuritzkes, D.R. (2016). Hematopoietic stem cell transplantation for HIV cure. *Journal of Clinical Investigation, 126*, 432–437. https://doi.org/10.1172/JCI80563

Kwon, M., Bautista, G., Balsalobre, P., Sánchez-Ortega, I., Serrano, D., Anguita, J., ... Cabrera, R. (2014). Haplo-cord transplantation using CD34+ cells from a third-party donor to speed engraftment in high-risk patients with hematologic disorders. *Biology of Blood and Marrow Transplantation, 20*, 2015–2022. https://doi.org/10.1016/j.bbmt.2014.08.024

Laberko, A., & Gennery, A.R. (2018). Clinical considerations in the hematopoietic stem cell transplant management of primary immunodeficiencies. *Expert Review of Clinical Immunology, 14*, 297–306. https://doi.org/10.1080/1744666X.2018.1459189

Lara, P.N., Jr., Higdon, R., Lim, N., Kwan, K., Tanaka, M., Lau, D.H.M., ... Lam, K.S. (2001). Prospective evaluation of cancer clinical trial accrual patterns: Identifying potential barriers to enrollment. *Journal of Clinical Oncology, 19*, 1728–1733. https://doi.org/10.1200/JCO.2001.19.6.1728

Lawitschka, A., Faraci, M., Yaniv, I., Veys, P., Bader, P., Wachowiak, J., ... Peters, C. (2015). Paediatric reduced intensity conditioning: Analysis of centre strategies on regimens and definitions by the EBMT Paediatric Diseases and Complications and Quality of Life WP. *Bone Marrow Transplantation, 50*, 592–597. https://doi.org/10.1038/bmt.2014.306

Lawson, L., Glennon, C., Fiscus, V., Harrell, V., Krause, K., Moore, A., & Smith, K. (2016). Effects of making art and listening to music on symptoms related to blood and marrow transplantation [Online exclusive]. *Oncology Nursing Forum, 43,* E56–E63. https://doi.org/10.1188/16.ONF.E56-E63

Lawson, L., Williams, P., Glennon, C., Carithers, K., Schnabel, E., Andrejack, A., & Wright, N. (2012). Effect of art making on cancer-related symptoms of blood and marrow transplantation recipients [Online exclusive]. *Oncology Nursing Forum, 39,* E353–E360. https://doi.org/10.1188/12.ONF.E353-E360

Leung, D., Fillion, L., Duval, S., Brown, J., Rodin, G., & Howell, D. (2012). Meaning in bone marrow transplant nurses' work: Experiences before and after a "meaning-centered" intervention. *Cancer Nursing, 35,* 374–381. https://doi.org/10.1097/NCC.0b013e318232e237

Lindsay, J.O., Allez, M., Clark, M., Labopin, M., Ricart, E., Rogler, G.R., ... Hawkey, C.J. (2017). Autologous stem-cell transplantation in treatment- refractory Crohn's disease: An analysis of pooled data from the ASTIC trial. *Lancet Gastroenterology and Hepatology, 2,* 399–406. https://doi.org/10.1016/S2468-1253(17)30056-0

Liu, Y.-M., Jaing, T.-H., Chen, Y.-C., Tang, S.-T., Li, C.-Y., Wen, Y.-C., ... Chen, M.-L. (2016). Quality of life after hematopoietic stem cell transplantation in pediatric survivors: Comparison with healthy controls and risk factors. *Cancer Nursing, 39,* 502–509. https://doi.org/10.1097/NCC.0000000000000339

Locatelli, F., Merli, P., & Strocchio, L. (2016). Transplantation for thalassemia major: Alternative donors. *Current Opinion in Hematology, 23,* 515–523. https://doi.org/10.1097/MOH.0000000000000280

Locatelli, F., & Stefano, P.D. (2004). New insights into haematopoietic stem cell transplantation for patients with haemoglobinopathies. *British Journal of Haematology, 125,* 3–11. https://doi.org/10.1111/j.1365-2141.2004.04842.x

London, S. (2013, July 25). Barriers to successful hematopoietic stem cell transplantation: A conversation with Mary M. Horowitz, MD, MS. *ASCO Post.* Retrieved from http://www.ascopost.com/issues/july-25-2013/barriers-to-successful-hematopoietic-stem-cell-transplantation

Lu, D.F., Hart, L., Lutgendorf, S., Oh, H., & Silverman, M. (2016). Effects of healing touch and relaxation therapy on adult patients undergoing hematopoietic stem cell transplant: A feasibility pilot study. *Cancer Nursing, 39,* E1–E11. https://doi.org/10.1097/NCC.0000000000000272

Lucarelli, G., Galimberti, M., Giardini, C., Polchi, P., Angelucci, E., Baronciani, D., ... Gaziev, D. (1998). Bone marrow transplantation in thalassemia: The experience of Pesaro. *Annals of the New York Academy of Sciences, 850,* 270–275. https://doi.org/10.1111/j.1749-6632.1998.tb10483.x

Lucarelli, G., Galimberti, M., Polchi, P., Angelucci, E., Baronciani, D., Giardini, C., ... Albertini, F. (1990). Bone marrow transplantation in patients with thalassemia. *New England Journal of Medicine, 322,* 417–421. https://doi.org/10.1056/NEJM199002153220701

Lucarelli, G., & Gaziev, J. (2008). Advances in the allogeneic transplantation for thalassemia. *Blood Reviews, 22,* 53–63. https://doi.org/10.1016/j.blre.2007.10.001

Lucas, W., Kennell, J., & Hanchett, S. (2018). CAR-T cell education for ICU and BMT nurses [Poster abstract No. 367]. *Oncology Nursing Forum, 45*(2), 51. https://doi.org/10.1188/18.ONF.E34

Mabed, M. (2011). The potential utility of bone marrow or umbilical cord blood transplantation for the treatment of type I diabetes mellitus. *Biology of Blood and Marrow Transplantation, 17,* 455–464. https://doi.org/10.1016/j.bbmt.2010.06.002

Madden, W., Dockery, J., Stapleton, E., & Hayes, T. (2018). Quality improvement initiative to reduce *Clostridium difficile* infections in a bone marrow transplant unit [Poster abstract No. 106]. *Oncology Nursing Forum, 45*(2), 137. https://doi.org/10.1188/18.ONF.E34

Madden, W., Johnson, K., & Rudolph, S. (2018). Pre-transplant education performed by a designated patient educator: Can this improve knowledge, behavior, comprehension, and satisfaction for bone marrow transplant patients? [Poster abstract No. 368]. *Oncology Nursing Forum, 45*(2), 51–52. https://doi.org/10.1188/18.ONF.E34

Malär, R., Sjöö, F., Rentsch, K., Hassan, M., & Güngör, T. (2011). Therapeutic drug monitoring is essential for intravenous busulfan therapy in pediatric hematopoietic stem cell recipients. *Pediatric Transplantation, 15,* 580–588. https://doi.org/10.1111/j.1399-3046.2011.01529.x

Mancardi, G., Sormani, M., Guslandi, F., Saiz, A., Carreras, E., Merelli, E., ... Saccardi, R. (2015). Autologous hematopoietic stem cell transplantation in multiple sclerosis: A phase II trial. *Neurology, 84,* 981–988. https://doi.org/10.1212/WNL.0000000000001329

Marshall, J.L. (2013, January 17). Why are only 3% of US cancer patients in clinical trials? *Medscape Oncology.* Retrieved from https://www.medscape.com/viewarticle/777662

Mathews, V., George, B., Deotare, U., Lakshmi, K., Viswahandya, A., Daniel, D., ... Srivastava, A. (2007). A new stratification strategy that identifies a subset of class III patients with an adverse prognosis among children with β thalassemia major undergoing a matched related allogeneic stem cell transplantation. *Biology of Blood and Marrow Transplantation, 13,* 889–894. https://doi.org/10.1016/j.bbmt.2007.05.004

McNinney, T., & Assalone, D. (2018). Can we give you some TIPS? Tailored interventions for patient safety on a hematopoietic stem cell transplant (HSCT) unit. Retrieved from https://ons.confex.com/ons/2018/meetingapp.cgi/Paper/3314

Meier, E.R., Dioguardi, J., & Kamani, N. (2015). Current attitudes of parents and patients toward hematopoietic stem cell transplantation for sickle cell anemia. *Pediatric Blood and Cancer, 62,* 1277–1284. https://doi.org/10.1002/pbc.25446

Morgan, R.A., Gray, D., Lomova, A., & Kohn, D.B. (2017). Hematopoietic stem cell gene therapy: Progress and lessons learned. *Cell Stem Cell, 21,* 574–590. https://doi.org/10.1016/j.stem.2017.10.010

Morrison, C.F., Martsolf, D., Borich, A., Coleman, K., Ramirez, P., Wehrkamp, N., ... Pai, A.L.H. (2018). Follow the yellow brick road: Self-management by adolescents and young adults after a stem cell transplant. *Cancer Nursing, 41,* 347–358. https://doi.org/10.1097/NCC.0000000000000566

Mulanovich, V.E., Desai, P.A., & Popat, U.R. (2016). Allogeneic stem cell transplantation for HIV-positive patients with hematologic malignancies. *AIDS, 30,* 2653–2657. https://doi.org/10.1097/QAD.0000000000001240

Nance, J., & Santacroce, S. (2017). Blogging during hematopoietic stem cell transplant [ICCN 2017 Oral Session Abstract No. O-163]. *Cancer Nursing, 40*(Suppl. 6), E48.

Nass, S.J., Moses, H.L., & Mendelsohn, J. (Eds.). (2010). *A national cancer clinical trials system for the 21st century: Reinvigorating the NCI Cooperative Group Program.* https://doi.org/10.17226/12879

Nathwani, A., Davidoff, A.M., & Linch, D.C. (2004). A review of gene therapy for haematological disorders. *British Journal of Haematology, 128,* 3–17. https://doi.org/10.1111/j.1365-2141.2004.05231.x

National Cancer Institute. (n.d.). NCI's role in cancer research. Retrieved from https://www.cancer.gov/research/nci-role

National Cancer Institute. (2007). *NCI's Clinical Trials Cooperative Groups national meetings report.* Retrieved from https://dctd.cancer.gov/NewsEvents/CoopGroupMeetingReport_dec07.pdf

National Cancer Institute. (2016). Phases of clinical trials. Retrieved from https://www.cancer.gov/about-cancer/treatment/clinical-trials/what-are-trials/phases

National Cancer Institute. (2019). NCTN: NCI's National Clinical Trials Network. Retrieved from https://www.cancer.gov/research/areas/clinical-trials/nctn

National Comprehensive Cancer Network. (n.d.). Phases of clinical trials. Retrieved from https://www.nccn.org/patients/resources/clinical_trials/phases.aspx

National Institute of Environmental Health Sciences. (2019, June). NIEHS Institutional Review Board. Retrieved from https://www.niehs.nih.gov/about/boards/irb/index.cfm

Ngwube, A., Hanson, C., Orange, J., Rider, N., Seeborg, F., Shearer, W., ... Martinez, C. (2018). Outcomes after allogeneic transplant in patients with Wiskott-Aldrich Syndrome. *Biology of Blood and Marrow Transplantation, 24,* 537–541. https://doi.org/10.1016/j.bbmt.2017.11.019

Nickel, R.S., & Kamani, N.R. (2018). Ethical challenges in hematopoietic cell transplantation for sickle cell disease. *Biology of Blood and Marrow Transplantation, 24,* 219–227. https://doi.org/10.1016/j.bbmt.2017.08.034

Nierengarten, M.B. (2017, June 14). Stem cell transplantation shown to improve outcomes in systemic sclerosis. Retrieved from https://www.the-rheumatologist.org/article/stem-cell-transplantation-shown-improve-outcomes-systemic-sclerosis

Nottingham Digestive Diseases Centre. (n.d.). ASTIC trial. Retrieved from https://www.nottingham.ac.uk/research/groups/giandliverdiseases/nddc-clinical-trials/astic-trial/index.aspx

NRG Oncology. (n.d.). Home. Retrieved from https://www.nrgoncology.org

O'Brien, M., Foster, J., Moore, H., & Schoeppner, K. (2018). Co-design of a hematopoietic cell transplant e-learning module for patients on fertility preservation and family planning. *Biology of Blood and Marrow Transplantation, 24*(Suppl. 3), S111. https://doi.org/10.1016/j.bbmt.2017.12.698

Ochs, H.D., & Petroni, D. (2018). From clinical observations and molecular dissection to novel therapeutic strategies for primary immunodeficiency disorders. *American Journal of Medical Genetics Part A, 176*, 784–803. https://doi.org/10.1002/ajmg.a.38480

Olausson, J., Hammer, M., & Brady, V. (2014). The impact of hyperglycemia on hematopoietic cell transplantation outcomes: An integrative review [Online exclusive]. *Oncology Nursing Forum, 41*, E302–E312. https://doi.org/10.1188/14.ONF.E302-E312

O'Nan, C.L. (2011). The effect of a journal club on perceived barriers to the utilization of nursing research in a practice setting. *Journal for Nurses in Staff Development, 27*, 160–164. https://doi.org/10.1097/NND.0b013e31822365f6

Otonkoski, T., Gao, R., & Lundin, K. (2005). Stem cells in the treatment of diabetes. *Annals of Medicine, 37*, 513–520. https://doi.org/10.1080/07853890500300279

Otsuka, A., Shomura, M., & Yanagihara, K. (2015). Search for meaning of hematopoietic stem cell transplantation in Japanese elderly [ICCN 2015 Abstract Book Manuscript Poster Abstract No. P-7]. *Cancer Nursing, 38*(Suppl. 4), S56. Retrieved from https://journals.lww.com/cancernursingonline/toc/2015/07001

Panasiuk, A., Nussey, S., Veys, P., Amrolia, P., Rao, K., Krawczuk-Rybak, M., & Leiper, A. (2015). Gonadal function and fertility in childhood after stem cell transplantation: Comparison of a reduced intensity conditioning regimen containing melphalan with a myeloablative regimen containing busulfan. *British Journal of Haematology, 170*, 719–726. https://doi.org/10.1111/bjh.13497

Peters, C. (2018). Allogeneic hematopoietic stem cell transplantation to cure transfusion dependent thalassemia: Timing matters! *Biology of Blood and Marrow Transplantation, 24*, 1107–1108. https://doi.org/10.1016/j.bbmt.2018.04.023

Pinto, F.O., & Roberts, I. (2008). Cord blood stem cell transplantation for haemoglobinopathies. *British Journal of Haematology, 141*, 309–324. https://doi.org/10.1111/j.1365-2141.2008.07016.x

Pintz, C., Zhou, Q.P., McLaughlin, M.K., Kelly, K.P., & Guzzetta, C.E. (2018). National study of nursing research characteristics at Magnet®-designated hospitals. *Journal of Nursing Administration, 48*, 247–258. https://doi.org/10.1097/NNA.0000000000000609

Platt, O.S., & Guinan, E.C. (1996). Bone marrow transplantation in sickle cell anemia—The dilemma of choice. *New England Journal of Medicine, 335*, 426–428. https://doi.org/10.1056/NEJM199608083350609

Porta, F., & Friedrich, W. (1998). Bone marrow transplantation in congenital immunodeficiency diseases. *Bone Marrow Transplantation, 21*(Suppl. 2), S21–S23.

Prasad, V.K., & Kurtzberg, J. (2008). Emerging trends in transplantation of inherited metabolic diseases. *Bone Marrow Transplantation, 41*, 99–108. https://doi.org/10.1038/sj.bmt.1705970

Re, A., Cattaneo, C., Skert, C., Balsalobre, P., Michieli, M., Bower, M., ... Rossi, G. (2013). Stem cell mobilization in HIV seropositive patients with lymphoma. *Haematologica, 98*, 1762–1768. https://doi.org/10.3324/haematol.2013.089052

Rein, L.A.M., Yang, H., & Chao, N.J. (2018). Applications of gene editing technologies to cellular therapies. *Biology of Blood and Marrow Transplantation, 24*, 1537–1545. https://doi.org/10.1016/j.bbmt.2018.03.021

Ritchie, D.S., Seymour, J.F., Roberts, A.W., Szer, J., & Grigg, A.P. (2001). Acute left ventricular failure following melphalan and fludarabine conditioning. *Bone Marrow Transplantation, 28*, 101–103. https://doi.org/10.1038/sj.bmt.1703098

Rimkus, C., & Trost, D. (2018). Tacrolimus dosing: Can we do it better? *Biology of Blood and Marrow Transplantation, 24*(Suppl. 3), S109–S110. https://doi.org/10.1016/j.bbmt.2017.12.027

Rodgers, C.C., Krance, R., Street, R.L., Jr., & Hockenberry, M.J. (2013). Feasibility of a symptom management intervention for adolescents recovering from a hematopoietic stem cell transplant. *Cancer Nursing, 36*, 394–399. https://doi.org/10.1097/NCC.0b013e31829629b5

Rodgers, C.C., Krance, R., Street, R.L., & Hockenberry, M.J. (2014). Symptom prevalence and physiologic biomarkers among adolescents using a mobile phone intervention following hematopoietic stem cell transplantation. *Oncology Nursing Forum, 42*, 229–236. https://doi.org/10.1188/14.ONF.229-236

Rodgers, C.C., Young, A., Hockenberry, M., Binder, B., & Symes, L. (2010). The meaning of adolescents' eating experiences during bone marrow transplant recovery. *Journal of Pediatric Oncology Nursing, 27*, 65–72. https://doi.org/10.1177/1043454209355984

Rodriguez, E., Brooks, C., LeStrange, N., Donofrio, L., & Hambright, K. (2017). A nursing led implementation of a homebound stem cell transplant program [Poster abstract No. 71]. *Oncology Nursing Forum, 44*(2), 26. https://doi.org/10.1188/17.ONF.E88

Romano, G., Micheli, P., Pacilio, C., & Giordano, A. (2000). Latest developments in gene transfer technology: Achievements, perspectives and controversies over therapeutic applications. *Stem Cells, 18*, 19–39. https://doi.org/10.1634/stemcells.18-1-19

Ruggeri, A., Eapen, M., Scaravadou, A., Cairo, M.S., Bhatia, M., Kurtzberg, J., ... Rocha, V. (2011). Umbilical cord blood transplantation for children with thalassemia and sickle cell disease. *Biology of Blood and Marrow Transplantation, 17*, 1375–1382. https://doi.org/10.1016/j.bbmt.2011.01.012

Russell, C., Harcourt, D., Henderson, L., & Marks, D.I. (2011). Patients' experiences of appearance changes following allogeneic bone marrow transplantation. *Cancer Nursing, 34*, 315–321. https://doi.org/10.1097/NCC.0b013e31181f8f884

Saba, N., & Flaig, T. (2002). Bone marrow transplantation for nonmalignant diseases. *Journal of Hematotherapy and Stem Cell Research, 11*, 377–387. https://doi.org/10.1089/152581602753658565

Sabloff, M., Chandy, M., Wang, Z., Logan, B.R., Ghavamzadeh, A., Li, C.-K., ... Walters, M.C. (2011). HLA-matched sibling bone marrow transplantation for β-thalassemia major. *Blood, 117*, 1745–1750. https://doi.org/10.1182/blood-2010-09-306829

Sabo, B., McLeod, D., & Couban, S. (2013). The experience of caring for a spouse undergoing hematopoietic stem cell transplantation: Opening Pandora's box. *Cancer Nursing, 36*, 29–40. https://doi.org/10.1097/NCC.0b013e31824fe223

Saccardi, R., Di Gioia, M., & Bosi, A. (2008). Haematopoietic stem cell transplantation for autoimmune disorders. *Current Opinion in Hematology, 15*, 594–600. https://doi.org/10.1097/MOH.0b013e3283136700

Saccardi, R., Freedman, M.S., Sormani, M.P., Atkins, H., Farge, D., Griffith, L.M., ... Muraro, P.A. (2012). A prospective, randomized, controlled trial of autologous haematopoietic stem cell transplantation for aggressive multiple sclerosis: A position paper. *Multiple Sclerosis Journal, 18*, 825–834. https://doi.org/10.1177/1352458512438454

Sams, K., Reich, R., Boyington, A.R., & Barilec, E. (2015). Community respiratory virus infection in hematopoietic stem cell transplantation recipients and household member characteristics. *Oncology Nursing Forum, 42*, 74–79. https://doi.org/10.1188/15.ONF.74-79

Sannes, T.S., Mikulich-Gilbertson, S.K., Natvig, C.L., Brewer, B.W., Simoneau, T.L., & Laudenslager, M.L. (2018). Caregiver sleep and patient neutrophil engraftment in allogeneic hematopoietic stem cell transplant: A secondary analysis. *Cancer Nursing, 41*, 77–85. https://doi.org/10.1097/NCC.0000000000000447

Sayre, C. (2015). Objective measure of strength in fall prevention for patients receiving hematopoietic stem cell transplant [ICCN 2015 Abstract Book Manuscript Poster Abstract No. O-25]. *Cancer Nursing, 38*(Suppl. 4), S8. Retrieved from https://journals.lww.com/cancernursingonline/toc/2015/07001

Schmitz, N., Dreger, P., Linch, D.C., Goldstone, A.H., Boogaerts, M.A., Demuynck, M.M.S., ... Borkett, K. (1996). Randomised trial of filgrastim-mobilised peripheral blood progenitor cell transplantation versus autologous bone-marrow transplantation in lymphoma patients. *Lancet, 347*, 353–357. https://doi.org/10.1016/S0140-6736(96)90536-X

Schoulte, J.A., Lohnberg, J.A., Tallman, B., & Altmaier, E.M. (2011). Influence of coping style on symptom interference among adult recipients of hematopoietic stem cell transplantation. *Oncology Nursing Forum, 38*, 582–586. https://doi.org/10.1188/11.ONF.582-586

Scleroderma Education Project. (n.d.). Scleroderma treatment: General – Experimental / alternate. Retrieved from https://sclerodermainfo.org/faq/treatments-experimental

Shalala, D.E., Bolton, L.B., Bleich, M.R., Brennan, T.A., Campbell, R.E., Devlin, L., … Vladeck, B.C. (2011). *The future of nursing: Leading change, advancing health.* https://doi.org/10.17226/12956

Shenoy, S. (2007). Has stem cell transplantation come of age in the treatment of sickle cell disease? *Bone Marrow Transplantation, 40,* 813–821. https://doi.org/10.1038/sj.bmt.1705779

Shenoy, S. (2013). Hematopoietic stem-cell transplantation for sickle cell disease: Current evidence and opinions. *Therapeutic Advances in Hematology, 4,* 335–344. https://doi.org/10.1177/2040620713483063

Shirey, M.R. (2005). Celebrating certification in nursing: Forces of magnetism in action. *Nursing Administration Quarterly, 29,* 245–253. https://doi.org/10.1097/00006216-200507000-00009

Sideri, A., Neokleous, N., Brunet De La Grange, P., Guerton, B., Le Bousse Kerdilles, M.-C., Uzan, G., … Gluckman, E. (2011). An overview of the progress on double umbilical cord blood transplantation. *Haematologica, 96,* 1213–1220. https://doi.org/10.3324/haematol.2010.038836

Siefker, S., & Vogelsang, N. (2018). Nursing interventions for the patient experiencing mucositis. *Biology of Blood and Marrow Transplantation, 24*(Suppl. 3), S111–S112. https://doi.org/10.1016/j.bbmt.2017.12.692

Sinclair, S., Booker, R., Fung, T., Raffin-Bouchal, S., Enns, B., Beamer, K., & Ager, N. (2016). Factors associated with post-traumatic growth, quality of life, and spiritual well-being in outpatients undergoing bone marrow transplantation: A pilot study. *Oncology Nursing Forum, 43,* 772–780. https://doi.org/10.1188/16.ONF.772-780

Singh, K., Warnock, C., Ireson, J., Strickland, S., Short, D., Seckl, M., & Hancock, B.W. (2017). Experiences of women with gestational trophoblastic neoplasia treated with high-dose chemotherapy and stem cell transplantation: A qualitative study. *Oncology Nursing Forum, 44,* 375–383. https://doi.org/10.1188/17.ONF.375-383

Slatter, M.A., Kanchan, R., Abd Hamid, I.J.A., Nademi, Z., Chiesa, R., Elfeky, R., … Veys, P. (2018). Treosulfan and fludarabine conditioning for hematopoietic stem cell transplantation in children with primary immunodeficiency: UK experience. *Biology of Blood and Marrow Transplantation, 24,* 529–536. https://doi.org/10.1016/j.bbmt.2017.11.009

Smiers, F.J., Krishnamurti, L., & Lucarelli, G. (2010). Hematopoietic stem cell transplantation for hemoglobinopathies: Current practice and emerging trends. *Pediatric Clinics of North America, 57,* 181–205. https://doi.org/10.1016/j.pcl.2010.01.003

Snowden, J.A., Badoglio, M., Labopin, M., Giebel, S., McGrath, E., Marjanovic, Z., … Farge, D. (2017). Evolution, trends, outcomes, and economics of hematopoietic stem cell transplantation in severe autoimmune diseases. *Blood Advances, 1,* 2742–2755. https://doi.org/10.1182/bloodadvances.2017010041

Snowden, J.A., Brooks, P.M., & Biggs, J.C. (1997). Haemopoietic stem cell transplantation for autoimmune diseases. *British Journal of Haematology, 99,* 9–22. https://doi.org/10.1046/j.1365-2141.1997.3273144.x

Snowden, J.A., Panés, J., Alexander, T., Allez, M., Ardizzone, S., Dierickx, D., … Ricart, E. (2018). Autologous haematopoietic stem cell transplantation (AHSCT) in severe Crohn's disease: A review on behalf of ECCO and EBMT. *Journal of Crohn's and Colitis, 12,* 476–488. https://doi.org/10.1093/ecco-jcc/jjx184

Snowden, J.A., Saccardi, R., Allez, M., Ardizzone, S., Arnold, R., Cervera, R., … Farge, D. (2012). Haematopoietic SCT in severe autoimmune diseases: Updated guidelines of the European Group for Blood and Marrow Transplantation. *Bone Marrow Transplantation, 47,* 770–790. https://doi.org/10.1038/bmt.2011.185

Sodani, P., Isgrò, A., Gaziev, J., Polchi, P., Paciaroni, K., Marziali, M., … Lucarelli, G. (2010). Purified T-depleted, CD34⁺ peripheral blood and bone marrow cell transplantation from haploidentical mother to child with thalassemia. *Blood, 115,* 1296–1302. https://doi.org/10.1182/blood-2009-05-218982

Son, T., Jakubowski, A., Lambert, S., & Loiselle, C. (2017). Adaptation of a coping intervention for stem cell transplantation patients and caregivers. *Cancer Nursing, 40*(Suppl. 6), E5.

Srivastava, A., & Shaji, R.V. (2017). Cure for thalassemia major—From allogeneic hematopoietic stem cell transplantation to gene therapy. *Haematologica, 102,* 214–223. https://doi.org/10.3324/haematol.2015.141200

Stanford Medicine. (n.d.). Scientific Review Committee. Retrieved from http://med.stanford.edu/cancer/research/trial-support/src.html

Statistics How To. (2016, August 20). Case-control study: Definition, real life examples. Retrieved from https://www.statisticshowto.datasciencecentral.com/case-control-study

Steele-Moses, S.K. (2010). The journey to Magnet®: Establishing a research infrastructure. *Clinical Journal of Oncology Nursing, 14,* 237–239. https://doi.org/10.1188/10.CJON.237-239

Steward, C.G. (2000). Stem cell transplantation for non-malignant disorders. *Best Practice and Research Clinical Haematology, 13,* 343–363. https://doi.org/10.1053/beha.2000.0082

Straathof, K.C., Rao, K., Eyrich, M., Hale, G., Bird, P., Berrie, E., … Amrolia, P. (2009). Haemopoietic stem-cell transplantation with antibody-based minimal-intensity conditioning: A phase 1/2 study. *Lancet, 374,* 912–920. https://doi.org/10.1016/S0140-6736(09)60945-4

Strocchio, L., & Locatelli, F. (2018). Hematopoietic stem cell transplantation in thalassemia. *Hematology/Oncology Clinics of North America, 32,* 317–328. https://doi.org/10.1016/j.hoc.2017.11.011

Strocchio, L., Romano, M., Cefalo, M.G., Vinti, L., Gaspari, S., & Locatelli, F. (2015). Cord blood transplantation in children with hemoglobinopathies. *Expert Opinion on Orphan Drugs, 3,* 1125–1136. https://doi.org/10.1517/21678707.2015.1076724

Sullivan, K.M., Goldmuntz, E.A., Keyes-Elstein, L., McSweeney, P.A., Pickney, A., Welch, B., … Furst, D.E. (2018). Myeloablative autologous stem-cell transplantation for severe scleroderma. *New England Journal of Medicine, 378,* 35–47. https://doi.org/10.1056/NEJMoa1703327

Sullivan, K.M., Muraro, P., & Tyndall, A. (2010). Hematopoietic cell transplantation for autoimmune disease: Updates from Europe and the United States. *Biology of Blood and Marrow Transplantation, 16*(Suppl. 1), S48–S56. https://doi.org/10.1016/j.bbmt.2009.10.034

Sullivan, K.M., Nelson, J.L., Arnason, B., Good, R., Burt, R., & Gratwohl, A. (1998). Evolving role of hematopoietic stem cell transplantation in autoimmune disease. In J.R. McArthur, G.P. Schechter, & S.L. Schrier (Eds.), *American Society of Hematology Educational Program Book* (pp. 198–214). Washington, DC: American Society of Hematology.

Sullivan, K.M., Parkman, R., & Walters, M.C. (2000). Bone marrow transplantation for non-malignant disease. *American Society of Hematology Education Book, 2000,* 319–338. https://doi.org/10.1182/asheducation-2000.1.319

Sundaramurthi, T., Wehrlen, L., Friedman, E., Thomas, S., & Bevans, M. (2017). Hematopoietic stem cell transplantation recipient and caregiver factors affecting length of stay and readmission. *Oncology Nursing Forum, 44,* 571–579. https://doi.org/10.1188/17.ONF.571-579

Sureda, A., Bader, P., Cesaro, S., Dreger, P., Duarte, R.F., Dufour, C., … Madrigal, A. (2015). Indications for allo- and auto-SCT for haematological diseases, solid tumours and immune disorders: Current practice in Europe, 2015. *Bone Marrow Transplantation, 50,* 1037–1056. https://doi.org/10.1038/bmt.2015.6

Swart, J., Delemarre, E., van Wijk, F., Boelens, J., Kuball, J., van Laar, J., & Wulffraat, N. (2017). Haematopoietic stem cell transplantation for autoimmune diseases. *Nature Reviews Rheumatology, 13,* 244–256. https://doi.org/10.1038/nrrheum.2017.7

SWOG Cancer Research Network. (n.d.). Welcome. Retrieved from https://www.swog.org/welcome

Thakkar, D., Katewa, S., Rastogi, N., Kohli, S., Nivargi, S., & Yadav, S.P. (2017). Successful reduced intensity conditioning alternate donor stem cell transplant for Wiskott-Aldrich syndrome. *Journal of Pediatric Hematology/Oncology, 39,* E493–E496. https://doi.org/10.1097/MPH.0000000000000959

Theroux, R. (2010). Systematic reviews: Strong evidence on which to base practice. *Nursing for Women's Health, 14,* 67–70. https://doi.org/10.1111/j.1751-486X.2010.01509.x

Thomas, E.D. (1999). A history of haemopoietic cell transplantation. *British Journal of Haematology, 105,* 330–339. https://doi.org/10.1111/j.1365-2141.1999.01337.x

Thomas, E.D., Buckner, C.D., Banaji, M., Clift, R.A., Fefer, A., Flournoy, N., … Weiden, P.L. (1977). One hundred patients with acute leukemia treated by chemotherapy, total body irradiation, and allogeneic marrow transplantation. *Blood, 49,* 511–533.

Thompson, A.A., Walters, M.C., Kwiatkowski, J., Rasko, J.E.J., Ribeil, J.-A., Hongeng, S., ... Cavazzana, M. (2018). Gene therapy in patients with transfusion-dependent β-thalassemia. *New England Journal of Medicine, 378*, 1479–1493. https://doi.org/10.1056/NEJMoa1705342

Tierney, D.K., Palesh, O., & Johnston, L. (2015). Sexuality, menopausal symptoms, and quality of life in premenopausal women in the first year following hematopoietic cell transplantation. *Oncology Nursing Forum, 42*, 488–497. https://doi.org/10.1188/15.ONF.488-497

Titler, M.G. (2008). The evidence for evidence-based practice implementation. In R.G. Hughes (Ed.), *Patient safety and quality: An evidence-based handbook for nurses Vol. 1*. Retrieved from https://archive.ahrq.gov/professionals/clinicians-providers/resources/nursing/resources/nurseshdbk/TitlerM_EEBPI.pdf

Tomblyn, M., & Drexler, R. (2008, December). RCI BMT—Another addition to the alphabet soup for clinical trials in transplantation! *CIBMTR Newsletter, 14*, 7. Retrieved from https://www.cibmtr.org/ReferenceCenter/Newsletters/Documents/Newsletter_Dec2008.pdf

Tyndall, A., & Gratwohl, A. (2000). Immune ablation and stem cell therapy in autoimmune disease–Clinical experience. *Arthritis Research, 2*, 276–280. https://doi.org/10.1186/ar102

Uggla, L., Svahn, B.-M., Wrangsjö, B., & Gustafsson, B. (2018). Music therapy effect health related quality of life in children undergoing HSCT; A randomized clinical study. *Biology of Blood and Marrow Transplantation, 24*(Suppl. 3), S114–S115. https://doi.org/10.1016/j.bbmt.2017.12.702

Uman, L.S. (2011). Systematic reviews and meta-analyses. *Journal of the Canadian Academy of Child and Adolescent Psychiatry, 20*, 57–59. Retrieved from https://www.ncbi.nlm.nih.gov/pmc/articles/PMC3024725

U.S. Food and Drug Administration. (2019, March 18). Institutional review boards frequently asked questions: Guidance for institutional review boards and clinical investigators. Retrieved from https://www.fda.gov/RegulatoryInformation/Guidances/ucm126420.htm

van Bekkum, D.W. (1999). Autologous stem cell transplantation for treatment of autoimmune diseases. *Stem Cells, 17*, 172–178. https://doi.org/10.1002/stem.170172

van Besien, K., Koshy, M., Anderson-Shaw, L., Talishy, N., Dorn, L., Devine, S., ... Kodish, E. (2001). Allogeneic stem cell transplantation for sickle cell disease: A study of patients' decisions. *Bone Marrow Transplantation, 28*, 545–549. https://doi.org/10.1038/sj.bmt.1703208

van der Lans, M.C.M., Witkamp, F.E., Oldenmenger, W.H., & Broers, A.E.C. (2019). Five phases of recovery and rehabilitation after allogeneic stem cell transplantation: A qualitative study. *Cancer Nursing, 42*, 50–57. https://doi.org/10.1097/NCC.0000000000000494

van Laar, J., Farge, D., Sont, J., Naraghi, K., Marjanovic, Z., Larghero, J., ... Tyndall, A. (2014). Autologous hematopoietic stem cell transplantation vs intravenous pulse cyclophosphamide in diffuse cutaneous systemic sclerosis: A randomized clinical trial. *JAMA, 311*, 2490–2498. https://doi.org/10.1001/jama.2014.6368

Velez, P., Latchford, T., & Tierney, D.K. (2018). A clinical nurses role in improving the care of the BMT recipient receiving high dose chemotherapy [Poster abstract No. 548]. *Oncology Nursing Forum, 45*(2), 21–22. https://doi.org/10.1188/18.ONF.E35

Vichinsky, E., Brugnara, C., Styles, L., & Wagner, J. (1998). Future therapy for sickle cell disease. In J.R. McArthur, G.P. Schechter, & S.L. Schrier (Eds.), *American Society of Hematology Educational Book* (pp. 1129–1135). Washington, DC: American Society of Hematology.

Voltarelli, J.C., & Couri, C.E.B. (2009). Stem cell transplantation for type 1 diabetes mellitus. *Diabetology and Metabolic Syndrome, 1*, 4. https://doi.org/10.1186/1758-5996-1-4

Voltarelli, J.C., Couri, C.E.B., Stracieri, A.B.P.L., Oliveira, M.C., Moraes, D.A., Pieroni, F., ... Burt, R.K. (2007). Autologous nonmyeloablative hematopoietic stem cell transplantation in newly diagnosed type 1 diabetes mellitus. *JAMA, 297*, 1568–1576. https://doi.org/10.1001/jama.297.14.1568

Von Ah, D., Spath, M., Nielsen, A., & Fife, B. (2016). The caregiver's role across the bone marrow transplantation trajectory [Online exclusive]. *Cancer Nursing, 39*, E12–E19. https://doi.org/10.1097/NCC.0000000000000242

Walters, M.C. (2005). Stem cell therapy for sickle cell disease: Transplantation and gene therapy. *American Society of Hematology Education Program Book, 2005*, 66–73. https://doi.org/10.1182/asheducation-2005.1.66

Walters, M. (2015). Update of hematopoietic cell transplantation for sickle cell disease. *Current Opinion in Hematology, 22*, 227–233. https://doi.org/10.1097/MOH.0000000000000136

Ward, J., Swanson, B., Fogg, L., & Rodgers, C.C. (2017). Pilot study of parent psychophysiologic outcomes in pediatric hematopoietic stem cell transplantation. *Cancer Nursing, 40*, E48–E57. https://doi.org/10.1097/NCC.0000000000000394

Watts, K.L., Adair, J., & Kiem, H.-P. (2011). Hematopoietic stem cell expansion and gene therapy. *Cytotherapy, 13*, 1164–1171. https://doi.org/10.3109/14653249.2011.620748

Wheatley, T. (2018). Implementing and evaluating a nurse-led educational intervention for bone marrow transplant patients in the acute care setting [Poster abstract No. 423]. *Oncology Nursing Forum, 45*(2), 81. https://doi.org/10.1188/18.ONF.E34

Wilkins, O., Keeler, A.M., & Flotte, T.R. (2017). CAR T-cell therapy: Progress and prospects. *Human Gene Therapy Methods, 28*, 61–66. https://doi.org/10.1089/hgtb.2016.153

Williams, L.A., Qazilbash, M.H., Shi, Q., Bashir, Q., Cleeland, C.S., & Champlin, R.E. (2018). Symptom monitoring and burden in autologous stem cell transplantation for multiple myeloma [Poster abstract No. 514]. *Oncology Nursing Forum, 45*(2), 287. https://doi.org/10.1188/18.ONF.E34

Wolff, D., Schleuning, M., von Harsdorf, S., Bacher, U., Gerbitz, A., Stadler, M., ... Holler, E. (2011). Consensus Conference on Clinical Practice in Chronic GVHD: Second-line treatment of chronic graft-versus-host disease. *Biology of Blood and Marrow Transplantation, 17*, 1–17. https://doi.org/10.1016/j.bbmt.2010.05.011

World Health Organization. (n.d.). Haematopoietic stem cell transplantation HSCtx. Retrieved from http://www.who.int/transplantation/hsctx/en

Wujcik, D. (2016). Scientific advances shaping the future roles of oncology nurses. *Seminars in Oncology Nursing, 32*, 87–98. https://doi.org/10.1016/j.soncn.2016.02.003

Wyant, T. (2018, January 18). A spirit of inquiry leads to evidence-based answers to practice questions. *ONS Voice*. Retrieved from https://voice.ons.org/news-and-views/a-spirit-of-inquiry-leads-to-evidence-based-answers-to-practice-questions

Zaia, J.A., & Forman, S.J. (2013). Transplantation in HIV-infected subjects: Is cure possible? *American Society of Hematology Education Program Book, 2013*, 389–393. https://doi.org/10.1182/asheducation-2013.1.389

CHAPTER 4

Considerations in Program Development and Sites of Care

Jody B. Acheson, RN, DNP, MPH, OCN®, BMTCN®, and Kelly A. Hofstra, RN, BSN, OCN®, BMTCN®

Introduction

Nurses play important roles in the multiple settings of transplantation: as inpatient and outpatient bedside staff, apheresis practitioners, program administrators, quality managers, educators, transplant coordinators, discharge planners, clinical nurse specialists, nurse practitioners, and researchers (Ford, Wickline, & Heye, 2016). Nurses have the unique opportunity to be involved in developing transplant programs in multiple ways. This chapter provides an overview of hematopoietic stem cell transplantation (HSCT) program considerations relevant to nurses, focusing on quality programs and the culture of caring.

Initial Program Development

HSCT program development began more than 50 years ago with transplants being performed at a few select locations. As the modality evolved, it became clear that the risks and complications associated with the treatment necessitated complex resources and planning to implement a transplant program. Now, programs are primarily located at large academic medical centers. However, in the past few years, a handful of new programs have been created in the United States, as well as several in developing countries ("Boise Woman Receives First Allogeneic Transplant in Idaho," 2018; Brandeis, 2016; Majolino et al., 2017; Mitchell et al., 2016; Yeh et al., 2018). This is likely due to improved regimens with decreased toxicity, improved infection and graft-versus-host disease (GVHD) prophylaxis, and expanded availability of donors, such as in haploidentical transplants (Henig & Zuckerman, 2014).

Although the transplant process has become more standardized, the infrastructure required to start a program remains significant. Organizational and financial support are needed to implement this complex treatment. Some programs, such as those in the Sarah Cannon network, have expanded using expertise from an existing program. Utilizing network or program affiliation was the first recommendation that came out of the experience of creating a program at Banner MD Anderson Cancer Center in Arizona (Mitchell et al., 2016). By partnering with an established program, the HSCT program can share its quality framework, order sets, standard operating procedures, and even established training.

However, if a program affiliation does not exist, new programs can still be established. It is helpful to look at the framework for programs that have recently been established and even new chimeric antigen receptor (CAR) T-cell therapy programs. The serious endeavor of starting a transplant program requires a dedicated interprofessional planning team, financial and organizational support, and internal and external analyses regarding feasibility of the program as part of the strategic plan for an organization. In addition, government agencies should be included in developing countries (Hashmi et al., 2017).

The first step in development is an evaluation of the feasibility of a transplant program. This includes an assessment of both the internal and external environments. The external environment includes the community at large, whereas assessment of the internal environment includes an evaluation of the organization, available resources, and commitment to the development and support of a transplant program. The purpose of the assessment is to provide a comprehensive and realistic review of the variables that will affect program development. Based on the information obtained from this process, the planning team and key members of the organization decide whether to proceed with a transplant program. Figure 4-1 presents questions to consider in a feasibility analysis. If this analysis indicates that the development and implementation of an HSCT program would be beneficial to the community without creating a financial burden for the organization, the planning process is ready to begin.

A preliminary financial analysis, or pro forma, for the HSCT program should include the capital and operating costs for startup and an ongoing assessment of costs and revenue for at least five years. The planning of the pro forma should include costs associated with infrastructure for air and water systems, apheresis, marrow harvest, cell processing, and laboratory facilities. It should include costs of staffing for providers and nurses, as well as quality management, laboratory, and apheresis staff. Other considerations include availability of transfusion services, diagnostic laboratories, pharmacy, intensive care unit (ICU) beds, and ancillary consult services (Yeh et al., 2018). A key factor to consider in this analysis is payer mix, which will influence the types and number of patients served and ultimately the financial sustainability of the program (Mitchell et al., 2016).

Once financial approval has been obtained, a stakeholder team should be formed. Key stakeholders of the planning team include the medical director, inpatient and outpatient hospital and nursing administrators, a payer reimbursement leader, a revenue cycle leader, an infectious disease physician, and a critical care or pulmonary physician. A project management model or framework can be used for planning and implementation. It often is helpful to utilize organizational project managers in conjunction with stakeholders to leverage area expertise. A CAR T-cell program was developed using a similar model and identified eight essential tasks in the workflow (Perica, Curran, Brentjens, & Girans, 2018): intake, consultation, collection, bridging, infusion, early care, late care, and regulation. Although planning for an HSCT program would differ in some areas, identifying the key tasks that define the workflow can facilitate the design outline for a program. Accounting for the aforementioned considerations in addition to understanding the need for the following components discussed in this chapter can lead to development of a high-quality, successful HSCT program.

Care Continuum

Historically, much of the care of HSCT recipients was performed in the traditional inpatient hospital setting. Advances in supportive care, the use of peripheral blood stem cells in place of bone marrow, the introduction of nonmyeloablative therapy, and cost-containment issues have brought alternative sites of care to the forefront. The role of professional nurses remains essential throughout all sites of care: to complete complex assessments, facilitate care planning, provide in-depth patient education, and help with patient management throughout the HSCT process (Bevans et al., 2009; Brown & Faltus, 2011; Thomson, Gorospe, Cooke, Giesie, & Johnson, 2015).

Inpatient Care

A core of knowledgeable interprofessional staff is essential to meet the special needs of transplant recipients. The program must have 24-hour access to ancillary services and critical care available either on the same unit or within the facility (Foundation for the Accreditation of Cellular Therapy [FACT] & Joint Accreditation Committee–International Society for Cellular Therapy and European Society for Blood and Marrow Transplantation [JACIE], 2018). Inpatient care in the autologous and allogeneic HSCT program may occur in designated rooms within a general oncology unit as a subset of the patient census. Most large transplant centers, however, have a dedicated transplant unit.

Intensive Care

The use of high-dose myeloablative therapy may cause complex side effects and complications that often require transfer to an ICU. All patients undergoing transplantation must have immediate access to intensive care services provided by physician consultants and nurses knowledgeable in the complications of this therapy (FACT & JACIE, 2018).

Studies report that critical care support in HSCT recipients has decreased from a high of 40% of patients in the 1980s to 8%–20% today (Afessa & Azoulay, 2010; Benz, Schanz, Maggiorini, Seebach, & Stussi, 2014; Pène et al., 2006; Shelton, 2010). Both autologous and allogeneic transplant recipients are at risk for life-threatening complications. The acuity of the allogeneic population has led some centers to provide critical care within the inpatient transplant unit. Toxicities associated with autologous and allogeneic HSCT have decreased, but significant treatment-related mortality and relapse rates remain (McArdle, 2009; Rimkus, 2010; Shelton, 2010).

Patients may require intensive care for a variety of complications that can affect multiple organ systems with potentially fatal outcomes. Pulmonary, cardiovascular, and neurologic complications and sepsis are some of the most common reasons for patients to require ICU care, as well as other complicating factors such as GVHD, renal failure, bleeding, or sinusoidal obstructive syndrome (Benz et al., 2014; Jenkins et al., 2015; Young, Mansfield, & Mandoza,

2017). These occur in the setting of marrow aplasia with subsequent infection risks. These treatment-related complications may persist for several weeks to months.

In a review article by Young et al. (2017), the average length of stay in the ICU was approximately 8 days, with a range of 4–14 days. In one center's report, the mean average length of stay in the ICU of 4.4 days accounted for 21% of the patient's hospital charges, and an average day of ICU charges was 2.1 times the average daily charges on the transplant unit (Jenkins et al., 2015).

The development of critical illness has historically been related to poor outcomes. Outcomes continue to be poor for some HSCT recipients; however, recent advances in the management and triage of patients who should receive critical care have led to an increase in survival (Lengliné et al., 2015). Some centers have found it beneficial to employ a risk stratification tool to guide decisions on whether a patient should be transferred to an ICU level of care (Jenkins et al., 2015). A focus on advance care planning prior to transplant and involvement of palliative care have decreased rates of admission to the ICU in adults. Programs should consider building advance care planning discussions into pretransplant evaluation (Cappell et al., 2018).

Approximately 17%–35% of pediatric HSCT recipients require critical care. Although the risk of mortality has improved, pediatric patients experience significant mortality risks if requiring intensive care treatment, with risk increasing with the need for mechanical ventilation, renal replacement therapy, or the presence of viral or fungal infections (Zinter, Dvorak, Spicer, Cowan, & Sapru, 2015).

Intensive care for HSCT recipients is delivered in a number of models: (a) provision of ventilator support, continuous renal replacement therapy, or invasive monitoring on the HSCT unit, (b) transfer of patients to a designated ICU, which may have designated HSCT beds, or (c) an HSCT specialty unit capable of one-to-one nursing care and frequent noninvasive monitoring with transfer of patients who require more monitoring and mechanical ventilation or continuous renal replacement therapy. The choice of model must be based on how best to meet patients' needs and the available institutional resources. In some cases, nursing staff may be cross-trained in critical care to accompany patients when transfer to an ICU is required. In other cases, nursing staff may be trained in critical care so that critical care measures can be implemented on the HSCT unit. The HSCT team continues to be involved in the clinical management and support of patients and families whether patients are receiving ICU care on the inpatient transplant unit or in an intensive care setting.

Focusing on continuity of care for patients and families regardless of changes in acuity requires a team approach. In their review, Young et al. (2017) discussed several interventions to improve patient and family outcomes of HSCT recipients in the ICU. Nurses caring for critically ill HSCT recipients should receive standardized training and ori-

entation to this population's unique needs, such as central line care and infection prevention, and education on the complications these patients experience. This education should be an ongoing process. The authors stressed the importance of communication and care coordination between the ICU staff and the HSCT staff (Young et al., 2017). Figure 4-2 demonstrates nursing's influence in the care of these patients and "how HSCT nurses are the thread that connects multiple disciplines with HSCT patients and families" (Young et al., 2017, p. 347).

Outpatient Care

Many programs are moving part or all of the management of transplant recipients to outpatient settings (Graff et al., 2015; Johnson, 2014; Lisenko et al., 2017; Solomon et al., 2009). With appropriate selection of patients with minimal comorbidities, autologous transplant for myeloma and lymphoma can be performed safely on an outpatient basis (Graff et al., 2015; Martino et al., 2016). Outpatient transplant is also a possibility in the allogeneic setting. The use of nonmyeloablative regimens has resulted in fewer days of neutropenia and less chemotherapy-related toxicity, which has allowed care to shift to the outpatient ambulatory care arena and resulted in decreased length of hospital stays and decreased cost. This has resulted in lower overall cost of care without increased risk of infection and no decrease in patient-reported quality of life or other adverse effects in selected populations (Graff et al., 2015; Holbro et al., 2013; McDiarmid et al., 2010; Schmit-Pokorny, Franco, Frappier, & Vyhlidal, 2003; Solomon et al., 2009; Svahn et al., 2008).

Several models exist for outpatient-based HSCT care. Mehta and Dulley (2009) described models that include a variety of settings:

- Entirely outpatient: Care is provided either at home or at the outpatient clinic. Patients are admitted to the hospital if complications arise that are unable to be managed in the outpatient setting.
- Early discharge: Patients are discharged from the hospital on a set day once the stem cell infusion is complete. Care is then continued as an outpatient at home or in the clinic. Patients are admitted if complications arise that are unable to be managed in the outpatient setting or can have a planned readmission with their anticipated nadir.

The Duke University Medical Center Bone Marrow Transplant Program led the nation in the late 1980s with the use of an early discharge model that administered high-dose therapy in the hospital and then discharged patients to a nearby cooperative residential hotel for housing following stem cell infusion (Peters et al., 1994). Patients were required to have a responsible caregiver staying with them and were followed at an outpatient clinic with extended hours. The program addressed administrative and logistic barriers. It also had the ability to provide emergency inpatient care, if required, by maintaining an open bed on

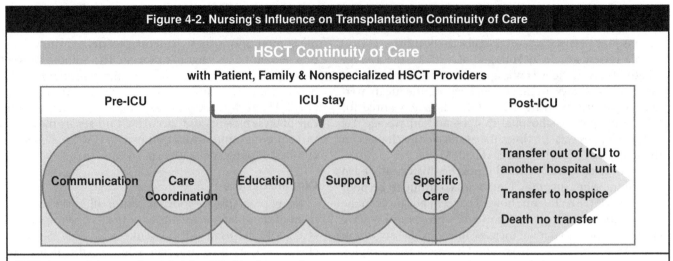

Figure 4-2. Nursing's Influence on Transplantation Continuity of Care

HSCT—hematopoietic stem cell transplantation; ICU—intensive care unit

Note. From "Nursing Care of Adult Hematopoietic Stem Cell Transplant Patients and Families in the Intensive Care Unit: An Evidence-Based Review," by L.K. Young, B. Mansfield, and J. Mandoza, 2017, *Critical Care Nursing Clinics of North America, 29,* p. 347. Copyright 2017 by Elsevier. Reprinted with permission.

the HSCT unit. This model was found to lower costs and increase patient satisfaction (Peters et al., 1994). Faucher et al. (2011) studied the early discharge model in a randomized trial. They demonstrated it was safe and feasible for patients to be discharged home on day 0 with a caregiver and outpatient clinic follow-up. The inpatient readmission rate was 86%. The overall length of hospital stay for those discharged early was decreased by five days, and costs were reduced by 19%. The authors stressed that readmissions should be expected and planned for in these patients.

The delayed admission model allows for administration of conditioning therapy and stem cell infusion in an outpatient setting. Patients are admitted for supportive care if they develop febrile neutropenia, have pain management issues secondary to mucositis, or require IV hydration and electrolyte replacement for vomiting or diarrhea. This model may or may not shorten inpatient stay (Mehta & Dulley, 2009).

The total outpatient model is a comprehensive approach whereby the conditioning therapy, hematopoietic stem cell infusion, and supportive care all occur in the outpatient setting. Studies indicate that autologous and allogeneic transplants performed in the outpatient setting result in short-term outcomes, including infectious complications, comparable to those achieved in the inpatient setting (McDiarmid et al., 2010).

Outpatient models require close proximity, with patients staying within 30–60 minutes of the center. When patients are referred from an outside facility or live more than 60 minutes away, nearby contracted residential hotels or on-campus housing facilities are used with frequent clinic visits or home health services (Mehta & Dulley, 2009). Insurance companies may provide a housing stipend for patients who travel to a referral center, thus saving patients the out-of-pocket housing costs (Stiff et al., 2006). All these

models have the ability to provide emergency inpatient care, if required, by having a bed reserved on the transplant unit.

Although eligibility criteria for outpatient care exist (see Figure 4-3), the most common limiting factor for outpatient care is the lack of a caregiver (Faucher et al., 2011; Rice & Bailey, 2009; Schmit-Pokorny et al., 2003). In a randomized study of early discharge compared to hospital care for autologous transplant recipients, 39% of otherwise eligible patients were not discharged early for social or psychological reasons, including lack of a caregiver (Faucher et al., 2011). Patients who do have a caregiver report similar levels of quality of life compared to inpatients. This article suggests that the quality of the caregiver may have more of an impact on patients' perceptions of their experience of outpatient transplant (Martino et al., 2018).

Figure 4-3. Outpatient Eligibility Criteria

Determining Eligibility
- Clinic eligibility—facilities available to determine disease staging, organ function, performance status, and comorbidities
- Psychosocial assessment
- Insurance review
- Dedicated/trained caregiver on a 24-hour basis
- Appropriate housing within proximity of 30–60 minutes
- Reliable transportation
- Access to 24-hour outpatient care

Continuation of Outpatient Care Status
- No evidence of active, ongoing, or uncontrolled infection
- Responsive to antiemetic and antibiotic regimens
- Ability to maintain fluid and electrolyte balance
- Appropriate level of pain control
- Performance status > 60%
- Homecare services to supplement trained caregiver (if required)

Note. Based on information from Rice & Bailey, 2009.

Community Setting

High-dose therapy with hematopoietic stem cell support in the community remains a high-risk intensive therapeutic process requiring interprofessional involvement and a structured program. Community cancer centers can successfully care for patients undergoing autologous and allogeneic HSCT with necessary laboratory and blood bank support and with careful preparation. FACT and JACIE will accredit autologous transplant programs that have had a dedicated team with a program director and at least one other trained or experienced physician in place for at least 12 months and that perform transplants on a minimum of five patients annually. Allogeneic transplant programs are required to perform transplants on 10 patients annually (FACT & JACIE, 2018). Extensive resources are necessary to implement a quality program regardless of the size of the institution. Many community sites are associated with regional medical centers that provide a full range of oncology services to a large area. Community programs have the ability to provide this treatment option in settings where patients can have maximum family and social support. Community oncology practices treat patients from the existing service area. Abou-Nassar et al. (2012) found that when patients had to drive further to their transplant center, they experienced worse overall survival. These patients also had notably fewer follow-up visits after transplant, which the authors felt contributed to the decrease in overall survival. Providing transplant resources in the community setting helps to increase access to care.

Home Care

Home care of HSCT recipients has been influenced by the growth and application of autologous and allogeneic transplant for a variety of disease processes, technologic advances, changing practice patterns, and managed care. Homecare providers for the transplant population can be part of a large tertiary care network or an independent, privately operated agency that offers services to the oncology or transplant population. The selection of a homecare agency requires an assessment of the agency's internal capabilities, resources, and commitment to the transplant population. An evaluation of the following will assist the transplant program or team in determining whether the homecare agency will meet the needs of the HSCT recipient: the agency's ability to complement existing services, understanding of the transplant process, scope of geographic coverage, ability to provide 24-hour care, timely responses to changes in therapy, and ability to educate the family or caregiver.

Standardized policies, procedures, and guidelines for discharge are essential for a smooth transition to the home. Centers must ensure discharges are planned and coordinated with community providers who are knowledgeable in post-transplant care (FACT & JACIE, 2018). After the return home and to referring physicians, patients may need home health services for infusion therapies such as antibiotics, antifungals, antiviral therapies, electrolytes, and total parenteral nutrition. Homecare agencies can assist in central venous catheter care and laboratory monitoring as needed.

An example from a Swedish hospital allowed for allogeneic transplant recipients who met the criteria for home care to choose to have the majority of their care provided in the home setting (Bergkvist, Fossum, Johansson, Mattsson, & Larsen, 2018). The study followed an early discharge model, with most patients being discharged home on day +1. The patients then had daily follow-up at home with an experienced transplant nurse in addition to a daily phone check-in with a transplant physician. If at any time patients had unstable vital signs or other complications that could not be managed at home, they were readmitted to the hospital. The authors discussed that the patients receiving most of their care in the home reported eating better, having more opportunities for physical activity, and deriving comfort from remaining in a familiar setting with their family (Bergkvist et al., 2018).

A Canadian center piloted home care in the pediatric population and found that parents reported fewer disruptions in daily routines, less need for child care, fewer days off from work, and reduced out-of-pocket costs from participating in the pilot (Lippert et al., 2017).

Referring Physician's Office

Reduction in the time that patients remain at the tertiary care center for outpatient monitoring has expanded the role of referring oncologists and other primary care practitioners in post-transplant monitoring and treatment. The expansion of reduced-intensity transplants and improved supportive care have resulted in more patients being offered transplant who are often older and sicker. The criteria for returning patients to referring physicians may depend on the physician's experience with transplant recipients and the HSCT recipient's clinical stability. Discharge plans for patients who have ongoing needs should be detailed to ensure availability of adequate post-transplant care (FACT & JACIE, 2018).

Patients may be required to return to the transplant center periodically for long-term follow-up or evaluation of specific post-transplant issues (Khera et al., 2017). The complex long-term follow-up needs are met in the community, where healthcare providers must be knowledgeable in assessment and treatment of the growing transplant population. Primary oncologists encounter chronic GVHD, long-term toxicities, secondary malignancies, and prolonged immunosuppression with the resulting need for prophylaxis, monitoring, and frequent visits. Khera et al. (2017) described the importance of quality care coordination among the transplant facility, referring hematology/oncology office, and primary care provider for this complex patient population.

Interprofessional Team

HSCT requires coordination and collaboration among disciplines and across settings. The *FACT-JACIE International*

Standards for Hematopoietic Cellular Therapy: Product Collection, Processing, and Administration defined a clinical transplant program as "an integrated medical team housed in a defined location that includes a Clinical Program Director and demonstrates common staff training, protocols, Standard Operating Procedures, quality management systems, clinical outcome analysis, and regular interaction among clinical sites" (FACT & JACIE, 2018, p. 8).

Systems are in place to foster regular interactions among team members, such as the formal committee structures in Figure 4-4. A variety of professionals support the transplant process and improve outcomes. Key team members include the program director, attending physicians, advanced practice providers, nurses, pharmacists, dietitians, psychosocial service providers, clinical laboratory scientists, rehabilitation therapists, data managers, and administrative and clerical staff. Nurses and nurse administrators formally educated and experienced in the management of HSCT recipients are essential. Pediatric transplantation is a specialty area that requires care provided by physicians, nurses, and consultants experienced in the management of pediatric patients. In many high-volume programs, physician specialists, dentists, psychologists, psychiatrists, child life specialists, and researchers are dedicated team members, whereas in other programs, they are available as consultants. Consulting physicians necessary for the appropriate care of the transplantation population include adult or pediatric specialists in surgery, pulmonary medicine, intensive care, gastroenterology, nephrology, infectious disease, cardiology, pathology, psychiatry, radiology, radiation oncology, transfusion medicine, neurology, ophthalmology, obstetrics/gynecology, dermatology, and palliative and end-of-life care (FACT & JACIE, 2018).

Program Director

Quality programs rely on the leadership of a designated transplant-trained physician to provide oversight of all program components (FACT & JACIE, 2018). Specialty education and dedication are required of the physician leader responsible for administrative and clinical operations, including compliance with established standards, applicable laws, and regulatory requirements. The program director is responsible for quality management, the selection and care of patients and donors, and cell collection and processing services. This includes responsibility for the clinical unit. The program director has oversight of the medical care provided by the clinical program. This includes responsibility for verifying the knowledge and skills of the transplant physicians and advanced practice practitioners. FACT publishes sample competency forms for the current FACT-JACIE standards at www.factwebsite.org/CTLibrary.

Although duties are frequently delegated, the director is ultimately responsible for the performance of the quality plan and monitoring all program elements (FACT & JACIE, 2018), as the sample organizational chart in Figure 4-5 demonstrates.

Physician Teams

In addition to the physician program director, HSCT programs need at least one attending physician licensed to practice medicine in the state with specialty certification or education in hematology, medical oncology, or immunology. Pediatric programs require physicians specialized in pediatric hematology/oncology or pediatric immunology (FACT & JACIE, 2018). Transplant physicians have specific knowledge in HSCT procedures. This includes bone marrow harvest, apheresis, cryopreservation, and product infusion. Ongoing annual education is required for physicians to provide appropriate care and keep up with the rapidly evolving field. Allogeneic transplantation requires physicians trained and competent in identification and selection of the stem cell source, use of donor registries, human leukocyte antigen typing, management of patients receiving ABO-incompatible products, diagnosis and management of infections common in immunocompromised patients, evaluation of chimerism, and management of post-transplant immunodeficiencies.

The American Society for Transplantation and Cellular Therapy (ASTCT, formerly the American Society for Blood and Marrow Transplantation) has expressed concern about the increased needs for complex follow-up care and impending shortages in the HSCT physician workforce. The National Marrow Donor Program and ASTCT formed the Physician Workforce Group to evaluate and discuss barriers and potential solutions to this projected physician shortage. One identified barrier was the perception of a poor work–life balance for transplant physicians. In a survey, 87% of transplant physicians reported working more than 50 hours per week. To help engage potential future transplant physicians, the Physician Workforce Group has developed educational outreach to students in fellowship training programs and an online HSCT training curriculum for fellows and medical students. Additionally, the Physician Workforce Group worked with the ASTCT Committee for Education and developed a new educational resource page on the ASTCT website. Future plans include working with hospital administrators to look at compensation and continued educational outreach to increase medical students' early exposure to the field of HSCT (Burns et al., 2014).

Figure 4-4. Blood and Marrow Transplant Program Committee Organization

Blood and Marrow Transplant (BMT) Operating Council
BMT Screening and Tumor Board
Systems Performance Improvement Team
Lead Performance Improvement Team
Patient Care Planning Team
BMT Inpatient Rounds Team

Note. Figure courtesy of St. Luke's Health System. Used with permission.

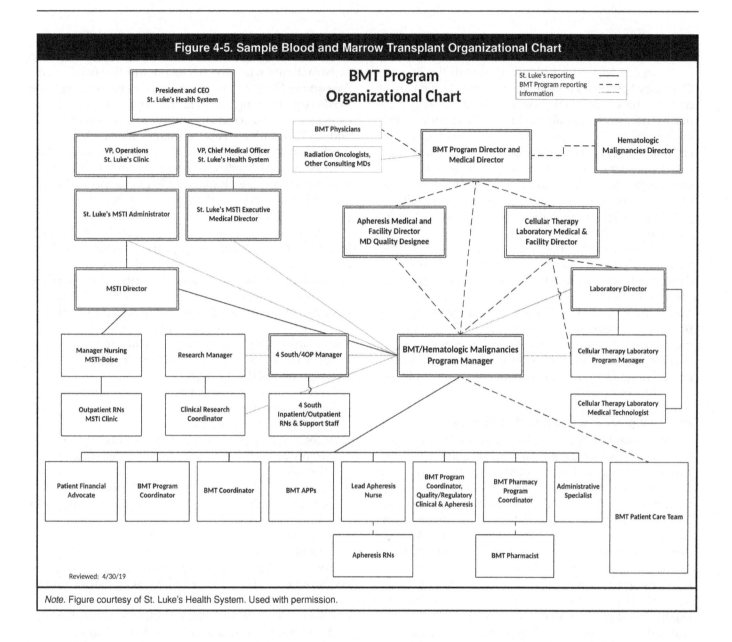

Figure 4-5. Sample Blood and Marrow Transplant Organizational Chart

BMT Program
Organizational Chart

St. Luke's reporting
BMT Program reporting
Information

President and CEO
St. Luke's Health System

BMT Physicians

Radiation Oncologists,
Other Consulting MDs

BMT Program Director and
Medical Director

Hematologic
Malignancies Director

VP, Operations
St. Luke's Clinic

VP, Chief Medical Officer
St. Luke's Health System

St. Luke's MSTI Administrator

St. Luke's MSTI Executive
Medical Director

Apheresis Medical and
Facility Director
MD Quality Designee

Cellular Therapy
Laboratory Medical &
Facility Director

MSTI Director

Laboratory Director

Manager Nursing
MSTI-Boise

Research Manager

4 South/4OP Manager

BMT/Hematologic Malignancies
Program Manager

Cellular Therapy Laboratory
Program Manager

Outpatient RNs
MSTI Clinic

Clinical Research
Coordinator

4 South
Inpatient/Outpatient
RNs & Support Staff

Cellular Therapy Laboratory
Medical Technologist

Patient Financial
Advocate

BMT Program
Coordinator

BMT Coordinator

BMT APPs

Lead Apheresis
Nurse

BMT Program
Coordinator,
Quality/Regulatory
Clinical & Apheresis

BMT Pharmacy
Program
Coordinator

Administrative
Specialist

BMT Patient Care Team

Apheresis RNs

BMT Pharmacist

Reviewed: 4/30/19

Note. Figure courtesy of St. Luke's Health System. Used with permission.

Nutrition Services

The transplant program dietitian is required to understand the nutritional needs of this patient population, be experienced with enteral and parenteral support, and provide counseling to avoid foodborne illnesses (FACT & JACIE, 2018). The nutrition plan is based on an assessment performed as part of the initial evaluation and includes ongoing monitoring of patients' nutrition status by using anthropometric, biochemical, and clinical data. The dietitian works collaboratively with the HSCT team by participating in daily rounds and making recommendations based on patients' diagnoses, comorbid conditions, and current clinical problems. An increased need exists for dietary advice on the use of vitamins, herbals, and nutritional supplements.

It is recommended that the dietitian be registered with the Academy of Nutrition and Dietetics, which offers board certification as a specialist in oncology nutrition through its credentialing agency, the Commission on Dietetic Registration (www.cdrnet.org).

Clinical Pharmacy

Clinical pharmacists are essential to provide for the multiple pharmaceutical needs of HSCT recipients. FACT recognizes the importance of the role and incorporates pharmacist involvement as a core requirement of a quality program (FACT & JACIE, 2018). The ASTCT Pharmacy Special Interest Group has published a summary of roles, responsibilities, and recommendations for HSCT pharmacists. Core competencies include medication management, chemotherapy and medication counseling, symptom management, therapeutic drug monitoring, discharge planning and transitions of care, policy and guideline development, evidence-based program development and evaluation, and education of team members, trainees, patients, and families (Clemmons, Alexander, DeGregory, & Kennedy, 2018).

Board certification for pharmacists with the Board of Pharmacy Specialties is offered as a board-certified oncology pharmacist, or BCOP. Board-certified oncology pharmacists have been identified as a potential resource to help address the predicted future shortage of oncology providers by assisting providers with aspects of care such as assessing chemotherapy toxicity; managing nausea, vomiting, and antiemetic therapy; managing symptoms and providing supportive care; managing pain; assisting with new patient consults; and providing medication reconciliation (Ignoffo et al., 2016).

Participation in interprofessional rounds allows pharmacists to educate the transplant team on prescribed drug therapies and make patient-specific therapeutic recommendations. Pharmacists play a key role in the post-transplant phase and have been shown to increase patient outcomes by monitoring for medication safety, including correct dosing, medication adherence, and recommendations for dose adjustments or other therapies to providers, and by providing patient education (Chieng et al., 2013; Ho et al., 2013).

Psychological and Psychiatric Services

Patients undergoing transplantation require team members skilled in social service, psychology, spiritual care, and psychiatry (FACT & JACIE, 2018). Programs performing allogeneic transplants often include a dedicated psychologist or have a collaborative relationship with a department of psychiatry. These specialists may be involved with patients from initial consultation to discharge. Programs depend on social workers, care coordinators, and chaplains as active team members and may maintain a consultative relationship with psychological and psychiatric services.

Cooke, Gemmill, Kravits, and Grant (2009) reviewed the psychological issues of stem cell transplant recipients and concluded that "the psychological impact after the experience of transplant can leave an indelible impression on the patient, caregiver, and nurse" (p. 139), and yet "often healthcare professionals forget or fail to understand the depth of trauma the patient may experience" (p. 140). Screening for psychosocial distress is a recommended standard of care for patients with cancer (Foster et al., 2009; National Comprehensive Cancer Network, 2019).

It is now well recognized that transplant survivors can experience psychological distress, anxiety, depression, and post-traumatic stress disorder, even several years after treatment (Baliousis, Rennoldson, & Snowden, 2016; Mosher, Redd, Rini, Burkhalter, & DuHamel, 2009). As transplant survival has increased, so have the demands on all teams to provide supportive and palliative care, long-term follow-up, and survivorship services (Bevans et al., 2006; Cooke, Gemmill, & Grant, 2011; Gajewski et al., 2009; Penalba, Asvat, Deshields, Vanderlan, & Chol, 2018; Wingard et al., 2010).

Oncology Social Work

Transplant programs assess and develop strategies to assist patients with diverse social and financial needs. Assessment for HSCT recipients includes tangible resource needs (e.g., housing, financial assistance, transportation, caregiver needs), screening of preexisting psychological and social problems (e.g., substance abuse, depression, psychiatric illness), ability to adhere to a treatment plan, legal competence, advance care planning, family interventions for those with high conflict or situational stressors, and coordination with the interprofessional care team (Cooke et al., 2009).

The National Marrow Donor Program/Be The Match Social Work Workforce Group (2017) developed a blood and marrow transplant (BMT) clinical social worker role description "to educate . . . about the specialty role of the BMT clinical social workers" (p. 1). Key points from the job description include that BMT clinical social workers:
- Are core members of the transplant team
- Implement standards of practice in the provision of psychosocial services for people with malignancy and nonmalignant life-threatening diseases
- Complete pretransplant psychosocial evaluation and high-risk screening for psychosocial factors that may negatively affect transplant outcomes
- Establish a therapeutic relationship and engage in problem solving and planning to develop caregiver and relocation plans
- Are experts in providing psychosocial care
- Facilitate family meetings and bridge communication with the care team
- Contribute to optimizing patient outcomes and quality of life

Board certification is available for oncology social workers through the Board of Oncology Social Work Certification (http://oswcert.org). The Association of Oncology Social Work (www.aosw.org) offers professional support and information and has a designated special interest group of BMT social workers. Other social services roles, such as patient financial advocates, navigators, and insurance case managers, make valuable contributions to the process of HSCT and can improve patient outcomes (Schmit-Pokorny, 2007). Early and continued involvement of these team members is essential. Additional patient resources include volunteers who can provide support to patients. Many newly referred patients find it helpful to network with transplant survivors and can find resources at the Blood and Marrow Transplant Information Network (www.bmtinfonet.org).

Spiritual Care and Chaplaincy Services

Another key component of the support team is chaplaincy services. Balboni et al. (2007) studied religiousness and spiritual support among patients with advanced cancer and found that although most considered religion to be important, 72% reported their needs were supported minimally or not at all by the medical system. In a prospective study of religious coping among patients with myeloma undergoing autologous transplantation, physical well-being was predicted by religious coping (Sherman, Plante, Simonton, Latif, & Anaissie, 2009). Patients with negative religious coping had worse post-transplant anxiety, depression, emotional well-being, and transplant-associated concerns (Sherman et al., 2009).

Spiritual assessment is important to the pretransplant evaluation and in the post-transplant and survivorship setting (Leeson et al., 2015). Chaplaincy care involves spiritual counseling according to the beliefs of patients and their families. Spiritual care may be provided through a hospital-based chaplaincy program or by the patient's own pastor, priest, or rabbi. Clearly defined referral systems and guidelines for chaplaincy services allow team members to facilitate patient and family access to spiritual care. Assessment of the needs for spiritual support includes the use of faith resources and devotional needs (e.g., prayer, meditation, guided imagery), sacramental needs (based on specific rituals of the patient's faith, tradition, and necessity for referral to specific clergy), and assessment of cultural, dietary, and medical care needs based on faith or belief systems (Cooke et al., 2009). Transplant center chaplains coordinate with the patient's own faith community, address general needs for spiritual support (either expressed or implied), and provide hope, strength, and support for effective coping. They strive to improve communications between patients and families and with the care team. Chaplains offer support during periods of medical, emotional, and spiritual crises, clarifying issues with grief, loss, or biomedical ethics. They may offer support to staff to address the emotional issues that arise while caring for transplant recipients (Cooke et al., 2009). Chaplaincy services participate in care teams to optimize patient and family support, improve communication, and assist staff members in addressing self-care needs.

Rehabilitation Services

The interprofessional rehabilitation care team offers "expertise in functional assessment, treatment of impairments and functional limitations, and disability prevention" (McNeely, Dolgoy, Onazi, & Suderman, 2016, p. 8). Physical therapy professionals provide expertise in patients' functional status to improve quality of life throughout the care continuum. Many patients enter the transplant process with impaired function associated with their disease state and prior treatments.

Physical therapy consultation focuses on preventive goals with early evaluation and instruction in an exercise program to minimize weakness and fatigue and enhance functional status. Recent studies of exercise programs in the pretransplant phase, the acute transplant phase, and the home setting have demonstrated that the programs are safe and well tolerated and result in improvements in strength, endurance, lung function, and quality-of-life measures such as fatigue,

mood, and sleep (Baumann, Kraut, Schüle, Bloch, & Fauser, 2010; Ibanez et al., 2018; Knols et al., 2011; McNeely et al., 2016; Oberoi et al., 2018; Silver, 2015; Steinberg, Asher, Bailey, & Fu, 2015). Additionally, many programs provide in-room exercise equipment to encourage activity.

Occupational therapists may develop restorative goals to assist post-transplant patients with issues of energy conservation, homemaking, work skills, and activities of daily living. Physical and occupational therapy assistance with chronic GVHD addresses myositis and prevents or decreases contractures. A treatment plan addressing range of motion, fine motor skills, and exercise is recommended. Integrating the work of multiple disciplines is crucial for the rehabilitation and adaptation of HSCT recipients prior to and following transplant. Recognition of the long-term recovery issues and late effects of HSCT demonstrates the need for ongoing assessment and intervention and requires the skills and expertise of multiple individuals in a team effort (Andrykowski et al., 2005; Syrjala, Langer, Abrams, Storer, & Martin, 2005; Wingard, 2007). Collaboration and coordination of care are essential to maintain quality patient outcomes and assist in developing a cohesive and comprehensive HSCT program (Rice & Bailey, 2009; Schmit-Pokorny, 2007).

Data Management Programs

The Stem Cell Therapeutic Outcomes Database (SCTOD) requires transplant centers in the United States to submit outcome data on allogeneic transplantation. Many centers also voluntarily report outcome data for autologous transplantation. This information is submitted through the Center for International Blood and Marrow Transplant Research (CIBMTR, 2019). Clinical data may be gathered by the BMT coordinator, a research coordinator, or a dedicated data manager, who may also enter information directly into a data management system.

With these reporting requirements, the BMT data manager has an increased role. The BMT data manager has expertise in data collection and management, clinical research trials, and reporting methods to the CIBMTR, as well as basic knowledge of HSCT (Hussain, Chaudhri, Alfraih, & Aljurf, 2017). The data manager acts as a liaison and reference for issues related to data collection and maintenance of complete and accurate donor and recipient records. The data manager prepares and submits required forms and selected research reports electronically to CIBMTR. The data manager continues to coordinate research and clinical data while helping the program meet reporting regulations of CIBMTR, FACT, and applicable regulatory agencies. FACT provides data management training and education resources on its website (www.factwebsite.org/DMWebsitePage).

Clinical Laboratory Scientists in the Cell Therapy Laboratory

The growth in cellular therapy is strongly based in laboratory science. Hematopoietic stem cell collection, processing, and storage activities interact with clinical team activities for quality programs. Transplant programs require 24-hour clinical laboratory services to provide crucial diagnostics and specialty blood product support for HSCT recipients (FACT & JACIE, 2018). Cellular therapy is an evolving field with scientific processes and significant technical requirements. Transplant centers may have integrated clinical, collection, and processing programs or may contract for collection and processing services.

Laboratory professionals in clinical programs are trained as medical technologists, now known as clinical laboratory scientists. The American Society for Clinical Pathology (www.ascp.org) provides education and certification in the various procedures of processing and cryopreservation of cellular products. Proficiency testing occurs at regular intervals, and documentation of formal training and continuing education is extremely important. The laboratory staff is involved in all phases of stem cell collection and processing: apheresis, cell counting techniques, progenitor cell assays, product manipulation, record maintenance, and quality control. The extensive experience of laboratory staff in quality assurance processes and frequent inspections by regulatory agencies are assets to the HSCT program (Leemhuis et al., 2014).

The clinical and administrative management of the cell processing facility is under the direction of the laboratory medical director. Day-to-day supervision of laboratory personnel working in the cellular processing facility is the responsibility of the laboratory manager or director. Hematopoietic stem cell processing standards address procedures according to the type of component collected and manipulation techniques needed.

Cellular processing requires standard operating procedures for component labeling, infection control, biochemical and radiologic safety measures, biohazard waste disposal, and emergency response systems; education and competency evaluation; and documentation procedures. Other aspects of the FACT accreditation standards include recommendations for storage, security, and transportation of product between centers and the disposal of unused stem cell components (FACT & JACIE, 2018).

Apheresis Practitioners and Collection Facilities

Apheresis for stem cell collection may be performed by nursing or trained clinical laboratory scientists (Pagano et al., 2017). The HSCT program may have integrated collection facilities or use a third-party facility. The collection facility for stem cells is affiliated with an accredited and licensed laboratory able to perform the diagnostic tests required for donors. A transfusion facility or blood bank is able to provide 24-hour blood component support, as well as emergency and intensive care services. The collection facility medical director must be a licensed physician who performs a minimum of 10 collection procedures and 1 marrow harvest annually. The collection facility medical director can be the same person as the director of the affil-

iated clinical program or a separate qualified physician (FACT & JACIE, 2018).

Apheresis practitioners have a unique role that involves multiple aspects of care of donors, such as in-depth knowledge of mobilization, medication administration, side effect management, and operation of the apheresis machine (Ikeda, Nollet, Vrielink, & Ohto, 2018; Nemec, 2017). The American Society for Apheresis partnered with the American Society for Clinical Pathology in 2016 to begin offering a Qualification in Apheresis examination. Topics covered include "basic science, clinical applications, donor/patient care, instrumentation, operational considerations, and standards, guidelines, and regulations" (American Society for Clinical Pathology Board of Certification, 2018, para. 1).

Nurse Leadership

Expert nursing leadership skills are required to manage the high complexity of the continuum of care in BMT programs. Outpatient care is emphasized, yet intensive clinical care demands remain. Long-term follow-up and survivorship care needs are increased. Transplant teams are facing workforce issues, escalating healthcare expenses, and consumer and regulatory demands in a time of economic uncertainty (Gajewski et al., 2009). In detailing the challenges for nurses in transplant programs, Rice and Bailey (2009) concluded:

> Nurses at all levels of practice must conceptualize and execute expert specialized care through all phases of transplantation. Attention must be paid to specialized functions such as care coordination and case management, as well as scope of practice. Focus must be given to quality assessment and improvement. (p. 151)

Nurses with expertise in transplant issues provide leadership in BMT programs as clinical specialists, nurse practitioners, coordinators, transplant unit managers, administrators, and researchers. In what have become classic references for transplant nursing, Buchsel and Whedon (1995) and Ezzone and Schmit-Pokorny (2007) have extensively reviewed nursing management and program development. Nurse leaders facilitate implementation of quality standards and coordination of multiple services in the evolving care environment. Nursing contributes to establishing standards for HSCT through active participation at national and international levels, including within CIBMTR, ASTCT, National Marrow Donor Program, and FACT-JACIE (Ezzone, Fliedner, & Sirilla, 2007). The HSCT program is resource intensive, and leadership is increasingly challenged to set priorities to achieve quality goals and promote a culture of caring (Cantrell, 2007). Nurse leaders must be role models of professional behavior, as well as motivate and empower staff. The management role entails understanding business principles for budgeting and resource management, overseeing special projects, facilitating staff performance, and monitoring quality indicators. Senior nurses, educators, and nurse managers in all settings provide direction, mentorship, and staff development while creating, maintaining, and expanding services to meet the demands of the care unit and the clinical transplant program (Brown & Faltus, 2011; Rice & Bailey, 2009).

Advanced Practice Practitioners

Advanced practice practitioner (APP) is used to describe the role of the nurse practitioner or physician assistant. The Oncology Nursing Society (ONS, 2019) defined core competencies for oncology nurse practitioners. APPs were involved in the development of the field of HSCT, providing continuity in settings where attending physicians and house staff rotated through clinical duties. ASTCT (n.d.) established a special interest group for nurse practitioners and physician assistants and provides a variety of resources for APPs, such as a document on recommended training and orientation as well as other educational resources.

Certification is available through the Oncology Nursing Certification Corporation for nurse practitioners as an advanced oncology certified nurse practitioner (AOCNP®). Nurse practitioners are also eligible for the blood and marrow transplant certified nurse (BMTCN®) certification. Information about these certifications is available at www.oncc.org/certifications.

APPs make vital contributions to the care team. They may provide 24-hour clinical coverage, often rotating between inpatient and outpatient services. APPs complete patient histories and physical examinations; order medications, blood products, and diagnostic studies; titrate immunosuppressive drugs; and participate in clinical research protocols (Knopf, 2011). APPs often initiate high-dose chemotherapy orders, providing an initial step in the quality assurance system to avoid medication errors. These providers can perform procedures such as bone marrow harvests, biopsies, and aspirations; skin biopsies; and lumbar punctures. APPs' education and competencies in transplant-related cognitive and procedure skills are similar to those required for attending physicians (FACT & JACIE, 2018).

Clinical Nurse Specialist and Educator

The oncology clinical nurse specialist role can be highly variable among institutions and may include many aspects, such as educator, researcher, and care coordinator. Clinical nurse specialists provide support and education to patients, families, and caregivers from initial evaluation and treatment to discharge teaching, follow-up, and long-term care. They also facilitate staff education programs and are involved in staff development. Clinical nurse specialists are viewed as the clinical practice experts and may be heavily involved in the development of policies and procedures and best nursing practices in the department (Cooke, Gemmill, & Grant, 2008; Gosselin, Dalton, & Penne, 2015; ONS, 2008).

ONS (2008) has defined core competencies for oncology clinical nurse specialists. Certification was available through the Oncology Nursing Certification Corporation as an advanced oncology certified clinical nurse specialist (AOCNS®) but is now only available for maintenance and renewal by current credential holders. Clinical nurse specialists are also eligible for the BMTCN® certification. Information about these certifications is available at www.oncc.org/certifications.

Nurse educators fulfill an important role in HSCT. They help with staff orientation and mentoring, competency development and tracking, and education on new procedures or medications. They may participate in the development of patient education materials or facilitate patient education classes. Educators may be designated to the department or may support other similar areas within the institution. Certification for nurse educators is available through two organizations: the National League for Nursing and the American Nurses Credentialing Center. The National League for Nursing offers the Certified Nurse Educator (CNE®) certification (see www.nln.org/Certification-for-Nurse-Educators). The American Nurses Credentialing Center offers the Nursing Professional Development Certification (RN-BC; see www.nursingworld.org/our-certifications/nursing-professional-development).

Blood and Marrow Transplant Coordinator and Nurse Navigator

Transplant coordinators may be baccalaureate-level nurses or advanced practice nurses. Other professionals experienced in HSCT may also hold this position. Coordinators are primarily involved in the patient evaluation and post-transplant phases. Education about the transplant process starts before patients arrive at the transplant center and is initiated by the coordinator. The BMT coordinator role is primarily behind the scenes starting at the time of referral, performing initial screening of patients and donors; gathering medical information, assisting with insurance issues, and confirming coverage; providing referral to social services; scheduling diagnostic tests and consultation; coordinating with the care team; and performing case review with referring physicians, case managers, and third-party payers. Coordinators arrange for post-transplant follow-up, including discharge planning for patients returning to their primary oncologists (Ford et al., 2016; Rice & Bailey, 2009; Thomson et al., 2015).

Nurse navigation is a growing field in oncology. An oncology nurse navigator (ONN) is

> a professional RN with oncology-specific clinical knowledge who offers individualized assistance to patients, families, and caregivers to help overcome healthcare system barriers. Using the nursing process, an ONN provides education and resources to facilitate informed decision making and timely access to quality health and psychosocial care throughout all phases of the cancer continuum. (ONS, 2017, p. 4)

BMT coordinators at many centers function as an ONN even though that may not be their official title (Khera et al., 2017). Oncology nurse navigation has been shown to provide many benefits, such as improved continuity of care, improved patient satisfaction, decreased barriers to care, and improved timeliness of care or evaluation (McMullen, 2013).

Transplant Nurses and Professional Development

As transplantation evolved, the role of the transplant nurse also expanded and became more complex. "Staff nurses manage the administration of complicated conditioning regimens (high-dose therapy); administer supportive care measures to prevent or treat side effects; and care for the complexities of psychosocial, familial, and spiritual needs of patients and families who are undergoing a long, arduous treatment" (Rice & Bailey, 2009, p. 154). Transplant nurses must understand general oncology and transplant principles. They must have detailed knowledge of high-dose chemotherapy and potential immediate and long-term side effects. They must be experts in the management of central venous catheters, blood product transfusions, and infection prevention and management. Additionally, transplant nurses frequently monitor the psychosocial needs of patients and their families, making referrals to psychiatrists, chaplains, social workers, integrative medicine providers, and other disciplines as needed. Nurses must continually update their knowledge in this ever-changing field and translate it into patient and family education. Nurses are frequently on the forefront of care delivery and must be the first to recognize problems and complete thorough assessments (Bevans et al., 2009; Brown & Faltus, 2011; Ford et al., 2016). To better understand how caring for this complex population affects the psychosocial health and well-being of transplant nurses, Sabo (2011) used an interpretative phenomenological design with interviews and focus groups. An overriding novel theme emerged: compassionate presence. This challenged the notion that working with patients who are suffering or at the end of life leads to adverse psychosocial effects in nurses. Sabo suggested that a potential buffering effect against adverse consequences of HSCT nursing work underscored the value of the relationship as an integral component of nursing work.

Orientation

Caring for the transplant population is highly complex and requires staff to complete a comprehensive orientation program. The program may extend for a period of six weeks to six months depending on the staff members' previous experience (Ford et al., 2016). Orientation programs must allow for variation in individual learning styles and previous work experience. Orientation should combine didactic content from the classroom with clinical experience at the bedside. Figure 4-6 addresses the recommended didac-

Figure 4-6. Orientation Content for Transplant Nurses

- Overview of hematopoietic stem cell transplantation
- History and development of transplantation
- Review of immunology
- Pathophysiology of diseases treated
- Common complications
- Terms and abbreviations
- Role of the interprofessional team
- Hematology/oncology patient care
- Administration of blood products and transfusion therapy
- Central venous catheter care
- Stem cell mobilization and collection
- Mobilization regimens
- Common side effects of collection by apheresis
- Marrow harvesting process
- Care needs and recovery following collection
- Transplant supportive care
- Administration of high-dose chemotherapy, growth factors, and immunosuppressive medications
- Side effects and complications of preparatory regimens, including radiation
- Infection prevention and control in the setting of compromised host defense mechanisms
- Administration of cellular therapy products and management of adverse reactions
- Neutropenic diet principles
- The role of exercise
- Evidence-based care in the management of common side effects, including diarrhea, nausea, vomiting, mucositis, and pain
- Knowledge and assessment of other complications, including anaphylaxis, cardiac dysfunction, cytokine release syndrome, disseminated intravascular coagulation, graft-versus-host disease, infectious and noninfectious processes, macrophage activation syndrome, neurotoxicity, neutropenic fever, renal and hepatic failure, respiratory distress, and tumor lysis syndrome
- Cellular therapy emergencies
- Ambulatory care after transplant
- Long-term effects and need for ongoing follow-up
- Palliative and end-of-life care
- Psychosocial issues
- Caregiver needs and support
- Emotional impact of transplant
- Sexuality changes
- Transplant nurse competency evaluation process, including annual review and skills updates

tic content. Orientation should be based on adult learning principles; therefore, content should be introduced in a variety of ways to enhance the learning process. The didactic portion should be provided in lecture format with audiovisuals, handouts, and reference articles. The clinical "hands-on" portion should include direct patient care and a variety of skills checkoffs or simulations. The nursing competencies required by FACT should be considered when planning nursing orientation (FACT & JACIE, 2018).

Continuing Education

Continuing education is required so that HSCT nurses can continue to develop and expand on the knowledge base and skills associated with advancing technology. The ultimate goal is to be able to provide up-to-date, cost-effective nursing care to HSCT recipients.

To help nurses meet this goal, ONS offers a self-paced, comprehensive online course on the fundamentals of blood and marrow transplant (see www.ons.org/courses/funda mentals-blood-and-marrow-transplant). The course covers program development, the transplant process, patient care, survivorship, accreditation, and many other topics.

Continuing education units are also available at conferences, such as the Transplant and Cellular Therapy Meetings of ASTCT and CIBMTR (formerly known as the BMT Tandem Meetings) and ONS national meetings. Employees' annual assessments can help program educators and leaders to evaluate learning needs for continuing education program development. Periodic in-services on pertinent clinical topics and mandatory in-services regarding research protocols keep staff up to date on current treatments. Staff must be required to attend in-services or view recorded instructional sessions on new research protocols that will be used for patient care on the unit. Recorded attendance and skills checklists demonstrate staff knowledge and competency and are required for programs to meet FACT guidelines.

Certification

The Oncology Nursing Certification Corporation now offers the BMTCN® certification (see www.oncc.org/certifi cations/blood-marrow-transplant-certified-nurse-bmtcn). Certification is valid for four years once obtained. Original certification is obtained by submitting an application and taking a multiple-choice test with 165 questions. Test content includes all aspects of HSCT nursing care for autologous and allogeneic transplants and pediatric and adult patients. The following is a high-level outline of the content covered (Oncology Nursing Certification Corporation, 2017):
- Foundations of transplant
- Cellular collection, preparative regimens, and infusion
- Early post-transplant management and education
- Late post-transplant management and education
- Quality of life
- Professional performance

Resource Utilization

As transplantation has evolved, management of resource utilization has been key. HSCT is an intensive treatment that involves resources throughout the hospital and outpatient settings. The cost is estimated to range from a median of $140,792 for autologous transplants to $289,283 for myeloablative allogeneic transplants for the first 100 days (Broder et al., 2017). Looking at the first year after transplant, the costs are as high as $500,000. Additionally, pediatric allogeneic transplantation is significantly more than transplantation in adults, with a median cost of $445,916, due predominantly to longer inpatient stays (Broder et al., 2017).

Because of the high cost of transplantation, many models of care have been tried to reduce resource utilization. Many of these models stem from patient-centered models of care coordination that reduce hospitalizations and ensure appropriate follow-up (Khera et al., 2017). Nurses have a unique opportunity to provide the key link in all of these models.

Khera et al. (2017) described a framework using the following components, all of which would involve nurses: patient navigation, telemedicine, survivorship clinics, self-management support and educational interventions, standardization, and psychosocial and financial support. Nurse navigators, as described earlier in this chapter, can help with many patient factors, including decreasing rates of hospitalization (Fillion et al., 2012). Telemedicine is new to the world of HSCT and has been successful in reducing geographic health disparities and improving long-term follow-up of patients with chronic GVHD (Khera et al., 2016). Further exploration of the use of telemedicine could help reduce the burden on patients traveling for follow-up. In survivorship, "significant and unique challenges confront survivors for decades after their underlying indication . . . has been cured" (Battiwalla, Tichelli, & Majhail, 2017, p. 184). During the survivorship time period, a significant number of resources continue to be used. Development of a survivorship clinic could improve the health and quality of life of patients and families and potentially eliminate unnecessary resource utilization (Fillion et al., 2012; Hashmi, Carpenter, Khera, Tichelli, & Savani, 2015). Educational interventions are one method of support that nurses can provide. Nurses can tailor education to patients and their caregivers. Educational interventions can reduce hospital utilization (Khera et al., 2017). The next component, standardization and application of evidence-based research, can reduce unnecessary testing and prescribing of expensive medications ("ASBMT and CBMTG Release Choosing Wisely BMT Recommendations," 2018). Finally, the framework described providing substantial support to reduce the burden of care of the mental and financial health of patients and caregivers (Khera et al., 2017).

Numerous reimbursement methodologies exist for transplant services, including fee for service, inpatient diagnosis-related group, bundled episode, case rates, disease-specific capitation, accountable care organization, and global capitation (LeMaistre & Farnia, 2015). The majority of methods involve some financial risk sharing between the transplant facility and the third-party payer. Risk sharing and the potential for financial exposure require accurate and reliable cost data for services provided throughout the transplant process. This information is necessary for a center to negotiate a reasonable contract for services (Ezzone et al., 2007; LeMaistre & Farnia, 2015; Potter, 2007).

Recently, the focus on pay for performance and value-based care has increased. Many of the larger insurance companies contract with a limited number of centers regionally or nationally for provision of specialty care. This allows the insurers to decrease cost variation and direct patients to programs with expertise. Sites included in the care network may be called Centers of Excellence (Ezzone et al., 2007; LeMaistre & Farnia, 2015). For providers to become part of the network, the process begins with the insurance carrier providing a request-for-proposal application to the transplant center. Requests for proposal differ from network to network, but they frequently include quality outcome data. Both patients and providers face challenges with this model, as insurers may direct patients to centers outside of their geographic area (LeMaistre & Farnia, 2015).

New and developing transplant programs usually do not meet the volume criterion and do not have the clinical outcome data required for the Centers of Excellence network. Additionally, the program may not be needed by the network because other comparable centers are available in the same service area. In developing a new program, it is important to assess not only the community's needs but also the predominant insurers in the market to determine if they mandate a Centers of Excellence facility for transplant services. This mandate will affect a new center's volume, and it could take several years for a new program to meet Centers of Excellence volume and outcome criteria.

Caregiver Support

Caregiver Burden and Needs

Caregivers are key members of the transplant team and are required for any patient undergoing HSCT. Caregivers are unpaid individuals caring for someone in the home environment. Typically, these individuals are family members. Informal caregivers assist with activities of daily living, basic medical care, social support, and advocacy. The caregiving can be a full-time job and can require that the caregiver quit a paying job or take extended leave (Beattie, Lebel, & Tay, 2013; Berry, Dalwadi, & Jacobson, 2017; Family Caregiver Alliance, 2016). These caregivers frequently experience caregiver burden. Caregiver burden is described as "difficulties assuming and functioning in the caregiver role as well as associated alterations in the caregiver's emotional and physical health" (Bevans, Coleman, Jadalla, Page, & Cagle, 2019, para. 1). The caregiver role for HSCT recipients is extremely important and also one of the most intensive. When patient care needs exceed the resources of the caregiver, caregivers can experience caregiver burden (Applebaum et al., 2016). Caregiver burden causes increased anxiety, depression, and lack of self-care in the caregiver, which, in turn, can affect the length of stay for HSCT recipients and their overall survival (Beattie et al., 2013; Foster et al., 2013; Kershaw et al., 2015; Sundaramurthi, Wehrlen, Friedman, Thomas, & Bevans, 2017).

Even as family caregivers are vital members of the transplant care team, they are experiencing the impact of cancer on their loved one and family system. Families will experience changes in family life they likely have not encountered before (Sundaramurthi et al., 2017). Several studies have explored the experience of spouses during the transplant process (Beattie et al., 2017; Wilson, Eilers, Heermann, & Million, 2009). Beattie et al. (2017) applied a theoretical framework to describe patient and caregiver distress but found that it did not entirely encompass the didactic experience during transplantation. They recommended providing pretransplant psychoeducation regarding role changes and proactively addressing any imbalances in the patient–caregiver dyad prior to transplantation.

Information and ongoing support during all phases of the transplant process are essential to the adjustment of patients and caregivers, who may experience role changes over the long term (Eilers & Breen, 2007). Interventions to support caregivers of HSCT recipients include massage, education, psychosocial interventions, and involvement of palliative care (El-Jawahri et al., 2016; Langer et al., 2012; Laudenslager et al., 2015; Ouseph, Croy, Natvig, Simoneau, & Laudenslager, 2014; Simoneau, Kilbourn, Spradley, & Laudenslager, 2017). One of the most successful interventions studied to date included eight one-on-one sessions with a master's-level social worker. The participants were randomized to treatment as usual or the intervention group, which consisted of psychoeducation, paced respiration, and relaxation. Utilizing validated tools—the Perceived Stress Scale, Center for Epidemiological Studies Depression Scale, State Anxiety Inventory, Caregiver Reaction Assessment, Profile of Mood States Total Mood Disturbance, Pittsburgh Sleep Quality Inventory, SF-36®, and Impact of Events Scale—the authors demonstrated statistically significant reduction in stress, anxiety, and depression when compared to the control group at one and three months after transplant (Laudenslager et al., 2015; Simoneau et al., 2017). Integrating evidence-based interventions such as this can decrease caregiver burden and ultimately improve patient health outcomes.

Caregiver Education

Transplant nurses often provide the initial and ongoing education to patients and their caregivers. They can reassure families that the changes and adjustments they are experiencing are an expected part of the process. Transplant nurses also can assess for increased burden, stress, or anxiety using validated tools. The transplant team should have resources available, such as referrals to medical social workers, marriage and family therapists, and other mental health professionals. It is important to give caregivers permission to seek and obtain help and support for themselves and to help them understand the benefit of self-care to the caregiving process (Applebaum et al., 2016).

Recognizing that different individuals learn best in different ways, transplant nurses can offer a variety of educational approaches, including written materials, videos, posters and flipcharts, individualized discussions, and group sessions. Health literacy assessments and materials developed at the appropriate reading level are especially important for written educational content (Ezzone, 2009; Spellecy et al., 2018). Emotional and educational needs can be overwhelming for both caregivers and the transplant patient, so programs should tailor information to suit the treatment phase as well as the learning style and emotional needs of family members (Eilers & Breen, 2007; Laudenslager et al., 2015; Ouseph et al., 2014; Simoneau et al., 2017). Centers may develop teaching materials or use nationally available resources through organizations such as Be The Match, BMT InfoNet, or the Family Caregiver Alliance (Ezzone et al., 2007).

The informational and psychological needs of patients and caregivers vary with each phase of treatment. The flow between treatment phases and sites of care can be confusing and must be explained. Education should begin at the pre-transplant evaluation and continue through the mobilization, collection, transplantation, discharge, and follow-up stages. A comprehensive and ongoing educational program is essential at each step of the transplant process. Runaas et al. (2017) implemented a health information technology road map for caregivers of HSCT pediatric transplant recipients that allowed real-time access to information and education. This ultimately resulted in caregivers reporting feeling more empowered and less anxious during patient rounds and patient care.

Professional Transplant Community

The broader professional transplant community is an exceptional resource. Professional associations provide specialty education, standards, and credentialing. Accrediting bodies validate important elements of transplant programs and their parent organizations. Patient support and survivor organizations are available to meet the needs of transplant recipients and their caregivers. Many organizations have developed patient education materials. Nurses also can learn informally through networking with colleagues, attending conferences, and visiting other transplant centers. The ASTCT houses a comprehensive list of organizations serving the transplant community (www.astct.org/practice-resources/external-organizations). Additional resources from professional organizations include the ASTCT special interest group communities (www.astct.org/special-interest-groups/about-sig-communities) and the ONS communities (https://communities.ons.org), including the Blood and Marrow Stem Cell Transplant Community. These forums allow nurses to connect with transplant nurses nationally and internationally and to ask questions regarding best practices and where to find information.

Quality Management

Quality management and continuous quality improvement must be the lifeblood of a transplant program because of the magnitude of risk that patients are exposed to while receiving this potentially lifesaving treatment. A well-defined quality program is required for accreditation by organizations such as the Joint Commission, FACT, the College of American Pathologists, and AABB. Regulatory bodies such as the U.S. Food and Drug Administration and the Centers for Medicare and Medicaid Services also have specific requirements for organizational quality measurement and reporting. The Health and Medicine Division of the National Academies of Sciences, Engineering, and Medicine (formerly the Institute of Medicine) defined *health care quality* as "the degree to which health services for individuals and populations increase the likelihood of desired health outcomes and are consistent with current professional knowledge"(Lohr, 1990, p. 4). Quality in transplant programs often is validated and confirmed by FACT-JACIE accreditation, which involves implementation and maintenance of a robust quality management program. In a study of 107,904 transplant recipients, Gratwohl et al. (2014) found that patient outcomes were significantly better when JACIE accreditation had been obtained. Insurers have recognized this link between quality and accreditation, with most denying coverage at centers that do not have FACT or JACIE accreditation.

Programs must develop meaningful quality programs. Figure 4-7 shows an example structure of a quality program. Many resources are available for developing quality management programs. The Alliance for Harmonisation of Cellular Therapy Accreditation developed a resource tool called "Essential Elements" that programs can use in developing or evaluating their quality program (Worel, 2017). It provides guidance based on several accrediting bodies in 15 areas: education and promotion, program organization, facility requirements, quality management, policies and procedures, donor issues, process controls, coding and labeling, product-related issues, storage, transportation, shipping and receipt, disposal, data management, and records. Another model of quality systems is based on concepts from Avedis Donabedian (Rodkey & Itani, 2009) and validated by Kunkel, Rosenqvist, and Westerling (2007). This model has three factors: process (culture and professional cooperation), structure (resources and administration), and outcomes (competence development and goal achievement). FACT's (2015) *Quality Handbook: A Guide to Implementing Quality Management in Cellular Therapy Organizations* provides a thorough overview of quality programs and the required elements, along with examples from many organizations.

Accreditation, Regulation, and the Quality Plan

The accreditation process not only offers the transplantation community's best consensus on quality indicators

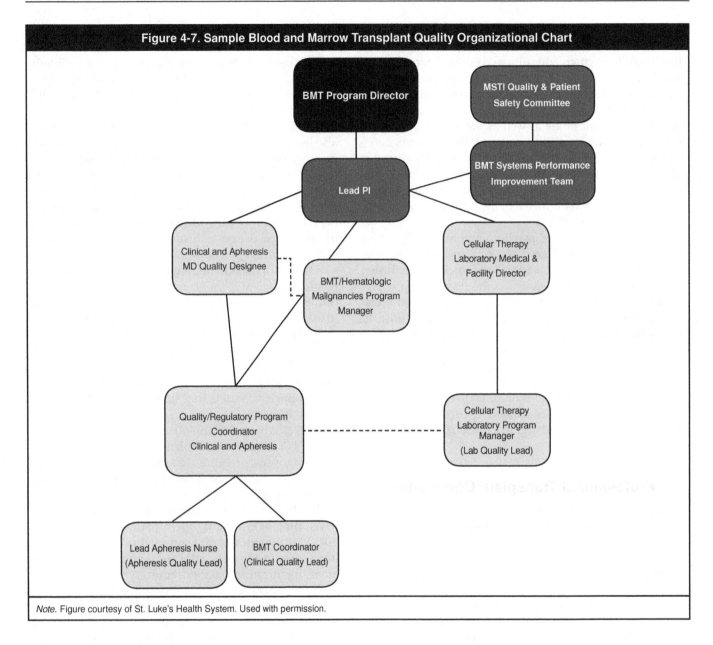

Figure 4-7. Sample Blood and Marrow Transplant Quality Organizational Chart

BMT Program Director

MSTI Quality & Patient Safety Committee

Lead PI

BMT Systems Performance Improvement Team

Clinical and Apheresis MD Quality Designee

BMT/Hematologic Malignancies Program Manager

Cellular Therapy Laboratory Medical & Facility Director

Quality/Regulatory Program Coordinator Clinical and Apheresis

Cellular Therapy Laboratory Program Manager (Lab Quality Lead)

Lead Apheresis Nurse (Apheresis Quality Lead)

BMT Coordinator (Clinical Quality Lead)

Note. Figure courtesy of St. Luke's Health System. Used with permission.

but also provides a structure and process for implementing the quality plan. Accreditation standards provide the minimum guidelines for facilities performing cellular therapy or cord blood banking or providing support services for such activities.

An active quality committee strengthens the transplant program (Rice & Bailey, 2009). "The committee can provide organization and structure to a program and be a key component in mitigating the many different institutional forces that can impact the HSCT program" (Rice & Bailey, 2009, p. 157). Additionally, the committee brings together the variety of disciplines and practice settings that must function as an integrated whole in the delivery of transplant care to focus each group's contribution to the overall program, such as the cytotherapy laboratory, apheresis services, social work and spiritual care, nursing, medicine, rehabilitative services,

food and nutrition services, and hospital administration (Rice & Bailey, 2009).

The regulatory environment is another important dimension of quality management and must be incorporated in quality management planning. National and international regulations are in place to ensure quality and safety of the final cell products intended for clinical use. Implementation of principles of good manufacturing practice and a quality control system is a major requirement. Good manufacturing practice regulations apply to all phases of cell collection, processing, and storage and to documentation, training of personnel, and cell processing equipment (Aktas et al., 2010; U.S. Food and Drug Administration, 2018). They must be followed by pharmaceutical companies and physicians involved in cell processing at academic institutions and cell therapy laboratories. The complex regulatory network for manufacturing cell products helps to standardize these procedures and ensure consistent quality and patient safety (Bailey, Arcidiacono, Benton, Taraporewala, & Winitsky, 2015).

Outcomes: Data, Reporting, and the Stem Cell Therapeutic Outcomes Database

As the FACT quality management standards make abundantly clear, data collection, analysis, and reporting are pivotal elements of quality management. In its 2006 *White Paper on Measurement of Quality Outcomes*, the ASTCT Committee on Hematopoietic Cell Therapy Quality Outcomes (Jones et al., 2006) developed recommendations for center-specific outcome reporting. These recommendations have guided both FACT accreditation standards and the federally mandated SCTOD, one component of the C.W. Bill Young Cell Transplantation Program (U.S. Department of Health and Human Services Health Resources and Services Administration, n.d.). The C.W. Bill Young Cell Transplantation Program legislation (Stem Cell Therapeutic and Research Act of 2005, as well as its reauthorization acts in 2010 and 2015) required analyses and reporting of transplant outcomes on a center-by-center basis and making those reports available to the public. Three transplant outcome reports are now provided: U.S. Patient Survival Report, U.S. Transplant Data by Center Report, and U.S. Transplant Data by Disease Report. CIBMTR developed a standard set of data elements to be collected for all transplant recipients to facilitate research, minimize the burden of data collection required by SCTOD, and ensure collection of the most relevant data. Their standardized data collection forms are available at www.cibmtr.org/Data Management/DataCollectionForms/Pages/index.aspx. ASTCT (2019) developed a standardized form for reporting transplant center information and treatment outcome data to third-party payers, containing additional measures to those required for reporting by FACT, CIBMTR, and/or the European Society for Blood and Marrow Transplantation. The request-for-information forms have been reviewed and accepted by many health insurance companies and often are required to gain approval as a Center of Excellence. Current versions of these forms should be consulted for data elements to incorporate into the collection and audit process (see www.astct.org/practice-resources/rfi-forms).

Effective and thorough quality management must be a cornerstone of the transplant program, comprehensive across all components of the program, integrated into the larger institution's quality program, and aligned with national quality and safety goals. Nurses in multiple roles are key in the development and ongoing refinement of the quality management plan and clinical policies and procedures. Accrediting bodies and national organizations offer a wealth of information and guidance on the best ways to accomplish this. Additional resources exist in the nursing literature that support the role of nursing in quality improvement and provide examples on methods of evaluating and implementing quality (Harris, Roussel, Dearman, & Thomas, 2020; Hickey & Brosnan, 2012).

Summary

HSCT is a constantly evolving and ever-changing field that has grown and matured over the past 50 years. Advances in scientific understanding have led to new stem cell technologies and to the new field of regenerative medicine with great promise for treating malignant and nonmalignant diseases. Expansion of HSCT to new groups of patients, innovations allowing outpatient care delivery, and increased complexities of treatment regimens have affected nursing practice. Transplant programs are no longer inpatient based. Nurses now provide comprehensive, coordinated care across settings to new patient groups with different needs. Along with scientific advances have come increasingly complex regulatory and reporting requirements, more intensive resource utilization, and greater economic demands. Quality standards have been developed, and transplant programs must demonstrate compliance through an international accreditation process. As transplant medicine and laboratory science have developed quality measures, so too must transplant nurses identify quality standards for education, patient care practices, and other pertinent areas of nursing science. Nurses at all levels make important contributions to this effort. Health care will continue to incorporate new information that will affect oncology and transplantation. Impending shortages of nurses, physicians, and other healthcare workers over the next 10 years will necessitate creative solutions. Nurses will continually be challenged to bridge new technologies with compassionate, caring environments.

The authors would like to acknowledge Kathleen Clifford, RN, MSN, FNP-BC, AOCNP®, and Julie Hall, MPH, RN, OCN®, for their contribution to this chapter that remains unchanged from the previous edition of this book.

References

Abou-Nassar, K.E., Kim, H.T., Blossom, J., Ho, V.T., Soiffer, R.J., Cutler, C.S., … Armand, P. (2012). The impact of geographic proximity to transplant center on outcomes after allogeneic hematopoietic stem cell transplantation. *Biology of Blood and Marrow Transplantation, 18*, 708–715. https://doi.org/10.1016/j.bbmt.2011.08.022

Afessa, B., & Azoulay, E. (2010). Critical care of the hematopoietic stem cell transplant recipient. *Critical Care Clinics, 26*, 133–150. https://doi.org/10.1016/j.ccc.2009.09.001

Aktas, M., Buchheiser, A., Houben, A., Reimann, V., Radke, T., Jeltsch, K., … Kogler, G. (2010). Good manufacturing practice-grade production of unrestricted somatic stem cell from fresh cord blood. *Cytotherapy, 12*, 338–348. https://doi.org/10.3109/14653241003695034

American Society for Clinical Pathology Board of Certification. (2018, September). *Qualification in Apheresis (QIA) examination topic outline.* Retrieved from https://www.ascp.org/content/docs/default-source/boc-pdfs/boc-us-guidelines/qia_topic_outline.pdf

American Society for Transplantation and Cellular Therapy. (n.d.). Nurse Practitioner and Physician Assistant SIG. Retrieved from https://www.astct.org/special-interest-groups/nurse-practitioner-and-physician-assistant-sig

American Society for Transplantation and Cellular Therapy. (2019). RFI forms. Retrieved from https://www.astct.org/practice-resources/rfi-forms

Andrykowski, M.A., Bishop, M.M., Hahn, E.A., Cella, D.F., Beaumont, J.L., Brady, M.J., … Wingard, J.R. (2005). Long-term health-related quality of life, growth, and spiritual well-being after hematopoietic stem-cell transplantation. *Journal of Clinical Oncology, 23*, 599–608. https://doi.org/10.1200/JCO.2005.03.189

Applebaum, A.J., Bevans, M., Son, T., Evans, K., Hernandez, M., Giralt, S., & DuHamel, K. (2016). A scoping review of caregiver burden during allogeneic HSCT: Lessons learned and future directions. *Bone Marrow Transplantation, 51*, 1416–1422. https://doi.org/10.1038/bmt.2016.164

ASBMT and CBMTG release Choosing Wisely BMT recommendations. (2018). *Biology of Blood and Marrow Transplantation, 24*, 880–881. https://doi.org/10.1016/j.bbmt.2018.03.020

Bailey, A.M., Arcidiacono, J., Benton, K.A., Taraporewala, Z., & Winitsky, S. (2015). United States Food and Drug Administration regulation of gene and cell therapies. In M. Galli & M. Serabian (Eds.), *Advances in Experimental Medicine and Biology: Regulatory aspects of gene therapy and cell therapy products* (Vol. 871, pp. 1–29). https://doi.org/10.1007/978-3-319-18618-4_1

Balboni, T.A., Vanderwerker, L.C., Block, S.D., Paulk, M.E., Lathan, C.S., Peteet, J.R., & Prigerson, H.G. (2007). Religiousness and spiritual support among advanced cancer patients and associations with end-of-life treatment preferences and quality of life. *Journal of Clinical Oncology, 25*, 555–560. https://doi.org/10.1200/JCO.2006.07.9046

Baliousis, M., Rennoldson, M., & Snowden, J.A. (2016). Psychological interventions for distress in adults undergoing hematopoietic stem cell transplantation: A systematic review with meta-analysis. *Psycho-Oncology, 25*, 400–411. https://doi.org/10.1002/pon.3925

Battiwalla, M., Tichelli, A., & Majhail, N.S. (2017). Long-term survivorship after hematopoietic cell transplantation: Roadmap for research and care. *Biology of Blood and Marrow Transplantation, 23*, 184–192. https://doi.org/10.1016/j.bbmt.2016.11.004

Baumann, F.T., Kraut, L., Schüle, K., Bloch, W., & Fauser, A.A. (2010). A controlled randomized study examining the effects of exercise therapy on patients undergoing haematopoietic stem cell transplantation. *Bone Marrow Transplantation, 45*, 355–362. https://doi.org/10.1038/bmt.2009.163

Beattie, S., Lebel, S., Petricone-Westwood, D., Wilson, K.G., Harris, C., Devins, G., … Tay, J. (2017). Balancing give and take between patients and their spousal caregivers in hematopoietic stem cell transplantation. *Psycho-Oncology, 26*, 2224–2231. https://doi.org/10.1002/pon.4340

Beattie, S., Lebel, S., & Tay, J. (2013). The influence of social support on hematopoietic stem cell transplantation survival: A systematic review of literature. *PLOS ONE, 8*, e61586. https://doi.org/10.1371/journal.pone.0061586

Benz, R., Schanz, U., Maggiorini, M., Seebach, J.D., & Stussi, G. (2014). Risk factors for ICU admission and ICU survival after allogeneic hematopoietic SCT. *Bone Marrow Transplantation, 49*, 62–65. https://doi.org/10.1038/bmt.2013.141

Bergkvist, K., Fossum, B., Johansson, U.-B., Mattsson, J., & Larsen, J. (2018). Patients' experiences of different care settings and a new life situation after allogeneic haematopoietic stem cell transplantation. *European Journal of Cancer Care, 27*, e12672. https://doi.org/10.1111/ecc.12672

Berry, L.L., Dalwadi, S.M., & Jacobson, J.O. (2017). Supporting the supporters: What family caregivers need to care for a loved one with cancer. *Journal of Oncology Practice, 13*, 35–41. https://doi.org/10.1200/JOP.2016.017913

Bevans, M.F., Coleman, M., Jadalla, A., Page, M., & Cagle, C.S. (2019, December 3). Symptom interventions: Caregiver strain and burden. Retrieved from https://www.ons.org/pep/caregiver-strain-and-burden

Bevans, M.F., Marden, S., Leidy, N.K., Soeken, K., Cusack, G., Rivera, P., … Barrett, A.J. (2006). Health-related quality of life in patients receiving reduced-intensity conditioning allogeneic hematopoietic stem cell transplantation. *Bone Marrow Transplantation, 38*, 101–109. https://doi.org/10.1038/sj.bmt.1705406

Bevans, M.F., Tierney, D.K., Bruch, C., Burgunder, M., Castro, K., Ford, R., … Schmit-Pokorny, K. (2009). Hematopoietic stem cell transplantation nursing: A practice variation study [Online exclusive]. *Oncology Nursing Forum, 36*, E317–E325. https://doi.org/10.1188/09.ONF.E317-E325

Boise woman receives first allogeneic transplant in Idaho. (2018, May 18). Retrieved from https://www.apnews.com/46706961bdd24441ae73dbbae325e3f6

Brandeis, A. (2016, October 24). Critical blood cancer treatment now available in Austin. Retrieved from https://www.kxan.com/news/critical-blood-cancer-treatment-now-available-in-austin

Broder, M.S., Quock, T.P., Chang, E., Reddy, S.R., Agarwal-Hashmi, R., Arai, S., & Villa, K.F. (2017). The cost of hematopoietic stem-cell transplantation in the United States. *American Health and Drug Benefits, 10*, 366–373. Retrieved from http://www.ahdbonline.com/issues/2017/october-2017-vol-10-no-7/2493-the-cost-of-hematopoietic-stem-cell-transplantation-in-the-united-states

Brown, S.L., & Faltus, K.J. (2011). Hematologic malignancy education for stem cell transplantation nurses. *Oncology Nursing Forum, 38*, 401–402. https://doi.org/10.1188/11.ONF.401-402

Buchsel, P.C., & Whedon, M.B. (Eds.). (1995). *Bone marrow transplantation: Administrative and clinical strategies*. Burlington, MA: Jones & Bartlett Learning.

Burns, L.J., Gajewski, J.L., Majhail, N.S., Navarro, W., Perales, M.-A., Shereck, E., … Litzow, M.R. (2014). Challenges and potential solutions for recruitment and retention of hematopoietic cell transplantation physicians: The National Marrow Donor Program's System Capacity Initiative Physician Workforce Group report. *Biology of Blood and Marrow Transplantation, 20*, 617–621. https://doi.org/10.1016/j.bbmt.2014.01.028

Cantrell, M.A. (2007). The art of pediatric oncology nursing practice. *Journal of Pediatric Oncology Nursing, 24*, 132–138. https://doi.org/10.1177/1043454206298842

Cappell, K., Sundaram, V., Park, A., Shiraz, P., Gupta, R., Jenkins, P., … Muffly, L. (2018). Advance directive utilization is associated with less aggressive end-of-life care in patients undergoing allogeneic hematopoietic cell transplantation. *Biology of Blood and Marrow Transplantation, 24*, 1035–1040. https://doi.org/10.1016/j.bbmt.2018.01.014

Center for International Blood and Marrow Transplant Research. (2019, June 25). What we do. Retrieved from http://www.cibmtr.org/About/WhatWeDo/Pages/index.aspx

Chieng, R., Coutsouvelis, J., Poole, S., Dooley, M.J., Booth, D., & Wei, A. (2013). Improving the transition of highly complex patients into the community: Impact of a pharmacist in an allogeneic stem cell transplant (SCT) outpatient clinic. *Supportive Care in Cancer, 21*, 3491–3495. https://doi.org/10.1007/s00520-013-1938-9

Clemmons, A.B., Alexander, M., DeGregory, K., & Kennedy, L. (2018). The hematopoietic cell transplant pharmacist: Roles, responsibilities, and recommendations from the ASBMT Pharmacy Special Interest Group. *Biology of Blood and Marrow Transplantation, 24*, 914–922. https://doi.org/10.1016/j.bbmt.2017.12.803

Cooke, L.D., Gemmill, R., & Grant, M.L. (2008). Advanced practice nurses core competencies: A framework for developing and testing an advanced practice nurse discharge intervention. *Clinical Nurse Specialist, 22*, 218–225. https://doi.org/10.1097/01.NUR.0000325366.15927.2d

Cooke, L.D., Gemmill, R., & Grant, M.L. (2011). Creating a palliative educational session for hematopoietic stem cell transplantation recipients at relapse. *Clinical Journal of Oncology Nursing, 15*, 411–417. https://doi.org/10.1188/11.CJON.411-417

Cooke, L.D., Gemmill, R., Kravits, K., & Grant, M.L. (2009). Psychological issues of stem cell transplant. *Seminars in Oncology Nursing, 25*, 139–150. https://doi.org/10.1016/j.soncn.2009.03.008

Eilers, J., & Breen, A. (2007). Family issues and perspectives. In S. Ezzone & K. Schmit-Pokorny (Eds.), *Blood and marrow stem cell transplantation: Principles, practice, and nursing insights* (3rd ed., pp. 339–367). Burlington, MA: Jones & Bartlett Learning.

El-Jawahri, A., LeBlanc, T., VanDusen, H., Traeger, L., Greer, J.A., Pirl, W.F., … Temel, J.S. (2016). Effect of inpatient palliative care on quality of life 2 weeks after hematopoietic stem cell transplantation: A randomized clinical trial. *JAMA, 316*, 2094–2103. https://doi.org/10.1001/jama.2016.16786

Ezzone, S.A. (2009). Patient and family caregiver teaching. In P.C. Buchsel & P.M. Kapustay (Eds.), *Stem cell transplantation: A clinical textbook* (pp. 6.1–6.10). Pittsburgh, PA: Oncology Nursing Society.

Ezzone, S.A., Fliedner, M., & Sirilla, J. (2007). Transplant networks and standards of care: International perspectives. In S.A. Ezzone &

K. Schmit-Pokorny (Eds.), *Blood and marrow stem cell transplantation: Principles, practice, and nursing insights* (3rd ed., pp. 441–462). Burlington, MA: Jones & Bartlett Learning.

Ezzone, S.A., & Schmit-Pokorny, K. (Eds.). (2007). *Blood and marrow stem cell transplantation: Principles, practice, and nursing insights* (3rd ed.). Burlington, MA: Jones & Bartlett Learning.

Family Caregiver Alliance. (2016). Caregiver statistics: Work and caregiving. Retrieved from https://www.caregiver.org/caregiver-statistics-work-and-caregiving

Faucher, C., Le Corroller Soriano, A.G., Esterni, B., Vey, N., Stoppa, A.M., Chabannon, C., … Blaise, D. (2011). Randomized study of early hospital discharge following autologous blood SCT: Medical outcomes and hospital costs. *Bone Marrow Transplantation, 47,* 549–555. https://doi.org/10.1038/bmt.2011.126

Fillion, L., Cook, S., Veillette, A., de Serres, M., Aubin, M., Rainville, F., … Doll, R. (2012). Professional navigation: A comparative study of two Canadian models. *Canadian Oncology Nursing Journal, 22,* 257–277. https://doi.org/10.5737/1181912x224257266

Ford, R.C., Wickline, M.M., & Heye, D. (2016). Nursing role in hematopoietic cell transplantation. In S.J. Forman, R.S. Negrin, J.H. Antin, & F.R. Appelbaum (Eds.), *Thomas' hematopoietic cell transplantation* (5th ed., pp. 362–374). https://doi.org/10.1002/9781118416426.ch30

Foster, L.W., McLellan, L., Rybicki, L., Dabney, J., Copelan, E., & Bolwell, B. (2013). Validating the positive impact of in-hospital lay care-partner support on patient survival in allogeneic BMT: A prospective study. *Bone Marrow Transplantation, 48,* 671–677. https://doi.org/10.1038/bmt.2012.208

Foster, L.W., McLellan, L., Rybicki, L., Dabney, J., Visnosky, M., & Bolwell, B. (2009). Utility of the Psychosocial Assessment of Candidates for Transplantation (PACT) scale in allogeneic BMT. *Bone Marrow Transplantation, 44,* 375–390. https://doi.org/10.1038/bmt.2009.37

Foundation for the Accreditation of Cellular Therapy. (2015). *FACT quality handbook: A guide to implementing quality management in cellular therapy organizations* (2nd ed.). Omaha, NE: Author.

Foundation for the Accreditation of Cellular Therapy & Joint Accreditation Committee–ISCT and EBMT. (2018). *FACT-JACIE international standards for hematopoietic cellular therapy product collection, processing, and administration* (7th ed.). Retrieved from https://www.ebmt.org/sites/default/files/2018-06/FACT-JACIE%207th%20Edition%20Standards.pdf

Gajewski, J.L., LeMaistre, C.F., Silver, S.M., Lill, M.C., Selby, G.B., Horowitz, M.M., … Maziarz, R.T. (2009). Impending challenges in the hematopoietic stem cell transplantation physician workforce. *Biology of Blood and Marrow Transplantation, 15,* 1493–1501. https://doi.org/10.1016/j.bbmt.2009.08.022

Gosselin, T.K., Dalton, K.A., & Penne, K. (2015). The role of the advanced practice nurse in the academic setting. *Seminars in Oncology Nursing, 31,* 290–297. https://doi.org/10.1016/j.soncn.2015.08.005

Graff, T.M., Singavi, A.K., Schmidt, W., Eastwood, D., Drobyski, W.R., Horowitz, M., … Fenske, T.S. (2015). Safety of outpatient autologous hematopoietic cell transplantation for multiple myeloma and lymphoma. *Bone Marrow Transplantation, 50,* 947–953. https://doi.org/10.1038/bmt.2015.46

Gratwohl, A., Brand, R., McGrath, E., van Biezen, A., Sureda, A., Ljungman, P., … Apperley, J. (2014). Use of the quality management system "JACIE" and outcome after hematopoietic stem cell transplantation. *Haematologica, 99,* 908–915. https://doi.org/10.3324/haematol.2013.096461

Harris, J.L., Roussel, L., Dearman, C., & Thomas, P. (2020). *Project planning and management: A guide for nurses and interprofessional teams* (3rd ed.). Burlington, MA: Jones & Bartlett Learning.

Hashmi, S., Carpenter, P., Khera, N., Tichelli, A., & Savani, B.N. (2015). Lost in transition: The essential need for long-term follow-up clinic for blood and marrow transplantation survivors. *Biology of Blood and Marrow Transplantation, 21,* 225–232. https://doi.org/10.1016/j.bbmt.2014.06.035

Hashmi, S.K., Srivastava, A., Rasheed, W., Adil, S., Wu, T., Jagasia, M., … Aljurf, M. (2017). Cost and quality issues in establishing hematopoietic cell transplant program in developing countries. *Hematology/Oncology and Stem Cell Therapy, 10,* 167–172. https://doi.org/10.1016/j.hemonc.2017.05.017

Henig, I., & Zuckerman, T. (2014). Hematopoietic stem cell transplantation—50 years of evolution and future perspectives

[Abstract]. *Rambam Maimonides Medical Journal, 5,* e0028. https://doi.org/10.5041/RMMJ.10162

Hickey, J.V., & Brosnan, C.A. (2012). *Evaluation of health care quality in advanced practice nursing.* New York, NY: Springer.

Ho, L., Akada, K., Messner, H., Kuruvilla, J., Wright, J., & Seki, J.T. (2013). Pharmacist's role in improving medication safety for patients in an allogeneic hematopoietic cell transplant ambulatory clinic. *Canadian Journal of Hospital Pharmacy, 66,* 110–117. https://doi.org/10.4212/cjhp.v66i2.1233

Holbro, A., Ahmad, I., Cohen, S., Roy, J., Lachance, S., Chagnon, M., … Kiss, T.L. (2013). Safety and cost-effectiveness of outpatient autologous stem cell transplantation in patients with multiple myeloma. *Biology of Blood and Marrow Transplantation, 19,* 547–551. https://doi.org/10.1016/j.bbmt.2012.12.006

Hussain, F., Chaudhri, N., Alfraih, F., & Aljurf, M. (2017). Current concepts on hematopoietic stem cell transplantation outcome registries; Emphases on resource requirements for new registries. *Hematology/Oncology and Stem Cell Therapy, 10,* 203–210. https://doi.org/10.1016/j.hemonc.2017.05.011

Ibanez, K., Espiritu, N., Souverain, R.L., Stimler, L., Ward, L., Riedel, E.R., … Stubblefield, M.D. (2018). Safety and feasibility of rehabilitation interventions in children undergoing hematopoietic stem cell transplant with thrombocytopenia. *Archives of Physical Medicine and Rehabilitation, 99,* 226–233. https://doi.org/10.1016/j.apmr.2017.06.034

Ignoffo, R., Knapp, K., Barnett, M., Barbour, S.Y., D'Amato, S., Iacovelli, L., … Trovato, J. (2016). Board-certified oncology pharmacists: Their potential contribution to reducing a shortfall in oncology patient visits. *Journal of Oncology Practice, 12,* e359–e368. https://doi.org/10.1200/JOP.2015.008490

Ikeda, K., Nollet, K.E., Vrielink, H., & Ohto, H. (2018). Apheresis education and certification for nurses. *Transfusion and Apheresis Science, 57,* 635–638. https://doi.org/10.1016/j.transci.2018.09.010

Jenkins, P., Johnston, L.J., Pickham, D., Chang, B., Rizk, N., & Tierney, D.K. (2015). Intensive care utilization for hematopoietic cell transplant recipients. *Biology of Blood and Marrow Transplantation, 21,* 2023–2027. https://doi.org/10.1016/j.bbmt.2015.07.026

Johnson, S. (2014). It takes a team: Creating a hematology/hematopoietic cell therapy day hospital. *Nursing Administration Quarterly, 38,* 206–213. https://doi.org/10.1097/NAQ.0000000000000038

Jones, R.B., Anasetti, C., Appel, P., DiPersio, J., Heslop, H., Lemaistre, F., … Stiff, P. (2006). White paper on measurement of quality outcomes. *Biology of Blood and Marrow Transplantation, 12,* 594–597. https://doi.org/10.1016/j.bbmt.2006.04.001

Kershaw, T., Ellis, K.R., Yoon, H., Schafenacker, A., Katapodi, M., & Northouse, L. (2015). The interdependence of advanced cancer patients' and their family caregivers' mental health, physical health, and self-efficacy over time. *Annals of Behavioral Medicine, 49,* 901–911. https://doi.org/10.1007/s12160-015-9743-y

Khera, N., Gooley, T., Flowers, M.E.D., Sandmaier, B.M., Loberiza, F., Lee, S.J., & Appelbaum, F. (2016). Association of distance from transplantation center and place of residence on outcomes after allogeneic hematopoietic cell transplantation. *Biology of Blood and Marrow Transplantation, 22,* 1319–1323. https://doi.org/10.1016/j.bbmt.2016.03.019

Khera, N., Martin, P., Edsall, K., Bonagura, A., Burns, L.J., Juckett, M., … Majhail, N.S. (2017). Patient-centered care coordination in hematopoietic cell transplantation. *Blood Advances, 22,* 1617–1627. https://doi.org/10.1182/bloodadvances.2017008789

Knols, R.H., de Bruin, E.D., Uebelhart, D., Aufdemkampe, G., Schanz, U., Stenner-Liewen, F., … Aaronson, N.K. (2011). Effects of an outpatient physical exercise program on hematopoietic stem-cell transplantation recipients: A randomized clinical trial. *Bone Marrow Transplantation, 46,* 1245–1255. https://doi.org/10.1038/bmt.2010.288

Knopf, K.E. (2011). Core competencies for bone marrow transplantation nurse practitioners. *Clinical Journal of Oncology Nursing, 15,* 102–105. https://doi.org/10.1188/11.CJON.102-105

Kunkel, S., Rosenqvist, U., & Westerling, R. (2007). The structure of quality systems is important to the process and outcome, an empirical study of 386 hospital departments in Sweden. *BMC Health Services Research, 7,* 104. https://doi.org/10.1186/1472-6963-7-104

Langer, S.L., Kelly, T.H., Storer, B.E., Hall, S.P., Lucas, H.G., & Syrjala, K.L. (2012). Expressive talking among caregivers of hematopoietic stem cell transplant survivors: Acceptability and concurrent subjective, objective, and physiologic indicators of emotion. *Journal of Psychosocial Oncology, 30,* 294–315. https://doi.org/10.1080/07347332.2012.664255

Laudenslager, M.L., Simoneau, T.L., Kilbourn, K., Natvig, C., Philips, S., Spradley, J., … Mikulich-Gilbertson, S.K. (2015). A randomized control trial of a psychosocial intervention for caregivers of allogeneic hematopoietic stem cell transplant patients: Effects on distress. *Bone Marrow Transplantation, 50,* 1110–1118. https://doi.org/10.1038/bmt.2015.104

Leemhuis, T., Padley, D., Keever-Taylor, C., Niederwieser, D., Teshima, T., Lanza, F., … Koh, M.B.C. (2014). Essential requirements for setting up a stem cell processing laboratory. *Bone Marrow Transplantation, 49,* 1098–1105. https://doi.org/10.1038/bmt.2014.104

Leeson, L.A., Nelson, A.M., Rathouz, P.J., Juckett, M.B., Coe, C.L., Caes, E.W., & Costanzo, E.S. (2015). Spirituality and the recovery of quality of life following hematopoietic stem cell transplantation. *Health Psychology, 34,* 920–928. https://doi.org/10.1037/hea0000196

LeMaistre, C.F., & Farnia, S.H. (2015). Goals for pay for performance in hematopoietic cell transplantation: A primer. *Biology of Blood and Marrow Transplantation, 21,* 1367–1372. https://doi.org/10.1016/j.bbmt.2015.04.014

Lengliné, E., Chevret, S., Moreau, A.-S., Péne, F., Blot, F., Bourhis, J.-H., … Azoulay, E. (2015). Changes in intensive care for allogeneic hematopoietic stem cell transplant recipients. *Bone Marrow Transplantation, 50,* 840–845. https://doi.org/10.1038/bmt.2015.55

Lippert, M., Semmens, S., Tacey, L., Rent, T., Defoe, K., Bucsis, M., … Lafay-Cousin, L. (2017). The Hospital at Home program: No place like home. *Current Oncology, 24,* 23–27. https://doi.org/10.3747/co.24.3326

Lisenko, K., Sauer, S., Bruckner, T., Egerer, G., Goldschmidt, H., Hillengass, J., … Wuchter, P. (2017). High-dose chemotherapy and autologous stem cell transplantation of patients with multiple myeloma in an outpatient setting. *BMC Cancer, 17,* 151. https://doi.org/10.1186/s12885-017-3137-4

Lohr, K.N. (Ed.). (1990). *Medicare: A strategy for quality assurance, volume I.* https://doi.org/10.17226/1547

Majolino, I., Othman, D., Rovelli, A., Hassan, D., Rasool, L., Vacca, M., … Girmenia, C. (2017). The start-up of the first hematopoietic stem cell transplantation center in the Iraqi Kurdistan: A capacity-building cooperative project by the Hiwa Cancer Hospital, Sulaymaniyah, and the Italian Agency for Development Cooperation: An innovative approach. *Mediterranean Journal of Hematology and Infectious Diseases, 9,* e2017031. https://doi.org/10.4084/mjhid.2017.031

Martino, M., Ciavarella, S., De Summa, S., Russo, L., Miliambro, N., Imbalzano, L., … Guarini, A. (2018). A comparative assessment of quality of life in patients with multiple myeloma undergoing autologous stem cell transplantation through an outpatient and inpatient model. *Biology of Blood and Marrow Transplantation, 24,* 608–613. https://doi.org/10.1016/j.bbmt.2017.09.021

Martino, M., Lemoli, R.M., Girmenia, C., Castagna, L., Bruno, B., Cavallo, F., … Olivieri, A. (2016). Italian consensus conference for the outpatient autologous stem cell transplantation management in multiple myeloma. *Bone Marrow Transplantation, 51,* 1032–1040. https://doi.org/10.1038/bmt.2016.79

McArdle, J.R. (2009). Critical care outcomes in the hematologic transplant recipient. *Clinics in Chest Medicine, 30,* 155–167. https://doi.org/10.1016/j.ccm.2008.10.002

McDiarmid, S., Hutton, B., Atkins, H., Bence-Bruckler, I., Bredeson, C., Sabri, E., & Huebsch, L. (2010). Performing allogeneic and autologous hematopoietic SCT in the outpatient setting: Effects on infectious complications and early transplant outcomes. *Bone Marrow Transplantation, 45,* 1220–1226. https://doi.org/10.1038/bmt.2009.330

McMullen, L. (2013). Oncology nurse navigators and the continuum of cancer care. *Seminars in Oncology Nursing, 29,* 105–117. https://doi.org/10.1016/j.soncn.2013.02.005

McNeely, M.L., Dolgoy, N., Onazi, M.A., & Suderman, K. (2016). The interdisciplinary rehabilitation care team and the role of physical therapy in survivor exercise. *Clinical Journal of Oncology Nursing, 20*(Suppl. 6), 8–16. https://doi.org/10.1188/16.CJON.S2.8-16

Mehta, J., & Dulley, F.L. (2009). Outpatient or inpatient stem cell transplantation: *Patria est ubicunque est bene? Leukemia and Lymphoma, 50,* 3–5. https://doi.org/10.1080/10428190802578858

Mitchell, S., Lindstrom, S.L., Jackson, M.I., Ulrickson, M.L., Wright, S., & Akpek, G. (2016). The challenges of opening a new stem cell trans-

plant program in today's healthcare environment [Abstract]. *Biology of Blood and Marrow Transplantation, 22*(Suppl.), S431–S432. https://doi.org/10.1016/j.bbmt.2015.11.989

Mosher, C.E., Redd, W.H., Rini, C.M., Burkhalter, J.E., & DuHamel, K.N. (2009). Physical, psychological, and social sequelae following hematopoietic stem cell transplantation: A review of the literature. *Psycho-Oncology, 18,* 113–127. https://doi.org/10.1002/pon.1399

National Comprehensive Cancer Network. (2019). *NCCN Clinical Practice Guidelines in Oncology (NCCN Guidelines®): Distress management* [v.3.2019]. Retrieved from https://www.nccn.org/professionals/physician_gls/pdf/distress.pdf

National Marrow Donor Program/Be The Match Social Work Workforce Group. (2017, June). BMT clinical social worker role description. Retrieved from https://higherlogicdownload.s3.amazonaws.com/ASBMT/43a1f41f-55cb-4c97-9e78-c03e867db505/UploadedImages/BMT_Clinical_Social_Worker_Role_Description_2017.pdf

Nemec, R. (2017). Apheresis education: One center curriculum design experience. *Transfusion and Apheresis Science, 56,* 263–267. https://doi.org/10.1016/j.transci.2017.03.012

Oberoi, S., Robinson, P.D., Cataudella, D., Culos-Reed, S.N., Davis, H., Duong, N., … Sung, L. (2018). Physical activity reduces fatigue in patients with cancer and hematopoietic stem cell transplant recipients: A systematic review and meta-analysis of randomized trials. *Critical Reviews in Oncology/Hematology, 122,* 52–59. https://doi.org/10.1016/j.critrevonc.2017.12.011

Oncology Nursing Certification Corporation. (2017). *Blood and Marrow Transplant Certified Nurse (BMTCN®) test content outline.* Retrieved from https://www.oncc.org/files/2018BMTCNTestContentOutline.pdf

Oncology Nursing Society. (2008). *Oncology clinical nurse specialist competencies.* Retrieved from https://www.ons.org/oncology-clinical-nurse-specialist-competencies

Oncology Nursing Society. (2017). *2017 oncology nurse navigator core competencies.* Retrieved from https://www.ons.org/oncology-nurse-navigator-competencies

Oncology Nursing Society. (2019). *Oncology nurse practitioner competencies.* Retrieved from https://www.ons.org/oncology-nurse-practitioner-competencies

Ouseph, R., Croy, C., Natvig, C., Simoneau, T., & Laudenslager, M.L. (2014). Decreased mental health care utilization following a psychosocial intervention in caregivers of hematopoietic stem cell transplant patients. *Mental Illness, 6,* 5120. https://doi.org/10.4081/mi.2014.5120

Pagano, M.B., Wehrli, G., Cloutier, D., Karr, E.G., Lopez-Plaza, I., Schwartz, J., … Zantek, N.D. (2017). Apheresis medicine education in the United States of America: State of the discipline. *Transfusion and Apheresis Science, 56,* 1–5. https://doi.org/10.1016/j.transci.2016.12.004

Penalba, V., Asvat, Y., Deshields, T.L., Vanderlan, J.R., & Chol, N. (2018). Rates and predictors of psychotherapy utilization after psychosocial evaluation for stem cell transplant. *Psycho-Oncology, 27,* 427–433. https://doi.org/10.1002/pon.4473

Pène, F., Aubron, C., Azoulay, E., Blot, F., Thiéry, G., Raynard, B., … Mira, J.P. (2006). Outcome of critically ill allogeneic hematopoietic stem-cell transplantation recipients: A reappraisal of indications for organ failure supports. *Journal of Clinical Oncology, 24,* 643–649. https://doi.org/10.1200/JCO.2005.03.9073

Perica, K., Curran, K.J., Brentjens, R.J., & Giralt, S.A. (2018). Building a CAR garage: Preparing for the delivery of commercial CAR T cell products at Memorial Sloan Kettering Cancer Center. *Biology of Blood and Marrow Transplantation, 24,* 1135–1141. https://doi.org/10.1016/j.bbmt.2018.02.018

Peters, W.P., Ross, M., Vredenburgh, J.J., Hussein, A., Rubin, P., Dukelow, K., … Kasprzak, S. (1994). The use of intensive clinic support to permit outpatient autologous bone marrow transplantation for breast cancer. *Seminars in Oncology, 21*(4, Suppl. 7), 25–31.

Potter, R. (2007). The bone marrow and blood stem cell transplant marketplace. In S. Ezzone & K. Schmit-Pokorny (Eds.), *Blood and marrow stem cell transplantation: Principles, practice, and nursing insights* (3rd ed., pp. 463–478). Burlington, MA: Jones & Bartlett Learning.

Rice, R.D., & Bailey, G. (2009). Management issues in hematopoietic stem cell transplantation. *Seminars in Oncology Nursing, 25,* 151–158. https://doi.org/10.1016/j.soncn.2009.03.009

Rimkus, C. (2010). Acute complications of stem cell transplant. *Seminars in Oncology Nursing, 25,* 129–138. https://doi.org/10.1016/j.soncn.2009.03.007

Rodkey, G.V., & Itani, K.M.F. (2009). Evaluation of healthcare quality: A tale of three giants. *American Journal of Surgery, 198*(Suppl. 5), S3–S8. https://doi.org/10.1016/j.amjsurg.2009.08.004

Runaas, L., Hanauer, D., Maher, M., Bischoff, E., Fauer, A., Hoang, T., ... Choi, S.W. (2017). BMT Roadmap: A user-centered design health information technology tool to promote patient-centered care in pediatric hematopoietic cell transplantation. *Biology of Blood and Marrow Transplantation, 23,* 813–819. https://doi.org/10.1016/j.bbmt.2017.01.080

Sabo, B.M. (2011). Compassionate presence: The meaning of hematopoietic stem cell transplant nursing. *European Journal of Oncology Nursing, 15,* 103–111. https://doi.org/10.1016/j.ejon.2010.06.006

Schmit-Pokorny, K. (2007). Blood and marrow transplantation: Indications, procedure, process. In S. Ezzone & K. Schmit-Pokorny (Eds.), *Blood and marrow stem cell transplantation: Principles, practice, and nursing insights* (3rd ed., pp. 339–367). Burlington, MA: Jones & Bartlett Learning.

Schmit-Pokorny, K., Franco, T., Frappier, B., & Vyhlidal, R.C. (2003). The Cooperative Care model: An innovative approach to deliver blood and marrow stem cell transplant care. *Clinical Journal of Oncology Nursing, 7,* 509–514, 556. https://doi.org/10.1188/03.CJON.509-514

Shelton, B.K. (2010). Admission criteria and prognostication in patients with cancer admitted to the intensive care unit. *Critical Care Clinics, 26,* 1–20. https://doi.org/10.1016/j.ccc.2009.10.003

Sherman, A.C., Plante, T.G., Simonton, S., Latif, U., & Anaissie, E.J. (2009). Prospective study of religious coping among patients undergoing autologous stem cell transplantation. *Journal of Behavioral Medicine, 32,* 118–128. https://doi.org/10.1007/s10865-008-9179-y

Silver, J.K. (2015). Cancer prehabilitation and its role in improving health outcomes and reducing health care costs. *Seminars in Oncology Nursing, 31,* 13–30. https://doi.org/10.1016/j.soncn.2014.11.003

Simoneau, T.L., Kilbourn, K., Spradley, J., & Laudenslager, M.L. (2017). An evidence-based stress management intervention for allogeneic hematopoietic stem cell transplant caregivers: Development, feasibility and acceptability. *Supportive Care in Cancer, 25,* 2515–2523. https://doi.org/10.1007/s00520-017-3660-5

Solomon, S.R., Matthews, R.H., Barreras, A.M., Bashey, A., Manion, K.L., McNatt, K., ... Holland, H.K. (2009). Outpatient myeloablative allo-SCT: A comprehensive approach yields decreased hospital utilization and low TRM. *Bone Marrow Transplantation, 45,* 468–475. https://doi.org/10.1038/bmt.2009.234

Spellecy, R., Tarima, S., Denzen, E., Moore, H., Abhyankar, S., Dawson, P., ... Majhail, N.S. (2018). Easy-to-read informed consent form for hematopoietic cell transplantation clinical trials: Results from the Blood and Marrow Transplant Clinical Trials Network 1205 study. *Biology of Blood and Marrow Transplantation, 24,* 2145–2151. https://doi.org/10.1016/j.bbmt.2018.04.014

Steinberg, A., Asher, A., Bailey, C., & Fu, J.B. (2015). The role of physical rehabilitation in stem cell transplantation patients. *Supportive Care in Cancer, 23,* 2447–2460. https://doi.org/10.1007/s00520-015-2744-3

Stem Cell Therapeutic and Research Act of 2005, Pub. L. No. 109-129.

Stiff, P., Mumby, P., Miler, L., Rodriguez, T., Parthswarthy, M., Kiley, K., ... Toor, A. (2006). Autologous hematopoietic stem cell transplants that utilize total body irradiation can safely be carried out entirely on an outpatient basis. *Bone Marrow Transplantation, 38,* 757–764. https://doi.org/10.1038/sj.bmt.1705525

Sundaramurthi, T., Wehrlen, L., Friedman, E., Thomas, S., & Bevans, M. (2017). Hematopoietic stem cell transplantation recipient and caregiver factors affecting length of stay and readmission. *Oncology Nursing Forum, 44,* 571–579. https://doi.org/10.1188/17.ONF.571-579

Svahn, B.-M., Remberger, M., Heijbel, M., Martell, E., Wikström, M., Eriksson, B., ... Ringdén, O. (2008). Case-control comparison of at-home and hospital care for allogeneic hematopoietic stem-cell transplantation: The role of nutrition. *Transplantation, 85,* 1000–1007. https://doi.org/10.1097/TP.0b013e3181 6a3267

Syrjala, K.L., Langer, S.L., Abrams, J.R., Storer, B.E., & Martin, P.J. (2005). Late effects of hematopoietic cell transplantation among 10-year adult survivors compared with case-matched controls. *Journal of Clinical Oncology, 23,* 6596–6606. https://doi.org/10.1200/JCO.2005.12.674

Thomson, B., Gorospe, G., Cooke, L., Giesie, P., & Johnson, S. (2015). Transitions of care: A hematopoietic stem cell transplantation nursing education project across the trajectory [Online exclusive]. *Clinical Journal of Oncology Nursing, 19,* E74–E79. https://doi.org/10.1188/15.CJON.E74-E79

U.S. Department of Health and Human Services Health Resources and Services Administration. (n.d.). Bone marrow and cord blood donation and transplantation. Retrieved from http://bloodcell.transplant.hrsa.gov/index.html

U.S. Food and Drug Administration. (2018, June 25). Facts about the current good manufacturing practices (CGMPs). Retrieved from https://www.fda.gov/Drugs/DevelopmentApprovalProcess/manufacturing/ucm169105.htm

Wilson, M.E., Eilers, J., Heermann, J.A., & Million, R. (2009). The experience of spouses as informal caregivers for recipients of hematopoietic stem cell transplants. *Cancer Nursing, 32,* E15–E23. https://doi.org/10.1097/NCC.0b013e31819962e0

Wingard, J.R. (2007). Bone marrow to blood stem cells past, present, future. In S. Ezzone & K. Schmit-Pokorny (Eds.), *Blood and marrow stem cell transplantation: Principles, practice, and nursing insights* (3rd ed., pp. 1–18). Burlington, MA: Jones & Bartlett Learning.

Wingard, J.R., Juang, I.-C., Sobocinski, K.A., Andrykowski, M.A., Cella, D., Rizzo, J.D., ... Bishop, M.M. (2010). Factors associated with self-reported physical and mental health after hematopoietic cell transplantation. *Biology of Blood and Marrow Transplantation, 16,* 1682–1692. https://doi.org/10.1016/j.bbmt.2010.05.017

Worel, N. (2017). Practical implementation—Essential elements resource tool. *Hematology/Oncology and Stem Cell Therapy, 10,* 198–202. https://doi.org/10.1016/j.hemonc.2017.05.023

Yeh, A.C., Khan, M.A., Harlow, J., Biswas, A.R., Akter, M., Ferdous, J., ... Dey, B.R. (2018). Hematopoietic stem-cell transplantation in the resource-limited setting: Establishing the first bone marrow transplantation unit in Bangladesh. *Journal of Global Oncology, 4,* 1–10. https://doi.org/10.1200/jgo.2016.006460

Young, L.K., Mansfield, B., & Mandoza, J. (2017). Nursing care of adult hematopoietic stem cell transplant patients and families in the intensive care unit: An evidence-based review. *Critical Care Nursing Clinics of North America, 29,* 341–352. https://doi.org/10.1016/j.cnc.2017.04.009

Zinter, M.S., Dvorak, C.C., Spicer, A., Cowan, M.J., & Sapru, A. (2015). New insights into multicenter PICU mortality among pediatric hematopoietic stem cell transplant patients. *Critical Care Medicine, 43,* 1986–1994. https://doi.org/10.1097/CCM.0000000000001085

CHAPTER 5

Stem Cell Collection

Kim Schmit-Pokorny, RN, MSN, OCN®, BMTCN®

Introduction

Stem cells may be collected for transplantation from bone marrow, peripheral blood, and umbilical cord blood (UCB). The previous chapters discussed the advantages and disadvantages to each method. Collecting stem cells from the blood has demonstrated several major advantages in comparison to surgically harvesting them from bone marrow. Patients who receive peripheral blood stem cells (PBSCs) may experience a more rapid hematopoietic recovery, have a lower risk of receiving a tumor cell–contaminated stem cell product, and experience a better overall outcome. In addition, PBSC collection may be performed in an outpatient setting without the use of general anesthesia. Patients who have tumors in the marrow or who have had pelvic irradiation resulting in bone marrow fibrosis may have stem cells collected from the blood. The use of bone marrow may offer the advantage of a decreased risk of chronic graft-versus-host disease (GVHD) (Anasetti et al., 2012). Potential advantages of UCB transplants are that the products contain many immature progenitor cells and may have the lowest incidence of GVHD. UCB products offer the additional advantages of permitting human leukocyte antigen (HLA) disparity and being readily available, versus having to wait for matched unrelated donor availability (Panch, Szymanski, Savani, & Stroncek, 2017).

Evaluation of Autologous and Allogeneic Donors for Collection

Prior to bone marrow harvest or PBSC collection, the transplant recipient must be evaluated to determine eligibility for transplantation (see Chapter 2). The recipient, if autologous stem cells are to be harvested, or the allogeneic donor must be evaluated prior to the harvest or collection procedure to determine eligibility and suitability for the procedure (Worel et al., 2015). Donor evaluation involves a history and physical, blood tests, possible radiologic tests, and questions to review health history. A thorough explanation of the bone marrow harvest or PBSC collection procedure must be provided (Foundation for the Accreditation of Cellular Therapy [FACT] & Joint Accreditation Committee–ISCT and EBMT [JACIE], 2018; Worel et al., 2015).

FACT and JACIE (2018) have outlined standards to protect the safety of the donor, recipient, and product. All donors, allogeneic and autologous, must be evaluated by trained medical personnel. Allogeneic donors should be evaluated by a physician who is not the primary healthcare provider overseeing the care of the recipient. Donors must be carefully evaluated and fully informed prior to donation. FACT and JACIE (2018) summarized the assessment process and regulatory issues associated with stem cell donation. A psychological evaluation may also be necessary to fully evaluate the donor. Legal and ethical aspects should be considered, especially when using minors as donors. Figure 5-1 lists evaluation elements recommended before bone marrow harvest or PBSC collection. In addition, written informed consent must be obtained from the donor. FACT and JACIE (2018) require the recipient's physician to write an order to collect and process the stem cells that includes recipient and donor information, treatment plan, collection protocol, processing and cryopreservation method, and any assays to be performed on the stem cell product. Figure 5-2 is an example of an order form for PBSC collection.

Bone Marrow Harvest

Bone marrow, which contains more pluripotent stem cells than peripheral blood, is harvested from the posterior iliac crests via multiple large-bore needle aspirations. Occasionally, the anterior iliac crest or the sternum may be used to obtain enough cells for transplant. The procedure usually is performed in an operating room with the patient under general or spinal anesthesia. Typically, the procedure lasts one to two hours, after which the patient may be admitted to the hospital, although most donors are discharged the same day as the surgery. The patient lies prone on the operating table, and bone marrow is collected from both posterior iliac crests by multiple needle aspirations. The minimum number of nucleated cells attempted to be harvested, based on the recipient's weight, ranges $1–2 \times 10^8$/kg for autologous transplant, and $2–6 \times 10^8$/kg for allogeneic transplant (Forman & Nakamura, 2011; Karakukcu & Unal, 2015). The total fluid volume obtained may be up to 1.5 L of blood (Panch et al., 2017). The National Marrow Donor Program (NMDP) bone marrow harvest guidelines allow up to 20 ml/kg of bone marrow to be safely har-

Figure 5-1. Evaluation of the Donor for Bone Marrow Harvest or Peripheral Blood Stem Cell Collection

Autologous Donor
- Complete blood count, differential, and platelet obtained within a 24-hour period prior to the first peripheral blood stem cell (PBSC) collection and within 24 hours before each subsequent PBSC collection
- Chemistries (liver and kidney function)
- Prothrombin time, partial thromboplastin time, and international normalized ratio
- Blood grouping and Rh typing (ABO and Rh)
- Evaluation for risk of hemoglobinopathy prior to mobilization agents
- Infectious disease tests (hepatitis B surface antigen, hepatitis B core antigen, hepatitis C antibody, HIV-1 antibody, HIV-2 antibody, HIV antigen, human T-cell lymphotropic viruses, syphilis, West Nile virus, *Trypanosoma cruzi* [Chagas disease])
- Electrocardiogram (consider for bone marrow donors only)
- Chest x-ray (consider for bone marrow donors only)
- Pregnancy assessment within 7 days prior to the start of growth factor
- History and physical
- Need for central venous access
- The following must be documented:
  - Suitability of donor to undergo stem cell collection
  - Abnormal findings and rationale for proceeding
  - Counseling of patient regarding abnormal findings
  - Patient informed of tests performed to protect the health of the patient
  - Patient informed of right to review test results
  - Need for central venous access
  - Informed consent

Allogeneic Donor
- Human leukocyte antigen (HLA)-A, HLA-B, and HLA-DRB1 typing (unrelated and related donors other than siblings should also be HLA-C typed)
- Anti-HLA antibody testing for mismatched donors and recipients
- Recipient evaluation to prove eligibility for transplant
- Complete blood count, differential, and platelet count obtained within a 24-hour period prior to the first PBSC collection and within 24 hours before each subsequent PBSC collection
- Chemistries (liver and kidney function)
- Prothrombin time, partial thromboplastin time, and international normalized ratio
- ABO group and Rh type, blood bank—bone marrow transplant evaluation (type and irregular antibody screen, red cell phenotype, red blood cell crossmatch between donor and recipient, anti-A and anti-B titers as appropriate)
- Evaluation for risk of hemoglobinopathy prior to mobilization agents
- Infectious disease tests (hepatitis B surface antigen, hepatitis B core antigen, hepatitis C antibody, HIV-1 antibody, HIV-2 antibody, HIV antigen, human T-cell lymphotropic viruses, syphilis, West Nile virus, *Trypanosoma cruzi* [Chagas disease], cytomegalovirus) performed within 30 days prior to collection
- Electrocardiogram (consider for bone marrow donors only)
- Chest x-ray (consider for bone marrow donors only)
- Pregnancy assessment within 7 days prior to the start of growth factor
- Screening questions for infectious disease and high-risk behavior (available at www.factwebsite.org)
- History and physical
- Need for central venous access
- The following must be documented:
  - Suitability of donor to undergo stem cell collection
  - Vaccination history
  - Travel history
  - Blood transfusion history
  - Risk of disease transmission, including a targeted screening history, physical, and laboratory testing as listed previously
  - Abnormal findings and rationale for proceeding
  - Counseling of patient regarding abnormal findings
  - Determination of whether recipient may be informed of abnormal findings and findings documented in recipient's chart
  - Recipient informed of abnormal findings and findings documented in recipient's chart
  - Donor informed of tests performed to protect the health of the patient
  - Donor informed of right to review test results
  - Need for central venous access
  - Informed consent

Note. Based on information from Foundation for the Accreditation of Cellular Therapy & Joint Accreditation Committee–ISCT and EBMT, 2018.

Figure 5-2. Cellular Therapy Product Order Form

Recipient Information

Affix hospital identification label here or legibly record: Name		Weight (kg)	ABO/Rh
		Birth date	Gender ☐ Male ☐ Female
		Diagnosis	
MRN or NMDP Recipient ID #			

Donor Information

☐ Autologous   ☐ Allogeneic, Unrelated   ☐ Allogeneic, Related   ☐ 1st degree or 2nd degree   ☐ Haplo

Affix hospital identification label here or legibly record: Name	Weight (kg)	ABO/Rh
	Birth date	Gender ☐ Male ☐ Female

☐ NA - Autologous

MRN or NMDP Recipient ID #

☐ HPC, Apheresis   ☐ HPC, Marrow   ☐ HPC, Cord Blood   ☐ MNC, Apheresis   ☐ MNC, Marrow

Anticipated Date of 1st Collection or Harvest Date	Collection Protocol_____ Clinical Trial _____

Cytokine Mobilization: ☐ None   ☐ Filgrastim   ☐ PEG-Filgrastim   ☐ Plerixafor   ☐ Sargramostim   ☐ Other _____

Chemotherapy Mobilization: ☐ No ☐ Yes _____ Date Started _____

Apheresis: Blood Volume to Process/collection: _____ L	Minimum CD34 dose/kg: _____ Target CD34 dose/kg: _____
Collection Consent Signed on:	Collection Site: ☐ Nebraska Medicine ☐ Other _____

Transplant Facility: ☐ Nebraska Medicine ☐ Other _____	HPC, Marrow Target Cell Dose: _____ x10^8 NC/kg recipient x _____ kg (recipient) = _____ TNC x 10^8

(Continued on next page)

Figure 5-2. Cellular Therapy Product Order Form *(Continued)*	
Cell Processing and Cryopreservation Information	

□ Fresh   □ 10% DMSO, controlled rate freezing; standard processing   □ Other_____

□ No Modification   □ RBC Reduced   □ Plasma Reduced   □ CD34 Enriched

□ Other _____ □ IRB _____ □ Volume-Reduced to _____ml/kg

CD3+ cell dose to be given FRESH _____/kg	Freeze in Even # bags: □ Yes □ No

Assays: □ Daily CD34 count on fresh collection   □ Haploidentical – CD3, CD4, CD8

□ CD3 count on Fresh Collection   □ Other _____

Anticipated Date of Infusion:	Research Sample Consent signed (IRB 214): □ Yes □ No
Care Team	
Physician Name (print)	Physician Phone #
Physician Signature Date	Recipient Case Manager Name _____ Recipient Case Manager Phone #_____ Donor Case Manager Name _____ Donor Case Manager Phone # _____

Additional Information _____

_____

Note. Copyright 2018 by Nebraska Medicine/University of Nebraska Medical Center, Hematopoietic Cell Transplantation Program, Omaha, Nebraska. Used with permission.

vested from unrelated donors (Furey et al., 2018; Panch et al., 2017). Furey et al. (2018) reported data supporting 3–5 × 10^6/kg cluster of differentiation (CD) 34+ cells as an optimum cell dose with an HLA-matched sibling donor, with higher doses having no effect on clinical outcomes. They suggested the volume harvested may be decreased and provided an algorithm based on donor age and weight, patient weight, and desired median CD34+ cell count. Harvesting lower amounts may lead to safer harvest procedures for pediatric donors (Furey et al., 2018).

Following the harvest, the bone marrow is filtered through progressively smaller screens to remove fat and bone particles, and it is then sent to a specialized laboratory for further processing. If the recipient and donor have a major ABO incompatibility, the product will be red cell or plasma depleted (AABB et al., 2018; Karakukcu & Unal, 2015). The marrow is ideally harvested the same day it will be infused into the patient, or it may be frozen until the recipient is ready to receive the transplant.

Side effects that donors may experience following bone marrow harvest include bleeding, infection, pain, hypovolemia, hypotension, hematoma, electrolyte imbalances, and side effects from general anesthesia. Nurses should assess harvest sites frequently for bleeding, drainage, or hematoma. Mild analgesics may be prescribed for pain. Following bone marrow harvest, donors may become anemic and require a blood transfusion, although this is unusual. Allogeneic donors should consider storing autologous red blood cells prior to the procedure, which may need to be infused at the time of the harvest. Autologous donors may need additional IV fluids or a transfusion of irradiated packed red blood cells. Typically, the bone marrow cells that were removed from the donor will regenerate within a few weeks (Chen, Wang, & Yang, 2013). Nurses should instruct donors to assess harvest sites daily for signs of bleeding or infection, avoid tub baths for several days (a shower within 24 hours may be permitted at some centers), and avoid heavy lifting.

Pulsipher et al. (2014) reviewed the early and late side effects from 2,726 unrelated bone marrow donors harvested between 2004 and 2009 through NMDP. They found that serious adverse events occurred in less than 1% of the procedures. The most common persistent side effect noted was mild localized pain at the harvest site. Some donors have described the pain as similar to a fall on ice. Chern, McCarthy, Hutchins, and Durrant (1999) assessed the duration and severity of pain following bone marrow harvest. They evaluated the effectiveness of a local analgesic, bupivacaine, which was infiltrated into one of the harvest sites, by having donors record the level of pain at each harvest site. The donors reported a significant reduction in pain at the harvest site that was injected with the analgesic. Thus, the authors recommended that bupivacaine be infiltrated into harvest sites routinely following harvest (Chern et al., 1999). This practice is currently being followed. Panch et al. (2017) reported that decreases in hemoglobin following harvest have taken up to six months to return to baseline. Bone marrow harvesting has been performed on many autologous and allogeneic donors; however, complications are possible, and the donors should be assessed following the harvest.

Switzer et al. (2014) described the quality of life that unrelated donors experienced during the harvest procedure and compared it to donors collecting PBSCs. They interviewed the people prior to donation, 48 hours after donation, weekly until recovered, and 6 and 12 months after donation. Overall, no long-term quality-of-life differences appeared to exist between the majority of bone marrow and PBSC donors. Bone marrow donors reported more physical side effects, including pain, within the 48 hours following harvest compared to PBSC donors. However, the authors found that the pain experienced by bone marrow donors 48 hours after donation was similar to that of the PBSC donors on day 4 of filgrastim. Although bone marrow donors reported greater impact on their social activities, they also reported more positive psychological status and were more likely to indicate that donation made their lives more meaningful. At 12 months following donation, approximately half of all donors had remaining concerns about the long-term impact of donation. Switzer et al. (2014) concluded that the long-term quality-of-life consequences for bone marrow and PBSC donation are similar.

Autologous bone marrow stem cell harvesting has been mostly replaced by PBSC collection. However, for allogeneic transplants, harvesting bone marrow is still appropriate. For pediatric patients undergoing an allogeneic transplant in 2015, bone marrow was used 81% of the time for related donor transplants and 76% of the time for unrelated donor transplants (D'Souza, Lee, Zhu, & Pasquini, 2017). Several authors indicated that the gold standard to achieve the best transplant outcomes in pediatric patients is to use stem cells harvested from the bone marrow of an HLA-matched sibling donor (Furey et al., 2018; Satwani, Kahn, & Jin, 2015).

Anasetti et al. (2012) conducted a phase 3 multicenter randomized study comparing transplantation of PBSCs to bone marrow from unrelated donors. A total of 551 patients at 48 transplant centers were enrolled in the study. The authors found that although PBSCs may decrease the risk of graft failure, bone marrow grafts may decrease the risk of chronic GVHD. They did not find any significant difference in acute GVHD, relapse, or survival between the two groups.

Peripheral Blood Stem Cell Collection

The use of stem cells collected from the peripheral blood for both autologous and allogeneic transplantation has grown since 1986, when six independent transplant centers reported successful autologous PBSC transplants (Bell, Figes, Oscier, & Hamblin, 1986; Castaigne et al., 1986; Kessinger, Armitage, Landmark, & Weisenburger, 1986; Körbling et al., 1986; Reiffers et al., 1986; Tilly et al., 1986). Kessinger et al. (1989) reported the first related allogeneic PBSC transplant in 1989.

Autologous PBSC transplants have mostly replaced the use of bone marrow. PBSCs are also the most common graft source for adult patients receiving allogeneic transplants: 89% of related transplant recipients and 87% of unrelated transplants in 2015 (D'Souza et al., 2017).

Collecting stem cells from the blood has demonstrated several advantages to transplant recipients, primarily more rapid hematopoietic recovery. An early report from Gale, Henon, and Juttner (1992) suggested that the difference is due to the increased number of mature granulocyte progenitors in the stem cell product. Other variables that may affect the rate of hematopoietic recovery include the dose of cells given, the intensity of the preparative regimen, and the amount of prior bone marrow damage. They stated that although a minimum number of cells may be required for transplant, many factors (e.g., infections, antibiotics) influence and obscure correlations between cell dose and hematopoietic recovery. The rapid hematopoietic recovery associated with PBSCs results in a decrease in infections, transfusions, hospital days, and overall cost compared to using bone marrow (Gale et al., 1992).

A second advantage of using PBSCs (discussed later in this chapter) for patients undergoing autologous transplantation is that the PBSC product may have a lower risk of contamination by tumor cells (Gale et al., 1992; Sharp et al., 1992). Also, patients who have a tumor in the marrow or who have had pelvic irradiation that caused bone marrow fibrosis may undergo successful PBSC collection. PBSC collections may be performed in an outpatient setting without general anesthesia, resulting in decreased cost and increased patient satisfaction. Anasetti et al. (2012) concluded that when compared to bone marrow, PBSCs may decrease the risk of graft failure, although patients may have a higher risk of chronic GVHD.

Mobilization of Stem Cells

The number of circulating stem cells in the blood is lower than that in the bone marrow. Stem cells may be collected from the blood while the bone marrow is in a steady state and after the patient has recovered from all chemotherapy or radiation. However, although this collection method will result in an adequate product, it may require multiple apheresis procedures. Mobilizing or stimulating stem cells that originate in bone marrow to move into the peripheral blood produces more stem cells in fewer apheresis collections and results in faster hematopoietic recovery after transplant (Panch et al., 2017; To, Levesque, & Herbert, 2011).

Methods currently used to mobilize circulating stem cells include the use of chemotherapy, hematopoietic growth factors, chemokine antagonists, or investigational agents. Initially, stem cells were collected in either the steady state or following chemotherapy mobilization. In 1988, two hematopoietic growth factors, filgrastim (Neupogen®), or granulocyte–colony-stimulating factor (G-CSF), and sargramostim (Leukine®), or granulocyte macrophage–colony-stimulating factor, were approved for use in mobilizing stem cells. Growth factors administered after chemotherapy for mobilization resulted in a greater number of stem cells (Socinski et al., 1988). Currently, chemotherapy alone is no longer used for mobilization and is combined with growth factors. A new class of agents, the chemokine antagonists, has also been shown to mobilize stem cells (DiPersio et al., 2009; Flomenberg et al., 2005). Plerixafor (AMD3100, Mozobil®), the first chemokine antagonist for stem cell mobilization, received U.S. Food and Drug Administration (FDA) approval in December 2008.

Chemotherapy

Following standard chemotherapy, a transient increase, or "overshoot," occurs in the number of circulating stem cells (Richman, Weiner, & Yankee, 1976). As white blood cells (WBCs) start to recover, the stem cells also recover and may be harvested during this transient increase. In one of the earliest reports, To et al. (1990) reported the use of cyclophosphamide at a dose of 4 g/m^2 to mobilize stem cells in 30 patients with lymphoma, myeloma, breast carcinoma, ovarian carcinoma, and sarcomas. They found that at approximately 16 days following the chemotherapy, the number of circulating colony-forming units–granulocyte macrophage (CFU-GM) increased approximately 14-fold above baseline, which lasted for approximately four to five days. Following this report, cyclophosphamide or chemotherapy regimens used for the treatment of the patient's malignancy became the most common mobilization methods. In another early study, Gianni et al. (1990) mobilized stem cells in patients with a combination of chemotherapy and growth factors. Because no growth factors were administered to patients after transplant, the accelerated hematopoietic recovery was attributed solely to the infusion of mobilized stem cells. Bishop (1994) indicated that the administration of chemotherapy for mobilization should be started when patients have recovered from prior chemotherapy or radiation. Patients should be closely monitored, and apheresis should begin when they start to recover from their neutrophil nadir, approximately 10–14 days following chemotherapy. Cyclophosphamide doses of 1.5–7 g/m^2 or chemotherapy used to treat the specific malignancy in conjunction with growth factors are currently used to mobilize stem cells.

Timing of filgrastim administration following chemotherapy treatment and the beginning of collection varies among centers. Kriegsmann et al. (2018) analyzed 11 chemotherapy mobilization regimens to determine mobilization and collection parameters for each. Chemotherapy regimens may be selected based on the patient's disease-specific treatment or given in addition to specific treatment. Determining when to start collections is less predictable than with growth factors alone. They summarized common chemotherapy regimens and developed a comprehensive schedule including the start of chemotherapy, growth factor administration, and monitoring to start collections (Kriegsmann et al., 2018).

Chemotherapy for mobilization may result in more rapid hematopoietic recovery following transplant, fewer apheresis collections, and reduced tumor burden (Kriegsmann et al., 2018). However, chemotherapy mobilization also has disadvantages. One of the early studies by To et al. (1990) reported that several patients who received myelosuppressive chemotherapy for mobilization developed neutropenic sepsis and required antibiotic therapy. One developed streptococcal septicemia due to neutropenia and died of a probable cardiac arrhythmia. Another disadvantage is that mobilization may fail in patients who have received multiple courses of chemotherapy or patients with tumor in their bone marrow (To et al., 1990). Using chemotherapy for mobilization requires additional time, as the patient must wait approximately 10–16 days after chemotherapy for the optimal time to collect, undergo collection over several days, and then completely recover from the toxicities. If an insufficient number of stem cells is collected, the process must be repeated.

Chemotherapy mobilization side effects are similar to those encountered with standard doses of chemotherapy, including pancytopenia, infection, hair loss, mucositis, nausea, vomiting, and other side effects associated with the specific chemotherapy agent. Patients should be closely monitored for side effects of the chemotherapy.

Hematopoietic Growth Factors

Another method to mobilize stem cells is using the hematopoietic growth factors filgrastim or sargramostim. In a pivotal report, Socinski et al. (1988) conducted a three-phase study in which patients with sarcoma received sargramostim. The study found that sargramostim alone increased the number of circulating progenitor cells by approximately 18-fold. In patients who received sargramostim and chemotherapy, the number of circulating progenitor cells increased by approximately 60-fold. This initial study concluded that the use of sargramostim may expedite collection of stem cells from the blood for transplantation.

In another original study, Haas et al. (1990) reported on the use of sargramostim to mobilize 12 patients with hematologic malignancies. Sargramostim was given as a continuous IV infusion. In these patients, an 8.5-fold increase was noted in progenitor cells. The researchers also noted a decrease in platelet count (median 21%, range 7%–67%) during sargramostim administration but prior to the start of the apheresis collection procedures.

In a sequential study involving hard-to-mobilize patients (i.e., those with extensive prior chemotherapy and/or bone marrow deficiencies, presence or history of morphologic tumor contamination, and/or hypocellularity), sargramostim mobilization allowed collection of adequate numbers of stem cells (Bishop et al., 1994). The authors also noted that transplantation with sargramostim-mobilized stem cells resulted in significantly earlier recovery for granulocytes and a shorter time to platelet and red blood cell transfusion independence. Following PBSC transplantation, growth factors did not affect the rate of engraftment in nonmobilized and mobilized groups of patients (Bishop et al., 1994).

Nademanee et al. (1994) compared patients transplanted with filgrastim-mobilized stem cells to patients who did not undergo mobilization. Mobilized patients received either filgrastim 5 mcg/kg or 10 mcg/kg. Only patients mobilized with filgrastim also received it following transplant. The authors concluded that the patients mobilized with filgrastim had a significantly faster hematopoietic recovery than those who received no mobilization.

Currently, sargramostim is rarely used, as it is less effective than filgrastim and has dose-related toxicities (Duong et al., 2014; Giralt et al., 2014; To et al., 2011). Mobilization using filgrastim results in higher doses of stem cells collected compared to sargramostim mobilization (H. Devine, Tierney, Schmit-Pokorny, & McDermott, 2010). Current practices for mobilization vary widely among institutions. A working group created by the Practice Guidelines Committee of the American Society for Blood and Marrow Transplantation (now the American Society for Transplantation and Cellular Therapy) summarized recommendations for mobilization (Duong et al., 2014). The most frequently used and preferred growth factor for mobilization is filgrastim 10 mcg/kg/day as a single or split dose (Duong et al., 2014; Panch et al., 2017; To et al., 2011). Bhamidipati et al. (2017) published the first randomized prospective study comparing the biosimilar tbo-filgrastim (Granix®) to filgrastim. The authors found no significant difference in how the patient mobilized, in toxicities, or in transplant outcomes. Although the authors did not perform a cost analysis, they predicted that using biosimilars will be more economical than using filgrastim (Bhamidipati et al., 2017).

Typically, growth factors are given as a subcutaneous injection, although initially, continuous IV infusion was commonly reported (Gianni et al., 1990; Haas et al., 1990; Socinski et al., 1988). They usually are given in a once-daily injection. However, Lee et al. (2000) gave filgrastim 5 mcg/kg twice daily to mobilize stem cells in healthy donors and pediatric patients for autologous backup before undergoing allogeneic stem cell transplantation. The group was compared to historical controls who had received filgrastim 10 mcg/kg daily. The authors concluded that the twice-daily dose of filgrastim was more efficient in mobilizing stem cells. Additional studies have not shown any advantage to twice-daily dosing (Duong et al., 2014). Also, split administration may not be commonly used because of the inconvenience of receiving—and increased cost of administering—two injections each day.

Many current mobilization protocols include chemotherapy and hematopoietic growth factors. The growth factors not only help to reduce cytopenia following chemotherapy but also dramatically increase the number of circulating progenitor cells (To et al., 2011). This combination method may produce the most stem cells possible, but patients may experience significant side effects from the chemotherapy.

The most common side effects associated with growth factors used for mobilization include bone pain, fever, and malaise. Other less common symptoms are chills, headache, nausea, vomiting, diarrhea, edema, rash, irritation at injection site, dyspnea, pleural or pericardial effusion, and nasal congestion (Behfar, Faghihi-Kashani, Hosseini, Ghavamzadeh, & Hamidieh, 2018). Most symptoms are minimal and easily treated and resolve upon discontinuation of the growth factor. Many centers stop filgrastim if the WBC count exceeds $100,000/mm^3$ (Duong et al., 2014).

Daily nursing assessments should include a discussion of symptoms and an evaluation of the patient's temperature, pulse, respirations, blood pressure, and weight. Patients may be instructed to take acetaminophen for bone pain or headache. Occasionally, patients will request a stronger pain reliever, such as acetaminophen with codeine. Other side effects should be assessed and treated symptomatically. More serious side effects (e.g., pleural or pericardial effusions) may necessitate stopping the growth factors.

Wei and Grigg (2001) and Adler et al. (2001) reported a rare but life-threatening sickle cell crisis in two patients with hemoglobin sickle cell disease who received filgrastim. One patient, who was a donor for her sister, was diagnosed with hemoglobin sickle cell disease six weeks prior to mobilization and had not had any complications related to the disease (Adler et al., 2001). Following filgrastim administration, she developed sickle cell crisis and died within 36 hours. Wei and Grigg (2001) reported on a patient with sickle cell/β+ thalassemia who developed sickle cell crisis and multiorgan dysfunction following filgrastim administration. A trial to evaluate the safety and feasibility of filgrastim mobilization in patients with the sickle cell trait reported no adverse events, including sickle cell crises, occurring in the study patients (Kang et al., 2002). However, the authors indicated that because of the increased symptoms and possibility for more serious adverse reactions, close monitoring is required.

Pegylated filgrastim (pegfilgrastim, Neulasta®), a modified form of filgrastim, may be administered as a single dose instead of daily injections of filgrastim. Kroschinsky et al. (2006) studied the use of pegfilgrastim and chemotherapy mobilization in patients with multiple myeloma or lymphoma. Following mobilization chemotherapy, patients received pegfilgrastim 6 mg subcutaneously daily. The target of 4×10^6 CD34+ cells/kg was reached in 70% of the patients. Patients who did not reach a peripheral blood CD34+ minimum of $10/mm^3$ were given daily doses of nonpegylated filgrastim 10 mcg/kg. The authors noted that those patients who were heavily pretreated with extensive chemotherapy regimens or mobilized with regimens containing platinum or melphalan needed the additional filgrastim. They concluded that using pegylated filgrastim is feasible but requires more investigation.

In another study, Bruns et al. (2006) compared two dose levels, 6 mg and 12 mg, of pegfilgrastim for mobilization. Patients with multiple myeloma received cyclophosphamide for mobilization, followed by a single dose of either 6 mg or 12 mg pegfilgrastim, or by daily doses of filgrastim 8 mcg/kg. Results from the study showed that pegfilgrastim at either dose yielded similar amounts of CD34+ cells. Pegfilgrastim appeared to work as well as filgrastim for mobilization. The authors suggested that even smaller doses of pegfilgrastim might mobilize stem cells. Duong et al. (2014) reported that pegylated filgrastim at a single dose of 12 mg is being used; however, not many transplant centers use pegylated filgrastim because of cost.

Several other types of growth factors have been used for mobilization of stem cells. Vose et al. (1992) examined the effect of interleukin-3 on the stem cell product. The conclusion was that although the progenitor cell content increased, the use of the cells for autologous transplantation did not result in quicker hematopoietic recovery.

Another study by Bishop et al. (1996) reported that the use of PIXY321, a fusion protein that consists of granulocyte macrophage–colony-stimulating factor and interleukin-3, successfully mobilized progenitors into the peripheral blood, and hematopoietic recovery was rapid following transplantation. The researchers concluded that PIXY321, if combined with other mobilization methods, might improve the quality of the stem cell product.

Recombinant human stem cell factor, usually in combination with filgrastim, is another growth factor that has been studied (Glaspy et al., 1997). Stem cell factor is active on early progenitor cells and on the erythroid and myeloid cell lines. Stem cell factor can synergize with other growth factors. Shpall (1999) reported on the use of stem cell factor with filgrastim compared to filgrastim alone to mobilize patients with breast cancer. Hard-to-mobilize patients who received stem cell factor plus filgrastim were able to reach the target CD34+ cell number and had a more sustained increase in the number of CD34+ cells, resulting in fewer apheresis collections.

Kessinger and Sharp (1996) reported on the administration of recombinant human erythropoietin (epoetin alfa) during PBSC collections for 12 patients. Patients received epoetin alfa at 200 units per day until an adequate product was obtained. In the 11 assessable patients, the peak mobilization effect occurred on the fourth day of growth factor administration. Nine of the patients received high-dose therapy and were transplanted with these PBSCs. Engraftment was comparable to patients who had received an autologous transplant. The authors concluded that the administration of epoetin alfa increased the number of circulating progenitor cells even from nonerythropoietic lineages. However, because of the need for more clinical trials, the clinical significance of epoetin alfa as a mobilizing agent is still undetermined.

Although other types of hematopoietic growth factors have been used in studies to mobilize stem cells, the use of chemotherapy and filgrastim or filgrastim alone for mobilization appears to result in the quickest collection time and the most rapid recovery time following transplant.

Chemokine Antagonists

The chemokine antagonist plerixafor has been used to mobilize stem cells into the bloodstream. Plerixafor, initially studied as an agent to inhibit entry of HIV into T cells, was found to produce leukocytosis in patients and healthy volunteers (Liles et al., 2003). H. Devine et al. (2010) summarized the biology and mechanism of action of chemokine antagonists and plerixafor. Clinical studies have shown that plerixafor in combination with filgrastim efficiently mobilizes stem cells (DiPersio et al., 2009; Flomenberg et al., 2005).

Flomenberg et al. (2005) described a phase 2 crossover study in which patients with multiple myeloma or non-Hodgkin lymphoma, serving as their own control, were randomized to receive either plerixafor with filgrastim followed by filgrastim alone, or filgrastim alone followed by plerixafor with filgrastim. The combination of plerixafor and filgrastim mobilized more stem cells than filgrastim alone. Side effects attributed to the plerixafor were upset stomach, flatulence, injection-site erythema, and paresthesias.

In a phase 3 study, plerixafor and filgrastim versus placebo and filgrastim were used to mobilize stem cells in patients with multiple myeloma (DiPersio et al., 2009). Significantly more patients in the plerixafor group reached the primary study endpoint of 6×10^6 CD34+ cells/kg or greater in less than two apheresis collections. Engraftment was similar between the two groups. The authors concluded that plerixafor and filgrastim allowed patients to collect the optimal dose of CD34+ cells in fewer apheresis procedures and that plerixafor was well tolerated.

Approved by FDA in December 2008, plerixafor is given in conjunction with filgrastim to mobilize hematopoietic stem cells (Genzyme, 2019). Patients are given filgrastim 10 mcg/kg for up to eight days. On the evening of the fourth day of the filgrastim, plerixafor 0.24 mg/kg is given as a subcutaneous injection. Plerixafor should be given approximately 11 hours before the apheresis procedure. Plerixafor may be repeated up to four consecutive days. Side effects related to plerixafor usually are gastrointestinal symptoms (e.g., nausea, vomiting, diarrhea), injection-site reactions, headache, fatigue, arthralgias, and dizziness. Because of the cost, many centers have created algorithms for using plerixafor as a salvage mobilization method (Duong et al., 2014). See Figure 5-3 for an example of a mobilization algorithm using filgrastim and salvage plerixafor.

Micallef et al. (2018) published the first follow-up observational report analyzing the long-term effects of plerixafor for mobilization. Results showed the use of plerixafor for stem cell mobilization did not affect five-year survival in patients with non-Hodgkin lymphoma or multiple myeloma.

S.M. Devine et al. (2008) reported on the use of plerixafor without filgrastim to mobilize related allogeneic donors. In the pilot study, 25 donors received 240 mcg/kg plerixafor and underwent apheresis four hours later. A single injection for two-thirds of the donors was adequate to mobilize enough stem cells for transplant. Donors experienced minimal side effects and no bone pain (typically associated with filgrastim mobilization). Doses of CD34+ cells were lower than what was expected for donors mobilized with filgrastim. However, recipients had rapid and long-lasting engraftment. S.M. Devine et al. (2008) concluded that using plerixafor to mobilize healthy donors is a strategy to decrease the length of time needed to obtain stem cells; however, more research is needed. Mobilization of healthy donors continues to be off-label, and only anecdotal reports describe its use.

Tumor Cell Mobilization

Circulating tumor cells have been detected in stem cell products from patients with lymphoma and metastatic breast cancer. Sharp et al. (1992) found that significantly fewer tumor cells were detected in PBSC products than in bone marrow products. They also found that patients with non-Hodgkin lymphoma with tumor in their bone marrow and who received PBSC products had a better survival outcome than patients who received bone marrow. Brugger et al. (1994) demonstrated that patients who had circulating tumor cells prior to mobilization showed an increase in the number of tumor cells present following mobilization. In patients who did not demonstrate any circulating tumor cells before mobilization, 21% (9 of 42) were found to have circulating tumor cells follow-

ing mobilization, especially in patients who had stage IV breast cancer or extensive-disease small cell lung cancer (Brugger et al., 1994).

A study by Kahn et al. (1997) demonstrated that as the number of apheresis procedures increased, the amount of tumor cell contamination in the product also increased. They noted that the incidence of tumor contamination dramatically increased from the first apheresis (5.4%) to the second apheresis (15.4%). The authors concluded that decreasing the number of apheresis collections would decrease the amount of tumor contamination for this patient population. The significance of harvesting tumor cells in the stem cell product is not verified, but infusing a product containing tumor cells might contribute to relapse (Micallef et al., 2018).

Mobilization Failure

Patients who have received multiple courses of chemotherapy or who have bone marrow metastases may not achieve an increased number of circulating stem cells with mobilization and may not be able to collect enough stem cells for transplant (Kessinger & Sharp, 2003; To et al., 2011). Stiff (1999) listed several chemotherapy agents (melphalan, nitrosoureas, procarbazine, nitrogen mustard, alkylating agents, and platinum compounds) that appear to be more toxic to the marrow and may cause difficulties in stem cell collection. Fludarabine has been shown to cause mobilization failure in up to 60% of patients (To et al., 2011). In patients with multiple myeloma, the use of lenalidomide has been associated with poor or failed stem cell mobilization (Popat et al., 2009). Other risk factors that may make it difficult to mobilize and collect an adequate number of stem cells are type of malignancy (breast cancer, Hodgkin lymphoma, non-Hodgkin lymphoma, and ovarian cancer), age older than 60 years, and prior radiation to marrow-producing sites (Duong et al., 2014; Giralt et al., 2014; Stiff, 1999; To et al., 2011). Giralt et al. (2014) reported that diabetes and smoking may be associated with poor mobilization. A platelet count less than $100,000/mm^3$ has been shown to predict poor mobilization (Duong et al., 2014). To et al. (2011) conservatively estimated that mobilization strategies fail in 5,000–10,000 patients each year, resulting in increased use of resources (e.g., growth factors, transfusions), and noted that mobilization strategies fail in up to 5% of healthy donors.

Strategies to maximize mobilization should be discussed prior to initiation. In patients who are receiving chemotherapy, mobilization and collection should be considered early in the treatment plan. Bone marrow disease should be minimal or absent. Collecting and storing cells prior to bone marrow irradiation should be considered.

In a compassionate-use study, patients with non-Hodgkin lymphoma, Hodgkin lymphoma, and multiple myeloma in whom a previous attempt at mobilization (chemotherapy and/or growth factors) had failed were eligible to receive plerixafor (then known as AMD3100) (Calandra

Figure 5-3. Mobilization Algorithm

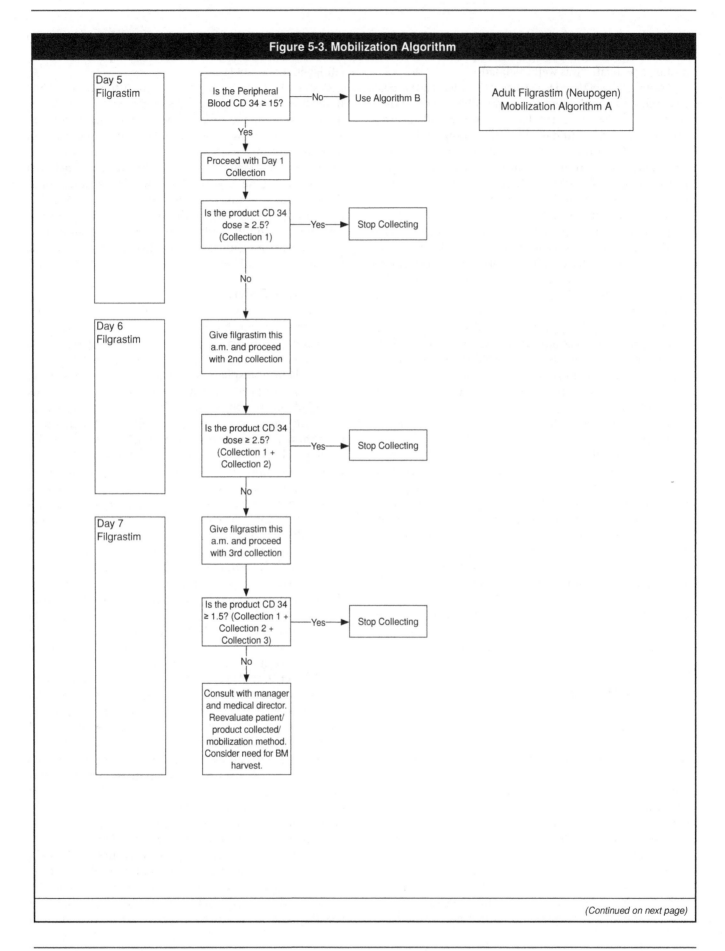

Day 5
Filgrastim

Is the Peripheral Blood CD 34 ≥ 15? —No→ Use Algorithm B

Adult Filgrastim (Neupogen) Mobilization Algorithm A

Yes

Proceed with Day 1 Collection

Is the product CD 34 dose ≥ 2.5? (Collection 1) —Yes→ Stop Collecting

No

Day 6
Filgrastim

Give filgrastim this a.m. and proceed with 2nd collection

Is the product CD 34 dose ≥ 2.5? (Collection 1 + Collection 2) —Yes→ Stop Collecting

No

Day 7
Filgrastim

Give filgrastim this a.m. and proceed with 3rd collection

Is the product CD 34 ≥ 1.5? (Collection 1 + Collection 2 + Collection 3) —Yes→ Stop Collecting

No

Consult with manager and medical director. Reevaluate patient/ product collected/ mobilization method. Consider need for BM harvest.

(Continued on next page)

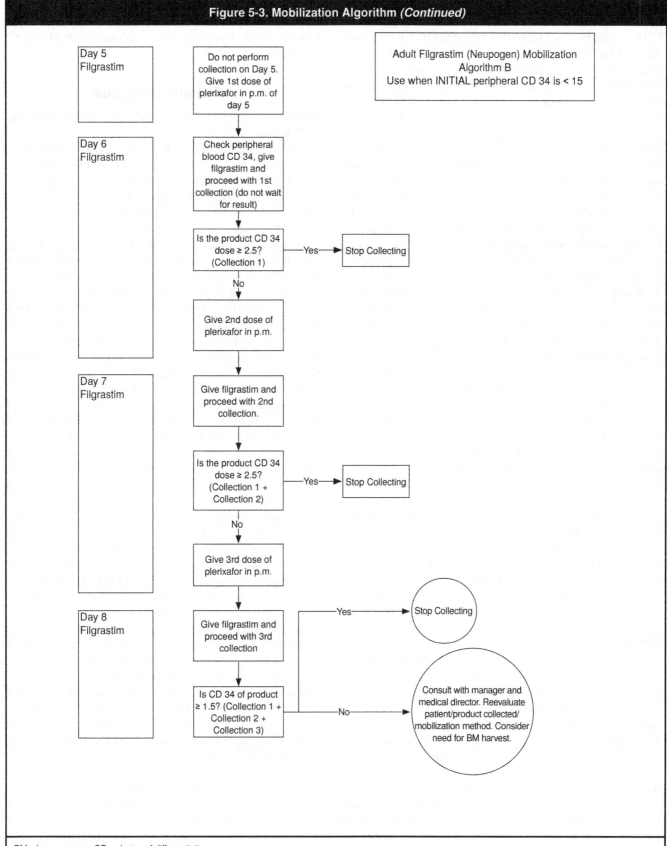

Figure 5-3. Mobilization Algorithm *(Continued)*

Adult Filgrastim (Neupogen) Mobilization Algorithm B
Use when INITIAL peripheral CD 34 is < 15

Day 5 Filgrastim

Do not perform collection on Day 5. Give 1st dose of plerixafor in p.m. of day 5

Day 6 Filgrastim

Check peripheral blood CD 34, give filgrastim and proceed with 1st collection (do not wait for result)

Is the product CD 34 dose ≥ 2.5? (Collection 1) —Yes→ Stop Collecting

No

Give 2nd dose of plerixafor in p.m.

Day 7 Filgrastim

Give filgrastim and proceed with 2nd collection.

Is the product CD 34 dose ≥ 2.5? (Collection 1 + Collection 2) —Yes→ Stop Collecting

No

Give 3rd dose of plerixafor in p.m.

Day 8 Filgrastim

Give filgrastim and proceed with 3rd collection

—Yes→ Stop Collecting

Is CD 34 of product ≥ 1.5? (Collection 1 + Collection 2 + Collection 3) —No→ Consult with manager and medical director. Reevaluate patient/product collected/ mobilization method. Consider need for BM harvest.

BM—bone marrow; CD—cluster of differentiation

Note. Copyright 2018 by Nebraska Medicine/University of Nebraska Medical Center, Hematopoietic Cell Transplantation Program, Omaha, Nebraska. Used with permission.

et al., 2008). Patients with a low peripheral blood CD34+ cell count or who were unable to collect at least 2×10^6 CD34+ cells/kg were eligible for this protocol. Patients then received filgrastim mobilization for four days. On the evening of day 4, the patients received plerixafor 240 mcg/kg. On day 5, they received another dose of filgrastim and then underwent apheresis (approximately 10 hours after the plerixafor injection). Apheresis was repeated daily, and plerixafor and filgrastim injections continued until the patient collected 2×10^6 CD34+ cells/kg or more or until failure to collect adequate cells. More than 200 patients were enrolled in the protocol; however, the authors focused their reporting on a subgroup of 115 patients. Many of the patients who had previously not produced enough stem cells for transplant were able to produce the minimum number of cells, greater than 2×10^6 CD34+ cells/kg, and proceed to transplant. Neutrophil and platelet engraftment in these patients occurred at medians of 11 days and 18 days, respectively. Most of the side effects (gastrointestinal effects, injection-site reactions, and paresthesias) were tolerable and resolved on their own. The authors concluded that plerixafor given with filgrastim is an option for patients who do not mobilize well.

Strategies to mobilize additional stem cells after initial failure to achieve the target CD34+ cell counts include increasing the dose of filgrastim and adding plerixafor, with or without chemotherapy (Giralt et al., 2014; To et al., 2011). A break of approximately two to four weeks is suggested between the failed mobilization attempt and remobilization. Currently, using plerixafor with filgrastim is the preferred remobilization approach (Duong et al., 2014). Many centers have created algorithms to start salvage mobilization strategies. Remobilizing patients who initially mobilized poorly may yield an adequate stem cell product. However, the costs involved in remobilization and the additional side effects must be considered. Attempting a salvage bone marrow harvest is also a consideration. However, patients with poor mobilization may also have an inadequate bone marrow harvest (Giralt et al., 2014; Stiff, 1999; To et al., 2011).

Future Directions of Mobilization

Since the approval of plerixafor, patients who would have typically been given chemotherapy for mobilization are now able to collect a high number of stem cells without the use of chemotherapy (Hari, 2018). Oyekunle et al. (2018) reviewed 236 patients who received chemotherapy mobilization. Disease response was evaluated prior to and following chemomobilization. They reported that chemomobilization did not improve remission status in patients with multiple myeloma. However, 28.4% of the patients in the study developed chemotherapy-related complications. Trends indicate that cytokine-only therapy is increasingly being used in the United States for mobilization (Hari, 2018). The Center for International Blood and Marrow Transplant Research has launched a large prospective observational study to compare clinical effectiveness, outcomes, and morbidity of mobilization practices in the United States (Hari, 2018). Novel agents to mobilize stem cells are needed, and increased understanding of the stem cell niche is necessary.

Apheresis Issues

Peripheral Venous Access Versus Central Venous Catheters

Antecubital veins may be used to collect PBSCs, but patients who have received multiple courses of chemotherapy may not have adequate venous access. Most centers use a thick-walled, large lumen (10–18.5 French) apheresis or hemodialysis catheter to withdraw blood, which allows flow rates up to 300–400 ml per hour or greater (Mackey, 2017). Apheresis catheters are usually inserted into the internal jugular vein and may be tunneled to provide long-term access. Other venous access sites that have been used include the subclavian vein, the femoral vein, and the inferior vena cava (Haire et al., 1990; Mackey, 2017). Pediatric patients may require a smaller catheter (6–8 French). Antecubital veins are most commonly used in allogeneic donors. However, if peripheral venous access cannot be obtained or maintained in allogeneic donors, a temporary nontunneled apheresis catheter may be placed in the internal jugular vein. Ultimately, the transplant team must consider the size and type of catheter that will yield the highest flow rate during apheresis, as well as patient or donor comfort. Often, the catheter used for apheresis may be used for venous access during the high-dose therapy, reinfusion of stem cells, and recovery phases.

Schulmeister (2017) described several adverse events that may occur during the placement of a catheter, including perforation of the vein, pneumothorax, or hemothorax. Other complications related to the catheter include infection, occlusion, thrombus, catheter rupture, and phlebitis. Table 5-1 describes the symptoms and management of some of these complications.

Care of the apheresis catheter varies widely from institution to institution, and no definitive recommendation can be made based on current evidence (Cope & Matey, 2017). Dressings should be changed if they become soiled or wet. Practices for flushing catheters also vary among institutions. Cope and Matey (2017) indicated that no definitive recommendation can be made for a specific flushing protocol; however, the practice standard is to flush with 0.9% normal saline following catheter access.

Timing and Initiation of Apheresis

Historically, the initiation of stem cell collection following chemotherapy mobilization was difficult to determine. Collection usually began when the WBC count reached $1,000/mm^3$. Once the WBC counts start to rise following nadir, the number of stem cells usually starts to increase. Stem cell collection following growth factor mobilization

Table 5-1. Complications of Central Venous Catheters

Complication	Time of Onset	Symptoms	Cause	Clinical Management	Nursing Management
Exit-site bleeding/ hematoma	Insertion	Oozing or frank bleeding from exit site; discoloration or bruising	Introducer sheath larger than catheter left in place or traumatic insertion. Patient may have coagulopathies or thrombocytopenia or be on anticoagulants.	Additional sutures, possible catheter removal	Apply local pressure. Change dressings as needed.
Pneumothorax or hemothorax	Insertion	Chest pain, tachypnea, dyspnea, decreased breath sounds	Air or blood in the pleural cavity because of pleura, vein, or thoracic duct injury	Chest x-ray, oxygen, needle aspirations, and chest tube drainage	Administer oxygen. Perform care of chest tube.
Exit-site infection	Duration of catheter placement	Fever, skin breakdown, local erythema, pain, tenderness at catheter insertion site, possible purulent drainage, sepsis	Neutropenia secondary to chemotherapy mobilization, poor catheter management techniques, commonly gram-positive organisms	Antibiotics	Obtain blood and exit-site cultures. Administer antibiotics if indicated. Teach aseptic technique in dressing changes and catheter flushing, signs and symptoms of infection, and emergency instructions.
Tunnel infection	Duration of catheter placement	Erythema, induration, tenderness along subcutaneous track of catheter, possible purulent exudate	Neutropenia secondary to chemotherapy mobilization, poor catheter management techniques, commonly gram-positive organisms	Antibiotics, possible catheter removal	Obtain blood cultures; culture exudate if present. Administer appropriate antibiotics.
Line infection	Duration of catheter placement	Cellulitis	Neutropenia secondary to chemotherapy mobilization, poor catheter management techniques, commonly gram-positive organisms, colonization of infecting organism (i.e., *Staphylococcus epidermis, Staphylococcus aureus*)	Antibiotics, possible catheter removal	Obtain blood cultures; culture exudate if present. Administer appropriate antibiotics.
Catheter occlusion	Duration of catheter placement, particularly during apheresis procedure	Inability to aspirate from or flush catheter, arm swelling, pain may be asymptomatic	Growth factors, thrombus, technical or mechanical problems, blood clotting, drug precipitate	Venogram, Doppler study, dye study, chest x-ray, alteplase (2 mg)	Perform gentle catheter flushing with heparin. Reposition patient. Consider possible catheter removal. Instill alteplase (2 mg) into lumen of catheter and let stand for 30 minutes. Attempt to aspirate; may repeat.
Catheter-related venous thrombus	Duration of catheter placement, particularly during mobilization and stem cell collection	Arm swelling, pain may be asymptomatic, venous congestion in neck on side of catheter	Venous collateral circulation	Venogram, Doppler study, dye study, chest x-ray, alteplase (2 mg)	Reposition patient. Perform gentle catheter flushing. Consider possible catheter removal. Monitor daily prothrombin time/ partial thromboplastin time.
Catheter rupture	Duration of catheter placement, particularly during mobilization and stem cell collection	Pain, shortness of breath, air and blood emboli, leakage from catheter, inability to aspirate catheter	Frequent catheter manipulation, forceful flushing against resistance	Replacement of catheter	Turn patient on left side and call physician. Clean and secure catheter; repair or exchange if possible. Consider possible catheter removal.

Note. Based on information from Schulmeister, 2017.

typically began when the WBC count reached $10,000/mm^3$ or greater, or approximately four to five days following the start of growth factor administration. If both chemotherapy and growth factors were used to mobilize stem cells, the collection began during the recovery of WBCs, approximately when the WBC count reached $1,000/mm^3$.

Assessing peripheral blood CD34+ cell counts to determine when to start collections has become the standard practice at many centers (Duong et al., 2014; Karakukcu & Unal, 2015; To et al., 2011). Using peripheral blood CD34+ cell counts has been shown to reduce apheresis costs (To et al., 2011). While starting apheresis has similar timing to historical practice, assessing the peripheral blood CD34+ count is the best predictor of the actual CD34+ count in the product. Monitoring peripheral blood CD34+ cell counts should begin on day 4 or 5 following filgrastim mobilization and generally about day 8–10 after chemotherapy and filgrastim (Duong et al., 2014; Karakukcu & Unal, 2015). Institutional practices vary on the minimal peripheral blood count to start apheresis. Counts ranging from $5–20/mm^3$ have been most routinely reported (Duong et al., 2014). Many centers have developed algorithms to guide mobilization in patients (Giralt et al., 2014; see Figure 5-3 for an example).

Healthy allogeneic donors who receive filgrastim for mobilization usually peak on day 5 (range 4–6) of growth factor (Karakukcu & Unal, 2015; To et al., 2011). Peripheral blood CD34+ cell counts may be assessed; however, starting collections on days 4–6 usually will achieve target counts.

Types of Apheresis Devices

Following mobilization, the PBSCs from the patient or donor are collected via a process called *apheresis*. This process involves using a commercial cell separator to centrifuge the blood and separate the components by density into various layers. The white cell and platelet layers are located between the red cell and plasma layers. Located in the white cell layer are the mononuclear cells and stem cells. The patient's or donor's blood is withdrawn through a central venous catheter into the apheresis machine and centrifuged. As the blood is drawn into the apheresis machine, the anticoagulant citrate dextrose solution (ACD-A) is added to prevent clotting. The ratio of ACD-A to blood is usually 1:12 to 1:15 (Lisenko et al., 2017). The apheresis machine centrifuges the blood, transfers the stem cell layer into a collection bag, and returns the remaining blood components to the patient or donor via the central venous catheter.

Several types of commercial cell separators are available. Deneys et al. (2017) compared the efficacy of three devices manufactured by Terumo BCT, Fenwal, and Fresenius Kabi. The authors reported that the median collection efficacy was similar among the three devices. A lower red cell contamination was found in the Terumo BCT and Fresenius Kabi machines, whereas a lower platelet contamination was found in the Fenwal device. However, further studies with a larger number of patients are recommended.

Amount of Blood to Process

In adults, approximately 12–15 L (2–3 times the patient's blood volume) of blood at a flow rate of 50–100 ml/min are commonly processed from a patient each day (Giralt et al., 2014). Each apheresis procedure takes two to four hours, and an adequate number of cells may be achieved in one collection. Improved mobilization methods, described previously, have decreased the number of collections to only one or very few apheresis procedures. However, some patients may need to undergo multiple collections to obtain adequate cells for transplant.

Apheresis procedures that process large volumes of blood (15–30 L, or 3–6 times the patient's blood volume) in a single collection result in the collection of large numbers of PBSCs (Giralt et al., 2014). Processing large blood volumes may result in increased side effects during the collection, such as hypocalcemia, hypomagnesemia, and thrombocytopenia (Giralt et al., 2014). Oral calcium may be given prophylactically, and administration of 1 g calcium gluconate IV every hour may be necessary to manage the toxicities associated with the large amount of citrate. Collecting adequate PBSCs in one collection enables transplantation to be a cost-effective option for patients. However, some patients may not be able to tolerate the lengthy procedure or the side effects. Reducing the number of collections results in a decrease in the amount of DMSO (dimethyl sulfoxide) necessary to preserve the product, thus potentially minimizing side effects during infusion of the stem cells.

Stem Cell Collection

The amount of stem cells collected is related to the rate of engraftment. Higher amounts of stem cells collected usually result in quicker engraftment, although complications associated with the high-dose therapy play a role (Giralt et al., 2014; Pusic et al., 2008; To et al., 2011). A variety of methods have been used to determine the adequate number of stem cells to collect for transplant. Initially, the number of mononuclear cells present in the product was used. Mononuclear cells are easy to measure, but these mature cells were not the most efficient method to determine the number of stem cells present. The colony assay, which detects committed progenitors, specifically CFU-GM, became the more common method to determine the number of cells required for transplant. To et al. (1992) reported that PBSC transplant recipients, who received a higher dose of CFU-GM in comparison to autologous and allogeneic bone marrow transplant recipients, recovered from neutropenia and thrombocytopenia significantly faster. The PBSC transplant recipients also required less supportive care. A disadvantage of using CFU-GM assays for determining adequate stem cell dosage is that the assays must incubate for approximately two weeks following each collection. After two weeks have passed, it may be determined that the product is inadequate, and the mobilization and collection process must be repeated. A second disadvantage to using CFU-GM assays is the different techniques used in laboratories and the lack of a consistent method, resulting in an inability to compare outcomes among centers (Bender, To, Williams, & Schwartzberg, 1992).

Currently, the most common method to determine an adequate dose of stem cells for transplant is the use of flow cytometric analysis to measure the number of cells expressing the CD34 antigen in the product (To et al., 2011). The CD34 antigen is present on committed hematopoietic progenitor cells and pluripotent stem cells (Golde, 1991). As PBSCs mature, expression of the CD34 antigen decreases, and these cells are no longer identified as CD34+ (Vescio et al., 1994). An advantage of flow cytometric analysis over colony assays is that the results are available in less than three hours after collection.

Siena et al. (1991) reported that the number of CD34+ cells correlated well with the number of circulating CFU-GM colonies in patients mobilized with chemotherapy and growth factors. Historically, the laboratory method of conducting the CD34+ assay varied from center to center, making it difficult to compare CD34+ numbers among centers. In 1995, the International Society of Hematotherapy and Graft Engineering (ISHAGE) created a committee to validate a standard method to quantitate CD34+ cells that is reproducible among transplant centers. The ISHAGE guidelines were published in 2009 (Sutherland, Anderson, Keeney, Nayar, & Chin-Yee, 2009) and have been adopted by many transplant centers.

The dose of CD34+ cells infused also varies widely among centers. Several studies in autologous transplantation indicated that a minimum dose of 2×10^6 CD34+ cells/kg ensures successful hematopoietic recovery (Duong et al., 2014; Forman & Nakamura, 2011; Giralt et al., 2014) and that a dose of 5×10^6 CD34+ cells/kg or greater ensures rapid engraftment (Giralt et al., 2014; To et al., 2011). However, doses less than $1-1.5 \times 10^6$ CD34+ cells/kg may result in delayed engraftment (Duong et al., 2014; Giralt et al., 2014; Pusic et al., 2008). In allogeneic (myeloablative and nonmyeloablative) transplantation, most centers use the minimum dose of 3×10^6 CD34+ cells/kg. However, doses greater than 5×10^6 CD34+ cells/kg have been shown to decrease resource utilization, result in quicker platelet engraftment, and achieve better survival for patients undergoing allogeneic transplantation (To et al., 2011). Doses of 10×10^6 CD34+ cells/kg or greater often are used for haploidentical transplants (To et al., 2011). Higher doses may result in faster engraftment, but they also may increase the risk of chronic GVHD (Duong et al., 2014).

Yamamoto et al. (2018) reported on the impact of a CD34+ dose less than 2×10^6 cells/kg on patients who received a related allogeneic transplant. They compared standard CD34+ doses ($2-5 \times 10^6$ cells/kg) to low doses ($1-2 \times 10^6$ cells/kg) and very low doses (less than 1×10^6 cells/kg). The low and very low CD34+ dose groups had delayed engraftment, both neutrophils and platelets. The two-year overall survival rate was similar in the standard and low dose groups and lower in the very low

dose group. However, a higher percentage of patients in the very low dose group had high-risk disease, were not in remission, or had undergone a previous transplant. No difference was found in relapse, nonrelapse mortality, or GVHD among the three groups. The authors concluded that low doses of CD34+ cells/kg are acceptable for transplant, whereas very low doses need further investigation (Yamamoto et al., 2018).

Side Effects of Collection

Common side effects encountered during the apheresis procedure are hypocalcemia, hypovolemia, thrombocytopenia, anemia, chilling, and headache. Usually these side effects are minimal and well tolerated. Table 5-2 describes potential complications of stem cell collections. Another complication frequently encountered during apheresis is catheter occlusion. Occlusion may result from the catheter resting against the wall of the vein, a kink in the catheter, or a clot or fibrin sheath around the end of the catheter.

Stephens, Haire, Schmit-Pokorny, Kessinger, and Kotulak (1993) compared patients who did not receive growth factors for mobilization with patients who were mobilized with continuous-infusion sargramostim. Although all patients received aspirin 325 mg daily as prophylaxis, the sargramostim-mobilized patients had a significantly higher rate of catheter occlusions. The exact mechanism for the formation of the clot is unknown, but the authors suggested that contributing factors may have included proliferation of "sticky" neutrophils, which aggregated at the catheter tip; the method of administration of the sargramostim; or changes in the coagulation and fibrinolytic systems caused by the sargramostim (Stephens et al., 1993).

Flushing the catheter with normal saline or repositioning the patient may correct the obstruction. A fibrinolytic agent, alteplase (Activase®), may be necessary to lyse or dissolve the clot. Occasionally, a cathetergram or dye injected into the catheter may be necessary to determine the exact cause of the obstruction. If a clot is noted at the end of the catheter, additional injections of alteplase may be necessary to dissolve it. The catheter may need to be repositioned or replaced if the clot cannot be corrected.

During the apheresis procedure, the platelet count or hemoglobin level may decrease because of removal of the cells into the product collection bag. Patients may need to receive irradiated packed red blood cells or platelets to replenish the cells removed. Patients who have received chemotherapy for mobilization may require blood products prior to apheresis to ensure a safe procedure. Transfusions should be considered for patients with a hemoglobin level less than 9 g/dl and a platelet count less than 80,000/mm³.

Allogeneic Blood Stem Cell Collection

The first reported related allogeneic PBSC transplant was in an 18-year-old man with acute lymphoblastic leukemia

Table 5-2. Potential Complications During Peripheral Blood Stem Cell Collection

Complication	Etiology	Assessment	Interventions
Hypocalcemia	Sodium citrate used to prevent blood from clotting in the apheresis machine binds ionized calcium.	Baseline serum calcium Hourly ionized calcium[a] Patient age Assess for paresthesias of the extremities or circumoral area during the procedure.	Notify physician if calcium is low. Slow flow rate and offer oral calcium, liquid or tablets. Increase calcium-containing foods. Advise patient to take oral calcium supplements. Administer IV calcium gluconate (for severe symptoms).
Hypovolemia	Extracorporeal volume greater than patient tolerance	Baseline pulse, blood pressure, hemoglobin/hematocrit, and health history Brief physical assessment and vital signs every 5 minutes initially, gradually decreasing frequency as patient's tolerance is established Assess for • Hypotension • Tachycardia • Light-headedness • Diaphoresis • Dysrhythmias	Notify physician of abnormal or unexpected findings before proceeding. Interrupt the procedure until the patient is stable, then resume at a slower flow rate and minimal extracorporeal volume. Monitor physical status and vital signs closely. Notify physician if symptoms persist or progress. Administer blood products. Administer fluid.
Thrombocytopenia	Collection of platelets into product	Baseline platelet count Determination of whether platelet-rich plasma will be returned at the procedure's completion	Notify physician if count is < 50,000/mm³. Monitor for signs of postprocedure bleeding. Administer platelet products.
Miscellaneous Effects			
Chilling	Cooling of blood while circulating in the apheresis machine	Observe for chilling.	Provide warmth (e.g., blankets, heating pad).
Severe headache	Growth factor side effect Intracranial metastases unique to patient with cancer	Pain relievers Computed tomography or magnetic resonance imaging of the brain in patients prone to intracranial metastases prior to beginning apheresis	Administer analgesics.
Prolonged cytopenia	Previous chemotherapy regimens Pediatric patients with less developed hematopoietic progenitor pool[a]	Observe for headache. Observe daily complete blood count, platelets, and differential.	Transfusion support

[a] Applies to pediatric patients

Note. Based on information from Cooling et al., 2017; Hsu & Cushing, 2016; Karakukcu & Unal, 2015; Lisenko et al., 2017.

From "Peripheral Blood Stem Cell Transplantation," by P.J. Hooper and E.J. Santos, 1993, *Oncology Nursing Forum, 20,* p. 1218. Copyright 1993 by Oncology Nursing Society. Adapted with permission.

(Kessinger et al., 1989). Stem cells were collected from his 21-year-old, HLA-identical sibling because he was unwilling to undergo general anesthesia and marrow harvesting. Ten apheresis collections were performed, and the product was T cell depleted. A bone marrow biopsy and cytogenetic studies on day +27 showed trilineage engraftment with donor cells. Unfortunately, the patient died from a fungal infection on day +32, and long-term engraftment could not be evaluated. Advantages of an allogeneic PBSC transplant include more rapid hematopoietic and immune recovery, avoidance of general anesthesia, and avoidance of the side effects associated with bone marrow harvest. Disadvantages may include an increased risk of GVHD (Anasetti et al., 2011).

Allogeneic donors usually are mobilized using filgrastim 5–10 mcg/kg, similar to patients undergoing autologous transplantation. Chemotherapy is not used to mobilize allogeneic donors. In an early study by Bishop et al. (1997), 41 donors were mobilized with filgrastim 5 mcg/kg who underwent a minimum of three apheresis procedures each. The clinical nurse coordinator and the apheresis nurse evaluated toxicities daily. Each donor maintained a diary to record adverse effects of filgrastim administration and apheresis procedures. The most common side effects were arthralgias/myalgias (83%), headache (44%), fever (27%), and chills (22%). Other side effects noted were nausea and vomiting, paresthesias, chest pain, cough, diarrhea, sore throat, and hypertension. Except for one, all recorded side effects were grade 1, according to the National Cancer Institute toxicity scale. One patient experienced grade 3 hypertension and was treated with nifedipine. The authors concluded that low doses of filgrastim can be effectively and safely used for mobilization.

In another early study, Wiesneth et al. (1998) reported the use of filgrastim 10–12 mcg/kg to mobilize 96 related donors. PBSC harvest was started on day 4 of the growth factor, and donors collected in an average of two days (range one to four). The researchers found that the peak level of CD34+ cells occurred between days 4 and 6 of filgrastim administration. They reported that female and older donors tended to have a decreased response to the filgrastim, but this was not statistically significant. Reinfusion of platelets collected during the apheresis procedure was necessary in 16% of the donors because of a platelet count less than 80,000/mm³ following apheresis.

A serious adverse event reported in an allogeneic donor possibly related to the mobilization technique was splenic rupture and pneumothorax that occurred in a 22-year-old man (Becker et al., 1997). The donor had received six days of filgrastim prior to apheresis. Four days after the completion of apheresis, the donor presented with left-sided abdominal pain, dyspnea, hypotension, and tachycardia. A computed tomography scan revealed a ruptured spleen, and emergency surgery was required. The authors concluded that although growth factors have proved to be advantageous for recipients, potentially serious adverse effects are possible in donors. In most circumstances, growth factor–mobilized stem cells can be safely collected from donors. However, because serious side effects may occur, donors should be thoroughly educated about potential complications.

Unrelated Blood Stem Cell Collection

NMDP, established in 1986, has facilitated more than 86,000 unrelated transplants through its Be The Match (n.d.-d) donor registry. Initially, all unrelated transplant patients received bone marrow transplants. In 1999, NMDP began to facilitate PBSC and UCB transplants. At the time of this writing, more than 19 million donors (Be The Match, n.d.-a) and 249,000 cord blood units were listed in the registry (Be The Match, n.d.-b).

Prior to 1999, the lack of knowledge regarding the long-term side effects of growth factors limited most unrelated transplants to the use of bone marrow. However, long-term follow-up studies showed no relationship between growth factor use and long-term effects. In a study reported by Pulsipher et al. (2014), 6,768 PBSC donors underwent collection between 2004 and 2009. All donors were mobilized with filgrastim 10 mcg/kg/day, and

cells were collected on day 5 or on days 5 and 6 of growth factor administration. Most side effects were associated with the filgrastim or apheresis procedure and resolved within a few days following the completion of apheresis. Extensive long-term follow-up (median 36 months, range 6 days to 89 months) was compared to 2,726 bone marrow donors (median 36 months, range 7 days to 86 months) who had not received filgrastim. The incidence of cancer, autoimmune disease, or thrombosis was similar between the groups. When compared to the general population, the PBSC donors showed a lower cancer incidence. The authors hoped their report provided reassurance to unrelated donors using filgrastim for mobilization followed by apheresis PBSC collection (Pulsipher et al., 2014).

The NMDP protocol for harvesting stem cells from an unrelated donor involves mobilizing and collecting the donor cells, similar to the process with related donors. Donors receive filgrastim for five consecutive days and then undergo apheresis to collect stem cells. Following stem cell collection, NMDP continues to follow the donors annually (Be The Match, n.d.-e).

Mismatched and Haploidentical Donors

Many candidates for high-dose therapy do not have an HLA-matched related sibling or are unable to locate an HLA-matched unrelated donor through national registries. In these cases, a partially mismatched related or unrelated haploidentical (half-matched) donor could be considered. One early study by Henslee-Downey et al. (1997) reported the use of partially mismatched related donors for 72 patients. The patients received total body irradiation and high-dose chemotherapy followed by transplantation of T-cell–depleted bone marrow. The authors concluded that a partially mismatched related donor transplant can be performed with acceptable rates of graft failure and GVHD, but more studies are needed.

Koh, Rizzieri, and Chao (2007) summarized several studies using mismatched or haploidentical donors. They concluded that haploidentical transplants provided an opportunity for patients to undergo transplantation when they did not have a matched sibling donor and found it difficult or time consuming to find a matched unrelated donor. Decreases in early transplant mortality and severe GVHD resulting from the use of T-cell depletion and reduced-intensity conditioning regimens have improved the benefits of haploidentical transplants. However, the authors indicated that post-transplant infections due to slow immune reconstitution and relapse were still issues, and continued studies are needed.

D'Souza et al. (2017) reported that mismatched related donor transplants are becoming more common, with 11% of all allogeneic transplants in 2015 coming from relatives with one or more HLA antigen mismatches compared to 9% in 2000. Haploidentical donor transplants are becoming more common because of greater availability of related donors (Panch et al., 2017).

Pediatric Blood Stem Cell Collection

Special consideration must be given to pediatric patients during the collection of PBSCs. Many children require a central venous catheter, which is placed with the patient under general anesthesia (Karakukcu & Unal, 2015). Pediatric allogeneic donors undergo mobilization and collection similar to adult allogeneic donors (Duong et al., 2014; Karakukcu & Unal, 2015). The most common growth factor is filgrastim 10 mcg/kg/day. The use of plerixafor in pediatric donors has been reported; however, no specific recommendations are available (Karakukcu & Unal, 2015), and its use in children is not FDA approved. Chemotherapy and filgrastim for mobilization in children have also been reported with good success (Karakukcu & Unal, 2015).

The volume of blood processed during the apheresis procedure must be based on the child's size. Commonly, 200–250 ml of blood per kilogram of body weight may be processed depending on the patient's tolerance of the procedure. Duong et al. (2014) and Karakukcu and Unal (2015) recommended transfusing red blood cells for low-weight pediatric patients whose hemoglobin level is below 12 g/dl. If more than 10%–15% of the child's total blood volume (a child weighing 20 kg or less) is needed for priming the apheresis machine, the machine and associated tubing may need to be preprimed with irradiated red blood cells or albumin to decrease the amount of blood loss (Duong et al., 2014; Karakukcu & Unal, 2015). Parents or family members may directly donate red blood cells. Another method to decrease the amount of blood loss is to dilute the red cells with albumin to approximate the same value as the patient's hematocrit, or slightly higher, prior to priming the apheresis machine. Calcium gluconate may be administered to prevent hypocalcemia (Cooling et al., 2017).

Cooling et al. (2017) reported a large prospective study of 62 pediatric patients undergoing apheresis for autologous transplant and their procedure-related adverse events. The median age was 4.5 years (range 1–17). The median weight of the patients was 18 kg (range 8–103), with 58% of the patients less than 20 kg. They found that 39% of the patients experienced procedural adverse events, including citrate reactions and venous access issues. Compared with earlier studies, older, larger children had more adverse events than the younger children.

Behfar et al. (2018) reported long-term follow-up (median 4.8 years, range 1.2–14.2 years) on 145 sibling donors whose median age at collection was 10 years (range 2–15 years). No serious adverse events, neoplastic disorders, or deaths were reported. The authors concluded that using filgrastim to mobilize healthy sibling donors is safe and well tolerated.

Pediatric donors often serve as a donor for their siblings. Rarely, children have been considered as a donor for their parent or other adult family member. Ethical considerations must be reviewed and addressed prior to mobilization and collection. Risks and benefits to the donor must be weighed with the risks and benefits to the recipient or family. Benefit to the donor is considered the psychosocial benefit of helping the recipient. However, reports show that children experience distress, and many pediatric donors believe they did not have a choice of whether to donate. The American Academy of Pediatrics has established ethical criteria so that children may be considered as donors (Karakukcu & Unal, 2015).

Psychological and Ethical Issues Related to Stem Cell Donation

Numerous feelings may accompany the donation of stem cells. Overall, the procedure is associated with minimal risks. Donors may feel proud to be a donor but may experience anxiety related to the donation. Occasionally, unknown medical conditions are discovered, or confidential personal issues become known by family members. Donors may experience a range of emotions, from ambivalence to jealousy to guilt. Wiener, Steffen-Smith, Fry, and Wayne (2007) summarized the available data related to the sibling donor experience. They stated that healthcare staff and the patient's family usually focused on the ill child. The authors summarized a variety of psychological manifestations, including anxiety, depression, post-traumatic stress reactions, low self-esteem, and other maladaptive responses. They found some positive response in sibling donors, such as increased maturity, better leadership skills, higher levels of social competence, and increased adaptive skills. The outcome of the transplant affected the sibling donor both positively and negatively. From the review of the literature, the authors concluded that donating stem cells is a stressful experience and may lead to long-term distress. They suggested that comprehensive preparation and follow-up after the donation may decrease the negative effects on the donor.

Stem cell donation is associated with various ethical issues. Consent for a minor child to donate stem cells to a sibling usually is given by the parent. The child may give consent or assent; however, the child may feel pressured to donate (Wiener et al., 2007). Ethical issues may arise when parents become desperate to find treatment options for a sick child or loved one. Neumann (2007) recommended extensive psychosocial and developmental assessments of donors who are minors. Another ethical issue might involve older donors with comorbidities, which may increase the risk of donation. A thorough medical assessment is crucial to identifying possible problems during the collection. Ethnic or religious beliefs of donors from other countries also may raise ethical issues.

An additional ethical issue may involve parents who choose to conceive a child through embryo selection to become a stem cell donor for an ill child. Kurtzberg, Lyerly, and Sugarman (2005) stated that although this may be successful, the baby may not be HLA matched or may have the same illness. Selecting embryos and conceiving a child to become a stem cell donor may raise numerous religious and philosophical issues.

Neumann (2007) gave several suggestions to protect the donor's rights, including establishment of program policies to ensure voluntary donation. A different physician than the recipient's physician should discuss donation and evaluate the donor. Detailed information on the risks associated with donation of stem cells should be discussed and reviewed with the donor. A formal ethics consult may be required to resolve ethical issues and safeguard the donor's rights and interests.

A report from van Walraven et al. (2018) recognized that although standards have been developed to ensure the safety of volunteer donors, organizations are frequently confronted with requests that cause adjustment of standard procedures. They provided guidance on ethical principles involved in donation and discussed nonstandard donations. They also discussed expectations and commitment of the donor, as well as the concepts of beneficence, autonomy, nonmaleficence, fairness, and honesty related to the donor. Informed consent and confidentiality were also reviewed. They gave case study examples that involved current concerns, including nonstandard product requests, multiple donations, genetic testing of donor samples, cryopreservation with and without consent, and recipient identification by the donor.

Cord Blood Stem Cell Transplantation

Another option for obtaining stem cells is the use of UCB and placental blood. UCB may be collected, cryopreserved, and stored for the donor (autologous transplant) or a family member (related allogeneic transplant) or donated to a UCB registry bank for an unrelated recipient (unrelated allogeneic transplant). The first report of a successful UCB transplant was a five-year-old boy with Fanconi anemia who was transplanted with his sibling's cord blood (Gluckman et al., 1989). Since that time, many UCB transplants have been reported, and determining the proper use of these stem cells has generated substantial research. HLA-matched or partially mismatched unrelated UCB transplants, primarily in pediatric patients, have shown to be comparable to transplanting with unrelated bone marrow (Dessels, Alessandrini, & Pepper, 2018). D'Souza et al. (2017) reported that in 2015, 33% of all pediatric unrelated donor transplants used UCB, compared to 25% in 2000.

Advantages for harvesting UCB seem to outweigh any disadvantages (see Figure 5-4). The potential for a low incidence of GVHD may be one of the most important advantages for using UCB. Because of the decreased effectiveness of the lymphocytes, UCB transplants result in signif-

Figure 5-4. Advantages and Disadvantages of Using Umbilical Cord Blood for Transplantation

Advantages
- Abundant source, usually discarded
- Ease and safety of collection
- May be stored for unrelated patients
- Potential for increased ethnic or minority participation
- Tolerant of mismatched human leukocyte antigen type
- Low incidence of acute and chronic graft-versus-host disease
- Low risk of viral contamination (e.g., cytomegalovirus, Epstein-Barr)
- Minimal ethical concerns

Disadvantages
- Potential maternal T-lymphocyte contamination
- Possible microbial contamination
- Limited number of stem cells harvested (may not be adequate for transplant)
- Potential for decreased graft-versus-tumor effect
- Possible delayed engraftment
- Potential for graft failure
- Impossible to obtain additional cells from unrelated donor
- Transmission of undiagnosed genetic diseases
- Transmission of infectious diseases
- Cost
- Ethical issues

Note. Based on information from Bertolini et al., 1995; Dessels et al., 2018; Kurtzberg et al., 2005; Lund, 2018; Panch et al., 2017.

icantly lower incidence and severity of GVHD compared to matched or mismatched transplants. Unfortunately, this may result in less graft-versus-tumor effect, increasing the potential for relapse (Panch et al., 2017).

Identifying a suitable cord blood match is much quicker than identifying an unrelated bone marrow or PBSC donor. The cord blood has already undergone viral testing, samples for confirmatory testing are already available, and the UCB, once identified, is already stored (Dessels et al., 2018; Panch et al., 2017). For ethnic or minority populations, the potential exists for increased participation in donating to a UCB bank. The risk of viral contamination (specifically cytomegalovirus and Epstein-Barr) may be lower with the use of UCB because few infants are infected with these viruses (Kline & Bertolone, 1998).

Initially, there were concerns that insufficient progenitor cells would be available for larger patients, and recipients were limited to 40 kg. Rubinstein et al. (1998) reported on 562 patients who received unrelated UCB transplants, of which 185 recipients weighed more than 40 kg. They noted that the heaviest patient (116 kg) received the lowest number of cells and still achieved successful engraftment. In a review article by Kamani et al. (2008), the authors indicated that the cell dose of the UCB unit is critical to hematopoietic recovery and survival after transplant, and evidence showed that HLA match also affects engraftment and survival. However, additional research is needed to determine the effect of cell dose and HLA match on transplant outcome. The authors summarized current data and indicated that a suitable cell dose is greater than 2.5–3 × 10^7 total precryopreserved nucleated cells per kilogram of recipient body weight.

Several methods have been studied to address the limitation of the UCB cell dose: infusion of 2 UCB units, expansion of the UCB in vitro, and expansion of the hematopoietic stem cells (Lund, 2018). In a study to address the low cell dose of one UCB unit, Ballen et al. (2007) transplanted adult patients with two partially matched UBC units to provide a higher cell dose and to decrease the risk of slow engraftment caused by a lower cell dose. Patients received a reduced-intensity conditioning regimen followed by 2 UCB units that were 4/6 HLA matched or better. The minimum precryopreservation cell dose was 3.7 × 10^7 nucleated cells/kg. Transplant-related mortality was low in this study, and the authors concluded that adult patients can tolerate a double UCB transplant. A double UCB transplant may be an option for patients who need an unrelated transplant.

A significant disadvantage of using UCB is the possible transfer of undiagnosed genetic diseases. Currently, cord blood donors are not followed past birth to determine if a congenital disease develops. However, extensive individual and family questionnaires are completed prior to birth to try to identify potential problems.

Other possible disadvantages include microbial or maternal T-lymphocyte contamination of the UCB product. Also, the amount of time a UCB product may be stored and still maintain its viability is unknown. Delayed immune reconstitution and the need for steroid-containing GVHD prophylaxis regimens are other possible disadvantages.

Collection of stem cells from an umbilical cord usually is accomplished by one of two methods. The main goal is to not disrupt the normal labor, delivery, and postpartum period. The most common method of collection is to remove the delivered placenta to a site outside the delivery room and, using aseptic technique, thoroughly cleanse and then puncture the umbilical vein with a 16- or 17-gauge needle (AABB et al., 2018; Kurtzberg et al., 2005). The blood then is drained by gravity into a blood bag or, less often, withdrawn into a 60 ml syringe containing anticoagulant. This method takes approximately 5–10 minutes and should be performed in a sterile fashion. Another option is to collect blood from the placenta while it is still in utero, after the baby has been delivered but prior to delivery of the placenta. Uterine contractions are used to force blood out of the placenta. Delay in delivery of the placenta may not be possible, and contamination with either maternal blood or infectious organisms is highly possible. Experienced staff collect an average of 110 ml from a placenta (AABB et al., 2018; Kurtzberg et al., 2005).

The two types of UCB banks are public and private. NMDP began facilitating unrelated UCB transplants in 1999. Since then, it has developed a central registry of more than 249,000 UCB units (Be The Match, n.d.-b). When international partners are included, NMDP has access to more than 712,000 cord blood units around the world (Be The Match, n.d.-c). Private UCB banks store cord blood units for use by the baby, family member, or relative.

Many ethical issues surround the use of UCB transplantation. First is the issue of for-profit companies that store UCB for potential future use by the donor or a family member versus donation of UCB to registries with the intended use for an unrelated UCB transplant. Several facilities offer cryopreservation and storage for a fee and are available around the country. Dessels et al. (2018) and Kurtzberg et al. (2005) questioned the ethics of marketing this service to new parents when the probability of using the cord blood is highly unlikely.

Another ethical issue involves informed consent. Consent is obtained from the mother for UCB banking. However, if the cells have not been used by the time the child reaches maturity, the question arises as to whether the cells belong to the child. The mother must provide additional information, both medical and personal, about the newborn and the family history for the product to be included in a public UCB bank. Figure 5-5 describes the informed consent process for UCB donation.

Ethical questions may arise when the parents of a sick child become pregnant with the hope of creating a compatible donor for their sick offspring. The potential also exists for liability issues arising from undiagnosed genetic diseases that may be transferred to a recipient of UCB from a public registry. UCB transplantation will continue to be evaluated to determine its place in stem cell transplantation.

Figure 5-5. Process for Consent to Donate Umbilical Cord Blood

- Information regarding umbilical cord blood collection and banking is given to and discussed (including opportunity for questions) with the mother.
- A consent form is signed with the following key statements:
  - Donation of the umbilical cord blood is voluntary.
  - The mother's blood and the umbilical cord blood unit may be tested for infectious diseases.
  - A detailed family medical history will be provided to the cord blood bank.
  - The cord blood is not being stored for personal use by the baby, family, or relatives.
  - The umbilical cord blood unit will be listed on a registry of unrelated donors and will be made available to patients.
  - In the future, the mother may be contacted by the cord blood bank to obtain follow-up information on the baby's health.
  - The mother's and the baby's identities will be protected.
- Timing of the consent is usually prior to collection of the cord blood, ideally prior to the beginning of active labor; however, in some circumstances, consent is obtained after collection.

Note. Based on information from Kurtzberg et al., 2005.

Stem Cell Processing

Once the stem cells from the bone marrow, blood, or umbilical cord are collected, they are further processed, possibly cryopreserved, and stored between –80°C and –196°C in a freezer. An autologous stem cell product is usually frozen until after the patient has received high-dose therapy and is ready for reinfusion or transplant. Allogeneic stem cell products may be infused immediately following collection and processing, stored in a refrigerator at 4°C, infused the day following collection, or frozen. Unrelated allogeneic stem cell products are collected at an NMDP-approved collection center and shipped via courier to the transplant center. At the transplant center, the stem cell product will undergo appropriate processing and then be transplanted.

All stem cell products require additional processing prior to freezing. The stem cells are tested for sterility and infectious diseases, and blood typing is completed to ensure a safe product. Usually the overall volume of each product is reduced to decrease the amount of cryoprotectant required. Increased volumes of cryoprotectant and cell lysis are associated with increased clinical toxicities during the reinfusion or transplant (Lecchi et al., 2016). Allogeneic related or unrelated products may be red cell– or plasma-depleted prior to infusing or freezing if ABO incompatibility exists between the recipient and the donor.

Following processing, the stem cells are cryopreserved. During this phase, a cryoprotectant is added to the cells to prevent cell damage during either freezing or thawing. Without some form of cryopreservation, ice crystals form in cells during the freezing and thawing processes. This results in ruptured cell membranes. The most common current method of cryopreservation is adding DMSO at 10% of the total product volume, followed by controlled-rate freezing, and then placing the product into a long-term storage freezer in liquid nitrogen or, more commonly, the vapor phase of liquid nitrogen (Lecchi et al., 2016).

Stem Cell Manipulation

Historically, manipulation of stem cells predominantly involved selection of the CD34+ cells, attempts to purge tumor cells from autologous stem cells, or depletion of T cells (Panch et al., 2017). Delays in engraftment were reported. Stem cell selection or purging is more labor intensive and costly than standard processing methods. T lymphocytes, the cells responsible for GVHD, may be depleted from the allogeneic stem cell product, thereby decreasing the incidence of GVHD (Cantilena et al., 2018). The goal in processing the cells is to remove enough of the T lymphocytes to decrease GVHD while still maintaining enough T lymphocytes to stimulate an immune response to the tumor (graft-versus-tumor response) and ensure engraftment. Both ex vivo and in vitro depletion methods involve elutriation (separates the cells based on size and density), monoclonal antibodies (bind to cell surface antigens), immunoaf-finity columns, and beads. The Blood and Marrow Transplant Clinical Trials Network is currently studying ex vivo CD34+ cell isolation using the CliniMACS® CD34 Reagent System for T-cell depletion (Cantilena et al., 2018; Kosuri et al., 2017).

Future Directions

Future directions lie in improving the stem cell graft, ex vivo expansion of stem cell products, gene manipulation, using hematopoietic stem cell transplantation in additional patient populations, and the manipulation of stem cells to differentiate into types of cells (e.g., bone, liver, heart) other than blood cells. Methods to reduce GVHD that have been reported include removal of select T-cell populations from the stem cell graft (Morgan, Gray, Lomova, & Kohn, 2017).

Stiff et al. (2018) reported on a multicenter study performing ex vivo expansion of UCB cells for 101 patients. They selected CD133+ cells from the UCB unit and expanded them in vitro using a copper chelator and cytokines. The outcomes, compared to patients who received a double UCB transplant, were faster engraftment and a reduced 100-day mortality rate. The authors suggested further study is needed. Lund (2018) indicated that several publications have described successful UCB cell expansion. Most of the studies showed earlier engraftment when compared to historical patients. These studies were not randomized, and the patients only had short-term follow-up. Currently, none of the products are available commercially. However, the studies indicated that UCB can be successfully expanded (Lund, 2018). Although progress in the expansion of stem cells has been made, research is still needed (Morgan et al., 2017).

Other areas of future interest include the use of high-dose therapy and PBSC transplant in patients with autoimmune diseases, such as multiple sclerosis, rheumatoid arthritis, scleroderma, type 1 diabetes, or systemic lupus erythematosus, in which standard therapy fails to cure or effectively treat the patient. High-dose therapy followed by transplantation may replace the immune system (allogeneic) or reset the immune system (autologous).

The use of PBSCs in gene therapy trials is currently under investigation (Morgan et al., 2017). Gene therapy involves the placement of a functioning gene into a patient's cells to correct a genetic error or to add a novel ability to those cells. Hematopoietic stem cells are being considered for use with gene therapy because they can differentiate into myeloid and lymphoid cell lines, have a long life span, and are capable of self-renewal. They are also easily accessible. UCB cells may be even more receptive than PBSCs to genetic engineering because of the immaturity of the cells. Three categories of targeted gene editing exist: gene disruption, gene correction, and gene insertion. Gene disruption may be accomplished by blocking or knocking out a regulatory element, viral receptor, or pathogenic gene. Genes may be corrected by providing a corrective gene sequence from a donor template for DNA repair. Gene insertion involves the targeted insertion of a corrective gene (Morgan et al., 2017). All methods are in current studies.

Summary

Hematopoietic stem cell transplantation is used to treat an extensive variety of diseases. Stem cells may be collected from multiple sources: bone marrow, blood, and UCB. Stem cells collected from the blood currently are the preferred autologous stem cell source for patients who receive high-dose therapy. PBSC transplant results in earlier hematologic recovery, which translates into a potential decrease in the number of transfusions, toxicities, and hospital days. Patients or donors usually are mobilized with chemotherapy and/or growth factors, and more recently, chemokine antagonists, to increase the number of circulating stem cells. The number of UCB transplants also may increase in the future because of the possibility of decreased GVHD incidence. Once stem cells are collected, they are either transplanted within 24 hours or are cryopreserved and stored in a freezer until transplanted.

As the applications for the use of stem cells expand, so will opportunities for nurses in all areas of patient care, research, and administration. Nurses must strive to keep up to date in this continuously evolving field to be able to provide appropriate care and education for patients and their families.

References

AABB, America's Blood Centers, American Red Cross, American Society for Apheresis, American Society for Blood and Marrow Transplantation, College of American Pathologists, … World Marrow Donor Association. (2018, October). *Circular of information for the use of cellular therapy products.* Retrieved from http://www.aabb.org/aabbcct/coi/Documents/CT-Circular-of-Information.pdf

Adler, B.K., Salzman, D.E., Carabasi, M.H., Vaughan, W.P., Reddy, V.V.B., & Prchal, J.T. (2001). Fatal sickle cell crisis after granulocyte colony-stimulating factor administration. *Blood, 97,* 3313–3314. https://doi.org/10.1182/blood.V97.10.3313

Anasetti, C., Logan, B.R., Lee, S.J., Waller, E.K., Weisdorf, D.J., Wingard, J.R., … Confer, D.L. (2011). Increased incidence of chronic graft-versus-host disease (GVHD) and no survival advantage with filgrastim-mobilized peripheral blood stem cells (PBSC) compared to bone marrow (BM) transplants from unrelated donors: Results of Blood and Marrow Transplant Clinical Trials Network (BMTCTN) protocol 0201, a phase III, prospective, randomized trial [Abstract]. *Blood, 118*(21), 1. https://doi.org/10.1182/blood.V118.21.1.1

Anasetti, C., Logan, B.R., Lee, S.J., Waller, E.K., Weisdorf, D.J., Wingard, J.R., … Confer, D.L. (2012). Peripheral-blood stem cells versus bone marrow from unrelated donors. *New England Journal of Medicine, 367,* 1487–1496. https://doi.org/10.1056/NEJMoa1203517

Ballen, K.K., Spitzer, T.R., Yeap, B.Y., McAfee, S., Dey, B.R., Attar, E., … Antin, J.H. (2007). Double unrelated reduced-intensity umbilical cord blood transplantation in adults. *Biology of Blood and Marrow Transplantation, 13,* 82–89. https://doi.org/10.1016/j.bbmt.2006.08.041

Be The Match. (n.d.-a). Be The Match registry. Retrieved from https://bethematchclinical.org/about-us/what-we-do/our-registry

Be The Match. (n.d.-b). Cord blood and transplants. Retrieved from https://bethematch.org/transplant-basics/cord-blood-and-transplants

Be The Match. (n.d.-c). Donor or cord blood unit search process. Retrieved from https://bethematchclinical.org/transplant-therapy-and-donor-matching/donor-or-cord-blood-search-process

Be The Match. (n.d.-d). Our story. Retrieved from https://bethematch.org/about-us/our-story

Be The Match. (n.d.-e). Steps of PBSC or bone marrow donation. Retrieved from https://bethematch.org/transplant-basics/how-marrow-donation-works/steps-of-bone-marrow-or-pbsc-donation

Becker, P.S., Wagle, M., Matous, S., Swanson, R.S., Pihan, G., Lowry, P.A., … Heard, S.O. (1997). Spontaneous splenic rupture following administration of granulocyte colony-stimulating factor (G-CSF): Occurrence in an allogeneic donor of peripheral blood stem cells. *Biology of Blood and Marrow Transplantation, 3,* 45–49.

Behfar, M., Faghihi-Kashani, S., Hosseini, A.S., Ghavamzadeh, A., & Hamidieh, A.A. (2018). Long-term safety of short-term administration of filgrastim (rhG-CSF) and leukopheresis procedure in healthy children: Application of peripheral blood stem cell collection in pediatric donors. *Biology of Blood and Marrow Transplantation, 24,* 866–870. https://doi.org/10.1016/j.bbmt.2017.12.786

Bell, A.J., Figes, A., Oscier, D.G., & Hamblin, T.J. (1986). Peripheral blood stem cell autografting. *Lancet, 327,* 1027. https://doi.org/10.1016/S0140-6736(86)91288-2

Bender, J.G., To, L.B., Williams, S., & Schwartzberg, L.S. (1992). Defining a therapeutic dose of peripheral blood stem cells. *Journal of Hematotherapy, 1,* 329–341. https://doi.org/10.1089/scd.1.1992.1.329

Bertolini, F., Battaglia, M., De Iulio, C., Sirchia, G., & Rosti, L. (1995). Placental blood collection: Effects on newborns [Letter to the editor]. *Blood, 85,* 3361–3362. https://doi.org/10.1182/blood.V85.11.3361.bloodjournal85113361

Bhamidipati, P.K., Fiala, M.A., Grossman, B.J., DiPersio, J.F., Stockerl-Goldstein, K., Gao, F., … Vij, R. (2017). Results of a prospective randomized, open-label, noninferiority study of tbo-filgrastim (Granix) versus filgrastim (Neupogen) in combination with plerixafor for autologous stem cell mobilization in patients with multiple myeloma and non-Hodgkin lymphoma. *Biology of Blood and Marrow Transplantation, 23,* 2065–2069. https://doi.org/10.1016/j.bbmt.2017.07.023

Bishop, M.R. (1994). Mobilization prior to the apheresis procedure. In A. Kessinger & J.D. McMannis (Eds.), *Practical considerations of apheresis in peripheral blood stem cell transplantation* (pp. 5–10). Lakewood, CO: COBE BCT.

Bishop, M.R., Anderson, J.R., Jackson, J.D., Bierman, P.J., Reed, E.C., Vose, J.M., … Kessinger, A. (1994). High-dose therapy and peripheral blood progenitor cell transplantation: Effects of recombinant human granulocyte-macrophage colony-stimulating factor on the autograft. *Blood, 83,* 610–616. https://doi.org/10.1182/blood.V83.2.610.610

Bishop, M.R., Jackson, J.D., O'Kane-Murphy, B., Schmit-Pokorny, K., Vose, J.M., Bierman, P.J., … Kessinger, A. (1996). Phase I trial of recombinant fusion protein PIXY321 for mobilization of peripheral-blood cells. *Journal of Clinical Oncology, 14,* 2521–2526. https://doi.org/10.1200/JCO.1996.14.9.2521

Bishop, M.R., Tarantolo, S.R., Jackson, J.D., Anderson, J.R., Schmit-Pokorny, K., Zacharias, D., … Kessinger, A. (1997). Allogeneic-blood stem-cell collection following mobilization with low-dose granulocyte colony-stimulating factor. *Journal of Clinical Oncology, 15,* 1601–1607. https://doi.org/10.1200/JCO.1997.15.4.1601

Brugger, W., Bross, K.J., Glatt, M., Weber, F., Mertelsmann, R., & Kanz, L. (1994). Mobilization of tumor cells and hematopoietic progenitor cells into peripheral blood of patients with solid tumors. *Blood, 83,* 636–640. https://doi.org/10.1182/blood.V83.3.636.636

Bruns, I., Steidl, U., Kronenwett, R., Fenk, R., Graef, T., Rohr, U.-P., … Kobbe, G. (2006). A single dose of 6 or 12 mg of pegfilgrastim for peripheral blood progenitor cell mobilization results in similar yields of CD34+ progenitors in patients with multiple myeloma. *Transfusion, 46,* 180–185. https://doi.org/10.1111/j.1537-2995.2006.00699.x

Calandra, G., McCarty, J., McGuirk, J., Tricot, G., Crocker, S.-A., Badel, K., … Bridger, G. (2008). AMD3100 plus G-CSF can successfully mobilize CD34+ cells from non-Hodgkin's lymphoma, Hodgkin's disease and multiple myeloma patients previously failing mobilization with chemotherapy and/or cytokine treatment: Compassionate use data. *Bone Marrow Transplantation, 41,* 331–338. https://doi.org/10.1038/sj.bmt.1705908

Cantilena, C.R., Ito, S., Tian, X., Jain, P., Chinian, F., Anandi, P., … Battiwalla, M. (2018). Distinct biomarker profiles in ex vivo T cell depletion graft manipulation strategies: CD34⁺ selection versus CD3⁺/19⁺ depletion in matched sibling allogeneic peripheral blood stem cell transplantation. *Biology of Blood and Marrow Transplantation, 24*, 460–466. https://doi.org/10.1016/j.bbmt.2017.11.028

Castaigne, S., Calvo, F., Douay, L., Thomas, F., Benbunan, M., Gerota, J., & Degos, L. (1986). Successful haematopoietic reconstitution using autologous peripheral blood mononucleated cells in a patient with acute promyelocytic leukaemia. *British Journal of Haematology, 63*, 209–211. https://doi.org/10.1111/j.1365-2141.1986.tb07513.x

Chen, S.-H., Wang, T.-F., & Yang, K.-L. (2013). Hematopoietic stem cell donation. *International Journal of Hematology, 97*, 446–455. https://doi.org/10.1007/s12185-013-1298-8

Chern, B., McCarthy, N., Hutchins, C., & Durrant, S.T.S. (1999). Analgesic infiltration at the site of bone marrow harvest significantly reduces donor morbidity. *Bone Marrow Transplantation, 23*, 947–949. https://doi.org/10.1038/sj.bmt.1701751

Cooling, L., Hoffmann, S., Webb, D., Meade, M., Yamada, C., Davenport, R., & Yanik, G. (2017). Procedure-related complications and adverse events associated with pediatric autologous peripheral blood stem cell collection. *Journal of Clinical Apheresis, 32*, 35–48. https://doi.org/10.1002/jca.21465

Cope, D.G., & Matey, L. (2017). Access device standards, recommendations, and controversies. In D. Camp-Sorrell & L. Matey (Eds.), *Access device standards of practice for oncology nursing* (pp. 3–24). Pittsburgh, PA: Oncology Nursing Society.

Deneys, V., Fabry, A., Van Hooydonk, M., Sonet, A., André, M., Bourgeois, M., & Botson, F. (2017). Efficiency of autologous stem cell collection: Comparison of three different cell separators. *Transfusion and Apheresis Science, 56*, 35–38. https://doi.org/10.1016/j.transci.2016.12.015

Dessels, C., Alessandrini, M., & Pepper, M.S. (2018). Factors influencing the umbilical cord blood stem cell industry: An evolving treatment landscape. *Stem Cells Translational Medicine, 7*, 643–650. https://doi.org/10.1002/sctm.17-0244

Devine, H., Tierney, D.K., Schmit-Pokorny, K., & McDermott, K. (2010). Mobilization of hematopoietic stem cells for use in autologous transplantation. *Clinical Journal of Oncology Nursing, 14*, 212–222. https://doi.org/10.1188/10.CJON.212-222

Devine, S.M., Vij, R., Rettig, M., Todt, L., McGlauchlen, K., Fisher, N., ... DiPersio, J.F. (2008). Rapid mobilization of functional donor hematopoietic cells without G-CSF using AMD3100, an antagonist of the CXCR4/SDF-1 interaction. *Blood, 112*, 990–998. https://doi.org/10.1182/blood-2007-12-130179

DiPersio, J.F., Stadtmauer, E.A., Nademanee, A., Micallef, I.N.M., Stiff, P.J., Kaufman, J.L., ... Calandra, G. (2009). Plerixafor and G-CSF versus placebo and G-CSF to mobilize hematopoietic stem cells for autologous stem cell transplantation in patients with multiple myeloma. *Blood, 113*, 5720–5726. https://doi.org/10.1182/blood-2008-08-174946

D'Souza, A., Lee, S., Zhu, X., & Pasquini, M. (2017). Current use and trends in hematopoietic cell transplantation in the United States. *Biology of Blood and Marrow Transplantation, 23*, 1417–1421. https://doi.org/10.1016/j.bbmt.2017.05.035

Duong, H.K., Savani, B.N., Copelan, E., Devine, S., Costa, L.J., Wingard, J.R., ... Carpenter, P.A. (2014). Peripheral blood progenitor cell mobilization for autologous and allogeneic hematopoietic cell transplantation: Guidelines from the American Society for Blood and Marrow Transplantation. *Biology of Blood and Marrow Transplantation, 20*, 1262–1273. https://doi.org/10.1016/j.bbmt.2014.05.003

Flomenberg, N., Devine, S.M., DiPersio, J.F., Liesveld, J.L., McCarty, J.M., Rowley, S.D., ... Calandra, G. (2005). The use of AMD3100 plus G-CSF for autologous hematopoietic progenitor cell mobilization is superior to G-CSF alone. *Blood, 106*, 1867–1874. https://doi.org/10.1182/blood-2005-02-0468

Forman, S.J., & Nakamura, R. (2011). Hematopoietic cell transplantation. In R. Pazdur, L.D. Wagman, K.A. Camphausen, & W.J. Hoskins (Eds.), *Cancer management: A multidisciplinary approach: Medical, surgical, and radiation oncology* [Online ed.]. Retrieved from https://www.cancernetwork.com/cancer-management/hematopoietic-cell-transplantation

Foundation for the Accreditation of Cellular Therapy & Joint Accreditation Committee–ISCT and EBMT. (2018). *FACT-JACIE international standards for hematopoietic cellular therapy product collection, processing, and administration* (7th ed.). Retrieved from https://www.ebmt.org/sites/default/files/2018-06/FACT-JACIE%207th%20Edition%20Standards.pdf

Furey, A., Rastogi, S., Prince, R., Jin, Z., Smilow, E., Briamonte, C., ... Satwani, P. (2018). Bone marrow harvest in pediatric sibling donors: Role of granulocyte colony-stimulating factor priming and CD34+ cell dose. *Biology of Blood and Marrow Transplantation, 24*, 324–329. https://doi.org/10.1016/j.bbmt.2017.10.031

Gale, R.P., Henon, P., & Juttner, C. (1992). Blood stem cell transplants come of age. *Bone Marrow Transplantation, 9*, 151–155.

Genzyme. (2019, May). *Mozobil® (plerixafor)* [Package insert]. Cambridge, MA: Author.

Gianni, A.M., Tarella, C., Siena, S., Bregni, M., Boccadoro, M., Lombardi, F., ... Pileri, A. (1990). Durable and complete hematopoietic reconstitution after autografting of rhGM-CSF exposed peripheral blood progenitor cells. *Bone Marrow Transplantation, 6*, 143–145.

Giralt, S., Costa, L., Schriber, J., DiPersio, J., Maziarz, R., McCarty, J., ... Devine, S. (2014). Optimizing autologous stem cell mobilization strategies to improve patient outcomes: Consensus guidelines and recommendations. *Biology of Blood and Marrow Transplantation, 20*, 295–308. https://doi.org/10.1016/j.bbmt.2013.10.013

Glaspy, J.A., Shpall, E.J., LeMaistre, C.F., Briddell, R.A., Menchaca, D.M., Turner, S.A., ... McNiece, I.K. (1997). Peripheral blood progenitor cell mobilization using stem cell factor in combination with filgrastim in breast cancer patients. *Blood, 90*, 2939–2951.

Gluckman, E., Broxmeyer, H.E., Auerbach, A.D., Friedman, H.S., Douglas, G.W., Devergie, A., ... Boyse, E.A. (1989). Hematopoietic reconstitution in a patient with Fanconi's anemia by means of umbilical-cord blood from an HLA-identical sibling. *New England Journal of Medicine, 321*, 1174–1175. https://doi.org/10.1056/NEJM198910263211707

Golde, D.W. (1991). The stem cell. *Scientific American, 265*, 86–93. https://doi.org/10.1038/scientificamerican1291-86

Haas, R., Ho, A.D., Bredthauer, U., Cayeux, S., Egerer, G., Knauf, W., & Hunstein, W. (1990). Successful autologous transplantation of blood stem cells mobilized with recombinant human granulocyte-macrophage colony-stimulating factor. *Experimental Hematology, 18*, 94–98.

Haire, W.D., Lieberman, R.P., Lund, G.B., Wieczorek, B.M., Armitage, J.O., & Kessinger, A. (1990). Translumbar inferior vena cava catheters: Safety and efficacy in peripheral blood stem cell transplantation. *Transfusion, 30*, 511–515. https://doi.org/10.1046/j.1537-2995.1990.30690333481.x

Hari, P. (2018). Chemo-mobilization in myeloma—Diminishing returns in the era of novel agent induction? *Biology of Blood and Marrow Transplantation, 24*, 203–206. https://doi.org/10.1016/j.bbmt.2017.12.781

Henslee-Downey, P.J., Abhyankar, S.H., Parrish, R.S., Pati, A.R., Godder, K.T., Neglia, W.J., ... Gee, A.P. (1997). Use of partially mismatched related donors extends access to allogeneic marrow transplant. *Blood, 89*, 3864–3872.

Hsu, Y.-M.S., & Cushing, M.M. (2016). Autologous stem cell mobilization and collection. *Hematology/Oncology Clinics of North America, 30*, 573–589. https://doi.org/10.1016/j.hoc.2016.01.004

Kahn, D.G., Prilutskaya, M., Cooper, B., Kennedy, M.J., Meagher, R., Pecora, A.L., ... Moss, T.J. (1997). The relationship between the incidence of tumor contamination and number of pheresis for stage IV breast cancer. *Blood, 90*(Suppl. 1), 565a.

Kamani, N., Spellman, S., Hurley, C.K., Barker, J.N., Smith, F.O., Oudshoorn, M., ... Confer, D.L. (2008). State of the art review: HLA matching and outcome of unrelated donor umbilical cord blood transplants. *Biology of Blood and Marrow Transplantation, 14*, 1–6. https://doi.org/10.1016/j.bbmt.2007.11.003

Kang, E.M., Areman, E.M., David-Ocampo, V., Fitzhugh, C., Link, M.E., Read, E.J., ... Tisdale, J.F. (2002). Mobilization, collection, and processing of peripheral blood stem cells in individuals with sickle cell trait. *Blood, 99*, 850–855. https://doi.org/10.1182/blood.V99.3.850

Karakukcu, M., & Unal, E. (2015). Stem cell mobilization and collection from pediatric patients and healthy children. *Transfusion and Apheresis Science, 53*, 17–22. https://doi.org/10.1016/j.transci.2015.05.010

Kessinger, A.M., Armitage, J.O., Landmark, J.D., & Weisenburger, D.D. (1986). Reconstitution of human hematopoietic function with autologous cryopreserved circulating stem cells. *Experimental Hematology, 14*, 192–196.

Kessinger, A.M., & Sharp, G. (1996). Mobilization of hematopoietic progenitor cells with epoetin alfa. *Seminars in Hematology, 33*(Suppl. 1), 10–15.

Kessinger, A.M., & Sharp, J.G. (2003). The whys and hows of hematopoietic progenitor and stem cell mobilization. *Bone Marrow Transplantation, 31,* 319–329. https://doi.org/10.1038/sj.bmt.1703837

Kessinger, A.M., Smith, D.M., Strandjord, S.E., Landmark, J.D., Dooley, D.C., Law, P., … Armitage, J.O. (1989). Allogeneic transplantation of blood-derived, T cell-depleted hemopoietic stem cells after myeloablative treatment in a patient with acute lymphoblastic leukemia. *Bone Marrow Transplantation, 4,* 643–646.

Kline, R.M., & Bertolone, S.J. (1998). Umbilical cord blood transplantation: Providing a donor for everyone needing a bone marrow transplant? *Southern Medical Journal, 91,* 821–828. https://doi.org/10.1097/00007611-199809000-00004

Koh, L.-P., Rizzieri, D.A., & Chao, N.J. (2007). Allogeneic hematopoietic stem cell transplant using mismatched/haploidentical donors. *Biology of Blood and Marrow Transplantation, 13,* 1249–1267. https://doi.org/10.1016/j.bbmt.2007.08.003

Körbling, M., Dörken, B., Ho, A.D., Pezzutto, A., Hunstein, W., & Fliedner, T.M. (1986). Autologous transplantation of blood-derived hemopoietic stem cells after myeloablative therapy in a patient with Burkitt's lymphoma. *Blood, 67,* 529–532.

Kosuri, S., Herrera, D.A., Scordo, M., Shah, G.L., Cho, C., Devlin, S.M., … Perales, M.-A. (2017). The impact of toxicities on first-year outcomes after ex vivo CD34⁺-selected allogeneic hematopoietic cell transplantation in adults with hematologic malignancies. *Biology of Blood and Marrow Transplantation, 23,* 2004–2011. https://doi.org/10.1016/j.bbmt.2017.07.012

Kriegsmann, K., Schmitt, A., Kriegsmann, M., Bruckner, T., Anyanwu, A., Witzens-Harig, M., … Wuchter, P. (2018). Orchestration of chemomobilization and G-CSF administration for successful hematopoietic stem cell collection. *Biology of Blood and Marrow Transplantation, 24,* 1281–1288. https://doi.org/10.1016/j.bbmt.2018.01.007

Kroschinsky, F., Hölig, K., Platzbecker, U., Poppe-Thiede, K., Ordemann, R., Blechschmidt, M., … Ehninger, G. (2006). Efficacy of single-dose pegfilgrastim after chemotherapy for the mobilization of autologous peripheral blood stem cells in patients with malignant lymphoma or multiple myeloma. *Transfusion, 46,* 1417–1423. https://doi.org/10.1111/j.1537-2995.2006.00911.x

Kurtzberg, J., Lyerly, A.D., & Sugarman, J. (2005). Untying the Gordian knot: Policies, practices, and ethical issues related to banking of umbilical cord blood. *Journal of Clinical Investigation, 115,* 2592–2597. https://doi.org/10.1172/JCI26690

Lecchi, L., Giovanelli, S., Gagliardi, B., Pezzali, I., Ratti, I., & Marconi, M. (2016). An update on methods for cryopreservation and thawing of hemopoietic stem cells. *Transfusion and Apheresis Science, 54,* 324–336. https://doi.org/10.1016/j.transci.2016.05.009

Lee, V., Li, C.K., Shing, M.M.K., Chik, K.W., Li, K., Tsang, K.S., … Yuen, P.M.P. (2000). Single vs. twice daily G-CSF dose for peripheral blood stem cells harvest in normal donors and children with non-malignant diseases. *Bone Marrow Transplantation, 25,* 931–935. https://doi.org/10.1038/sj.bmt.1702338

Liles, W.C., Broxmeyer, H.E., Rodger, E., Wood, B., Hübel, K., Cooper, S., … Dale, D.C. (2003). Mobilization of hematopoietic progenitor cells in healthy volunteers by AMD3100, a CXCR4 antagonist. *Blood, 102,* 2728–2730. https://doi.org/10.1182/blood-2003-02-0663

Lisenko, K., Pavel, P., Bruckner, T., Puthenparambil, J., Hundemer, M., Schmitt, A., … Wuchter, P. (2017). Comparison between intermittent and continuous Spectra Optia leukapheresis systems for autologous peripheral blood stem cell collection. *Journal of Clinical Apheresis, 32,* 27–34. https://doi.org/10.1002/jca.21463

Lund, T.C. (2018). Umbilical cord blood expansion: Are we there yet? *Biology of Blood and Marrow Transplantation, 24,* 1311–1312. https://doi.org/10.1016/j.bbmt.2018.05.002

Mackey, H.T. (2017). Apheresis catheters. In D. Camp-Sorrell & L. Matey (Eds.), *Access device standards of practice for oncology nursing* (pp. 75–78). Pittsburgh, PA: Oncology Nursing Society.

Micallef, I.N., Stiff, P.J., Nademanee, A.P., Maziarz, R.T., Horwitz, M.E., Stadtmauer, E.A., … DiPersio, J.F. (2018). Plerixafor plus granulocyte colony-stimulating factor for patients with non-Hodgkin lymphoma and multiple myeloma: Long-term follow-up report. *Biology of Blood and Marrow Transplantation, 24,* 1187–1195. https://doi.org/10.1016/j.bbmt.2018.01.039

Morgan, R.A., Gray, D., Lomova, A., & Kohn, D.B. (2017). Hematopoietic stem cell gene therapy: Progress and lessons learned. *Cell Stem Cell, 21,* 574–590. https://doi.org/10.1016/j.stem.2017.10.010

Nademanee, A., Sniecinski, I., Schmidt, G.M., Dagis, A.C., O'Donnell, M.R., Snyder, D.S., … Molina, A. (1994). High-dose therapy followed by autologous peripheral-blood stem-cell transplantation for patients with Hodgkin's disease and non-Hodgkin's lymphoma using unprimed and granulocyte colony-stimulating factor-mobilized peripheral-blood stem cells. *Journal of Clinical Oncology, 12,* 2176–2186. https://doi.org/10.1200/JCO.1994.12.10.2176

Neumann, J. (2007). Ethical issues inherent to blood and marrow transplantation. In S. Ezzone & K. Schmit-Pokorny (Eds.), *Blood and marrow stem cell transplantation: Principles, practice, and nursing insights* (3rd ed., pp. 369–390). Burlington, MA: Jones & Bartlett Learning.

Oyekunle, A., Shumilov, E., Kostrewa, P., Burchert, A., Trümper, L., Wuchter, P., … Kröger, N. (2018). Chemotherapy-based stem cell mobilization does not result in significant paraprotein reduction in myeloma patients in the era of novel induction regimens. *Biology of Blood and Marrow Transplantation, 24,* 276–281. https://doi.org/10.1016/j.bbmt.2017.10.008

Panch, S.R., Szymanski, J., Savani, B.N., & Stroncek, D.F. (2017). Sources of hematopoietic stem and progenitor cells and methods to optimize yields for clinical cell therapy. *Biology of Blood and Marrow Transplantation, 23,* 1241–1249. https://doi.org/10.1016/j.bbmt.2017.05.003

Popat, U., Saliba, R., Thandi, R., Hosing, C., Qazilbash, M., Anderlini, P., … Giralt, S. (2009). Impairment of filgrastim-induced stem cell mobilization after prior lenalidomide in patients with multiple myeloma. *Biology of Blood and Marrow Transplantation, 15,* 718–723. https://doi.org/10.1016/j.bbmt.2009.02.011

Pulsipher, M.A., Chitphakdithai, P., Logan, B.R., Navarro, W.H., Levine, J.E., Miller, J.P., … Confer, D.L. (2014). Lower risk for serious adverse events and no increased risk for cancer after PBSC vs BM donation. *Blood, 123,* 3655–3663. https://doi.org/10.1182/blood-2013-12-542464

Pusic, I., Jiang, S.Y., Landua, S., Uy, G.L., Rettig, M.P., Cashen, A.F., … DiPersio, J.F. (2008). Impact of mobilization and remobilization strategies on achieving sufficient stem cell yields for autologous transplantation. *Biology of Blood and Marrow Transplantation, 14,* 1045–1056. https://doi.org/10.1016/j.bbmt.2008.07.004

Reiffers, J., Bernard, P., David, B., Vezon, G., Sarrat, A., Marit, G., … Broustet, A. (1986). Successful autologous transplantation with peripheral blood hemopoietic cells in a patient with acute leukemia. *Experimental Hematology, 14,* 312–315.

Richman, C.M., Weiner, R.S., & Yankee, R.A. (1976). Increase in circulating stem cells following chemotherapy in man. *Blood, 47,* 1031–1039.

Rubinstein, P., Carrier, C., Scaradavou, A., Kurtzberg, J., Adamson, J., Migliaccio, A.R., … Stevens, C.E. (1998). Outcomes among 562 recipients of placental-blood transplants from unrelated donors. *New England Journal of Medicine, 339,* 1565–1577. https://doi.org/10.1056/NEJM199811263392201

Satwani, P., Kahn, J., & Jin, Z. (2015). Making strides and meeting challenges in pediatric allogeneic hematopoietic cell transplantation clinical trials in the United States: Past, present and future. *Contemporary Clinical Trials, 45,* 84–92. https://doi.org/10.1016/j.cct.2015.06.011

Schulmeister, L. (2017). Complications of long-term venous access devices. In D. Camp-Sorrell & L. Matey (Eds.), *Access device standards of practice for oncology nursing* (pp. 79–98). Pittsburgh, PA: Oncology Nursing Society.

Sharp, J.G., Kessinger, A., Vaughan, W.P., Mann, S., Crouse, D.A., Dicke, K., … Weisenburger, D.D. (1992). Detection and clinical significance of minimal tumor cell contamination of peripheral stem cell harvests. *International Journal of Cell Cloning, 10*(Suppl. 1), 92–94. https://doi.org/10.1002/stem.5530100731

Shpall, E.J. (1999). The utilization of cytokines in stem cell mobilization strategies. *Bone Marrow Transplantation, 23*(Suppl. 2), S13–S19. https://doi.org/10.1038/sj.bmt.1701669

Siena, S., Bregni, M., Brando, B., Belli, N., Ravagnani, F., Gandola, L., … Gianni, A.M. (1991). Flow cytometry for clinical estimation of circulating hematopoietic progenitors for autologous transplantation in cancer patients. *Blood, 77,* 400–409.

Socinski, M.A., Elias, A., Schnipper, L., Cannistra, S.A., Antman, K.H., & Griffin, J.D. (1988). Granulocyte-macrophage colony stimulating factor expands the circulating haemopoietic progenitor cell compartment in man. *Lancet, 331*, 1194–1198. https://doi.org/10.1016/S0140-6736(88)92012-0

Stephens, L.C., Haire, W.D., Schmit-Pokorny, K., Kessinger, A., & Kotulak, G. (1993). Granulocyte macrophage colony stimulating factor: High incidence of apheresis catheter thrombosis during peripheral stem cell collection. *Bone Marrow Transplantation, 11*, 51–54.

Stiff, P.J. (1999). Management strategies for the hard-to-mobilize patient. *Bone Marrow Transplantation, 23*(Suppl. 2), S29–S33.

Stiff, P.J., Montesinos, P., Peled, T., Landau, E., Goudsmid, N.R., Mandel, J., ... Sanz, G. (2018). Cohort-controlled comparison of umbilical cord blood transplantation using carlecortemcel-L, a single progenitor-enriched cord blood, to double cord blood unit transplantation. *Biology of Blood and Marrow Transplantation, 24*, 1463–1470. https://doi.org/10.1016/j.bbmt.2018.02.012

Sutherland, D.R., Anderson, L., Keeney, M., Nayar, R., & Chin-Yee, I. (2009). The ISHAGE guidelines for CD34+ cell determination by flow cytometry. *Journal of Hematotherapy, 5*, 213–226. https://doi.org/10.1089/scd.1.1996.5.213

Switzer, G.E., Bruce, J.G., Harrington, D., Haagenson, M., Drexler, R., Foley, A., ... Wingard, J.R. (2014). Health-related quality of life of bone marrow versus peripheral blood stem cell donors: A prespecified subgroup analysis from a phase III RCT–BMTCTN protocol 0201. *Biology of Blood and Marrow Transplantation, 20*, 118–127. https://doi.org/10.1016/j.bbmt.2013.10.024

Tilly, H., Bastit, D., Lucet, J.-C., Esperou, H., Monconduit, M., & Piguet, H. (1986). Haemopoietic reconstitution after autologous peripheral blood stem cell transplantation in acute leukaemia [Letter to the editor]. *Lancet, 328*, 154–155. https://doi.org/10.1016/S0140-6736(86)91962-8

To, L.B., Levesque, J.-P., & Herbert, K.E. (2011). How I treat patients who mobilize hematopoietic stem cells poorly. *Blood, 118*, 4530–4540. https://doi.org/10.1182/blood-2011-06-318220

To, L.B., Roberts, M.M., Haylock, D.N., Dyson, P.G., Branford, A.L., Thorp, D., ... Davy, M.L. (1992). Comparison of haematological recovery times and supportive care requirements of autologous recovery phase peripheral blood stem cell transplants, autologous bone marrow transplants and allogeneic bone marrow transplants. *Bone Marrow Transplantation, 9*, 277–284.

To, L.B., Shepperd, K.M., Haylock, D.N., Dyson, P.G., Charles, P., Thorp, D.L., ... Sage, R.E. (1990). Single high doses of cyclophosphamide enable the collection of high numbers of hemopoietic stem cells from the peripheral blood. *Experimental Hematology, 18*, 442–447.

van Walraven, S.M., Egeland, T., Borrill, V., Nicoloso-de Faveri, G., Rall, G., & Szer, J. (2018). Addressing ethical and procedural principles for unrelated allogeneic hematopoietic progenitor cell donation in a changing medical environment. *Biology of Blood and Marrow Transplantation, 24*, 887–894. https://doi.org/10.1016/j.bbmt.2018.01.018

Vescio, R.A., Hong, C.H., Cao, J., Kim, A., Schiller, G.J., Lichtenstein, A.K., ... Berenson, J.R. (1994). The hematopoietic stem cell antigen, CD34, is not expressed on the malignant cells in multiple myeloma. *Blood, 84*, 3283–3290.

Vose, J.M., Kessinger, A., Bierman, P.J., Sharp, G., Garrison, L., & Armitage, J.O. (1992). The use of rhIL-3 for mobilization of peripheral blood stem cells in previously treated patients with lymphoid malignancies. *International Journal of Cell Cloning, 10*(Suppl. 1), 62–65. https://doi.org/10.1002/stem.5530100722

Wei, A., & Grigg, A. (2001). Granulocyte colony-stimulating factor-induced sickle cell crisis and multiorgan dysfunction in a patient with compound heterozygous sickle cell/β+ thalassemia. *Blood, 97*, 3998–3999. https://doi.org/10.1182/blood.V97.12.3998

Wiener, L.S., Steffen-Smith, E., Fry, T., & Wayne, A.S. (2007). Hematopoietic stem cell donation in children: A review of the sibling donor experience. *Journal of Psychosocial Oncology, 25*, 45–66. https://doi.org/10.1300/J077v25n01_03

Wiesneth, M., Schreiner, T., Friedrich, W., Bunjes, D., Duncker, C., Krug, E., ... Kubanek, B. (1998). Mobilization and collection of allogeneic peripheral blood progenitor cells for transplantation. *Bone Marrow Transplantation, 21*(Suppl. 3), S21–S24.

Worel, N., Buser, A., Greinix, H.T., Hägglund, H., Navarro, W., Pulsipher, M., ... Halter, J.P. (2015). Suitability criteria for adult related donors: A consensus statement from the Worldwide Network for Blood and Marrow Transplantation Standing Committee on Donor Issues. *Biology of Blood and Marrow Transplantation, 21*, 2052–2060. https://doi.org/10.1016/j.bbmt.2015.08.009

Yamamoto, C., Ogawa, H., Fukuda, T., Igarashi, A., Okumura, H., Uchida, N., ... Kanda, Y. (2018). Impact of a low CD34+ cell dose on allogeneic peripheral blood stem cell transplantation. *Biology of Blood and Marrow Transplantation, 24*, 708–716. https://doi.org/10.1016/j.bbmt.2017.10.043

CHAPTER 6

Transplant Treatment Course and Acute Complications

Katherine Byar, MSN, APN, BC, BMTCN®

Introduction

Hematopoietic stem cell transplantation (HSCT) is a treatment used to control or cure many conditions, but primarily malignant diseases. The side effects and toxicities of this treatment can vary depending on the type of transplant, regimen, and overall health of the patient. The transplant treatment course consists of three parts: the conditioning regimen, the hematopoietic stem cell (HSC) infusion, and post-transplant engraftment. This chapter discusses the conditioning regimens, cellular infusion, acute complications, and the post-transplant engraftment phase.

Conditioning Regimens for Hematopoietic Stem Cell Transplantation

The transplant treatment course begins with the preparative or conditioning regimen. Conditioning regimens may have various combinations of chemotherapy, radiation therapy, and immunotherapeutic agents (Antin & Raley, 2013). The choice of conditioning regimen administered to patients prior to transplant can vary in the drugs used, doses, and schedules based on the patient's disease and overall health, type of transplant, and goal of therapy (Forman, Negrin, Antin, & Appelbaum, 2016).

For patients with malignant diseases, the purposes of standard conditioning regimens are to eliminate or reduce the tumor burden and suppress the recipient's immune system to allow engraftment of HSCs (Forman et al., 2016; Olsen, LeFebvre, & Brassil, 2019). Patients with severe combined immunodeficiency disease often do not require a conditioning regimen before transplantation because there are no abnormal cells that need to be eradicated and the immune system is so compromised that the infused human leukocyte antigen (HLA)-matched donor cells rarely are rejected by the recipient's cells (Marlein & Rushworth, 2018). In contrast, patients with aplastic anemia have a minimally competent immune system. Therefore, conditioning is required to prevent rejection of the donor hematopoietic cells. A commonly used preparative regimen for aplastic anemia consists of high-dose cyclo-

phosphamide given alone or in combination with antithymocyte globulin (ATG) (Marlein & Rushworth, 2018). Over the past decade, newer high-dose regimens have been developed specifically for patients with hematologic malignancies and solid tumors (Atilla, Atilla, & Demirer, 2017).

The intensity of the conditioning regimen will vary depending on the goal of the therapy and the type of transplant. Regimens may be administered in an inpatient or outpatient setting depending on the specific drugs and the institution. Conditioning regimens are either myeloablative or nonmyeloablative. *Myeloablative* regimens are used for both allogeneic and autologous transplants, whereas *nonmyeloablative* regimens are only for allogeneic transplants (McAdams & Burgunder, 2013).

Myeloablative conditioning regimens require the administration of lethal doses of chemotherapy, with or without total body irradiation (TBI), with the goal of eradicating tumor cells and creating a state of profound immunosuppression (Forman et al., 2016; Niess, 2013; Olsen et al., 2019). The ablated marrow space must be repopulated with progenitor cells (AABB et al., 2018), and the resulting immunosuppression lessens the recipient's ability to reject a transplanted donor graft and reduces the likelihood of the donor cells attacking the host, known as graft-versus-host disease (GVHD).

Myeloablative regimens with allogeneic transplants were the first treatment approach in transplantation for malignant diseases because of the antitumor effects from the graft-versus-tumor response (Niess, 2013). Unlike allogeneic transplants, autologous transplants are associated with fewer complications because of the absence of GVHD and requisite post-transplant immunosuppression, resulting in fewer infectious complications. The incidence of sinusoidal obstruction syndrome is also lower. Autologous transplants are used in the treatment of most lymphomas, myelomas, and other tumors in which the marrow is not overtly involved with disease. Autologous transplants have also been explored as a treatment option for patients with leukemia but are associated with higher relapse rates (Niess, 2013).

The observation that donor cells possess antitumor effects, referred to as *graft-versus-leukemia response*, led to the question of whether harnessing this mechanism along with nonmyeloablative regimens might be as effective as myeloablative regimens but with significantly fewer toxicities (Niess, 2013).

Nonmyeloablative regimens use agents that do not cause severe myelosuppression (e.g., fludarabine), with or without TBI, and reduced-intensity conditioning regimens rely on lower doses of chemotherapy (Olsen et al., 2019). The terms *nonmyeloablative* and *reduced-intensity conditioning* often are used interchangeably, yet they are different. Nonmyeloablative regimens cause minimal marrow suppression, whereas reduced-intensity conditioning regimens cause pancytopenia of intermediate duration (Niess, 2013). The primary goal of reduced-intensity conditioning is to suppress the immune system enough to allow engraftment of the donor's progenitor and immune system cells. This, in turn, creates a graft-versus-leukemia effect in which the immune cells of the graft eliminate tumor cells (Koniarczyk & Ferraro, 2016; Niess, 2013). This approach relies on the graft-versus-leukemia response instead of high-dose chemotherapy to kill tumor cells. Chimerism is evaluated by testing genetic markers to distinguish between the recipient and the donor and to determine the percentage of donor and host cells. The goal of myeloablative HSCT is to obtain 100% donor cells. However, for reduced-intensity conditioning and nonmyeloablative HSCT, host and donor cells need to coexist in what is termed a *mixed chimerism* (Spinks, 2016). Compared with high-dose preparative regimens, nonmyeloablative and reduced-intensity regimens result in a shorter duration of pancytopenia with reduced transfusion needs, fewer bacterial infections, and a lower incidence of direct toxicities to the lung and liver (Storb et al., 2013).

In general, myeloablative conditioning is preferred in patients who are suitable candidates because relapse rates are generally higher with reduced-intensity regimens (Niess, 2013). Data support improved five-year overall survival and quality of life in the use of nonmyeloablative regimens in patients older than 60 years who may have been previously deemed ineligible for an allogeneic HSCT because of age or comorbidities (e.g., renal, hepatic, or cardiac disease) (Bodge, Culos, Haider, Thompson, & Savani, 2014; Bodge, Reddy, Thompson, & Savani, 2014; Koniarczyk & Ferraro, 2016).

Two conventional myeloablative regimens commonly used in the preparative phase for myeloablative transplantation are cyclophosphamide and TBI (known as Cy/TBI) or the combination of IV busulfan and fludarabine (known as Bu/Flu) (McAdams & Burgunder, 2013). Nonmyeloablative regimens usually contain low-dose (2 Gy) TBI, with or without fludarabine (Atilla et al., 2017). These conditioning regimens may cause mild myelosuppression and antitumor responses for an extended period but are thought to have fewer toxicities than with myeloablative regimens. A conditioning regimen that does not fulfill a myeloablative or nonmyeloablative regimen is defined as reduced-intensity conditioning. The dose of alkylating agents or TBI for reduced-intensity conditioning is at least 30% less than normally used in myeloablative regimens (Atilla et al., 2017). Most regimens use a combination of fludarabine along with an alkylating agent, such as melphalan, busulfan, or thiotepa, or reduced-dose TBI (Atilla et al., 2017). The known complications of allogeneic HSCT, such as pancytopenia, mucositis, and organ damage, occur less frequently with reduced-intensity conditioning. It also has been suggested that reduced-intensity conditioning might be associated with improved survival and lower incidence of relapse compared to nonmyeloablative conditioning (Spinks, 2016). A study compared the outcomes of nonmyeloablative conditioning regimens (n = 323) versus reduced-intensity conditioning regimens (n = 877) in acute myeloid leukemia and found similar two-year disease-free survival rates in the two groups (50% vs. 53%, respectively) (Gurman et al., 2016).

For the autologous setting, high-dose therapy with stem cell rescue is frequently administered as a salvage treatment for relapse or persistent disease, as well as consolidation for patients with high-risk disease. Sequential or tandem transplants are used for some diseases to prolong survival (Bubalo, 2015).

The preparative regimen may include planned days of rest that allow chemotherapy to be eliminated from the body. The scheduled days of the preparative regimen are counted as minus days, with transplant day as day 0. For example, Cy/TBI comprises two days of cyclophosphamide followed by four days of TBI with chemotherapy beginning on day –7. A treatment road map would consist of the following schedule: day –6, high-dose chemotherapy; day –5, high-dose chemotherapy; day –4, TBI; day –3, TBI; day –2, TBI; day –1, rest; day 0, transplant. Figure 6-1 provides an example of a road map.

High-Dose Chemotherapy

High-dose conditioning regimens use combinations of the most effective agents for a disease while delivering total myeloablation (McAdams & Burgunder, 2013; Olsen et al., 2019). See Table 6-1 for common conditioning regimens and diseases treated. The Bu/Cy regimen, which may be used in allogeneic or autologous transplants for patients with hematologic malignancies, consists of cyclophosphamide 60 mg/kg IV on two consecutive days and busulfan 3.2 mg/kg IV for four consecutive days, or 4 mg/kg orally for four consecutive days (McAdams & Burgunder, 2013). The absorption of oral busulfan is variable, with low absorption correlating to relapse and high absorption inducing toxicity. The IV formulation is more stable, less toxic, and associated with good survival in the transplant setting (Forman et al., 2016; McAdams & Burgunder, 2013). Although high-dose chemotherapy is often effective at eradicating disease and preventing relapse, it is associated with significant adverse effects and mortality, requiring intensive nursing care and supportive therapies (Olsen et al., 2019).

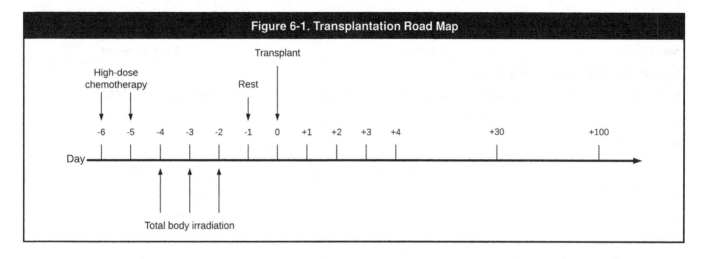

Figure 6-1. Transplantation Road Map

Other common high-dose regimens used in the preparative phase for myeloablative transplantation are Cy/TBI and fractionated TBI (divided doses) and etoposide (Koniarczyk & Ferraro, 2016; McAdams & Burgunder, 2013). The combination of IV busulfan and fludarabine (IV Bu/Flu) is well tolerated when given at high doses and demonstrates decreased nonrelapse mortality. Some drugs, such as cyclophosphamide, may cause adverse effects at high doses (e.g., cardiotoxicity, hemorrhagic cystitis) not typically seen at lower doses (Koniarczyk & Ferraro, 2016; McAdams & Burgunder, 2013). It is critical for nurses to know what to anticipate and monitor in patients receiving high-dose chemotherapy (Olsen et al., 2019). For most conditioning agents, the dose used for myeloablative regimens is associated with pancytopenia, sterility, and alopecia. Breakdown of the entire gastrointestinal tract may result in stomatitis, esophagitis, nausea, vomiting, and diarrhea. Nurses caring for patients during this acute phase need to address the toxicities daily because of the additional supportive care and attention needed to minimize morbidity.

Common myeloablative regimens used for autologous transplants to treat lymphoma or multiple myeloma include BEAM (carmustine, etoposide, cytarabine, and melphalan) and busulfan, etoposide, and cyclophosphamide (Koniarczyk & Ferraro, 2016). Other regimens include TBI, cyclophosphamide, and etoposide; busulfan, melphalan, and thiotepa (BuMelTT); cyclophosphamide, carmustine, and etoposide (CBV); and busulfan and cyclophosphamide (Bu/Cy). Studies are evaluating the efficacy of using radioimmunotherapy (e.g., ibritumomab, tositumomab) and monoclonal antibodies (e.g., rituximab) with high-dose chemotherapy regimens for the treatment of B-cell lymphoma (Koniarczyk & Ferraro, 2016). Carboplatin, ifosfamide, and etoposide, and etoposide and carboplatin are regimens used for relapsed or refractory germ cell tumors (Koniarczyk & Ferraro, 2016).

Multiple myeloma is commonly treated with autologous HSCT using high-dose melphalan (200 mg/m²) with or without bortezomib (1 mg/m²), or melphalan (140 mg/m²) and TBI (Gleason & Kaufman, 2017). These prepara-

tive regimens are ideal because melphalan is highly active in myeloma and amyloidosis, and myeloma is sensitive to radiation therapy. Thus, as previously noted, the patient's underlying disease dictates the preparative regimen (Gleason & Kaufman, 2017). See Table 6-2 for toxicities of preparative regimens.

Conditioning regimens are designed to allow for higher doses of chemotherapy from different classes of drugs to be administered without having similar side effect profiles. These chemotherapies are similar in that they attack fast-growing cells, such as tumor cells, but can affect other fast-growing cells in the body, such as those in the gastrointestinal tract and skin. This can lead to breakdown of tissues, producing nausea, vomiting, diarrhea, constipation, alopecia, dermatitis, and mucositis, colitis, or proctitis. Symptoms vary depending on the specific agents used and the intensity of the regimen (Koniarczyk & Ferraro, 2016).

Total Body Irradiation

The use of TBI for conditioning was developed in the 1970s, evolving from experience with survivors of radiation exposure after World War II. Advantages of using TBI as part of a conditioning regimen include the ability to create profound immunosuppression, deliver dose homogeneity to the whole body regardless of blood supply, and kill tumor cells. The possibility of cross-resistance with other antineoplastic agents is lower, and there are no concerns regarding excretion or detoxification. Dose distribution can be individualized by using shields or, conversely, by providing treatment boosts for specific anatomic sites known to harbor tumor cells, such as the central nervous system, testes, and ovaries (Forman et al., 2016; Ishibashi et al., 2016; Koniarczyk & Ferraro, 2016).

The preparative regimens for HSCT and TBI vary among facilities, and no consensus exists as to the most suitable regimen (Ishibashi et al., 2016). The patient's age, disease, and type of HSCT are the determining factors for the best regimen for any given patient.

Toxicities are increased when TBI is delivered in one myeloablative dose; therefore, fractionated (divided) doses are

Table 6-1. Common Conditioning Regimens[a]

Abbreviation	Regimen	Disease Treated
Common Autologous Conditioning Regimens		
BEAM ± R	Carmustine/etoposide/cytarabine/melphalan ± rituximab	Hodgkin lymphoma, NHL
Bu/E	Busulfan/etoposide	AML
Bu/etoposide/Cy	Busulfan/etoposide/cyclophosphamide	AML, NHL
BuMelTT	Busulfan/melphalan/thiotepa	Hodgkin lymphoma, NHL
Carbo/etoposide	Carboplatin/etoposide	Germ cell (may be done as a tandem)
Carbo/etoposide/Cy	Carboplatin/etoposide/cyclophosphamide	Germ cell (may be done as a tandem)
CBV ± R	Cyclophosphamide/carmustine/etoposide ± rituximab	Hodgkin lymphoma, NHL
Cy/etoposide/TBI	Cyclophosphamide/etoposide/total body irradiation	Hodgkin lymphoma, NHL
Melphalan	High-dose melphalan	Amyloidosis, MM
Melphalan ± B	High-dose melphalan ± bortezomib	MM
Common Myeloablative Conditioning Regimens		
Bu/Cy	Oral busulfan/cyclophosphamide	Myeloid leukemia, MDS
BuMel	Busulfan/melphalan	MM
Cy/TBI	Cyclophosphamide/total body irradiation	Leukemias, MDS, NHL
Flu/Bu	Fludarabine/busulfan	Leukemias, MDS, NHL
Flu/Mel	Fludarabine/melphalan	Leukemias, MDS, NHL
IV Bu/Cy	IV busulfan/cyclophosphamide	Myeloid leukemia, MDS
TBI/VP	Total body irradiation/etoposide	Leukemias
Common Reduced-Intensity Conditioning Regimens		
Bu/Cy	IV busulfan/cyclophosphamide	Leukemias
Bu/Flu/TBI	Busulfan/fludarabine/total body irradiation	Leukemias
Flu/Mel	Fludarabine/melphalan	MM, NHL
Flu/TBI	Fludarabine/total body irradiation	Leukemias
TBI/200 cGy	Low-dose total body irradiation	Leukemias

[a] This list is not all-inclusive and serves only as examples of conditioning regimens.

AML—acute myeloid leukemia; MDS—myelodysplastic syndromes; MM—multiple myeloma; NHL—non-Hodgkin lymphoma

Note. Based on information from Bensinger, 2016; Bubalo, 2015; de Lima et al., 2008; Forman & Nakamura, 2011; Lazarus et al., 2019; Riddell & Warren, 2019.

used (Ishibashi et al., 2016). For myeloablative HSCT, a total TBI dose of 12–15 Gy delivered in 8–12 fractions over three to four days is the most conventional (McAdams & Burgunder, 2013). However, if TBI is fractionated in two to three treatments per day, the patient will experience less toxicity. Low-dose TBI, such as 2–8 Gy in one to four fractions, may be used in a non-myeloablative preparative regimen (Ishibashi et al., 2016).

Indications for Total Body Irradiation

TBI is used mostly in the management of malignancies that exhibit a high sensitivity to irradiation, such as leuke-mias and lymphomas, and is more widely used in alloge-neic HSCT than autologous HSCT. In allogeneic HSCT, TBI provides powerful immunosuppression to prevent rejec-tion of the donor cells and to eradicate tumor cells. Most patients also receive chemotherapy drugs, such as cyclo-phosphamide or etoposide (McAdams & Burgunder, 2013; see Table 6-1 for common regimens).

Administration of Total Body Irradiation

An interprofessional team, including radiation and med-ical oncologists, medical physicists, dosimetrists, radiation

Table 6-2. Side Effects of Preparative Regimens by Agent and System

System	Busulfan	Carboplatin	Carmustine	Cyclophosphamide	Cytarabine	Etoposide	Fludarabine	Melphalan	Mitoxantrone	TBI	Thiotepa
Cardiovascular											
Cardiotoxicity	X			X					X	X	
Hypo- or hypertension	X					X					
Gastrointestinal											
Constipation		X			X		X				
Diarrhea		X		X	X	X	X	X	X	X	
Hepatotoxicity, HSOS	X		X	X	X	X					X
Mucositis, stomatitis	X	X		X	X	X	X	X	X	X	X
Nausea, vomiting	X	X	X	X	X	X	X	X	X	X	X
Genitourinary											
Electrolyte imbalances		X		X		X					
Hemorrhagic cystitis				X							X
Nephrotoxicity		X	X	X			X			X	X
Hematologic											
Anemia	X	X	X	X	X	X	X	X	X	X	X
Leukopenia	X	X	X	X	X	X	X	X	X	X	X
Thrombocytopenia	X	X	X	X	X	X	X	X	X	X	X
Immunologic											
Fever/chills					X	X	X		X	X	X
Hypersensitivity, allergic reaction, anaphylaxis	X	X		X	X	X	X	X			X
Integumentary											
Alopecia	X	X	X	X	X	X	X	X	X	X	X
Dermatitis		X			X	X	X	X	X	X	X
Erythema	X		X	X	X	X			X	X	X
Hyperpigmentation	X		X	X		X		X		X	

(Continued on next page)

Table 6-2. Side Effects of Preparative Regimens by Agent and System (Continued)

System	Busulfan	Carboplatin	Carmustine	Cyclophosphamide	Cytarabine	Etoposide	Fludarabine	Melphalan	Mitoxantrone	TBI	Thiotepa
Miscellaneous											
Cataracts	X									X	
Conjunctivitis	X		X	X	X				X		
Nasal congestion			X								
Parotitis										X	
Secondary malignancy	X	X	X	X		X		X		X	X
Thyroid disorders										X	
Neurologic											
Headache, altered mental status	X		X	X	X		X	X	X		X
Ototoxicity		X									
Peripheral neuropathy		X				X	X	X			
Seizures	X		X						X		
Pulmonary											
Fibrosis	X		X			X		X		X	
Pneumonitis	X		X			X	X		X	X	
Reproductive											
Infertility	X		X	X				X		X	X

HSOS—hepatic sinusoidal obstruction syndrome; TBI—total body irradiation

Note. Based on information from Forman & Nakamura, 2011; Iwamoto et al., 2012; Olsen et al., 2019.

therapists, and nurses, coordinates the delivery of TBI (Iwamoto, Haas, & Gosselin, 2012). Because TBI has the potential to cause fatal toxicity, team members adhere to stringent policies and guidelines to ensure the best possible patient outcomes (McAdams & Burgunder, 2013).

A medical physicist considers prior radiation when planning dose calculations for TBI, as well as parameters including but not limited to field size, collimator rotation, treatment distance, dose per fraction, dose rate, total dose, number of fractions per day, interval between fractions, beam energy, shielding, and boost specifications (McAdams & Burgunder, 2013). The calculations are confirmed by another physicist or dosimetrist and approved by the radiation oncologist. The treatment suite is set up by the radiation therapists, who also deliver the TBI, follow the treatment prescription exactly, and monitor patients during the treatment (McAdams & Burgunder, 2013). The usual amount of time for TBI treatment to be delivered is 20–30 minutes (Iwamoto et al., 2012). Nurses should educate patients and families about TBI and what to expect during, shortly after, and months after treatment. They should inform patients of any procedures to promote comfort and safety and monitor patients' tolerance of the TBI treatments. Nurses also should share information with the rest of the team regarding special precautions for the care of immunosuppressed patients to ensure patients are treated in a supportive environment (McAdams & Burgunder, 2013).

A variety of patient positioning techniques have been used to deliver TBI, such as standing, sitting, and lying flat. The daily positioning needs to be reproducible. This is achieved using frameless devices such as foam or vacuum devices, depending on the patient's position. Special TBI stands, treatment couches, or treatment tables also assist in immobilizing patients, holding organ shields, and providing support for patients (McAdams & Burgunder, 2013).

Acute Side Effects of Conditioning Regimens

Fractionated and hyperfractionated TBI programs generally are well tolerated. As most patients receive both high-dose chemotherapy and TBI, it can be difficult to distinguish among the side effects. TBI side effects can be acute and long term, and most are manageable. The most common side effects of TBI are listed in Table 6-2.

Gastrointestinal toxicity is an acute toxicity of TBI that includes nausea, vomiting, enteritis, and mucositis (Koniarczyk & Ferraro, 2016; McAdams & Burgunder, 2013). However, treatment with IV fluids, electrolytes, antidiarrheal agents, antiemetics, and antibiotics help to protect the gastrointestinal tract and minimize this toxicity. Nursing care includes meticulous mouth care with rinses (e.g., saline with sodium bicarbonate, water, saline), which dilute and help remove mucus, decrease acidity, and discourage the growth of yeast while providing moisture (Forman et al., 2016). TBI, as well as high-dose chemotherapy, is considered moderately to highly emetogenic, and prophylaxis

with antiemetic therapy is necessary. Sedation is commonly required for young children receiving TBI (McAdams & Burgunder, 2013). See Chapter 9 for additional information.

Pulmonary complications are reported to occur in 25%–55% of all transplant recipients (Stephens, 2013) and can be due to infections (viral, bacterial, and fungal) or a direct insult from the conditioning. Other complications include pneumothorax, hemorrhage, and edema. Treatments are based on the underlying cause: antibiotics for infections, high-dose corticosteroids and platelet support for hemorrhage, and diuretics for pulmonary edema (Forman et al., 2016).

Idiopathic pneumonia syndrome occurs 30–90 days after transplant in up to 5% of patients (Forman et al., 2016; Ishibashi et al., 2016). As with other toxicities, the incidence is dependent, in part, on the preparative regimen, occurring more frequently following administration of regimens that include high doses of TBI. Preexisting lung disease, prior radiation therapy to the chest, and increased age also seem to be associated with an increased risk of idiopathic pneumonia syndrome, whereas fractionated radiation, instead of single-dose radiation, appears to decrease this risk. The mortality rate associated with idiopathic pneumonia syndrome is approximately 50%, and no available treatments are clearly effective, although early results with tumor necrosis factor blockade may be favorable (Forman et al., 2016; Ishibashi et al., 2016). Additional information on pulmonary complications can be found in Chapter 11.

Hepatic sinusoidal obstruction syndrome (HSOS), previously termed *veno-occlusive hepatic disease*, can develop within one to four weeks of conditioning and is believed to be caused by TBI/cyclophosphamide, with a higher incidence historically reported in patients receiving high doses of TBI (Chao, 2014; Forman et al., 2016; Ishibashi et al., 2016). Carreras et al. (2011) reviewed 845 allogeneic HSCT patient records and reported a decline in the incidence of HSOS from 11.5% to 6.5% over a 24-year period. The researchers attributed the decline to the increased use of reduced-intensity conditioning and a decrease in myeloablative conditioning with transplant using unrelated donors. Risk factors for HSOS include myeloablative conditioning, prior hepatic disease, poor performance status, and transplant from unrelated donors (Anderson-Reitz & Clancy, 2013; Forman et al., 2016). Symptoms include weight gain, ascites, tender hepatomegaly, and jaundice. Prophylaxis with ursodeoxycholic acid may decrease the incidence of HSOS, although it remains controversial. Mild HSOS typically does not require treatment; however, defibrotide should be initiated for severe HSOS (Anderson-Reitz & Clancy, 2013; Chao, 2014; Forman et al., 2016; see Chapter 10 for more detailed information on HSOS).

Long-term side effects of TBI include but are not limited to bone necrosis, bronchiolitis obliterans, cardiotoxicity, cataracts, endocrine disorders caused by hypopituitarism and bone growth disorders, GVHD, hypothyroidism, infertility, and neurotoxicity (Ishibashi et al., 2016; see Chapter 14 for more information).

Immunotherapeutic Agents

Biologic agents, such as alemtuzumab or ATG, may be added to enhance immunosuppression. Immunosuppressants destroy thymus-dependent human T cells and other immune cells (e.g., natural killer cells, dendritic cells) responsible for cellular-mediated immunity. ATG is indicated for the treatment of aplastic anemia and is also used in other regimens for malignancies to facilitate depletion of residual host T cells (Antin & Raley, 2013; Kröger et al., 2016). ATG is initially administered at a slow rate because reactions are common. Nurses must carefully monitor the patient's response before incrementally titrating the rate in a similar fashion to rituximab or IV immunoglobulin (IVIG). Patients are premedicated with diphenhydramine and/or corticosteroids. Immediate toxicities include rare, but fatal, allergic reaction. More common side effects include chills, fever, hypotension, and third spacing with pulmonary edema and prerenal azotemia. A syndrome of delayed skin rash and joint pains (known as serum sickness) also can occur.

Nonmyeloablative Regimens

Despite the curative potential of HSCT for a wide range of malignancies, transplant-related mortality increases with patient age and the presence of comorbidities. Over the past decade, nonmyeloablative and reduced-intensity conditioning regimens have been designed to decrease toxicity and allow HSCT to be an option in populations historically deemed ineligible (e.g., older adults, medically infirm individuals) for this transplant (Koniarczyk & Ferraro, 2016; McAdams & Burgunder, 2013). As many as 30 different nonmyeloablative and reduced-intensity regimens exist. Some of the more common are fludarabine/melphalan, with or without alemtuzumab or ATG; fludarabine/TBI, with or without ATG; cladribine/cytarabine; and fludarabine/cyclophosphamide (Koniarczyk & Ferraro, 2016; Kröger et al., 2016; McAdams & Burgunder, 2013).

Nursing Management of Preparative Regimens

All institutions should have specific policies and procedures for the administration of chemotherapy. Guidelines, such as those available from the Oncology Nursing Society (ONS, www.ons.org), provide a wealth of information for both patient and nursing safety. High-dose chemotherapy and TBI present many unique issues. An important component of nursing management is recognizing, preventing, and treating both expected and unexpected toxicities.

TBI, as well as most high-dose chemotherapy, is considered moderately to highly emetogenic, and prophylaxis with antiemetic therapy is necessary. Sedation is commonly required for young children receiving TBI (McAdams & Burgunder, 2013).

Many regimens contain bladder-toxic drugs, such as cyclophosphamide and ifosfamide, which can result in hemorrhagic cystitis (Forman et al., 2016). Prophylaxis includes a combination of vigorous IV hydration, placement of a Foley catheter with bladder irrigation, forced diuresis, and mesna (McAdams & Burgunder, 2013). Additional information on hemorrhagic cystitis can be found in Chapter 10.

Nephrotoxic drugs often require hyperhydration with IV fluids (Forman et al., 2016). Diuretics may be necessary to avoid fluid overload, although caution is required when administered concomitantly with other nephrotoxic agents. Frequent assessment for signs of fluid overload, including congestive heart failure and pulmonary edema, and electrolyte imbalance is necessary. Accurate intake and output should be recorded every four to eight hours along with daily or twice-daily weights. As many chemotherapy agents are excreted in the urine, nurses should refer to the ONS *Safe Handling of Hazardous Drugs* (Polovich & Olsen, 2018) for proper precautions. Managing complex chemotherapy regimens and associated side effects, along with careful assessment of fluid volume status, creates a busy and challenging situation for even the most experienced nurses. Familiarity with regimens and associated toxicities is paramount. See Chapter 10 for additional information on hepatorenal complications.

Patient and Caregiver Education

Patient and caregiver education should be initiated during the pretransplant workup and continued throughout the entire transplant course. Many centers have an HSCT patient education handbook containing a wealth of information, including post-transplant guidelines. Support groups or specialized education departments also may be available in some centers to assist with educational needs (McAdams & Burgunder, 2013). Important educational topics start with the conditioning regimen and include its purpose and the names, doses, schedules, and side effects of each chemotherapy agent. For patients receiving TBI, important information includes the treatment schedule, patient positioning, and short- and long-term side effects. It is important to discuss the differences between HSCT conditioning and previous chemotherapy treatments. Although some of the same agents may be used, patients and family members must understand the differences associated with myeloablative therapies.

Many centers perform various types of transplants in the outpatient setting, which requires specific caregiver education and places high demands on caregivers. Education should be in-depth and ongoing (McAdams & Burgunder, 2013). Often, centers have formal classes for caregivers that include central venous catheter care, intake and output measurement, and emergency procedures and contacts. Written materials and support services for caregivers also should be provided. Outpatient transplant often requires patients to reside within a specific distance from the transplant center to accommodate acute changes and ensure patient safety.

Cellular Infusion of Hematopoietic Stem Cells

The infusion of HSCs occurs on day 0. Autologous cells may be infused in one or more days depending on the number of bags and total number of nucleated cells, and to minimize the side effects of the cryoprotectant DMSO (dimethyl sulfoxide) (AABB et al., 2018; McAdams & Burgunder, 2013). HSCs may be infused without delay after TBI but usually are infused 48–72 hours after the last dose of chemotherapy to ensure no residual cytotoxic drugs remain that could harm the reinfused cells (McAdams & Burgunder, 2013). With the increase in the number of haploidentical transplants being performed, reports exist of an increased incidence of high-grade fever that mimics cytokine release syndrome 24–48 hours after infusion of haploidentical HSCs (Solomon, Solh, Morris, Holland, & Bashey, 2016).

Infusion of Cryopreserved Hematopoietic Stem Cells

HSCs can be cryopreserved to be infused at a later date. Both peripheral blood stem cells and bone marrow can be cryopreserved or infused fresh depending on donor availability and specific patient requirements. Cryopreserved HSCs and marrow can be successfully stored for many years, primarily limited by the inherent financial aspects of maintaining the product.

To prevent cell damage during freezing and thawing, a cryoprotectant is required. The most commonly used cryoprotectant is 10% DMSO, although concentrations as low as 5% have been used (Forman et al., 2016). Cryopreserved HSCs and marrow are rapidly thawed at the bedside and infused immediately (AABB et al., 2018). HSC laboratory personnel transport the product to the bedside. Sterile saline or sterile water is heated in a disinfected water bath to 37°C–45°C (98.6°F–113°F) at the bedside. Patient and bag identification are verified by two staff members (e.g., nurse, physician, HSC laboratory personnel) prior to thawing (AABB et al., 2018). Bags are then placed into the water bath. A secondary bag may be used to protect the cells in the event that breakage or leakage occurs. The cells are immediately infused by gravity or syringe, although some facilities may use a pump. The actual time for infusion can vary from 10–120 minutes depending on the patient, number of bags collected, and institutional policy (McAdams & Burgunder, 2013). Patients should be monitored frequently for adverse events during the infusion that may require adjustment of the infusion rate for the product. The thawing process for the second bag should not be initiated until infusion of the first bag is completed because prolonged exposure of thawed stem cells to DMSO has been shown to decrease colony formation of cryopreserved HSCs. Unless the thawed cells have been washed to remove DMSO (a common practice with umbilical cord blood), it is recommended to limit DMSO content to no more than 1 ml per kilogram of recipient weight per day of administration (AABB et al., 2018). Therefore, some autologous patients may have multiple days of infusion, with "day 0" being adjusted based on institutional policy.

Little research has been conducted comparing infusion methods (IV drip vs. IV bolus) or infusion rates. Theoretically, bolus methods result in shorter exposure of thawed stem cells to the DMSO, whereas drip methods may allow better patient tolerance of the emetogenic and arrhythmogenic effects of the DMSO. However, one pilot study looking at nausea and vomiting associated with DMSO showed no decrease in these symptoms with longer versus shorter infusions (Eisenberg, Wickline, Linenberger, Gooley, & Holmberg, 2013).

DMSO has several unique toxicities, some of which increase with each bag of HSCs. Red cells contained within a cryopreserved product do not survive the thawing process, and their breakdown can cause hemoglobinuria for 24–48 hours following the infusion (AABB et al., 2018). DMSO induces hemolysis, which may lead to pigment nephropathy and acute renal failure. Aggressive IV hydration is initiated before transplant to increase renal perfusion and minimize renal compromise (McAdams & Burgunder, 2013). Pre- and post-transplant hydration, along with advances in cryopreservation techniques, have helped to reduce the incidence of renal failure. Depending on the institution, hydration may include mannitol and sodium bicarbonate to promote osmotic diuresis. Diuretics may be indicated to manage fluid volume excess (McAdams & Burgunder, 2013). Education should include an explanation to patients and families regarding pink or red urine. They should be assured that the discolored urine is not caused by bleeding but rather from the breakdown of the red cells in the stem cell infusion product.

DMSO can induce a cholinergic response that causes bradycardia and abdominal cramping (Forman et al., 2016). It also is believed to release histamine, resulting in hives, nausea, vomiting, abdominal cramping, diarrhea, facial flushing, hypertension, hypotension, bradycardia, tachycardia, cardiac arrhythmias, tachypnea, dyspnea, cough, chest tightness, fever, and chills (Eisenberg et al., 2013; Potter, Eisenberg, Cain, & Berry, 2011). Premedication with acetaminophen and diphenhydramine is commonly used (McAdams & Burgunder, 2013).

Scant nursing research has been published on relieving some symptoms associated with cryopreserved infusions. Nausea and vomiting, typically occurring during and immediately after infusion, can be a source of patient distress. No guidelines exist for prevention in this setting, although a study of 49 patients receiving autologous infusions reported a significant decrease in both nausea and vomiting (p = 0.03) with the addition of ondansetron to acetaminophen and diphenhydramine (Eisenberg et al., 2013). Lorazepam, if ordered, should be used cautiously because of potential synergistic effects with DMSO, which may cause extreme drowsiness.

DMSO is converted to dimethyl sulfone ($DMSO_2$), which is excreted via the kidneys, and dimethyl sulfide, which is excreted via the respiratory system. Both compounds produce a unique, unpleasant garlic-like smell in the urine and breath, respectively. The strong odor also is associated with a foul taste, which can potentially worsen nausea (Forman et al., 2016; McAdams & Burgunder, 2013; Potter et al., 2011). Pulmonary excretion (and the associated odor) begins shortly after initiating the infusion and typically lasts for 24–48 hours. DMSO has a serum half-life of 20 hours. However, because the half-life of $DMSO_2$ is approximately 72 hours, nurses should discuss this unique side effect with patients and family members (AABB et al., 2018; Forman et al., 2016; Runckel & Swanson, 1980).

It has been theorized that the accompanying throat "tickle" is due to irritation of the upper respiratory membranes by DMSO as the compound is exhaled (Potter et al., 2011). Although it is not life threatening, patients may have a sensation of choking with difficulty swallowing, speaking, and catching their breath. Institutions have employed different methods to minimize these sensations, including having patients suck on hard candies and strawberry lollipops and smell oranges. A pilot study (N = 60) compared the smelling of oranges to orange aromatherapy and a control group (receiving neither intervention) to determine whether throat tickle, coughing, nausea, and vomiting could be decreased. Although the results did not reach statistical significance because of the small sample size, a trend in decreased symptoms was reported for the orange inhalation cohort but not the orange aromatherapy or control cohorts. The authors concluded that further research in this area is warranted (Potter et al., 2011).

HSCs cryopreserved with DMSO are normally administered via a central venous catheter because 10% DMSO is hyperosmotic and can cause endothelial cell damage (Glass, Perrin, Pocock, & Bates, 2006). Although not common practice, a study using a low volume of DMSO for cryopreserved lymphocytes demonstrated safety using a 20-gauge peripheral IV catheter (Gladstone et al., 2014). A variety of different central venous catheters, including peripherally inserted central catheters, large- and small-bore tunneled catheters, and temporary large-bore catheters (e.g., Mahurkar™), can be used depending on the transplant center.

Prior to and after infusion, nurses must assess for adequate urine output. Some centers monitor patients' cardiac rhythm and oxygenation throughout the infusion. Cardiac monitoring equipment and oxygen support should be available at the bedside. Vital signs should be checked prior to the start of the infusion, at least every 10–30 minutes during the infusion, and after the infusion. Severe reactions to DMSO may occur despite prophylactic medications, and frequent assessment should be performed for at least four hours after the infusion (Forman et al., 2016). See Table 6-3 for management of adverse events related to infusion of cryopreserved frozen stem cells.

Table 6-3. Management of Adverse Events of Cryopreserved Hematopoietic Stem Cells

Signs and Symptoms	Management Strategies
Cough, flushing, rash, chest tightness, wheezing, nausea and vomiting, bradycardia, tachycardia, hypertension, garlic or creamed-corn odor on breath	Premedicate with antihistamines. Wash the cells before administering them. Maintain adequate hydration. Slow the rate of administration. Monitor vital signs frequently throughout infusion. Monitor oxygen saturation. Consider diuretics to prevent fluid overload. Keep emergency equipment at bedside should cardiorespiratory support be needed.
Chills, fever, headache, unstable blood pressure, facial flushing, burning sensation along vein, dyspnea, chest or back pain, abnormal bleeding, possible signs of disseminated intravascular coagulation, shock	Stop infusion.[a] Maintain or correct blood pressure. Promote and maintain urine flow. Administer oxygen as needed. Correct coagulopathy. Keep emergency equipment at bedside should cardiorespiratory support be needed.
Urticaria, pruritus, facial or glottal edema	Stop infusion.[a] Administer antihistamines. Consider administering corticosteroids or epinephrine for severe reactions. Keep emergency equipment at bedside should cardiorespiratory support be needed.
Bronchospasm/laryngospasm, hypotension, severe dyspnea, pulmonary/laryngeal edema, facial burning/flushing, abdominal pain, diaphoresis, diarrhea, dizziness	Stop infusion.[a] Monitor volume status and correct fluids as required. Consider administering corticosteroids or epinephrine. Administer oxygen as needed. Keep emergency equipment at bedside should cardiorespiratory support be needed.

[a] Follow institutional protocol.

Note. Based on information from AABB et al., 2018; Gregory, 2017.

Patient and family education ideally begins at least a day before the infusion and is repeated on the day of infusion. This can help decrease patient anxiety. Education should cover room setup and equipment, use of premedications, the thawing process, infusion of the stem cells, and potential adverse reactions.

Fresh Hematopoietic Stem Cell Infusion

Allogeneic HSCs usually are infused as soon as possible after apheresis collection or marrow harvest. Under some circumstances, they can be stored overnight or cryopreserved for infusion at a later date. Fresh allogeneic stem cells are taken from the donor to the processing laboratory (AABB et al., 2018). If the donor and recipient have incompatible red cell phenotype, processing may include red cell depletion or plasma reduction (AABB et al., 2018). Other processing may include T-cell depletion to reduce the incidence of GVHD (AABB et al., 2018). Once processing is completed, the cells are delivered at the bedside and infused via gravity or a pump. Unlike cryopreserved HSCs, fresh cells do not require a central venous catheter, although one is typically in place for other reasons. There is disagreement as to whether filtered tubing is required for fresh HSCs, and each organization should have a clearly written policy. When used, filters typically are the same size as those used for blood products (e.g., 170–260 micron). Infusions are started slowly and increased after 30 minutes, based on the patient's calculated maximum rate (McAdams & Burgunder, 2013).

Vital signs are monitored before the start of the infusion and then every 10–30 minutes depending on the organization's protocol. Cardiac monitoring and/or pulse oximetry to monitor oxygenation may be indicated. ABO-compatible HSCs should be infused over two to four hours via pump, based on the volume. Because they are plasma reduced, the infusion time may be shorter because of decreased volume. However, ABO hemolytic reactions can still occur, and patients should be closely monitored for signs and symptoms of a reaction (e.g., flank or back pain, fever, feeling of impending doom). Upon completion of the infusion, the catheter should be flushed with preservative-free saline to prevent damage to the stem cells.

Fresh HSC infusions tend to have fewer adverse effects than cryopreserved infusions because of the absence of DMSO. Patients who have a history of transfusion reactions require premedication, although some institutions may elect to administer prophylactic acetaminophen and diphenhydramine even in the absence of a transfusion reaction history. In addition to ABO incompatibility, other major risks associated with infusion of fresh HSCs include nonhemolytic transfusion reactions and volume overload. Febrile reactions can occur and are due to cytokine release. However, because fresh HSCs are stored at 4°C (39.2°F) or room temperature, product contamination must be eliminated as a potential source of fever.

Treatment of fresh HSC reactions can include slowing the rate of the infusion and administering medications such as hydrocortisone and diphenhydramine. Serious allergic reactions may require epinephrine and oxygen, as well as diuretics for volume overload (AABB et al., 2018; Forman et al., 2016; McAdams & Burgunder, 2013). Although not common, aggressive cardiopulmonary support may be necessary. Therefore, emergency equipment should be readily available (Forman et al., 2016).

The fresh HSC infusion process should be reviewed with patients and families prior to and again on the day of the infusion. Providing information early may help to decrease patient and family anxiety. Education should include the equipment (e.g., cardiac monitor), medications, vital sign frequency, and potential adverse reactions. Patients should be encouraged to report all symptoms experienced and to ask questions throughout the infusion. Related family donors also may be present during the infusion and may require emotional support from transplant nurses.

After Stem Cell Infusion

The first day after HSC infusion is referred to as day +1, and subsequent days are numbered accordingly. The first few weeks following infusion are the most critical, as patients can begin to experience multiple toxicities from the preparative regimen while having little or no bone marrow function. If not recognized and treated immediately, these complications can lead to significant morbidity and mortality. In addition to the conditioning-related toxicities (see Table 6-2), several other adverse effects may occur.

Many organs can be affected by the conditioning regimen, and complications are described in more detail in other chapters. Validated comorbidity scales are reliable at predicting transplant-related mortality (McAdams & Burgunder, 2013). In general, patients with preexisting renal, hepatic, pulmonary, or cardiac disease have an increased risk for developing conditioning-related complications. Other risk factors include older age, obesity, donor type, and disease (Forman et al., 2016; McAdams & Burgunder, 2013).

Acute Complications

Acute complications are defined as those occurring from conditioning to day +100. Both the nature and the degree of complications associated with the transplant depend on the patient's age and health, the specific preparative regimen, and, to a lesser degree, the source of stem cells. The frequency of complications is higher in patients with Karnofsky performance scores less than 80% and in those with significant preexisting comorbidities (Sorror et al., 2014). For allogeneic recipients, GVHD is associated with an increased incidence of infection due to requisite immunosuppression.

Following most preparative regimens, toxicities such as nausea, vomiting, diarrhea, fever, and mild skin erythema are common. High-dose cyclophosphamide can cause hemorrhagic cystitis and HSOS. These toxicities are discussed in detail in Chapter 10. Parotitis, commonly seen in patients undergoing TBI, and mucositis, which can occur with either chemotherapy or TBI, can range from mild to severe. Mucositis may require narcotic analgesia and can be an emotionally stressful and potentially life-threatening complication. Refer to Chapter 9 for additional information.

Tumor Lysis Syndrome

Tumor lysis syndrome (TLS) is a metabolic emergency that occurs during conditioning, typically within one to five days of chemotherapy or radiation (Brown, 2015; Koniarczyk & Ferraro, 2016; McBride, Trifilio, Baxter, Gregory, & Howard, 2017; Wilson & Berns, 2014). Although uncommon in patients who are in remission or with minimal disease, patients with high tumor burden (e.g., leukemia, high-grade lymphoma) or with an elevated lactate dehydrogenase or renal dysfunction are at an increased risk (Brown, 2015; Koniarczyk & Ferraro, 2016; Wilson & Berns, 2014).

Acute TLS is characterized by the rapid development of hyperuricemia, hyperkalemia, hyperphosphatemia, hypocalcemia, azotemia, or acute renal failure. These abnormalities may occur alone or together and are commonly accompanied by acute elevation in blood urea nitrogen and serum phosphorus. Hypocalcemia and increases in lactate dehydrogenase are frequently seen. These biochemical alterations are related to the release of intracellular products into the circulation from the lysis of tumor cells (McBride et al., 2017). Acute renal insufficiency results from the precipitation of uric acid or calcium phosphate crystals in the renal tubules. When the release of uric acid occurs more slowly, uric acid stones can form in the renal pelvis and occasionally lead to ureteral obstruction.

Prevention of TLS is the primary goal. The use of allopurinol prior to chemotherapy has reduced the incidence of acute renal failure related to uric acid nephropathy. Urate oxidase (uricase) therapy may be used to reduce uric acid levels. Marked hyperphosphatemia is the usual precipitating factor of renal failure following chemotherapy. Despite the use of allopurinol or recombinant urate (rasburicase), hyperhydration with sodium bicarbonate may be instituted to facilitate urinary alkalization with the goal of increasing pH to at least 7 (Brown, 2015; Koniarczyk & Ferraro, 2016; McBride et al., 2017; Wilson & Berns, 2014). Acetazolamide, given orally or intravenously, also may be used to alkalinize the urine, especially in patients with metabolic acidosis or decreased renal function. Nurses should be aware that vigorous urinary alkalization may increase the risk of calcium phosphate precipitation in the renal tubules. Therefore, sodium bicarbonate should be discontinued once serum uric acid is normalized (McBride et al., 2017). Frequent monitoring of potassium, uric acid, calcium, phosphorus, lactate dehydrogenase, and renal function is essential (Wilson & Berns, 2014). Laboratory studies are commonly monitored at least twice daily for patients at high risk (Koniarczyk & Ferraro, 2016).

Hyperkalemia is the most life-threatening component of TLS and should be acted upon immediately. The usual treatment includes hypertonic glucose with insulin and sodium–potassium exchange resin. Furosemide is useful and acts by increasing urinary potassium excretion. Calcium should not be administered unless evidence of neuromuscular irritability is present. It is common for patients who are at risk for developing acute TLS to have some degree of renal insufficiency, because of either lymphomatous infiltration of the kidneys or urinary obstruction before starting the chemotherapy. Treatment of the underlying malignancy may improve renal function by correcting the underlying cause of the renal failure. Hemodialysis may be required to correct hyperkalemia, hyperuricemia, hyperphosphatemia, and hypocalcemia, if supportive care measures fail (Brown, 2015; Koniarczyk & Ferraro, 2016; McBride et al., 2017; Wilson & Berns, 2014).

Nursing management involves identifying patients at risk for developing acute TLS and monitoring for electrolyte abnormalities, fluid balance, and response to treatment. Early recognition of signs and symptoms of hyperuricemia, hyperkalemia, hyperphosphatemia, and hypocalcemia will promote prompt initiation of preventive therapy and minimize additional complications.

Hypercalcemia

Hypercalcemia is uncommon in the HSCT setting but may occur in patients with multiple myeloma because of extensive bone destruction or in patients with lymphoma (Koniarczyk & Ferraro, 2016; McAdams & Burgunder, 2013). Hypercalcemia occurs when more calcium is released from the bones than the kidneys can excrete or that the bones can reabsorb. Bone resorption is increased by parathyroid hormone–related protein and osteoclast-activating factors secreted from myeloma cells. In addition, related substances that possess osteoclast-activating factor properties, such as the cytokines tumor necrosis factor-beta, interleukin-1, and interleukin-6, are potent inhibitors of osteoblastic bone formation (Koniarczyk & Ferraro, 2016; McAdams & Burgunder, 2013).

Ninety-nine percent of the body's calcium is combined with phosphorus and is concentrated in the skeletal system, which serves as the body's calcium reservoir. The remaining 1% is in the serum, half of which is freely ionized, and the other half bound primarily by albumin (Koniarczyk & Ferraro, 2016; McAdams & Burgunder, 2013). The freely ionized form is biologically active and must be maintained within a narrow range. Homeostasis of normal calcium levels involves a balance of several body processes, including bone remodeling, renal calcium reabsorption, and gastrointestinal absorption. Hormonal factors influence the interchange of calcium between the gut, kidney, bone, and extracellular fluid. Parathyroid hormone and calcitonin are the primary hormones that regulate extracellular calcium homeostasis. In turn, each substance is controlled by the level of serum ionized calcium (Koniarczyk & Ferraro, 2016; McAdams & Burgunder, 2013).

Humoral hypercalcemia and local osteolytic hypercalcemia are the two main mechanisms that contribute to the occurrence of hypercalcemia in malignancy. These mechanisms disrupt the balance of calcium by producing hormones, cytokines, or growth factors that interfere with the normal physiologic functioning of the bone, kidneys, and gut (Koniarczyk & Ferraro, 2016; McAdams & Burgunder, 2013). Another humoral mediator of malignancy-related hypercalcemia is vitamin D. Although vitamin D–related hypercalcemia is not common, it has been seen in human T-cell leukemia virus–related T-cell lymphomas and Hodgkin lymphoma (Koniarczyk & Ferraro, 2016; McAdams & Burgunder, 2013). Calcium plays a role in maintaining cell membrane permeability, which affects the cellular activity of multiple body systems, and disruption of this permeability results in the signs and symptoms of hypercalcemia (Koniarczyk & Ferraro, 2016; McAdams & Burgunder, 2013).

Common symptoms of hypercalcemia include fatigue, anorexia, weight loss, bone pain, constipation, polydipsia, muscle weakness, nausea, vomiting, confusion, polyuria, diarrhea, lethargy, muscle cramps, oliguria, acute renal failure, kidney stones, headache, dehydration, and dysrhythmias (Koniarczyk & Ferraro, 2016; McAdams & Burgunder, 2013). In symptomatic patients with a serum calcium level of 12–14 mg/dl, the finding is serious because any event that causes volume depletion or a decrease in the glomerular filtration rate may lead to severe hypercalcemia. Urgent treatment is required for patients with a corrected serum calcium greater than 14 mg/dl and for patients with symptomatic moderate hypercalcemia (McAdams & Burgunder, 2013).

Hypercalcemia is diagnosed by the corrected serum calcium level. The total serum calcium level is a poor indicator of freely ionized calcium; therefore, the use of a correction formula that considers the effect of an altered albumin concentration is important. The following formula is used: corrected serum calcium (mg/dl) = measured total serum calcium (mg/dl) + [0.8 × (4 – serum albumin level [g/dl])] (Kaplan, 2018). Other important laboratory values include serum electrolytes, ionized calcium, blood urea nitrogen, and creatinine. Potassium and calcium have an inverse relationship, and hypokalemia has been reported in more than half of patients with hypercalcemia whose renal function is normal (Koniarczyk & Ferraro, 2016; McAdams & Burgunder, 2013). Magnesium levels also may decrease, aggravating the neuromuscular effects. Hypercalcemia resulting from direct bone involvement (e.g., breast cancer, myeloma, renal cell carcinoma) often results in increased serum phosphorus levels (Koniarczyk & Ferraro, 2016; McAdams & Burgunder, 2013).

Treatment of malignancy-induced hypercalcemia is aimed at treating the underlying disease as well as the mechanisms causing hypercalcemia. The two mechanisms of hypercalcemia (accelerated bone resorption and increased calcium reabsorption in the kidneys) are treated by initiating hydration with saline diuresis to increase calcium excretion from the kidneys followed by antiresorptive therapy to decrease bone resorption (McAdams & Burgunder, 2013). Once rehydration has been established, bisphosphonates are effective when administered orally or intravenously, depending on the severity of the hypercalcemia. Treatment includes a review of medications that might contribute to hypercalcemia, such as thiazide diuretics, vitamins A and D, or any type of calcium supplements, including additives in hyperalimentation (McAdams & Burgunder, 2013).

Nursing management of hypercalcemia of malignancy is directed at prevention, early detection, treatment, management, and patient and family support. It is important to identify patients who are at risk, assess for signs and symptoms, and monitor laboratory values (Koniarczyk & Ferraro, 2016; McAdams & Burgunder, 2013).

Disseminated Intravascular Coagulation

Disseminated intravascular coagulation (DIC) is the simultaneous development of thrombosis and hemorrhage as the result of overstimulation of the clotting cascade. This syndrome can develop suddenly or be a chronic complication and can progress to other conditions such as microangiopathic hemolytic anemia. DIC can occur due to septic shock but also can be seen in patients with TLS, liver failure, vascular injuries, or leukemia.

DIC results from injury to the vascular endothelium and activation of platelets and clotting factors. Depending on severity, the syndrome may be chronic, acute, or fulminating. In DIC, coagulation is overstimulated and there is an inability to control intravascular thrombin that can activate both coagulation and fibrinolysis. The initial event in acute DIC is a thrombotic diathesis, in which clotting factors and platelets are consumed (Koniarczyk & Ferraro, 2016; McAdams & Burgunder, 2013). Excess circulating thrombin separates fibrinogen, which combines with circulating fibrin degradation products (FDPs) to form an insoluble form of fibrin. These insoluble clots may become deposited in the microvasculature of various organs, with resultant multisystem failure (Koniarczyk & Ferraro, 2016). The lodged clots further trap circulating platelets, leading to a worsening of the thrombocytopenic state. The trapped platelets also impede blood flow, leading to hypoxia, tissue ischemia, and necrosis of affected organs, along with consumption of clotting factors (Gobel, 2018). Once clotting factors and platelets drop below critical levels, hemorrhage occurs. Excess thrombin assists in the conversion of plasminogen to plasmin, resulting in fibrinolysis that leads to increased FDPs. FDPs have strong anticoagulant properties and thus interfere with fibrin clot formation and aid in the consumption of clotting factors and platelets. Plasmin can activate the complement and kinin systems. Activation of these systems leads to shock, hypotension, and increased vascular permeability (McAdams & Burgunder, 2013). The clinical presentation generally is a combination of extreme thrombosis and bleeding.

Bleeding is the most obvious sign of DIC. Most patients with DIC bleed from at least three unrelated sites (Koniarczyk & Ferraro, 2016). A less evident but equally dramatic sign of DIC is thrombosis. Both microvascular and large-vessel thrombosis may occur, which may result in end-organ damage and ischemic changes. Subtle signs and symptoms of thrombi include red, indurated areas in multiple organ sites (Koniarczyk & Ferraro, 2016).

Laboratory testing for DIC can be variable and complex based on the pathophysiology. In DIC, the prothrombin time may be normal or even reduced because of interference from activating clotting factors or FDPs. The activated partial thromboplastin time is normal in approximately 40%–50% of patients with DIC. The platelet count usually is decreased but the presence of thrombocytopenia is neither sensitive nor specific for DIC. At the same time, a continuous drop, even within a normal range, may indicate the active generation of thrombin (Koniarczyk & Ferraro, 2016).

One of the most reliable tests to assess DIC is the D-dimer assay. D-dimer is a neoantigen formed when plasmin digests fibrin. The D-dimer test is specific for FDPs. Another test for DIC is the FDP titer; a positive FDP titer indicates DIC. DIC is almost always associated with increased fibrinolysis, which may result in increased levels of FDPs. The diagnosis of DIC may be supported by tests that reveal accelerated fibrinolysis. A decreased level of antithrombin III demonstrates accelerated coagulation (Gobel, 2018). More recently, an atypical light transmittance profile on the activated partial thromboplastin time has been associated with DIC (Koniarczyk & Ferraro, 2016). Referred to as the *biphasic wave form*, this abnormality occurs independently of prolongation in the clotting times and, through prospective studies, has been shown to be a simple, rapid, robust indicator of DIC (Koniarczyk & Ferraro, 2016; McAdams & Burgunder, 2013). However, its performance is limited to specific photo-optical analyzers that display clot formation over time.

The basic principle of treating DIC is to treat the underlying cause (Koniarczyk & Ferraro, 2016; McAdams & Burgunder, 2013). If the process of DIC continues after measures aimed at treating the underlying stimulus have been attempted, treating the intravascular clotting process is the next step. The reason for treating the clotting process next is that thrombosis is the process with the most impact on the morbidity and mortality associated with DIC. Heparin may inhibit coagulation pathways but must be used with caution in patients at risk for bleeding. Transfusion of platelets or plasma is indicated in patients with DIC and bleeding and those at high risk for bleeding.

Nursing management involves early detection, with the goal of early diagnosis, and treatment. Although thrombosis is the strongest contributor to morbidity and mortality, bleeding is the most observable sign. Routine physical assessment should focus on evidence of bleeding or thrombosis. Daily weights and strict monitoring of intake and output every shift are important in preventing dehydration and fluid overload. Providing care in a calm and reassuring environment may help to decrease patient and family anxiety (Koniarczyk & Ferraro, 2016).

Syndrome of Inappropriate Antidiuretic Hormone Secretion

Syndrome of inappropriate antidiuretic hormone secretion (SIADH) is a potentially life-threatening oncologic emergency. SIADH is an endocrine-mediated syndrome causing abnormal production or secretion of antidiuretic hormone. Normally, the posterior pituitary gland releases antidiuretic hormone in response to increased plasma osmolality or decreased plasma volume and sends signals to the collecting ducts of the kidneys to reabsorb water,

concentrate the urine, and normalize serum osmolality (Brown, 2015).

The hallmark of SIADH in euvolemic patients is hyponatremia with increased urine osmolality, decreased plasma osmolality, and elevated urine sodium (Brown, 2015; Koniarczyk & Ferraro, 2016). Hyponatremia is a direct result of excess water, rather than a deficiency in sodium (Brown, 2015). The most common cause in the HSCT setting is medications. SIADH is mediated through enhanced action of antidiuretic hormone on the renal tubules by various drugs, particularly cyclophosphamide. Other drugs, such as melphalan, vincristine, morphine, nicotine, monoamine oxidase inhibitors, selective serotonin reuptake inhibitors, and tricyclic antidepressants, are less frequently implicated in this population.

Symptoms usually correlate with the rate of onset and severity of the hyponatremia (Koniarczyk & Ferraro, 2016). Patients often are asymptomatic if the hyponatremia is mild or chronic. If SIADH develops acutely (i.e., within one to three days), patients may complain of a headache, fatigue, anorexia, difficulty concentrating, weakness, muscle cramps, or weight gain. Unfortunately, these nonspecific signs and symptoms are observed frequently in patients with cancer. Moderate signs and symptoms may include thirst, impaired taste, confusion, lethargy, nausea, vomiting, diarrhea, oliguria, incontinence, depressed deep tendon reflexes, and personality changes. Severe signs and symptoms may progress to coma and seizure activity. The development of cyclophosphamide-induced SIADH in the outpatient setting usually requires emergent admission to correct the hyponatremia and monitor for associated side effects.

Diagnostic studies include a serum hyponatremia of sodium less than 135 mg/dl, serum osmolality less than 270 mOsm/kg, and inappropriately concentrated urine (urine osmolality greater than 1,000 mOsm/kg, specific gravity greater than 1.015, urine sodium greater than 20 mEq/L) (Koniarczyk & Ferraro, 2016).

Treatment is based on the underlying cause. Although mild hyponatremia may respond to fluid restriction of 500–1,000 ml/day to promote a negative water balance, this may not be practical immediately following the administration of cyclophosphamide, for which hyperhydration is indicated for preventing hemorrhagic cystitis (Brown, 2015). It is important to correct the sodium no faster than 12 mEq in 24 hours or 0.5 mEq/L per hour to avoid cerebral edema from developing as a result of sudden fluid and electrolyte shifting (Brown, 2015; Koniarczyk & Ferraro, 2016).

In the transplant setting, mild to moderate hyponatremia can be treated with conservative doses of furosemide. Inducing excess diuresis in patients receiving cyclophosphamide can cause hypovolemia, leading to orthostasis and an increased risk of hemorrhagic cystitis. Nursing management involves monitoring serum sodium levels per institution guidelines, performing accurate intake and output measurements, recording daily weights, and taking orthostatic vital signs to help assess volume status. The substantial hydration necessary with cyclophosphamide may worsen SIADH and result in fluid retention. Diuresis can result in decreases in weight of up to 2–3 kg over several days, reflecting excretion of excess water. Measurements of urine-specific gravity, taken every four to eight hours depending on specific guidelines, can help assess the kidneys' ability to concentrate urine (Koniarczyk & Ferraro, 2016).

If diuresis is ineffective or neurologic symptoms are present, pharmacologic therapy with demeclocycline is typically initiated. Demeclocycline inhibits the action of antidiuretic hormone at the renal tubules, therefore allowing secretion of water. Correction of hyponatremia should not exceed 0.5 mEq/L per hour and not more than 12 mEq in any 24-hour period (Koniarczyk & Ferraro, 2016). Patients with life-threatening hyponatremia (i.e., severe neurologic symptoms) require aggressive therapy with hypertonic saline (3%) and IV furosemide (Brown, 2015; Koniarczyk & Ferraro, 2016). During reversal of hyponatremia, especially in severe cases, nurses must be aware of overcorrection. If normal sodium levels are exceeded, it may be necessary to slow or discontinue therapy.

Sepsis and Infectious Complications

Infection is a major risk for nearly all transplant patients. Recipients of autologous transplants are at risk for early bacterial and fungal infections common to all patients with granulocytopenia. Allogeneic patients, particularly those who develop GVHD, have an increased risk for late-onset bacterial, fungal, and viral diseases. See Chapter 7 for more information.

Sepsis is a condition characterized by a systemic inflammatory response syndrome and the presence of infection (McAdams & Burgunder, 2013). The normal host response to infection is a complex process that serves to localize and control pathogen invasion and initiate repair of injured tissue.

Patients with sepsis will present with fever and either vasodilation and relative vascular volume deficiency, or vasoconstriction and myocardial depression (McAdams & Burgunder, 2013). Failure to develop a febrile response and the presence of leukopenia are characteristic of severe disease and probably represent anomalies in inflammatory response (McAdams & Burgunder, 2013). The most important management strategies for suspected sepsis in any HSCT recipient with cancer are early detection and prompt initiation of antimicrobial therapy (Forman et al., 2016). Unless patients exhibit signs or symptoms of impending shock, the antimicrobial regimen usually is not changed for 72 hours (McAdams & Burgunder, 2013).

The process of sepsis involves neurologic, endocrine, immunologic, and cardiovascular compensatory responses that produce an integrated attempt to reject and destroy the pathogen. When compensation is present, inflammatory mediators are predominant, and a "warm hyperdynamic" clinical presentation is typical. When compensatory mecha-

nisms fail and myocardial depression prevails, a "cold hypodynamic" (myocardial failure and perfusion deficit) clinical picture is evident. Patients with sepsis develop a cluster of symptoms that signal the onset of septic shock, such as shaking chills, temperature increase, skin flushing, galloping pulse, and alternating rise and fall of blood pressure. A thorough physical examination focusing on high-risk sites of infection, such as the skin and oral cavity, is necessary (McAdams & Burgunder, 2013).

Risk factors for infection in transplant recipients include the underlying disease, preexisting comorbidities (e.g., history of pulmonary *Aspergillus*), and treatment modalities (see Table 6-4). Recipients of allogeneic

Table 6-4. Factors Affecting the Risk of Infection

Factor	Risk of Infection
Type of transplant	Higher risk with allogeneic, lower risk with autologous or syngeneic, depending on graft manipulation and clinical setting, including previous therapies
Time from transplant	Lower risk with more time elapsed from transplant
Pretransplant factors	Higher risk with extensive pretransplant immunosuppressive therapy (e.g., fludarabine, clofarabine), prolonged pretransplant neutropenia, or pretransplant infection
Graft-versus-host disease (GVHD)	Higher risk with grade III–IV acute GVHD or extensive chronic GVHD
Human leukocyte antigen (HLA) match	Higher risk with HLA-mismatched donors, particularly with haploidentical donors
Disease (e.g., leukemia) status	Higher risk with more advanced disease at the time of transplant
Donor type	Higher risk with unrelated marrow donor than with a fully matching sibling donor
Graft type	Highest risk with cord blood, intermediate risk with bone marrow, and lowest risk with colony-stimulating factor–mobilized blood stem cells. Higher risk with T-cell–depleted grafts (depending upon method used)
Immunosuppression after transplant	Higher with immunosuppressive drugs, in particular with corticosteroids, antithymocyte globulin, alemtuzumab
Conditioning intensity	Lower risk in the first 1–3 months posttransplant with low-dose chemo/radiotherapy
Neutrophil engraftment	Higher risk with delayed engraftment/nonengraftment

Note. From "Guidelines for Preventing Infectious Complications Among Hematopoietic Cell Transplantation Recipients: A Global Perspective," by M. Tomblyn, T. Chiller, H. Einsele, R. Gress, K. Sepkowitz, J. Storek, … M.A. Boeckh, 2009, *Biology of Blood and Marrow Transplantation, 15*, p. 1152. Copyright 2009 by American Society for Blood and Marrow Transplantation. Retrieved from https://doi.org/10.1016/j.bbmt.2009.06.019. Licensed under CC BY-NC-ND 4.0 (https://creativecommons.org/licenses/by-nc-nd/4.0).

HSCT are at increased risk for a variety of infections based on their degree and duration of immunosuppression. The types of infections to which these individuals are the most vulnerable can be roughly divided into three time periods beginning with day 0: pre-engraftment (less than three weeks), immediate postengraftment (three weeks to three months), and late postengraftment (more than three months). Although the division into time periods is somewhat arbitrary, it is helpful in the management of allogeneic transplant recipients. By contrast, autologous transplant recipients typically are vulnerable to infection during the pre-engraftment and immediate postengraftment periods. All patients can develop bacterial, fungal, viral, or parasitic infections, although specific pathogens tend to cause disease during some periods more than others (McAdams & Burgunder, 2013; Tomblyn et al., 2009; see Figure 6-2).

The diagnosis of sepsis is based on clinical indicators, laboratory tests, and a variety of other diagnostic procedures, such as radiology or sonography. The most important and sensitive of these tests is the culture and sensitivity of body fluids (Koniarczyk & Ferraro, 2016; McAdams & Burgunder, 2013). Blood cultures are a vital part of any fever workup and can determine the pathogenic organisms responsible for the septic condition. A minimum of two sets of cultures should be drawn initially. Many organizations require at least two sets, which may include one from the vascular access catheter and one obtained peripherally (Taplitz et al., 2018).

The single most important method of preventing infection in immunocompromised patients is recognizing risk factors and altering them whenever possible. Immunocompromised patients develop infection from environmental exposures, through reactivation of latent organisms, from

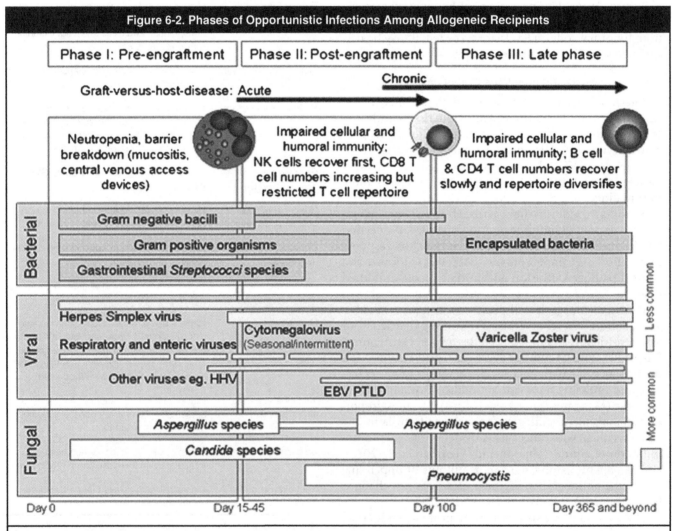

Figure 6-2. Phases of Opportunistic Infections Among Allogeneic Recipients

EBV—Epstein-Barr virus; HHV6—human herpesvirus 6; PTLD—post-transplant lymphoproliferative disease

Note. From "Guidelines for Preventing Infectious Complications Among Hematopoietic Cell Transplantation Recipients: A Global Perspective," by M. Tomblyn, T. Chiller, H. Einsele, R. Gress, K. Sepkowitz, J. Storek, … M.A. Boeckh, 2009, *Biology of Blood and Marrow Transplantation, 15*, p. 1152. Copyright 2009 by American Society for Blood and Marrow Transplantation. Retrieved from https://doi.org/10.1016/j.bbmt.2009.06.019. Licensed under CC BY-NC-ND 4.0 (https://creativecommons.org/licenses/by-nc-nd/4.0).

normal flora, and through nosocomial exposures during hospitalization.

Prophylactic antibiotics are used in the effort to prevent infection. Fevers are common during the early neutropenic post-transplant period, and approximately 50% of these infections are bacterial (Lewis, 2017). Therefore, most transplant centers initiate antibiotics once patients become neutropenic, even if they are afebrile. Studies comparing infection rates with and without prophylactic antibiotics in high-risk patients receiving high-dose therapy have demonstrated that prophylactic antibiotics reduce infection morbidity (Lewis, 2017; McAdams & Burgunder, 2013). For patients with acute leukemia or those who undergo HSCT, prophylaxis with fluoroquinolones diminishes the risk of death from any cause by 33% (McAdams & Burgunder, 2013). Excessive local levels of resistance to fluoroquinolones or high local incidence of infections caused by *Clostridium difficile* and related to fluoroquinolones should prompt reconsideration of prophylaxis with ciprofloxacin or levofloxacin (McAdams & Burgunder, 2013).

Prophylaxis against fungal pathogens has been shown to reduce rates of fungal infection and improve overall survival. Fluconazole is generally recommended for patients with standard risk. An agent active against molds, such as voriconazole or posaconazole, should be considered for patients with higher-risk disease, including those with a prior fungal infection, recipients of cord blood, or recipients of unrelated donor transplants (Girmenia et al., 2014). Although having a prior invasive fungal infection increases transplant risk, with current methods of prophylaxis, it should not be considered a contraindication for transplant (Maziarz et al., 2017). Patients who become or remain febrile despite treatment with broad-spectrum antibiotics and who have no obvious source of infection are usually treated with additional antifungal agents (e.g., voriconazole, micafungin, amphotericin), depending on the clinical situation. Recipients of cord blood transplants sometime develop "cord colitis," a syndrome of diarrhea responsive to metronidazole alone or in combination with a fluoroquinolone (Herrera et al., 2011). Molecular studies have suggested *Bradyrhizobium enterica* as the causative pathogen (Bhatt et al., 2013).

Although laminar airflow isolation and prophylactic granulocyte transfusions can prevent early infection, neither action influences overall survival; thus, neither approach is recommended. With current methods of supportive care, the risk of death due to infections during the early granulocytopenia period is less than 3% for recipients of either allogeneic or autologous transplants (McAdams & Burgunder, 2013).

Herpes simplex infection, which can contribute to the severity of oral mucositis, can be prevented with the use of systemic acyclovir and continued post-transplant for one to six months (Erard et al., 2007).

In the past, symptomatic cytomegalovirus (CMV) infection, which typically involves either the gastrointestinal tract or the lungs, occurred in approximately 25% of patients who received an allogeneic transplant. Death, typically from CMV pneumonia, occurred in 10%–15% of patients (McAdams & Burgunder, 2013). Primary CMV infection, in which both the donor and recipient are without latent CMV infection (as evidenced by having no detectable antibodies to CMV before transplantation), can be prevented by only using blood products from CMV-negative donors who have undergone leukocyte reduction. In CMV-positive donors or recipients, weekly CMV polymerase chain reaction is performed to ensure initiation of timely treatment. For patients with evidence of latent CMV before transplantation, the use of prophylactic ganciclovir, starting at either initial engraftment or CMV reactivation, can substantially reduce the risk of CMV disease (McAdams & Burgunder, 2013).

Pneumocystis jirovecii pneumonia can be prevented with the treatment of trimethoprim-sulfamethoxazole (TMP-SMX), beginning before transplant and continuing until six months after, or until immunosuppression has been discontinued. TMP-SMX should be discontinued during the pre-engraftment period because it can cause pancytopenia. Allergic reactions to TMP-SMX are common but usually can be managed with desensitization, or, instead, pentamidine inhalation can be administered monthly. Sometimes, dapsone or atovaquone may be prescribed as a substitute for patients with a TMP-SMX allergy (McAdams & Burgunder, 2013).

Commonly acquired viral infections, including respiratory syncytial virus (RSV), influenza, and parainfluenza, can cause lethal pneumonias in the transplant population. Patients with upper respiratory symptoms before transplant should be screened by nasopharyngeal lavage for viral infections before proceeding. If RSV, influenza, adenovirus, or parainfluenza is found, the transplant should be delayed. Ribavirin and anti-RSV antibody may be effective in treating established RSV infection in the transplant patient (McAdams & Burgunder, 2013).

Hematopoietic growth factors are used to accelerate cell regeneration and differentiation in patients with bone marrow aplasia. In the transplant setting, the current standard of care is to administer colony-stimulating factors (CSFs) after autologous, but not allogeneic, peripheral blood stem cell transplantation (McAdams & Burgunder, 2013). The American Society of Clinical Oncology 2015 clinical practice guideline cautioned that reports of an increase in the incidence of severe GVHD and a reduction in survival have been linked to the use of CSFs after allogeneic transplantation (McAdams & Burgunder, 2013; Smith et al., 2015). The use of granulocyte–colony-stimulating factor (G-CSF) for autologous patients resulted in decreased hospitalization and overall medical costs. However, the same was not observed in allogeneic recipients (McAdams & Burgunder, 2013; Smith et al., 2015).

Research has revealed that immunosuppressed HSCT recipients become immunoglobulin deficient. When immunoglobulin G deficiency is present, response to polysaccharide encapsulated bacteria is impaired, making infections with pneumococci and *Haemophilus influenzae* more common (McAdams & Burgunder, 2013). IVIG therapy has been shown to be effective in the prevention of some viral infections. Provan (2004) reported that infection rates and survival are similar, regardless of whether IVIG is given, and a Cochrane analysis of 40 studies showed similar results (Raanani et al., 2008). Still, about one-third of HSCT recipients continue to receive IVIG because of hypogammaglobulinemia in the context of protein-losing enteropathy, GVHD, or rituximab pretreatment (Cantoni et al., 2009).

IVIG generally is well tolerated but, as with all foreign proteins, hypersensitivity reaction is possible. Therefore, infusions are started slowly, and the rate titrated incrementally while the patient is monitored. A number of different IVIG preparations are currently U.S. Food and Drug Administration approved, and although administration and side effects are similar, the drugs are not without significant differences. Nurses unfamiliar with a specific IVIG product should use available resources (e.g., clinical pharmacist, Micromedex® or prescribing information sheets). While IVIG contains nonspecific antibodies, a product specifically intended for CMV infection (known as CMVIG) has also been used for prophylaxis and treatment.

Other Complications

Delayed complications attributable to the preparative regimen include decreased growth velocity in children and delayed development of secondary sexual characteristics. Most postpubescent women will experience ovarian failure, and few men regain spermatogenesis following HSCT using high-dose preparative regimens. Cataracts occur in as many as one-third of patients, with an increased risk among patients receiving myeloablative doses of TBI and patients requiring steroids for treatment of GVHD. Thyroid dysfunction also can occur. Patients treated with high-dose chemotherapy, with or without TBI, are at increased risk for developing secondary cancers and post-transplant lymphoproliferative disorders (Rasche, Kapp, Einsele, & Mielke, 2014). See Chapter 14 for additional information regarding late effects and long-term survivorship issues.

Engraftment Phase

Following the administration of a myeloablative preparative regimen and the infusion of HSCs, a period of profound myelosuppression ensues. Within one to two weeks after transplantation, the peripheral leukocyte count begins to increase, signifying the beginning of engraftment. *Engraftment* refers to the state of acceptance of infused HSCs as evidenced by a gradual but steady increase in blood counts. The first sign of engraftment is the return of circulating white blood cells to a sufficient level, defined as an absolute neutrophil count of greater than 500/mm³ for three consecutive days. Another indication is an increased platelet count without transfusion support, which typically occurs

after recovery of the absolute neutrophil count (Koniarczyk & Ferraro, 2016).

When stem cells are procured from marrow and no hematopoietic growth factors are used after transplantation, the granulocyte count reaches 100/mm³ by approximately day 16 and 1,000/mm³ by day 26. Administration of G-CSF to the recipient accelerates the recovery of the peripheral granulocyte count by one week. The platelet count recovers simultaneously with or shortly after recovery of granulocytes. When the peripheral blood is the source of stem cells, engraftment is more rapid, with a granulocyte count of 500/mm³ and platelet count of 20,000/mm³ achieved by day 12, on average. Engraftment following cord blood transplantation is typically delayed by approximately one week compared with marrow. Engraftment of allogeneic stem cells can be documented using fluorescence in situ hybridization of sex chromosomes if the donor and recipient are of opposite sex, or DNA-based assays of short tandem repeat loci. With these techniques, the donor-versus-recipient origin of cell populations can now be determined in virtually all cases (McAdams & Burgunder, 2013).

Migration or homing of transplanted cells to the bone marrow for engraftment is a complex process that is not fully understood. After infusion, these cells pass through a blood–marrow barrier, which appears to be facilitated by five families of adhesion molecules: integrins, immunoglobulins, selectins, mucins, and proteoglycans. The cell membranes of CD34+ cells have multiple receptors for these adhesion molecules. The cell membrane receptors are highly specific but have regulatable levels of affinity, allowing them to bind and then release the molecules, enabling the adhesion molecule receptors found on CD34+ cells to direct stem cells to move along a particular pathway. This pathway has been called the *adhesion cascade* (Koniarczyk & Ferraro, 2016; McAdams & Burgunder, 2013). In the process of migration, stem cells first adhere to the inner surface of the blood–marrow barrier, the endothelial cells lining the vascular sinuses in the bones. After forming a migration pore in the endothelial cell cytoplasm, stem cells penetrate the basement membrane and then pass through gaps in the adventitial reticular layer. Once stem cells pass through the barrier and into the extravascular space, components of the marrow stroma interact with the cells to direct them into their appropriate niches. Here, presumably, they are retained or trapped (Koniarczyk & Ferraro, 2016; McAdams & Burgunder, 2013).

Following the transplantation, infused stem cells give rise to a new hematopoietic and immune system. A consistent rise in the white blood cell count heralds hematopoietic and immune recovery. Early evidence of engraftment is seen as the white blood cell count rises and the cell population shifts from lymphocytes to neutrophils. Red blood cells, platelets, and neutrophils are all capable of functioning effectively as soon as they are generated. This is not the case, however, for T and B cells, whose effectiveness returns slowly and may never return to pretransplant levels (McAdams & Burgunder, 2013).

In autologous HSCT, white blood cells appear in the circulation 7–10 days following transplant. When using bone marrow as the stem cell source, white blood cells appear about two weeks later. Faster recovery sometimes allows the entire transplant procedure to be performed in the outpatient arena, eliminating the need for hospitalization and resulting in considerable cost savings. Faster recovery also results in improved quality of life. This rapid recovery is the major reason why autologous transplants using marrow are rarely performed today and peripheral blood progenitor cells are the standard of care for patients needing autologous HSC rescue (Lazarus, Hamadani, & Hari, 2019).

Engraftment Following Allogeneic Hematopoietic Stem Cell Transplantation

Following myeloablative conditioning, HSCT recipients typically experience a period of severe neutropenia spanning days to weeks, depending on the donor source. In the allogeneic setting, successful engraftment of donor cells in marrow is known as a *chimeric state* (meaning that only donor cells exist within the patient), which is the intent of the transplant (Koniarczyk & Ferraro, 2016; McAdams & Burgunder, 2013). In some patients, a mix of donor and recipient cells, referred to as *mixed chimerism*, may exist after transplant. Ideally, in myeloablative transplants, only the donor cells will populate the patient's marrow. For nonmyeloablative transplants, a mixed chimerism is expected, as it is the relationship between donor and host cells that results in eradicating disease and preventing relapse. If available, a backup infusion of stem cells may be given in the event of graft failure. Donor lymphocyte infusions may be administered to the patient if donor chimerism is delayed or the patient's underlying disease relapses (McAdams & Burgunder, 2013).

Although the increase of peripheral cell counts suggests engraftment, cytogenetic studies such as chromosomal analysis may help to signify successful transplant by identifying the origin of the new marrow. If the donor and recipient are not of the same gender, engraftment is confirmed by the presence of the donor's sex chromosomes in the recipient's new bone marrow. Cytogenetic studies detect disease remission by monitoring the disappearance of unique chromosomal abnormalities specific to the patient's malignancy. If the recipient and donor are the same sex, erythrocyte typing, HLA typing, complement typing, and immunoglobulin allele typing may confirm engraftment. However, complex methods of DNA typing tests are commonly used to confirm engraftment.

The rapidity of neutrophil recovery varies with the type of graft: approximate recovery time is two weeks for G-CSF–mobilized peripheral blood grafts, three weeks with marrow grafts, and four weeks with umbilical cord blood (UCB) grafts. Nonmyeloablative allogeneic transplant recipients exhibit substantial heterogeneity in the duration and timing of pancytopenia, with some regimens not exhibiting any significant clinical myelosuppression (Tomblyn et al., 2009). In general, hematopoietic recovery is more rapid following transplantation using peripheral blood stem cells than bone marrow (McAdams & Burgunder, 2013). Although the exact mechanisms are not fully understood, a number of factors most likely contribute. A larger number of progenitor cells are collected peripherally than from marrow. A higher percentage of progenitor cells are committed to a line of differentiation, so less time is needed for these cells to traverse the differentiation compartments. The number of peripheral cells in cycle is greater than the number of cells in cycle that are collected directly from the marrow. It is not completely clear whether this is because of the differences between HSCs collected from the peripheral blood and those harvested directly from the marrow (McAdams & Burgunder, 2013).

The tempo of immune reconstitution following transplant depends on several factors: the rate at which the patient's cells disappear after preparation, the rate of engraftment of new cells, and the survival and longevity of mature lymphocytes present in the graft at the time of transplantation. When stem cells are collected by apheresis, the product typically contains 10 times more T cells than the product of a marrow harvest. This may lead to better engraftment but increases the possibility of developing GVHD (McAdams & Burgunder, 2013).

Four evidence-based principles associated with successful nonmyeloablative stem cell engraftment include a conditioning regimen with sufficient immunomodulation to overcome host immunity not eradicated by the regimen, host and donor hematopoietic cells that are able to coexist, higher stem cell and lymphocyte dose to facilitate engraftment, and dependence on immune reactivity, versus the conditioning regimen, to control residual disease (McAdams & Burgunder, 2013).

Engraftment Syndrome

Engraftment syndrome typically presents with fever and hypoxia that coincide with white blood cell recovery. This can progress to diffuse alveolar hemorrhage. High-dose steroids are used for initial therapy. An increased platelet transfusion parameter may be required for patients with diffuse alveolar hemorrhage. Recombinant factor VIIa or aminocaproic acid may be considered for persistent bleeding (McAdams & Burgunder, 2013).

Stability and Sustainment

The most conventional way to monitor immediate hematopoietic recovery is through granulocyte recovery. Granulocyte recovery is more rapid with blood versus bone marrow autografts, regardless of whether mobilization is achieved with chemotherapy or with hematopoietic growth factors.

In 2012, Bensinger reported updated data on the results of a multicenter randomized trial that compared allogeneic transplantation of bone marrow with matched

HLA-identical, G-CSF–mobilized peripheral stem cells in patients with hematologic cancers. Patients receiving peripheral blood cells experienced faster recovery of neutrophils and platelets and required fewer platelet transfusions than patients receiving bone marrow. Specifically, absolute neutrophil counts exceeded 500/mm³ five days earlier in the peripheral blood cell group than the bone marrow group. Platelet counts exceeded 20,000/mm³ without the need for transfusions six days earlier in the peripheral blood cell group than in the bone marrow group, even though the two groups received a similar number of red cell units. The findings of the trial demonstrated that peripheral blood stem cells are a preferred source for many types of allogeneic transplant for which matched related donors are available. Determining whether the same benefits are true with unrelated donors will require further research (Bensinger, 2012).

Umbilical Cord Blood Transplants

The successful transplantation of unrelated UCB cells from central storage facilities was one of the most exciting developments of the 1990s. Part of the interest in UCB as a stem cell source is that before its widespread collection for cryopreservation and banking, it had no known use and was usually discarded. However, cord blood provides a potentially unlimited source of hematopoietic progenitor cells. These cells appear to possess an immature (and therefore more tolerant) immune component, which allows for a greater degree of mismatch between the donor and recipient (AABB et al., 2018). Two drawbacks of using UCB include delayed engraftment and a relatively low number of cells. As a result, the majority of successful UCB transplants have been in small children (McAdams & Burgunder, 2013). Although engraftment after unrelated UCB transplantation has improved in recent years as a result of better HLA matching, several approaches are being investigated to enhance use of UCB units. These include the use of double (unrelated) units and reduced-intensity conditioning regimens (Petropoulou & Rocha, 2011). Research is also looking into ways of increasing the number of hematopoietic progenitor cells in the laboratory prior to infusion for adult recipients because larger patients require more cells. Improving engraftment and accelerating hematopoietic recovery are crucial for the effective use of UCB transplantation in adult patients.

Patient and Caregiver Education

The site of care during the transplant period influences the required patient and caregiver education. Nurses caring for transplant recipients should be well equipped to answer questions within their scope of practice. Because each transplant center is unique, institution-specific educational materials must be developed. These materials must provide detailed information on the preparative regimen, including the drugs, dose, route, frequency, duration, side effects, and side effect management. The anticipated time of engraftment and monitoring of transplant-related complications should be discussed, with an emphasis on patient and caregiver reporting of symptoms to the transplant team.

Instructions regarding protective precautions recommended during the period of myelosuppression include dietary restrictions, infection prevention, and bleeding precautions. Eligibility criteria for discharge vary according to the site of care, time frame after transplant, and follow-up care required. Because the site of care varies among transplant centers at each phase following transplant, specific criteria must be developed to ensure consistent care. If partial or complete outpatient transplant is performed, medical and nursing care may need to be coordinated through a homecare agency. Patient and family caregiver education may include detailing IV infusions, central venous catheter care, medication administration, and total parenteral nutrition; obtaining, reporting, and documenting vital signs; following oral care regimens; symptom management strategies; obtaining emergency care; and providing transportation to outpatient appointments (Niess, 2013).

Patients usually are discharged from the transplant center to the care of the referring physician one to two months after transplant. Each transplant center may have unique requirements for continued follow-up care that depend on protocols and the type of transplant the patient received. The expected frequency of outpatient visits both at the transplant center and at the referring physician's office should be explained to patients and family members. Some medications and protective precautions may be continued on a long-term basis and should be explained. Successful methods of providing education are individualized patients' and caregivers' education levels, reading levels, attentiveness, and stated preferences (Niess, 2013).

Summary

HSCT is oftentimes used to control or cure primarily malignant conditions. The conditioning regimen administered to patients prior to transplant can vary in drugs used, doses, and schedules based on the patient's disease, type of transplant, goal of therapy, and the patient's overall health. Adverse effects from the conditioning regimen and infusion of the cellular products can vary among patients depending on the regimen and type of product being infused. Care of patients during the post-transplant engraftment phase requires oncology nurses to understand the process and be able to provide support for patients and families during a complex and potentially traumatic time.

The author would like to acknowledge Frances Walker McAdams, RN, MSN, AOCNS®, and Mary Reilly Burgunder, MSN, RN, OCN®, for their contribution to this chapter that remains unchanged from the previous edition of this book.

References

AABB, America's Blood Centers, American Red Cross, American Society for Apheresis, American Society for Blood and Marrow Transplantation, College of American Pathologists, ... World Marrow Donor Association. (2018, October). *Circular of information for the use of cellular therapy products.* Retrieved from http://www.aabb.org/aabbcct/coi/Documents/CT-Circular-of-Information.pdf

Anderson-Reitz, L., & Clancy, C. (2013). Hepatorenal complications. In S.A. Ezzone (Ed.), *Hematopoietic stem cell transplantation: A manual for nursing practice* (2nd ed., pp. 191–200). Pittsburgh, PA: Oncology Nursing Society.

Antin, J.H., & Raley, D.Y. (2013). *Manual of stem cell and bone marrow transplantation* (2nd ed). New York, NY: Cambridge University Press.

Atilla, E., Atilla, P.A., & Demirer, T. (2017). A review of myeloablative vs reduced intensity/non-myeloablative regimens in allogeneic hematopoietic stem cell transplantations. *Balkan Medical Journal, 34,* 1–9. https://doi.org/10.4274/balkanmedj.2017.0055

Bensinger, W.I. (2012). Allogeneic transplantation: Peripheral blood versus bone marrow. *Current Opinion in Oncology, 24,* 191–196. https://doi.org/10.1097/CCO.0b013e32834f5c27

Bhatt, A.S., Freeman, S.S., Herrera, A.F., Pedamallu, C.S., Gevers, D., Duke, F., ... Meyerson, M. (2013). Sequence-based discovery of *Bradyrhizobium enterica* in cord colitis syndrome. *New England Journal of Medicine, 369,* 517–528. https://doi.org/10.1056/NEJMoa1211115

Bodge, M.N., Culos, K.A., Haider, S.N., Thompson, M.S., & Savani, B.N. (2014). Preparative regimen dosing for hematopoietic stem cell transplantation in patients with chronic hepatic impairment: Analysis of the literature and recommendations. *Biology of Blood and Marrow Transplantation, 20,* 622–629. https://doi.org/10.1016/j.bbmt.2014.01.029

Bodge, M.N., Reddy, S., Thompson, M.S., & Savani, B.N. (2014). Preparative regimen dosing for hematopoietic stem cell transplantation in patients with chronic kidney disease: Analysis of the literature and recommendations. *Biology of Blood and Marrow Transplantation, 20,* 908–919. https://doi.org/10.1016/j.bbmt.2014.02.013

Brown, C.G. (Ed.). (2015). *A guide to oncology symptom management* (2nd ed.). Pittsburgh, PA: Oncology Nursing Society.

Bubalo, J.S. (2015). Conditioning regimens. In R.T. Maziarz & S.S. Slater (Eds.), *Blood and marrow transplant handbook: Comprehensive guide for patient care* (2nd ed., pp. 67–80). Basel, Switzerland: Springer International.

Cantoni, N., Weisser, M., Buser, A., Arber, C., Stern, M., Heim, D., ... Gratwohl, A. (2009). Infection prevention strategies in a stem cell transplant unit: Impact of change of care in isolation practice and routine use of high dose intravenous immunoglobulins on infectious complications and transplant related mortality. *European Journal of Haematology, 83,* 130–138. https://doi.org/10.1111/j.1600-0609.2009.01249.x

Carreras, E., Díaz-Beyá, M., Rosiñol, L., Martínez, C., Fernández-Avilés, F., & Rovira, M. (2011). The incidence of veno-occlusive disease following allogeneic hematopoietic stem cell transplantation has diminished and the outcome improved over the last decade. *Biology of Blood and Marrow Transplantation, 17,* 1713–1720. https://doi.org/10.1016/j.bbmt.2011.06.006

Chao, N. (2014). How I treat sinusoidal obstruction syndrome. *Blood, 123,* 4023–4026. https://doi.org/10.1182/blood-2014-03-551630

de Lima, M., Alousi, A., & Giralt, S. (2008). Preparative regimens for hematopoietic cell transplantation. In R. Hoffman, B. Furie, E.J. Benz Jr., P. McGlave, L.E. Silberstein, & S.J. Shattil (Eds.), *Hematology: Basic principles and practice* (5th ed., pp. 1665–1675). Philadelphia, PA: Elsevier Churchill Livingstone.

Eisenberg, S., Wickline, M., Linenberger, M., Gooley, T., & Holmberg, L. (2013). Prevention of dimethylsulfoxide-related nausea and vomiting by prophylactic administration of ondansetron for patients receiving autologous cryopreserved peripheral blood stem cells. *Oncology Nursing Forum, 40,* 285–292. https://doi.org/10.1188/13.ONF.285-292

Erard, V., Guthrie, K.A., Varley, C., Heugel, J., Wald, A., Flowers, M.E.D., ... Boeckh, M. (2007). One-year acyclovir prophylaxis for preventing varicella-zoster virus disease after hematopoietic cell transplantation: No evidence of rebound varicella-zoster virus disease after drug discontinuation. *Blood, 110,* 3071–3077. https://doi.org/10.1182/blood-2007-03-077644

Forman, S.J., & Nakamura, R. (2011). Hematopoietic cell transplantation. In R. Pazdur, L.D. Wagman, K.A. Camphausen, & W.J. Hoskins (Eds.), *Cancer management: A multidisciplinary approach: Medical, surgical, and radiation oncology* [Online ed.]. Retrieved from https://www.cancernetwork.com/cancer-management/hematopoietic-cell-transplantation

Forman, S.J., Negrin, R.S., Antin, J.H., & Appelbaum, F.R. (Eds.). (2016). *Thomas' hematopoietic cell transplantation: Stem cell transplantation* (5th ed.). https://doi.org/10.1002/9781118416426

Girmenia, C., Barosi, G., Piciocchi, A., Arcese, W., Aversa, F., Bacigalupo, A., ... Rambaldi, A. (2014). Primary prophylaxis of invasive fungal diseases in allogeneic stem cell transplantation: Revised recommendations from a consensus process by Gruppo Italiano Trapianto Midollo Osseo (GITMO). *Biology of Blood and Marrow Transplantation, 20,* 1080–1088. https://doi.org/10.1016/j.bbmt.2014.02.018

Gladstone, D.E., Davis-Sproul, J., Campian, J., Lemas, M.V., Malatyali, S., Borrello, I., ... Grossman, S.A. (2014). Infusion of cryopreserved autologous lymphocytes using a standard peripheral i.v. catheter. *Bone Marrow Transplantation, 49,* 1119–1120. https://doi.org/10.1038/bmt.2014.98

Glass, C.A., Perrin, R.M., Pocock, T.M., & Bates, D.O. (2006). Transient osmotic absorption of fluid in microvessels exposed to low concentrations of dimethyl sulfoxide. *Microcirculation, 13,* 29–40. https://doi.org/10.1080/10739680500383464

Gleason, C., & Kaufman, J. (2017). New treatment strategies making an impact in multiple myeloma. *Journal of the Advanced Practitioner in Oncology, 8,* 285–290. Retrieved from https://www.ncbi.nlm.nih.gov/pmc/articles/PMC6003754/pdf/jadp-08-285.pdf

Gobel, B.H. (2018). Disseminated intravascular coagulation. In C.H. Yarbro, D. Wujcik, & B.H. Gobel (Eds.), *Cancer nursing: Principles and practice* (8th ed., pp. 1095–1106). Burlington, MA: Jones & Bartlett Learning.

Gregory, S.J. (2017). Hematopoietic stem cell transplantation. In J. Eggert (Ed.), *Cancer basics* (2nd ed., pp. 323–353). Pittsburgh, PA: Oncology Nursing Society.

Gurman, G., Guloksuz, G.A., Atilla, E., Atilla, P.A., Bozdag, S.C., Yüksel, M.K., ... Beksac, M. (2016). Comparison of reduced intensity conditioning (RIC) regimen and myeloablative conditioning (MAC) regimen in allogeneic hematopoietic stem cell transplantation (allo-HSCT) for adult patients with acute leukemia. *Blood, 128,* 5757. https://doi.org/10.1182/blood.V128.22.5757.5757

Herrera, A.F., Soriano, G., Bellizzi, A.M., Hornick, J.L., Ho, V.T., Ballen, K.K., ... Marty, F.M. (2011). Cord colitis syndrome in cord-blood stem-cell transplantation. *New England Journal of Medicine, 365,* 815–824. https://doi.org/10.1056/NEJMoa1104959

Ishibashi, N., Maebayashi, T., Aizawa, T., Sakaguchi, M., Abe, O., Sakanishi, K., ... Tanaka, Y. (2016). Various regimens of total body irradiation for hematopoietic stem cell transplant. *Experimental and Clinical Transplantation, 14,* 670–675. https://doi.org/10.6002/ect.2016.0014

Iwamoto, R.R., Haas, M.L., & Gosselin, T.K. (Eds.). (2012). *Manual for radiation oncology nursing practice and education* (4th ed.). Pittsburgh, PA: Oncology Nursing Society.

Kaplan, M. (2018). Hypercalcemia of malignancy. In C.H. Yarbro, D. Wujcik, & B.H. Gobel (Eds.), *Cancer nursing: Principles and practice* (7th ed., pp. 1107–1134). Burlington, MA: Jones & Bartlett Learning.

Koniarczyk, H., & Ferraro, C. (2016). Transplant preparative regimens, cellular infusion, acute complications, and engraftment. In B. Faiman (Ed.), *BMTCN® certification review manual* (pp. 37–68). Pittsburgh, PA: Oncology Nursing Society.

Kröger, N., Solano, C., Wolschke, C., Bandini, G., Patriarca, F., Pini, M., ... Bonifazi, F. (2016). Antilymphocyte globulin for prevention of chronic graft-versus-host disease. *New England Journal of Medicine, 374,* 43–53. https://doi.org/10.1056/NEJMoa1506002

Lazarus, H.M., Hamadani, M., & Hari, P.N. (2019). Autologous hematopoietic cell transplantation. In V.T. DeVita Jr., T.S. Lawrence, & S.A. Rosenberg (Eds.), *DeVita, Hellman, and Rosenberg's cancer: Principles and practice of oncology* (11th ed., pp. 2008–2019). Philadelphia, PA: Wolters Kluwer.

Lewis, J.S., II. (2017). Best practices in the management of infectious complications for patients with cancer. *Journal of the Advanced Practitioner in Oncology, 8,* 291–295.

Marlein, C.R., & Rushworth, S.A. (2018). Bone marrow. In *eLS*. https://doi.org/10.1002/9780470015902.a0000505.pub2

Maziarz, R.T., Brazauskas, R., Chen, M., McLeod, A.A., Martino, R., Wingard, J.R., … Riches, M.L. (2017). Pre-existing invasive fungal infection is not a contraindication for allogeneic HSCT for patients with hematologic malignancies: A CIBMTR study. *Bone Marrow Transplantation, 52*, 270–278. https://doi.org/10.1038/bmt.2016.259

McAdams, F.W., & Burgunder, M.R. (2013). Transplant treatment course and acute complications. In S.A. Ezzone (Ed.), *Hematopoietic stem cell transplantation: A manual for nursing practice* (2nd ed., pp. 47–66). Pittsburgh, PA: Oncology Nursing Society.

McBride, A., Trifilio, S., Baxter, N., Gregory, T.K., & Howard, S.C. (2017). Managing tumor lysis syndrome in the era of novel cancer therapies. *Journal of the Advanced Practitioner in Oncology, 8*, 705–720. https://doi.org/10.6004/jadpro.2017.8.7.4

Niess, D. (2013). Basic concepts of transplantation. In S.A. Ezzone (Ed.), *Hematopoietic stem cell transplantation: A manual for nursing practice* (2nd ed., pp. 13–21). Pittsburgh, PA: Oncology Nursing Society.

Olsen, M.M., LeFebvre, K.B., & Brassil, K.J. (Eds.). (2019). *Chemotherapy and immunotherapy guidelines and recommendations for practice.* Pittsburgh, PA: Oncology Nursing Society.

Petropoulou, A.D., & Rocha, V. (2011). Risk factors and options to improve engraftment in unrelated cord blood transplantation. *Stem Cells International, 2011*, 1–8. https://doi.org/10.4061/2011/610514

Potter, P., Eisenberg, S., Cain, K., & Berry, D. (2011). Orange interventions for symptoms associated with dimethyl sulfoxide during stem cell reinfusions: A feasibility study. *Cancer Nursing, 35*, 361–368. https://doi.org/10.1097/NCC.0b013e31820641a5

Provan, D. (2004). The use of intravenous immunoglobulin in hematology and transplantation. In M.C. Dalakas & P.J. Späth (Eds.), *Intravenous immunoglobulins in the third millennium* (pp. 356–360). Boca Raton, FL: Parthenon.

Raanani, P., Gafter-Gvili, A., Paul, M., Ben-Bassat, I., Leibovici, L., & Shpilberg, O. (2008). Immunoglobulin prophylaxis in hematological malignancies and hematopoietic stem cell transplantation. *Cochrane Database of Systematic Reviews, 2008*(4). https://doi.org/10.1002/14651858.CD006501.pub2

Rasche, L., Kapp, M., Einsele, H., & Mielke, S. (2014). EBV-induced post-transplant lymphoproliferative disorders: A persisting challenge in allogeneic hematopoietic SCT. *Bone Marrow Transplantation, 49*, 163–167. https://doi.org/10.1038/bmt.2013.96

Riddell, S.R., & Warren, E.H. (2019). Allogeneic stem cell transplantation. In V.T. DeVita Jr., T.S. Lawrence, & S.A. Rosenberg (Eds.), *DeVita, Hellman, and Rosenberg's cancer: Principles and practice of oncology* (11th ed.). Philadelphia, PA: Wolters Kluwer.

Runckel, D.N., & Swanson, J.R. (1980). Effect of dimethyl sulfoxide on serum osmolality. *Clinical Chemistry, 26*, 1745–1747.

Smith, T.J., Bohlke, K., Lyman, G.H., Carson, K.R., Crawford, J., Cross, S.J., … Armitage, J.O. (2015). Recommendations for the use of WBC growth factors: American Society of Clinical Oncology clinical practice guideline update. *Journal of Clinical Oncology, 33*, 3199–3212. https://doi.org/10.1200/JCO.2015.62.3488

Solomon, S.R., Solh, M., Morris, L.E., Holland, H.K., & Bashey, A.(2016). Myeloablative conditioning with PBSC grafts for T-cell-replete haploidentical donor transplantation using posttransplant cyclophosphamide. *Advances in Hematology, 2016*, 9736564. https://doi.org/10.1155/2016/9736564

Sorror, M.L., Martin, P.J., Storb, R.F., Bhatia, S., Maziarz, R.T., Pulsipher, M.A., … Gooley, T.A. (2014). Pretransplant comorbidities predict severity of acute graft-versus-host disease and subsequent mortality. *Blood, 124*, 287–295. https://doi.org/10.1182/blood-2014-01-550566

Spinks, R. (2016). Pretransplant issues. In B. Faiman (Ed.), *BMTCN® certification review manual* (pp. 15–36). Pittsburgh, PA: Oncology Nursing Society.

Stephens, J.M.L. (2013). Cardiopulmonary complications. In S.A. Ezzone (Ed.), *Hematopoietic stem cell transplantation: A manual for nursing practice* (2nd ed., pp. 201–230). Pittsburgh, PA: Oncology Nursing Society.

Storb, R., Gyurkocza, B., Storer, B.E., Sorror, M.L., Blume, K., Niederwieser, D., … Sandmaier, B.M. (2013). Graft-versus-host disease and graft-versus-tumor effects after allogeneic hematopoietic cell transplantation. *Journal of Clinical Oncology, 31*, 1530–1538. https://doi.org/10.1200/JCO.2012.45.0247

Taplitz, R.A., Kennedy, E.B., Bow, E.J., Crews, J., Gleason, C., Hawley, D.K., … Flowers, C.R. (2018). Outpatient management of fever and neutropenia in adults treated for malignancy: American Society of Clinical Oncology and Infectious Diseases Society of America clinical practice guidelines update. *Journal of Clinical Oncology, 36*, 1443–1453. https://doi.org/10.1200/JCO.2017.77.6211

Tomblyn, M., Chiller, T., Einsele, H., Gress, R., Sepkowitz, K., Storek, J., … Boeckh, M.J. (2009). Guidelines for preventing infectious complications among hematopoietic cell transplantation recipients: A global perspective. *Biology of Blood and Marrow Transplantation, 15*, 1143–1238. https://doi.org/10.1016/j.bbmt.2009.06.019

Wilson, F.P., & Berns, J.S. (2014). Tumor lysis syndrome: New challenges and recent advances. *Advances in Chronic Kidney Disease, 21*, 18–26. https://doi.org/10.1053/j.ackd.2013.07.001

CHAPTER 7

Acute and Chronic Graft-Versus-Host Disease

Sandra A. Mitchell, PhD, CRNP, AOCN®, and Pamela D. Paplham, DNP, AOCNP®, FNP-BC, FAANP

Introduction

Early human transplants of allogeneic marrow were often complicated by graft-versus-host disease (GVHD), which remains one of the most serious transplant-related complications. GVHD adversely affects the overall success of allogeneic hematopoietic stem cell transplantation (HSCT) (Bhatia et al., 2007). As the treatment of infections and procedure-related complications has improved, GVHD has emerged as the main factor limiting wider application of allogeneic HSCT. Despite advances in prophylaxis, GVHD is estimated to occur in up to 40% of sibling transplant recipients and 80% of unrelated transplant recipients (Harris et al., 2016). The incidence of acute GVHD varies with respect to several clinical variables.

Strategies to reduce the risk of developing GVHD include use of a histocompatible hematopoietic stem cell donor, T-cell depletion of the stem cell product, and post-transplant immunosuppression and immunomodulation. Although GVHD can be a major cause of morbidity and mortality in allogeneic HSCT and may significantly affect the quality of life of long-term survivors, strategies aimed at eliminating GVHD also can have devastating side effects, resulting in an increased incidence of disease relapse, fatal infections, and graft failure. The goal of ongoing and future research is to design immunomodulatory and graft engineering approaches that achieve rapid and durable engraftment and limit the development of severe GVHD while preserving a graft-versus-tumor effect (Blazar, MacDonald, & Hill, 2018; Zeiser, 2018; Zeiser, Socié, & Blazar, 2016).

Definitions

GVHD occurs when immunologically competent donor-derived T lymphocytes (the graft) recognize the antigens and cells in the transplant recipient (or host) as foreign and mount an immunologic attack. The attack of these donor-derived T lymphocytes causes damage of varying degrees of severity to recipient tissues (disease). Thus, the term *graft-versus-host disease* is used to describe the result of this immunologic assault.

As first proposed by Rupert E. Billingham almost 60 years ago, three conditions are required for the development of GVHD (Vriesendorp & Heidt, 2016). First, the graft must contain a sufficient number of immunologically competent cells. Second, the recipient must possess tissue antigens that are not present in the donor so that the recipient appears foreign to the graft. Third, the recipient must be incapable of mounting an effective immunologic response to destroy the transplanted cells.

Historically, a clear distinction was drawn between an early acute form of GVHD and a delayed chronic form of GVHD, with the distinction based predominantly on the time of onset after transplant (less than or more than 100 days, respectively) (Vriesendorp & Heidt, 2016). However, more recent observations in patients receiving cord blood transplants, reduced-intensity conditioning regimens, and post-transplant donor lymphocyte infusions (DLIs) have confirmed that acute GVHD can occur several months after transplant and that the classic characteristics of chronic GVHD can occur as early as two months after transplant (Jagasia et al., 2015). The current consensus is that the clinical manifestations must determine whether the GVHD is acute, chronic, or an overlap syndrome (wherein diagnostic or distinctive features of acute and chronic disease occur together), not the temporal relationship to transplant (S.J. Lee, 2017).

Clinical features, and in some circumstances the histopathologic features, can distinguish acute from chronic GVHD regardless of the time frame in which they develop: *acute GVHD* is used to describe a distinctive syndrome affecting the liver, skin, gastrointestinal tract, and immune system that typically occurs within 100 days of allogeneic HSCT, whereas *chronic GVHD* describes a syndrome that is variable in its manifestations, involving multiple organ systems (Jagasia et al., 2015). It can include abnormalities of the skin, conjunctiva, oral mucosa, lung, gastrointestinal tract, liver, genitalia, and muscles/fascia, as well as cytopenias and immunodeficiency (Flowers & Martin, 2015). At least one distinctive manifestation (e.g., oral or vaginal lichenoid findings, cutaneous sclerosis, ocular sicca, bronchiolitis obliterans) is required for a diagnosis of chronic GVHD. Biopsy and other diagnostic tests (e.g., pulmonary function studies, laboratory studies) are recommended to confirm the diagnosis (S.J. Lee, 2017) and exclude other possible complications such as infection, drug toxicities, recurrent malignancy, or residual postinflammatory scarring (Flowers & Martin, 2015).

Since the criteria for GVHD were first identified (Vries-endorp & Heidt, 2016), they have been revised to incorporate the current understanding that a syndrome analogous to GVHD can also occur with autologous and syngeneic HSCT (Hammami et al., 2018; Latif et al., 2003), or following the transfusion of nonirradiated blood products in immunocompetent individuals (Kopolovic et al., 2015).

Acute Graft-Versus-Host Disease

Pathogenesis

Much has been learned about the pathogenesis of acute GVHD. This improved understanding has expanded research into therapies for prevention and treatment while preserving the beneficial antitumor aspects (Zeiser & Blazar, 2017).

GVHD occurs when T lymphocytes contained in an allogeneic hematopoietic stem cell graft proliferate and differentiate in vivo in response to antigens present on host tissue recognized by the graft as foreign. Directly, and through the secretion of inflammatory cytokines (Cooke et al., 2017), these donor T lymphocytes attack host tissues and produce the signs and symptoms of acute GVHD. The pathogenesis is multifaceted and thought to occur in three sequential phases involving both complex cellular interactions and inflammatory cascades (Kuba & Raida, 2018; see Figure 7-1).

The first phase involves tissue damage secondary to the conditioning regimen, which causes the release of pro-inflammatory cytokines and imbalances in the intestinal microbiota. The second phase consists of donor T-cell activation, proliferation, differentiation, and migration. In the third phase, donor T cells produce, either directly or indirectly, damage to tissues within the target organs. Common sites include the skin, liver, gastrointestinal tract, and hematopoietic system. Emerging evidence suggests GVHD-related immune dysregulation further disrupts the intestinal epithelium, specifically intestinal stem cells, Paneth cells, and goblet cells, producing a vicious circle exacerbating inflammation and bacterial translocation (Naymagon et al., 2017; Shono & van den Brink, 2018). This three-phase model allows understanding of the pathways that can be targeted to prevent or treat the disease (Zeiser, 2018).

Phase One: Host Tissue Damage and Antigen Presentation

The first phase in GVHD development is initiated even before donor cells are infused. The transplant conditioning regimen of chemotherapy and radiation therapy damages and activates host tissues, including the intestinal mucosa, liver, and skin. In response to this tissue damage and the resultant bacterial translocation, inflammatory cytokines are secreted, including tumor necrosis factor-alpha (TNF-α), interleukin (IL)-1, IL-12, transforming growth factor-beta, and others (Qayed & Horan, 2016). These cytokines cause the damaged tissues to attract and retain white blood cells.

They also upregulate major histocompatibility complex and minor histocompatibility antigens present on host tissues. This upregulation makes it easier for the mature donor T cells contained in the stem cell graft to recognize the host's tissues as foreign and mount an inflammatory response (Zeiser & Blazar, 2017).

Phase Two: Donor T-Cell Activation and Cytokine Production

In the second phase, the donor T lymphocytes contained in the stem cell graft recognize recipient or host tissues as foreign and mount a series of responses. These responses include recruitment of donor and residual host antigen-presenting cells, activation and stimulation of T lymphocytes, and proliferation and differentiation of these activated T cells (Zeiser et al., 2016).

The stem cell transplant graft contains both pluripotent stem cells, which are necessary to establish engraftment, and mature T lymphocytes. The donor-derived mature T lymphocytes circulate in the recipient's bloodstream, coming into extensive contact with many minor antigens expressed on the surface of the recipient's cells.

Even in related transplants in which the major histocompatibility complex antigens are matched, the donor T cells will recognize one or more of the recipient's minor antigens as foreign and will bind to the antigen. Subsequently, costimulatory signals direct a subset of T lymphocytes (helper T or Th-1 lymphocytes) to begin producing several proinflammatory cytokines, including TNF-α, IL-2, and interferon gamma (IFN-γ), and increase expression of receptors for these cytokines on the surface of the T cell. These cytokines recruit cytotoxic T lymphocytes and natural killer (NK) cell responses and stimulate both donor and residual host monocytes to produce IL-1 and TNF-α. The activated T cells expand and differentiate over three to five days following antigen recognition, producing the specific cytokines that result in the recruitment of cytotoxic T lymphocytes and NK cells to enact the cell and tissue destruction in target organs that is postulated to occur in the final phase of the GVHD process (Ghimire et al., 2017).

Phase Three: Destruction of Target Tissues

The tissue destruction and end-organ dysfunction that produce the signs and symptoms of GVHD are hypothesized to result from several additive and synergistic mechanisms. First, direct cytolytic damage occurs in the target organs of the skin, gut, and liver caused by cytotoxic T lymphocytes that are recruited by the Th-1 cytokines (IL-2 and IFN-γ) released by the lymphocytes in phase two. The Th-1 lymphocytes stimulate cytotoxic T lymphocytes and NK cells to increase secretion of inflammatory cytokines, including TNF-α and IL-1. TNF-α plays an important role in the pathophysiology of acute GVHD, and studies have demonstrated elevated levels in the serum of patients with acute GVHD (Zeiser & Blazar, 2017). TNF-α can cause direct tissue damage by inducing necrosis of target cells, or it may

Figure 7-1. Pathophysiology of Graft-Versus-Host Disease

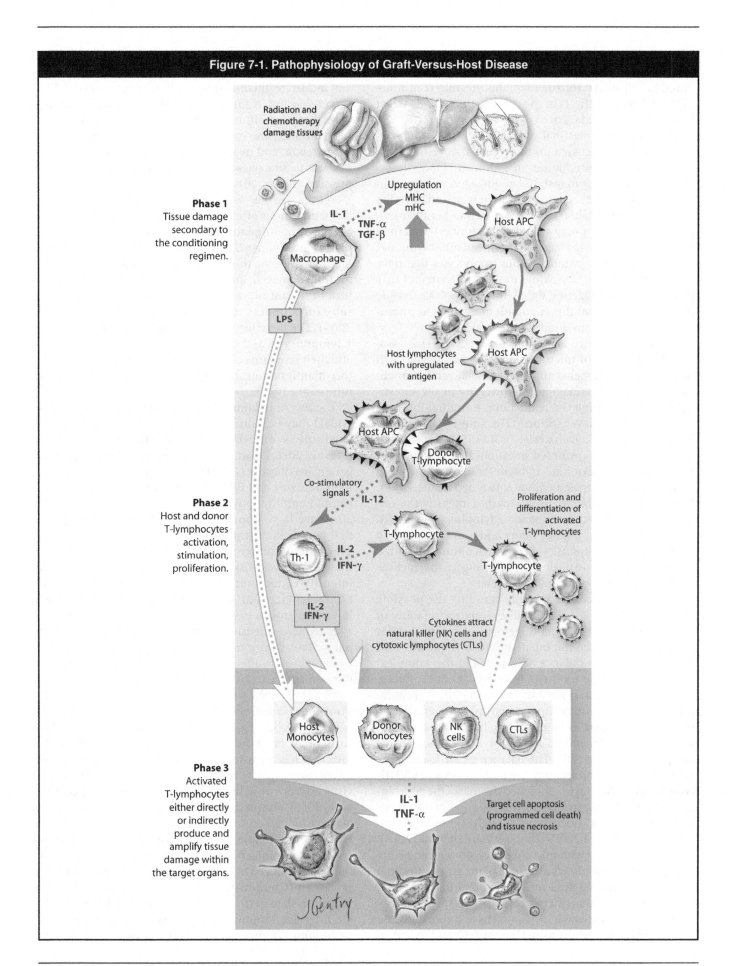

Phase 1
Tissue damage secondary to the conditioning regimen.

Radiation and chemotherapy damage tissues

Upregulation MHC mHC

IL-1

TNF-α
TGF-β

Host APC

Macrophage

LPS

Host lymphocytes with upregulated antigen

Host APC

Phase 2
Host and donor T-lymphocytes activation, stimulation, proliferation.

Host APC

Donor T-lymphocyte

Co-stimulatory signals
IL-12

Th-1

IL-2
IFN-γ

T-lymphocyte

Proliferation and differentiation of activated T-lymphocytes

T-lymphocyte

IL-2
IFN-γ

Cytokines attract natural killer (NK) cells and cytotoxic lymphocytes (CTLs)

Host Monocytes

Donor Monocytes

NK cells

CTLs

Phase 3
Activated T-lymphocytes either directly or indirectly produce and amplify tissue damage within the target organs.

IL-1
TNF-α

Target cell apoptosis (programmed cell death) and tissue necrosis

JGentry

induce tissue destruction through apoptosis. In addition to these proinflammatory cytokines, excess nitric oxide produced by activated cytotoxic T lymphocytes may contribute to the deleterious effects of the cytokines on GVHD target tissues (Kuba & Raida, 2018).

The damage to intestinal cells caused by the conditioning regimen, as discussed for phase one, may result in the release of lipopolysaccharide, an endotoxin. Lipopolysaccharide subsequently may stimulate gut-associated lymphocytes and macrophages to increase their secretion of TNF-α and IL-1 (Kuba & Raida, 2018). Lipopolysaccharide reaching skin tissues also may stimulate keratinocytes, dermal fibroblasts, and macrophages to produce similar cytokines in the dermis and epidermis. Thus, monocytes that have been primed by Th-1 cytokines to secrete TNF-α and IL-1 receive a second triggering signal from lipopolysaccharide to increase secretion; this is a result of damage to intestinal cells caused by the conditioning regimen.

Emerging evidence also indicates that GVHD is associated with a loss of microbial diversity and overgrowth of intestinal pathogens, and that these adverse changes cause synergistic damage to the integrity of the intestinal barrier, including the epithelium, intestinal immune cells, and mucus layer (Shono, Docampo, Peled, Perobelli, & Jenq, 2015; Zama et al., 2017). Translocation of bacteria across the disrupted intestinal barrier reinforces GVHD-associated cytokine and cellular inflammatory signaling (Staffas, Burgos da Silva, & van den Brink, 2017). In phase three, inflammatory cytokines intensify the cellular damage caused by cytotoxic T lymphocytes and NK cells, amplifying local tissue injury and further promoting an inflammatory response—all of which ultimately lead to the observed target tissue destruction to organs that include the liver, skin, and gastrointestinal tract.

Recent developments in understanding the possible role for regulatory T cells, Toll-like receptors (a family of proteins that recognize pathogen-associated molecular patterns and activate the innate immune response), and Th-1/Th-2 cytokine balance have added further complexity to the three-step model (Ghimire et al., 2017; Zeiser, 2018; Zeiser & Blazar, 2017; Zeiser et al., 2016). Regulatory T cells function to suppress both innate and adaptive immune responses by producing inhibitory cytokines and by contact-dependent inhibition and cytotoxicity of antigen-presenting cells. The balance of Th-1 and Th-2 cytokines is also important in the pathogenesis of GVHD. Numerous studies have highlighted the role of the gastrointestinal microbiome in shaping the responses of the mucosal immune system associated with GVHD (Kumari, Palaniyandi, & Hildebrandt, 2018; Shono & van den Brink, 2018). GVHD is associated with microbial diversity loss, and early use of systemic antibiotics after transplant, gastrointestinal infection (including viral infections), and the decreased oral dietary intake that often occurs post-transplant all contribute to the overgrowth of pathogens and other adverse changes in microbial diversity (Ferrara & Chaudhry, 2018;

Shono & van den Brink, 2018). As new data emerge and the understanding of the inhibitory pathways that regulate and moderate inflammation evolves, approaches to GVHD prevention and treatment will increasingly emphasize therapies that promote tolerance, amplify regulatory immunologic mechanisms, mitigate target tissue damage, enhance tissue repair, and modulate the intestinal microbiome, in contrast to strategies that cause nonspecific immunosuppression (Zeiser, 2018).

Ferrara, Levine, Reddy, and Holler (2009) summarized the pathogenesis of acute GVHD as an exaggerated and dysregulated manifestation of a normal physiologic inflammatory mechanism. When donor cells are transplanted into the recipient, they encounter a host that has been profoundly damaged, and they react in a fashion that would foster the control or resolution of an invasion of foreign substances under ordinary circumstances (Ferrara et al., 2009). The net effects of this complex interaction among T lymphocytes and other inflammatory cells, cytokines, and their resultant cellular targets are the severe inflammatory manifestations recognized clinically as GVHD (Ghimire et al., 2017).

The role of inflammatory cytokines and chemokines in GVHD may explain several unique and seemingly unrelated aspects of the disease (Toubai, Mathewson, Magenau, & Reddy, 2016; Zeiser, 2018). For example, the principal target organs of acute GVHD all share an extensive exposure to endotoxins and other bacterial products that can trigger and amplify local inflammation. These target organs also have large populations of antigen-presenting cells that may facilitate the graft-versus-host reaction (Ghimire et al., 2017). Furthermore, a number of studies have noted that an increased risk of GVHD is associated with certain intensive conditioning regimens and with viral infection (Zeiser & Blazar, 2017). The reduction in acute GVHD seen in certain groups of patients undergoing transplantation after reduced-intensity conditioning regimens or in laminar airflow environments with gut decontamination may be explained by the reduction of bacterial endotoxins in the skin and gut.

Viral infections are commonly associated with GVHD. Viral infections not only are more frequent in patients with GVHD, but also may cause the initiation of GVHD or worsening of established disease. Cytomegalovirus (CMV) infection has a particularly close and potentially bidirectional association with GVHD, as does the herpes simplex virus and possibly human herpesvirus 6 (Tong & Worswick, 2015). The precise pathophysiology of the association between viral infection and acute GVHD remains uncertain. It may be that cellular damage to the intestines or liver as a result of these infections causes a release of endotoxins, or that virus-induced activated T cells or NK cells attack target tissues (Ghimire et al., 2017). It also may be that viral infections flare in the setting of GVHD as a result of either the intensified immunosuppressive therapy or the intrinsic immunosuppression of GVHD (Szyska & Na, 2016).

An understanding of the roles postulated for donor T lymphocytes; IL-1, IL-2, TNF-α, and Th-1/Th-2 cytokine balance; and cytokine, chemokine, and intracellular signaling pathways, together with greater appreciation of the potential role played by the microbiome, points to numerous targets that might be therapeutically exploited for prevention or to attain better disease control (Hill et al., 2018; Magenau & Reddy, 2014).

A wide array of immunomodulatory approaches have been designed, are undergoing clinical trials, or are in development (Im, Hakim, & Pavletic, 2017; MacDonald, Betts, & Couriel, 2017; Teshima, Reddy, & Zeiser, 2016; Zeiser, 2018). For example, corticosteroids interfere with antigen processing and presentation and induce apoptosis of activated lymphocytes. Monoclonal antibodies have been developed that target activated T lymphocytes with overexpression of TNF-α receptor (infliximab) or IL-2 receptors (daclizumab). T-cell depletion strategies attempt to remove T lymphocytes from the stem cell product prior to transplantation or to remove T lymphocytes from the circulation through the use of a monoclonal antibody that destroys lymphocytes. Cyclosporine A and tacrolimus are potent inhibitors of early phases of T-cell activation, and antimetabolites, such as mycophenolate mofetil, interfere with T-lymphocyte proliferation. These and other approaches are discussed in more detail later in this chapter.

Incidence and Predictive Factors

Even with intensive immunosuppression, clinically significant acute GVHD, defined as grades 2–4, occurs in approximately 40% of patients who receive an human leukocyte antigen (HLA)-identical sibling HSCT, and the incidence in unrelated HLA-matched HSCT is approximately 50% (Jamil & Mineishi, 2015). The development of grade 3–4 acute GVHD significantly affects the outcome of HSCT, with only 40%–50% of patients experiencing long-term survival (El-Jawahri et al., 2016).

Factors associated with a greater incidence and severity of GVHD include donor–recipient incompatibilities in HLA and minor HLA peptides, use of more than 1,200 cGy of total body irradiation in the conditioning regimen, early engraftment, viral serology in the donor or recipient (higher risk when the recipient is CMV or Epstein-Barr virus seropositive; higher risk when the donor is herpes simplex virus or CMV seropositive or Epstein-Barr virus seronegative), older donor age, parous donors, and male recipients of grafts from female donors (Nassereddine, Rafei, Elbahesh, & Tabbara, 2017; Petersdorf, 2017; Socié & Ritz, 2014). The effects of graft source (i.e., peripheral blood stem cells vs. bone marrow) on outcomes, including the incidence of GVHD, remain a topic of intense debate (Amouzegar, Dey, & Spitzer, 2019). Although studies suggest that the use of peripheral blood stem cells is associated with more rapid engraftment and possibly a lower risk of disease relapse, recent evidence suggests it is also associated with a higher incidence of both acute and chronic

GVHD (Byrne, Savani, Mohty, & Nagler, 2016; Holtick et al., 2014). One theory is that less GVHD is associated with reduced-intensity conditioning because these regimens produce less-extensive tissue injury and less GVHD in a state of mixed chimerism, in which both donor and patient immune systems "coexist" (Nakamura & Forman, 2014). Reduced-intensity conditioning regimens may be associated with a reduced incidence of acute GVHD (Abdul Wahid et al., 2014). However, data also indicate that a high degree of donor T-cell chimerism in the early post-transplant period may be associated with an increased risk of GVHD (Mahr, Granofszky, Muckenhuber, & Wekerle, 2018). The factors associated with a higher risk of acute GVHD are summarized in Table 7-1. Many of the risk factors are characteristics of the donor–recipient pair and not amenable to modification, particularly if only one HLA-matched donor is available.

Clinical and Histopathologic Features

The onset of acute GVHD generally occurs 14–60 days after transplant. However, if methotrexate is not used for GVHD prophylaxis, the onset may be as early as the first week after stem cell infusion (Nassereddine et al., 2017). Neutrophil recovery is not necessary for GVHD to occur, and the signs of GVHD may be noted prior to hematopoietic engraftment. In the setting of reduced-intensity conditioning regimens, acute GVHD can occur several months after transplant, and it commonly occurs after DLI for the prevention or treatment of disease relapse after transplant. The median time to onset of GVHD is approximately one month after DLI (Chang, Zang, & Xia, 2016). With few exceptions, the manifestations of acute GVHD following DLI are generally comparable to post-transplant GVHD (Scarisbrick et al., 2015). Signs and symptoms of acute GVHD also can develop after withdrawal of immunosuppression.

The classic target organs of acute GVHD are the skin, intestinal tract, and liver. Any one organ or combination of these organs may be affected. Involvement of each organ system is assessed clinically and pathologically, and staging is generally summarized in the form of an overall grade, as discussed later in this chapter.

Cutaneous

An erythematous maculopapular skin rash, usually occurring at or near the time of white blood cell engraftment, is the first and most common clinical manifestation of acute GVHD. The exanthema may be red to violaceous in color. Early stages of the rash may be pruritic or painful and may be described as a sunburn. Classically, the first areas involved include the nape of the neck, ears, and shoulders, as well as the palms of the hands and soles of the feet. The rash may spread, becoming more confluent and involving the whole integument. In severe GVHD, the maculopapular rash can evolve into generalized erythroderma and bullous lesions, often progressing to desquamation and epi-

Table 7-1. Risk Factors Influencing Incidence and Severity of Acute Graft-Versus-Host Disease

Factor	Lower Risk and/or Lesser Severity	Higher Risk and/or Greater Severity
Degree of donor–recipient histocompatibility	Human leukocyte antigen (HLA)-identical related donors	HLA-matched unrelated donor HLA-mismatched related donors (haploidentical, 1 or 2 antigen mismatches), with increasing degrees of histoincompatibility associated with more graft-versus-host disease (GVHD)
Type of pretransplant conditioning regimen	Reduced-intensity conditioning regimens associated with a lower incidence or severity of GVHD	Regimens that include intense, myeloablative conditioning chemotherapy and total body irradiation > 1,200 cGy associated with more GVHD
Source of stem cells	Bone marrow Umbilical cord blood	Peripheral blood
CD34+ count and T-cell dose in the graft	–	Studies are inconclusive, but higher CD34+ count and higher T-cell dose in the stem cell graft possibly associated with more acute GVHD
Cellular composition of the graft	T cell depleted	Unmanipulated T cell repleted
Intensity of GVHD prophylaxis used	Broader prophylaxis with 1 or more agents at full doses Tacrolimus possibly more effective than cyclosporine A for prevention of acute GVHD	Prophylaxis with single-agent or reduced-dose/attenuated course of prophylaxis (e.g., reduced dose of cyclosporine A or tacrolimus, omission of 1 or more post-transplant methotrexate doses) associated with increased GVHD
Cytokine gene polymorphisms	–	Numerous polymorphisms in recipient or donor associated with acute GVHD
ABO group	–	ABO mismatch
Donor–recipient sex match	Male to male Male to female	Female to male
Donor viral serologies	–	Donor cytomegalovirus seropositivity
Donor parity	Nulliparous female	Parous female
Donor transfusion status	Donor never received blood transfusions	Donor previously transfused
Age of recipient/donor	Younger	Older
Host microenvironment	Protective environment, including skin and gut decontamination	No special protective environment; no skin and gut decontamination
History of prior splenectomy	–	Possibly increased GVHD risk with splenectomy before transplantation

Note. Based on information from Jagasia et al., 2012; S.-E. Lee et al., 2013; Zeiser & Blazar, 2017.

dermal necrolysis (Strong Rodrigues, Oliveira-Ribeiro, de Abreu Fiuza Gomes, & Knobler, 2018; see Figure 7-2).

Differential diagnoses of a post-transplant skin rash include chemotherapy and radiation effects, drug allergy, and viral infection. Careful history and physical examination, consultation with dermatology, and skin biopsy are helpful in establishing the diagnosis. Biopsy of the skin rash will reveal classic dermal and epidermal changes, including exocytosed lymphocytes, dyskeratotic epidermal keratinocytes, follicular involvement, satellite lymphocytes adjacent to or surrounding dyskeratotic epidermal keratinocytes, and dermal perivascular lymphocytic infiltration (Strong Rodrigues

et al., 2018). However, histopathologic confirmation may be limited because similar changes can be seen within the first few months after chemotherapy or radiation therapy and may occur with infection (Strong Rodrigues et al., 2018). Serial biopsies and careful observation of the rash features help to establish the diagnosis and severity of GVHD. Viral studies for CMV and human herpesvirus 6 may help to differentiate GVHD from a viral exanthem.

Gastrointestinal

The second most affected organ system in acute GVHD is the gut, and it often is the most severe. Symptoms of acute

Figure 7-2. Acute Graft-Versus-Host Disease of the Skin

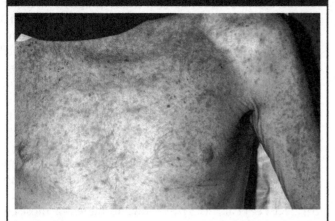

Photograph depicts fine, discrete, and confluent erythematous, as well as blanchable macules and papules involving the upper trunk. Lesions may be pruritic or slightly tender with palpation. Earliest skin findings usually are seen on the face, palms and soles, and upper trunk.

Note. Image courtesy of Steven Pavletic. Used with permission.

GVHD of the distal small bowel and colon include profuse watery diarrhea, intestinal bleeding, crampy abdominal pain, distension, and paralytic ileus. The diarrhea often is green, mucoid, watery, and mixed with exfoliated cells and tissue shreds.

Paralytic ileus may develop in association with GVHD or the increased use of narcotics and antimotility agents to control abdominal pain and diarrhea. Voluminous secretory diarrhea may persist even with cessation of oral intake and can exceed 10 L per day (McDonald, 2016). The diarrhea initially may be watery but often becomes progressively bloody, with increasing transfusion requirements. Hypoalbuminemia, at times severe, can occur secondary to GVHD-associated intestinal protein leak and negative nitrogen balance. Patients also may present with upper gastrointestinal symptoms, including nausea, vomiting, anorexia, food intolerance, and dyspepsia (Naymagon et al., 2017).

GVHD of the gut should be considered among the differential diagnoses when an HSCT recipient experiences abdominal pain, nausea, vomiting, diarrhea, or hyperbilirubinemia (Sung et al., 2018). Other possible etiologies for these symptoms include residual effects of chemotherapy and radiation therapy, and intestinal infection, primarily CMV, *Candida* species, or *Clostridium difficile* in the lower gastrointestinal tract and CMV, *Candida* species, or herpes simplex virus in the upper gastrointestinal tract (McDonald, 2016; Naymagon et al., 2017). Other etiologies of diarrhea can include malabsorption, lactose intolerance, or exocrine pancreatic insufficiency (Robak, Zambonelli, Bilinski, & Basak, 2017). Lower or upper endoscopy or both may be required to evaluate symptoms and to exclude other diag-

noses, such as gastroesophageal ulceration. Enteric cultures are needed to rule out infection.

Endoscopic findings suggestive of GVHD include mucosal erythema, edema, and mucosal sloughing involving the cecum, ileum, ascending colon, stomach, duodenum, and rectum (Naymagon et al., 2017; see Figure 7-3). Whole areas may be denuded, similar to the loss of epithelium observed in the skin (Naymagon et al., 2017). Histopathologic confirmation of enteric GVHD includes crypt cell (the epithelial cells lining the tubular invaginations of the small intestine) apoptosis, degeneration, and loss; accumulation of cellular debris within crypts; variable lymphocytic infiltration of the epithelium; and, in severe cases, total epithelial denudation (Ferrara & Chaudhry, 2018).

Figure 7-3. Acute Graft-Versus-Host Disease of the Gastrointestinal Tract

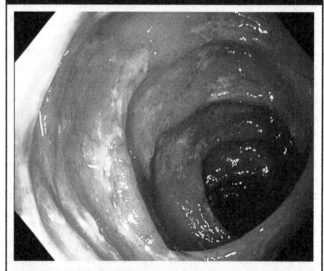

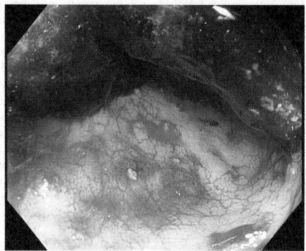

Photographs depict endoscopic findings in acute graft-versus-host disease of the gastrointestinal tract. Mucosal tissues show edema, friability, exudates, areas of necrosis, erythematous lesions, and loss of normal vascularity.

Note. Images courtesy of Kevin Robillard. Used with permission.

Imaging of the bowel with computed tomography scanning typically reveals diffuse mucosal enhancement and fluid-filled dilated bowel loops (Lubner et al., 2017). Bowel wall thickening may be patchy, diffuse, or absent in acute GVHD but more focal and prominent in chronic GVHD. Strictures or webbing may occur in the esophagus, small bowel, or colon, with associated luminal narrowing (Lubner et al., 2017). High-resolution ultrasonography and color Doppler imaging may be useful tools in following patients' therapeutic response to immunosuppressive therapy (Nishida et al., 2015).

Hepatic

Hepatic involvement with GVHD occurs in less than 20% of cases (McDonald, 2016) and can be challenging to diagnose because of nonspecific clinical signs and symptoms and the overlap of histopathologic features with other conditions commonly seen following transplantation (Matsukuma, Wei, Sun, Ramsamooj, & Chen, 2016). The earliest and most common abnormalities include a rise in direct bilirubin, alkaline phosphatase two or more times the upper limits of normal, and elevations in aminotransferases, reflecting a nonspecific cholestatic picture (Matsukuma et al., 2016). Patients may have jaundice; skin and diarrhea may have preceded the onset of liver function abnormalities (Matsukuma et al., 2016). Differential diagnoses include hepatic sinusoidal obstruction syndrome, the effects of the preparatory regimen, total parenteral nutrition, viral infection, gram-negative sepsis, biliary obstruction, and toxicity to drugs, including cyclosporine A, tacrolimus, and methotrexate, which are used for GVHD prophylaxis (McDonald, 2016).

Hepatotoxicity caused by tacrolimus or cyclosporine A usually improves within several days of modifying the dose. Transvenous liver biopsy may be performed, revealing bile duct atypia and degeneration, cholestasis, lymphocytic infiltration of portal tracts, degeneration and destruction of small bile ducts, periportal fibrosis, and hepatocyte degeneration (Salomao, Dorritie, Mapara, & Sepulveda, 2016). A hepatitic variant of GVHD of the liver, characterized by markedly elevated transaminases and histologic evidence of lobular hepatitis, has been described following DLI (Matsukuma et al., 2016). A third presentation of liver GVHD, characterized by slow progressive increases in alkaline phosphatase and gamma-glutamyl transpeptidase levels with subsequent development of jaundice, has also been described (Matsukuma et al., 2016).

Other Manifestations

Although the issue of whether acute GVHD involves other organs has remained controversial, subtle effects on hematopoiesis and immune functioning co-occur with acute GVHD. These include hypogammaglobulinemia; decline in white blood cell count, hematocrit level, and platelet count; and increased risk of infection, especially CMV (Szyska & Na, 2016). Other findings include photophobia, hemorrhagic conjunctivitis, scleritis, infectious and noninfectious pneumonia, and serositis (Seber, Khan, & Kersey, 1996; Tung, 2017).

Although rare in the setting of GVHD prophylaxis, hyperacute GVHD is a severe fulminant form of acute GVHD that is frequently fatal. It develops 7–14 days after transplantation with manifestations including fever, generalized erythroderma, desquamation, severe hepatitis, noncardiogenic pulmonary edema, and vascular leakage (Saliba et al., 2007). Hyperacute GVHD may be difficult to distinguish from preengraftment syndrome (Y.-H. Lee & Rah, 2016).

Diagnosis, Classification, and Severity Grading

The National Institutes of Health has developed standardized terminologies and criteria to aid in the diagnosis and classification of GVHD (Jagasia et al., 2015; S.J. Lee, 2017; S.J. Lee et al., 2015). As shown in Table 7-2, those criteria recognize two diagnostic categories of GVHD. The first is acute GVHD without any features consistent with chronic GVHD, subdivided into (a) classic acute GVHD (occurring before day +100) and (b) persistent, recurrent, or late acute GVHD (occurring after day +100, often in association with immunosuppression tapering or DLI) (Jagasia et al., 2015). The second is chronic GVHD, subdivided into (a) classic chronic GVHD (manifested by diagnostic clinical features of chronic GVHD occurring any time after transplantation) and (b) an overlap syndrome in which features of both acute and chronic GVHD are present (Jagasia et al., 2015). Thus, for example, a patient with secretory diarrhea along with classic features of chronic GVHD, such as ocular sicca and esophageal webbing or liver function abnormalities, would be classified as having overlap syndrome, and a patient who develops erythematous maculopapular dermatitis after DLI would be classified as having late acute GVHD.

The severity of acute GVHD is determined both histologically and clinically. The Glucksberg staging and grading criteria assign a stage reflecting the degree of skin, liver, and gut involvement, and the resultant stages are summarized in the form of an overall grade (see Table 7-2). Approximating the daily amount of diarrhea, identifying the level of hyperbilirubinemia, and distinguishing maculopapular rashes from erythroderma with bullous formation are the factors considered in determining the stage and grade of GVHD (Harris et al., 2016; Schoemans, Lee, et al., 2018).

As illustrated in Figure 7-4, the Rule of Nines is used to estimate the extent of skin involvement. Clinically significant acute GVHD usually is defined as overall grades 2–4. Although the hematopoietic and immune systems may also be target organs for acute GVHD manifestations, they are not included in the grading schemas.

Several problems have been identified with the reproducibility and validity of the staging and grading system for acute GVHD. Some limitations include a failure to consider the kinetics of GVHD (e.g., subclinical disease); the interobserver variability in assigning a stage or grade; the requirement that patients with different patterns of skin, liver, and gut involvement (who also have significantly

Table 7-2. Updated Glucksberg Criteria for Clinical Staging and Grading of Acute Graft-Versus-Host Disease

Extent of Organ Involvement

Stage	Skin	Liver	Gut
1	Rash on < 25% of skin[a]	Bilirubin 2–3 mg/dl[b]	Diarrhea > 500 ml/day[c] or persistent nausea[d]
2	Rash on 25%–50% of skin	Bilirubin 3–6 mg/dl	Diarrhea > 1,000 ml/day
3	Rash on > 50% of skin	Bilirubin 6–15 mg/dl	Diarrhea > 1,500 ml/day
4	Generalized erythroderma with bullous formation involving ≥ 5% of body surface area	Bilirubin > 15 mg/dl	Diarrhea > 2,000 ml/day, severe abdominal pain with or without ileus, or grossly bloody stools (regardless of stool volume)

Grade[e]

	Skin	Liver	Gut
I	Stages 1–2	–	–
II	Stage 3 or	Stage 1 or	Stage 1
III	–	Stages 2–3 or	Stages 2–3
IV[f]	Stage 4	Stage 4	Stage 4

[a] Use "Rule of Nines" or burn chart to determine extent of rash.
[b] Range given as total bilirubin. Downgrade one stage if an additional cause of elevated bilirubin has been documented.
[c] Volume of diarrhea applies to adults. For pediatric patients, the volume of diarrhea should be based on body surface area. Downgrade one stage if an additional cause of diarrhea has been documented.
[d] Persistent nausea with histologic evidence of graft-versus-host disease exist in the stomach or duodenum.
[e] Criteria for grading is given as a minimum degree of organ involvement required to confer that grade.
[f] Grade IV may also include lesser organ involvement with an extreme decrease in performance status.

Note. Based on information from Schoemans, Lee, et al., 2018.

From "1994 Consensus Conference on Acute GVHD Grading," by D. Przepiorka, D. Weisdorf, P. Martin, H.-G. Klingemann, P. Beatty, J. Hows, and E.D. Thomas, 1995, *Bone Marrow Transplantation, 15,* p. 826. Copyright 1995 by Nature Publishing Group. Adapted with permission.

different risks of treatment-related mortality and treatment failure) may be assigned the same summary grade; and the fact that additional target organs, such as the conjunctivae and immune system, are not addressed (Goyal, Goyal, & Sankaranarayan, 2015). Work is ongoing to evaluate current systems for grading and staging and develop consensus definitions and digital tools to improve grading and staging (Harris et al., 2016; Levine et al., 2014) and to advance valid and reliable endpoints for risk prediction (Caulier et al., 2018; MacMillan et al., 2015) and therapeutic response (Inamoto, Martin, et al., 2014; Sengsayadeth et al., 2014).

Efforts also are underway to identify and validate serum biomarkers that can estimate individual risk, identify sub-clinical acute GVHD before the onset of symptoms such as diarrhea, confirm the diagnosis, and help guide treatment decision making (He & Holtan, 2018; Major-Monfried et al., 2018). Several categories of biomarkers are being studied for use prior to transplant in the early transplant period or at the onset of acute GVHD symptoms, including microRNAs, proteins, cellular subsets, gene polymorphisms, and markers of gut barrier physiology (He & Holtan, 2018; Rashidi et al., 2018; Rashidi & Weisdorf, 2017). Clinical trials testing novel therapeutic approaches as either preemptive or primary treatment of acute GVHD in high-risk patients, as well as deintensified GVHD therapies (including early tapering) that avoid some of the toxicities of steroid-based immunosuppression, are ongoing (Ferrara & Chaudhry, 2018).

Chronic Graft-Versus-Host Disease

Chronic GVHD remains the most common late complication of allogeneic HSCT. Although significant improvements have been achieved in the prevention and treatment of acute GVHD, these advancements have not substantially reduced the incidence of chronic GVHD. Depending on stem cell source (peripheral blood stem cells vs. bone marrow vs. umbilical cord blood), the degree of donor matching (matched sibling vs. haploidentical related donor vs. unrelated donor), and the diagnostic criteria used, studies estimate that the incidence of chronic GVHD is 20%–60% (Ferrara & Chaudhry, 2018; Socié & Ritz, 2014). Factors influencing the rising rates of chronic GVHD include the increased use of peripheral blood stem cells, decreased early transplant-related mortality, transplantation in older recipients, and use of DLI after transplantation (Afram et al., 2018; Amouzegar et al., 2019; Scarisbrick et al., 2015).

Pathogenesis

Although less is known about the pathogenesis of chronic GVHD, the hypothesis is that it includes all the mechanisms outlined previously for acute GVHD plus self-reactive and alloreactive mechanisms. These mechanisms include thymic dysfunction, regulatory T-cell deficiencies, autoantibody production by B cells, and a variety of cytokines and chemokines (including IL-17, B-cell activating factor, and others) that are involved in the humoral immune response, B-cell activation, and upregulation of helper T-17 cells, resulting in an inflammatory response and formation of fibrotic lesions (Fisher et al., 2017; Presland, 2017).

In chronic GVHD, the T lymphocytes come to recognize as foreign not only the minor histocompatibility antigens (those antigens that are not able to be matched between recipient and donor) but also the major histocompatibility antigens (those antigens that generally are completely matched between recipient and donor) (Cooke et al., 2017). The development of these self-reactive or autoreactive T cells is thought to be related to impaired thymus functioning (Alho et al., 2016).

Figure 7-4. Rule of Nines

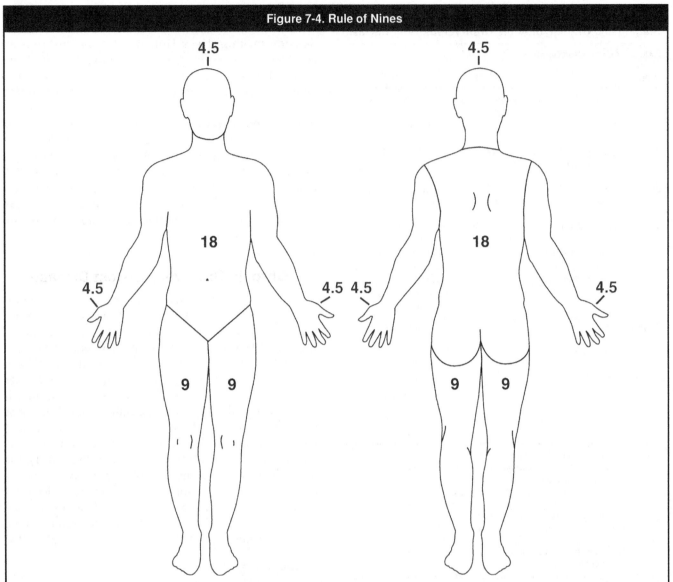

The Rule of Nines body surface area diagram is used to estimate the percentage of body surface involved with graft-versus-host disease of the skin.

When the thymus is functioning normally, it can eliminate autoreactive T lymphocytes before they can mount a response against the host. However, when the thymus is damaged, whether by age, injury from the chemotherapy and radiation therapy used in the conditioning regimen, or acute GVHD, its ability to delete these autoreactive T cells may be impaired. This can result in circulating T lymphocytes programmed to recognize the host as foreign and stimulate the cytokine cascade similar to that described for acute GVHD (Im et al., 2017; Li, Gao, Feng, & Zhang, 2019). Thymic damage also permits the maturation of autoreactive donor B lymphocytes that produce autoantibodies, such as antinuclear antibody, similar to those noted in other chronic autoimmune disorders. Research has indicated that the balance of T and B lymphocyte subsets, as well as T- and B-cell receptor

signaling, is important for the development and maintenance of immune tolerance and in the inflammatory response, tissue destruction, and fibrosis that occurs in chronic GVHD (Cutler, Koreth, & Ritz, 2017).

Incidence and Predictive Factors

Chronic GVHD occurs in up to 85% of patients who survive beyond day +100 after stem cell transplantation, depending on stem cell source, degree of HLA matching, the use of DLI (Scarisbrick et al., 2015), and potentially the use of post-transplant chimeric antigen receptor T-cell therapy (M. Smith, Zakrzewski, James, & Sadelain, 2018) to treat minimal residual disease or disease relapse. Risk factors for chronic GVHD include reduced-intensity conditioning, previous acute GVHD, older recipient age, and female donor to male recipient (Afram et al., 2018). The incidence of chronic GVHD also is thought to be higher in recipients of peripheral blood stem cells versus recipients of bone marrow stem cells (Holtick et al., 2014).

Clinical and Histopathologic Features

Clinical manifestations of chronic GVHD resemble those of progressive systemic sclerosis, systemic lupus erythematosus, lichen planus, Sjögren syndrome, and rheumatoid arthritis. Manifestations are seen in the skin, liver, eyes, oral cavity, lungs, gastrointestinal system, neuromuscular system, and a variety of other body systems.

Cutaneous

The skin is the most involved organ in chronic GVHD. Two types of cutaneous involvement have been described: sclerodermatous (similar to scleroderma) and lichenoid (similar to lichen planus) (Strong Rodrigues et al., 2018). The onset of skin involvement may be generalized erythema with plaques and extensive areas of desquamation. Without treatment, this can progress to skin that is hyper- or hypopigmented with tightening (hide-like skin), atrophy, and telangiectasias. Joint contractures similar to scleroderma can occur as a result. Skin involvement can occur anywhere and does not show the typical distribution of acute GVHD. Localized chronic GVHD of the skin demonstrates nodular induration and dyspigmentation, whereas the generalized type frequently exhibits severe poikiloderma (atrophy of the skin with associated pigmentation changes, erythema, and telangiectasias) with diffuse areas of hypo- and hyperpigmentation and, if progressive, contractures, alopecia, damage to or loss of nails, and skin ulcerations (Strong Rodrigues et al., 2018; see Figures 7-5 through 7-8). Skin damaged from acute GVHD, sun exposure, or herpes zoster infection may be more susceptible to chronic GVHD.

Although the diagnosis of cutaneous chronic GVHD is based mostly on clinical features, skin biopsy may be helpful in excluding other causes of rash and establishing the diagnosis (Kavand, Lehman, Hashmi, Gibson, & El-Azhary, 2017), particularly in cases of atypical presentation (Cornejo, Kim, Rosenbach, & Micheletti, 2015). Histomorphologically, in early-phase chronic GVHD, the features are similar to those seen with acute GVHD. With increasing deposition of collagen, the changes acquire a scleroderma-like appearance with thickening and homogenization of collagen bundles (Filipovich et al., 2005). The overlying epidermis becomes diffusely atrophic, and the rete ridges disappear (Villarreal, Alanis, Perez, & Candiani, 2016). Atrophy and fibrosis of adnexal structures also develops. In contrast to acute GVHD, involvement of the eccrine glands is a characteristic of chronic GVHD (Shulman et al., 2015).

Gastrointestinal

The esophagus, small bowel, and colon may demonstrate involvement in chronic GVHD. Diarrhea, abdominal pain, and cramping may be present, but the more common manifestations are wasting syndrome with malabsorption, weight loss, poor performance status, and increasing gastrointestinal symptoms, such as dysphagia and early satiety, suggestive of GVHD progression (Akpek et al., 2003; Kida & McDonald, 2012). Esophageal involvement with chronic GVHD results in dysphagia, odynophagia, and retrosternal pain from mucosal desquamation and peptic esophagitis with resultant fibrosis, esophageal webs, and stricture (Lubner et al., 2017). Endoscopy may reveal diffuse muco-

Figure 7-5. Lichen Sclerosus–Like Chronic Graft-Versus-Host Disease

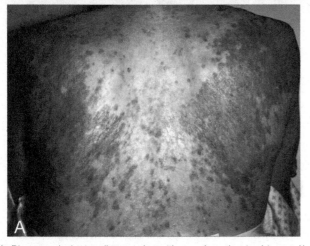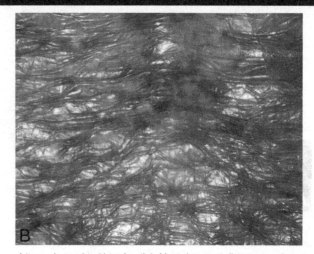

A: Photograph depicts flat papules with a surface that is shiny and/or lacy white and atrophic (thin, fragile). Note the postinflammatory hyperpigmentation that has developed in some areas.
B: Photograph depicts "cigarette-paper" wrinkling.

Note. Images courtesy of Edward Cowen. Used with permission.

sal sloughing, with histologic examination demonstrating fibrosis and significant crypt distortion, or features more characteristic of acute GVHD of the intestine with apoptosis—with or without cryptitis (Naymagon et al., 2017; Salomao et al., 2016). Pancreatic insufficiency may accompany

or complicate chronic GVHD of the gastrointestinal tract or liver (Kida & McDonald, 2012).

Hepatic

As discussed previously, hepatic involvement with GVHD is recognized as having two forms after day +100. The first form reflects persistent, recurrent, or late-onset acute GVHD of the liver. The features of recurrent or late-onset acute GVHD of the liver are identical to those of classic acute GVHD of the liver, and no accompanying clinical features of chronic GVHD are present (e.g., ocular manifestations, sclerotic skin changes). Recurrent or late-onset acute GVHD of the liver often occurs in association with DLI, steroid taper, or withdrawal of immunosuppression. The second classification is overlap GVHD in which specific clinical findings diagnostic of chronic GVHD (e.g., ocular manifestations, oral ulcerations, obstructive pulmonary changes) are present, together with hepatic features of acute GVHD. Typically, liver function tests reveal predominantly cholestatic abnormalities with moderate elevations in alkaline phosphatase, bilirubin, and transaminases. Clinically, patients typically have few symptoms referable to their liver, such as jaundice, until their hepatic disease becomes severe. The differential diagnosis of late hepatic abnormalities is broad and includes viral infection, hepatotoxic drug reactions, gallstones, and fungal infection (McDonald, 2016).

Liver biopsies are helpful in establishing the diagnosis, although they carry the risk of complications such as bleeding (Matsukuma et al., 2016). Pathology demonstrates a marked reduction or complete absence of small bile ducts, cholestasis, and a dense plasmacytic infiltration in por-

Figure 7-6. Lichen Planus–Like Chronic Graft-Versus-Host Disease

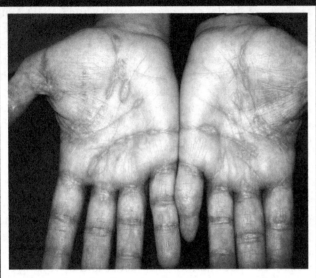

Photograph depicts hyperpigmented/violaceous purple papules, which may coalesce into annular (ring-like) small plaques. These lesions closely resemble the dermatologic disease lichen planus.

Note. Image courtesy of Edward Cowen. Used with permission.

Figure 7-7. Features Associated With Cutaneous Graft-Versus-Host Disease

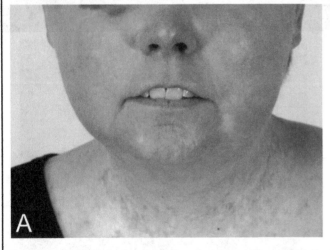 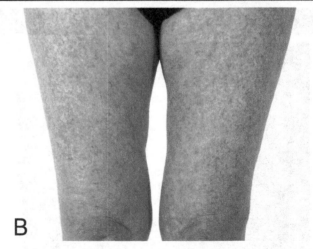

A: Photograph depicts sclerotic skin manifestations in the supraclavicular region, with a thickened, shiny, tight appearance to the skin, and prominence of the small blood vessels visible just beneath the skin surface. Note the thinning of the lips and slight effacement of the oral aperture, as well as cushingoid facial features.
B: Photograph depicts poikiloderma—the classic features of patchy hypopigmentation and hyperpigmentation, dermal atrophy, and telangiectasias (small-diameter linear blood vessels seen on the skin's surface).

Note. Images courtesy of Edward Cowen. Used with permission.

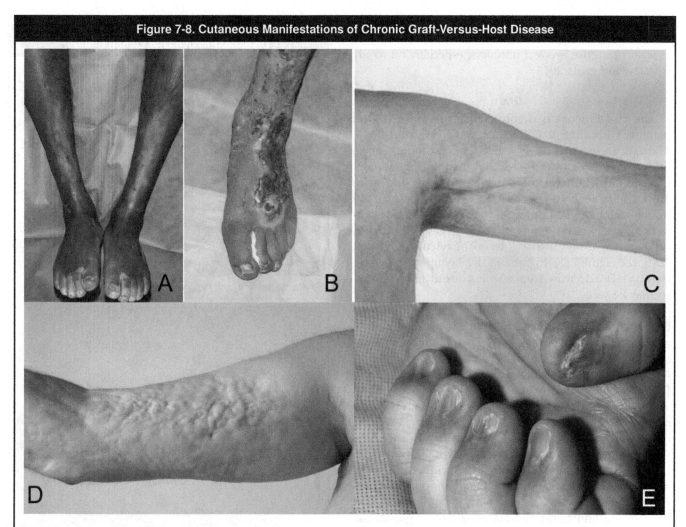

Sclerotic manifestations include skin that is shiny and tight (hidebound) (A), skin ulcerations (B), rippling/grooving (groove sign) (C), or dimpling, cellulite-like appearance (D). Also seen here are the nail changes (onychodystrophy) typical of chronic graft-versus-host disease (E). These may include splitting, nail fragility and roughness, longitudinal striations/ridging, periungual erythema and edema, and onycholysis (separation of the nail plate starting at the distal free margin and progressing proximally).

Note. Images courtesy of Edward Cowen. Used with permission.

tal areas (Salomao et al., 2016). Differential diagnosis of GVHD of the liver from viral infections such as CMV and hepatitis is important because immunosuppressive therapy following an erroneous diagnosis of chronic GVHD is likely to alleviate the clinical manifestations of both processes and mask an underlying viral hepatitis infection or reactivation (Matsukuma et al., 2016). Histopathologic features such as cytologically atypical, damaged, or destroyed bile ducts and portal inflammation favor the diagnosis of chronic GVHD (Salomao et al., 2016), whereas mononuclear cell infiltration of portal tracts and sinusoids and spotty hepatocellular necrosis suggest viral infection (Matsukuma et al., 2016).

Ocular

Ocular involvement occurs in approximately 50%–80% of patients with chronic GVHD and produces significant effects on quality of life (Munir & Aylward, 2017). Ophthalmic symptoms of keratoconjunctivitis sicca include burning, irritation, photophobia, excessive tearing (an early manifestation), mucoid secretion, decreased visual acuity, foreign body sensation, and pain (Nassiri et al., 2013). Tear function is evaluated by Schirmer testing and fluorescein biomicroscopy of the cornea. Findings typically noted in patients with chronic GVHD of the eye include lacrimal deficiency manifested as a Schirmer tear test showing less than 5 mm of wetting, hyperemic sclerae and conjunctivae, and blepharitis (erythema of the eyelids with edema) (Munir & Aylward, 2017). Slit-lamp biomicroscopy may reveal pseudomembranous conjunctivitis that can progress to corneal slough, sterile corneal ulcers, and nonhealing epithelial defects of the cornea (Inamoto et al., 2019). Even in the absence of symptoms, for at least five years after transplant, patients should be screened annually for ocular sicca and started on artificial tear replacement if indicated (Inamoto et al., 2019). Patients should be advised to wear protective eyewear outdoors, especially on windy days (Nassiri et al., 2013).

Oral

The oral mucosa is involved in more than 80% of patients with chronic GVHD (Mawardi, Hashmi, Elad, Aljurf, & Treister, 2019). Patients develop dryness, sensitivity to acidic or spicy foods, and increasing oral pain. Lichenoid reactions range from fine, white, lace-like striae on buccal surfaces to large plaques on the buccal surface or the lateral tongue (Mawardi et al., 2018). Mucosal surfaces may become atrophic with resultant gingival and buccal stippling (Mays, Fassil, Edwards, Pavletic, & Bassim, 2013; see Figure 7-9). In patients displaying sclerodermatous GVHD, a decreased oral opening due to perioral fibrosis may be seen.

Patients with chronic GVHD often report oral pain (either continuous or occurring with the stimulation of eating or performing oral hygiene), which may be one of the first symptoms associated with the onset of chronic GVHD of the oral cavity or may herald a flare-up of disease (Margaix-Muñoz, Bágan, Jiménez, Sarrión, & Poveda-Roda, 2015). Xerostomia is associated with chronic GVHD, and studies of patients more than one year after HSCT have demonstrated that chronic GVHD adversely influences salivary flow rates (Mays et al., 2013). However, in the first four to six months after HSCT, it may be difficult to differentiate GVHD-related oral dryness from radiation-induced salivary gland dysfunction. Xerostomia is uncomfortable, may interfere with nutrition, and places patients at greater risk for dental caries. Patients with GVHD involving the oral cavity benefit from regular, thorough evaluation of the oral mucosa and close follow-up because they are at greater risk for dental caries and second malignancies involving the oral mucosa (Inamoto et al., 2015). Fluoride treatments may be beneficial in patients at increased risk for dental caries because of xerostomia (Mawardi et al., 2019).

Sinopulmonary

Obstructive lung disease, called bronchiolitis obliterans, is a clinical feature of chronic GVHD. In bronchiolitis obliterans, progressive obstruction of small bronchioles occurs because of proliferation of the peribronchiolar tissue. This can progress to pulmonary fibrosis that often is related to cofactors such as the long-term pulmonary toxicity of total body irradiation or chemotherapy, or interstitial fibrosis resulting from viral infection (Grønning-saeter et al., 2017). Bronchodilator-resistant decrements may be noted prior to the onset of symptoms. Decreased diffusing capacity of the lung for carbon monoxide and forced expiratory volume in one second less than 75% of predicted, in combination with an increased residual volume greater than 120% and ratio of forced expiratory volume in one second/forced vital capacity less than 0.70 on

Figure 7-9. Manifestations of Oral Graft-Versus-Host Disease: Erosive Oral Lichen Planus

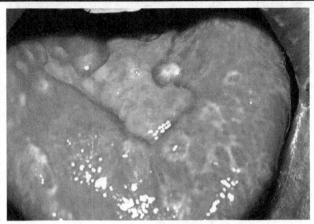

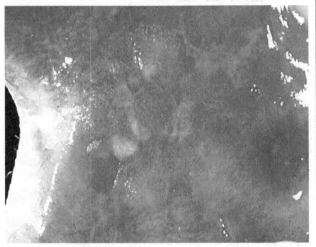

Erythema, edema, and hyperkeratotic plaques

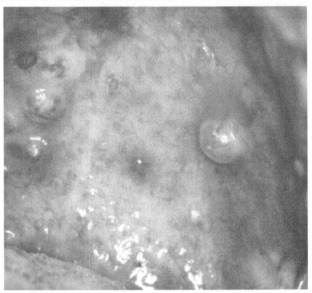

Lichenoid lesions and shallow ulcerations

Mucoceles (inflamed salivary glands)

Note. Images courtesy of Steven Pavletic. Used with permission.

pulmonary function tests, suggests the obstructive pattern typical of bronchiolitis obliterans (Hakim et al., 2018). High-resolution computed tomography of the chest with inspiratory and expiratory sequences showing air trapping, bronchiectasis, or small airway thickening also may be used to confirm the diagnosis (Grønningsaeter et al., 2017). Accompanying symptoms may include dry cough, dyspnea, and wheezing. Because of the high prevalence of sinusitis in patients with GVHD who are on immunosuppression, radiographic assessment of the paranasal sinuses is recommended (Hakim et al., 2018). Video-assisted thoracoscopic lung biopsy is required to make a definitive histologic diagnosis. Lung biopsies show small airway involvement with fibrinous obliteration of the lumen. Peribronchiolar inflammatory cellular infiltrates consisting of neutrophils and lymphocytes also may be present (Grønningsaeter et al., 2017). In patients with mild airway obstruction, consideration should be given to treatment with montelukast and low-dose azithromycin (Grønningsaeter et al., 2017; Hakim et al., 2018). First-line treatment of moderate to severe bronchiolitis obliterans syndrome consists of systemic steroids, either alone or in combination with other systemic immunosuppressive or immunomodulatory approaches, including rituximab, extracorporeal photopheresis (ECP), or sirolimus. Emerging treatments currently being tested in clinical trials include bortezomib, etanercept, imatinib, ofatumumab, and ruxolitinib (Grønningsaeter et al., 2017).

Musculoskeletal

Myositis, fasciitis, and myopathy have been described in patients with chronic GVHD (Ganta, Chatterjee, Pohlman, & Hojjati, 2015; Meng, Ji, Wang, & Bu, 2018; New-Tolley et al., 2018). Patients with GVHD frequently report muscle cramps, although the exact etiology of these cramps remains unclear. Patients may develop limited range of motion of joints secondary to involvement of the deeper fascia or because of thickening or sclerosis of the skin (Inamoto, Pidala, et al., 2014; Vukiç et al., 2016). The involvement of the deeper fascia can be appreciated on magnetic resonance imaging (Oda et al., 2009).

Immunosuppressive therapy with corticosteroids plus a calcineurin inhibitor is often not fully effective in the treatment of fasciitis. Other options include rituximab, low-dose methotrexate, imatinib, and ECP (Marks et al., 2011). Physical therapy for stretching, strengthening, thermal modalities, lymphatic drainage, and joint mobilization is essential to manage limb edema, prevent contractures, and maintain functional performance (Mohammed et al., 2019).

Neurologic

Neurologic conditions have been reported in patients with chronic GVHD, including peripheral neuropathy (Bilic et al., 2016), myasthenia gravis, and immune-mediated sensory-motor neuropathies or encephalitis (Grauer et al., 2010). Nerve conduction studies, nerve biopsy, and autoantibody studies may help in diagnosing these complications. Neuropathy is frequently associated with the treatment of GVHD with immunosuppressive or immunomodulating agents, including thalidomide analogs and occasionally tacrolimus or cyclosporine A (Anghel et al., 2013). Patients with chronic GVHD are also at risk for opportunistic infections of the central nervous system, such as toxoplasmosis.

Hematopoietic

The hematopoietic system is increasingly recognized as a GVHD target organ, resulting in cytopenias, immunodeficiencies, and immune dysregulation (Szyska & Na, 2016). Suppression of peripheral blood counts is a common occurrence in patients with chronic GVHD, and sometimes eosinophilia is seen (Cromvik, Johnsson, Vaht, Johansson, & Wenneras, 2014). It is not clear whether these hematopoietic and immunologic abnormalities are a direct result of chronic GVHD or if they represent a specific autoimmune manifestation.

Autoimmune Manifestations

Nearly all known autoimmune syndromes have been reported as part of chronic GVHD. Aspects of GVHD may mimic autoimmune hemolytic anemia, eosinophilic fasciitis, idiopathic thrombocytopenic purpura, lichen planus, myasthenia gravis, polymyositis, progressive systemic sclerosis, rheumatoid arthritis, scleroderma, sicca syndrome, Sjögren syndrome, and systemic lupus erythematosus (Holbro, Abinun, & Daikeler, 2012). In patients with chronic GVHD, autoantibodies such as antinuclear antibody can be detected similarly to those found in connective tissue diseases, and some evidence supports that antibodies perpetuate chronic GVHD and promote fibrogenesis (Li et al., 2019).

Effects on Immunologic Reconstitution

Multiple deficiencies in immune system reconstitution and functioning are observed in patients with chronic GVHD (Ogonek et al., 2016). Thymic injury, impaired mucosal defense, chemotactic defects, functional asplenia, T-cell alloreactivity, and qualitative and quantitative B-cell abnormalities contribute to prolonged immunodeficiency, immune dysregulation, and susceptibility to infection in patients with chronic GVHD (Li et al., 2019; Szyska & Na, 2016).

Other Findings

Vaginal sicca, stenosis, and stricture and the formation of vaginal synechiae have been noted in women with chronic GVHD (Hamilton, Goje, Savani, Majhail, & Stratton, 2017). Lichenoid nail changes (Palencia, Rodríguez-Peralto, Castaño, Vanaclocha, & Iglesias, 2002) and recurrent sterile effusions, including polyserositis and pericardial effusion (Leonard et al., 2015), also are reported manifestations of chronic GVHD.

Diagnosis, Classification, and Severity Grading

Chronic GVHD may occur as an extension of acute GVHD (progressive chronic GVHD), after resolution of acute GVHD (quiescent onset), or without preceding acute GVHD (de novo onset). Although progressive chronic GVHD is the most common pattern of onset, the increasing use of DLIs and reduced-intensity conditioning regimens has increased the incidence of quiescent and de novo onset chronic GVHD (Nakamura & Forman, 2014; Scarisbrick et al., 2015).

Patients with chronic GVHD can be classified based on the organs involved and the severity of involvement as mild, moderate, or severe (Jagasia et al., 2015). Criteria developed by the National Institutes of Health grade chronic GVHD based on the number of organs involved and the severity of involvement (S.J. Lee, 2017). Each organ is scored on a 0–3 scale, from no involvement or symptoms (0) to severe involvement or functional compromise (3). Patients also may be classified according to their primary clinical and histologic pattern as having lichenoid or sclerodermatous disease. These three models for categorizing patients with chronic GVHD are summarized in Table 7-3. Similar to testing for acute GVHD, biopsies of the skin, oral cavity, and sometimes liver may be used in the differential diagnosis.

The spectrum, character, and timing of onset of abnormalities in chronic GVHD may be affected by newer treatment approaches, including nonmyeloablative conditioning (Nakamura & Forman, 2014), use of DLI (Scarisbrick et al., 2015), and new regimens for the prevention and treatment of acute GVHD. Table 7-4 summarizes the clinical features, screening and evaluation tests, and interventions recommended for patients with chronic GVHD.

Preventing and Treating Acute and Chronic Graft-Versus-Host Disease

Advances in the development of medications and other therapies to prevent and treat GVHD have played a key role in improving the outcomes of allogeneic transplantation. Knowledge of the optimal combinations and sequencing of GVHD therapies is continuing to evolve (Cutler et al., 2017; Flowers & Martin, 2015; Hill et al., 2018). With the availability of biomarkers of subclinical disease and potentially disease response, a more precise, risk-adapted approach to the treatment of acute and chronic GVHD is on the horizon (Holtan & MacMillan, 2016; Martínez-Laperche et al., 2018; Rashidi et al., 2018; Rashidi & Weisdorf, 2017). The wide range of therapeutic options available to prevent and treat acute and chronic GVHD is presented in Figure 7-10.

These therapies and modalities are used in different combinations and sequences with the goal of either preventing or treating GVHD. Selection of the optimal therapy is as much an art as it is an evolving science, as there is a fine balance between too much or too little immunosuppression, and treatment with immunosuppression can be complicated by significant side effects, including diabetes, hypertension, myopathy, osteoporosis, and avascu-

Table 7-3. Models for Classifying Graft-Versus-Host Disease

Model	Classification	Features
Pattern of onset	De novo	No antecedent acute GVHD
	Quiescent	Onset after complete resolution of acute GVHD
	Progressive	Direct evolution from acute GVHD
National Institutes of Health disease severity (determined by the number of organs affected and the severity of involvement)	Mild	1 or 2 organ systems (excluding lung) affected; mild manifestations with no effect on organ function
	Moderate	More than 2 organ systems (with or without mild lung manifestations); mild impairment of organ function
	Severe	More than 2 organ systems involved, or moderate or severe lung manifestations, with disease manifestations causing significant impairment in organ function
National Institutes of Health classification system	Classic acute GVHD	Onset occurs < 100 days after HSCT. Manifestations include rash, nausea, vomiting, anorexia, diarrhea, ileus, or cholestatic hepatitis.
	Persistent, recurrent, late-onset acute GVHD	Features of acute GVHD persist, recur, or present > 100 days after HSCT; features of classic acute GVHD occur without diagnostic and distinctive features of chronic GVHD.
	Classic chronic GVHD	Diagnostic or distinctive manifestations of chronic GVHD present any time after HSCT; at least 1 diagnostic or distinctive manifestation of chronic GVHD occurs without features of acute GVHD. Diagnostic and distinctive features of chronic GVHD include poikiloderma, lichen planus–like changes, sclerotic changes, morphea, fasciitis, joint contractures secondary to cutaneous sclerosis, hyperkeratotic plaques involving the oral mucosa, and restriction of mouth opening from circumoral sclerosis. Additional diagnostic and distinctive features include lichen planus lesions involving the genitalia, vaginal scarring or stenosis, esophageal webbing and strictures, and obstructive changes on pulmonary function studies.
	Overlap	Features of acute GVHD and diagnostic/distinctive manifestations of chronic GVHD occur together.

GVHD—graft-versus-host disease; HSCT—hematopoietic stem cell transplantation

Note. Based on information from Jagasia et al., 2015; S.J. Lee, 2017.

Table 7-4. Chronic Graft-Versus-Host Disease: Clinical Manifestations, Screening and Evaluation, and Interventions

System	Clinical Manifestations	Screening/Evaluation	Interventions
Dermal	Dyspigmentation, xerosis (dryness), erythema, hyperkeratosis, pruritus, scleroderma, lichenification, onychodystrophy (nail ridging/nail loss), alopecia, second malignancies	Clinical examination, skin biopsy—3 mm punch biopsy from forearm and posterior iliac crest areas	Consider immunosuppressive therapy. Perform PUVA or extracorporeal photopheresis. Apply topical tacrolimus ointment (Prograf® ointment). Apply topical steroid creams, moisturizers/emollients, and antibacterial ointments to prevent superinfection; aggressively lubricate the skin. If sweat glands are affected, avoid overheating because heat prostration and heat stroke can occur. Avoid sunlight exposure; use sunblock lotion and a large hat that shades the face when outdoors.
Oral	Lichen planus, xerostomia, ulceration, second malignancies	Oral biopsy from inner lower lip	Use steroid mouth rinses, topical clobetasol ointment, effervescent budesonide, tacrolimus or cyclosporine A ointments/topical preparations, oral PUVA, pilocarpine and anethole trithione for xerostomia, and fluoride gels/rinses to decrease caries. Pay careful attention to oral hygiene, perform regular dental evaluations, and screen oral cavity for squamous cell carcinoma of the oral cavity and monitor for development of bisphosphonate-related osteonecrosis of the jaw in at-risk individuals.
Ocular	Keratitis, sicca syndrome; increased risk for cataracts secondary to protracted use of post-transplant steroids	Schirmer test, ophthalmic evaluation	Perform regular ophthalmologic follow-up. Use preservative-free tears and moisturizing ophthalmic ointments. Consider temporary or permanent lacrimal duct occlusion. Consider trial of topical anti-inflammatory agents, including topical corticosteroids, cyclosporine A, or tacrolimus ophthalmic emulsion, or a trial of autologous serum eye drops or scleral lenses.
Hepatic	Jaundice, abdominal pain	Liver function tests—ALT and AST, alkaline phosphatase, bilirubin	Consider bile acid displacement therapy with ursodeoxycholic acid (Actigall®) 300 mg PO TID.
Pulmonary	Obstructive/restrictive pulmonary disease, shortness of breath, cough, dyspnea, wheezing, fatigue, hypoxia, pleural effusion	Pulmonary function studies, peak flow, arterial blood gas, CT of the chest	Prevent and treat pulmonary infections, including *Pneumocystis jirovecii* and *Streptococcus pneumoniae*. Aggressively investigate changes in pulmonary function, as these may represent GVHD of the lung/bronchiolitis obliterans. Encourage tobacco cessation; avoid smoking of marijuana.
Gastrointestinal	Nausea, odynophagia, dysphagia, anorexia, early satiety, malabsorption, diarrhea, weight loss	Stool cultures, esophagogastroduodenoscopy, colonoscopy, nutritional assessment, fecal fat excretion studies, serum amylase, D-xylose absorption test, CT of the abdomen	Refer to gastroenterologist; consult with nutritionist; suggest nutrition support. Consider empirical trial of pancreatic enzyme supplementation. Perform aggressive management of gastrointestinal symptoms, such as nausea, vomiting, diarrhea, and abdominal pain. Consider the use of cholestyramine, pancrelipase, tincture of opium, octreotide, diphenoxylate-atropine, or loperamide in the management of diarrhea. Consider a trial of oral beclomethasone.
Nutritional	Protein and calorie deficiency, malabsorption, dehydration, weight loss, muscle wasting	Weight, fat store measurement, prealbumin	Implement nutritional monitoring, supplementation, and symptom-specific interventions. Institute trial of megestrol acetate or other approaches to appetite stimulation (e.g., mirtazapine or similar antidepressants, dronabinol).

(Continued on next page)

Table 7-4. Chronic Graft-Versus-Host Disease: Clinical Manifestations, Screening and Evaluation, and Interventions *(Continued)*

System	Clinical Manifestations	Screening/Evaluation	Interventions
Genitourinary	Vaginal sicca, vaginal atrophy, stenosis or inflammation	Pelvic examination	Consider trial of mucosal application of corticosteroid ointment, cyclosporine A ointment, or tacrolimus ointment. Suggest use of vaginal lubricants and dilators. Low-dose topical estrogen (e.g., Estring® vaginal ring) may be helpful in reducing vaginal tissue atrophy and vaginal synechiae. Suggest sexual counseling. Recommend annual gynecologic evaluation. Consider human papillomavirus vaccination, in accordance with nationally recommended guidelines based on age.
Immunologic	Hypogammaglobulinemia, autoimmune syndromes, recurrent infections, including cytomegalovirus, herpes simplex virus, varicella zoster virus, fungus, *Pneumocystis jirovecii* pneumonia, and encapsulated bacteria	Quantitative immunoglobulin levels, CD4/CD8 lymphocyte subsets	Implement IV immunoglobulin supplementation, as indicated, and prophylactic antimicrobials (rotating antibiotics for recurrent sinopulmonary infections, *Pneumocystis jirovecii* pneumonia prophylaxis, topical antifungals). Screen for cytomegalovirus and other opportunistic infection with frequent surveillance cultures and antigen detection. Consider vaccination against influenza and pneumococcus.
Musculoskeletal	Contractures, debility, muscle cramps/aches, carpal spasm	Performance status, formal quality-of-life evaluation (e.g., FACT-BMT), formal evaluation of rehabilitation needs, performance-based measures of physical function such as range-of-motion measurement, and 2- and 6-minute walk tests	Provide referral to physical therapy. Correct electrolyte imbalances. Consider clonazepam or magnesium supplementation for treatment of muscle cramping or myalgias.

ALT—alanine aminotransferase; AST—aspartate aminotransferase; CT—computed tomography; FACT-BMT—Functional Assessment of Cancer Therapy–Bone Marrow Transplant; GVHD—graft-versus-host disease; PO—by mouth; PUVA—psoralen and ultraviolet A irradiation; TID—three times a day

Note. Based on information from Carpenter et al., 2015; Flowers & Martin, 2015; Majhail et al., 2012.

lar necrosis (McCune & Bemer, 2016; McCune, Bemer, & Long-Boyle, 2016). Improved understanding of the underlying immune pathways that have been activated in chronic GVHD will support the development of more effective therapeutic regimens. As will be discussed later in the chapter, the therapeutic regimen selected will vary based on whether the goal is prevention or treatment, whether the patient has acute or chronic GVHD, the organ systems involved, and the patient's response to alternative therapies (Flowers & Martin, 2015; Holtan, Pasquini, & Weisdorf, 2014; Im et al., 2017; Jamil & Mineishi, 2015; Zhang, Yu, & Wei, 2018). Each transplant center follows center-specific protocols for the prophylaxis and treatment of acute and chronic GVHD, as well as for the supportive care management. Table 7-5 summarizes the mechanism of action for the major categories of immunosuppressive agents used in GVHD treatment.

Systemic Immunosuppression

A wide variety of systemic immunosuppressive therapies may be used to prevent or treat GVHD, including nonspecific immunosuppressive agents (e.g., corticosteroids, methotrexate), specific T-cell and B-cell immunosuppressive drugs (e.g., cyclosporine A, mycophenolate mofetil, siro-

limus, tacrolimus), monoclonal or polyclonal antibodies, and molecularly targeted agents, including kinase inhibitors, proteasome inhibitors, and agents that favorably alter the cytokine profile (Hill et al., 2018).

Corticosteroids have broad immunosuppressive effects, including induction of apoptosis of activated lymphocytes, downregulation of cytokine expression in lymphocytes and phagocytes, decreased antigen processing and presentation, and decreased phagocytosis (Allison, 2016). As single agents, corticosteroids are not effective in preventing GVHD. Furthermore, although they may be used in combination regimens for GVHD prophylaxis, they are of uncertain efficacy and may increase the morbidity of allogeneic HSCT and the frequency of chronic GVHD (Villa, Rahman, McFadden, & Cogle, 2016). However, corticosteroids are an important component of the treatment of both acute and chronic GVHD and often are given at high doses (Martin et al., 2012). Side effects of corticosteroids include hyperglycemia, hypertension, edema, myopathy, headaches, psychiatric disturbances, nausea, and gastric ulceration or bleeding. In addition, they may accelerate the development of cataracts, osteoporosis, and avascular necrosis (Malat & Culkin, 2016). In patients receiving high-dose corticoste-

Figure 7-10. Options for Graft-Versus-Host Disease Prevention and Treatment

Systemic Immunosuppression
- Corticosteroids
- Cyclophosphamide
- Cyclosporine A
- Methotrexate
- Mycophenolate mofetil
- Pentostatin
- Sirolimus
- Tacrolimus

Polyclonal or Monoclonal Antibody–Based Therapies
- Alemtuzumab
- Antithymocyte globulin
- Basiliximab
- Daclizumab
- Etanercept
- Infliximab
- Rituximab

Molecularly Targeted Immunomodulatory Agents
- Baricitinib
- Bortezomib
- Imatinib
- Pomalidomide
- Ruxolitinib

Phototherapy
- 8-Methoxypsoralen plus ultraviolet A irradiation
- Extracorporeal photopheresis
- Ultraviolet B narrow band or broadband phototherapy

Local and Topical Therapies
- Beclomethasone
- Budesonide
- Corticosteroid creams or ointments
- Corticosteroids or calcineurin inhibitors compounded for vaginal administration
- Cyclosporine A eye drops
- Dexamethasone mouthwash
- Intralesional steroid injections (mouth only)
- Prednisone eye drops
- Topical tacrolimus

Other
- Low-dose interleukin-2
- Mesenchymal stromal cell infusion
- Regulatory T-cell infusion
- Total lymphoid irradiation

rin inhibitor concentrations in the early post-transplant period may result in unfavorable outcomes, particularly in patients receiving cyclosporine A (Nasu, Nannya, Shinohara, Ichikawa, & Kurokawa, 2014).

Sirolimus (rapamycin) is structurally similar to the calcineurin inhibitors; however, it exerts its mechanisms of action by binding with the mammalian target of rapamycin (mTOR) (McCune et al., 2016; Villa et al., 2016). The sirolimus–mTOR complex inhibits multiple cytokine-stimulated inflammatory pathways and works synergistically with calcineurin inhibitors to enhance T-cell immunosuppression (McCune et al., 2016). It has minimal nephrotoxicity and has shown effectiveness in preventing and treating acute GVHD when used in combination with tacrolimus (Abouelnasr, Roy, Cohen, Kiss, & Lachance, 2013). Studies are ongoing to further clarify its role in combination with calcineurin inhibitors or cyclophosphamide (McCune et al., 2016).

Commonly encountered side effects of cyclosporine A include glucose intolerance, hirsutism, hyperkalemia, hypertension, magnesium wasting, renal insufficiency, and tremor (Malat & Culkin, 2016). Other side effects include confusion, cortical blindness, gingival hyperplasia, headache, hemolytic uremic syndrome, hyperchloremic metabolic acidosis, hyperlipidemia, hyperuricemia, microangiopathic hemolytic anemia, palmar-plantar dysesthesia, and seizures (Malat & Culkin, 2016). The side effect profile of tacrolimus is similar to that of cyclosporine A except that tacrolimus does not cause gingival hyperplasia, hirsutism, or hyperlipidemia and is associated with less hypertension. Some toxic events are idiosyncratic or precipitated by rapid infusion of the drug, but the risk of nephrotoxicity is increased with elevated blood concentrations of either cyclosporine A or tacrolimus (McCune & Bemer, 2016). The clearance of both drugs is through hepatic metabolism. Cyclosporine A– and tacrolimus-induced liver dysfunction can mimic hepatic sinusoidal obstruction syndrome or acute GVHD of the liver, resulting in jaundice, hepatorenal syndrome, elevated transaminases, and hepatic encephalopathy (McCune & Bemer, 2016). Sirolimus has several specific adverse reactions that require careful monitoring, including cutaneous reactions, hyperlipidemia, interstitial pneumonitis, mucosal ulcers, and reversible cytopenias, as well as impaired wound healing (Jamil & Mineishi, 2015; Malat & Culkin, 2016). When sirolimus is combined with calcineurin inhibitors, an increased incidence of thrombotic microangiopathy and possibly sinusoidal obstruction syndrome also has been reported (Abouelnasr et al., 2013).

Tacrolimus, cyclosporine A, and sirolimus require therapeutic monitoring, but no consensus exists on the target drug levels to be achieved (Ruutu et al., 2014). Some emerging evidence suggests that higher concentrations of calcineurin inhibitor early after nonmyeloablative HSCT may be associated with reduced nonrelapse mortality (McCune & Bemer, 2016; Nasu et al., 2014). The target range for tacro-

roids, consideration should be given to the need for gastric cytoprotection with a proton pump inhibitor, such as omeprazole, and for antimicrobial prophylaxis.

Cyclosporine A and tacrolimus inhibit calcineurin, thereby preventing transcription of the earliest activation genes in T lymphocytes (Villa et al., 2016). In addition, cyclosporine A attenuates the expression of IL-2 and IL-2R in activated T lymphocytes (Malat & Culkin, 2016). Studies comparing cyclosporine A to tacrolimus have suggested that tacrolimus is slightly more effective in preventing acute GVHD. Evidence has suggested that inadequate calcineu-

limus whole blood concentrations is usually 10–20 ng/ml, although some centers use a range of 5–15 ng/ml (McCune & Bemer, 2016). Cyclosporine A should be dosed to achieve a target concentration of 200–300 ng/ml during the first three to four weeks after transplant, and then 100–200 ng/ml until three months after HSCT if no GVHD or toxicity is present (McCune & Bemer, 2016). It is important to note that the different oral preparations of cyclosporine A are not bioequivalent, and the conversion ratio from the IV to the oral route depends on which formulation is used. Sirolimus is typically dosed to achieve trough levels of 3–12 ng/ml. In contrast to cyclosporine A and tacrolimus, sirolimus has a long half-life; thus, dose adjustments based on blood concentrations should not be undertaken more often than approximately every 7–10 days after maintenance dosing has been established. As cyclosporine A adheres to

Table 7-5. Side Effects and Nursing Implications of Selected Immunosuppressants Used in Allogeneic Stem Cell Transplantation

Mechanism of Action	Dosing/Administration	Side Effects	Nursing Implications
Alemtuzumab			
Monoclonal antibody directed against the cell surface antigen CD52, which is expressed on B and T lymphocytes	Institutional protocols vary; usual dose is 20 mg/day IV given over several hours for 5 days, beginning before transplant.	Infusional toxicities may be severe and include fever and rigors in more than 80% of patients. Other adverse effects include anemia, fatigue, hypotension, nausea, neutropenia, rash, thrombocytopenia, and vomiting.	Premedicate patients with acetaminophen and diphenhydramine. Medications for treating hypersensitivity reactions (e.g., acetaminophen, antihistamines, corticosteroids, epinephrine) and supplemental oxygen should be available for immediate use in the event of a reaction. Consider treatment with meperidine to control infusional rigors. Administer fluid bolus as ordered to treat hypotension. Produces profound and rapid lymphopenia; therefore, patients require broad antifungal, antibacterial, antiviral, and antiprotozoal prophylaxis for at least 4 months following treatment and ongoing surveillance for cytomegalovirus and adenovirus infection.
Antithymocyte Globulin (ATGAM®, equine; Thymoglobulin®, rabbit)			
Polyclonal immunoglobulin composed of horse or rabbit antibodies capable of destroying human leukocytes	Institutional protocols vary; usual dose is 10–40 mg/kg/day for equine ATG and 2.5 mg/kg/day for rabbit ATG.	Adverse reactions include anaphylaxis, chills, fever, laryngospasm, leukopenia, pulmonary edema, seizures, and thrombocytopenia. Because ATG is a foreign xenogeneic protein and an antibody, serum sickness can occur, including arthralgias, dysphagia, fever, hand and facial edema, myalgias, rash, and sore throat.	Monitor patients closely, both during and following infusion, for signs of serum sickness and anaphylaxis. Consider premedication with corticosteroids, acetaminophen, and H_1 and H_2 blockers. Medications for treating hypersensitivity reactions (e.g., acetaminophen, antihistamines, corticosteroids, epinephrine) and supplemental oxygen should be available for immediate use in the event of a reaction. Because transient and at times severe thrombocytopenia may occur following ATG administration in patients with platelet counts < 100,000/mm³, monitor platelet count 1 hour following ATG administration and transfuse platelets as indicated.
Azathioprine			
Antimetabolite that selectively inhibits proliferation of T and B lymphocytes by interfering with purine nucleotide synthesis	Usual dose is 2–2.5 mg/kg/day. Oral and IV doses are the same.	Alopecia, hepatotoxicity, infection, myelosuppression, nausea	Dose decrement is required when given with allopurinol. Use may lead to anemia and leukopenia when given with angiotensin-converting enzyme inhibitors. Drug is synergistic with other bone marrow suppressants. Use with caution in patients with hepatic or renal impairment. Drug is teratogenic; advise patients and their partners about the need for contraception.

(Continued on next page)

Mechanism of Action	Dosing/Administration	Side Effects	Nursing Implications
Cyclosporine A			
Prevents IL-2 gene expression, thus impairs IL-2 synthesis and activation of T lymphocytes	Total daily dosage is usually 1.5 mg/kg IV every 12 hrs, 0.75 mg/kg every 6 hrs, or 3 mg/kg/day as a continuous infusion, with dosage adjusted to achieve therapeutic levels. IV to oral conversion is approximately 1:3. Dosage is dependent on achieving and sustaining therapeutic blood levels based on laboratory evaluation. Therapeutic monitoring is not required once drug is being tapered.	Cardiovascular: chest pain, hypertension Cutaneous: acneform rash, striae GI: abdominal pain, anorexia, ascites, constipation, diarrhea, elevated liver function tests, nausea, vomiting Hematologic: anemia Metabolic: diabetes mellitus, hyperkalemia and hyperglycemia, hypomagnesemia, hyperlipidemia, hyperuricemia Neurotoxicity: dizziness, headache, insomnia, paresthesia, seizures, tremor Renal: elevated creatinine, nephrotoxicity Other: flushing, gingival hyperplasia, hirsutism, impaired wound healing, infection, osteoporosis, peripheral edema, sweating	Bioavailability differs between oral solution and capsule formulation. Once a regimen is established, patients should be instructed not to change the formulation or brand. Drug should be taken with food. Instruct patients on importance of strict adherence to the administration schedule and to notify the healthcare team immediately if unable to take because of GI side effects. Monitor serum creatinine, blood urea nitrogen, potassium, magnesium, glucose, and triglyceride levels. Avoid potassium-sparing diuretics. Replete electrolytes as indicated. Coadministration with grapefruit juice may increase cyclosporine A levels and should be avoided. Drug–drug interactions can lead to subtherapeutic or toxic cyclosporine A levels. Drugs that inhibit or induce cytochrome P450 are most responsible. Cyclosporine A trough levels are to be drawn prior to administration of morning dose. Therefore, doses are usually timed for 10 am and 10 pm to allow trough blood draw at morning clinic visit. Instruct patients to bring dose to clinic and to administer once trough level is drawn. Drug should not be used simultaneously with tacrolimus.
Daclizumab			
Monoclonal antibody against the IL-2 receptor expressed on activated T cells Binds to the IL-2 receptor in a nonactivating fashion, competing with IL-2 and thereby inhibiting IL-2–driven proliferation of the activated T lymphocyte. IL-2–induced proliferation of activated (antigen-stimulated) T lymphocytes critical step in proliferation and, ultimately, tissue destruction	Institutional protocols vary; usual dose is 1 mg/kg by IV administration.	Abdominal distension, abdominal pain, back pain, chest pain, constipation, coughing, diarrhea, dizziness, dyspnea, edema, fatigue, fever, headache, hypertension, hypotension, musculoskeletal pain, nausea, nephrotoxicity, pain, pulmonary edema, tachycardia, tremor, vomiting	Anaphylactoid reactions following the administration of daclizumab have not been observed but can occur following the administration of proteins. Medications for the treatment of severe hypersensitivity reactions should be available for immediate use. The calculated volume of daclizumab should be mixed with 50 ml of sterile 0.9% sodium chloride solution and administered via a peripheral or central vein over a 15-minute period. Once the infusion is prepared, it should be administered intravenously within 4 hours. If it must be held longer, it should be refrigerated between 2°–8°C (36°–46°F) for up to 24 hours. After 24 hours, the prepared solution should be discarded. No incompatibility between daclizumab and PVC or polyethylene bags or infusion sets has been observed. No dosage adjustment is necessary for patients with severe renal impairment.

(Continued on next page)

Table 7-5. Side Effects and Nursing Implications of Selected Immunosuppressants Used in Allogeneic Stem Cell Transplantation *(Continued)*

Mechanism of Action	Dosing/Administration	Side Effects	Nursing Implications
Infliximab			
Monoclonal antibody against TNF-α Binds to soluble and membrane-bound TNF-α, producing reduction in serum IL-1 and reduced levels of nitric oxide synthase	Institutional protocols vary; usual dose is 10 mg/kg by IV administration. Administer over at least 2 hours. Give with a low-protein-binding filter of ≤ 1.2 mcm.	Abdominal pain, coughing, fatigue, fever, headache, nausea Infusion reactions including chest pain, chills, fever, headache, hypotension, and urticaria can occur during the infusion and for up to 2 hours after the infusion is complete. There was no increase in the incidence of reactions after the initial infusion. Delayed serum sickness–like reactions, including arthralgias, dysphagia, fever, hand and facial edema, myalgias, rash, and sore throat, can be seen 3–12 days after infusion. Patients may develop human antichimeric antibody (known as HACA).	Monitor patients for development of infusional toxicities. Consider premedication with acetaminophen and diphenhydramine. Initiate therapy at 10 ml/hr × 15 minutes, increase to 20 ml/hr × 15 minutes, and then increase to 40 ml/hr × 15 minutes, then 80 ml/hr × 15 minutes, then 150 ml/hr × 30 minutes, and then 250 ml/hr × 30 minutes to complete infusion in 2 hours. Stop or slow infusion and give diphenhydramine, acetaminophen, or Solu-Cortef® to treat mild to moderate infusion reaction. Resume infusion at 10 ml/hour once reaction is controlled or abated. Medications for treating hypersensitivity reactions (e.g., acetaminophen, antihistamines, corticosteroids, epinephrine) and supplemental oxygen should be available for immediate use in the event of a reaction. Drug is incompatible with PVC equipment or devices. Use glass infusion bottles and polyethylene-lined administration sets.
Methotrexate			
Antimetabolite that inhibits dihydrofolate reductase, thereby hindering DNA synthesis and cell reproduction and inhibiting lymphocyte proliferation	Institutional protocols vary; usual dose is 5–15 mg/m² via IV on days +1, +3, +6, and +11 after transplant.	Interstitial pneumonitis, hepatotoxicity, mucositis, myelosuppression, nephrotoxicity, photosensitivity	Dose and schedule for methotrexate prophylaxis for GVHD varies by institution. A common regimen is methotrexate 5–15 mg/m² on days +1, +3, +6, and +11 post-transplant. Doses may be adjusted or held for severe mucositis and renal or liver insufficiency. Doses may need to be adjusted for hypoalbuminemia. Wait until at least 24 hours following stem cell infusion to give day +1 dose.
Methoxsalen			
When photoactivated by UV light exposure, inhibits mitosis by binding covalently to pyrimidine bases in DNA	Usual dose is 400 mcg/kg PO 1.5–2 hrs prior to exposure to UV light.	–	Patients who have received cytotoxic chemotherapy or radiation and who are taking methoxsalen are at increased risk for skin cancers, and long-term use may increase the risk of skin cancer. Toxicity increases with concurrent use of phenothiazines, thiazides, and sulfanilamides. Severe burns may occur from sunlight or UVA exposure if dose or treatment frequency is exceeded. Pretreatment eye examinations are indicated to evaluate for the presence of cataracts. Repeat eye examinations should be performed every 6 months while patients are undergoing treatment with psoralen and UVA irradiation.

(Continued on next page)

Table 7-5. Side Effects and Nursing Implications of Selected Immunosuppressants Used in Allogeneic Stem Cell Transplantation *(Continued)*

Mechanism of Action	Dosing/Administration	Side Effects	Nursing Implications
N-Acetylcysteine			
Inhibits B7-1/CD28 expression in vitro; thought to interfere with T-cell/antigen-presenting cell costimulator pathways May also counterbalance tissue damage from free radicals and oxidative stress	Bolus of 150 mg/kg IV is followed by continuous IV infusion of 50 mg/kg/day over at least 7–21 days.	–	Monitor vital signs every 15 minutes during initial bolus infusion. Compatibilities with other therapies such as total parenteral nutrition are unknown. Should be infused on separate IV access.
Rapamycin			
Structurally similar to tacrolimus and cyclosporine A; however, has a distinct immunosuppressant activity Inhibits response of B and T lymphocytes to cytokine stimulation by IL-2 and inhibits antibody production by B cells	Initial dosing should be low (e.g., 0.25–0.5 mg/day), owing to the long half-life of rapamycin. In patients receiving concomitant voriconazole, the starting dose should be reduced by 90% (0.1 mg/day). Long half-life permits once daily dosing.	Anorexia, dizziness, headache, hyperlipidemia, leukopenia, nausea, thrombocytopenia, oral ulceration, impaired wound healing	Drug may suppress hematopoietic recovery if used in patients who have recently undergone high-dose therapy. Oral bioavailability is variable and improved with high-fat meals. As with tacrolimus and cyclosporine A, it is metabolized through the cytochrome P450 3A system. Monitor trough blood levels.
Rituximab			
Chimeric monoclonal antibody that targets the B-cell CD20 antigen and causes rapid and specific B-cell depletion	Institutional protocols vary; usual dose is 375 mg/m² weekly × 4 doses by IV administration.	Infusion-related side effects; persistent immunosuppression and resultant risk for opportunistic infection, including sepsis and Epstein-Barr virus or cytomegalovirus reactivation, due to B-cell elimination	Infusion reaction may occur; risk is greatest with first infusion. Premedication and a slow infusion rate may mitigate severity of infusion reaction. Medications for the treatment of severe hypersensitivity reactions should be available for immediate use.
Tacrolimus			
Impaired synthesis of IL-2 prevents T-lymphocyte proliferation; interferes with gene transcription for a variety of cytokines, including interferon gamma and TNF-α	Total daily dose is usually 1–2 mg PO every 12 hrs; administer 0.05–0.1 mg/kg/day as a continuous infusion, with dosage adjusted to achieve therapeutic levels. IV to PO conversion is approximately 1:4. Dosage is dependent on achieving and sustaining therapeutic blood levels based on laboratory evaluation. Therapeutic monitoring is not required once drug is tapered.	Cardiovascular: chest pain, hypertension GI: abdominal pain, anorexia, ascites, constipation, diarrhea, elevated liver function tests, nausea, vomiting Hematologic: anemia, leukocytosis, thrombocytopenia Metabolic: diabetes mellitus, hyperglycemia, hyperkalemia and hypokalemia, hyperlipidemia, hypomagnesemia, hypophosphatemia Neurotoxicity: dizziness, headache, insomnia, paresthesia, seizures, tremor Renal: elevated creatinine, nephrotoxicity	Drug should be taken on an empty stomach. Instruct patients on importance of strict adherence to the administration schedule and to notify the healthcare team immediately if unable to take because of GI side effects. Monitor serum creatinine, blood urea nitrogen, potassium, magnesium, phosphorus, glucose, and triglyceride levels. Avoid potassium-sparing diuretics. Replete electrolytes as indicated. Coadministration with grapefruit juice may increase tacrolimus levels and should be avoided. Drug–drug interactions can lead to subtherapeutic or toxic tacrolimus levels. Drugs that inhibit or induce cytochrome P450 are most responsible. Tacrolimus trough levels are to be drawn prior to administration of morning dose. Therefore, doses usually are timed for 10 am and 10 pm to allow trough blood draw at morning clinic. Tacrolimus should be discontinued 24 hours prior to starting cyclosporine A. In the presence of increased tacrolimus levels, initiation of cyclosporine A usually should be further delayed. Doses should be adjusted for renal dysfunction. Monitor levels carefully in patients with renal or hepatic dysfunction.

(Continued on next page)

Table 7-5. Side Effects and Nursing Implications of Selected Immunosuppressants Used in Allogeneic Stem Cell Transplantation *(Continued)*

Mechanism of Action	Dosing/Administration	Side Effects	Nursing Implications
Thalidomide			
Immunosuppressive and anti-inflammatory properties include impaired neutrophil phagocytosis and chemotaxis; reduced antibody production in response to antigenic stimulation; increased suppressor T cells and reduced helper T cells; inhibition of TNF-α production by monocytes	Usual dose is 100 mg PO daily at bedtime, increasing gradually to 400–600 mg daily at bedtime. Total daily dose may also be given in 3–4 divided doses per day.	Bradycardia, constipation, hypotension, hypothyroidism, light-headedness, neutropenia, peripheral neuropathy, skin rash, skin ulceration, somnolence/sedation	Thalidomide is a potent teratogen and is contraindicated in patients who are, or are likely to become, pregnant. A systematic counseling and education program, written informed consent, and participation in a confidential survey program at the start of treatment and throughout treatment is required for all patients receiving thalidomide. Both men and women who are of childbearing potential must practice protected sex while on this drug. Perform pregnancy test prior to initiating treatment with thalidomide. The combination of thalidomide with certain antibiotics, HIV protease inhibitors, rifampin, griseofulvin, phenytoin, or carbamazepine may decrease the effectiveness of oral contraceptives. Obtain baseline electrocardiogram prior to treatment. Thalidomide should not be started if ANC is < 750/mm³, and therapy should be reevaluated if ANC drops below this level. Always administer doses in the evening to minimize the impact of drowsiness on lifestyle and safety. Teach patients to use caution when taking thalidomide with other drugs that can cause drowsiness or neuropathy. Teach patients to rise slowly from a supine position to avoid light-headedness. Teach patients to immediately report signs or symptoms suggestive of peripheral neuropathy, including numbness or tingling in the hands or feet, or the development of skin rash or skin lesion. These may require immediate cessation of the drug until the patient can be evaluated for the neuropathy or skin rash. Teach patients to use protective measures (e.g., sunscreens, protective clothing) against exposure to UV light or sunlight. Control/manage constipation with a stool softener or mild laxative.

ANC—absolute neutrophil count; ATG—antithymocyte globulin; GI—gastrointestinal; GVHD—graft-versus-host disease; IL—interleukin; PVC—polyvinyl chloride; TNF-α—tumor necrosis factor-alpha; UV—ultraviolet

Note. Based on information from Allison, 2016; Enderby & Keller, 2015; Malat & Culkin, 2016; McCune & Bemer, 2016; McCune et al., 2016; Wolff, Schleuning et al. 2011.

the lumen of central venous catheters, it should always be infused through the same designated lumen (e.g., white), with drug levels drawn through another lumen.

Doses of tacrolimus, cyclosporine A, and sirolimus should be modified for renal toxicity, with changes made for as little as a 25% increase from baseline creatinine (Malat & Culkin, 2016). When cyclosporine A, tacrolimus, or sirolimus are used as second-line treatment for chronic GVHD, long-term renal toxicity could result. Therefore, dosing to maintain a plasma trough level in the lower therapeutic range often is advised (McCune & Bemer, 2016).

Because cyclosporine A, tacrolimus, and sirolimus are metabolized mainly by the CYP3A enzyme systems, substances known to inhibit these enzymes may decrease the metabolism of cyclosporine A, tacrolimus, or sirolimus, with resultant increases in whole blood or plasma concentrations (Enderby & Keller, 2015). Drugs known to induce these enzyme systems may result in an increased metabolism of cyclosporine A, tacrolimus, or sirolimus, with resultant decreases in whole blood or plasma concentrations. Monitoring of blood concentrations and appropriate dosage adjustments are essential when such drugs are used concomitantly, as is often the case in HSCT (McCune & Bemer, 2016). It also is important to note that discontinuation of agents such as fluconazole that inhibit CYP3A can result in a decline in blood concentrations of cyclosporine A, tacrolimus, or sirolimus, leaving patients at risk for GVHD. Drugs that may alter cyclosporine A, tacrolimus, and sirolimus levels are presented in Table 7-6. Care also should be exercised when drugs that are nephrotoxic or metabolized by CYP3A (e.g., ritonavir) are administered concomitantly with cyclosporine A, tacrolimus, or sirolimus. In addition, grapefruit juice affects CYP3A-mediated metabolism and should be avoided in patients taking these agents. Dose adjustment of tacrolimus, cyclosporine A, and methotrexate is required in patients with renal or liver dysfunction. These dose adjustments can be found in Table 7-7.

The schedules for tapering tacrolimus or cyclosporine A post-transplant are typically protocol specific or institutionally derived and vary from 5% per week starting on day +50 to 10% per week starting on day +180. Early discontinuation of cyclosporine A or tacrolimus generally is reserved for patients at high risk for relapse, with HLA-identical donors, and in the absence of acute GVHD, but carries with it the risk for the onset of potentially severe chronic GVHD. It is important to follow patients carefully during tapering to avoid missing a flare of acute GVHD or the onset of chronic GVHD.

Methotrexate inhibits T-lymphocyte function by blocking purine synthesis and DNA replication. The most common toxic events associated with methotrexate are hepatotoxicity, mucositis, and myelosuppression (Malat & Culkin, 2016). Routine use of leucovorin does not abrogate the immunosuppressive effect of methotrexate and may reduce toxicity. Methotrexate is cleared renally, and dose modification is required in patients with renal insufficiency, as illustrated in Table 7-7. Doses of methotrexate

may need to be reduced or omitted if the patient develops severe oral mucositis or liver function abnormalities prior to completing a planned course of methotrexate prophylaxis. Unfortunately, attenuating a planned course of methotrexate prophylaxis increases a patient's risk of acute GVHD (McCune & Bemer, 2016). Sample guidelines for methotrexate dose modification in patients with hyperbilirubinemia are given in Table 7-7. Low-dose methotrexate also may be used to treat chronic GVHD that has not responded to first-line treatments (Flowers & Martin, 2015) and may also be tried alone or in combination with other immunosuppressive agents to treat cutaneous chronic GVHD or sole organ involvement with chronic GVHD in patients without thrombocytopenia (Nassar et al., 2014).

Cyclophosphamide given post-transplant for the prevention of acute GVHD eliminates alloreactive T lymphocytes while sparing regulatory T cells and has shown promising results in both HLA-matched and HLA-mismatched related transplantation (Anasetti, 2015; Lutz & Mielke, 2016; Mussetti, Greco, Peccatori, & Corradini, 2017). Typically, post-transplant cyclophosphamide is used in combination with other immunosuppressive agents, such as mycophenolate mofetil, tacrolimus or sirolimus, and T-cell antibodies (Al-Homsi, Roy, Cole, Feng, & Duffner, 2015; Anasetti, 2015). When used in the setting of reduced-intensity conditioning regimens, post-transplant cyclophosphamide has been associated with a higher risk of leukemia relapse. This association has not been observed when post-transplant cyclophosphamide is used as GVHD prophylaxis in conjunction with myeloablative conditioning regimens. Further research is needed to clarify the use of cyclophosphamide in the context of varying conditioning regimen intensities, donor type, and graft source (Mussetti et al., 2017). Phase 3 trials are ongoing to determine the role of cyclophosphamide, alone

Table 7-6. Pharmacologic Agents That May Alter Tacrolimus, Cyclosporine A, and Sirolimus Levels

Action	Agents
May increase blood concentrations	Antibiotics: clarithromycin, doxycycline, erythromycin, norfloxacin, troleandomycin Antifungal agents: clotrimazole, fluconazole, itraconazole, ketoconazole Calcium channel blockers: diltiazem, nicardipine, nifedipine, verapamil Prokinetic agents: metoclopramide Other agents: acyclovir, allopurinol, aprepitant, bromocriptine, cimetidine, danazol, estrogens, methylprednisolone, mycophenolate mofetil, protease inhibitors, sertraline hydrochloride
May decrease blood concentrations	Antibiotics: isoniazid, nafcillin, rifampin, IV trimethoprim-sulfamethoxazole Anticonvulsants: carbamazepine, phenobarbital, phenytoin Other agents: octreotide
May have synergistic nephrotoxicity	Antibiotics: aminoglycosides, amphotericin B, cephalosporins, erythromycin Diuretics: furosemide, thiazides Ganciclovir Melphalan Nonsteroidal anti-inflammatory agents

Note. Based on information from McCune & Bemer, 2016.

Table 7-7. Sample Dose Adjustments of Tacrolimus, Cyclosporine A, and Methotrexate in Patients With Renal or Hepatic Dysfunction

Function	Tacrolimus/Cyclosporine Dosage	Methotrexate Dosage
Renal Function (Creatinine, mg/dl)		
< 1.5	100%	100%
1.5–1.7	75%	75%
1.8–2	50%	50%
> 2	Hold dose.	Hold dose.
Hepatic Function (Bilirubin, mg/dl)		
< 2	–	100%
2.1–3	–	75%
3.1–5	–	50%
> 5	–	Hold dose.

Note. Based on information from McCune & Bemer, 2016.

or in combination with other therapies for prevention of GVHD, and to better define short- and long-term outcomes with respect to acute and chronic GVHD incidence and severity, infectious complications, and relapse (Lutz & Mielke, 2016; Mussetti et al., 2017). These studies will help to establish whether post-transplant cyclophosphamide should be the standard of care for GVHD prevention in HLA-matched and HLA-mismatched related donor transplantation.

Mycophenolate mofetil blocks purine synthesis and is used both for prophylaxis of acute GVHD (Ruutu et al., 2014) and as a salvage therapy for refractory chronic GVHD (Flowers & Martin, 2015). Absorption is variable, and coadministration with magnesium oxide, aluminum- or magnesium-containing antacids, or cholestyramine decreases mycophenolate mofetil absorption. In patients with renal dysfunction, therapeutic monitoring of mycophenolate mofetil metabolite levels may be helpful in directing therapy. Although mycophenolate mofetil has been shown to be both effective and well tolerated, it is associated with a high rate of opportunistic or serious viral or bacterial infections (McCune et al., 2016).

Systemic immunosuppressive agents have many long-term effects, including hypertension, renal insufficiency, hyperlipidemia, metabolic complications (e.g., hyperglycemia, electrolyte abnormalities), and osteoporosis. Nurses working in HSCT should be skilled in the assessment, prevention, and management of these complications (Allison, 2016; Enderby & Keller, 2015; Malat & Culkin, 2016). The side effects and nursing implications of the systemic immunosuppressive agents commonly used in allogeneic HSCT are presented in Table 7-5.

Monoclonal or Polyclonal Antibody Therapies

Based on the understanding of the role of various cellular and cytokine effectors in the evolution of GVHD, monoclonal or polyclonal antibodies directed against specific cellular components of the immune system or the cytokines implicated in the pathogenesis of GVHD are now increasingly being used in the prevention and treatment of GVHD.

Daclizumab is a humanized monoclonal antibody directed against the alpha chain of the IL-2 receptor. Daclizumab binds to the IL-2 receptor in a nonactivating fashion, competing with IL-2 and thereby inhibiting IL-2–driven proliferation of the activated T lymphocyte. IL-2–induced proliferation of activated (antigen stimulated) T lymphocytes is a critical step in proliferation and, ultimately, tissue destruction. Studies have shown that daclizumab in combination with infliximab has substantial activity for the treatment of acute GVHD (Tan et al., 2017; Zeiser, 2018; Zhang et al., 2018), although its use is not recommended to treat chronic GVHD (Flowers & Martin, 2015).

Basiliximab, daclizumab, etanercept, infliximab, and inolimomab are monoclonal antibodies being studied as single or multiagent combination treatment of acute GVHD, particularly in the context of steroid-refractory disease (Nadeau et al., 2016; Socié et al., 2017; Tan et al., 2017; van Groningen et al., 2016). Alemtuzumab is a humanized immunoglobulin G1 monoclonal antibody directed against the cell surface antigen CD52, which is expressed on B and T lymphocytes. It is a potent immunosuppressive agent that diminishes B and T lymphocytes, NK cells, and dendritic cells. It currently is being studied for the prevention of acute GVHD in both myeloablative and reduced-intensity conditioning regimens (Ali, Ramdial, Algaze, & Beitinjaneh, 2017) and for the treatment of severe acute GVHD refractory to conventional immunosuppressive therapy (Martin et al., 2012; Tey et al., 2016). It is given daily for five days beginning before transplant. The most common side effects of alemtuzumab are infusion-related toxicities, such as rigors and chills, fever, and headache. Neutropenia and thrombocytopenia can occur, and a profound, long-lasting immunosuppression can result in a markedly increased risk for infections, especially viral infection (Ali et al., 2017).

Rituximab is a monoclonal antibody that targets CD20 on the surface of B lymphocytes, thereby eliminating them or potently suppressing their function. It is being evaluated as a method to prevent acute GVHD (Rezvani & Storb, 2012) and as both first- and second-line treatment of chronic GVHD, particularly in patients with bronchiolitis obliterans syndrome, cutaneous sclerosis, or myofascial manifestations (Solomon et al., 2019). Rituximab causes persistent and profound hypogammaglobulinemia. Patients should be monitored closely for this effect, and immunoglobulin repletion in accordance with guidelines should be provided (Majhail et al., 2012).

Antithymocyte globulin (ATG) is a polyclonal antibody directed primarily against circulating T lymphocytes, although it does contain antibodies against other formed elements of the blood, such as platelets and red blood cells. It is used as a component of GVHD prophylaxis regimens and is very effective in reducing the incidence of severe acute GVHD following HSCT (Busca & Aversa, 2017; Nishihori, Al-Kadhimi, Hamadani, & Kharfan-Dabaja, 2016). However, inclusion of ATG in the prophylaxis regimen has been shown to result in an increased risk of lethal fungal and viral infections (Arai, Jo, Matsui, Kondo, & Takaori-Kondo, 2017). Three different ATG preparations are available, although the two derived from rabbits are typically used (Gagelmann, Ayuk, Wolschke, & Kröger, 2017). The optimal dose, timing, and schedule of ATG administration have not been empirically defined (McCune & Bemer, 2016). Adverse reactions include anaphylaxis, fever and chills, laryngospasm, leukopenia, pulmonary edema, seizures, and thrombocytopenia.

Because ATG is a foreign xenogeneic protein and an antibody, serum sickness can occur. Symptoms include arthralgias, dysphagia, fever, hand and facial edema, myalgias, rash, and sore throat (Storek, Mohty, & Boelens, 2015). Longer-term complications of GVHD prophylaxis with ATG include graft failure and Epstein-Barr virus–associated lymphoproliferative disorder (Arai et al., 2017). Little evidence exists to support the use of ATG in the treatment of GVHD, either as a salvage therapy for steroid-refractory acute GVHD or as a second-line therapy for chronic GVHD (Ali et al., 2017).

Molecularly Targeted Agents

A better understanding of the pathobiology of GVHD has allowed for the emergence of many new therapeutic strategies for prevention and treatment. These strategies are not directly immunosuppressive, but target immunomodulation and cytokine inhibition or effect an increase in the relative proportion or distribution of T cells while preserving graft-versus-tumor effects (Al-Homsi et al., 2016; Kekre & Antin, 2016; Rahmat & Logan, 2018). Many of these agents are actively being studied in clinical trials to determine which subpopulations (based on underlying malignant disease and stem cell source) and what sequencing and combination of therapies for prevention and treatment optimize GVHD-related outcomes, including GVHD control, tolerability, and graft-versus-tumor effects (da Silva, da Cunha, Terra, & Camara, 2017; Kekre & Antin, 2016; Yeshurun et al., 2015).

Cytokine inhibitors, including tocilizumab and alpha-1 antitrypsin, generally are well tolerated and have demonstrated favorable effects on IL-6, IL-10, and IL-Ra in murine and human models. Prospective clinical trials of these agents are underway. Therapies such as natalizumab, which mitigates T-cell homing to the gastrointestinal tract, and IL-2, which supports the development, activity, and survival of regulatory T cells needed for the development of tolerance, are currently being studied in phase 2 safety and efficacy trials (Kekre & Antin, 2016).

Other Systemic Therapies

IV immunoglobulin (IVIG) given post-transplant at a dosage of 500 mg/kg per week until day +90 has been associated with a reduced incidence of acute GVHD, fewer CMV infections, and less interstitial pneumonia (Ahn et al., 2018). Its immunomodulatory properties may be partially explained by understanding that when immunoglobulin G is bound to macrophages, IL-1 receptor antagonist production is preferentially increased over the production of IL-1, one of the cytokines responsible for GVHD (Issekutz, Rowter, & MacMillan, 2011). Data from both animal models and human studies also indicate that IVIG may induce apoptosis of donor-derived Th-1 cytokine-producing T lymphocytes and may enhance the activation of regulatory T cells (Kaufman et al., 2015).

Because IVIG has been hypothesized to inhibit these inflammatory mechanisms that mediate GVHD, some transplant programs have used it to reduce or modulate the severity of acute GVHD and to address hypogammaglobulinemia in patients with frequent infectious events (Gea-Banacloche et al., 2017; Sánchez-Ramón, Dhalla, & Chapel, 2016). However, rigorous scientific data supporting its use to prevent or treat GVHD are lacking (Ahn et al., 2018), and significant practice variations exist in transplant settings (Bourassa-Blanchette et al., 2017). A meta-analysis has suggested that IVIG was associated with an increased risk of disease relapse, although such results should be interpreted cautiously (Ahn et al., 2018; Tjon, van Gent, Geijtenbeek, & Kwekkeboom, 2015). Prospective trials examining outcomes associated with the use of IVIG in the setting of GVHD are needed (Gea-Banacloche et al., 2017).

Thalidomide and its analogs lenalidomide and pomalidomide have been found to have immunosuppressive and immunomodulating properties and may be useful in patients with chronic GVHD who do not respond to other therapies, especially patients with sclerotic skin or musculoskeletal involvement (Linhares, Pavletic, & Gale, 2013). These agents are thought to function by downregulating TNF-α and suppressing programmed cell death-ligand 1 upregulation on antigen-presenting cells, and they also may have antifibrotic effects. With all these agents, therapy typically is initiated at a lower dose and titrated up. Side effects include constipation, neutropenia, peripheral neuropathy, skin rash, somnolence, thrombocytopenia, and thrombosis. Pomalidomide appears to be more potent and better tolerated, and preliminary evidence shows it may have a role in treating steroid-refractory chronic GVHD, though trials are ongoing (Im et al., 2016).

Octreotide, a synthetic somatostatin analog, is useful in managing severe diarrhea caused by intestinal acute GVHD (McDonald, 2016). Octreotide decreases gastropancreatic secretions, stool volume, intestinal motility, and luminal fluids. It also inhibits electrolyte secretion and stimulates water, chloride, and sodium reabsorption. Potential side effects include abdominal cramps, constipation, flatulence, nausea, and, rarely, ileus. Biliary sludge and cholestasis, as well as hyperglycemia or hypoglycemia, may occur. A dosage of 100–150 mcg every eight hours may be given as initial therapy, titrated up to 500 mcg IV every eight hours until symptom control is achieved (McDonald, 2016). Octreotide should be tapered over three to five days, depending on tolerance, to prevent rebound of the diarrhea.

Ultraviolet Phototherapy

Several therapeutic approaches to the treatment of acute and chronic GVHD, all of which involve the use of ultraviolet (UV) A or B irradiation, may have an important role as an adjunct to systemic immunosuppression, particularly in patients who are refractory to corticosteroids, intolerant of corticosteroids, or would benefit from steroid sparing (Greinix, Worel, Just, & Knobler, 2014). These phototherapy approaches include ECP, psoralen and UVA irradiation (PUVA), UVB (narrowband or broadband) irradiation, and UVA1 irradiation (Bittenbring & Reichrath, 2016; Gandelman et al., 2018; Greinix & Tanew, 2012; Greinix et al., 2014; Hashimoto et al., 2016; Kitko & Levine, 2015; Sakellari et al., 2018; Vieyra-Garcia & Wolf, 2018). The precise mechanisms of action of this diverse group of strategies for the treatment of GVHD are still under study. Mechanisms may include apoptotic and antiproliferative effects on T lymphocytes; moderating effects on cell activation, antigen presentation, and cytokine release; and immunomodulatory effects on lymphocyte subsets and Th-1/Th-2 balance (Garbutcheon-Singh & Fernández-Peñas, 2015; Rafei, Kharfan-Dabaja, & Nishihori, 2017). All these phototherapies have the advantage of being relatively nontoxic, particularly when compared to systemic immunosuppression, and may allow for a reduction in systemic immunosuppression, thus sparing patients some of the associated side effects of immunosuppressive agents.

ECP is a therapeutic approach based on the biologic effect of methoxypsoralen and UV light on mononuclear cells collected by apheresis and reinfused into the patient (Radojcic, Pletneva, & Couriel, 2015). It is performed using a standard apheresis procedure whereby 150–200 ml of buffy coat is collected, and 200 mcg of methoxypsoralen is injected into the bag containing the white blood cells that have been diluted with plasma or Plasma-Lyte®. The cell solution then is exposed to UV light and reinfused into the patient. Patients usually are treated on two consecutive days at two- to four-week intervals (Schneiderman, 2017). The mechanism of action of ECP appeared to involve a shift in cytokine profiles from a Th-1 to a Th-2 response, inactivation and apoptosis of T lymphocytes, and induction of donor-derived regulatory T cells (A. Cho, Jantschitsch, & Knobler, 2018). Although no treatment schedule (e.g., weekly, two consecutive days every two weeks) has proved to be superior, in general, patients demonstrating a response to ECP continue to receive treatment every two weeks for an extended period, with progressively longer intervals between treatments once maximal response has been achieved (Das-Gupta et al., 2014). The optimal duration of ECP treatment for GVHD is unclear; however, reports have indicated that more than six months of ECP treatment may be necessary to attain an optimal clinical improvement (Rafei et al., 2017). Abrupt termination of ECP is avoided because symptoms may rebound. Studies examining the effectiveness of ECP for the treatment of acute and chronic GVHD have shown variable outcomes and are confounded by differences in patient selection, entry criteria, additive immunosuppressive treatment, and differing ECP treatment frequency (Schneiderman, 2017). However, substantial therapeutic responses in cutaneous, gastrointestinal, liver, oral, and pulmonary manifestations of acute and chronic GVHD have been described in adult and pediatric patients, allowing reduction or even discontinuation of steroids (Das-Gupta et al., 2014; Del Fante et al., 2016; Greinix & Tanew, 2012; Greinix et al., 2014; Kitko & Levine, 2015; Rafei et al., 2017). In general, ECP is well tolerated, although complications such as transient hypotension during the procedure and catheter infection and thrombosis, related to the long-term indwelling central venous apheresis catheters needed to maintain the vascular access required for the treatment, may occur (Mohammadi et al., 2017; Schneiderman, 2017). ECP also poses logistical challenges for patients in terms of access to ECP programs, reimbursement, and travel and time commitment.

Phototherapy using UVA or UVB irradiation has been used for many years to treat a variety of dermatologic diseases, including vitiligo, lichen planus, atopic dermatitis, and eczema. Although the photobiologic effects of phototherapy and the mechanisms involved in the generation of immunosuppression are not fully understood, UV irradiation has profound effects that can prevent or inhibit allorecognition between donor and host cells and tissues (Garbutcheon-Singh & Fernández-Peñas, 2015). UVA or UVB phototherapy may be used to treat both acute and chronic GVHD of the skin (Garbutcheon-Singh & Fernández-Peñas, 2015) and oral manifestations of chronic GVHD (Mays et al., 2013). It can be highly effective in some patients, although response may be difficult to predict. Several weeks of treatment may be required until improvement is noted. Patients are given the photosensitizing medication methoxypsoralen approximately two hours before controlled exposure to the UV light. PUVA is given three to four times per week until symptoms resolve and is slowly tapered thereafter (Garbutcheon-Singh & Fernández-Peñas, 2015). Serious side effects such as severe phototoxicity are rare, although many patients experience slight redness, dryness, burning, and peeling and may be at greater risk for development of cutaneous malignancies (Garbutcheon-Singh & Fernández-Peñas, 2015).

Local or Topical Therapy

Although virtually all patients with extensive disease require systemic therapy, many patients will derive symptomatic relief from local or topical therapy (Carpenter et al., 2015; Flowers & Martin, 2015). Topical oral immunosuppressants such as clobetasol, beclomethasone, dexamethasone, or tacrolimus can be compounded for application via a gel, ointment, or mouthwash. Such approaches may control oral manifestations of chronic GVHD and can help to reduce oral mucosal pain and irritation (Albuquerque et al., 2016).

Betamethasone enemas have shown some effect in improving diarrhea and abdominal pain in patients with refractory or severe intestinal GVHD (Wada et al., 2001). Additionally, the use of the oral topical glucocorticoids beclomethasone or budesonide has been described in the treatment of intestinal GVHD (Ibrahim et al., 2009; McDonald, 2016). Tacrolimus ointment and topical steroids of varying potencies are effective in treating cutaneous erythema and pruritus and vulvovaginal manifestations of chronic GVHD and may be a useful therapeutic bridge to other therapies that have a slower onset, such as PUVA or ECP (Hamilton et al., 2017; Marks et al., 2011; Strong Rodrigues et al., 2018). Topical cyclosporine A and corticosteroid eye drops may be helpful in controlling ocular inflammation, and punctal occlusion, autologous serum eye drops, or scleral lenses provide significant symptom improvement in patients experiencing ocular dryness, grittiness, and sensitivity (Dietrich-Ntoukas et al., 2012; Inamoto et al., 2019; Munir & Aylward, 2017).

Other Strategies for Prevention

Ex vivo T-cell depletion is an approach to prevent GVHD, in which T lymphocytes are removed from the stem cell graft prior to infusion. It is an attractive and highly effective method of preventing acute GVHD because it offers the potential for prevention of GVHD without the morbidity associated with immunosuppressive drugs (Busca & Aversa, 2017).

Several ex vivo approaches have been developed to deplete donor T cells from the allogeneic hematopoietic stem cell graft, including physical separation methods, immunologic separation methods, and combined physical and immunologic separation methods (C. Cho & Perales, 2019). Physical separation techniques may be divided into negative and positive selection techniques. Negative selection techniques are designed to select the unwanted components out of the graft. Examples include density gradient fractionation or soybean lectin agglutination followed by rosetting with sheep red blood cells. Positive selection techniques are designed to select only the desired components out of the graft, thereby eliminating the undesired components. Immunoadsorption columns for CD34+ cell separation are an example of a positive selection technique to physically remove CD34+ lymphocytes from the stem cell graft product.

Immunologic methods include monoclonal antibodies directed against T-cell antigens. Examples of immunologic methods of T-cell depletion include immunotoxins (e.g., anti-CD5-ricin) and the set of antibodies known as CAMPATH-1. Sometimes both physical and immunologic methods are combined; for example, soybean agglu-

tination may be followed by treatment of the graft with a monoclonal antibody.

Although T-cell depletion reduces the incidence of GVHD, it also is associated with several adverse effects, including delayed engraftment or graft failure or loss, increased risk of relapse, delayed immune reconstitution, opportunistic infections (e.g., CMV, adenovirus), and the potential development of secondary malignancies in the post-transplant period (Anasetti, 2015). Newer approaches to the evaluation of chimerism hold the potential to predict individuals at the greatest risk for disease relapse following a T-cell-depleted transplant, thus permitting earliest intervention with strategies such as DLI to treat minimal residual disease (Mo, Lv, & Huang, 2017). Despite the limitations associated with current approaches to T-cell depletion, significant progress has occurred in the biologic, technical, and clinical development of these graft manipulation approaches, particularly for recipients of HLA-mismatched grafts (Busca & Aversa, 2017; Hamilton, 2018). Studies are testing redesigned stem cell grafts that have been manipulated to contain only a small number of mature T cells that are enough to reconstitute immunity and mediate antitumor activity. These manipulated stem cell grafts may also be depleted of B cells and include a post-transplant add-back of regulatory T cells, or have had the T cells in the graft manipulated with a suicide gene that can trigger their immediate cell death if GVHD develops (Fisher et al., 2017; Saad & Lamb, 2017; Zhou & Brenner, 2016).

Strategies for Prophylaxis and Treatment

Prophylaxis of Acute Graft-Versus-Host Disease

Two major approaches to the prophylaxis of acute GVHD following HSCT exist: T-cell depletion of the graft (discussed in the previous section) and pharmacologic therapy. Prevention of acute GVHD may be achieved with single-agent immunosuppression (often tacrolimus or cyclosporine A) or with multiagent immunosuppression (methotrexate, tacrolimus, cyclosporine A, sirolimus, steroids, ATG, cyclophosphamide, and mycophenolate mofetil), sometimes in combination with T-cell depletion and/or IVIG administration (Choi & Reddy, 2014; Servais et al., 2016; Villa & McFadden, 2018). More intensive strategies for acute GVHD prevention are required for patients who are at higher risk, especially those undergoing matched unrelated HSCT.

Prospective randomized trials have demonstrated that combination therapy is superior to single-agent therapy in preventing acute GVHD. However, to date, no one regimen of prophylaxis has consistently shown superiority in preventing acute GVHD or improving overall outcomes (Choi & Reddy, 2014; Servais et al., 2016). The most widely used pharmacologic regimen for the prophylaxis of acute GVHD is a combination of methotrexate, cyclosporine A, tacrolimus, and sirolimus (Ruutu et al., 2014). Other pharmacologic agents included in some acute GVHD prophylaxis regimens are alemtuzumab, ATG, corticosteroids, cyclophosphamide, daclizumab, and mycophenolate mofetil. Examples of some commonly used drug regimens for prevention of acute GVHD are shown in Table 7-8.

Treatment of Acute Graft-Versus-Host Disease

Despite preventive measures, 30%–60% of patients will still develop some degree of acute GVHD that must be treated (Martin et al., 2012). Treatment generally is required for grade 2–4 acute GVHD and often involves many of the same agents used for prophylaxis. Along with continuing the drugs used for prophylaxis (e.g., tacrolimus or cyclosporine A), high doses of methylprednisolone are used, varying from 1–50 mg/kg/day. These regimens are associated with fatal opportunistic infections and consequently cannot be administered for more than a few days. Most clinicians reduce the corticosteroid dose rapidly to 2 mg/kg/day in divided doses. Once maximal improvement is achieved, the steroids are tapered over 8–20 weeks depending on patient response. Concomitant prophylactic antibiotic, antiviral, and antifungal therapy is recommended.

For patients in whom initial therapy has failed (commonly defined as progression after 3 days, no change after 7 days, or incomplete response after 14 days of steroid treatment), a variety of salvage or secondary regimens are implemented (Baron et al., 2014; Garnett, Apperley, & Pavlů, 2013; Jamil & Mineishi, 2015; Martin et al., 2012; Mohammadi et al., 2017; Zhang et al., 2018). Therapeutic options include ATG, alemtuzumab, basiliximab, daclizumab, ECP, etanercept, infliximab, methotrexate, mesenchymal stromal cells, mycophenolate mofetil, pentostatin, rituximab, and sirolimus. Recommendations for second- and third-line therapy for acute GVHD have been published (Dignan et al., 2012; Martin et al., 2012).

The outcome of treatment is predicted by the overall grade of acute GVHD, with higher grades associated with a poorer prognosis (Martin et al., 2012). Response to treatment is another key determinant of outcome, with mortality and morbidity highest in patients who do not achieve a complete response to the initial treatment strategy (Jamil & Mineishi, 2015). Opportunistic infections, including CMV disease, invasive aspergillosis, and disseminated varicella zoster infection, are a particular risk in patients who have received second- and third-line treatment of acute GVHD (García-Cadenas et al., 2017).

Treatment of Chronic Graft-Versus-Host Disease

The diversity of organ involvement with chronic GVHD, in addition to the hematologic and immunologic dysfunction associated with the syndrome, contributes to whether treatment is successful (Hill et al., 2018; Im et al., 2017). Limited chronic GVHD generally is not treated or is managed with topical therapies alone, whereas a variety of therapies can be used for extensive chronic GVHD (Jamil & Mineishi, 2015). Patients with limited chronic GVHD at presentation require careful follow-up because they may progress to a more extensive category (Flowers & Martin, 2015).

The current standard treatment for extensive chronic GVHD in high-risk patients is a combination of alternate-day cyclosporine A or tacrolimus and prednisone. In patients with newly diagnosed extensive chronic GVHD, initial treatment consists of prednisone 1 mg/kg/day and daily cyclosporine A or tacrolimus. Treatment is continued until objective evidence of improvement, in manifestations of chronic GVHD, is observed. Tapering of prednisone by 25%–50% per week should begin within two weeks after the first evidence of improvement, even if manifestations have not resolved entirely. Tapering should continue to achieve a dose of 1 mg/kg every other day if there is no exacerbation of chronic GVHD manifestations (Flowers & Martin, 2015). After reach-

---

Table 7-8. Examples of Commonly Used Drug Regimens for Prevention of Acute Graft-Versus-Host Disease

Regimen	Dosing Schedule
Cyclosporine A and steroids	Cyclosporine A[a] 3 mg/kg/day IV infusion from day –2, taper 10% weekly starting day +180 Methylprednisolone 0.25 mg/kg BID days +7 to +14, 0.5 mg/kg BID days +15 to +28, 0.4 mg/kg BID days +29 to +42, 0.25 mg/kg BID days +59 to +119, and 0.1 mg/kg daily days +120 to +180
Cyclosporine A, methotrexate, and steroids	Cyclosporine A[a] 5 mg/kg/day IV infusion from day –2, taper 20% every two weeks starting day +84 Methotrexate 15 mg/m^2 on day +1, 10 mg/m^2 on days +3 and +6 Methylprednisolone 0.25 mg/kg BID days +7 to +14, 0.5 mg/kg BID days +15 to +28, 0.4 mg/kg BID days +29 to +42, 0.25 mg/kg BID days +59 to +119, and 0.1 mg/kg daily days +120 to +180
Tacrolimus and mini-methotrexate	Tacrolimus[a] 0.03 mg/kg/day infusion from day –2, taper 20% every two weeks starting day +180 Methotrexate 5 mg/m^2 on days +1, +3, +6, and +11
ATG, cyclosporine A, and methotrexate	ATG 20 mg/kg IV days –3, –2, and –1 Cyclosporine A[a] 5 mg/kg/day IV infusion from day –1, taper 10% weekly starting day +180 Methotrexate 10 mg/m^2 on days +1, +3, +6, and +11

[a] Tacrolimus and cyclosporine A have been used interchangeably with this methotrexate or steroid dose schedule.

ATG—antithymocyte globulin; BID—twice daily

Note. Based on information from Ruutu et al., 2014.

---

ing an every-other-day dosing schedule, the prednisone dose is held constant until all reversible manifestations of chronic GVHD have resolved. The prednisone taper schedule can then be resumed, and prednisone subsequently discontinued after at least two weeks of treatment at a dose of 0.15 mg/kg every other day (Wolff et al., 2010). The calcineurin inhibitor can then be tapered slowly. A sample tapering schedule using these concepts is illustrated in Table 7-9.

For chronic GVHD that is refractory to steroids and calcineurin inhibitors or is not well controlled, a variety of secondary and investigational therapies are available (Cutler et al., 2017; Dignan et al., 2012; Flowers & Martin, 2015; Hill et al., 2018; Im et al., 2017; Jamil & Mineishi, 2015; Mohammadi et al., 2017; Villa et al., 2016). These include baricitinib, bortezomib, ECP, ibrutinib, imatinib, sirolimus, low-dose IL-2, methotrexate, mycophenolate mofetil, pentostatin, rituximab, ruxolitinib, thalidomide analogs, or a cell-based therapy such as regulatory T-cell infusion or mesenchymal stromal cell infusion. A wide variety of novel immunomodulatory approaches are currently under development (Cutler et al., 2017; Hill et al.,

2018; Im et al., 2017; Villa & McFadden, 2018). Dignan et al. (2012) presented an algorithm for controlling active chronic GVHD by combining high-dose steroids with one or more of these approaches.

For patients with liver GVHD and associated cholestasis, administration of ursodeoxycholic acid (Actigall®) has shown effectiveness in improving liver function (McDonald, 2016). The mechanisms underlying the beneficial effects of ursodeoxycholic acid in liver GVHD are not well understood but may include protection of cholangiocytes against cytotoxicity of bile acids, stimulation of hepatobiliary secretion, and protection against bile acid–induced hepatocyte cell death. When used prophylactically from the day preceding conditioning until day +90 after transplant, it has been shown to be effective in reducing the overall severity of acute GVHD, possibly mediated by inhibiting production of IL-2, IL-4, and IFN-γ by peripheral blood mononuclear cells (Ruutu et al., 2002). Ursodeoxycholic acid is inexpensive, given orally, and extremely well tolerated. Diarrhea, the most common side effect, occurs in less than 5% of patients (Ruutu et al., 2002). The optimal dosage is unknown, although 12 mg/kg/day in a divided dose

Table 7-9. Sample Tapering Schedule for the Management of Extensive Chronic Graft-Versus-Host Disease

Treatment Week of Therapy	Prednisone (mg/kg/day PO)[a]		Tacrolimus (mg/kg/day PO)[b,c]		Cyclosporine A (mg/kg/day PO)[b,c]	
	Day A	Day B	Day A	Day B	Day A	Day B
1	1	1	0.12	0.12	10	10
2	1	1	0.12	0.12	10	10
3[d]	1	0.75	0.12	0.12	10	10
4	1	0.50	0.12	0.12	10	10
5	1	0.25	0.12	0.12	10	10
6	1	0.12	0.12	0.12	10	10
7	1	0.06	0.12	0.12	10	10
After Resolution of All Clinical Manifestations						
↓	1	0	0.12	0.12	10	10
20	0.7	0	0.12	0.12	10	10
22	0.55	0	0.12	0.12	10	10
24	0.35	0	0.12	0.12	10	10
26	0.25	0	0.12	0.12	10	10
28	0.20	0	0.12	0.12	10	10
30	0.15	0	0.12	0.12	10	10
32	0.15	0	0.12	0.12	10	10
34	Discontinue prednisone.	Discontinue prednisone.	May begin tapering tacrolimus.	May begin tapering tacrolimus.	May begin tapering cyclosporine A.	May begin tapering cyclosporine A.

[a] Prednisone is given as a single morning dose.
[b] Monitor tacrolimus or cyclosporine levels.
[c] Dose is given in a divided dose and based on ideal weight or actual weight, whichever is less.
[d] Prednisone taper begins within 2 weeks of objective improvement.

has been shown to be effective. Coadministration with food may enhance absorption.

For pulmonary manifestations of chronic GVHD, including bronchiolitis obliterans and bronchiolitis obliterans organizing pneumonia, corticosteroids along with intensified immunosuppression with ECP, mycophenolate mofetil, rituximab, or tacrolimus may be necessary (Grønningsaeter et al., 2017). Inhaled corticosteroids plus beta-agonists, together with montelukast and macrolide antibiotics such as azithromycin, may be helpful in modifying the disease course and improving symptoms (Hakim et al., 2018).

Topical immunosuppressive interventions (corticosteroids or calcineurin-inhibiting agents applied to the skin, oral cavity, eyes, or vulvovaginal area or inhaled or targeted to the intestine) may be helpful in improving symptoms (Wolff et al., 2010). Oral GVHD manifestations can be managed with a variety of topical therapies applied to the oral mucosa or lips via rinses or ointments including budesonide, clobetasol, dexamethasone, or tacrolimus (Elsaadany, Ahmed, & Aghbary, 2017), or oral UV phototherapy (Strong Rodrigues et al., 2018). In patients with oral and ocular dryness, pilocarpine 5 mg orally every six hours can reduce dryness and may be beneficial in treating these symptoms (Mays et al., 2013). Oral beclomethasone or budesonide may be helpful in the management of enteritis (Ibrahim et al., 2009). As with acute GVHD treatment, tacrolimus ointment, corticosteroid ointment, or cyclosporine A ointment can be helpful in the management of vaginal sicca and stricture formation. Ocular sicca symptoms may benefit from the insertion of punctal plugs, ophthalmic cyclosporine A or tacrolimus, autologous serum eye drops, or scleral lenses (Dietrich-Ntoukas et al., 2012; Inamoto et al., 2019).

It should be noted that in patients with oral manifestations of GVHD who are on immunosuppression, oral infections caused by herpes simplex virus and *Candida* species can occur simultaneously (Mawardi et al., 2019). Careful evaluation of the oral cavity and cultures of any lesions are key to accurate diagnosis and treatment of oral cavity infections. Good oral hygiene, prevention of tissue trauma, and topical fluoride applications are also important (Carpenter et al., 2015).

Although systemic immunosuppression is the basis of chronic GVHD treatment, there is a delicate balance between controlling symptoms and increasing susceptibility to infections, a major cause of death in these patients. Central to managing chronic GVHD is the ability to recognize its initial manifestations and establish the diagnosis; assess its severity, trajectory, and response to therapy; and gauge its impact on survival and quality of life (Krupski & Jagasia, 2015). The presentation of chronic GVHD is varied, and its symptoms may mimic other disease entities, including adrenal insufficiency, infections, drug effects, or iron overload (Flowers & Martin, 2015; Strong Rodrigues et al., 2018). Furthermore, because the therapy for chronic GVHD can have significant toxicities, accurate and prompt recognition is essential for optimal management and to avoid under- or overtreatment (S.J. Lee, Nguyen, et al., 2018). Data suggest that major practice variation exists in the diagnosis of chronic GVHD, assessment of disease severity, and management of immunosuppression (Pidala et al., 2011). Significant progress is occurring in the development of improved diagnostic strategies, as well as criteria and classification systems for diagnosis and staging (Schoemans, Goris, et al., 2018; Schoemans, Lee, et al., 2018). These will ultimately improve risk prediction and enhance the ability to offer targeted and tailored therapies.

Components of Supportive Care

Both acute and chronic GVHD are a cause of significant morbidity, mortality, and increased use of healthcare resources. Supportive care measures to manage pain and other symptoms, infection prophylaxis, nutritional management, interprofessional team involvement, and coordination and continuity of care are essential to improving the length and quality of life for patients with GVHD (Carpenter et al., 2015; Clark, Savani, Mohty, & Savani, 2016; Dignan et al., 2012).

Supportive and Rehabilitative Care

Both the manifestations and treatment of GVHD produce a wide range of distressing symptoms, including oral and ocular pain, abdominal pain, muscular pain from myositis, neuropathy, and muscle cramping. Treatment with calcineurin inhibitors can amplify pain (Ma, El-Jawahri, LeBlanc, & Roeland, 2018). Joint pain is common, particularly in association with steroid tapering. Additional concerns that cause pain and other distressing symptoms include peripheral neuropathy and avascular necrosis.

The diverse symptoms experienced by this patient population require a tailored interprofessional approach to achieve best results (Mitchell, 2018; Roeland et al., 2010). Directed and general strategies to optimize the management of pain and other symptoms, and to mitigate the impact of symptom distress on functional performance and quality of life, have been integrated throughout this chapter. Patients should understand the importance of using topical and local immunosuppressive medications for the skin, eyes, mouth, gastrointestinal tract, and vulvovaginal area to reduce symptoms (Elsaadany et al., 2017; Hamilton et al., 2017; Wolff et al., 2010). Muscle and joint pains may be relieved with acupuncture, heat, long-acting narcotics, and physical therapy (Marks et al., 2011). Proper management of abdominal pain, diarrhea, gastrointestinal bleeding, nausea, and vomiting are paramount (McDonald, 2016). Opioid analgesics often are needed to control abdominal pain but should be used with caution because they may hinder gut motility and exacerbate pain (Naymagon et al., 2017). Loperamide, octreotide, or tincture of opium should be trialed for diarrhea management and titrated to effect. Diphenoxylate-atropine also may be used to treat diarrhea, although patients require close monitoring for the development of ileus (Naymagon et al., 2017). Options for managing neuropathic pain include tricyclic antidepressants and anticonvulsants (Carpenter et al., 2015).

Acute and chronic GVHD can have significant and persistent negative effects on functional status and quality of life (Krupski & Jagasia, 2015). Early referral to interprofessional teams that specialize in symptom management, supportive care, and rehabilitation is essential (Bakhsh, Mohammed, & Hashmi, 2018; Mohammed et al., 2018).

Early Detection and Prophylaxis Against Infection

Patients with GVHD are more susceptible to bacterial, fungal, and viral infections because of the immunosuppressive effects of GVHD itself and its treatment (Gea-Banacloche et al., 2017; Sahin, Toprak, Atilla, Atilla, & Demirer, 2016). In the presence of GVHD, immune defects involving both cellular and humoral immunity lead to poor secondary immune responses and failure of interaction between helper T and B cells. Immunosuppression with corticosteroids and other potent immunosuppressive agents intensifies this immune dysregulation (Flowers & Martin, 2015). Infections including *Pneumocystis jirovecii* pneumonia (formerly *Pneumocystis carinii* pneumonia), viral infections (e.g., adenovirus, CMV, polyomavirus), pneumococcal infections, and the common pathogens found in the oropharynx and upper airways such as *Moraxella catarrhalis* and *Haemophilus influenzae* are a major cause of morbidity and mortality (Gea-Banacloche et al., 2017; Sahin et al., 2016; Ullmann et al., 2016). Guidelines for antimicrobial prophylaxis of patients with GVHD tend to be institution or protocol specific. Although much new information on prevention and treatment of infection is emerging, many of the HSCT-specific guidelines for prophylaxis of infections have not been recently updated (Rubinstein, Culos, Savani, & Satyanarayana, 2018; Ullmann et al., 2016). Thus, recommendations tend to be institution or protocol specific. Controversy remains in several areas, particularly with regard to routine prophylaxis for bacterial infections (Horton, Haste, & Taplitz, 2018) and vaccination against infectious diseases (Conrad, Alcazer, Valour, & Ader, 2018). Flowers and Martin (2015) and Ullmann et al. (2016) recommended that patients with chronic GVHD receive prophylaxis for *Pneumocystis jirovecii* with trimethoprim-sulfamethoxazole (Bactrim DS®) twice daily two to three times per week. Inhaled atovaquone, dapsone, or pentamidine may be used in patients with an allergy to sulfa agents or for those who cannot tolerate treatment with trimethoprim-sulfamethoxazole. Prophylaxis continues for at least six months following the completion of GVHD therapy. Topical antifungal prophylaxis with clotrimazole troches or nystatin swishes should be used in all patients receiving local steroid therapy. Highly immunosuppressed transplant recipients in whom mold-active prophylaxis is deemed necessary should receive posaconazole; voriconazole may increase the risk for phototoxicity and cutaneous second malignancies (Cowen et al., 2010; Kuklinski, Li, Karagas, Weng, & Kwong, 2017; Rubinstein et al., 2018). Because many patients with chronic GVHD have low serum immunoglobulin G levels, additional infection protection may be afforded by supplemental IVIG. The goal of such therapy is to keep the immunoglobulin G level greater than 500 mg/dl (Gea-Banacloche et al., 2017). The usual dosage is 500 mg/kg administered weekly or twice monthly.

CMV antigen surveillance should be performed weekly or at least twice monthly while patients are receiving GVHD treatment (Camargo & Komanduri, 2017; Flowers & Martin, 2015). Preemptive antiviral therapy should be initiated at the first signs of viral reactivation (Sandherr et al., 2015). Patients with previous CMV reactivation or infection may require closer surveillance and may be maintained on foscarnet, ganciclovir, or valganciclovir prophylaxis while receiving intensive systemic immunosuppression or when they have active GVHD (Camargo & Komanduri, 2017). In patients with previous varicella zoster virus infection, long-term administration of acyclovir, famciclovir, or valacyclovir is recommended to prevent varicella zoster virus reactivation (Sandherr et al., 2015). Patients with acute or chronic GVHD with a history of hepatitis B or hepatitis C coinfection should receive careful prospective surveillance for viral reactivation. Sarmati et al. (2017) recommended that all HSCT recipients infected with hepatitis B should be monitored for viral reactivation beginning two weeks after transplant. Early initiation of preemptive antiviral therapy may suppress viral replication during the post-transplant window when patients are intensively immunosuppressed and limit hepatocellular damage at the critical time of immune recovery and immunosuppressive therapy withdrawal (Sarmati et al., 2017).

Consideration should be given to vaccination against pneumococcus and *Haemophilus influenzae* type B and seasonal immunization against influenza to establish pathogen-specific immunity, although vaccination does not diminish the need for close follow-up and antimicrobial prophylaxis, particularly in patients with chronic GVHD and those on immunosuppressive therapies (L'Huillier & Kumar, 2015). In hepatitis B–seronegative transplant survivors, consideration should be given to hepatitis B vaccination. Vaccination of patients with active chronic GVHD requires an individualized approach but should be pursued once GVHD is resolved and the steroid dose is less than 5 mg/day (Conrad et al., 2018). Annual gynecologic examination and consideration of human papillomavirus vaccination also are important aspects of routine health maintenance, particularly given the increased risk of cervical dysplasia in long-term allogeneic HSCT survivors (L'Huillier & Kumar, 2015).

Patients and families should be educated about the importance of taking prophylactic antimicrobials as ordered and contacting the healthcare team immediately if they experience fever or malaise. To minimize morbidity and mortality in chronic GVHD, healthcare providers must have a high index of suspicion for and aggressively investigate potential infections in patients with chronic GVHD.

Nutrition Management

The clinical manifestations of gastrointestinal GVHD, including nausea, vomiting, severe abdominal pain and cramping, voluminous diarrhea, and intestinal bleeding, can affect nutritional intake, digestion and absorption of nutrients, and enjoyment of food. Malabsorption and intestinal protein losses are characteristic of the mucosal degeneration and resultant diarrhea associated with intestinal GVHD (McDonald, 2016). Multiple coexisting nutrition-related problems are associated with chronic GVHD, including oral sensitivity and stomatitis, xerostomia, anorexia/poor oral intake, altered taste, fatigue, reflux symptoms, dysgeusia, weight loss and steroid-induced nitrogen loss, weight gain, diabetes, and fluid retention (Fuji, Einsele, Savani, & Kapp, 2015; Verdi Schumacher & Moreira Faulhaber, 2017). The weight loss noted in patients with GVHD may be related to a higher resting energy expenditure and elevated serum level of TNF-α (van der Meij et al., 2013; Zatarain & Savani, 2012). Moreover, many of the medications used to prevent or treat GVHD have nutritional implications (Allison, 2016; Jomphe, Lands, & Mailhot, 2018). Close monitoring of nutritional status and optimal support are important complements to the therapy (Baumgartner et al., 2017; El-Ghammaz, Ben Matoug, Elzimaity, & Mostafa, 2017). Post-transplant supplementation of micronutrients and vitamins A and D has shown favorable effects on several body systems, including the immune system and bone health, and should be considered in all HSCT recipients, especially those with acute or chronic GVHD (X. Chen & Mayne, 2018; Kendler et al., 2018; Ros-Soto, Anthias, Madrigal, & Snowden, 2019; Zheng, Taylor, & Chen, 2018).

A five-phase dietary regimen is outlined in Table 7-10 and should be instituted with the onset of clinical signs consistent with intestinal GVHD (e.g., more than 500 ml of watery diarrhea) (Koc et al., 2016; van der Meij et al., 2013). The first phase consists of bowel rest with complete reliance on total parenteral nutrition to meet the needs for energy, protein, and micronutrients. Advancement through the stages from gut rest to the resumption of normal diet is based on improvement of clinical symptoms and diet tolerance. Clinical symptoms of diet intolerance include increased stool volume or diarrhea, increased emesis, and increased abdominal cramping (van der Meij et al., 2013). Lactose intolerance is common in patients with intestinal GVHD because lactose is one of the last disaccharidases to return following villous atrophy (Naymagon et al., 2017). In severe intestinal GVHD, the majority of a patient's calories and protein may need to be provided parenterally. Protein-losing enteropathy may require increased protein administration to improve nitrogen balance and maintain lean body mass (Naymagon et al., 2017).

Even when total parenteral nutrition is needed to support nutritional status, in general, some enteral nutrition should be maintained if possible. Enteral nutrition has a trophic effect on the intestinal mucosa, reducing bacterial translocation into the bloodstream (Baumgartner et al., 2017), stimulating gallbladder function, and supporting normal gut microflora. It also stimulates gallbladder function, reducing cholestatic complications (Beckerson et al., 2019). Nutrition interventions should be tailored to the patient's specific problems and symptoms (Baumgartner et al., 2017). Consultation and ongoing follow-up with a clinical dietitian should be part of the standard of care for these patients (Dignan et al., 2012). Further research is needed to determine the impact of nutrition interventions, such as glutamine supplementation, lipid supplementation, administration of N-acetylcysteine and selenium, and enteral feeding on GVHD and the outcomes of HSCT (Fuji et al., 2015; Kota & Chamberlain, 2017; van der Meij et al., 2013). The development of evidence-based guidelines for nutritional management of patients with gastrointestinal GVHD would help to reduce practice variation (Botti, Liptrott, Gargiulo, & Orlando, 2015).

Avoidance of Sun Exposure

Sun exposure may activate or exacerbate GVHD of the skin. UV radiation exposure may damage epidermal cells, leading to increased antigen expression or increased cytokine release (Hardy et al., 2016). Moreover, a number of the medications patients commonly require following HSCT have photosensitivity as part of their side effect profile, including the azole antifungals, trimethoprim-sulfamethoxazole, and the fluoroquinolones (Kim et al., 2018). Patients should be advised about appropriate methods for minimizing sun exposure (see Figure 7-11).

Interprofessional Team Involvement

Frequent interprofessional interventions, including dentistry or oral medicine, endocrinology, gynecology, ophthalmology, pulmonology, rheumatology, nutrition support, physical and occupational therapy, and psychosocial oncology, are essential in caring for patients with acute and chronic GVHD (Carpenter et al., 2015; Dignan et al., 2012; Wolff, Bertz, et al., 2011). Because GVHD may affect the skin, eyes, mouth, and genitourinary tract, regular follow-up with dermatology, ophthalmology, dentistry, and gynecology for surveillance and treatment is an important component of supportive care. Ophthalmologic follow-up is important to prevent long-term damage to the eyes in patients with ocular sicca syndrome and to ensure a successful outcome should surgery for cataracts (a common complication of long-term steroid use and total body irradiation) be needed (Inamoto et al., 2019; Munir & Aylward, 2017). Patients with oral sicca syndrome are

Table 7-10. Graft-Versus-Host Disease Progressive Diet Regimen

Stage	Diet Principles	Suggested Foods
1	Rest bowel.	Nothing by mouth (NPO); consider need for total parenteral nutrition (TPN).
2	Allow liquids (isotonic, lactose free, low residue, no caffeine) at 60 ml every 2–3 hours. If diarrhea or cramps recur or persist, return to bowel rest. Continue TPN.	Water, decaffeinated tea, decaffeinated coffee, caffeine-free diet soft drinks, caffeine-free and sugar-free imitation fruit drinks (e.g., Crystal Light®), sugar-free gelatin, sugar-free ice pops, clear broth, consommé, bouillon, sugar-free or dietetic hard candy that does not contain sorbitol or xylitol
3	Introduce solid foods, choosing low-fiber, lactose-free, fat-free, starchy foods. Sugar is introduced during this phase. Small portions only. No meat or meat products are allowed. Low total acidity; no gastric irritants such as caffeine. Introduce 1 food at a time. Each new food may be tried with foods taken previously. Discontinue the most recently added food if diarrhea or abdominal pain increases. If symptoms persist, return to bowel rest. Continue TPN until calorie and protein counts and fluid intake are adequate. Patient may drink water, decaffeinated tea, decaffeinated coffee, caffeine-free diet soft drinks, and caffeine-free and sugar-free imitation fruit drinks (e.g., Crystal Light), in addition to foods chosen from list.	Plain white bread/toast, bagel, English muffin, soda crackers, melba toast, matzo, graham crackers Cream of Wheat®, crisped rice, cornflakes, oat cereals, white rice, plain noodles Arrowroot cookies, social tea cookies Fruit juices (< 60 ml serving; may try half-strength): apple, cranberry, grape, pineapple, orange, grapefruit, or tomato juice (no more than 2 servings/day) Mashed or boiled potato without skin or butter Clear chicken, beef, or vegetable broth; consommé; broth containing noodles or rice Gelatin, ice pops
4	Allow solid foods as in stage 3 but with fat intake slowly increased.	Lactose-free milk Plain white bread/toast, bagel, English muffin, soda crackers, melba toast, matzo, graham crackers Cream of Wheat, crisped rice, cornflakes, oat cereals, white rice, plain noodles Arrowroot cookies, social tea cookies Fruit juices (half-strength or < 60 ml serving): apple, cranberry, grape, pineapple, orange, grapefruit, or tomato juice (may increase to 4 servings/day) Mashed or boiled potato without skin or butter Trimmed lean meats, fish, and poultry baked, broiled, poached, boiled, roasted, or stewed Maximum 1 egg per day, boiled or poached tuna or salmon packed in water or broth Cooked vegetables (e.g., asparagus, carrots), 1–2 servings/day Clear chicken, beef, or vegetable broth; consommé; broth containing noodles or rice Cream soups prepared with lactose-free milk Natural hard, low-fat cheese (skim-milk mozzarella, parmesan) Gelatin, ice pops, peaches or pears canned in juice or water (maximum of half-cup or two halves)
5	Advance to regular diet by adding restricted foods, 1 per day, to assess tolerance.	Last foods to be added: high-fiber foods, food or drinks that contain caffeine (e.g., coffee, chocolate, soft drinks with caffeine), and lactose-containing foods (e.g., ice cream, custard, milk, cottage cheese)

Note. Based on information from Henry & Loader, 2009; Koc et al., 2016.

at increased risk for dental caries; therefore, close dental follow-up is essential.

Consultation with specialists in endocrinology is an important role given the high prevalence of endocrine dysfunction in long-term survivors of HSCT, including gonadal dysfunction in men and women, adrenal insufficiency, thyroid dysfunction, and bone complications as a result of the conditioning therapy, immunosuppressive treatments, and immune system derangement (Akirov, Sawka, Ben-Baruch, Lipton, & Ezzat, 2019; Kendler et al., 2018). Physical therapy is important to prevent the limitations in range of motion, joint contractures, and impaired functional status that can result from sclerodermatous skin changes (Mohammed et al., 2019) and to minimize the proximal muscle weakness that results from long-term corticosteroid therapy. Support groups, individual and fam-

Figure 7-11. Counseling Guidelines for Limiting Sun Exposure

- Limit outdoor activities between the hours of 10 am and 4 pm. Stay in the shade.
- Do not visit tanning salons.
- Routinely and liberally use a sunscreen with a sun protection factor (SPF) of 15 or higher. Apply the lotion one half-hour before going out in the sun. Apply a generous amount and cover all exposed skin. Reapply at least every 2 hours and after swimming or perspiring.
- Use a lip balm with an SPF 15 sunscreen. Apply sunscreen to the face, even if wearing a hat.
- Some sunscreens may cause allergic reactions. If a sunscreen irritates the skin, change to another brand or consult a physician.
- Always apply sunscreen or cover your skin if any sun exposure will occur. Remember that sun exposure occurs even on cloudy or hazy days. Water, sand, snow, and concrete can all reflect large amounts of sunlight onto the skin.
- Wear a wide-brimmed hat and sunglasses and cover all exposed areas of skin. Dark-colored, long-sleeved shirts and slacks with tightly woven fabrics offer the most protection.
- The risk of sunburn is greater at high altitudes. The thinner atmosphere at high altitudes absorbs lesser amounts of damaging UV rays than at sea level.
- Some drugs and cosmetics may increase susceptibility to sunburn. These "photosensitivity reactions" may be caused by some antibiotics and by several other medications that transplant recipients commonly take.

ily psychotherapy, physical therapy, occupational therapy, and preventive and preemptive rehabilitation measures may help to mitigate functional decline, cognitive dysfunction, and emotional distress, thereby improving quality of life (Krupski & Jagasia, 2015; S.R. Smith & Asher, 2016; Syrjala, Martin, & Lee, 2012).

There is growing recognition that a patient-centered interprofessional approach is fundamental to optimizing outcomes in patients with GVHD (Bevans et al., 2017). No single healthcare profession has all the knowledge needed to provide total patient-centered care because the needs of patients with GVHD are both multidimensional and complex. Nurse coordinators, outpatient clinic nurses, and advanced practice nurses have key responsibilities in the coordination and leadership of the interprofessional team (Mueller, 2016). These responsibilities include performing intake activities; fostering collaboration among team members; contributing to the development of measures, standards, procedures, and care protocols that improve clinical and operational outcomes; and developing systems to ensure all patients with GVHD have access to relevant services (Majhail, 2017; Rioth, Warner, Savani, & Jagasia, 2016).

Coordination and Continuity of Care

Chronic GVHD is a primary factor in late transplant-related morbidity, including abnormalities of growth and development in children, quality of life, functional performance status, somatic symptoms, psychological functioning, sexual satisfaction, and employment in adults (El-Jawahri et al., 2018; Krupski & Jagasia, 2015; S.J. Lee, Onstad, et al., 2018). Nurses have an important role in coordinating interprofessional involvement, assessing and managing symptoms, and ensuring continuity of care. Providing supportive care and symptom management is a key nursing role. A standard of care for patients with GVHD is presented in Figure 7-12.

Ongoing monitoring of patients for the rest of their lives is critical for the prevention of late complications and disability (Inamoto & Lee, 2017). At the time that chronic GVHD often develops, patients may be back in their local communities, at a distance from healthcare providers with expertise in the identification and management of the diverse manifestations of chronic GVHD. Although much of the care required by survivors with chronic GVHD can be effectively delivered by clinicians who are generalists, effective management requires periodic access to providers with specific expertise. Such access is particularly essential for patients with a new diagnosis of chronic GVHD, those with refractory manifestations or with serious adverse effects of treatment (e.g., life-threatening infection, severe myodystrophy), and those who demonstrate high-risk features and poor prognostic signs. Long-term follow-up contact by telephone, fax, or mail to patients and contact with primary care physicians, combined with regular evaluations at the transplant center, is crucial. Documentation of the development, features, severity, course, and management of GVHD is important to ensure quality of care and outcome evaluation. Figure 7-13 provides a tool for documenting the risk factors, features, severity, prevention, and management of GVHD.

Care coordination for patients with GVHD occurs across settings and geographic distances and often must incorporate a transplant team, private oncologist, general practitioner, and subspecialists (e.g., dermatology, endocrinology, ophthalmology). Reimbursement issues may constrain the delivery of needed services to survivors who have lost insurance as a result of persistent unemployment or exceeded lifetime reimbursement caps because of the need for treatment of late effects such as chronic GVHD (Syrjala et al., 2012). A further challenge to optimal care of HSCT survivors is that many healthcare professionals in general oncology practice or primary care may have limited knowledge of the survivorship phase of allogeneic HSCT, including chronic GVHD, and standards of care for this population are lacking. The National Marrow Donor Program (https://bethematch.org) and the Center for International Blood and Marrow Transplant Research (www.cibmtr.org) endorsed guidelines for screening and evaluation of late effects of transplant, including chronic GVHD (Inamoto & Lee, 2017; Majhail et al., 2012; Schoemans, Lee, et al., 2018). Evidence-based guidelines for the long-term follow-up care of allogeneic HSCT survivors, including surveillance and preventive and preemptive management of long-term and late effects, and for supportive care of survivors with chronic GVHD have also been advanced (Carpenter et al., 2015; Dignan et al., 2012; Majhail

Goals and Outcome Standards
- Patient will exhibit the absence or control of signs and symptoms of potential physiologic and psychosocial problems listed subsequently.
- Patient or significant other will verbalize an understanding of graft-versus-host disease (GVHD) and its potential impact on lifestyle and present and future health status:
  - State the signs and symptoms of common potential complications and the appropriate action to be taken.
  - Describe risk factors for GVHD and measures that the patient can take to reduce the risk of GVHD.
  - Describe measures to minimize the complications of GVHD, including altered skin integrity, nausea and vomiting, diarrhea, liver function abnormalities, fluid and electrolyte abnormalities, malnutrition, infection, pain, body image changes, weakness and activity intolerance, and inadequate or impaired self-monitoring, health maintenance, or treatment adherence.
  - Describe the rationale for the diagnostic tests used to evaluate the signs and symptoms of GVHD.
  - State the name, purpose, scheduling, and major side effects of the treatment approach currently being used to manage GVHD.
  - State appropriate resources for support in coping with GVHD.

Nursing Interventions and Process Standards
Assess, monitor, and detect the following:
- Risk factors for the development of acute and chronic GVHD
- The impact of other preexisting health problems

Prevent the following potential problems and implement nursing interventions as appropriate:
- Altered skin integrity, as evidenced by erythematous, macular, papular skin rash involving the palms, soles, trunk, ears, face, and extremities; bullae, desquamation, and epidermal necrosis may occur, with progression to generalized desquamation of the skin. The skin rash may be painful, burning, or itchy.
  - Monitor skin daily for the development of findings suggestive of GVHD of skin and for the development of infection in areas of skin involved with GVHD.
  - Keep skin lubricated with gentle moisturizing lotions.
  - Consider use of antipruritic or steroid topical agents to manage symptoms.
  - If skin breakdown occurs, consult enterostomal therapist or wound management specialist concerning nonadherent, absorptive dressings and the role of special beds/mattresses.
  - Monitor patient for dehydration if there are increased insensible losses of fluid through skin with bullae and desquamation.
  - Provide patient and family education regarding skin biopsy.
  - Teach patient and family the importance of avoiding direct sun exposure and the importance of using sunblock and protective clothing when outdoors.
  - Consider the need for antimicrobial prophylaxis or topical antimicrobial ointments to minimize secondary infection of open skin lesions.
- Anorexia, nausea, and vomiting, as evidenced by lack of appetite; vague uneasiness/discomfort in the epigastrium, throat, or abdomen; forceful expulsion of stomach contents through the mouth; taste alteration
  - Provide a calm, well-ventilated, aesthetic environment.
  - Discuss approaches to use when experiencing taste changes, early satiety, nausea, or mucositis.
  - Maintain hydration; consider need for total parenteral nutrition.
  - Provide antiemetics.
  - Modify diet to eliminate hot and spicy foods; offer cool, bland foods; provide small, frequent feedings.
  - Absorption of oral medications may be severely impaired. Monitor blood levels of medications carefully and consider switching patient to parenteral formulation.
  - Provide patient and family education regarding endoscopy.
- Diarrhea, as evidenced by profuse, green, mucoid, watery stools mixed with exfoliated cells and tissue shreds, hypoalbuminemia, electrolyte imbalance, fluid imbalance, intestinal bleeding, crampy abdominal pain, and ileus
  - Evaluate history of onset and duration of diarrhea, description of the number of stools, and stool composition; review medication profile and dietary intake to identify any diarrheagenic agents/foods. Review pretreatment history, including usual bowel pattern, usual stool characteristics, and any history of recent travel or family members with diarrhea.
  - Measure the amount of daily diarrhea and assess for the presence of hematochezia, abdominal cramping, and bowel sounds.
  - Evaluate for dehydration, including weight loss, fluid balance, urine-specific gravity, blood urea nitrogen and creatinine (BUN/Cr), and the presence of symptoms such as dizziness or lethargy.
  - Absorption of oral medications may be severely impaired. Monitor blood levels of medications carefully and/or consider switching patient to parenteral formulation, if available.
  - Stop all lactose-containing products and high-osmolar food supplements, such as Ensure Plus®, laxatives, bulk fiber, and stool softeners.
  - Instruct patient to avoid caffeine and alcohol and to consume a low-fat, low-fiber diet. Implement the five-phase diet outlined in Table 7-10, as appropriate.
  - Encourage adequate oral fluids; consider the need for IV fluids to prevent dehydration.
  - Check stool workup, including presence of blood, fecal leukocytes, *Clostridium difficile* toxin, *Salmonella* species, *Campylobacter* species, vancomycin-resistant *Enterococcus*, and viruses.
  - Administer loperamide (two capsules) after every loose stool (maximum daily dose 16 mg or 8 capsules), or 2 every 6 hours around the clock.
  - If symptoms persist, consider tincture of opium at 0.3–1 ml PO every 2–6 hrs as needed (maximum daily dose 6 ml). May titrate upward, as needed.

(Continued on next page)

- If persistent diarrhea, consider octreotide 100–150 mcg three times daily. Consider escalating dose if no response.
- Other pharmacologic agents to consider include diphenoxylate-atropine, cholestyramine, and pancrelipase.
- Consider a trial of oral beclomethasone.
- For chronic diarrhea, consider a trial of pancreatic enzyme replacement or lactase enzyme replacement.
- Consider antibiotic prophylaxis against infection with organisms commonly found in the gut.
- Assess perirectal skin integrity every shift and provide water-barrier ointment to areas to limit skin breakdown.
- Consider enterostomal therapy consultation for input regarding measures to prevent or treat perirectal skin breakdown.
- Provide patient and family education regarding endoscopy procedures.
- Liver function abnormalities, as evidenced by increased bilirubin, alkaline phosphatase, aspartate transaminase, alanine aminotransferase, gamma-glutamyl transpeptidase, 5'-nucleotidase, hepatomegaly, jaundice, and ascites
    - Monitor liver function tests and drug levels of cyclosporine A or tacrolimus at regular intervals.
    - Use caution when prescribing multiple hepatotoxic medications, or, where possible, select medications that are less likely to cause hepatotoxicity.
    - Provide patient and family education regarding invasive procedures, such as liver biopsy.
    - Administer ursodeoxycholic acid as ordered.
- Fluid and electrolyte abnormalities, as evidenced by hypokalemia, hypoalbuminemia, hypomagnesemia, orthostatic hypotension, orthostatic tachycardia, and increased BUN/Cr
    - Reinforce the importance of oral hydration of 2–3 L/day, if not currently on bowel rest. If patient is NPO (nothing by mouth), administer IV fluids as ordered.
    - Rehydrate with 3–4 L of normal saline over a 24-hour period.
    - During aggressive hydration, monitor for fluid overload and pulmonary edema through careful intake and output, serial weights, and clinical assessment.
    - Ensure adequate replacement of fluid lost through diarrhea, third spacing, or desquamation of skin.
    - Replete electrolytes lost through diarrhea.
- Malnutrition, as evidenced by inadequate carbohydrate, protein, or fat intake for needs; weight loss; low prealbumin levels
    - Ensure regular and comprehensive evaluation of nutrition status. Follow GVHD diet, as outlined in Table 7-10, or as per institutional standards or recommendations from clinical dietitian.
    - Monitor calorie counts and fluid intake to assess adequacy of nutrition intake.
    - Discuss approaches to use when experiencing taste changes, thick/viscous saliva and mucus, xerostomia, early satiety, nausea/vomiting, mucositis or esophagitis, and other troubling symptoms.
    - If patient is receiving high-dose steroids, ensure increased protein intake, calcium, and vitamin D supplementation. Consider restricted concentrated carbohydrate intake if hyperglycemia is present. Consider restricted sodium intake if fluid retention is especially problematic.
    - Administer multiple vitamins without iron (to prevent iron overload), folic acid 1 mg by mouth daily.
    - Consider repletion of zinc and supplemental vitamin C if patient presents with extensive skin or gastrointestinal GVHD. Increase protein intake in patients with extensive skin or gastrointestinal GVHD.
- Infection, as evidenced by fever, chills, cough, dyspnea, shortness of breath, chest pain, diarrhea, dysuria, frequency, swelling, drainage, odor, perirectal pain, and change in mental status
    - Teach patient and family self-care strategies that can minimize the risk of infection. Administer prophylactic and empiric antibiotics, as ordered.
    - Consider IV immunoglobulin therapy, if recurrent, life-threatening infections occur.
    - Consider immunization against influenza and *Pneumococcus*, particularly for patients with chronic GVHD.
- Pain, as evidenced by verbalization or expression of pain/discomfort; may report abdominal cramping, muscle aches, oral mucosal pain, or skin pain
    - Reduce diarrhea and associated cramping with loperamide or octreotide.
    - Consider codeine, morphine, dicyclomine hydrochloride, belladonna, and opium or deodorized tincture of opium in the management of spasmodic abdominal pain.
    - Consider the role of a special bed/mattress to reduce pressure if skin is painful to touch. Administer narcotic analgesics as indicated.
- Body image changes, as evidenced by guilt, shame, denial, anger, hostility, despair, avoidance of social interactions, depression, inactivity, and verbalized disgust with body
    - Assess/build upon patient's strengths, appropriate socialization patterns, and coping skills. Encourage maintenance of role responsibilities.
    - Encourage therapeutic interactions with others.
    - Provide for continuity of care with minimal changes in caregiver.
    - Provide privacy to discuss feelings of self-esteem, body image, role performance, and personal identity. Encourage discussion about condition, treatment, and prognosis.
    - Assist with personal grooming.
- Weakness and activity intolerance, as evidenced by focal muscle weakness, fatigue, and dyspnea/shortness of breath
    - Refer to physical and occupational therapy for assessment and treatment.
    - Encourage focus exercises that provide proximal muscle strengthening to reduce proximal muscle weakness that occurs secondary to treatment with corticosteroids.
    - Encourage patient to maintain maximal independence in activities of daily living and self-care.
    - Assess which activities are most important, rewarding, and the patient's priority.
    - Determine a schedule that allows adequate rest by coordinating all activities and treatments (e.g., activities of daily living, medications, health team rounds, patient's habits).
    - Discuss parameters of assessment for tolerance and set goals for improving tolerance/endurance in activities.

(Continued on next page)

- Inadequate or impaired self-monitoring, health maintenance, or treatment adherence, as evidenced by missed appointments, unused/overused medications, questioning need for further treatment, depression, difficulty problem solving, difficulty demonstrating desired skills, inadequate knowledge base, and nonadherence/noncompliance with nursing and/or medical recommendations
  – Establish trust and congruence in goals and objectives.
  – Provide information in a timely and specific manner.
  – Serve as liaison between the physician and patient in interpreting medical jargon and helping patient to acquire needed information.
  – Use positive reinforcement.
  – Allow patient as much choice and control as appropriate and feasible.
  – Encourage self-care whenever possible. Involve patient and family in problem-solving process.
  – Demonstrate care, respect, and concern for the patient.
  – Avoid the use of approaches that foster dependency (e.g., coercion, persuasion, manipulation).

Note. Based on information from Murray et al., 2018; Neumann, 2017.

et al., 2012; Wolff, Bertz, et al., 2011). Innovations including videoconferencing, digital imaging, touchscreen assessments, and other telehealth strategies can strengthen collaboration between tertiary care centers and community-based healthcare providers and reinforce transplant survivor self-management (Hashmi et al., 2017; Schoemans, Goris, et al., 2018). The potential role of these technologies and others in the delivery of risk-adapted, guideline-concordant post-transplant care is currently being explored (Morello, Malagola, Bernardi, Pristipino, & Russo, 2018; Muhsen, Elhassan, & Hashmi, 2018; Rioth et al., 2016). In addition to improving clinical outcomes, such technologies also may reduce healthcare costs and improve patient satisfaction and adherence (Dyer et al., 2016).

Evaluating Outcomes

Outcome evaluation in acute and chronic GVHD is important to provide data concerning the effectiveness of interventions at the individual level and to systematically develop and test new approaches to management in clinical trials. To comprehensively appreciate the health outcomes and patient experience consequent to acute and chronic GVHD and its treatment requires a framework that integrates traditional biomedical indicators, such as disease response, morbidity, and mortality, with performance-based and patient-reported outcome indicators.

Performance-based and instrumented measures assess the characteristics of an individual's performance of a task in daily life. These measures can be used to evaluate outcomes such as physical or cognitive functioning. Examples of performance-based and instrumented indicators include the 2-, 6-, and 12-minute walk tests, grip strength, Timed Up and Go Test, actigraphy, and the Trail Making Test. Although they have had limited application to date in HSCT, evidence suggests that performance-based measures offer complementary and nonredundant information to that gathered by self-report (Douma, Verheul, & Buffart, 2018; Pidala et al., 2013). Performance-based indicators are reproducible, detect clinically meaningful change, predict mortality, and are safe to perform using prescribed procedures (Ferriolli et al., 2012; Pidala et al.,

2013). Patient-reported outcome measures are evaluated by self-report domains that include self-rated health status and perception of disease and treatment effects, such as symptoms and health-related quality of life (Shaw, 2019). Such outcomes are complementary to clinician-assessed outcomes derived from physical examination and diagnostic testing. The inclusion of performance-based and patient-reported outcome indicators adds clinically meaningful context and provides information about the factors that mediate outcome disparities relative to endpoints such as disease response, morbidity, and overall survival. Performance-based and patient-reported outcomes also can help identify impairments that would otherwise remain undetected (Morishita et al., 2017). Such indicators are essential for comparative effectiveness research, thus producing a more complete determination of what interventions work best for whom.

The National Institutes of Health criteria for evaluating therapeutic response in chronic GVHD were published in 2006 and updated in 2015 (S.J. Lee et al., 2015). As shown in Table 7-11, the criteria include core and ancillary measures and encompass objective indicators, clinician-assessed indicators, and patient-reported outcomes. Measurement domains were conceptually defined, and measures were specifically selected to represent each of those domains—namely, chronic GVHD signs, symptoms, global ratings, functional status, and quality of life. Outcome evaluation should occur at three-month intervals and whenever a major change in treatment occurs. Provisional definitions of complete response, partial response, and disease progression for each organ and for overall response also have been proposed (S.J. Lee et al., 2015). Standardized terminologies and guidance for standardized assessment of acute and chronic GVHD and clinical data collection have been endorsed as well (Harris et al., 2016; Schoemans, Lee, et al., 2018).

Preclinical and Developmental Strategies for Prophylaxis, Treatment, and Control

A wide variety of approaches to the prevention, treatment, and control of GVHD are currently in development

Figure 7-13. Summary Record of Graft-Versus-Host Disease Prophylaxis and Treatment

Type of transplant:

☐ Related, 12/12 matched   ☐ Haploidentical   ☐ Matched, unrelated   ☐ Other: _____

Stem cell source:

☐ Peripheral blood   ☐ Bone marrow   ☐ Cord blood

Disease:

☐ Acute myeloid leukemia   ☐ Acute lymphoblastic leukemia   ☐ Chronic myeloid leukemia   ☐ Aplastic anemia   ☐ Hodgkin lymphoma

☐ Non-Hodgkin lymphoma   ☐ Multiple myeloma

Other:_____

Conditioning regimen:

☐ Ablative   ☐ Nonmyeloablative

☐ T-cell depleted   ☐ T-cell repleted

Cell dose: _____ CD34+ cells/kg: _____ CD3+ cells/kg _____ Date of transplant: _____

Donor CMV status: ☐ Reactive   ☐ Non-reactive

Recipient ABO:_____

Donor ABO: _____

Date of initial engraftment of WBC (ANC > 1,000 for two days): _____

Dates and dose of donor lymphocyte infusion:

_____ cells/kg

_____ cells/kg

_____ cells/kg

_____ cells/kg

Initial GVHD Prophylaxis:

☐ Cyclosporine A   ☐ Tacrolimus   ☐ Methotrexate ___ mg/m² on days _____, _____, _____

Methylprednisolone/Methylprednisolone sodium succinate: _____

Other: _____

Extent of GVHD

Date	Site(s) of GVHD	Biopsy Findings	Stage/Grade Acute/Chronic	Performance Status

GVHD Management Plan

Therapy/Treatment	Date Therapy Initiated/ Modified	Reason Initiated/ Modified	Maximum Overall GVHD Grade	Other Findings/ Comments

ANC—absolute neutrophil count; CMV—cytomegalovirus; GVHD—graft-versus-host disease; WBC—white blood cell

Table 7-11. National Institutes of Health Therapeutic Response Criteria Measures

Measure	Clinician Reported	Patient Reported
Core Domains/Measures		
Signs	Organ-specific measures	–
Symptoms	Clinician assessed	Lee Symptom Scale
Global ratings	7-point rating of change in chronic GVHD severity	7-point rating of change in chronic GVHD severity
	Chronic GVHD severity (mild, moderate, severe)	Chronic GVHD severity (mild, moderate, severe)
	0–10 chronic GVHD symptom severity scale	0–10 chronic GVHD symptom severity scale
Ancillary Domains/Measures		
Function	Grip strength 2-minute walk time	Human Activity Profile
Performance status	Karnofsky or Lansky Performance Status Scale	–
Health-related quality of life	–	Functional Assessment of Cancer Therapy–Bone Marrow Transplant Medical Health Outcomes Study Short Form-36® v.2

GVHD—graft-versus-host disease

Note. Based on information from Jagasia et al., 2015; S.J. Lee, 2017.

(Baron et al., 2014; Cutler et al., 2017; Hill et al., 2018; Im et al., 2017; Servais et al., 2016; Villa & McFadden, 2018; Zeiser, 2018; Zeiser & Blazar, 2017; Zeiser, Sarantopoulos, & Blazar, 2018). Strategies currently in preclinical and clinical testing include the use of regulatory T cells, mesenchymal stromal cells, or microbiome manipulation; agents that inhibit B cells or achieve in vivo B-cell depletion; cellular suicide gene therapy to prevent or control GVHD; novel agents for cytokine modulation; new monoclonal antibodies; and agents that prevent or treat GVHD by inhibiting key immunologic pathways including the proteasome, the JAK/STAT pathway, or the Rho-associated protein kinase (Hill et al., 2018; Im et al., 2017; Villa et al., 2016).

The ability to predict which patients are at greatest risk for GVHD or to identify patients with only biochemical serologic evidence of developing GVHD is important both for clinical trial design and clinical management. Although patients at higher risk for acute GVHD may benefit from special treatment or intensified immunosuppression, at present, the degree of GVHD that will occur in an individual patient cannot be precisely anticipated. Research efforts are ongoing to develop in vitro testing methods and sensitive predictive assays that can estimate an individual patient's likelihood of developing GVHD and provide a clinically useful early indicator of evolving GVHD and a biologic measure of response to treatment (Ferrara & Chaudhry, 2018; Paczesny, 2018).

Increasingly, graft engineering and immune regulatory cell infusion approaches may be a component of the prevention or control of GVHD (Blazar et al., 2018). For example, in animal models, the addition to the graft of a subset of regulatory (CD4+, CD25+) donor T cells that were exposed to recipient antigens and then expanded ex vivo delayed or even prevented the onset of GVHD without altering post-transplant immune reconstitution (Filippini & Rutella, 2014). Investigators are focused on attempts to remove from the graft only the alloreactive T cells—the ones presumed to be major effectors of GVHD (Villa et al., 2016). Efforts also are underway to develop methods of deactivating, rather than removing, T cells within the graft, thus inducing a state of tolerance. Researchers are exploring whether GVHD can be controlled through insertion of a suicide gene into donor T cells at the time of engraftment. With this method, donor T cells are transfected with a gene-encoding herpes simplex type 1 thymidine kinase (TK) prior to transplant, and patients are then given a short course of ganciclovir. In this system, ganciclovir selectively kills dividing but not quiescent TK-gene-transfected T cells. When the TK-gene-transfected donor T cells proliferate and divide to create GVHD, they are selectively eliminated by the ganciclovir. The pool of nonreactive, nondividing T cells is spared, thus contributing to recipient immune system reconstitution and graft-versus-tumor effect (Villa et al., 2016).

The expanding knowledge of the cellular and molecular pathways that initiate and sustain GVHD provides a foundation for preclinical and clinical testing of immune regulatory cell infusions to prevent or treat acute and chronic GVHD. Mesenchymal stromal cells are multipotent cells that can develop into connective tissue (e.g., bone or cartilage), but they also have immunomodulatory and anti-inflammatory properties (Castro-Manrreza & Montesinos, 2015; Dunavin, Dias, Li, & McGuirk, 2017). Mesenchymal stromal cells can be isolated from several different tissue sources (e.g., bone marrow, fat, umbilical cord) and then culture-expanded in large numbers in the laboratory. In addition, an off-the-shelf preparation (remestemcel-L) manufactured using bone marrow from healthy human donors has been developed (Locatelli, Algeri, Trevisan, & Bertaina, 2017). The mesenchymal stromal cell product is infused intravenously in single or multiple doses, either concurrent with infusion of the stem cell transplant (as GVHD prophylaxis) (Kallekleiv, Larun, Bruserud, & Hatfield, 2016), or following stem cell transplantation, as treatment for GVHD. Research in both animal models and in humans is ongoing to define the biologic effects, mechanisms of action, and efficacy of mesenchymal stromal cells with respect to the prevention and treatment of acute or chronic GVHD. Some encouraging evidence supports their use in the treatment of steroid-refractory acute GVHD (Bozdağ, Tekgündüz, & Altuntaş, 2016; Munneke et al., 2016), and these cellular products appear to be well tolerated with no infusion-related toxicity (Fisher et al., 2019). However, while some studies suggest that cotransplantation of mesenchymal stromal cells may reduce the risk of chronic but not acute GVHD, overall the quality of evidence is low (Fisher et al., 2019; Kallekleiv et al., 2016). More than a dozen ongoing trials are examining the effects of differing mesenchymal stromal cell product sources, timing of infusion, cell dosage, administration schedule, and production protocol for the prevention and treatment of acute and chronic GVHD (Bozdağ et al., 2016; Fisher et al., 2019).

The success of DLI for the treatment of post-transplant relapse of chronic myeloid leukemia has led researchers to explore the role of combining T-cell depletion with a preplanned course of DLI post-transplant (Chang et al., 2016). This approach is potentially attractive in that one can reap the benefits of T-cell depletion early after transplant by minimizing acute GVHD yet be able to restore the graft-versus-tumor effect at a later time with DLI (Yan et al., 2020). In nonmyeloablative transplantation, early patterns of chimerism may allow clinicians to predict the time frame following HSCT at which the individual is at greatest risk for GVHD. This information can be used to guide decisions about post-transplant immunosuppression and the dose and timing of post-transplant DLI (Mo et al., 2017). Currently, however, GVHD remains a major complication of DLI even when DLI is administered at a time when the patient is removed from the conditioning therapy and its associated inflammatory cytokine milieu (Scarisbrick et al., 2015).

Induction of Graft-Versus-Host Disease: Preserving the Graft-Versus-Tumor Effect

Strategies for preventing GVHD are designed to limit the capacity of the newly grafted immune system to mount an immunologic response. These strategies have reduced the severity of GVHD; however, they are associated with higher rates of graft failure and disease relapse (Chang et al., 2016). It is now apparent that patients who develop GVHD have a lower risk of recurrent disease than patients without GVHD. Indirect evidence of a graft-versus-tumor effect includes the observations that T-cell depletion of the HSCT graft and syngeneic HSCT are associated with a higher risk of relapse than allogeneic HSCT. It has been demonstrated clinically that graft-versus-tumor responses occur with DLI in 60%–80% of patients with chronic myeloid leukemia and to a lesser extent with acute myeloid leukemia, chronic lymphocytic leukemia, multiple myeloma, non-Hodgkin lymphoma, and renal cell carcinomas (Chang et al., 2016). Both GVHD and the graft-versus-tumor effect are thought to be mediated by alloreactive donor T cells and NK cells recognizing host histocompatibility antigens. This hypothesis has subsequently led to the use of DLI as well as other methods to augment the graft-versus-host response in an effort to prevent or treat disease relapse.

The initial step in promoting a graft-versus-tumor response to treat disease relapse involves immediate withdrawal of immunosuppressants. The allogeneic stem cell donor then is contacted for collection of lymphocytes by leukapheresis. The lymphocytes are infused into the patient, often as an outpatient procedure. DLI has few immediate effects; however, it has a 20% incidence of treatment-related mortality, mainly because of life-threatening GVHD and pancytopenia (Scarisbrick et al., 2015). Severe acute GVHD (grades 2–4) following DLI occurs in 40%–55% of patients, and pancytopenia occurs in approximately 20% of patients (Orti et al., 2017). Pancytopenia may resolve spontaneously but may require an infusion of donor stem cells to reestablish hematopoiesis. Following DLI, patients require close follow-up to monitor their disease response to DLI, determine the need for escalating DLI doses, ensure the earliest identification and appropriate treatment of signs of GVHD, and receive comprehensive supportive care to prevent and manage the effects of pancytopenia.

Escalating doses of DLI, as measured by the DLI product's CD34+ cell dose per kilogram of the patient's body weight, may be used to achieve an adequate graft-versus-tumor effect without producing life-threatening GVHD (de Witte et al., 2017). Studies have suggested that patients with greater tumor cell burdens, as in the case of a hematologic relapse, require greater DLI cell doses than do patients in cytogenetic or molecular relapse (Castagna et al., 2016).

It is possible for patients to have an allogeneic graft-versus-tumor effect that is not associated with clinically evident GVHD. Research is ongoing to identify strategies to augment the graft-versus-tumor effect while minimizing or separating it from GVHD (Chang et al., 2016). These approaches include selective depletion of allo-activated donor T lymphocytes from the DLI, escalating the lymphocyte cell dose infused to establish a dose that will stimulate graft-versus-tumor effect but that is below the threshold that produces severe GVHD, and combining DLI with pharmacologic treatment of relapse (Chang et al., 2016; Y.-B. Chen et al., 2018).

Summary

GVHD is a direct result of one of the principal functions of the immune system: the distinction of self from nonself. The pathophysiology of GVHD involves recognition of epithelial target tissues within the host as foreign by immunocompetent cells contained in the graft, resulting in an inflammatory response and eventual apoptotic death of the target tissue. Despite an improved understanding of the pathogenesis of GVHD and the new and more targeted approaches to immunosuppression, graft engineering, and adoptive immunotherapy that are emerging at a rapid pace, GVHD remains a major cause of morbidity and mortality after HSCT.

Oncology and HSCT nurses have important roles in the care of patients experiencing this complication. Key nursing responsibilities include (a) safely and effectively administering a multidrug regimen to prevent or treat GVHD, (b) monitoring patients for the effectiveness and side effects of GVHD-directed treatment, (c) providing patient and family education to ensure adherence to therapy and effective self-management of expected side effects, (d) assessing and managing symptoms such as infection risk, fluid and electrolyte imbalance, nutritional compromise, altered skin integrity, and discomfort, and (e) facilitating coordination and continuity of care and appropriate ongoing follow-up.

References

Abdul Wahid, S.F., Ismail, N.-A., Mohd-Idris, M.-R., Jamaluddin, F.W., Tumian, N., Sze-Wei, E.Y., ... Nai, M.L. (2014). Comparison of reduced-intensity and myeloablative conditioning regimens for allogeneic hematopoietic stem cell transplantation in patients with acute myeloid leukemia and acute lymphoblastic leukemia: A meta-analysis. *Stem Cells and Development, 23*, 2535–2552. https://doi.org/10.1089/scd.2014.0123

Abouelnasr, A., Roy, J., Cohen, S., Kiss, T., & Lachance, S. (2013). Defining the role of sirolimus in the management of graft-versus-host disease: From prophylaxis to treatment. *Biology of Blood and Marrow Transplantation, 19*, 12–21. https://doi.org/10.1016/j.bbmt.2012.06.020

Afram, G., Simón, J.A.P., Remberger, M., Caballero-Velázquez, T., Martino, R., Piñana, J.L., ... Hägglund, H. (2018). Reduced intensity conditioning increases risk of severe cGVHD: Identification of risk factors for cGVHD in a multicenter setting. *Medical Oncology, 35*, 79. https://doi.org/10.1007/s12032-018-1127-2

Ahn, H., Tay, J., Shea, B., Hutton, B., Shorr, R., Knoll, G.A., ... Cowan, J. (2018). Effectiveness of immunoglobulin prophylaxis in reducing clinical complications of hematopoietic stem cell transplantation: A systematic review and meta-analysis. *Transfusion, 58*, 2437–2452. https://doi.org/10.1111/trf.14656

Akirov, A., Sawka, A.M., Ben-Baruch, S., Lipton, J., & Ezzat, S. (2019). Endocrine complications in patients with GVHD. *Endocrine Practice, 25*, 485–490. https://doi.org/10.4158/ep-2018-0529

Akpek, G., Chinratanalab, W., Lee, L.A., Torbenson, M., Hallick, J.P., Anders, V., & Vogelsang, G.B. (2003). Gastrointestinal involvement in chronic graft-versus-host disease: A clinicopathologic study. *Biology of Blood and Marrow Transplantation, 9*, 46–51. https://doi.org/10.1053/bbmt.2003.49999

Albuquerque, R., Khan, Z., Poveda, A., Higham, J., Richards, A., Monteiro, L., ... Warnakulasuriya, S. (2016). Management of oral graft versus host disease with topical agents: A systematic review. *Medicina Oral, Patología Oral y Cirugía Bucal, 21*, e72–e81. https://doi.org/10.4317/medoral.20968

Alho, A.C., Kim, H.T., Chammas, M.J., Reynolds, C.G., Matos, T.R., Forcade, E., ... Ritz, J. (2016). Unbalanced recovery of regulatory and effector T cells after allogeneic stem cell transplantation contributes to chronic GVHD. *Blood, 127*, 646–657. https://doi.org/10.1182/blood-2015-10-672345

Al-Homsi, A.S., Feng, Y., Duffner, U., Al Malki, M.M., Goodyke, A., Cole, K., ... Abdel-Mageed, A. (2016). Bortezomib for the prevention and treatment of graft-versus-host disease after allogeneic hematopoietic stem cell transplantation. *Experimental Hematology, 44*, 771–777. https://doi.org/10.1016/j.exphem.2016.05.005

Al-Homsi, A.S., Roy, T.S., Cole, K., Feng, Y., & Duffner, U. (2015). Post-transplant high-dose cyclophosphamide for the prevention of graft-versus-host disease. *Biology of Blood and Marrow Transplantation, 21*, 604–611. https://doi.org/10.1016/j.bbmt.2014.08.014

Ali, R., Ramdial, J., Algaze, S., & Beitinjaneh, A. (2017). The role of anti-thymocyte globulin or alemtuzumab-based serotherapy in the prophylaxis and management of graft-versus-host disease. *Biomedicines, 5*, 1–22. https://doi.org/10.3390/biomedicines5040067

Allison, T.L. (2016). Immunosuppressive therapy in transplantation. *Nursing Clinics of North America, 51*, 107–120. https://doi.org/10.1016/j.cnur.2015.10.008

Amouzegar, A., Dey, B.R., & Spitzer, T.R. (2019). Peripheral blood or bone marrow stem cells? Practical considerations in hematopoietic stem cell transplantation. *Transfusion Medicine Reviews, 33*, 43–50. https://doi.org/10.1016/j.tmrv.2018.11.003

Anasetti, C. (2015). Use of alternative donors for allogeneic stem cell transplantation. *American Society of Hematology Education Program Book, 2015*, 220–224. https://doi.org/10.1182/asheducation-2015.1.220

Anghel, D., Tanasescu, R., Campeanu, A., Lupescu, I., Podda, G., & Bajenaru, O. (2013). Neurotoxicity of immunosuppressive therapies in organ transplantation. *Maedica, 8*, 170–175.

Arai, Y., Jo, T., Matsui, H., Kondo, T., & Takaori-Kondo, A. (2017). Efficacy of antithymocyte globulin for allogeneic hematopoietic cell transplantation: A systematic review and meta-analysis. *Leukemia and Lymphoma, 58*, 1840–1848. https://doi.org/10.1080/10428194.2016.1266624

Bakhsh, H.R., Mohammed, J., & Hashmi, S.K. (2018). Are graft-versus-host-disease patients missing out on the vital occupational therapy services? A systematic review. *International Journal of Rehabilitation Research, 41*, 110–113. https://doi.org/10.1097/mrr.0000000000000275

Baron, F., Humblet-Baron, S., Ehx, G., Servais, S., Hannon, M., Belle, L., ... Beguin, Y. (2014). Thinking out of the box—New approaches to controlling GVHD. *Current Hematologic Malignancy Reports, 9*, 73–84. https://doi.org/10.1007/s11899-013-0187-9

Baumgartner, A., Bargetzi, A., Zueger, N., Bargetzi, M., Medinger, M., Bounoure, L., ... Schuetz, P. (2017). Revisiting nutritional support for allogeneic hematologic stem cell transplantation—A systematic review. *Bone Marrow Transplantation, 52*, 506–513. https://doi.org/10.1038/bmt.2016.310

Beckerson, J., Szydlo, R.M., Hickson, M., Mactier, C.E., Innes, A.J., Gabriel, I.H., ... Pavlu, J. (2019). Impact of route and adequacy of nutritional intake on outcomes of allogeneic haematopoietic cell transplantation for haematologic malignancies. *Clinical Nutrition, 38*, 738–744. https://doi.org/10.1016/j.clnu.2018.03.008

Bevans, M., El-Jawahri, A., Tierney, D.K., Wiener, L., Wood, W.A., Hoodin, F., ... Syrjala, K.L. (2017). National Institutes of Health Hematopoietic Cell Transplantation Late Effects Initiative: The Patient-Centered Outcomes Working Group report. *Biology of Blood and Marrow Transplantation, 23*, 538–551. https://doi.org/10.1016/j.bbmt.2016.09.011

Bhatia, S., Francisco, L., Carter, A., Sun, C.-L., Baker, K.S., Gurney, J.G., ... Weisdorf, D.J. (2007). Late mortality after allogeneic hematopoietic cell transplantation and functional status of long-term survivors: Report from the Bone Marrow Transplant Survivor Study. *Blood, 110*, 3784–3792. https://doi.org/10.1182/blood-2007-03-082933

Bilic, E., Delimar, V., Desnica, L., Pulanic, D., Bilic, E., Bakovic, M., ... Pavletic, S.Z. (2016). High prevalence of small- and large-fiber neuropathy in a prospective cohort of patients with moderate to severe chronic GvHD. *Bone Marrow Transplantation, 51,* 1513–1517. https://doi.org/10.1038/bmt.2016.158

Bittenbring, J., & Reichrath, J. (2016). Extracorporeal photopheresis for non-skin GvHD. *Anticancer Research, 36,* 1395–1396.

Blazar, B.R., MacDonald, K.P.A., & Hill, G.R. (2018). Immune regulatory cell infusion for graft-versus-host disease prevention and therapy. *Blood, 131,* 2651–2660. https://doi.org/10.1182/blood-2017-11-785865

Botti, S., Liptrott, S.J., Gargiulo, G., & Orlando, L. (2015). Nutritional support in patients undergoing haematopoietic stem cell transplantation: A multicentre survey of the Gruppo Italiano Trapianto Midollo Osseo (GITMO) transplant programmes. *Ecancermedicalscience, 9,* 545. https://doi.org/10.3332/ecancer.2015.545

Bourassa-Blanchette, S., Knoll, G., Tay, J., Bredeson, C., Cameron, D.W., & Cowan, J. (2017). A national survey of screening and management of hypogammaglobulinemia in Canadian transplantation centers. *Transplant Infectious Disease, 19,* e12706. https://doi.org/10.1111/tid.12706

Bozdağ, S.C., Tekgündüz, E., & Altuntaş, F. (2016). Treatment of acute graft versus host disease with mesancyhmal stem cells: Questions and answers. *Transfusion and Apheresis Science, 54,* 71–75. https://doi.org/10.1016/j.transci.2016.01.016

Busca, A., & Aversa, F. (2017). In-vivo or ex-vivo T cell depletion or both to prevent graft-versus-host disease after hematopoietic stem cell transplantation. *Expert Opinion on Biological Therapy, 17,* 1401–1415. https://doi.org/10.1080/14712598.2017.1369949

Byrne, M., Savani, B.N., Mohty, M., & Nagler, A. (2016). Peripheral blood stem cell versus bone marrow transplantation: A perspective from the Acute Leukemia Working Party of the European Society for Blood and Marrow Transplantation. *Experimental Hematology, 44,* 567–573. https://doi.org/10.1016/j.exphem.2016.04.005

Camargo, J.F., & Komanduri, K.V. (2017). Emerging concepts in cytomegalovirus infection following hematopoietic stem cell transplantation. *Hematology/Oncology and Stem Cell Therapy, 10,* 233–238. https://doi.org/10.1016/j.hemonc.2017.05.001

Carpenter, P.A., Kitko, C.L., Elad, S., Flowers, M.E., Gea-Banacloche, J.C., Halter, J.P., ... Couriel, D.R. (2015). National Institutes of Health Consensus Development Project on Criteria for Clinical Trials in Chronic Graft-versus-Host Disease: V. The 2014 Ancillary Therapy and Supportive Care Working Group report. *Biology of Blood and Marrow Transplantation, 21,* 1167–1187. https://doi.org/10.1016/j.bbmt.2015.03.024

Castagna, L., Sarina, B., Bramanti, S., Perseghin, P., Mariotti, J., & Morabito, L. (2016). Donor lymphocyte infusion after allogeneic stem cell transplantation. *Transfusion and Apheresis Science, 54,* 345–355. https://doi.org/10.1016/j.transci.2016.05.011

Castro-Manrreza, M.E., & Montesinos, J.J. (2015). Immunoregulation by mesenchymal stem cells: Biological aspects and clinical applications. *Journal of Immunology Research, 2015,* 1–20. https://doi.org/10.1155/2015/394917

Caulier, A., Drumez, E., Gauthier, J., Robin, M., Blaise, D., Beguin, Y., ... Yakoub-Agha, I. (2018). Scoring system based on post-transplant complications in patients after allogeneic hematopoietic cell transplantation for myelodysplastic syndrome: A study from the SFGM-TC. *Current Research in Translational Medicine, 67,* 8–15. https://doi.org/10.1016/j.retram.2018.08.003

Chang, X., Zang, X., & Xia, C.-Q. (2016). New strategies of DLI in the management of relapse of hematological malignancies after allogeneic hematopoietic SCT. *Bone Marrow Transplantation, 51,* 324–332. https://doi.org/10.1038/bmt.2015.288

Chen, X., & Mayne, C.G. (2018). The role of micronutrients in graft-vs.-host disease: Immunomodulatory effects of vitamins A and D. *Frontiers in Immunology, 9,* 2853. https://doi.org/10.3389/fimmu.2018.02853

Chen, Y.-B., McCarthy, P.L., Hahn, T., Holstein, S.A., Ueda, M., Kröger, N., ... de Lima, M. (2018). Methods to prevent and treat relapse after hematopoietic stem cell transplantation with tyrosine kinase inhibitors, immunomodulating drugs, deacetylase inhibitors, and hypomethylating agents. *Bone Marrow Transplantation, 54,* 497–507. https://doi.org/10.1038/s41409-018-0269-3

Cho, A., Jantschitsch, C., & Knobler, R. (2018). Extracorporeal photopheresis—An overview. *Frontiers in Medicine, 5,* 236. https://doi.org/10.3389/fmed.2018.00236

Cho, C., & Perales, M.-A. (2019). Expanding therapeutic opportunities for hematopoietic stem cell transplantation: T cell depletion as a model for the targeted allograft. *Annual Review of Medicine, 70,* 381–393. https://doi.org/10.1146/annurev-med-120617-041210

Choi, S.W., & Reddy, P. (2014). Current and emerging strategies for the prevention of graft-versus-host disease. *Nature Reviews Clinical Oncology, 11,* 536–547. https://doi.org/10.1038/nrclinonc.2014.102

Clark, C.A., Savani, M., Mohty, M., & Savani, B.N. (2016). What do we need to know about allogeneic hematopoietic stem cell transplant survivors? *Bone Marrow Transplantation, 51,* 1025–1031. https://doi.org/10.1038/bmt.2016.95

Conrad, A., Alcazer, V., Valour, F., & Ader, F. (2018). Vaccination post-allogeneic hematopoietic stem cell transplantation: What is feasible? *Expert Review of Vaccines, 17,* 299–309. https://doi.org/10.1080/14760584.2018.1449649

Cooke, K.R., Luznik, L., Sarantopoulos, S., Hakim, F.T., Jagasia, M., Fowler, D.H., ... Blazar, B.R. (2017). The biology of chronic graft-versus-host disease: A task force report from the National Institutes of Health Consensus Development Project on Criteria for Clinical Trials in Chronic Graft-versus-Host Disease. *Biology of Blood and Marrow Transplantation, 23,* 211–234. https://doi.org/10.1016/j.bbmt.2016.09.023

Cornejo, C.M., Kim, E.J., Rosenbach, M., & Micheletti, R.G. (2015). Atypical manifestations of graft-versus-host disease. *Journal of the American Academy of Dermatology, 72,* 690–695. https://doi.org/10.1016/j.jaad.2014.12.022

Cowen, E.W., Nguyen, J.C., Miller, D.D., McShane, D., Arron, S.T., Prose, N.S., ... Fox, L.P. (2010). Chronic phototoxicity and aggressive squamous cell carcinoma of the skin in children and adults during treatment with voriconazole. *Journal of the American Academy of Dermatology, 62,* 31–37. https://doi.org/10.1016/j.jaad.2009.09.033

Cromvik, J., Johnsson, M., Vaht, K., Johansson, J.-E., & Wenneras, C. (2014). Eosinophils in the blood of hematopoietic stem cell transplanted patients are activated and have different molecular marker profiles in acute and chronic graft-versus-host disease. *Immunity, Inflammation and Disease, 2,* 99–113. https://doi.org/10.1002/iid3.25

Cutler, C.S., Koreth, J., & Ritz, J. (2017). Mechanistic approaches for the prevention and treatment of chronic GVHD. *Blood, 129,* 22–29. https://doi.org/10.1182/blood-2016-08-686659

Das-Gupta, E., Dignan, F., Shaw, B., Raj, K., Malladi, R., Gennery, A., ... Scarisbrick, J. (2014). Extracorporeal photopheresis for treatment of adults and children with acute GVHD: UK consensus statement and review of published literature. *Bone Marrow Transplantation, 49,* 1251–1258. https://doi.org/10.1038/bmt.2014.106

da Silva, M.B., da Cunha, F.F., Terra, F.F., & Camara, N.O. (2017). Old game, new players: Linking classical theories to new trends in transplant immunology. *World Journal of Transplantation, 7,* 1–25. https://doi.org/10.5500/wjt.v7.i1.1

Del Fante, C., Galasso, T., Bernasconi, P., Scudeller, L., Ripamonti, F., Perotti, C., & Meloni, F. (2016). Extracorporeal photopheresis as a new supportive therapy for bronchiolitis obliterans syndrome after allogeneic stem cell transplantation. *Bone Marrow Transplantation, 51,* 728–731. https://doi.org/10.1038/bmt.2015.324

de Witte, T., Bowen, D., Robin, M., Malcovati, L., Niederwieser, D., Yakoub-Agha, I., ... Kröger, N. (2017). Allogeneic hematopoietic stem cell transplantation for MDS and CMML: Recommendations from an international expert panel. *Blood, 129,* 1753–1762. https://doi.org/10.1182/blood-2016-06-724500

Dietrich-Ntoukas, T., Cursiefen, C., Westekemper, H., Eberwein, P., Reinhard, T., Bertz, H., ... Wolff, D. (2012). Diagnosis and treatment of ocular chronic graft-versus-host disease: Report from the German-Austrian-Swiss Consensus Conference on Clinical Practice in chronic GVHD. *Cornea, 31,* 299–310. https://doi.org/10.1097/ico.0b013e318226bf97

Dignan, F.L., Scarisbrick, J.J., Cornish, J., Clark, A., Amrolia, P., Jackson, G., ... Shaw, B.E. (2012). Organ-specific management and supportive care in chronic graft-versus-host disease. *British Journal of Haematology, 158,* 62–78. https://doi.org/10.1111/j.1365-2141.2012.09131.x

Douma, J.A.J., Verheul, H.M.W., & Buffart, L.M. (2018). Are patient-reported outcomes of physical function a valid substitute for objective measurements? *Current Oncology, 25,* e475–e479. https://doi.org/10.3747/co.25.4080

Dunavin, N., Dias, A., Li, M., & McGuirk, J. (2017). Mesenchymal stromal cells: What is the mechanism in acute graft-versus-host disease? *Biomedicines, 5*, 1–16. https://doi.org/10.3390/biomedicines5030039

Dyer, G., Gilroy, N., Brown, L., Hogg, M., Brice, L., Kabir, M., ... Kerridge, I. (2016). What they want: Inclusion of blood and marrow transplantation survivor preference in the development of models of care for long-term health in Sydney, Australia. *Biology of Blood and Marrow Transplantation, 22*, 731–743. https://doi.org/10.1016/j.bbmt.2015.12.019

El-Ghammaz, A.M.S., Ben Matoug, R., Elzimaity, M., & Mostafa, N. (2017). Nutritional status of allogeneic hematopoietic stem cell transplantation recipients: Influencing risk factors and impact on survival. *Supportive Care in Cancer, 25*, 3085–3093. https://doi.org/10.1007/s00520-017-3716-6

El-Jawahri, A., Li, S., Antin, J.H., Spitzer, T.R., Armand, P.A., Koreth, J., ... Chen, Y.-B. (2016). Improved treatment-related mortality and overall survival of patients with grade IV acute GVHD in the modern years. *Biology of Blood and Marrow Transplantation, 22*, 910–918. https://doi.org/10.1016/j.bbmt.2015.12.024

El-Jawahri, A., Pidala, J., Khera, N., Wood, W.A., Arora, M., Carpenter, P.A., ... Lee, S.J. (2018). Impact of psychological distress on quality of life, functional status, and survival in patients with chronic graft-versus-host disease. *Biology of Blood and Marrow Transplantation, 24*, 2285–2292. https://doi.org/10.1016/j.bbmt.2018.07.020

Elsaadany, B.A., Ahmed, E.M., & Aghbary, S.M.H. (2017). Efficacy and safety of topical corticosteroids for management of oral chronic graft versus host disease. *International Journal of Dentistry, 2017*, 1908768. https://doi.org/10.1155/2017/1908768

Enderby, C., & Keller, C.A. (2015). An overview of immunosuppression in solid organ transplantation. *American Journal of Managed Care, 21*(Suppl. 1), s12–s23.

Ferrara, J.L.M., & Chaudhry, M.S. (2018). GVHD: Biology matters. *Blood Advances, 2*, 3411–3417. https://doi.org/10.1182/bloodadvances.2018020214

Ferrara, J.L.M., Levine, J.E., Reddy, P., & Holler, E. (2009). Graft-versus-host disease. *Lancet, 373*, 1550–1561. https://doi.org/10.1016/s0140-6736(09)60237-3

Ferriolli, E., Skipworth, R.J., Hendry, P., Scott, A., Stensteth, J., Dahele, M., ... Fearon, K.C. (2012). Physical activity monitoring: A responsive and meaningful patient-centered outcome for surgery, chemotherapy, or radiotherapy? *Journal of Pain and Symptom Management, 43*, 1025–1035. https://doi.org/10.1016/j.jpainsymman.2011.06.013

Filipovich, A.H., Weisdorf, D., Pavletic, S., Socie, G., Wingard, J.R., Lee, S.J., ... Flowers, M.E.D. (2005). National Institutes of Health Consensus Development Project on Criteria for Clinical Trials in Chronic Graft-Versus-Host Disease: I. Diagnosis and Staging Working Group report. *Biology of Blood and Marrow Transplantation, 11*, 945–956. https://doi.org/10.1016/j.bbmt.2005.09.004

Filippini, P., & Rutella, S. (2014). Recent advances on cellular therapies and immune modulators for graft-versus-host disease. *Expert Review of Clinical Immunology, 10*, 1357–1374. https://doi.org/10.1586/1744666x.2014.955475

Fisher, S.A., Cutler, A., Dorée, C., Brunskill, S.J., Stanworth, S.J., Navarrete, C., & Girdlestone, J. (2019). Mesenchymal stromal cells as treatment or prophylaxis for acute or chronic graft-versus-host disease in haematopoietic stem cell transplant (HSCT) recipients with a haematological condition. *Cochrane Database of Systematic Reviews, 2019*(1). https://doi.org/10.1002/14651858.cd009768.pub2

Fisher, S.A., Lamikanra, A., Dorée, C., Gration, B., Tsang, P., Danby, R.D., & Roberts, D.J. (2017). Increased regulatory T cell graft content is associated with improved outcome in haematopoietic stem cell transplantation: A systematic review. *British Journal of Haematology, 176*, 448–463. https://doi.org/10.1111/bjh.14433

Flowers, M.E.D., & Martin, P.J. (2015). How we treat chronic graft-versus-host disease. *Blood, 125*, 606–615. https://doi.org/10.1182/blood-2014-08-551994

Fuji, S., Einsele, H., Savani, B.N., & Kapp, M. (2015). Systematic nutritional support in allogeneic hematopoietic stem cell transplant recipients. *Biology of Blood and Marrow Transplantation, 21*, 1707–1713. https://doi.org/10.1016/j.bbmt.2015.07.003

Gagelmann, N., Ayuk, F., Wolschke, C., & Kröger, N. (2017). Comparison of different rabbit anti-thymocyte globulin formulations in allogeneic stem cell transplantation: Systematic literature review and network meta-analysis. *Biology of Blood and Marrow Transplantation, 23*, 2184–2191. https://doi.org/10.1016/j.bbmt.2017.08.027

Gandelman, J.S., Song, D.J., Chen, H., Engelhardt, B.G., Chen, Y.-B., Clark, W.B., ... Jagasia, M. (2018). A prospective trial of extracorporeal photopheresis for chronic graft-versus-host disease reveals significant disease response and no association with frequency of regulatory T cells. *Biology of Blood and Marrow Transplantation, 24*, 2373–2380. https://doi.org/10.1016/j.bbmt.2018.06.035

Ganta, C.C., Chatterjee, S., Pohlman, B., & Hojjati, M. (2015). Chronic graft-versus-host disease presenting as eosinophilic fasciitis: Therapeutic challenges and an additional case. *Journal of Clinical Rheumatology, 21*, 86–94. https://doi.org/10.1097/rhu.0000000000000212

Garbutcheon-Singh, K.B., & Fernández-Peñas, P. (2015). Phototherapy for the treatment of cutaneous graft versus host disease. *Australasian Journal of Dermatology, 56*, 93–99. https://doi.org/10.1111/ajd.12191

García-Cadenas, I., Rivera, I., Martino, R., Esquirol, A., Barba, P., Novelli, S., ... Sierra, J. (2017). Patterns of infection and infection-related mortality in patients with steroid-refractory acute graft versus host disease. *Bone Marrow Transplantation, 52*, 107–113. https://doi.org/10.1038/bmt.2016.225

Garnett, C., Apperley, J.F., & Pavlů, J. (2013). Treatment and management of graft-versus-host disease: Improving response and survival. *Therapeutic Advances in Hematology, 4*, 366–378. https://doi.org/10.1177/2040620713489842

Gea-Banacloche, J., Komanduri, K.V., Carpenter, P., Paczesny, S., Sarantopoulos, S., Young, J.-A., ... Wingard, J.R. (2017). National Institutes of Health Hematopoietic Cell Transplantation Late Effects Initiative: The Immune Dysregulation and Pathobiology Working Group report. *Biology of Blood and Marrow Transplantation, 23*, 870–881. https://doi.org/10.1016/j.bbmt.2016.10.001

Ghimire, S., Weber, D., Mavin, E., Wang, X.N., Dickinson, A.M., & Holler, E. (2017). Pathophysiology of GvHD and other HSCT-related major complications. *Frontiers in Immunology, 8*, 79. https://doi.org/10.3389/fimmu.2017.00079

Goyal, R.K., Goyal, M., & Sankaranarayan, K. (2015). Grading acute graft-versus-host disease: Time to reconsider. *Pediatric Transplantation, 19*, 252–254. https://doi.org/10.1111/petr.12433

Grauer, O., Wolff, D., Bertz, H., Greinix, H., Kühl, J.S., Lawitschka, A., ... Kleiter, I. (2010). Neurological manifestations of chronic graft-versus-host disease after allogeneic haematopoietic stem cell transplantation: Report from the Consensus Conference on Clinical Practice in chronic graft-versus-host disease. *Brain, 133*, 2852–2865. https://doi.org/10.1093/brain/awq245

Greinix, H.T., & Tanew, A. (2012). UV treatment of chronic skin graft-versus-host disease—Focus on UVA1 and extracorporeal photopheresis. *Current Problems in Dermatology, 43*, 116–131. https://doi.org/10.1159/000335404

Greinix, H.T., Worel, N., Just, U., & Knobler, R. (2014). Extracorporeal photopheresis in acute and chronic graft-versus-host disease. *Transfusion and Apheresis Science, 50*, 349–357. https://doi.org/10.1016/j.transci.2014.04.005

Grønningsaeter, I.S., Tsykunova, G., Lilleeng, K., Ahmed, A.B., Bruserud, O., & Reikvam, H. (2017). Bronchiolitis obliterans syndrome in adults after allogeneic stem cell transplantation—Pathophysiology, diagnostics and treatment. *Expert Review of Clinical Immunology, 13*, 553–569. https://doi.org/10.1080/1744666x.2017.1279053

Hakim, A., Cooke, K.R., Pavletic, S.Z., Khalid, M., Williams, K.M., & Hashmi, S.K. (2018). Diagnosis and treatment of bronchiolitis obliterans syndrome accessible universally. *Bone Marrow Transplantation, 54*, 383–392. https://doi.org/10.1038/s41409-018-0266-6

Hamilton, B.K. (2018). Current approaches to prevent and treat GVHD after allogeneic stem cell transplantation. *American Society of Hematology Education Program Book, 2018*, 228–235. https://doi.org/10.1182/asheducation-2018.1.228

Hamilton, B.K., Goje, O., Savani, B.N., Majhail, N.S., & Stratton, P. (2017). Clinical management of genital chronic GvHD. *Bone Marrow Transplantation, 52*, 803–810. https://doi.org/10.1038/bmt.2016.315

Hammami, M.B., Talkin, R., Al-Taee, A.M., Schoen, M.W., Goyal, S.D., & Lai, J.-P. (2018). Autologous graft-versus-host disease of the gastrointestinal tract in patients with multiple myeloma and hematopoietic stem cell transplantation. *Gastroenterology Research, 11*, 52–57. https://doi.org/10.14740/gr925w

Hardy, J.M., Marguery, M.-C., Huynh, A., Borel, C., Apoil, P.A., Lamant, L., ... Bulai Livideanu, C. (2016). Photo-induced graft-versus-host disease. *Photodermatology, Photoimmunology and Photomedicine, 32*, 291–295. https://doi.org/10.1111/phpp.12273

Harris, A.C., Young, R., Devine, S., Hogan, W.J., Ayuk, F., Bunworasate, U., ... Levine, J.E. (2016). International, multicenter standardization of acute graft-versus-host disease clinical data collection: A report from the Mount Sinai Acute GVHD International Consortium. *Biology of Blood and Marrow Transplantation, 22*, 4–10. https://doi.org/10.1016/j.bbmt.2015.09.001

Hashimoto, A., Sato, T., Iyama, S., Yoshida, M., Ibata, S., Tatekoshi, A., ... Kato, J. (2016). Narrow-band ultraviolet B phototherapy ameliorates acute graft-versus-host disease of the intestine by expansion of regulatory T cells. *PLOS ONE, 11*, e0152823. https://doi.org/10.1371/journal.pone.0152823

Hashmi, S.K., Bredeson, C., Duarte, R.F., Farnia, S., Ferrey, S., Fitzhugh, C., ... Majhail, N.S. (2017). National Institutes of Health Blood and Marrow Transplant Late Effects Initiative: The Healthcare Delivery Working Group report. *Biology of Blood and Marrow Transplantation, 23*, 717–725. https://doi.org/10.1016/j.bbmt.2016.09.025

He, F.C., & Holtan, S.G. (2018). Biomarkers in graft-versus-host disease: From prediction and diagnosis to insights into complex graft/host interactions. *Current Hematologic Malignancy Reports, 13*, 44–52. https://doi.org/10.1007/s11899-018-0433-2

Henry, L., & Loader, G. (2009). Nutrition support. In J. Treleaven & A.J. Barrett (Eds.), *Hematopoietic stem cell transplantation* (pp. 344–354). Edinburgh, Scotland: Elsevier Limited.

Hill, L., Alousi, A., Kebriaei, P., Mehta, R., Rezvani, K., & Shpall, E. (2018). New and emerging therapies for acute and chronic graft versus host disease. *Therapeutic Advances in Hematology, 9*, 21–46. doi:10.1177/2040620717741860

Holbro, A., Abinun, M., & Daikeler, T. (2012). Management of autoimmune diseases after haematopoietic stem cell transplantation. *British Journal of Haematology, 157*, 281–290. https://doi.org/10.1111/j.1365-2141.2012.09070.x

Holtan, S.G., & MacMillan, M.L. (2016). A risk-adapted approach to acute GVHD treatment: Are we there yet? *Bone Marrow Transplantation, 51*, 172–175. https://doi.org/10.1038/bmt.2015.261

Holtan, S.G., Pasquini, M., & Weisdorf, D.J. (2014). Acute graft-versus-host disease: A bench-to-bedside update. *Blood, 124*, 363–373. https://doi.org/10.1182/blood-2014-01-514786

Holtick, U., Albrecht, M., Chemnitz, J.M., Theurich, S., Skoetz, N., Scheid, C., & von Bergwelt-Baildon, M. (2014). Bone marrow versus peripheral blood allogeneic haematopoietic stem cell transplantation for haematological malignancies in adults. *Cochrane Database of Systematic Reviews, 2014*(4). https://doi.org/10.1002/14651858.cd010189.pub2

Horton, L.E., Haste, N.M., & Taplitz, R.A. (2018). Rethinking antimicrobial prophylaxis in the transplant patient in the world of emerging resistant organisms—Where are we today? *Current Hematologic Malignancy Reports, 13*, 59–67. https://doi.org/10.1007/s11899-018-0435-0

Ibrahim, R.B., Abidi, M.H., Cronin, S.M., Lum, L.G., Al-Kadhimi, Z., Ratanatharathorn, V., & Uberti, J.P. (2009). Nonabsorbable corticosteroids use in the treatment of gastrointestinal graft-versus-host disease. *Biology of Blood and Marrow Transplantation, 15*, 395–405. https://doi.org/10.1016/j.bbmt.2008.12.487

Im, A., Hakim, F.T., & Pavletic, S.Z. (2017). Novel targets in the treatment of chronic graft-versus-host disease. *Leukemia, 31*, 543–554. https://doi.org/10.1038/leu.2016.367

Inamoto, Y., & Lee, S.J. (2017). Late effects of blood and marrow transplantation. *Haematologica, 102*, 614–625. https://doi.org/10.3324/haematol.2016.150250

Inamoto, Y., Martin, P.J., Storer, B.E., Mielcarek, M., Storb, R.F., & Carpenter, P.A. (2014). Response endpoints and failure-free survival after initial treatment for acute graft-versus-host disease. *Haematologica, 99*, 385–391. https://doi.org/10.3324/haematol.2013.093062

Inamoto, Y., Pidala, J., Chai, X., Kurland, B.F., Weisdorf, D., Flowers, M.E.D., ... Carpenter, P.A. (2014). Assessment of joint and fascia manifestations in chronic graft-versus-host disease. *Arthritis and Rheumatology, 66*, 1044–1052. https://doi.org/10.1002/art.38293

Inamoto, Y., Shah, N.N., Savani, B.N., Shaw, B.E., Abraham, A.A., Ahmed, I.A., ... Majhail, N.S. (2015). Secondary solid cancer screening following hematopoietic cell transplantation. *Bone Marrow Transplantation, 50*, 1013–1023. https://doi.org/10.1038/bmt.2015.63

Inamoto, Y., Valdés-Sanz, N., Ogawa, Y., Alves, M., Berchicci, L., Galvin, J., ... Petriček, I. (2019). Ocular graft-versus-host disease after hematopoietic cell transplantation: Expert review from the Late Effects and Quality of Life Working Committee of the CIBMTR and Transplant Complications Working Party of the EBMT. *Bone Marrow Transplantation, 54*, 662–673. https://doi.org/10.1038/s41409-018-0340-0

Issekutz, A.C., Rowter, D., & MacMillan, H.F. (2011). Intravenous immunoglobulin G (IVIG) inhibits IL-1- and TNF-α-dependent, but not chemotactic-factor-stimulated, neutrophil transendothelial migration. *Clinical Immunology, 141*, 187–196. https://doi.org/10.1016/j.clim.2011.08.003

Jagasia, M.H., Arora, M., Flowers, M.E.D., Chao, N.J., McCarthy, P.L., Cutler, C.S., ... Hahn, T. (2012). Risk factors for acute GVHD and survival after hematopoietic cell transplantation. *Blood, 119*, 296–307. https://doi.org/10.1182/blood-2011-06-364265

Jagasia, M.H., Greinix, H.T., Arora, M., Williams, K.M., Wolff, D., Cowen, E.W., ... Flowers, M.E.D. (2015). National Institutes of Health Consensus Development Project on Criteria for Clinical Trials in Chronic Graft-versus-Host Disease: I. The 2014 Diagnosis and Staging Working Group report. *Biology of Blood and Marrow Transplantation, 21*, 389–401.e1. https://doi.org/10.1016/j.bbmt.2014.12.001

Jamil, M.O., & Mineishi, S. (2015). State-of-the-art acute and chronic GVHD treatment. *International Journal of Hematology, 101*, 452–466. https://doi.org/10.1007/s12185-015-1785-1

Jomphe, V., Lands, L.C., & Mailhot, G. (2018). Nutritional requirements of lung transplant recipients: Challenges and considerations. *Nutrients, 10*, 790. https://doi.org/10.3390/nu10060790

Kallekleiv, M., Larun, L., Bruserud, O., & Hatfield, K.J. (2016). Co-transplantation of multipotent mesenchymal stromal cells in allogeneic hematopoietic stem cell transplantation: A systematic review and meta-analysis. *Cytotherapy, 18*, 172–185. https://doi.org/10.1016/j.jcyt.2015.11.010

Kaufman, G.N., Massoud, A.H., Dembele, M., Yona, M., Piccirillo, C.A., & Mazer, B.D. (2015). Induction of regulatory T cells by intravenous immunoglobulin: A bridge between adaptive and innate immunity. *Frontiers in Immunology, 6*, 469. https://doi.org/10.3389/fimmu.2015.00469

Kavand, S., Lehman, J.S., Hashmi, S., Gibson, L.E., & El-Azhary, R.A. (2017). Cutaneous manifestations of graft-versus-host disease: Role of the dermatologist. *International Journal of Dermatology, 56*, 131–140. https://doi.org/10.1111/ijd.13381

Kekre, N., & Antin, J.H. (2016). Emerging drugs for graft-versus-host disease. *Expert Opinion on Emerging Drugs, 21*, 209–218. https://doi.org/10.1517/14728214.2016.1170117

Kendler, D.L., Body, J.J., Brandi, M.L., Broady, R., Cannata-Andia, J., Cannata-Ortiz, M.J., ... Ebeling, P.R. (2018). Bone management in hematologic stem cell transplant recipients. *Osteoporosis International, 29*, 2597–2610. https://doi.org/10.1007/s00198-018-4669-4

Kida, A., & McDonald, G.B. (2012). Gastrointestinal, hepatobiliary, pancreatic, and iron-related diseases in long-term survivors of allogeneic hematopoietic cell transplantation. *Seminars in Hematology, 49*, 43–58. https://doi.org/10.1053/j.seminhematol.2011.10.006

Kim, W.B., Shelley, A.J., Novice, K., Joo, J., Lim, H.W., & Glassman, S.J. (2018). Drug-induced phototoxicity: A systematic review. *Journal of the American Academy of Dermatology, 79*, 1069–1075. https://doi.org/10.1016/j.jaad.2018.06.061

Kitko, C.L., & Levine, J.E. (2015). Extracorporeal photopheresis in prevention and treatment of acute GVHD. *Transfusion and Apheresis Science, 52*, 151–156. https://doi.org/10.1016/j.transci.2015.02.001

Koç, N., Gündüz, M., Azık, M.F., Tavil, B., Gürlek-Gökçebay, D., Özaydin, E., ... Uçkan, D. (2016). Stepwise diet management in pediatric gastrointestinal graft versus host disease. *Turkish Journal of Pediatrics, 58*, 145–151. https://doi.org/10.24953/turkjped.2016.02.004

Kopolovic, I., Ostro, J., Tsubota, H., Lin, Y., Cserti-Gazdewich, C.M., Messner, H.A., ... Callum, J. (2015). A systematic review of transfusion-associated graft-versus-host disease. *Blood, 126*, 406–414. https://doi.org/10.1182/blood-2015-01-620872

Kota, H., & Chamberlain, R.S. (2017). Immunonutrition is associated with a decreased incidence of graft-versus-host disease in bone marrow transplant recipients: A meta-analysis. *Journal of Parenteral and Enteral Nutrition, 41*, 1286–1292. https://doi.org/10.1177/0148607116663278

Krupski, C., & Jagasia, M. (2015). Quality of life in the Chronic GVHD Consortium cohort: Lessons learned and the long road ahead. *Current Hematologic Malignancy Reports, 10*, 183–191. https://doi.org/10.1007/s11899-015-0265-2

Kuba, A., & Raida, L. (2018). Graft versus host disease: From basic pathogenic principles to DNA damage response and cellular senescence. *Mediators of Inflammation, 2018*, 9451950. https://doi.org/10.1155/2018/9451950

Kuklinski, L.F., Li, S., Karagas, M.R., Weng, W.-K., & Kwong, B.Y. (2017). Effect of voriconazole on risk of nonmelanoma skin cancer after hematopoietic cell transplantation. *Journal of the American Academy of Dermatology, 77*, 706–712. https://doi.org/10.1016/j.jaad.2017.06.032

Kumari, R., Palaniyandi, S., & Hildebrandt, G.C. (2018). Microbiome: An emerging new frontier in graft-versus-host disease. *Digestive Diseases and Sciences, 64*, 669–677. https://doi.org/10.1007/s10620-018-5369-9

Latif, T., Pohlman, B., Kalaycio, M., Sobecks, R., Hsi, E.D., Andresen, S., & Bolwell, B.J. (2003). Syngeneic graft-versus-host disease: A report of two cases and literature review. *Bone Marrow Transplantation, 32*, 535–539. https://doi.org/10.1038/sj.bmt.1704171

Lee, S.-E., Cho, B.-S., Kim, J.-H., Yoon, J.-H., Shin, S.-H., Yahng, S.-A., … Park, C.-W. (2013). Risk and prognostic factors for acute GVHD based on NIH consensus criteria. *Bone Marrow Transplantation, 48*, 587–592. https://doi.org/10.1038/bmt.2012.187

Lee, S.J. (2017). Classification systems for chronic graft-versus-host disease. *Blood, 129*, 30–37. https://doi.org/10.1182/blood-2016-07-686642

Lee, S.J., Nguyen, T.D., Onstad, L., Bar, M., Krakow, E.F., Salit, R.B., … Flowers, M.E. (2018). Success of immunosuppressive treatments in patients with chronic graft-versus-host disease. *Biology of Blood and Marrow Transplantation, 24*, 555–562. https://doi.org/10.1016/j.bbmt.2017.10.042

Lee, S.J., Onstad, L., Chow, E.J., Shaw, B.E., Jim, H.S.L., Syrjala, K.L., … Flowers, M.E. (2018). Patient-reported outcomes and health status associated with chronic graft-versus-host disease. *Haematologica, 103*, 1535–1541. https://doi.org/10.3324/haematol.2018.192930

Lee, S.J., Wolff, D., Kitko, C., Koreth, J., Inamoto, Y., Jagasia, M., … Pavletic, S. (2015). Measuring therapeutic response in chronic graft-versus-host disease. National Institutes of Health Consensus Development Project on Criteria for Clinical Trials in Chronic Graft-Versus-Host Disease: IV. The 2014 Response Criteria Working Group report. *Biology of Blood and Marrow Transplantation, 21*, 984–999. https://doi.org/10.1016/j.bbmt.2015.02.025

Lee, Y.-H., & Rah, W.-J. (2016). Pre-engraftment syndrome: Clinical significance and pathophysiology. *Blood Research, 51*, 152–154. https://doi.org/10.5045/br.2016.51.3.152

Leonard, J.T., Newell, L.F., Meyers, G., Hayes-Lattin, B., Gajewski, J., Heitner, S., … Holtan, S.G. (2015). Chronic GvHD-associated serositis and pericarditis. *Bone Marrow Transplantation, 50*, 1098–1104. https://doi.org/10.1038/bmt.2015.105

Levine, J.E., Hogan, W.J., Harris, A.C., Litzow, M.R., Efebera, Y.A., Devine, S.M., … Ferrara, J.L.M. (2014). Improved accuracy of acute graft-versus-host disease staging among multiple centers. *Best Practice and Research. Clinical Haematology, 27*, 283–287. https://doi.org/10.1016/j.beha.2014.10.011

L'Huillier, A.G., & Kumar, D. (2015). Immunizations in solid organ and hematopoeitic stem cell transplant patients: A comprehensive review. *Human Vaccines and Immunotherapeutics, 11*, 2852–2863. https://doi.org/10.1080/21645515.2015.1078043

Li, X., Gao, Q., Feng, Y., & Zhang, X. (2019). Developing role of B cells in the pathogenesis and treatment of chronic GVHD. *British Journal of Haematology, 184*, 323–336. https://doi.org/10.1111/bjh.15719

Linhares, Y.P.L., Pavletic, S., & Gale, R.P. (2013). Chronic GVHD: Where are we? Where do we want to be? Will immunomodulatory drugs help? *Bone Marrow Transplantation, 48*, 203–209. https://doi.org/10.1038/bmt.2012.76

Locatelli, F., Algeri, M., Trevisan, V., & Bertaina, A. (2017). Remestemcel-L for the treatment of graft versus host disease. *Expert Review of Clinical Immunology, 13*, 43–56. https://doi.org/10.1080/1744666x.2016.1208086

Lubner, M.G., Menias, C.O., Agrons, M., Alhalabi, K., Katabathina, V.S., Elsayes, K.M., & Pickhardt, P.J. (2017). Imaging of abdominal and pelvic manifestations of graft-versus-host disease after hematopoietic stem cell transplant. *American Journal of Roentgenology, 209*, 33–45. https://doi.org/10.2214/ajr.17.17866

Lutz, M., & Mielke, S. (2016). New perspectives on the use of mTOR inhibitors in allogeneic haematopoietic stem cell transplantation and graft-versus-host disease. *British Journal of Clinical Pharmacology, 82*, 1171–1179. https://doi.org/10.1111/bcp.13022

Ma, J.D., El-Jawahri, A.R., LeBlanc, T.W., & Roeland, E.J. (2018). Pain syndromes and management in adult hematopoietic stem cell transplantation. *Hematology/Oncology Clinics of North America, 32*, 551–567. https://doi.org/10.1016/j.hoc.2018.01.012

MacDonald, K.P.A., Betts, B.C., & Couriel, D. (2017). Emerging therapeutics for the control of chronic graft-versus-host disease. *Biology of Blood and Marrow Transplantation, 24*, 19–26. https://doi.org/10.1016/j.bbmt.2017.10.006

MacMillan, M.L., Robin, M., Harris, A.C., DeFor, T.E., Martin, P.J., Alousi, A., … Weisdorf, D.J. (2015). A refined risk score for acute graft-versus-host disease that predicts response to initial therapy, survival, and transplant-related mortality. *Biology of Blood and Marrow Transplantation, 21*, 761–767. https://doi.org/10.1016/j.bbmt.2015.01.001

Magenau, J., & Reddy, P. (2014). Next generation treatment of acute graft-versus-host disease. *Leukemia, 28*, 2283–2291. https://doi.org/10.1038/leu.2014.195

Mahr, B., Granofszky, N., Muckenhuber, M., & Wekerle, T. (2018). Transplantation tolerance through hematopoietic chimerism: Progress and challenges for clinical translation. *Frontiers in Immunology, 8*, 1762. https://doi.org/10.3389/fimmu.2017.01762

Majhail, N.S. (2017). Long-term complications after hematopoietic cell transplantation. *Hematology/Oncology and Stem Cell Therapy, 10*, 220–227. https://doi.org/10.1016/j.hemonc.2017.05.009

Majhail, N.S., Rizzo, J.D., Lee, S.J., Aljurf, M., Atsuta, Y., Bonfim, C., … Tichelli, A. (2012). Recommended screening and preventive practices for long-term survivors after hematopoietic cell transplantation. *Biology of Blood and Marrow Transplantation, 18*, 348–371. https://doi.org/10.1016/j.bbmt.2011.12.519

Major-Monfried, H., Renteria, A.S., Pawarode, A., Reddy, P., Ayuk, F., Holler, E., … Levine, J.E. (2018). MAGIC biomarkers predict long-term outcomes for steroid-resistant acute GVHD. *Blood, 131*, 2846–2855. https://doi.org/10.1182/blood-2018-01-822957

Malat, G., & Culkin, C. (2016). The ABCs of immunosuppression: A primer for primary care physicians. *Medical Clinics of North America, 100*, 505–518. https://doi.org/10.1016/j.mcna.2016.01.003

Margaix-Muñoz, M., Bagán, J.V., Jiménez, Y., Sarrión, M.-G., & Poveda-Roda, R. (2015). Graft-versus-host disease affecting oral cavity. A review. *Journal of Clinical and Experimental Dentistry, 7*, e138–e145. https://doi.org/10.4317/jced.51975

Marks, C., Stadler, M., Häusermann, P., Wolff, D., Buchholz, S., Stary, G., … Bertz, H. (2011). German-Austrian-Swiss Consensus Conference on clinical practice in chronic graft-versus-host disease (GVHD): Guidance for supportive therapy of chronic cutaneous and musculoskeletal GVHD. *British Journal of Dermatology, 165*, 18–29. https://doi.org/10.1111/j.1365-2133.2011.10360.x

Martin, P.J., Rizzo, J.D., Wingard, J.R., Ballen, K., Curtin, P.T., Cutler, C., … Carpenter, P.A. (2012). First- and second-line systemic treatment of acute graft-versus-host disease: Recommendations of the American Society of Blood and Marrow Transplantation. *Biology of Blood and Marrow Transplantation, 18*, 1150–1163. https://doi.org/10.1016/j.bbmt.2012.04.005

Martínez-Laperche, C., Buces, E., Aguilera-Morillo, M.C., Picornell, A., González-Rivera, M., Lillo, R., … Buño, I. (2018). A novel predictive approach for GVHD after allogeneic SCT based on clinical variables and cytokine gene polymorphisms. *Blood Advances, 2*, 1719–1737. https://doi.org/10.1182/bloodadvances.2017011502

Matsukuma, K.E., Wei, D., Sun, K., Ramsamooj, R., & Chen, M. (2016). Diagnosis and differential diagnosis of hepatic graft versus host disease (GVHD). *Journal of Gastrointestinal Oncology, 7*(Suppl. 1), S21–S31. https://doi.org/10.3978/j.issn.2078-6891.2015.036

Mawardi, H., Hashmi, S.K., Elad, S., Aljurf, M., & Treister, N. (2019). Chronic graft-versus-host disease: Current management paradigm and future perspectives. *Oral Diseases, 25,* 931–948. https://doi.org/10.1111/odi.12936

Mays, J.W., Fassil, H., Edwards, D.A., Pavletic, S.Z., & Bassim, C.W. (2013). Oral chronic graft-versus-host disease: Current pathogenesis, therapy, and research. *Oral Diseases, 19,* 327–346. https://doi.org/10.1111/odi.12028

McCune, J.S., & Bemer, M.J. (2016). Pharmacokinetics, pharmacodynamics and pharmacogenomics of immunosuppressants in allogeneic haematopoietic cell transplantation: Part I. *Clinical Pharmacokinetics, 55,* 525–550. https://doi.org/10.1007/s40262-015-0339-2

McCune, J.S., Bemer, M.J., & Long-Boyle, J. (2016). Pharmacokinetics, pharmacodynamics, and pharmacogenomics of immunosuppressants in allogeneic hematopoietic cell transplantation: Part II. *Clinical Pharmacokinetics, 55,* 551–593. https://doi.org/10.1007/s40262-015-0340-9

McDonald, G.B. (2016). How I treat acute graft-versus-host disease of the gastrointestinal tract and the liver. *Blood, 127,* 1544–1550. https://doi.org/10.1182/blood-2015-10-612747

Meng, L., Ji, S., Wang, Q., & Bu, B. (2018). Polymyositis as a manifestation of chronic graft-versus-host disease after allo-HSCT. *Clinical Case Reports, 6,* 1723–1726. https://doi.org/10.1002/ccr3.1709

Mitchell, S.A. (2018). Palliative care during and following allogeneic hematopoietic stem cell transplantation. *Current Opinion in Supportive and Palliative Care, 12,* 58–64. https://doi.org/10.1097/spc.0000000000000327

Mo, X.-D., Lv, M., & Huang, X.-J. (2017). Preventing relapse after haematopoietic stem cell transplantation for acute leukaemia: The role of post-transplantation minimal residual disease (MRD) monitoring and MRD-directed intervention. *British Journal of Haematology, 179,* 184–197. https://doi.org/10.1111/bjh.14778

Mohammadi, S., Mohammadi, A.M., Norooznezhad, A.H., Heshmati, F., Alimoghaddam, K., & Ghavamzadeh, A. (2017). Extra corporeal photochemotherapy in steroid refractory graft versus host disease: A review of guidelines and recommendations. *Transfusion and Apheresis Science, 56,* 376–384. https://doi.org/10.1016/j.transci.2017.01.006

Mohammed, J., Savani, B.N., El-Jawahri, A., Vanderklish, J., Cheville, A.L., & Hashmi, S.K. (2018). Is there any role for physical therapy in chronic GvHD? *Bone Marrow Transplantation, 53,* 22–28. https://doi.org/10.1038/bmt.2017.155

Mohammed, J., Smith, S.R., Burns, L., Basak, G., Aljurf, M., Savani, B.N., … Hashmi, S.K. (2019). Role of physical therapy before and after hematopoietic stem cell transplantation—White paper report. *Biology of Blood and Marrow Transplantation, 25,* e191–e198. https://doi.org/10.1016/j.bbmt.2019.01.018

Morello, E., Malagola, M., Bernardi, S., Pristipino, C., & Russo, D. (2018). The role of allogeneic hematopoietic stem cell transplantation in the four P medicine era. *Blood Research, 53,* 3–6. https://doi.org/10.5045/br.2018.53.1.3

Morishita, S., Kaida, K., Yamauchi, S., Wakasugi, T., Ikegame, K., Ogawa, H., & Domen, K. (2017). Relationship of physical activity with physical function and health-related quality of life in patients having undergone allogeneic haematopoietic stem-cell transplantation. *European Journal of Cancer Care, 26,* e12669. https://doi.org/10.1111/ecc.12669

Mueller, S.K. (2016). Transdisciplinary coordination and delivery of care. *Seminars in Oncology Nursing, 32,* 154–163. https://doi.org/10.1016/j.soncn.2016.02.009

Muhsen, I.N., Elhassan, T., & Hashmi, S.K. (2018). Artificial intelligence approaches in hematopoietic cell transplantation: A review of the current status and future directions. *Turkish Journal of Haematology, 35,* 152–157. https://doi.org/10.4274/tjh.2018.0123

Munir, S.Z., & Aylward, J. (2017). A review of ocular graft-versus-host disease. *Optometry and Vision Science, 94,* 545–555. https://doi.org/10.1097/opx.0000000000001071

Munneke, J.M., Spruit, M.J., Cornelissen, A.S., van Hoeven, V., Voermans, C., & Hazenberg, M.D. (2016). The potential of mesenchymal stromal cells as treatment for severe steroid-refractory acute graft-versus-host disease: A critical review of the literature. *Transplantation, 100,* 2309–2314. https://doi.org/10.1097/tp.0000000000001029

Murray, J., Stringer, J., & Hutt, D. (2018). Graft-versus-host disease (GvHD). In M. Kenyon & A. Babic (Eds.), *The European blood and marrow transplantation textbook for nurses* (pp. 221–251). https://doi.org/10.1007/978-3-319-50026-3_11

Mussetti, A., Greco, R., Peccatori, J., & Corradini, P. (2017). Post-transplant cyclophosphamide, a promising anti-graft versus host disease prophylaxis: Where do we stand? *Expert Review of Hematology, 10,* 479–492. https://doi.org/10.1080/17474086.2017.1318054

Nadeau, M., Perreault, S., Seropian, S., Foss, F., Isufi, I., & Cooper, D.L. (2016). The use of basiliximab-infliximab combination for the treatment of severe gastrointestinal acute GvHD. *Bone Marrow Transplantation, 51,* 273–276. https://doi.org/10.1038/bmt.2015.247

Nakamura, R., & Forman, S.J. (2014). Reduced intensity conditioning for allogeneic hematopoietic cell transplantation: Considerations for evidence-based GVHD prophylaxis. *Expert Review of Hematology, 7,* 407–421. https://doi.org/10.1586/17474086.2014.898561

Nassar, A., Elgohary, G., Elhassan, T., Nurgat, Z., Mohamed, S.Y., & Aljurf, M. (2014). Methotrexate for the treatment of graft-versus-host disease after allogeneic hematopoietic stem cell transplantation. *Journal of Transplantation, 2014,* 980301. https://doi.org/10.1155/2014/980301

Nassereddine, S., Rafei, H., Elbahesh, E., & Tabbara, I. (2017). Acute graft versus host disease: A comprehensive review. *Anticancer Research, 37,* 1547–1555. https://doi.org/10.21873/anticanres.11483

Nassiri, N., Eslani, M., Panahi, N., Mehravaran, S., Ziaei, A., & Djalilian, A.R. (2013). Ocular graft versus host disease following allogeneic stem cell transplantation: A review of current knowledge and recommendations. *Journal of Ophthalmic and Vision Research, 8,* 351–358. Retrieved from https://www.ncbi.nlm.nih.gov/pmc/articles/PMC3957042/pdf/JOVR-08-351.pdf

Nasu, R., Nannya, Y., Shinohara, A., Ichikawa, M., & Kurokawa, M. (2014). Favorable outcomes of tacrolimus compared with cyclosporine A for GVHD prophylaxis in HSCT for standard-risk hematological diseases. *Annals of Hematology, 93,* 1215–1223. https://doi.org/10.1007/s00277-014-2027-y

Naymagon, S., Naymagon, L., Wong, S.-Y., Ko, H.M., Renteria, A., Levine, J., … Ferrara, J. (2017). Acute graft-versus-host disease of the gut: Considerations for the gastroenterologist. *Nature Reviews Gastroenterology and Hepatology, 14,* 711–726. https://doi.org/10.1038/nrgastro.2017.126

Neumann, J. (2017). Nursing challenges caring for bone marrow transplantation patients with graft versus host disease. *Hematology/Oncology and Stem Cell Therapy, 10,* 192–194. https://doi.org/10.1016/j.hemonc.2017.06.001

New-Tolley, J., Smith, C., Koszyca, B., Otto, S., Maundrell, A., Bardy, P., … Limaye, V. (2018). Inflammatory myopathies after allogeneic stem cell transplantation. *Muscle and Nerve, 58,* 790–795. https://doi.org/10.1002/mus.26341

Nishida, M., Shigematsu, A., Sato, M., Kudo, Y., Omotehara, S., Horie, T., … Teshima, T. (2015). Ultrasonographic evaluation of gastrointestinal graft-versus-host disease after hematopoietic stem cell transplantation. *Clinical Transplantation, 29,* 697–704. https://doi.org/10.1111/ctr.12570

Nishihori, T., Al-Kadhimi, Z., Hamadani, M., & Kharfan-Dabaja, M.A. (2016). Antithymocyte globulin in allogeneic hematopoietic cell transplantation: Benefits and limitations. *Immunotherapy, 8,* 435–447. https://doi.org/10.2217/imt.15.128

Oda, K., Nakaseko, C., Ozawa, S., Nishimura, M., Saito, Y., Yoshiba, F., … Okamoto, S. (2009). Fasciitis and myositis: An analysis of muscle-related complications caused by chronic GVHD after allo-SCT. *Bone Marrow Transplantation, 43,* 159–167. https://doi.org/10.1038/bmt.2008.297

Ogonek, J., Kralj Juric, M., Ghimire, S., Varanasi, P.R., Holler, E., Greinix, H., & Weissinger, E. (2016). Immune reconstitution after allogeneic hematopoietic stem cell transplantation. *Frontiers in Immunology, 7,* 1–15. https://doi.org/10.3389/fimmu.2016.00507

Orti, G., Barba, P., Fox, L., Salamero, O., Bosch, F., & Valcarcel, D. (2017). Donor lymphocyte infusions in AML and MDS: Enhancing the graft-versus-leukemia effect. *Experimental Hematology, 48,* 1–11. https://doi.org/10.1016/j.exphem.2016.12.004

Paczesny, S. (2018). Biomarkers for posttransplantation outcomes. *Blood, 131,* 2193–2204. https://doi.org/10.1182/blood-2018-02-791509

Palencia, S.I., Rodríguez-Peralto, J.L., Castaño, E., Vanaclocha, F., & Iglesias, L. (2002). Lichenoid nail changes as sole external manifestation of graft vs. host disease. *International Journal of Dermatology, 41,* 44–45. https://doi.org/10.1046/j.0011-9059.2001.01399.x

Petersdorf, E.W. (2017). Which factors influence the development of GVHD in HLA-matched or mismatched transplants? *Best Practice and*

Research in Clinical Haematology, 30, 333–335. https://doi.org/10.1016/j.beha.2017.09.003

Pidala, J., Chai, X., Martin, P., Inamoto, Y., Cutler, C., Palmer, J., … Lee, S.J. (2013). Hand grip strength and 2-minute walk test in chronic graft-versus-host disease assessment: Analysis from the Chronic GVHD Consortium. *Biology of Blood and Marrow Transplantation, 19,* 967–972. https://doi.org/10.1016/j.bbmt.2013.03.014

Pidala, J., Lee, S.J., Quinn, G., Jim, H., Kim, J., & Anasetti, C. (2011). Variation in management of immune suppression after allogeneic hematopoietic cell transplantation. *Biology of Blood and Marrow Transplantation, 17,* 1528–1536. https://doi.org/10.1016/j.bbmt.2011.03.006

Presland, R.B. (2017). Application of proteomics to graft-versus-host disease: From biomarker discovery to potential clinical applications. *Expert Review of Proteomics, 14,* 997–1006. https://doi.org/10.1080/14789450.2017.1388166

Qayed, M., & Horan, J.T. (2016). The role of intestinal microbiota in graft versus host disease. *Mini Reviews in Medicinal Chemistry, 16,* 193–199. https://doi.org/10.2174/1389557515666150722110547

Radojcic, V., Pletneva, M.A., & Couriel, D.R. (2015). The role of extracorporeal photopheresis in chronic graft-versus-host disease. *Transfusion and Apheresis Science, 52,* 157–161. https://doi.org/10.1016/j.transci.2015.02.002

Rafei, H., Kharfan-Dabaja, M.A., & Nishihori, T. (2017). A critical appraisal of extracorporeal photopheresis as a treatment modality for acute and chronic graft-versus-host disease. *Biomedicines, 5,* 60. https://doi.org/10.3390/biomedicines5040060

Rahmat, L.T., & Logan, A.C. (2018). Ibrutinib for the treatment of patients with chronic graft-versus-host disease after failure of one or more lines of systemic therapy. *Drugs Today, 54,* 305–313. https://doi.org/10.1358/dot.2018.54.5.2807865

Rashidi, A., Shanley, R., Holtan, S.G., MacMillan, M.L., Blazar, B.R., Khoruts, A., & Weisdorf, D.J. (2018). Pretransplant serum citrulline predicts acute graft-versus-host disease. *Biology of Blood and Marrow Transplantation, 24,* 2190–2196. https://doi.org/10.1016/j.bbmt.2018.06.036

Rashidi, A., & Weisdorf, D. (2017). Association between single nucleotide polymorphisms of tumor necrosis factor gene and grade II–IV acute GvHD: A systematic review and meta-analysis. *Bone Marrow Transplantation, 52,* 1423–1427. https://doi.org/10.1038/bmt.2017.144

Rezvani, A.R., & Storb, R.F. (2012). Prevention of graft-vs.-host disease. *Expert Opinion on Pharmacotherapy, 13,* 1737–1750. https://doi.org/10.1517/14656566.2012.703652

Rioth, M.J., Warner, J., Savani, B.N., & Jagasia, M. (2016). Next-generation long-term transplant clinics: Improving resource utilization and the quality of care through health information technology. *Bone Marrow Transplantation, 51,* 34–40. https://doi.org/10.1038/bmt.2015.210

Robak, K., Zambonelli, J., Bilinski, J., & Basak, G.W. (2017). Diarrhea after allogeneic stem cell transplantation: Beyond graft-versus-host disease. *European Journal of Gastroenterology and Hepatology, 29,* 495–502. https://doi.org/10.1097/meg.0000000000000833

Roeland, E., Mitchell, W., Elia, G., Thornberry, K., Herman, H., Cain, J., … von Gunten, C.F. (2010). Symptom control in stem cell transplantation: A multidisciplinary palliative care team approach. Part 1: Physical symptoms. *Journal of Supportive Oncology, 8,* 100–116.

Ros-Soto, J., Anthias, C., Madrigal, A., & Snowden, J.A. (2019). Vitamin D: Is it important in haematopoietic stem cell transplantation? A review. *Bone Marrow Transplantation, 54,* 810–820. https://doi.org/10.1038/s41409-018-0377-0

Rubinstein, S.M., Culos, K.A., Savani, B., & Satyanarayana, G. (2018). Foiling fungal disease post hematopoietic cell transplant: Review of prophylactic strategies. *Bone Marrow Transplantation, 53,* 123–128. https://doi.org/10.1038/bmt.2017.222

Ruutu, T., Eriksson, B., Remes, K., Juvonen, E., Volin, L., Remberger, M., … Ringdén, O. (2002). Ursodeoxycholic acid for the prevention of hepatic complications in allogeneic stem cell transplantation. *Blood, 100,* 1977–1983. https://doi.org/10.1182/blood-2001-12-0159

Ruutu, T., Gratwohl, A., de Witte, T., Afanasyev, B., Apperley, J., Bacigalupo, A., … Niederwieser, D. (2014). Prophylaxis and treatment of GVHD: EBMT-ELN working group recommendations for a standardized practice. *Bone Marrow Transplantation, 49,* 168–173. https://doi.org/10.1038/bmt.2013.107

Saad, A., & Lamb, L.S. (2017). Ex vivo T-cell depletion in allogeneic hematopoietic stem cell transplant: Past, present and future. *Bone Marrow Transplantation, 52,* 1241–1248. https://doi.org/10.1038/bmt.2017.22

Sahin, U., Toprak, S.K., Atilla, P.A., Atilla, E., & Demirer, T. (2016). An overview of infectious complications after allogeneic hematopoietic stem cell transplantation. *Journal of Infection and Chemotherapy, 22,* 505–514. https://doi.org/10.1016/j.jiac.2016.05.006

Sakellari, I., Gavriilaki, E., Batsis, I., Mallouri, D., Panteliadou, A.-K., Lazaridou, A., … Anagnostopoulos, A. (2018). Favorable impact of extracorporeal photopheresis in acute and chronic graft versus host disease: Prospective single-center study. *Journal of Clinical Apheresis, 33,* 654–660. https://doi.org/10.1002/jca.21660

Saliba, R.M., de Lima, M., Giralt, S., Andersson, B., Khouri, I.F., Hosing, C., … Couriel, D.R. (2007). Hyperacute GVHD: Risk factors, outcomes, and clinical implications. *Blood, 109,* 2751–2758. https://doi.org/10.1182/blood-2006-07-034348

Salomao, M., Dorritie, K., Mapara, M.Y., & Sepulveda, A. (2016). Histopathology of graft-vs-host disease of gastrointestinal tract and liver: An update. *American Journal of Clinical Pathology, 145,* 591–603. https://doi.org/10.1093/ajcp/aqw050

Sánchez-Ramón, S., Dhalla, F., & Chapel, H. (2016). Challenges in the role of gammaglobulin replacement therapy and vaccination strategies for hematological malignancy. *Frontiers in Immunology, 7,* 317. https://doi.org/10.3389/fimmu.2016.00317

Sandherr, M., Hentrich, M., von Lilienfeld-Toal, M., Massenkeil, G., Neumann, S., Penack, O., … Cornely, O.A. (2015). Antiviral prophylaxis in patients with solid tumours and haematological malignancies—Update of the Guidelines of the Infectious Diseases Working Party (AGIHO) of the German Society for Hematology and Medical Oncology (DGHO). *Annals of Hematology, 94,* 1441–1450. https://doi.org/10.1007/s00277-015-2447-3

Sarmati, L., Andreoni, M., Antonelli, G., Arcese, W., Bruno, R., Coppola, N., … Gentile, G. (2017). Recommendations for screening, monitoring, prevention, prophylaxis and therapy of hepatitis B virus reactivation in patients with haematologic malignances and patients who underwent haematologic stem cell transplantation—A position paper. *Clinical Microbiology and Infection, 23,* 935–940. https://doi.org/10.1016/j.cmi.2017.06.023

Scarisbrick, J.J., Dignan, F.L., Tulpule, S., Gupta, E.D., Kolade, S., Shaw, B., … Raj, K. (2015). A multicentre UK study of GVHD following DLI: Rates of GVHD are high but mortality from GVHD is infrequent. *Bone Marrow Transplantation, 50,* 62–67. https://doi.org/10.1038/bmt.2014.227

Schneiderman, J. (2017). Extracorporeal photopheresis: Cellular therapy for the treatment of acute and chronic graft-versus-host disease. *American Society of Hematology Education Program Book, 2017,* 639–644. https://doi.org/10.1182/asheducation-2017.1.639

Schoemans, H.M., Goris, K., Van Durm, R., Fieuws, S., De Geest, S., Pavletic, S.Z., … Dobbels, F. (2018). The eGVHD App has the potential to improve the accuracy of graft-versus-host disease assessment: A multicenter randomized controlled trial. *Haematologica, 103,* 1698–1707. https://doi.org/10.3324/haematol.2018.190777

Schoemans, H.M., Lee, S.J., Ferrara, J.L., Wolff, D., Levine, J.E., Schultz, K.R., … Pavletic, S.Z. (2018). EBMT-NIH-CIBMTR Task Force position statement on standardized terminology and guidance for graft-versus-host disease assessment. *Bone Marrow Transplantation, 53,* 1401–1415. https://doi.org/10.1038/s41409-018-0204-7

Seber, A., Khan, S.P., & Kersey, J.H. (1996). Unexplained effusions: Association with allogeneic bone marrow transplantation and acute or chronic graft-versus-host disease. *Bone Marrow Transplantation, 17,* 207–211. https://doi.org/10.1038/sj.bmt.1700764

Sengsayadeth, S., Savani, B.N., Jagasia, M., Goodman, S., Greer, J.P., Chen, H., … Engelhardt, B.G. (2014). Six-month freedom from treatment failure is an important end point for acute GVHD clinical trials. *Bone Marrow Transplantation, 49,* 236–240. https://doi.org/10.1038/bmt.2013.157

Servais, S., Beguin, Y., Delens, L., Ehx, G., Fransolet, G., Hannon, M., … Baron, F. (2016). Novel approaches for preventing acute graft-versus-host disease after allogeneic hematopoietic stem cell transplantation. *Expert Opinion on Investigational Drugs, 25,* 957–972. https://doi.org/10.1080/13543784.2016.1182498

Shaw, B.E. (2019). Graft versus host disease clinical trials: Is it time for patients centered outcomes to be the primary objective? *Current Hema-*

tologic Malignancy Reports, 14, 22–30. https://doi.org/10.1007/s11899
-019-0494-x

Shono, Y., Docampo, M.D., Peled, J.U., Perobelli, S.M., & Jenq, R.R. (2015). Intestinal microbiota-related effects on graft-versus-host disease. *International Journal of Hematology, 101,* 428–437. https://doi.org/10.1007/s12185-015-1781-5

Shono, Y., & van den Brink, M.R.M. (2018). Gut microbiota injury in allogeneic haematopoietic stem cell transplantation. *Nature Reviews Cancer, 18,* 283–295. https://doi.org/10.1038/nrc.2018.10

Shulman, H.M., Cardona, D.M., Greenson, J.K., Hingorani, S., Horn, T., Huber, E., … Kleiner, D.E. (2015). NIH Consensus Development Project on Criteria for Clinical Trials in Chronic Graft-Versus-Host Disease: II. The 2014 Pathology Working Group report. *Biology of Blood and Marrow Transplantation, 21,* 589–603. https://doi.org/10.1016/j.bbmt.2014.12.031

Smith, M., Zakrzewski, J., James, S., & Sadelain, M. (2018). Posttransplant chimeric antigen receptor therapy. *Blood, 131,* 1045–1052. https://doi.org/10.1182/blood-2017-08-752121

Smith, S.R., & Asher, A. (2016). Rehabilitation in chronic graft-versus-host disease. *Physical Medicine and Rehabilitation Clinics of North America, 28,* 143–151. https://doi.org/10.1016/j.pmr.2016.08.009

Socié, G., & Ritz, J. (2014). Current issues in chronic graft-versus-host disease. *Blood, 124,* 374–384. https://doi.org/10.1182/blood-2014-01-514752

Socié, G., Vigouroux, S., Yakoub-Agha, I., Bay, J.-O., Fürst, S., Bilger, K., … Vernant, J.-P. (2017). A phase 3 randomized trial comparing inolimomab vs usual care in steroid-resistant acute GVHD. *Blood, 129,* 643–649. https://doi.org/10.1182/blood-2016-09-738625

Solomon, S.R., Sizemore, C.A., Ridgeway, M., Zhang, X., Brown, S., Holland, H.K., … Bashey, A. (2019). Safety and efficacy of rituximab-based first line treatment of chronic GVHD. *Bone Marrow Transplantation, 54,* 1218–1226. https://doi.org/10.1038/s41409-018-0399-7

Staffas, A., Burgos da Silva, M., & van den Brink, M.R.M. (2017). The intestinal microbiota in allogeneic hematopoietic cell transplant and graft-versus-host disease. *Blood, 129,* 927–933. https://doi.org/10.1182/blood-2016-09-691394

Storek, J., Mohty, M., & Boelens, J.J. (2015). Rabbit anti-T cell globulin in allogeneic hematopoietic cell transplantation. *Biology of Blood and Marrow Transplantation, 21,* 959–970. https://doi.org/10.1016/j.bbmt.2014.11.676

Strong Rodrigues, K., Oliveira-Ribeiro, C., de Abreu Fiuza Gomes, S., & Knobler, R. (2018). Cutaneous graft-versus-host disease: Diagnosis and treatment. *American Journal of Clinical Dermatology, 19,* 33–50. https://doi.org/10.1007/s40257-017-0306-9

Sung, A.D., Hassan, S., Cardona, D.M., Wild, D., Nichols, K.R., Mehdikhani, H., … Sullivan, K.M. (2018). Late gastrointestinal complications of allogeneic hematopoietic stem cell transplantation in adults. *Biology of Blood and Marrow Transplantation, 24,* 734–740. https://doi.org/10.1016/j.bbmt.2017.12.772

Syrjala, K.L., Martin, P.J., & Lee, S.J. (2012). Delivering care to long-term adult survivors of hematopoietic cell transplantation. *Journal of Clinical Oncology, 30,* 3746–3751. https://doi.org/10.1200/jco.2012.42.3038

Szyska, M., & Na, I.-K. (2016). Bone marrow GvHD after allogeneic hematopoietic stem cell transplantation. *Frontiers in Immunology, 7,* 118. https://doi.org/10.3389/fimmu.2016.00118

Tan, Y., Xiao, H., Wu, D., Luo, Y., Lan, J., Liu, Q., … Huang, H. (2017). Combining therapeutic antibodies using basiliximab and etanercept for severe steroid-refractory acute graft-versus-host disease: A multi-center prospective study. *Oncoimmunology, 6,* e1277307. https://doi.org/10.1080/2162402x.2016.1277307

Teshima, T., Reddy, P., & Zeiser, R. (2016). Acute graft-versus-host disease: Novel biological insights. *Biology of Blood and Marrow Transplantation, 22,* 11–16. https://doi.org/10.1016/j.bbmt.2015.10.001

Tey, S.K., Vuckovic, S., Varelias, A., Martins, J.P., Olver, S., Samson, L., … Hill, G.R. (2016). Pharmacokinetics and immunological outcomes of alemtuzumab-based treatment for steroid-refractory acute GvHD. *Bone Marrow Transplantation, 51,* 1153–1155. https://doi.org/10.1038/bmt.2016.83

Tjon, A.S.W., van Gent, R., Geijtenbeek, T.B., & Kwekkeboom, J. (2015). Differences in anti-inflammatory actions of intravenous immuno-globulin between mice and men: More than meets the eye. *Frontiers in Immunology, 6,* 197. https://doi.org/10.3389/fimmu.2015.00197

Tong, L.X., & Worswick, S.D. (2015). Viral infections in acute graft-versus-host disease: A review of diagnostic and therapeutic approaches. *Journal of the American Academy of Dermatology, 72,* 696–702. https://doi.org/10.1016/j.jaad.2014.12.002

Toubai, T., Mathewson, N.D., Magenau, J., & Reddy, P. (2016). Danger signals and graft-versus-host disease: Current understanding and future perspectives. *Frontiers in Immunology, 7,* 539. https://doi.org/10.3389/fimmu.2016.00539

Tung, C.I. (2017). Graft versus host disease: What should the oculoplastic surgeon know? *Current Opinion in Ophthalmology, 28,* 499–504. https://doi.org/10.1097/icu.0000000000000400

Ullmann, A.J., Schmidt-Hieber, M., Bertz, H., Heinz, W.J., Kiehl, M., Krüger, W., … Maschmeyer, G. (2016). Infectious diseases in allogeneic haematopoietic stem cell transplantation: Prevention and prophylaxis strategy guidelines 2016. *Annals of Hematology, 95,* 1435–1455. https://doi.org/10.1007/s00277-016-2711-1

van der Meij, B.S., de Graaf, P., Wierdsma, N.J., Langius, J.A.E., Janssen, J.J., van Leeuwen, P.A., & Visser, O.J. (2013). Nutritional support in patients with GVHD of the digestive tract: State of the art. *Bone Marrow Transplantation, 48,* 474–482. https://doi.org/10.1038/bmt.2012.124

van Groningen, L.F., Liefferink, A.M., de Haan, A.F., Schaap, N.P., Donnelly, J.P., Blijlevens, N.M., & van der Velden, W.J. (2016). Combination therapy with inolimomab and etanercept for severe steroid-refractory acute graft-versus-host disease. *Biology of Blood and Marrow Transplantation, 22,* 179–182. https://doi.org/10.1016/j.bbmt.2015.08.039

Verdi Schumacher, M., & Moreira Faulhaber, G.A. (2017). Nutritional status and hyperglycemia in the peritransplant period: A review of associations with parenteral nutrition and clinical outcomes. *Revista Brasileira de Hematologia e Hemoterapia, 39,* 155–162. https://doi.org/10.1016/j.bjhh.2016.09.016

Vieyra-Garcia, P.A., & Wolf, P. (2018). From early immunomodulatory triggers to immunosuppressive outcome: Therapeutic implications of the complex interplay between the wavebands of sunlight and the skin. *Frontiers in Medicine, 5,* 232. https://doi.org/10.3389/fmed.2018.00232

Villa, N.Y., & McFadden, G. (2018). Virotherapy as potential adjunct therapy for graft-vs-host disease. *Current Pathobiology Reports, 6,* 247–263. https://doi.org/10.1007/s40139-018-0186-6

Villa, N.Y., Rahman, M.M., McFadden, G., & Cogle, C.R. (2016). Therapeutics for graft-versus-host disease: From conventional therapies to novel virotherapeutic strategies. *Viruses, 8,* 85. https://doi.org/10.3390/v8030085

Villarreal, C.D., Alanis, J.C.S., Perez, J.C., & Candiani, J.O. (2016). Cutaneous graft-versus-host disease after hematopoietic stem cell transplant—A review. *Anais Brasileiros de Dermatologia, 91,* 336–343. https://doi.org/10.1590/abd1806-4841.20164180

Vriesendorp, H.M., & Heidt, P.J. (2016). History of graft-versus-host disease. *Experimental Hematology, 44,* 674–688. https://doi.org/10.1016/j.exphem.2016.05.011

Vukic, T., Robinson Smith, S., Ljubas Kelečić, D., Desnica, L., Prenc, E., Pulanic, D., … Pavletic, S.Z. (2016). Joint and fascial chronic graft-vs-host disease: Correlations with clinical and laboratory parameters. *Croatian Medical Journal, 57,* 266–275. https://doi.org/10.3325/cmj.2016.57.266

Wada, H., Mori, A., Okada, M., Takatsuka, H., Tamura, A., Seto, Y., … Kakishita, E. (2001). Treatment of intestinal graft-versus-host disease using betamethasone enemas. *Transplantation, 72,* 1451–1453. https://doi.org/10.1097/00007890-200110270-00020

Wolff, D., Bertz, H., Greinix, H., Lawitschka, A., Halter, J., & Holler, E. (2011). The treatment of chronic graft-versus-host disease: Consensus recommendations of experts from Germany, Austria, and Switzerland. *Deutsches Ärzteblatt International, 108,* 732–740. https://doi.org/10.3238/arztebl.2011.0732

Wolff, D., Gerbitz, A., Ayuk, F., Kiani, A., Hildebrandt, G.C., Vogelsang, G.B., … Greinix, H. (2010). Consensus conference on clinical practice in chronic graft-versus-host disease (GVHD): First-line and topical treatment of chronic GVHD. *Biology of Blood and Marrow Transplantation, 16,* 1611–1628. https://doi.org/10.1016/j.bbmt.2010.06.015

Wolff, D., Schleuning, M., von Harsdorf, S., Bacher, U., Gerbitz, A., Stadler, M., … Holler, E. (2011). Consensus conference on clinical practice in chronic GVHD: Second-line treatment of chronic graft-versus-host disease. *Biology of Blood and Marrow Transplantation, 17*, 1–17. https://doi.org/10.1016/j.bbmt.2010.05.011

Yan, C.-H., Liu, Q.-F., Wu, D.-P., Zhang, X., Xu, L.-P., Zhang, X.-H., ... Huang, X.-J. (2020). Corrigendum to 'prophylactic donor lymphocyte infusion (DLI) followed by minimal residual disease and graft-versus-host disease guided multiple DLIs could improve outcomes after allogeneic hematopoietic stem cell transplantation in patients with refractory/relapsed acute leukemia' [Biology of Blood and Marrow Transplantation 23/8 (2017) 1311-1319]. *Biology of Blood and Marrow Transplantation, 23*, 1311–1319. https://doi.org/10.1016/j.bbmt.2019.03.006

Yeshurun, M., Shpilberg, O., Herscovici, C., Shargian, L., Dreyer, J., Peck, A., ... Ram, R. (2015). Cannabidiol for the prevention of graft-versus-host-disease after allogeneic hematopoietic cell transplantation: Results of a phase II study. *Biology of Blood and Marrow Transplantation, 21*, 1770–1775. https://doi.org/10.1016/j.bbmt.2015.05.018

Zama, D., Biagi, E., Masetti, R., Gasperini, P., Prete, A., Candela, M., ... Pession, A. (2017). Gut microbiota and hematopoietic stem cell transplantation: Where do we stand? *Bone Marrow Transplantation, 52*, 7–14. https://doi.org/10.1038/bmt.2016.173

Zatarain, L., & Savani, B.N. (2012). The role of nutrition and effects on the cytokine milieu in allogeneic hematopoietic stem cell transplantation. *Cell Immunology, 276*, 6–9. https://doi.org/10.1016/j.cellimm.2012.05.003

Zeiser, R. (2018). Biology-driven developments in the therapy of acute graft-versus-host disease. *American Society of Hematology Education Program Book, 2018*, 236–241. https://doi.org/10.1182/asheducation-2018.1.236

Zeiser, R., & Blazar, B.R. (2017). Acute graft-versus-host disease—Biologic process, prevention, and therapy. *New England Journal of Medicine, 377*, 2167–2179. https://doi.org/10.1056/nejmra1609337

Zeiser, R., Sarantopoulos, S., & Blazar, B.R. (2018). B-cell targeting in chronic graft-versus-host disease. *Blood, 131*, 1399–1405. https://doi.org/10.1182/blood-2017-11-784017

Zeiser, R., Socié, G., & Blazar, B.R. (2016). Pathogenesis of acute graft-versus-host disease: From intestinal microbiota alterations to donor T cell activation. *British Journal of Haematology, 175*, 191–207. https://doi.org/10.1111/bjh.14295

Zhang, L., Yu, J., & Wei, W. (2018). Advance in targeted immunotherapy for graft-versus-host disease. *Frontiers in Immunology, 9*, 1087. https://doi.org/10.3389/fimmu.2018.01087

Zheng, J., Taylor, B., & Chen, X. (2018). Role of vitamin A in modulating graft-versus-host disease. *Journal of Immunology Research and Therapy, 3*, 124–128.

Zhou, X., & Brenner, M.K. (2016). Improving the safety of T-cell therapies using an inducible caspase-9 gene. *Experimental Hematology, 44*, 1013–1019. https://doi.org/10.1016/j.exphem.2016.07.011

CHAPTER 8

Hematologic Effects

Robin Rosselet, DNP, APRN-CNP, AOCN®

Introduction

The most common hematologic effects that occur following hematopoietic stem cell transplantation (HSCT) include neutropenia, immunosuppression, thrombocytopenia, anemia, graft failure, and delayed engraftment. Although these effects typically result as complications from the transplant preparative regimen, other risk factors should be considered. This chapter explores the effects of preparative regimens as well as factors that lead to hematologic abnormalities. Less-toxic preparative regimens that allow for engraftment of donor stem cells with lower risks for treatment-related toxicity are now used. This chapter discusses the pathophysiology, etiology, management, and nursing implications of each hematologic complication related to the effects of the conditioning or preparatory regimen as well as T-cell dysregulation seen in HSCT.

Neutropenia

Chemotherapy and radiation cause myelosuppression and decrease the number of neutrophils. This results in a condition known as neutropenia, which is a major dose-limiting side effect of cancer treatment. Table 8-1 shows the Common Terminology Criteria for Adverse Events (CTCAE) grading system for neutropenia (National Cancer Institute Cancer Therapy Evaluation Program [NCI CTEP], 2017). Profound neutropenia with an absolute neutrophil count less than $100/mm^3$ is common in HSCT recipients as a result of high-dose chemotherapy and radi-

ation therapy administered during the pretransplant preparative regimen (Koniarczyk & Ferraro, 2016). The duration of neutropenia depends on several factors, including prior chemotherapy and radiation, preparative regimen, stem cell source, number of CD34+ cells per kilogram infused, use of growth factors following transplant, and post-transplant complications. Prolonged periods of neutropenia combined with other transplant complications (e.g., impaired skin and mucosal integrity, graft-versus-host disease [GVHD], graft rejection, steroid therapy, malnutrition, invasive venous catheters [central venous catheters]) increase the risk of morbidity and mortality related to severe infections (Koniarczyk & Ferraro, 2016).

Substantial progress has occurred over the past several decades in limiting the toxicities associated with allogeneic HSCT, particularly with myeloablative conditioning regimens (Sandmaier & Storb, 2016). Pancytopenia can lead to life-threatening infections and damage to the liver, kidneys, and lungs. Organ damage can complicate the ability to successfully perform a myeloablative transplant (Sandmaier & Storb, 2016). Findings in the 1970s and 1980s led to a greater understanding of the graft-versus-tumor effects of allogeneic transplant and greater relapse-free survival (Bensinger, 2016; Sandmaier & Storb, 2016). From these findings, investigators have developed reduced-intensity conditioning, which has decreased regimen-related toxicities (Bensinger, 2016; Sandmaier & Storb, 2016).

Neutropenia and its associated infections are the most common complications of HSCT. Improvements in supportive care management have decreased the number of

Table 8-1. Common Terminology Criteria for Adverse Events Grading of Neutropenia

Adverse Event	Grade				
	1	2	3	4	5
Neutrophil count decreased	< LLN–1,500/mm³; < LLN–1.5 × 10⁹/L	< 1,500–1,000/mm³; < 1.5–1 × 10⁹/L	< 1,000–500/mm³; < 1–0.5 × 10⁹/L	< 500/mm³; < 0.5 × 10⁹/L	–

Definition: A finding based on laboratory test results that indicate a decrease in the number of neutrophils in a blood specimen.

LLN—lower limit of normal

Note. From *Common Terminology Criteria for Adverse Events* [v.5.0], by National Cancer Institute Cancer Therapy Evaluation Program, 2017. Retrieved from https://ctep.cancer.gov/protocolDevelopment/electronic_applications/docs/CTCAE_v5_Quick_Reference_8.5x11.pdf.

transplant-associated infections during the neutropenic phase; however, infection remains the leading cause of post-transplant mortality and morbidity (Norton, Garcia, & Noonan, 2016).

The body has two basic lines of defense against invasion of infection-causing pathogens. The first is the skin and mucosal linings; the second is the white blood cell (WBC). The WBC community contains granulocytes (which consist of neutrophils, basophils, and eosinophils), monocytes (which mature into macrophages), and lymphocytes (which include various T cells and B cells). Neutrophils are phagocytes that contain lytic enzymes in their cytoplasm and are the first to respond to invading organisms and produce the inflammatory response (Devine, 2016). They represent approximately 60% of the WBC population, making them a prominent component of an adequate immune system (Devine, 2016).

The duration of neutropenia is directly related to the risk of infection in transplant recipients. Infections typically are discussed in the context of the time after transplant in which they occur. Different risk factors and organisms are associated with different phases of the transplant process and are described elsewhere in this book. Yet, despite improvements in management and supportive care over the past decade driven by new anti-infective agents and novel conditioning regimens, infection remains the primary cause of death in 8% of autologous and 17%–20% of allogeneic HSCT recipients (Devine, 2016; Norton et al., 2016).

The transplant process may be defined in phases beginning with pretransplant, followed by the immediate post-transplant or pre-engraftment phase (0–15 days), the intermediate post-transplant or postengraftment phase (15–100 days), and the late post-transplant phase (after day +100) (Devine, 2016; Norton et al., 2016). Table 8-2 describes infectious complications common during each phase of the transplant process.

Pre-Engraftment Infections (0–15 Days)

During the pre-engraftment phase, transplant recipients are at risk for infection because of severe myelosuppression-causing neutropenia and gastrointestinal mucosal toxicity, which occur as expected side effects of the preparative regimen. The skin is the largest organ in the body and serves as a barrier to infection. However, it is colonized with bacteria that aid in the body's defense against pathogens. The resident bacteria can become opportunistic and gain access through skin breakdown (Devine, 2016; Koniarczyk & Ferraro, 2016). In addition, placement of a central venous catheter impairs skin integrity. Previous exposure to infections, such as herpes simplex virus and cytomegalovirus (CMV), poses an additional risk, as reactivation is possible during the neutropenic phase. Other factors contributing to the overwhelming risk for infections include the type of transplant, pretransplant recipient factors, disease status, human leukocyte antigen (HLA) match, donor source, and conditioning intensity (see Table 8-3).

Bacterial Infections

Bacteria are the most common cause of infection during this period, accounting for 90% of neutropenic infections (Devine, 2016; Koniarczyk & Ferraro, 2016; Leather & Wingard, 2016). Common bacterial infection-causing pathogens include gram-negative (*Escherichia coli*, *Klebsiella pneumoniae*, and *Pseudomonas aeruginosa*) and gram-positive (*Staphylococcus epidermidis*, *Staphylococcus aureus*, and *Streptococci*) species (Devine, 2016; Leather & Wingard, 2016). The most common sites for infection are the oral mucosa and those associated with central venous catheters.

Guidelines for preventing infectious complications among HSCT recipients were published in 2009 as a joint effort of 10 expert groups and agencies and more recently updated in 2016 (Tomblyn et al., 2009; Wingard, 2020). The 2009 guidelines were an update to guidelines published in 2000 by the Centers for Disease Control and Prevention, the Infectious Diseases Society of America, and the American Society for Transplantation and Cellular Therapy (formerly the American Society for Blood and Marrow Transplantation). The goal was to compile infection prevention guidelines based on a summary of current data, provide evidence-based recommendations, and publish a worldwide reference (Tomblyn et al., 2009; Wingard, 2020). Although the 2000 edition did not recommend prophylactic bacterial coverage for afebrile transplant recipients, the 2009 guidelines recommended quinolone prophylaxis for adult HSCT recipients who were expected to be neutropenic for at least seven days (Tomblyn et al., 2009). The 2016 update suggested that antibacterial prophylaxis with a fluoroquinolone has been shown in randomized trials and meta-analyses to reduce all-cause mortality, infection-related mortality, fever, and infections in high-risk neutropenic patients and supported its use up through engraftment (Wingard, 2020). However, no evidence exists to support this practice in the pediatric transplant population.

With the first febrile episode, fluoroquinolone should be discontinued, and coverage for gram-positive and gram-negative organisms should be instituted. Commonly used antibiotic classes include third- and fourth-generation cephalosporins, carbapenems, penicillinase-resistant penicillins, quinolones, aminoglycosides, and vancomycin (for staphylococcal infections). Antibiotic selection should be guided by local antibiotic resistance patterns. Because of the emergence of vancomycin-resistant *Enterococcus*, vancomycin should not be used as prophylaxis and should be discontinued if culture sensitivity is not documented (Tomblyn et al., 2009; Wingard, 2020). In conjunction with any change or implementation of antibiotic therapy, nurses should expect other diagnostic tests, including blood cultures, chest x-ray, and stool and urine cultures.

Fungal Infections

Yeast and fungal infections may be problematic during the pre-engraftment phase and include *Candida albicans*, primarily as stomatitis, and *Aspergillus* species. Infections

Table 8-2. Infectious Complications and Occurrence in Hematopoietic Stem Cell Transplantation Recipients

Organism	Common Sites	Treatment
Prophylaxis		
Bacterial	Blood, sinopulmonary	Fluoroquinolone for adults with anticipated neutropenia for > 7 days
Fungal	Esophageal, oral, sinopulmonary, skin	Fluconazole for invasive candidiasis before engraftment Micafungin or posaconazole for patients at high risk for infections from molds or fluconazole-resistant *Candida* species; alternative: voriconazole
Viral	Esophageal, gastrointestinal (GI) tract, genital, oral, sinopulmonary, skin	Acyclovir for all herpes simplex virus–seropositive allogeneic recipients Ganciclovir for cytomegalovirus (CMV)-seropositive recipients or seronegative recipients with seropositive donors
Bacterial		
Gram negative (*Escherichia coli, Pseudomonas aeruginosa, Klebsiella*)	Blood, GI tract, oral, perirectal	Antibiotic selection guided by local antibiotic resistance patterns
Gram positive (*Staphylococcus epidermidis, Staphylococcus aureus, Streptococci*)	Blood, sinopulmonary, skin	Aminoglycosides, third- and fourth-generation cephalosporins, quinolones, vancomycin
Fungal		
Aspergillus (fumigata, flavum)	Sinopulmonary	Liposomal amphotericin, micafungin, posaconazole, voriconazole
Candida (albicans, glabrata, krusei)	Esophageal, oral, skin	Fluconazole, itraconazole, micafungin, posaconazole, voriconazole
Viral		
Epstein-Barr virus	Esophageal, GI tract, oral, skin	Rituximab
Herpes simplex virus	Esophageal, GI tract, genital, oral, skin	First line: acyclovir Alternative: valacyclovir
Respiratory syncytial virus (RSV)	Sinopulmonary	Aerosolized ribavirin Prophylaxis: palivizumab during RSV season
1–4 Months Post-Transplant		
Bacterial		
Gram positive	Sinopulmonary	Aminoglycosides, third- and fourth-generation cephalosporins, quinolones, vancomycin
Fungal		
Candida species	Hepatosplenic, integument, oral	Fluconazole, itraconazole, micafungin, posaconazole, voriconazole
Aspergillus species	Central nervous system (CNS), sinopulmonary	–
Protozoan		
Pneumocystis jirovecii (carinii)	Pulmonary	Standard: trimethoprim-sulfamethoxazole (TMP-SMX) Alternatives: atovaquone, dapsone, pentamidine
Toxoplasma gondii	CNS, pulmonary	Standard: TMP-SMX Alternatives: pyrimethamine plus leucovorin may be combined with clindamycin
Viral		
Adenovirus	Blood, GI tract, urinary	Standard: cidofovir Alternative: ribavirin
CMV	GI tract, hepatic, pulmonary	First line: ganciclovir Alternatives: acyclovir, foscarnet, valacyclovir
Enteric viruses (rotavirus, *Coxsackie*, adenovirus)	GI tract, hepatic, pulmonary, urinary	No specific treatment

(Continued on next page)

Table 8-2. Infectious Complications and Occurrence in Hematopoietic Stem Cell Transplantation Recipients (Continued)

Organism	Common Sites	Treatment
1–4 Months Post-Transplant *(cont.)*		
Viral *(cont.)*		
Parainfluenza	Pulmonary	Possibly ribavirin, but no standard treatment
RSV	Sinopulmonary	Aerosolized ribavirin Prophylaxis: palivizumab during RSV season
4–12 Months Post-Transplant		
Bacterial		
Gram positive (*Streptococcus pneumoniae, Haemophilus influenzae, Pneumococci*)	Blood, sinopulmonary	Aminoglycosides, third- and fourth-generation cephalosporins, quinolones, vancomycin
Fungal		
Aspergillus	Sinopulmonary	Liposomal amphotericin, micafungin, posaconazole, voriconazole
Protozoan		
Pneumocystis jirovecii (carinii)	Pulmonary	Standard: TMP-SMX Alternatives: atovaquone, dapsone, pentamidine
Toxoplasma gondii	CNS, pulmonary	Standard: TMP-SMX Alternative: pyrimethamine plus leucovorin may be combined with clindamycin
Viral		
Adenovirus	Blood, GI tract, urinary	Standard: cidofovir Alternative: ribavirin
CMV, echoviruses, RSV, varicella-zoster virus (VZV)	Hepatic, pulmonary, skin	CMV: acyclovir, foscarnet, ganciclovir, valacyclovir Echoviruses: no specific treatment, IV immunoglobulins RSV: aerosolized ribavirin VZV: acyclovir, famciclovir, valacyclovir
> 12 Months Post-Transplant		
Bacterial		
Gram positive (*Streptococci, H. influenzae*, encapsulated bacteria)	Blood, sinopulmonary	Aminoglycosides, third- and fourth-generation cephalosporins, quinolones, vancomycin
Viral		
VZV	Skin	Post-exposure prophylaxis: VZV immunoglobulin (if available) Standard: acyclovir Alternative: valacyclovir

Note. Based on information from Norton et al., 2016; Tomblyn et al., 2009.

caused by less common amphotericin-resistant molds have been described, including non-*fumigatus Aspergillus* species, *Fusarium* species, and *Scedosporium* species (Marr et al., 2009). Prophylaxis for fungal infection may include medications such as fluconazole for invasive candidiasis before engraftment and an "azole" such as posaconazole or voriconazole for patients at high risk for infections from mold post-transplant (e.g., patients on post-transplant immunosuppression such as prednisone for GVHD) (Devine, 2016; Koniarczyk & Ferraro, 2016; Leather & Wingard, 2016; Tomblyn et al., 2009; Wingard, 2020). Patients who are most at risk for fungal infections are those who are neutropenic, are on prolonged immunosuppression, or have chronic GVHD.

Common treatment of invasive fungal infections such as *Aspergillus* includes micafungin, liposomal amphotericin, posaconazole, and voriconazole (Tomblyn et al., 2009; Wingard, 2020). Oral treatments such as nystatin and clotrimazole troches may reduce colonization by *Candida* albicans; however, these agents have not been proved to prevent invasion or dissemination of yeast or mold, and their prophylactic use is unclear (Tomblyn et al., 2009; Wingard, 2020). Patients should be instructed to prevent exposure to molds by avoiding construction sites, building renovation areas, and gardening activities (Tomblyn et al., 2009; Wingard, 2020).

In hospitals with transplant units, it is important to minimize exposure of immunocompromised patients to fungal risk factors. The following are recommendations for infection prevention (Devine, 2016; Norton et al., 2016; Wingard, 2020):

- Allogeneic patients should be placed in protective isolation during hospitalization, especially during the neutropenic phases after HSCT. It also can be used for autologous HSCT recipients, depending on room availability.
- Protective isolation room ventilation should have 12 or more air exchanges per hour using HEPA filters with 99.7% efficiency for removing particles 0.3 mcm or larger, directed airflow, positive air pressure differential between the patient's room and the hallway, well-sealed rooms, continuous pressure monitoring, and self-closing doors to maintain constant pressure differentials.
- The use of laminar airflow remains controversial because its possible benefit remains unclear, and it is not recommended for newly constructed patient rooms. During construction or renovation, intensified mold control measures should be put into place to minimize fungal spore counts in patient rooms.
- HSCT patient rooms should be cleaned at least daily with special attention to dust control. Selection of furnishings should focus on creating and maintaining a dust-free environment.

Viral Infections

HSCT recipients, particularly those who have undergone allogeneic transplants, are at an increased risk for contracting a variety of viruses, including herpes simplex virus, varicella zoster virus, CMV, Epstein-Barr virus, respiratory viruses (e.g., influenza, parainfluenza, respiratory syncytial virus, adenovirus), human herpesvirus 6, hepatitis B, and hepatitis C (Wingard, 2020). Prophylaxis or pre-emptive therapy against some of these is recommended and will be discussed here.

Patients and donors should be evaluated for latent viruses known to reactivate following HSCT before conditioning chemotherapy is initiated. During the neutropenic and later phases, patients are susceptible not only to community-acquired respiratory viral infections but also reactivation of one of the many herpes families of viruses. Reactivation of herpes simplex virus 1 and 2, human herpesvirus 6, and CMV may occur during the immediate post-transplant phase. Herpes simplex most often manifests as stomatitis. Prophylaxis with acyclovir or valacyclovir is commonly used in the pre-engraftment phase (Devine, 2016).

Allogeneic HSCT recipients have a much higher incidence of CMV antigenemia (presence of CMV in the blood) than autologous HSCT recipients. Of allogeneic patients, those with acute GVHD beyond grade 1 have a higher incidence of CMV (Devine, 2016; Norton et al., 2016; Wingard, 2020). With the use of leukocyte filters for platelet and red blood cell (RBC) transfusions and proper management, CMV-seronegative patients have a low risk of contracting CMV infections (Seifried & Schmidt, 2016). Sero-

Table 8-3. Risk Factors for Post-Transplant Infection

Factor	Lower Risk of Infection	Higher Risk of Infection
Type of transplant	Autologous or syngeneic	Allogeneic, graft manipulation
Time from transplant	> 100 days post-HSCT	Pre-engraftment and first 100 days post-HSCT
Pretransplant host factors	–	Extensive pre-HSCT immunosuppression (fludarabine, clofarabine), prolonged pre-HSCT neutropenia, and pre-HSCT infection
GVHD	–	Grade 3–4 acute GVHD; extensive chronic GVHD
HLA match	Matched donors	Mismatched, particularly haploidentical
Disease status	Disease in first remission	Advanced or refractory disease at time of HSCT
Donor type	Matched sibling	Unrelated donor
Graft type	Intermediate with bone marrow	Highest with UCB
Post-HSCT immunosuppression	–	Use of immunosuppression, especially corticosteroids, antithymocyte globulin, or alemtuzumab
Conditioning intensity	Reduced-intensity conditioning for 1–3 months	Myeloablative conditioning
Neutrophil engraftment	Intermediate with bone marrow, highest with UCB	Bone marrow, UCB, delayed engraftment, or nonengraftment

GVHD—graft-versus-host disease; HLA—human leukocyte antigen; HSCT—hematopoietic stem cell transplantation; UCB—umbilical cord blood

Note. Based on information from Tomblyn et al., 2009.

positive patients and seronegative patients with seropositive donors should be placed on CMV disease surveillance and/or prevention starting at engraftment (approximately day +10) until a minimum of 100 days post-HSCT (Seifried & Schmidt, 2016). CMV disease prevention varies among transplant centers, but the minimum should include weekly surveillance with the use of sensitive and specific laboratory tests that enable rapid diagnosis of viral replication (Seifried & Schmidt, 2016). Most centers favor a preemptive (based on screening with a sensitive assay [e.g., polymerase chain reaction] to detect early infection) approach rather than a prophylactic approach. CMV prophylaxis has been studied using a variety of agents including acyclovir, foscarnet, ganciclovir, letermovir, valacyclovir, and valganciclovir (Wingard, 2020). Of the available agents, IV ganciclovir has been the most effective but must be used cautiously because it causes bone marrow suppression. High-dose acyclovir and valacyclovir have less bone marrow toxicity but have inferior in vitro activity against CMV (Wingard, 2020). Therefore, treatment generally is held immediately before transplant and restarted after successful engraftment. Seropositive autologous patients who are at high risk are those who have received total body irradiation; those who have received recent alemtuzumab, cladribine, or fludarabine; or those who received manipulated grafts (Wingard, 2020). Most centers will test patients weekly for CMV reactivation until 60 days after transplant.

Testing for CMV is primarily performed through one of three methods: CMV pp65 antigen in leukocytes (antigenemia), CMV DNA by quantitative polymerase chain reaction, or the detection of CMV RNA (Wingard, 2020). Centers that perform allogeneic transplants should have the capability to perform these tests.

Varicella zoster virus–seropositive patients should receive prophylaxis with oral acyclovir (800 mg twice daily) or valacyclovir (500 mg twice daily) for at least a year, and immunocompromised patients with GVHD should remain on prophylaxis until six months after immunosuppression has been discontinued (Wingard, 2020).

For patients who are herpes simplex virus seropositive (herpes simplex virus immunoglobulin G positive), antiviral prophylaxis is recommended using oral acyclovir (800 mg twice daily) or oral valacyclovir (500 mg twice daily) if not tolerated, then IV acyclovir (5 mg/kg every 12 hours or 250 mg/m² every 12 hours). Prophylaxis should be given from conditioning until engraftment or until mucositis resolves (Wingard, 2020).

Prophylaxis of Pneumocystis Jirovecii Pneumonia

Pneumocystis jirovecii pneumonia (PJP; formerly referred to as *Pneumocystis carinii* pneumonia) is uncommon (less than 1%) in HSCT recipients receiving prophylaxis with trimethoprim-sulfamethoxazole (TMP-SMX) (Wingard, 2020). The diagnosis should be considered in HSCT recipients with the following symptoms: high fever, dry cough, hypoxemia, and interstitial pneumonitis who are at risk but are not being given prophylaxis, who are being given suboptimal agents (aerosolized pentamidine or dapsone given on alternate days), or who are nonadherent with PJP prophylaxis. The efficacy of daily dapsone in preventing PJP appears to be similar to that observed in patients able to remain on TMP-SMX, although aerosolized pentamidine is less effective than either TMP-SMX or dapsone (Wingard, 2020). Patients at greatest risk include those with prolonged administration of immunosuppressive therapies (high-dose glucocorticoids), chronic GVHD, therapy with purine analogs or rituximab, a CD4+ T-cell count less than 200 cells/mm³, and relapse of hematologic malignancy (Wingard, 2020).

Other Infection Prevention Measures

The changing healthcare landscape has resulted in some patients now receiving part or all of their care in outpatient clinics and at home. Selected patients treated outside of filtered hospital rooms may be at higher risk for infection during the pre-engraftment phase (Wingard, 2020). Likewise, it has been reported that carefully selected patients treated in the outpatient environment may use approximately the same amount of antibiotics and develop fevers at approximately the same rate as those in inpatient settings (Bergkvist, Fossum, Johansson, Mattsson, & Larsen, 2018). Allowing treatment in the outpatient setting or sending patients out of the hospital prior to engraftment may improve their emotional and social outlook without compromising safety. It is important that patients be carefully selected for programs allowing this flexibility.

Perhaps more important than air filtration systems is the patient's and family's understanding of interventions to prevent infections: appropriate hygiene, oral and central venous catheter care, appropriate low-bacterial diets, and avoidance of crowds, fresh flowers or plants, and other sources of infectious contamination. Nurses play a unique role in providing education regarding infection prevention irrespective of whether the patient is treated in the inpatient or outpatient setting.

Neutrophil Engraftment

The point at which the neutrophil count is maintained at greater than 500/mm³ is considered neutrophil engraftment (Antin & Raley, 2013; Koniarczyk & Ferraro, 2016). The most recognized and important factors in the fight against early infectious complications after transplant are the use of colony-stimulating factors, mobilized peripheral blood stem cells (PBSCs), and the number of stem cells (CD34+ cells per kilogram) transplanted. Transplants using PBSCs mobilized with hematopoietic growth factors (specifically filgrastim, granulocyte–colony-stimulating factor) have improved hematologic recovery for autologous and allogeneic recipients (Antin & Raley, 2013; Koniarczyk & Ferraro, 2016; Wingard, 2020). A 2014 Cochrane review of five studies (n = 662) demonstrated that neutrophil and platelet engraftment was faster with PBSCs versus bone marrow (p < 0.00001) (Holtick et al., 2014). In the autologous transplant population, using mobilized PBSCs rather than bone marrow decreases the duration of neutropenia (Devine, 2016; Koniarczyk & Ferraro, 2016). A variety of studies have shown the engraftment time is related to type of transplant, source of stem cells, use of filgrastim, and type of immunosuppression (Antin & Raley, 2013; Koniarczyk & Ferraro, 2016).

Nonmyeloablative preparative regimens are becoming more common in the allogeneic HSCT setting. Because of a shorter neutropenic phase and less mucosal tissue damage, the incidence of bacterial infections may be decreased during the early phase of transplant (Sandmaier & Storb, 2016). However, patients undergoing nonmyeloablative transplant regimens have not had fewer infections in later phases of the transplant process.

The dose of infused cells contributes to the duration of neutropenia. Cell dose is commonly calculated based on the number of CD34+ cells. CD34+ is a molecule on the surface of primitive progenitor cells. These earliest cells are most valuable in reestablishing hematopoiesis after transplant. Therefore, the number of CD34+ cells to be transplanted has become a marker for engraftment potential. Kiss et al. (1997) and Schulman, Birch, Zhen, Pania, and Weaver (1999) reported research indicating that faster neutrophil engraftment time was associated with CD34+ cell infusions greater than 5×10^6 cells/kg in autologous transplant. Both groups also reported a decrease of one day (p = 0.004, p = 0.0001, respectively) in the median number of days to neutrophil engraftment. Schulman et al. (1999) equated a CD34+ cell dose of greater than 5×10^6 cells/kg with a reduction in patient resource utilization, including fewer platelet and RBC infusions, decreased length of hospitalization, decreased use of IV antibiotics and antifungal agents, and decreased days of filgrastim administration. More recently, a dose of 3×10^6 CD34+ cells/kg was associated with not only rapid hematopoietic recovery but also a decrease in the incidence of fungal infections and improved overall survival (Antin & Raley, 2013; Wingard, 2020). Bittencourt et al. (2002) reported that a CD34+ cell dose of at least 3×10^6 cells/kg significantly decreased the neutropenic duration (p = 0.04). Neutrophil engraftment occurred prior to day +60 in 97.1% of patients.

Umbilical cord blood is sometimes used as a source of stem cells for allogeneic transplant. Although it contains a rich source of stem cells, the quantity of cells available for transplant from a single umbilical cord is small, resulting in a delayed engraftment until day +40. However, if a second cord unit is infused, the time to engraftment decreases significantly to an average of 12–24 days (Antin & Raley, 2013).

The use of colony-stimulating factors such as filgrastim and sargramostim (granulocyte macrophage–colony-stimulating factor) has decreased the duration of neutropenia following both allogeneic and autologous HSCT. Early studies with autologous transplants showed that neutrophil recovery was accelerated in granulocyte-colony-stimulating factor–treated patients compared to historical controls: 11 versus 18 (Finke & Mertelsmann, 2016). A plethora of biosimilars and nonoriginator biologics of filgrastim have been approved or are in development. Recent studies by the World Marrow Donor Association found no evidence of an increased risk of filgrastim antibody formation (Pahnke et al., 2019). Based on these studies, the association therefore recommended that stem cell donor registries can use filgrastim biosimilars for mobilization in healthy donors (Pahnke et al., 2019). Initially it was thought that use of colony-stimulating factors after allogeneic HSCT may potentiate GVHD or increase the rate of relapse in patients with myeloid leukemia. However, colony-stimulating factors have essentially the same effects after autologous transplantation as they do after an allogeneic transplant (Finke & Mertelsmann, 2016).

A study in children and adolescents receiving an allogeneic HSCT showed that filgrastim improved the number of days to neutrophil engraftment. The added cost of using filgrastim was largely offset by a trend toward reduced use of antimicrobials (O'Rafferty et al., 2016). Another study in a pediatric population comparing the administration of filgrastim on day +6 versus day +1 found that delayed administration had no adverse effect on time to neutrophil engraftment or clinical outcomes and significantly decreased costs by requiring administration of less drug overall (p = 0.003) (Pai, Fernandez, Laudick, Rosselet, & Termuhlen, 2010).

Additional benefits of using granulocyte–colony-stimulating factor include a decrease in the number of hospital days and transfusion requirements. However, disadvantages include potential cytokine-induced engraftment syndromes, increased rates of GVHD, and additional costs (Finke & Mertelsmann, 2016).

Postengraftment Infections (15–100 Days)

HSCT recipients remain at high risk for infections even late after transplantation and may require extended follow-up. Risk factors for late infectious complications include extensive chronic GVHD and intensive immunosuppressive therapy for GVHD, with delayed immune reconstitution; CMV seronegative donor status and seropositive recipient status; and high-dose (myeloablative) and radiation-based conditioning regimens (Wingard, 2020).

Upper respiratory tract infections, sinusitis, pneumonia, and meningitis are most frequently caused by the encapsulated bacteria (*Streptococcus pneumoniae*, *Haemophilus influenzae*, *Neisseria meningitidis*) during this late postengraftment period (Wingard, 2020). Late bacterial sepsis is not uncommon after allogeneic HSCT and encapsulated bacteria staphylococci, and gram-negative bacteria such as *Pseudomonas* species are the most frequent pathogens (Wingard, 2020).

In the postengraftment phase, differences between allogeneic and autologous transplants become more evident. For autologous patients, the risk of developing infectious complications decreases during the intermediate post-transplant or postengraftment phase. However, for allogeneic patients, risk factors such as GVHD, graft rejection, prolonged neutropenia, and continued immunosuppressive therapy increase susceptibility to infection (Antin & Raley, 2014; Wingard, 2020). During this time, patients are especially at risk for viral and fungal infections, although the threat of bacterial infection continues.

Prior to the routine use of prophylactic or preemptive anti-CMV treatment, CMV-seropositive allogeneic HSCT recipients had a 70%–80% risk of reactivation, and 33% developed CMV disease, mostly pneumonia (Zaia, 2016). With more sophisticated detection assays and preemptive treatment, CMV reactivation occurred in only 45% of autologous or syngeneic HSCT recipients, yet CMV disease rarely occurs (Zaia, 2016). In allogeneic recipients who are CMV seropositive, with either donor CMV seropositivity, recipient CMV seropositivity, donor CMV seronegativity, or recipient CMV seropositivity, the incidence of CMV infection is 20%–75%, and the risk for CMV-associated disease is significant (Zaia, 2016).

With the advent of early detection, preventive treatment, and prophylaxis, CMV pneumonia is infrequent, occurring in less than 5% of allogeneic recipients (Afessa, Badley, & Peters, 2010). However, because it is fatal if untreated, evaluation of pneumonia should include tests to exclude or confirm CMV as a possible etiology. The major risk factors for CMV reactivation and disease are GVHD, the use of high-dose glucocorticoids, and prior CMV viremia. Surveillance per institutional policy is recommended. Interstitial pneumonia often is caused by community-acquired viruses and is more common between days +30 and +100 (Wingard, 2020). Refer to Chapter 11 for more information on interstitial pneumonia. Localized or disseminated varicella zoster virus infections also can occur during this time. Treatment for zoster infections caused by reactivation or a primary infection includes the use of high-dose acyclovir.

It is vitally important for nurses who care for transplant recipients to understand the neutropenic process and the diagnosis and treatment of infections often associated with neutropenia. One of the main roles of HSCT nurses is monitoring patients for neutropenic infections and administering treatments as ordered. To be successful, nurses must understand each patient's risk for infection based on past medical history and the treatment plan. Second, nurses must be aware of the HSCT timeline during which patients will most likely be neutropenic and the types of infections that may occur.

Nursing care of patients during the postengraftment phase includes frequent and thorough assessment, encompassing the central venous catheter site, respiratory status, and vital signs. Interventions include obtaining blood, urine, and catheter site cultures and administering antibiotics, antifungals, and antiviral medications. Historically, patients with post-HSCT infections have been hospitalized. However, it now is common for non-neutropenic patients to be managed in the outpatient setting or cared for in the home by homecare nurses and family members. Nursing care also involves education of patients and caregivers. Teaching the importance of hand hygiene, as well as personal hygiene, for infection control is imperative (Norton et al., 2016). Other important educational topics include recognizing the signs and symptoms of infection by monitoring temperature and assessing the skin, mucosal linings, and catheter insertion site.

Thrombocytopenia

Megakaryocytes typically are the last cell line to engraft following transplantation, although the period is shorter when using PBSCs as compared to bone marrow (Devine, 2016; Norton et al., 2016). Platelets are small fragments derived from megakaryocytes in the bone marrow and have a life span of 9–10 days. They are crucial for preventing bleeding and maintaining vascular integrity (Tormey & Rinder, 2016). The production of platelets is regulated by a hormone-like substance called thrombopoietin, which is produced by the kidneys. A normal platelet count for healthy individuals is in the range of 150,000–450,000/mm^3. Thrombocytopenia generally is defined as a platelet count less than 100,000/mm^3 (Norton et al., 2016) and commonly is seen in myeloablative transplant recipients.

Approximately 15,000–45,000 platelets must be produced per day to maintain hemostasis (Tormey & Rinder, 2016). In healthy individuals, an estimated one-third of the total number of platelets is sequestered within the spleen and released when needed (Murphy, Stanworth, & Estcourt, 2016). Splenomegaly, seen with myelofibrosis, various types of lymphomas, and certain types of leukemia, can result in an abnormally high number of platelets being sequestered, thus reducing the number of available platelets in circulation (Murphy et al., 2016). Immune-mediated thrombocytopenia may occur later in the post-transplant phase after an initial recovery and can be caused by viral or bacterial infections and medications (e.g., antibiotics, antivirals, heparin) (Norton et al., 2016). Severity of thrombocytopenia is graded using CTCAE (NCI CTEP, 2017; see Table 8-4).

Causes of Thrombocytopenia

As they age and die, platelets are removed from the circulation through the reticuloendothelial system. In healthy individuals, they are released from the bone marrow to maintain homeostasis (Devine, 2016; Norton et al., 2016). However, suppressed production of platelets is a common sequela of chemotherapy or radiation used in preparative conditioning regimens (Devine, 2016; Norton et al., 2016). This results in a delay of approximately one to three months before platelet counts normalize and transfusion support is no longer necessary (Devine, 2016; Norton et al., 2016).

In addition to the conditioning regimen, destruction or consumptive processes can cause thrombocytopenia. Viral infections including CMV, Epstein-Barr virus, human her-

Table 8-4. Common Terminology Criteria for Adverse Events Grading of Thrombocytopenia

Adverse Event	Grade				
	1	2	3	4	5
Platelet count decreased	< LLN–75,000/mm³; < LLN–75 × 10⁹/L	< 75,000–50,000/mm³; < 75–50 × 10⁹/L	< 50,000–25,000 mm³; < 50–25 × 10⁹/L	< 25,000/ mm³; < 25 × 10⁹/L	–

Definition: A finding based on laboratory test results that indicate a decrease in the number of platelets in a blood specimen.

LLN—lower limit of normal

Note. From *Common Terminology Criteria for Adverse Events* [v.5.0], by National Cancer Institute Cancer Therapy Evaluation Program, 2017. Retrieved from https://ctep.cancer.gov/protocolDevelopment/electronic_applications/docs/CTCAE_v5_Quick_Reference_8.5x11.pdf.

pesvirus 6, hantavirus, and HIV commonly cause thrombocytopenia. Other infectious diseases include mycoplasma and mycobacteria (Murphy et al., 2016). Nonsteroidal anti-inflammatory drugs, aspirin, and aspirin-containing products cause disorders of platelet function. Other medications such as TMP-SMX, quinine, and quinidine are thought to cause thrombocytopenia through an immune-mediated complex (Murphy et al., 2016). Quinine, quinidine, sulfonamides, sulfonamide derivatives such as furosemide, vancomycin, and the anticonvulsants valproic acid and gabapentin also have been associated with autoantibody formation (Murphy et al., 2016).

Immune-mediated thrombocytopenia commonly is associated with the use of heparin (Estcourt et al., 2015). Heparin-induced thrombocytopenia is a special class of immune-mediated thrombocytopenia defined as a prothrombotic drug reaction caused by immunoglobulin G antibodies to platelet factor 4 (responsible for activating platelets) (Estcourt et al., 2015). The differential diagnosis for heparin-induced thrombocytopenia includes suppressed platelet production, abnormal distribution of platelets, accelerated platelet destruction, or consumption of greater than 50% (Estcourt et al., 2015). Treatment includes discontinuing the use of heparin and initiating other methods of maintaining central venous catheter patency (e.g., sodium citrate).

Studies have examined the risk of serious bleeding based on specific platelet count targets, with the goal of preventing hemorrhage while minimizing the number of transfusions. A 2015 Cochrane review of prophylactic platelet transfusions after HSCT compared a trigger of 10,000/mm³ (referred to as a standard trigger) versus a trigger of 20,000/mm³ or 30,000/mm³ (Estcourt et al., 2015). Three trials were included in the review (N = 499), which showed no difference in the number of patients with clinically significant bleeding between the standard and higher trigger groups. Not surprisingly, the standard trigger group showed significant reduction in the number of transfusions per participant (Estcourt et al., 2015). It has been suggested that indiscriminate prophylactic transfusions may lead to sensitizing patients to antigens found on platelets (alloimmunization), with subsequent inability to control hemorrhage when it occurred (McFarland, 2016). Other reasons for limiting the number of platelet transfusions include reducing unnecessary costs and minimizing potential exposure to pathogens.

Platelet refractoriness, defined as the inability to achieve a desired increment after successive transfusions, can occur in the HSCT setting. It can be caused by immune and nonimmune mechanisms (Eisenberg, 2010). Both mechanisms may be present simultaneously, treating one will have no effect on the other. Refractoriness can take weeks to develop but may occur in as few as four days after a transfusion (Eisenberg, 2010). Refractoriness due to alloimmunization is associated with multiple transfusions and can be caused by HLA antigens or human platelet antigens (Eisenberg, 2010). When alloimmunization occurs, antibodies attack transfused platelets and cause platelet levels to decrease. A dose–response pattern appears to exist for the development of alloimmunization: the more antigens the recipient is exposed to through multiple units of blood and platelets, the greater the risk of developing alloimmunization (McFarland, 2016). Patients in whom alloimmunization is suspected should be tested by determining platelet count levels with serial blood draws after platelet transfusions. Blood tests are available to detect antiplatelet cytotoxic antibodies and anti-HLA antibodies. The use of special filters that remove leukocytes from blood products before transfusion can minimize or delay alloimmunization risk (McFarland, 2016). Most blood banks leukoreduce blood products before sending to the unit/clinic for transfusion.

Management strategies for platelet refractoriness are based on the likely source. Immune-related refractoriness can be alleviated by using only ABO-identical, HLA-compatible platelet products (Eisenberg, 2010). Evidence suggests that better HLA matches can produce better post-transfusion platelet counts, and up to 40% of alloimmunized refractory patients may lose their refractoriness over a period of weeks to months (Eisenberg, 2010).

Prevention and Treatment

First-generation thrombopoietic agents, recombinant and pegylated human megakaryocytic growth factors, were introduced in the 1990s for the prevention of severe thrombocytopenia following myelosuppressive chemotherapy (McCullough, 2016). However, these agents have limited use in the transplant setting because of significant side effects, which include dyspnea, edema, and tachycardia. Although the threshold for prophylactic platelet transfusions remains controversial (McCullough, 2016), most transplant programs designate a minimum threshold as a trigger for platelet transfusion. A Cochrane review of clinical trials conducted between 1991 and 2001 indicated that hemorrhage was seen more frequently and with greater severity when platelet counts were less than 10,000/mm³ (Estcourt et al., 2015). This review also indicated that gross visible hemorrhage rarely occurred with platelet counts greater than 20,000/mm³. Thus, the 20,000/mm³ threshold served as a trigger for initiating prophylactic platelet transfusion to prevent hemorrhage (Estcourt et al., 2015).

Patients with thrombocytopenia who are actively bleeding require an aggressive approach to platelet transfusions. Patients on defibrotide for hepatic sinusoidal occlusive disease (veno-occlusive disease) prophylaxis may be kept at a higher threshold, because of an increased incidence of bleeding (McCullough, 2016). See Chapter 10 for additional information on defibrotide.

Three major types of platelet products exist based on the methods used for procurement. Pooled platelets (formerly referred to as *random donor platelets*) are obtained from multiple units of whole blood. Although historically as many as 10 units of blood were used, blood banks in the United States have decreased that number to four, although six may still be available in some areas. Regardless of the number of whole blood units used, a bag of pooled platelets provides approximately the same number of cells as a single bag of platelets collected from one donor, known as apheresis platelets (Murphy et al., 2016). Pooled platelets are more readily available and less expensive than apheresis platelets but expose the patient to multiple donors, which increases the risk of alloimmunization and transfusion-transmitted disease (Murphy et al., 2016).

Apheresis platelets, formerly referred to as *single-donor platelets*, are obtained from a random donor through apheresis. This process yields greater than or equal to 3×10^{11} platelets in approximately 250 ml of plasma (Murphy et al., 2016). Patients who have suspected refractoriness often are only transfused with single-donor and/or HLA-matched platelets (McFarland, 2016).

Platelets collected from an HLA-matched family member or community donor are referred to as *HLA-matched* or *directed platelets*. Because of its inherent limited availability, this product usually is reserved for refractory patients.

Nursing Management

Management of thrombocytopenia includes preventive measures, supportive care, and platelet transfusions. Prevention of bleeding, although not always possible, is the first goal. Ensuring a safe hospital and clinic environment can reduce accidental trauma from falls. Head injuries in thrombocytopenic patients can have catastrophic and even fatal consequences. Protocols for falls should be instituted

as appropriate and may include teaching patients to wear slippers at all times when out of bed (Norton et al., 2016). In the setting of thrombocytopenia, the most common sites of bleeding are the mucous membranes, skin, gastrointestinal system, genitourinary system, respiratory tract, and intracranial compartment. Preventive nursing management for transplant recipients during this time includes teaching patients to use very soft bristle toothbrushes or sponges when performing mouth care to prevent trauma and bleeding of the mucous membranes. Maintenance of skin integrity using a good emollient lotion minimizes dryness and potential skin tears (Norton et al., 2016). Other measures to prevent trauma to mucous membranes include avoiding the use of rectal thermometers and rectal suppositories. Stool softeners may be used, and patients are encouraged to increase their fluid intake to prevent constipation. Patients should be routinely monitored for nosebleeds, black tarry stools, and hematuria, as well as occult bleeding. Menstruating females typically are started on hormone therapy to prevent bleeding.

Some transplant recipients may need a higher threshold trigger for prophylactic platelet transfusions. This would include patients who are on chronic anticoagulation therapy, are receiving an invasive procedure (e.g., lumbar puncture), or are on mechanical ventilation with frequent suctioning, as well as those who have a history of bleeding or brain injury. In addition, patients undergoing apheresis for hematopoietic stem cell collection are kept at a higher threshold because platelets are lost during the procedure.

It is important that a platelet pre-count (within four hours) and a post-count be drawn for patients receiving HLA-matched platelets. The pre-count is necessary in determining the increment. If the anticipated increment is not achieved, the transplant team will decline to use that donor for this patient. This prevents wasting a limited resource, as the donor may be needed for another HLA-matched patient.

Thrombotic Thrombocytopenia Purpura/Hemolytic Uremic Syndrome

Thrombotic thrombocytopenia purpura/hemolytic uremic syndrome (TTP/HUS) is a form of thrombotic microangiopathy accompanied by renal failure and hemolytic anemia and severe thrombocytopenia that generally occurs three months to one year post-HSCT (Norton et al., 2016). Clinical distinction between TTP/HUS and disseminated intravascular coagulation (discussed in detail in Chapter 6) is critical, as the management for these complications differs (Arnold, Patriquin, & Nazy, 2017). Post-HSCT thrombocytopenia can be associated with thrombotic TTP/HUS. TTP/HUS can be defined as "a disorder characterized by a form of thrombotic microangiopathy with renal failure, hemolytic anemia, and severe thrombocytopenia" (NCI CTEP, 2017, p. 4; see Table 8-5). This syndrome has become more widely recognized in the post-transplant population in recent years, and the presence of thrombocytopenia and microangiopathic hemolytic anemia, without another clin-

Table 8-5. Common Terminology Criteria for Adverse Events Grading of Hemolytic Uremic Syndrome

Adverse Event	Grade				
	1	2	3	4	5
Hemolytic uremic syndrome	–	–	Laboratory findings with clinical consequences (e.g., renal insufficiency, petechiae)	Life-threatening consequences (e.g., central nervous system hemorrhage or thrombosis/embolism or renal failure)	Death

Definition: A disorder characterized by a form of thrombotic microangiopathy with renal failure, hemolytic anemia, and severe thrombocytopenia.

Note. From *Common Terminology Criteria for Adverse Events* [v.5.0], by National Cancer Institute Cancer Therapy Evaluation Program, 2017. Retrieved from https://ctep.cancer.gov/protocolDevelopment/electronic_applications/docs/CTCAE_v5_Quick_Reference_8.5x11.pdf.

ically apparent cause, is sufficient to establish this diagnosis (O'Donnell, 2016).

TTP/HUS is a vascular endothelial injury resulting in the release of von Willebrand factors and vascular microthrombi. Symptoms result from reversible platelet thrombus formation within the microvasculature leading to transient ischemia of the brain, kidneys, and other organs (Arnold et al., 2015). The disorder is most commonly seen as a subacute chronic process that occurs 3–12 months following HSCT (Arnold et al., 2015). TTP/HUS may have multiple etiologies, including drug toxicity, infection, and autoimmune processes (Arnold et al., 2015; Koniarczyk & Ferraro, 2016).

TTP/HUS has been difficult to recognize because complications in critically ill HSCT recipients can be similar (Koniarczyk & Ferraro, 2016). The factors that positively correlate with TTP/HUS include recipients of transplants from matched unrelated donors and HLA-mismatched donors, GVHD, total body irradiation as part of the preparative regimen, and infections. Nephrotoxicity and neurotoxicity associated with cyclosporine use may be a complicating finding in making the diagnosis of TTP/HUS (Koniarczyk & Ferraro, 2016).

Although the diagnosis of TTP/HUS should be suspected in the presence of microangiopathic hemolytic anemia and thrombocytopenia, most patients also present with renal and neurologic abnormalities. Symptoms may include aphasia, confusion, memory loss, paresis, and behavioral changes. Clinical manifestations of HUS are bleeding, bruising, central nervous system changes, fatigue, fever, increased diastolic blood pressure, pallor, petechiae, and renal failure. Patients may complain of abdominal symptoms such as pain, nausea, vomiting, and diarrhea. A diagnosis of HUS is not made by any one laboratory test; it is a clinical diagnosis supported by several laboratory tests showing increased serum creatinine and lactate dehydrogenase (LDH); decreased platelets, hemoglobin, and hematocrit; and a negative Coombs test with no evidence of disseminated intravascular coagulation with normal prothrombin time and partial thromboplastin time.

If not recognized and treated promptly, TTP/HUS can be fatal. Treatment often requires plasma exchange and elimination of the underlying cause. Once the diagnosis is made, emergency plasma volume exchange is performed daily until the platelet count and LDH levels normalize and are stable for three days (O'Donnell, 2016). Unless severe, life-threatening bleeding occurs, platelet transfusions are contraindicated because they may contribute to the formation of microthrombi (Murphy et al., 2016).

Thrombotic Microangiopathy

Thrombotic microangiopathy is an infrequent but severe complication that involves vascular damage post-HSCT (Koniarczyk & Ferraro, 2016; Murphy et al., 2016). Risk factors include the calcineurin inhibitors cyclosporine and tacrolimus, female sex, use of total body irradiation, unrelated or haploidentical donor transplant, GVHD, and infections (Koniarczyk & Ferraro, 2016; Murphy et al., 2016). Miano, Faraci, Dini, and Bordigoni (2008) described the diagnostic criteria and staging for thrombotic microangiopathy, which were established by an international working group consensus. The diagnostic criteria include (a) more than 4% schistocytes in blood, (b) de novo, prolonged, or progressive thrombocytopenia, (c) sudden reduction in LDH, (d) a decrease in hemoglobin or sudden increase in transfusion needs, and (e) a decrease in serum haptoglobin. Withdrawal of cyclosporine or tacrolimus and substitution with another immunosuppressive agent generally is the first step to treating thrombotic microangiopathy. The efficacy of plasmapheresis has not been demonstrated. Supportive care is based on the symptoms demonstrated by the individual patient.

Anemia

Anemia is defined as a decrease in RBCs or hemoglobin level that results in reduction of the oxygen-carrying capacity of blood (Carson & Hébert, 2016). Erythropoietin, an erythrocyte growth factor, is produced or suppressed based on a feedback mechanism involving oxygen tension. Erythropoietin is produced primarily in the kidneys in response to hypoxia (Koury, 2016). When oxygen tension drops, interstitial renal cell and central vein hepatocyte receptors signal expression of an erythropoietin gene resulting in erythropoietin production. As erythropoietin enters the systemic circulation, it quickly stimulates erythrocyte precursor cells in the bone marrow to accelerate RBC production and maturation (Koury, 2016).

The life span of an RBC is approximately 120 days. The severity of anemia can be graded using the CTCAE (NCI CTEP, 2017; see Table 8-6).

Causes of Anemia

Anemia may result from several factors, including decreased RBC production, increased RBC destruction, or hemorrhage (see Figure 8-1). Other risk factors include hemolysis, malignancy type, suppression of bone marrow function from antineoplastic agents and radiation therapy, nutritional deficiency, HUS, thrombotic microangiopathy, and kidney failure.

The suppressive effects of intensive chemotherapy and radiation on the hematopoietic function of bone marrow are well documented. Chemotherapy agents used in preparative regimens suppress erythropoiesis, and gastrointestinal toxicities can lead to poor dietary intake of iron and vitamins and cause RBC lysis and microangiopathic bleeding. For transplant recipients, these factors are complex and can overlap.

Radiation exposure results in decreased production of RBCs when marrow-producing areas, such as the pelvis, sternum, and proximal ends of long bones, are included in the radiation field. Many drugs aside from chemotherapy are toxic to the kidneys, further compromising erythropoiesis (Norton et al., 2016; Shelton, 2016).

An acute hemolytic transfusion reaction is one of the most serious complications of bone marrow or PBSC infusion (Norton et al., 2016; Shelton, 2016). Most reactions are due to major ABO antigen incompatibilities between the donor and recipient (see Table 8-7). Clinical features include a feeling of impending doom, increased temperature and pulse rate, chills, dyspnea, chest or back pain, abnormal bleeding, or shock. Laboratory tests may reveal hemoglobinemia or hemoglobinuria followed by an increased serum bilirubin (Norton et al., 2016; Shelton, 2016). Hemolytic anemia may occur in as many as one-third of allogeneic stem cell transplants (Norton et al., 2016).

Donor–recipient ABO incompatibility is not a contraindication to successful transplantation and has no significant adverse impact on the incidence of graft rejection, GVHD, or survival. However, patients receiving an ABO-incompatible transplant are at risk for developing several other complications (see Figure 8-2). Incompatibilities could lead to delayed erythropoiesis, persistent hemolysis, and pure red cell aplasia (Carson & Hébert, 2015; Koniarczyk & Ferraro, 2016; Norton et al., 2016; Shelton, 2016). ABO incompatibility can be defined as the presence of alloantibodies in the recipient that react against donor RBC antigens; this is what causes prolonged donor-derived RBC destruction. Pure red cell aplasia can last months to years and is influenced by factors such as HLA disparity, recipient anti-donor antibody titers, RBC incompatibility that involves donor A antigens, the conditioning regimen, the stem cell source, and GVHD (Carson & Hébert, 2015; Koniarczyk & Ferraro, 2016; Norton et al., 2016; Shelton, 2016).

Delayed hemolysis, on the other hand, results from infusion of viable donor lymphocytes after minor ABO-incompatible allogeneic transplantation. Recent cases of severe life-threatening hemolysis are thought to be explained by increased numbers of lymphocytes in PBSC apheresis products (Koniarczyk & Ferraro, 2016; Norton et al., 2016; Shelton, 2016). The use of reduced-intensity conditioning regimens is thought to be responsible for the increased incidence of pure red cell aplasia secondary to delayed disappearance of alloantibody-producing plasma cells of host origin (Koniarczyk & Ferraro, 2016; Norton et al., 2016; Shelton, 2016).

Prevention and Treatment

Prevention strategies include removal of incompatible RBCs from donated bone marrow and RBC depletion of PBSCs before infusion. The RBC content in PBSCs is less than in marrow but may be sufficient to cause hemolysis at the time of the infusion (Koniarczyk & Ferraro, 2016). Nurses infusing ABO-incompatible products must remain vigilant in monitoring and assessing patients during the infusion. Patient education must include signs and symptoms of a hemolytic reaction.

Leukemias, lymphomas, multiple myelomas, and myelodysplastic syndromes are the cancers most frequently asso-

Table 8-6. Common Terminology Criteria for Adverse Events Grading of Anemia

Adverse Event	Grade				
	1	2	3	4	5
Anemia	Hemoglobin (Hgb), LLN–10 g/dL; < LLN–6.2 mmol/L; < LLN–100 g/L	Hgb < 10–8 g/dL; < 6.2–4.9 mmol/L; < 100–80 g/L	Hgb < 8 g/dL; < 4.9 mmol/L; < 80 g/L; transfusion indicated	Life-threatening consequences; urgent intervention indicated	Death

Definition: A disorder characterized by a reduction in the amount of hemoglobin in 100 ml of blood. Signs and symptoms of anemia may include pallor of the skin and mucous membranes, shortness of breath, palpitations of the heart, soft systolic murmurs, lethargy, and fatigability.

Note. From *Common Terminology Criteria for Adverse Events* [v.5.0], by National Cancer Institute Cancer Therapy Evaluation Program, 2017. Retrieved from https://ctep.cancer.gov/protocolDevelopment/electronic_applications/docs/CTCAE_v5_Quick_Reference_8.5x11.pdf.

Figure 8-1. Bleeding Complications and Etiologies That May Contribute to Anemia in Transplant Recipients

Pathophysiology	Etiology	Signs/Symptoms	Management
• Myelosuppression induced by preparative regimen • Delayed platelet engraftment • Marrow suppressive medications • Coagulation abnormalities • Platelet autoantibodies • Graft rejection	• Graft-versus-host disease • Cyclosporine • Veno-occlusive disease • Altered mucosal barriers • Delayed/failed engraftment • Viral infection • ABO-incompatible bone marrow transplantation	• Skin/mucosa: petechiae, ecchymoses, bruising, scleral hemorrhage, epistaxis • Genitourinary: hematuria, menorrhagia • Gastrointestinal: guaiac-positive stool or emesis, abdominal distension or discomfort • Pulmonary: epistaxis, hemoptysis, change in breathing pattern • Intracranial: headache, restlessness, change in pupil response, seizure, change in mental status or level of consciousness	• Perform frequent assessment. • Monitor hemoglobin/hematocrit, platelets, and coagulation studies. • Minimize blood loss. • Administer blood products. • Avoid medications that inhibit platelet production or function. • Avoid invasive procedures. • Follow bleeding precautions.

Note. Based on information from Devine, 2016.

---

ciated with anemia and are among the most frequently transplanted malignant diseases (Lassiter, 2016). A history of prior myelosuppressive drug therapy, particularly platinum-derived agents, may cause a cumulative impairment of erythropoiesis (Norton et al., 2016; Shelton, 2016). The intensive preparative conditioning regimens in the transplant setting create a hypoproliferative anemia because of the myelosuppressive effects on the bone marrow (Norton et al., 2016; Shelton, 2016).

Transplant recipients commonly experience nausea and/or vomiting and mucositis as side effects of preparative conditioning regimens. The intake of essential nutrients, including iron, folate, and vitamin B_{12}, for normal differentiation and proliferation of erythroid progenitor cells thus is insufficient. The ability to take in adequate nutrients is compromised, adding another complicating factor for the development of anemia (Cunningham, 2018).

Finally, acute hemolysis can be caused by cyclosporine A, tacrolimus, or sirolimus. An ABO-incompatible graft, infection, or HUS can cause bleeding and subsequent anemia (Arnold et al., 2015; Norton et al., 2016; Shelton, 2016). The clinical features of anemia include fatigue, pallor, shortness of breath, headaches, dizziness, decreased cognition, sleep disorders, and sexual dysfunction (Arnold et al., 2015; Norton et al., 2016; Shelton, 2016). Hypotension and orthostasis may be present in the setting of an acute drop in hematocrit (Norton et al., 2016; Shelton, 2016). HUS is a clinical syndrome that has features of thrombocytopenia, hematuria, hypertension, renal failure, and microangiopathic hemolytic anemia (Arnold et al., 2015; Norton et al., 2016; Shelton, 2016).

Nursing Management

Management of anemia in transplant recipients includes anticipation of risk factors and initiation of strategies to minimize patient risk. RBC transfusions should be anticipated to correct hemoglobin during the acute phases of the transplant. Hemoglobin and hematocrit should be moni-

tored regularly throughout the period of aplasia and more frequently if patients are actively bleeding. Testing of emesis, stool, and urine for blood are important nursing interventions. The hemolysis workup includes urinalysis, complete blood count, haptoglobin, LDH, direct and indirect Coombs test, and fractionated bilirubin (Norton et al., 2016; Shelton, 2016).

Tachycardia, tachypnea, hypotension, dyspnea at rest, and other symptoms of tissue hypoxia may occur as anemia becomes more severe (Norton et al., 2016; Shelton, 2016).

As with platelets, RBCs should be transfused only when necessary. The decision to transfuse RBCs is based on hemoglobin concentration and signs and symptoms of anemia. Overtransfusing has the disadvantages of exposing patients to more donors, increasing the risk of a transfusion reaction and potential volume overload. Generally, patients

Table 8-7. ABO-Incompatible Hematopoietic Stem Cell Transplantation

Type of Incompatibility	Recipient ABO	Donor ABO
Major	O	A
		B
		AB
	A	AB
	B	AB
Minor	A	O
	B	O
	AB	A
		B
		O
Bidirectional	A	B
	B	A

Note. Based on information from Daniel-Johnson & Schwartz, 2011.

Figure 8-2. Types of ABO Incompatibility and Potential Adverse Effects in Stem Cell Transplantation

Major ABO Incompatibility
- Definition: recipient isoagglutinins (anti-A, anti-B, anti-AB) incompatible with donor red blood cells (RBCs)
- Donor–recipient ABO pairs
  - Group A, B, and AB donor and group O recipient
  - Group AB donor and group A and B recipient
- Potential adverse effects
  - Immediate hemolysis of RBCs infused with donor marrow (acute hemolytic reaction)
  - Delayed hemolysis of RBCs produced by engrafted marrow
  - Delayed onset of erythropoiesis
  - Pure red cell aplasia

Minor ABO Incompatibility
- Definition: recipient RBCs incompatible with donor isoagglutinins
- Donor–recipient ABO pairs
  - Group O donor and group A, B, or AB recipient
- Potential adverse effects
  - Immediate hemolysis of recipient RBCs by infused marrow
  - Passenger lymphocyte syndrome causing delayed hemolysis

Major and Minor ABO Incompatibility (Bidirectional)
- Definition: combination of both incompatibilities
- Donor–recipient ABO pairs
  - Group A donor and B recipient
  - Group B donor and A recipient
- Potential adverse effects
  - Immediate hemolysis caused by recipient and/or donor
  - Passenger lymphocyte syndrome causing delayed hemolysis

Note. Based on information from Daniel-Johnson & Schwartz, 2011.

---

with a hemoglobin of 10 g/dl do not need a transfusion, but when hemoglobin is less than 7–8 g/dl and signs and symptoms of anemia are present, transfusion is required (McCullough, 2016; Norton et al., 2016; Shelton, 2016). However, patients with underlying cardiopulmonary compromise and older adults may require transfusions at higher hemoglobin thresholds (McCullough, 2016). One unit of packed RBCs (10–15 ml/kg in pediatric patients) can raise the hemoglobin increment by approximately 1 g/dl (Hillman, Ault, Leporrier, & Rinder, 2011).

Blood Product Transfusions

HSCT recipients will require multiple transfusions of blood products during the period of aplasia following the transplant until stable recovery of hematopoiesis. Although component therapy is significantly safer now than it was in the past, notable risks are still associated with transfusion therapy (Norton et al., 2016). Complications include infectious disease transmission, alloimmunization, acute hemolytic transfusion reactions, febrile nonhemolytic transfusion reactions, allergic transfusion reactions, transfusion-related acute lung injury, and transfusion-associated circulatory overload (Eisenberg, 2018).

Infectious Disease Transmission

Viruses with the potential for transmission include HIV, human T-cell leukemia virus-1, parvovirus B19, Epstein-Barr virus, CMV, and hepatitis A, B, and C (McCullough, 2016). Bacterial and protozoal agents have potential transmission through the blood supply (McCullough, 2016). With the current methods employed and advances in recruiting, screening, and testing of donor blood, the risk for viral infection by transfusion of screened blood products has been dramatically reduced (McCullough, 2016; Seifried & Schmidt, 2016).

Leukocytes are unintended contaminants in blood products and are associated with alloimmunization, febrile nonhemolytic transfusion reactions, histamine-mediated allergic reactions, immunosuppression, and transmission or reactivation of intracellular viruses (e.g., CMV) (Eisenberg, 2018; Singh & Kumar, 2009). Leukocyte reduction has been shown to be clinically effective in reducing the incidence of transfusion-related complications, which can significantly decrease the cost of medical care (Singh & Kumar, 2009).

Transfusion Reactions

Febrile nonhemolytic reactions are defined as an unexplained increase in temperature of 1°C from baseline and oral temperature of 38°C or higher, or rigors or chills occurring within four hours of completion of transfusion (Ellsworth, Ellsworth, & Stevens, 2016). Most febrile reactions are caused by cytokines. These pyrogenic mediators include the interleukins IL-1β, IL-6, and IL-8 and tumor necrosis factor-alpha and are released from captive WBCs contained in the blood product. The reactions can occur during, shortly after, or up to several hours after the transfusion and can be difficult to distinguish from sepsis, although the latter generally is associated with hypotension and tachypnea. Patients are treated symptomatically with acetaminophen. Widespread use of leukocyte reduction of all transfused blood products decreases the incidence of febrile nonhemolytic transfusion reactions (Eisenberg, 2018). Although extremely rare (estimated incidence of 1 in 500 for platelet transfusions), febrile nonhemolytic reactions also can be caused by bacterial contamination in the product (Eisenberg, 2018). Astute nursing assessment is required, and blood cultures may be ordered to aid in differentiation.

Transfusion-related acute lung injury is defined as acute hypoxemia with partial pressure of oxygen/fraction of inspired oxygen ratio of 300 mm Hg or less combined and chest x-ray showing bilateral infiltrates in the absence of circulatory overload (Ellsworth et al., 2016). Onset of transfusion-related acute lung injury is abrupt and thought to be caused by HLA antigens.

Transfusion-associated circulatory overload is defined as an infusion volume that cannot be effectively processed by the recipient, likely due to either high infusion rate or volume or an underlying cardiac or pulmonary pathology (Ellsworth et al., 2016). Signs and symptoms include acute respiratory distress (dyspnea, orthopnea, cough), evidence of positive fluid balance, radiographic evidence of pulmonary edema, evidence of left-sided heart failure, and elevated central venous pressure (Ellsworth et al., 2016).

HSCT nurses should be knowledgeable about the signs and symptoms of transfusion reactions (Eisenberg, 2018). If a reaction is suspected, the transfusion should immediately be stopped, as severity can be related to the amount of blood product transfused. The medical provider should be promptly notified with the following information reported: vital signs, oxygen saturation, volume of product transfused, rate of transfusion when the reaction occurred, and list of premedications, if administered (Eisenberg, 2018).

Delayed Engraftment

Delayed engraftment and *graft failure* refer to the lack of functional hematopoiesis after stem cell transplantation. The terminology used to describe problems with engraftment includes *delayed engraftment, graft failure, graft rejection,* and *primary and secondary graft failure.* Primary graft failure is the failure to establish hematopoiesis or a defined number of neutrophils by 21–28 days after transplant. Incidence is 1%–20%, and prognosis is poor (Martin, 2016; Norton et al., 2016). In autologous transplants, this may be due to an inadequate number of cells, a defect in the quality of stem cells, the cryopreservation process, or damage during collection (Martin, 2016; Norton et al., 2016).

In allogeneic transplants, graft failure is more commonly seen with HLA-mismatched donor bone marrow, umbilical cord blood transplant, or T-cell–depleted bone marrow but also may be related to primary disease, inadequate dose of stem cells, immunosuppression, immune-mediated processes, septicemia, ABO incompatibility, viral infections, and drug toxicity (Martin, 2016; Norton et al., 2016). Secondary or late graft failure occurs when the recipient engrafts initially but later the donor graft is unable to be maintained (Martin, 2016; Norton et al., 2016). Primary graft failure occurs in less than 5% of recipients with a hematologic malignancy; however, it is estimated to occur in 10%–20% of recipients with hereditary nonmalignant diseases, such as aplastic anemia or thalassemia (Martin, 2016; Norton et al., 2016). Diagnostic studies include at least daily complete blood counts with differential and platelets to follow engraftment trends and evaluate transfusion needs. Bone marrow aspirate and biopsy and cytogenetic studies often are used to evaluate engraftment and disease status (Koniarczyk & Ferraro, 2016).

Management of graft failure may include discontinuation of drugs known to be myelosuppressive (e.g., ganciclovir, TMP-SMX). Other possible strategies include reinfusion of allogeneic hematopoietic stem cells or marrow, infusion of backup bone marrow with or without further conditioning, or attempted stimulation with colony-stimulating factors (Koniarczyk & Ferraro, 2016).

In HSCT, *chimerism* indicates the presence of donor lymphohematopoietic cells in the recipient (Martin, 2016). The origin of marrow and blood cells after HSCT can be identified by testing genetic markers that distinguish donor from recipient (Martin, 2016). Full or complete chimerism indicates that all hematopoietic cells are of donor origin; in contrast, a mixed chimerism indicates the presence of both donor and recipient cells. Chimerism testing can be useful in determining how well a patient has engrafted after HSCT or to determine reasons for delayed or failed engraftment and can aid in early detection of relapse of hematologic malignancies. Several methods are used to detect chimerism. Cytogenetic analysis with the use of fluorescence in situ hybridization is used in sex-mismatched transplants, which determines whether the hematopoietic cells contain Y versus XY markers (Koniarczyk & Ferraro, 2016; Martin, 2016). Analysis used for sex-matched transplants includes RFLP (restriction fragment length polymorphism), STR (short tandem repeats), VNTR (variable number tandem repeats), and SNP (single nucleotide polymorphism) (Koniarczyk & Ferraro, 2016; Martin, 2016). DNA amplification and molecular testing using in situ hybridization have made chimerism testing widely available for many post-HSCT applications (Martin, 2016).

Immune recovery after HSCT has two phases: recovery of stem cells (e.g., WBCs, RBCs, platelets) and functional recovery of the immune system (e.g., B and T cells, NK cells) (Devine, 2016). The use of T-cell–depleting agents such as antithymocyte globulin or alemtuzumab may delay immune recovery (Devine, 2016; Koniarczyk & Ferraro, 2016). While other hematopoietic cell lines recover within weeks of transplant, lymphocyte recovery is more prolonged and requires at least several months and up to several years (Lassiter, 2016).

Late Post-Transplant Infections (More Than 100 Days)

The final phase of the HSCT process is the late post-transplant phase. At this point, most patients will have engraftment of WBCs, healing of mucosal linings, and adequate skin integrity. Patients without ongoing complications of HSCT are not significantly at risk for major infectious complications. Patients with ongoing complications, such as GVHD, graft rejection or failure, or relapse or progression of disease may continue to be at greater risk for infectious complications. Common infections during this time are *Streptococcus pneumoniae, Haemophilus influenzae, Neisseria meningitidis,* sinusitis, and varicella zoster virus (Devine, 2016; Koniarczyk & Ferraro, 2016; see Figure 6-2 and Table 8-2).

Nursing Management

During the final phase of transplant, ongoing patient and caregiver education continues to be important. Depending on the transplant center and geographic location, patients may be seen infrequently by the transplant team because of financial constraints, distance from the transplant center, or transportation limitations. Education for caregivers and patients should include assessment for infectious complications. HSCT nurses must share details of the patient's transplant course and information concerning monitoring and referral with the nurses and physicians who will resume care of the patient after the patient leaves the transplant center. For patients still being seen by the transplant team, nursing care continues to include education, assessment, administration of appropriate medications, and provision of a care plan patients can take home.

Immune Recovery After Transplantation

Full immune recovery after HSCT requires at least a few months to several years. NK cells are the first lymphocytes to recover, and next are CD8+ T cells, which return to normal in two to eight months (Devine, 2016; Koniarczyk & Ferraro, 2016). Lymphocyte regeneration involves two pathways: using the first pathway, lymphocytes regenerate from bone marrow lymphoid progenitors, and in the second pathway, it is driven by a thymic-independent pathway (Devine, 2016; Koniarczyk & Ferraro, 2016). NK cells use the first pathway, whereas B cells are regenerated primarily from lymphoid progenitors but also are dependent on the bone marrow microenvironment, which is affected by conditioning regimens as well as GVHD (Devine, 2016; Koniarczyk & Ferraro, 2016). The thymus is damaged by normal aging, as well as conditioning regimens and GVHD. As a result, adult patients show little T-cell recovery for months to years after transplantation. Therefore, CD4+ counts may be one of the most predictive markers of immune recovery after HSCT (Dudakov, Perales, & van den Brink, 2016). For a year or longer after HSCT, recipients are at risk for infections from encapsulated bacteria and viruses (Devine, 2016; Koniarczyk & Ferraro, 2016). Graft types are a risk factor for poor immune recovery. PBSC graft recipients have a more rapid immune recovery, whereas umbilical cord blood and T-cell–depleted haploidentical graft recipients have poor immune recovery and high rates of infection (Devine, 2016; Koniarczyk & Ferraro, 2016).

Summary

Hematologic and infectious complications are complex and common occurrences in patients undergoing HSCT. Nurses traditionally have held the key responsibility for symptom identification and management. Aggressive, proactive nursing care is critical in helping patients through these dangerous phases of the post-transplant period. A well-rounded grasp of current knowledge is essential to maintaining the skills required to anticipate these complications and intervene early and effectively. Patient and caregiver education is an essential role of HSCT nurses for ongoing infection prevention and detection as patients move across the transplant trajectory, from inpatient care on the HSCT unit, to self-care at home, and to care by their local healthcare team.

References

Afessa, B., Badley, A.D., & Peters, S.G. (2010). Pulmonary complications of bone-marrow and stem-cell transplantation. In P. Camus & E.C. Rosenow III (Eds.), *Drug-induced and iatrogenic respiratory disease* (pp. 172–191). Boca Raton, FL: CRC Press.

Antin, J., & Raley, D. (2013). *Manual of stem cell and bone marrow transplantation* (2nd ed.). New York, NY: Cambridge University Press.

Arnold, D.M., Patriquin, C.J., & Nazy, I. (2017). Thrombotic microangiopathies: A general approach to diagnosis and management. *CMAJ, 189*, E153–E159. https://doi.org/10.1503/cmaj.160142.

Bensinger, W.I. (2016). High-dose preparatory regimens. In S.J. Forman, R.S. Negrin, J.H. Antin, & F.R. Appelbaum (Eds.), *Thomas' hematopoietic cell transplantation: Stem cell transplantation* (5th ed., pp. 223–231). https://doi.org/10.1002/9781118416426.ch20

Bergkvist, K., Fossum, B., Johansson, U.-B., Mattsson, J., & Larsen, J. (2018). Patients' experiences of different care settings and a new life situation after allogeneic haematopoietic stem cell transplantation. *European Journal of Cancer Care, 27*, e12672. https://doi.org/10.1111/ecc.12672

Bittencourt, H., Rocha, V., Chevret, S., Socié, G., Espérou, H., Devergie, A., … Gluckman, E. (2002). Association of CD34 cell dose with hematopoietic recovery, infections, and other outcomes after HLA-identical sibling bone marrow transplantation. *Blood, 99*, 2726–2733. https://doi.org/10.1182/blood.V99.8.2726

Carson, J.L., & Hébert, P. (2016). Anemia and red blood cell transfusion. In T.L. Simon, J. McCullough, E.L. Snyder, B.G. Solheim, & R.G. Strauss (Eds.), *Rossi's principles of transfusion medicine* (5th ed., pp. 110–125). https://doi.org/10.1002/9781119013020.ch10

Cunningham, R.S. (2018). Nutritional disturbances. In C.H. Yarbro, D. Wujcik, & B.H. Gobel (Eds.), *Cancer nursing: Principles and practice* (8th ed., pp. 941–970). Burlington, MA: Jones & Bartlett Learning.

Daniel-Johnson, J., & Schwartz, J. (2011). How do I approach ABO-incompatible hematopoietic progenitor cell transplantation? *Transfusion, 51*, 1143–1149. https://doi.org/10.1111/j.1537-2995.2011.03069.x

Devine, B.H. (2016). Blood and marrow stem cell transplantation. In B.H. Gobel, S. Triest-Robertson, & W.H. Vogel (Eds.), *Advanced oncology nursing certification review and resource manual* (2nd ed., pp. 293–344). Pittsburgh, PA: Oncology Nursing Society.

Dudakov, J.A., Perales, M.-A., & van den Brink, M.R.M. (2016). Immune reconstitution following hematopoietic cell transplantation. In S.J. Forman, R.S. Negrin, J.H. Antin, & F.R. Appelbaum (Eds.), *Thomas' hematopoietic cell transplantation: Stem cell transplantation* (5th ed., pp. 160–165). https://doi.org/10.1002/9781118416426.ch15

Eisenberg, S. (2010). Refractory response to platelet transfusion therapy. *Journal of Infusion Nursing, 33*, 89–97. https://doi.org/10.1097/nan.0b013e3181cfd392

Eisenberg, S. (2018). Infusion reactions, extravasation, and transfusion reactions. In M. Kaplan (Ed.), *Understanding and managing oncologic emergencies: A resource for nurses* (3rd ed., pp. 327–414). Pittsburgh, PA: Oncology Nursing Society.

Ellsworth, B., Ellsworth, P., & Stevens, W.T. (2016, May 4). Adverse reaction case definition criteria from appendix A of the Biovigilance Component of the National Healthcare Safety Network (NHSN) Manual. Retrieved from http://www.aabb.org/research/hemovigilance/Documents/Forms/AllItems.aspx

Estcourt, L.J., Stanworth, S.J., Doree, C., Hopewell, S., Trivella, M., & Murphy, M.F. (2015). Comparison of different platelet count thresholds to guide administration of prophylactic platelet transfusion for preventing bleeding in people with haematological disorders after myelosuppressive chemotherapy or stem cell transplantation. *Cochrane Database of Systematic Reviews, 2015*(11). https://doi.org/10.1002/14651858.cd010983.pub2

Finke, J., & Mertelsmann, R. (2016). Use of recombinant growth factors after hematopoietic cell transplantation. In S.J. Forman, R.S. Negrin, J.H. Antin, & F.R. Appelbaum (Eds.), *Thomas' hematopoietic cell transplantation: Stem cell transplantation* (5th ed., pp. 480–488). https://doi.org/10.1002/9781118416426.ch43'

Hillman, R.S., Ault, K.A., Leporrier, M., & Rinder, H.M. (2011). *Hematology in clinical practice* (5th ed.). New York, NY: McGraw-Hill.

Holtick, U., Albrecht, M., Chemnitz, J.M., Theurich, S., Skoetz, N., Scheid, C., & von Bergwelt-Baildon, M. (2014). Bone marrow versus peripheral blood allogeneic haematopoietic stem cell transplantation for haematological malignancies in adults. *Cochrane Database of Systematic Reviews, 2014*(4). https://doi.org/10.1002/14651858.CD010189.pub2

Kiss, J.E., Rybka, W.B., Winkelstein, A., deMagalhaes-Silverman, M., Lister, J., D'Andrea, P., & Ball, E.D. (1997). Relationship of CD34⁺ cell dose to early and late hematopoiesis following autologous peripheral blood stem cell transplantation. *Bone Marrow Transplantation, 19*, 303–310. https://doi.org/10.1038/sj.bmt.1700671

Koniarczyk, H., & Ferraro, C. (2016). Transplant preparative regimens, cellular infusion, acute complications, and engraftment. In B. Faiman (Ed.), *BMTCN® certification review manual* (pp. 37–68). Pittsburgh, PA: Oncology Nursing Society.

Koury, M. (2016). Red blood cell production and kinetics. In T.L. Simon, J. McCullough, E.L. Snyder, B.G. Solheim, & R.G. Strauss (Eds.), *Rossi's principles of transfusion medicine* (5th ed., pp. 87–96). https://doi.org/10.1002/9781119013020.ch9

Lassiter, M. (2016). Basic concepts and indications for transplantation. In B. Faiman (Ed.), *BMTCN® certification review manual* (pp. 1–8). Pittsburgh, PA: Oncology Nursing Society.

Leather, H.L., & Wingard, J.R. (2016). Bacterial infections. In S.J. Forman, R.S. Negrin, J.H. Antin, & F.R. Appelbaum (Eds.), *Thomas' hematopoietic cell transplantation: Stem cell transplantation* (5th ed., pp. 1038–1062). https://doi.org/10.1002/9781118416426.ch85

Marr, K.A., Bow, E., Chiller, T., Maschmeyer, G., Ribaud, P., Segal, B., ... Nucci, M. (2009). Fungal infection prevention after hematopoietic cell transplantation. *Bone Marrow Transplantation, 44*, 483–487. https://doi.org/10.1038/bmt.2009.259

Martin, P.J. (2016). Documentation of engraftment and characterization of chimerism after hematopoietic cell transplantation. In S.J. Forman, R.S. Negrin, J.H. Antin, & F.R. Appelbaum (Eds.), *Thomas' hematopoietic cell transplantation: Stem cell transplantation* (5th ed., pp. 272–280). https://doi.org/10.1002/9781118416426.ch24

McCullough, J. (2016). Principles of transfusion support before and after hematopoietic cell transplantation. In S.J. Forman, R.S. Negrin, J.H. Antin, & F.R. Appelbaum (Eds.), *Thomas' hematopoietic cell transplantation: Stem cell transplantation* (5th ed., pp. 961–975). https://doi.org/10.1002/9781118416426.ch79

McFarland, J.G. (2016). Platelet immunology and alloimmunization. In T.L. Simon, J. McCullough, E.L. Snyder, B.G. Solheim, & R.G. Strauss (Eds.), *Rossi's principles of transfusion medicine* (5th ed., pp. 215–227). https://doi.org/10.1002/9781119013020.ch18

Miano, M., Faraci, M., Dini, G., & Bordigoni, P. (2008). Early complications following haematopoietic SCT in children. *Bone Marrow Transplantation, 41*, S39–S42. https://doi.org/10.1038/bmt.2008.53

Murphy, M.F., Stanworth, S.J., & Estcourt, L. (2016). Thrombocytopenia and platelet transfusion. In T.L. Simon, J. McCullough, E.L. Snyder, B.G. Solheim, & R.G. Strauss (Eds.), *Rossi's principles of transfusion medicine* (5th ed., pp. 235–244). https://doi.org/10.1002/9781119013020.ch20

National Cancer Institute Cancer Therapy Evaluation Program. (2017). *Common terminology criteria for adverse events* [v.5.0]. Retrieved from https://ctep.cancer.gov/protocolDevelopment/electronic_applications/docs/CTCAE_v5_Quick_Reference_8.5x11.pdf

Norton, R., Garcia, I.N., & Noonan, K. (2016). Post-transplant issues. In B. Faiman (Ed.), *BMTCN® certification review manual* (pp. 125–231). Pittsburgh, PA: Oncology Nursing Society.

O'Donnell, M. (2016). Blood group incompatibilities and hemolytic complications of hematopoietic cell transplantation. In S.J. Forman, R.S. Negrin, J.H. Antin, & F.R. Appelbaum (Eds.), *Thomas' hematopoietic cell transplantation: Stem cell transplantation* (5th ed., pp. 955–960). https://doi.org/10.1002/9781118416426.ch78

O'Rafferty, C., O'Brien, M., Smyth, E., Keane, S., Robinson, H., Lynam, P., ... Smith, O.P. (2016) Administration of G-CSF from day +6 post-allogeneic hematopoietic stem cell transplantation in children and adolescents accelerates neutrophil engraftment but does not appear to have an impact on cost savings. *Pediatric Transplantation, 20*, 432–437. https://doi.org/10.1111/petr.12670

Pahnke, S., Egeland, T., Halter, J., Hägglund, H., Shaw, B.E., Woolfrey, A.E., & Szer, J. (2019). Current use of biosimilar G-CSF for haematopoietic stem cell mobilisation. *Bone Marrow Transplantation, 54*, 858–866. https://doi.org/10.1038/s41409-018-0350-y

Pai, V., Fernandez, S.A., Laudick, M., Rosselet, R., & Termuhlen, A. (2010). Delayed administration of filgrastim (G-CSF) following autologous peripheral blood stem cell transplantation (APBSCT) in pediatric patients does not change time to neutrophil engraftment and reduces use of G-CSF. *Pediatric Blood and Cancer, 54*, 728–733. https://doi.org/10.1002/pbc.22394

Sandmaier, B.M., & Storb, R. (2016). Reduced-intensity allogeneic transplantation regimens. In S.J. Forman, R.S. Negrin, J.H. Antin, & F.R. Appelbaum (Eds.), *Thomas' hematopoietic cell transplantation: Stem cell transplantation* (5th ed., pp. 232–243). https://doi.org/10.1002/9781118416426.ch21

Schulman, K.A., Birch, R., Zhen, B., Pania, N., & Weaver, C.H. (1999). Effect of CD34⁺ cell dose on resource utilization in patients after high-dose chemotherapy with peripheral-blood stem-cell support. *Journal of Clinical Oncology, 17*, 1227–1233. https://doi.org/10.1200/JCO.1999.17.4.1227

Seifried, E., & Schmidt, M. (2016). Transfusion-transmitted virus infections. In T.L. Simon, J. McCullough, E.L. Snyder, B.G. Solheim, & R.G. Strauss (Eds.), *Rossi's principles of transfusion medicine* (5th ed., pp. 583–598). https://doi.org/10.1002/9781119013020.ch51

Shelton, B.K. (2016). Myelosuppression and second malignancies. In B.H. Gobel, S. Triest-Robertson, & W.H. Vogel (Eds.), *Advanced oncology nursing certification review and resource manual* (2nd ed., pp. 451–490). Pittsburgh, PA: Oncology Nursing Society.

Singh, S., & Kumar, A.K. (2009). Leukocyte depletion for safe blood transfusion. *Biotechnology Journal, 4*, 1140–1151. https://doi.org/10.1002/biot.200800182

Tomblyn, M., Chiller, T., Einsele, H., Gress, R., Sepkowitz, K., Storek, J., ... Boeckh, M.A. (2009). Guidelines for preventing infectious complications among hematopoietic cell transplantation recipients: A global perspective. *Biology of Blood and Marrow Transplantation, 15*, 1143–1238. https://doi.org/10.1016/j.bbmt.2009.06.019

Tormey, C.A., & Rinder, H.M. (2016). Platelet production and kinetics. In T.L. Simon, J. McCullough, E.L. Snyder, B.G. Solheim, & R.G. Strauss (Eds.), *Rossi's principles of transfusion medicine* (5th ed., pp. 206–214). https://doi.org/10.1002/9781119013020.ch17

Wingard, J.R. (2020). Prevention of viral infections in hematopoietic cell transplant recipients. In S. Bond (Ed.), *UpToDate*. Retrieved February 6, 2020, from https://www.uptodate.com/contents/prevention-of-viral-infections-in-hematopoietic-cell-transplant-recipients

Zaia, J.A. (2016). Cytomegalovirus infection. In S.J. Forman, R.S. Negrin, J.H. Antin, & F.R. Appelbaum (Eds.), *Thomas' hematopoietic cell transplantation: Stem cell transplantation* (5th ed., pp. 1069–1078). https://doi.org/10.1002/9781118416426.ch87

CHAPTER 9

Gastrointestinal Complications

Rebecca Martin, BSN, RN, OCN®, BMTCN®, and Kimberly A. Noonan, DNP, ANP-BC, AOCN®

Introduction

Autologous and allogeneic hematopoietic stem cell transplantation (HSCT) can cause many gastrointestinal (GI) complications in pediatric and adult transplant recipients. These complications include mucositis, salivary gland dysfunction and xerostomia, taste changes, nausea and vomiting, diarrhea, perineal-rectal skin alterations, and malnutrition. Graft-versus-host disease (GVHD) is discussed fully in Chapter 7 and is only mentioned in this chapter when appropriate.

Mucositis

Damage to blood cells, the use of immunosuppression, and the effects of cytotoxic therapies can result in oral complications, including mucositis, xerostomia, and dysgeusia (Elad et al., 2015). Patients undergoing HSCT are at risk for oral complications that can cause significant morbidity and mortality.

Mucositis refers to inflammatory, erosive, and ulcerative lesions of any part of the GI tract and can be separated into oral mucositis and GI mucositis. For patients receiving high-dose chemotherapy prior to HSCT, oral mucositis has been reported to be the single most debilitating complication of transplantation (Elad et al., 2015). The incidence of oral mucositis has been reported as high as 80% of patients undergoing HSCT, with 21.6% developing severe mucositis (Bowen & Wardill, 2017; Vagliano et al., 2011). The intensity of the conditioning regimen, in addition to the use of methotrexate or cyclophosphamide for GVHD prophylaxis, influences both the incidence and severity of oral mucositis. Patients who have significant oral mucositis require supportive care measures, such as total parenteral nutrition, fluid replacement, and prophylaxis against infections, which adds substantially to the total cost of care.

Mucositis occurs as a result of the direct and indirect effects of chemotherapy and radiation therapy, myelosuppression, and GVHD and affects the oral mucosa, esophagus, pharynx, and the rest of the GI tract. Oropharyngeal mucositis receives much of the attention because of its clinically obvious symptoms of ulceration and severe pain. However, it is important to identify and understand the effects of mucositis on the rest of the GI tract as well. These effects may include nausea and vomiting, abdominal cramping, and profuse watery diarrhea. Mucositis complications may cause poor nutrition, dehydration, fluid and electrolyte imbalances, local infection or inflammation (e.g., typhlitis), systemic infection, and hemorrhage.

Complications of mucositis are associated with an increased risk of morbidity and mortality. The morbidity of oral mucositis is primarily due to pain associated with the oral mucosal inflammation and ulceration. Mucositis pain negatively affects oral dietary intake, adherence with oral medications, oral hygiene, and quality of life. Mucositis of the oropharynx and esophagus results in loss of the protective mucosal barrier, which can lead to colonization of oral ulcerations by microbial flora. Although mucositis is not infectious, secondary microbial colonization of the oral lesions can cause clinically relevant local or systemic infection, which potentially increases mucositis severity. The occurrence of streptococcal and enterococcal bacteremia has been associated with oral mucositis (Vanhoecke, De Ryck, Stinger, Van de Wiele, & Keefe, 2015). As with oral mucositis, mucositis of the GI mucosa causes disruption of endogenous microflora and allows for the overgrowth of microbial pathogens. Although similar to the oral cavity, the GI tract harbors a much more complex endogenous microflora with a greater variety of aerobic and anaerobic bacteria (Vanhoecke et al., 2015). Mucosal injury allows for bacterial translocation through the disrupted mucosal epithelium, allowing microbial pathogens to spread to extraintestinal sites and the blood.

Pathophysiology

The pathophysiology associated with mucositis has been attributed to oxidative stress resulting from exposure to chemotherapy or radiation therapy, leading to DNA damage, cell death, presence of proinflammatory cytokines, and ulceration followed by healing (Van Sebille et al., 2015). Sonis (2004) described five phases of mucositis: initiation, primary damage response, signaling and amplification, ulceration, and healing. During the ulcerative phase, pain, edema, and bleeding occur (Sonis, 2004).

Endogenous and nonendogenous microbial pathogens colonize oral submucosal tissues, which further stimulates cytokine release from the surrounding tissues and increases the risk of systemic infections. A decrease in the quantity and quality of mucus and saliva impair local immune defenses of the oral cavity. During this phase, GI permeability increases, allowing for microbial pathogens to pass through the intestinal wall to extraintestinal sites and the blood (bacterial translocation). Healing begins to occur with neutrophil recovery. Epithelial proliferation and differentiation repair the tissues of the oral mucosa, usually within two to three weeks. The extent of oral mucositis in any particular patient depends on factors such as age, sex, underlying disease, and race, as well as tissue-specific factors (e.g., epithelia types, local microbial environment and function).

Risk Factors

Many therapy-related and patient-related risk factors contribute to the development and severity of mucositis. Knowledge and recognition of these risk factors can ensure prompt initiation of preventive therapies and patient education (see Figure 9-1).

Assessment of Oral Mucositis

Nursing assessments of oral status are an essential part of mucositis management. As oral mucositis progresses, patients may exhibit ropy or absent saliva; ulcerations on the lips, tongue, gingiva, and mucous membranes of the mouth, pharynx, and esophagus; severe pain; difficulty or inability to talk and swallow; large areas of plaque and debris; and xerostomia (Van Sebille et al., 2015).

During assessments, nurses must be aware of common infections and their presenting signs and symptoms. Infections of the oropharynx and esophagus may be bacterial, viral, or fungal in origin. Mucosal breakdown offers the perfect entry portal for the systemic spread of oral pathogens, and all attempts at prevention should be employed. It is important to note that immunocompromised patients may not display the same signs and symptoms of inflam-

---

Figure 9-1. Oral Mucositis Risk Factors

Patient Related
- Age: < 20 years, > 65 years
- Sex: females at greater risk
- Preexisting oral problems: Drug-related xerostomia or infections caused by disease or myelosuppressive treatments
- Excessive tobacco or alcohol consumption
- Type of tumor
- Genetic factors
- Poor oral care

Treatment Related
- Chemotherapy and radiation directly assault the oral mucosa.
- Many chemotherapies are known to cause oral mucositis even at standard doses.
- Risk level depends on the antineoplastic therapy, as well as on the dose and treatment schedule.
- Risk increases in cases of combined chemoradiation.

Note. Based on information from Chaudhry et al., 2016.

---

mation and infection as immunocompetent patients. See Chapter 8 for general infection control practices.

Reactivation of the herpes simplex virus is the most common cause of early oropharyngeal and esophageal viral infections. Oral herpes simplex virus infections appear mainly on the hard palate, gingiva, and lip as multiple painful vesicles or ulcers with raised, erythematous borders. Occasionally, the virus may present as a single painful lesion. Cytomegalovirus gastroenteritis is a major infectious complication of the GI tract after allogeneic HSCT (Bhat, Joshi, Sarode, & Chavan, 2015). The infection can be virulent and may be refractory to treatment in the HSCT population.

Oral bacterial infections have been associated with systemic bacteremia in immunocompromised patients. Close follow-up of the results of culture and sensitivity testing and biopsy is imperative. Bacterial infections may present as raised, ulcerative, yellow or yellow-white, painful lesions. Erythema may or may not be present. The most common pathogens include gram-positive *Streptococci* and *Staphylococci* and gram-negative *Pseudomonas*, *Klebsiella*, *Enterobacter*, *Escherichia coli*, *Serratia*, and *Fusobacterium* (Al-Dasooqi et al., 2013). Prophylaxis and treatment are dependent on institutional culture and sensitivity patterns and may include topical and systemic oral or IV therapy.

Oral fungal infections may develop from endogenous yeast flora. Fungal infections may present as white patches on the inner cheeks, tongue, roof of mouth, and throat; redness or soreness; loss of taste; pain while swallowing or eating; or cracking and redness at the corners of the mouth (Pappas et al., 2016).

Patients and caregivers should be taught how to assess the oral cavity to identify and accurately report early changes. This is particularly important as more transplants are shifted to the outpatient arena. A detailed oral assessment and history should be performed at the time of admission or presentation for HSCT. Thereafter, a thorough oral assessment documenting any new patient complaints should be performed at least daily during myelosuppression. Initial signs and symptoms include erythema, generalized tenderness, easy bleeding, difficulty or pain with swallowing and talking, and dry, cracked lips.

The use of an oral assessment instrument is helpful in documenting baseline oral status and evaluating the changes and responses to interventions. A variety of scales have been developed that focus on symptomatic and functional outcomes, such as pain or ability to eat, clinical manifestations based on visualization of the oral mucosa, or a combination of both. Each tool has advantages and limitations—some are more appropriate for research, whereas others are more useful in clinical management (see Table 9-1).

Prevention and Management

No single, scientifically proven intervention can prevent or treat the numerous complications associated with muco-

Table 9-1. Summary of Oral Mucositis Grading Scales

Grading Scale	Grade					
	0	1	2	3	4	5
ECOG	None	Mild: soreness	Moderate: ulcers—can eat	Severe: ulcers—cannot eat	Life threatening	Lethal
NCI CTCAE	Absence of other criteria	Asymptomatic or mild symptoms; intervention not indicated	Moderate pain; not interfering with oral intake; modified diet intake	Severe pain; interfering with oral intake	Life-threatening consequences; urgent intervention	Death
SWOG	None	Painless ulcers, erythema or mild soreness	Painful erythema, edema or ulcers; can eat	Painful erythema, edema or ulcers; cannot eat	Requires parenteral or enteral support	N/A
WHO Scale	Absence of other criteria	Oral soreness, erythema	Ulcers but able to eat solid foods	Oral ulcers and able to take liquids only	Oral alimentation not possible	N/A

ECOG—Eastern Cooperative Oncology Group; NCI CTCAE—National Cancer Institute Common Terminology Criteria for Adverse Events version 3.0; WHO—World Health Organization

Note. Based on information from Green & Weiss, 1992; Lalla et al., 2014; National Cancer Institute Cancer Therapy Evaluation Program, 2017; World Health Organization, 2017.

From "The Incidence and Severity of Oral Mucositis Among Allogeneic Hematopoietic Stem Cell Transplantation Patients: A Systematic Review," by H.M. Chaudhry, A.J. Bruce, R.C. Wolf, M.R. Litzow, W.J. Hogan, M.S. Patnaik, … S.K. Hashmi, 2016, *Biology of Blood and Marrow Transplantation, 22*, p. 607. Copyright 2016 by American Society of Blood and Marrow Transplantation. Retrieved from https://doi.org/10.1016/j.bbmt.2015.09.014. Licensed under CC BY-NC-ND 4.0 (https://creativecommons.org/licenses/by-nc-nd/4.0).

sitis. Detailed assessments and early multimodal interventions that prevent trauma and infection and control pain are the most important factors for the prevention and treatment of severe mucositis. In 2014, a systematic review was completed to update the Multinational Association of Supportive Care in Cancer and International Society of Oral Oncology (MASCC/ISOO) clinical practice guidelines for mucositis (Lalla et al., 2014). These guidelines are outlined in Figure 9-2 and Table 9-2. The Oncology Nursing Society mucositis resource (Eilers et al., 2019) states the following recommendations for practice.

Cryotherapy

The use of ice chips or ice-cold water has been studied for its efficacy in the prevention of oral mucositis. Oral cryotherapy protocols have resulted in a lower incidence and severity of oral mucositis for chemotherapy with a short half-life (e.g., melphalan). This leads to decreased severity and duration of oral mucositis, resulting in a decrease in parenteral narcotics (J. Chen, Seabrook, Fulford, & Rajakumar, 2017). Cryotherapy is based on the theory that vasoconstriction caused by cold temperatures decreases the exposure of the oral cavity mucous membranes to mucotoxic agents. Patients suck on ice or hold ice-cold water in their mouths prior to, during, and after infusions of mucotoxic agents with a short half-life. Outside of transplant, 30 minutes of oral cryotherapy is suggested for patients receiving bolus 5-fluorouracil (Lalla et al., 2014). Within the context of transplant, cryotherapy has been used in patients receiving high-dose melphalan (J. Chen et al., 2017). Unfortunately, other mucotoxic

agents, such as cyclophosphamide and etoposide, have relatively long half-lives, making the application of cryotherapy largely impractical.

Low-Level Laser Therapy

Low-level laser therapy (LLLT) uses a wavelength at 650 nm, power of 40 mW, and each square centimeter treated with sufficient time to deliver a tissue energy dose of 2 J/cm^2 (Lalla et al., 2014). For more than a decade, LLLT has been used to prevent and treat mucositis in patients receiving HSCT conditioning or radiation therapy to the oral cavity. Handheld infrared lasers affect cells and physical symptoms often related to inflammation by exerting an anti-inflammatory effect; promoting wound healing and the activation of local microcirculation; stimulating the production of collagen, serotonin, cortisol, and endorphins (reducing pain); and regulating interleukins IL-1β and IL-6 and tumor necrosis factor-alpha (Ferreira, da Motta Silveira, & de Orange, 2016; Migliorati et al., 2013). LLLT has also been successfully used in combination with cryotherapy (de Paula Eduardo et al., 2015). Studies using LLLT have shown up to an 80% reduction in the incidence of severe mucositis in HSCT. Most of these studies, however, are small, and more research is necessary to solidify its place in oral mucositis prophylaxis and treatment (Migliorati et al., 2013).

Oral Care Protocol

The foundation of an oral care protocol is good oral hygiene. A protocol should include brushing the teeth with a soft toothbrush. Patients who routinely floss should con-

RECOMMENDATIONS IN FAVOR OF AN INTERVENTION (ie, strong evidence supports effectiveness in the treatment setting listed):

1. The panel *recommends* that 30 min of oral cryotherapy be used to *prevent* oral mucositis in patients receiving bolus 5-fluorouracil chemotherapy (II).
2. The panel *recommends* that recombinant human keratinocyte growth factor-1 (KGF-1/palifermin) be used to *prevent* oral mucositis (at a dose of 60 mcg/kg per day for 3 days prior to conditioning treatment and for 3 days after transplant) in patients receiving high-dose chemotherapy and total body irradiation, followed by autologous stem cell transplantation, for a hematologic malignancy (II).
3. The panel *recommends* that low-level laser therapy (wavelength at 650 nm, power of 40 mW, and each square centimeter treated with the required time to a tissue energy dose of 2 J/cm^2), be used to *prevent* oral mucositis in patients receiving HSCT conditioned with high-dose chemotherapy, with or without total body irradiation (II).
4. The panel *recommends* that patient-controlled analgesia with morphine be used to *treat* pain due to oral mucositis in patients undergoing HSCT (II).
5. The panel *recommends* that benzydamine mouthwash be used to *prevent* oral mucositis in patients with head and neck cancer receiving moderate dose radiation therapy (up to 50 Gy), without concomitant chemotherapy (I).

SUGGESTIONS IN FAVOR OF AN INTERVENTION (ie, weaker evidence supports effectiveness in the treatment setting listed):

1. The panel *suggests* that oral care protocols be used to *prevent* oral mucositis in all age groups and across all cancer treatment modalities (III).
2. The panel *suggests* that oral cryotherapy be used to *prevent* oral mucositis in patients receiving high-dose melphalan, with or without total body irradiation, as conditioning for HSCT (III).
3. The panel *suggests* that low-level laser therapy (wavelength around 632.8 nm) be used to *prevent* oral mucositis in patients undergoing radiotherapy, without concomitant chemotherapy, for head and neck cancer (III).
4. The panel *suggests* that transdermal fentanyl may be effective to *treat* pain due to oral mucositis in patients receiving conventional or high-dose chemotherapy, with or without total body irradiation (III).
5. The panel *suggests* that 2% morphine mouthwash may be effective to *treat* pain due to oral mucositis in patients receiving chemoradiation for head and neck cancer (III).
6. The panel *suggests* that 0.5% doxepin mouthwash may be effective to *treat* pain due to oral mucositis (IV).
7. The panel *suggests* that systemic zinc supplements administered orally may be of benefit to *prevent* oral mucositis in oral cancer patients receiving radiation therapy or chemoradiation (III).

RECOMMENDATIONS AGAINST AN INTERVENTION (ie, strong evidence indicates lack of effectiveness in the treatment setting listed):

1. The panel *recommends* that PTA (polymyxin, tobramycin, amphotericin B) and BCoG (bacitracin, clotrimazole, gentamicin) antimicrobial lozenges and PTA paste *not* be used to *prevent* oral mucositis in patients receiving radiation therapy for head and neck cancer (II).
2. The panel *recommends* that iseganan antimicrobial mouthwash *not* be used to *prevent* oral mucositis in patients receiving high-dose chemotherapy, with or without total body irradiation, for HSCT (II), or in patients receiving radiation therapy or concomitant chemoradiation for head and neck cancer (II).
3. The panel *recommends* that sucralfate mouthwash *not* be used to *prevent* oral mucositis in patients receiving chemotherapy for cancer (I), or in patients receiving radiation therapy (I) or concomitant chemoradiation (II) for head and neck cancer.
4. The panel *recommends* that sucralfate mouthwash *not* be used to *treat* oral mucositis in patients receiving chemotherapy for cancer (I), or in patients receiving radiation therapy (II) for head and neck cancer.
5. The panel *recommends* that intravenous glutamine *not* be used to *prevent* oral mucositis in patients receiving high-dose chemotherapy, with or without total body irradiation, for HSCT (II).

SUGGESTIONS AGAINST AN INTERVENTION (ie, weaker evidence indicates lack of effectiveness in the treatment setting listed):

1. The panel *suggests* that chlorhexidine mouthwash *not* be used to *prevent* oral mucositis in patients receiving radiation therapy for head and neck cancer (III).
2. The panel *suggests* that granulocyte macrophage–colony-stimulating factor mouthwash *not* be used to *prevent* oral mucositis in patients receiving high-dose chemotherapy, for autologous or allogeneic stem cell transplantation (II).
3. The panel *suggests* that misoprostol mouthwash *not* be used to *prevent* oral mucositis in patients receiving radiation therapy for head and neck cancer (III).
4. The panel *suggests* that systemic pentoxifylline, administered orally, *not* be used to *prevent* oral mucositis in patients undergoing bone marrow transplantation (III).
5. The panel *suggests* that systemic pilocarpine, administered orally, *not* be used to *prevent* oral mucositis in patients receiving radiation therapy for head and neck cancer (III), or in patients receiving high-dose chemotherapy, with or without total body irradiation, for HSCT (II).

Gy—grays; HSCT—hematopoietic stem cell transplantation; MASCC/ISOO—Multinational Association of Supportive Care in Cancer and International Society of Oral Oncology; mW—milliwatt; nm—nanometers

[a] Level of evidence for each guideline is in brackets after the guideline statement.

Table 9-2. Summary of Recommendations for the Prevention of Oral Mucositis in Pediatric Patients Receiving Treatment for Cancer or Undergoing Hematopoietic Stem Cell Transplantation

Health Question and Recommendations	Strength of Recommendation/ Level of Evidence
What prophylactic interventions are effective at preventing or reducing the severity of oral and oro-pharyngeal mucositis in children (0–18 years) receiving treatment for cancer or undergoing hemato-poietic stem cell transplantation (HSCT)?	
Recommendation 1.1: We suggest that cryotherapy may be offered to cooperative children receiving chemotherapy or HSCT conditioning with regimens associated with a high rate of mucositis. *Remarks:* This recommendation places high value on the possible reduction in mucositis with an intervention with a low risk of harm. It is a weak recommendation because of the lack of pediatric-specific evidence, because the majority of studies that demonstrated the benefit of cryotherapy were conducted using chemotherapy regimens not commonly given to children and because of the methodologic limitations of the conducted trials. Regimens appropriate for cryotherapy are restricted to agents with a short infusion time and a short half-life.	Weak recommendation Moderate-quality evidence
Recommendation 1.2: We suggest that low-level light therapy may be offered to cooperative children receiving chemotherapy or HSCT conditioning with regimens associated with a high rate of mucositis. *Remarks:* This recommendation places high value on the possible reduction in mucositis with an intervention with a low risk of harm. It is a weak recommendation because this strategy requires specialized equipment and expertise, and it is unknown whether it is feasible to deliver this modality in routine clinical practice, particularly in a pediatric population. The ideal treatment parameters and cost-effectiveness of this approach are unknown.	Weak recommendation High-quality evidence
Recommendation 1.3: We suggest that keratinocyte growth factor (KGF) may be offered to children receiving HSCT conditioning with regimens associated with a high rate of severe mucositis. *Remarks:* This recommendation places high value on the evidence of efficacy of KGF in adult populations. It is a weak recommendation because of the lack of efficacy and toxicity data in children, a theoretical concern that young children may be at increased risk for adverse effects related to mucosal thickening and the lack of long-term follow-up data in pediatric cancers.	Weak recommendation High-quality evidence

Note. From "Guideline for the Prevention of Oral and Oropharyngeal Mucositis in Children Receiving Treatment for Cancer or Undergoing Haematopoietic Stem Cell Transplantation," by L. Sung, P. Robinson, N. Treister, T. Baggott, P. Gibson, W. Tissing, … L.L. Dupuis, 2017, *BMJ Supportive and Palliative Care, 7*, p. 9. Copyright 2017 by British Medical Journal. Retrieved from https://doi.org/10.1136/bmjspcare-2014-000804. Licensed under CC BY-NC-ND 4.0 (https://creativecommons.org/licenses/by-nc-nd/4.0).

tinue unless there is a risk of bleeding because of thrombocytopenia or other clotting abnormalities. Dentures must be removed to avoid additional mucosal irritation. Oral care protocols may include different cleansing and treatment regimens. Although no evidence exists to show superiority, saline is commonly used because of its isotonic nature. However, the singular component of any oral care protocol is consistency, which has a positive effect on mucositis prevention and management. In addition to saline, some institutions may use sodium bicarbonate (baking soda). It is mildly alkaline and may buffer the pH of the rinse solution, promoting adherence. In addition to routine oral care, the Oncology Nursing Society mucositis resource (Eilers et al., 2019) has stated the following interventions are likely to be effective.

Palifermin With High-Dose Chemotherapy

Palifermin (Kepivance®), a truncated form of recombinant human keratinocyte growth factor-1, demonstrated its ability to reduce mucositis after chemoradiation therapy in preclinical models and human studies. It received U.S. Food and Drug Administration (FDA) approval in 2004. Palifermin is administered as a short IV push three times prior to transplant and again three times upon completion of stem cell transfusion. The third administration of the pretransplant doses should be given 24–48 hours prior to beginning the conditioning regimen. The last three doses are administered after completion of the conditioning regimen, with the first of these doses on the same day but after the HSCT infusion and at least seven days after the most recent dose of palifermin. When palifermin is being administered through a heparinized line, the line should be flushed with saline prior to and after infusion. The updated MASCC/ISOO clinical practice guidelines recommend the use of palifermin only for total body irradiation–based autologous HSCT; no recommendation could be given in the allogeneic setting because of conflicting results and insufficient evidence (Schmidt et al., 2018). A meta-analysis conducted by Mozaffari et al. (2017) showed palifermin was associated with reduction in the incidence and severity of oral mucositis and also was effective and safe on oral mucositis after allogeneic or autologous HSCT. Palifermin had no effect on the incidence and severity of acute skin GVHD, which has been of particular concern because rash is the most common side effect of the drug (Mozaffari et al., 2017).

Other interventions for the prevention and management of oral mucositis have been tried, and many were found to not be effective: Caphosol® was not shown to reduce severe oral mucositis when compared with placebo (Sung et al., 2017). Although commonly used in practice, "Magic Mouthwash," chlorhexidine, and sucralfate also are not recommended because of lack of efficacy (Eilers et al., 2019).

Dental Evaluation and Management

The Centers for Disease Control and Prevention, along with other organizations, published guidelines for preventing opportunistic infections among HSCT recipients (Tomblyn et al., 2009). Its recommendation stated all patients should have a thorough dental consultation before conditioning therapy and that all likely sources of dental infection and trauma should be vigorously eliminated.

Dental caries should be treated with permanent restoration whenever possible. Teeth with endodontic infections or abscesses need to be treated by endodontic therapy, when time permits, or extracted. Nonrestorable teeth should be extracted (Tomblyn et al., 2009). Healing and resolution of infection must occur 10–14 days prior to conditioning therapy. Culture and sensitivity results of wound or abscess drainage should determine antibiotic use (Tomblyn et al., 2009).

Periodontal infections (gingivitis/periodontitis) are a frequent cause of dental infections in transplant recipients. Optimally, dental prophylaxis, scaling, and curettage should be performed when medically possible (Tomblyn et al., 2009). To decrease the risk of mechanical trauma, secondary infection, and radiation backscatter, fixed orthodontic appliances (e.g., bands, brackets, arch wires) and space maintainers should not be worn from the start of conditioning until stomatitis resolves. Other sources of trauma, such as sharp teeth, should be remedied prior to conditioning therapy.

Following transplantation, elective dental treatments should be postponed until full immune recovery has occurred. During dental procedures, aerosolization of bacteria can cause aspiration pneumonias. When dental procedures are required, prophylactic antibiotics and medical support with platelet transfusions may be necessary (Tomblyn et al., 2009).

Pain Management

The primary symptom of oral mucositis is pain, which can significantly affect nutritional intake, mouth care, and quality of life. Pain occurs as a result of ulceration, edema, and denuding of the epithelial lining. Mucositis pain varies in location, duration, and intensity from patient to patient but generally is described initially as a burning sensation that progresses over time to a continuous tender, sharp, aching feeling. The use of age-appropriate self-reports is the most reliable means of assessing pain intensity because patients are best able to determine acceptable levels of pain intensity and distress. Instruments used for pain assessments vary among transplant centers because of institutional and protocol preference. However, all instruments should be simple, easily understood by patients, and age appropriate and have documented validity and reliability. Pain should be assessed as often as necessary to ensure optimal patient comfort and safety. Comprehensive nursing assessments are imperative for effective pain management, especially in nonverbal and critically ill children and adults.

The majority of transplant recipients who experience moderate to severe oral mucositis require IV opioid therapy by continuous infusion or patient-controlled analgesia. Dosing of opioids should be individualized. All patients receiving opioids should be observed closely for signs and symptoms of overdose, including hypotension, bradycardia, decreased respirations, and oversedation (Brown, 2015). Opioid doses should be increased until comfort is achieved or until side effects prohibit further dose escalation.

Nutritional Support

Nutritional intake can be significantly compromised by the pain associated with oral mucositis, along with the taste changes secondary to chemotherapy or radiation therapy. Nutritional intake should be monitored by a dietitian or other professionals. This is best achieved when working in combination with the patient and caregiver. A soft diet and liquid supplements are better tolerated and reduce the likelihood of increasing trauma to friable mucous membranes. In patients with severe oral mucositis, enteral or parenteral nutrition should be considered.

Route of nutrition (enteral vs. parenteral) continues to be controversial, as research remains inconclusive and both have advantages and disadvantages. Enteral nutrition can cause nausea, vomiting, and diarrhea. Infusion of enteral nutrition is also difficult, as tube placement in the setting of oral mucositis can cause significant discomfort to patients. However, enteral nutrition is associated with reduced infectious complications by preventing translocation of intestinal bacteria and promoting gut function. Parenteral nutrition is an appropriate route if nutritional support is needed and oral or enteral intake is not an option. Parenteral nutrition requires central venous access, as well as close monitoring of metabolic panels. In the setting of oral mucositis, parenteral nutrition typically is advised because the GI tract often is unable to tolerate enteral nutrition (Cotogni, 2016).

Salivary Gland Dysfunction and Xerostomia

Pathophysiology

Xerostomia (dryness of the oral mucosa) and salivary gland dysfunction occur as a result of chemotherapy and radiation toxicity. Mouth breathing, GVHD, and medications with anticholinergic effects may contribute to the severity. Xerostomia occurs approximately 7–10 days after the conditioning regimen and may persist for several months as a result of treatment-related damage to the salivary glands. Saliva becomes thick and ropy with decreased flow rates, leading to a sensation of oral dryness. Xerostomia increases the risk of *Candida* infections, and antifungal therapy should be instituted as clinically indicated (Daikeler et al., 2013).

Management

Treatment focuses on strategies to reduce symptoms. Bland mouth rinses (saltwater with or without baking soda), frequent sips of water, and commercially produced artificial saliva can help to ease the sensation of severe dryness. Sodium bicarbonate rinses can reduce the viscosity of saliva and neutralize the acidic oral environment associated with xerostomia. Aggressive oral hygiene practices that include topical fluorides, sealants, and a reduced dietary intake of refined carbohydrates, such as soda and juice, can help to prevent dental decay. Cautious use of oral suction, specifically soft-tip flexible suction catheters, may be comforting to patients with thick, ropy secretions. Commercial products include gum, alcohol-free mouthwash, and gel developed to provide oral lubrication and protect the oral mucosa from irritation. These products may relieve dry mouth symptoms of burning, soreness, and swallowing difficulties. However, they have not been evaluated in randomized clinical trials involving HSCT recipients. Toothpaste should be used with caution, as strong flavors can irritate mucous membranes and increase discomfort.

Taste Changes

Pathophysiology

Toxicity to oropharyngeal taste receptors from conditioning regimens is a common cause of taste changes, which include hypogeusia (loss of taste), dysgeusia (distorted taste), and ageusia (absence of taste). Taste and smell changes can lead to altered food preferences and thereby contribute to loss of appetite, reduced food intake, and weight changes. When food is eaten, smell, taste, and somatosensory (irritation, texture, and temperature) signals, as well as psychological elements including emotions and behavior, determine the overall flavor of food. Systemic chemotherapy induces taste and odor changes due to cytotoxic damage to the rapidly dividing taste and smell receptor cells. Lower quantity or quality of saliva also interferes. Furthermore, HSCT recipients often receive supportive medications, such as antibiotics, which can affect taste and smell. Decreased saliva, a common side effect of chemotherapy, affects taste perception. Too little saliva causes dry mouth, but it also disrupts taste perception, as saliva plays a major role in taste transfer (van Oort, Kramer, de Groot, & Visser, 2018).

Management

Strategies to improve taste changes include practicing frequent oral hygiene, sucking on hard candy, and using artificial saliva. Patients may improve the overall taste, smell, and appearance of food by increasing seasoning; eating small, frequent portions; and avoiding fatty foods. The majority of HSCT recipients will regain their sense of taste; however, the time to full recovery varies and is based on the degree of oral mucositis and xerostomia, as well as continued treatment with supportive medications.

Nutrition

Malnutrition in patients undergoing HSCT is related to a series of factors, including the underlying disease, pretransplant nutritional state, conditioning regimen used, and complications such as GVHD. Nutritional intake decrease of up to 60% frequently is observed in HSCT recipients (Botti, Liptrott, Gargiulo, & Orlando, 2015). Malnutrition can occur rapidly in the absence of nutritional support and may have a severe negative impact on mortality and morbidity, with persistent serious long-term effects. Methods to improve or maintain nutritional intake include oral nutritional supplements, parenteral nutrition, or tube feeding. Several studies have shown that malnutrition is an independent negative prognostic indicator for the survival of pediatric and adult HSCT recipients (Lemal et al., 2015).

An interprofessional approach to nutritional support is imperative and should include patients, caregivers, doctors, nutritionists/dietitians, pharmacists, and nurses. Prolonged symptoms such as nausea and vomiting may occur in some clinical situations, affecting nutritional status. During periods of severe oropharyngeal and esophageal mucositis and severe diarrhea, patients may be unable to tolerate foods and oral fluids. Because mucositis resolves with neutrophil recovery, autologous transplant recipients usually will resume adequate oral intake within one to two weeks after transplant. However, allogeneic transplant recipients may be neutropenic for three to four weeks and also may experience severe diarrhea from GI GVHD. Parenteral nutrition often is necessary in these circumstances; however, whenever possible, refeeding via the GI tract is the first choice for nutrition (Wędrychowicz, Spodaryk, Krasowska-Kwiecień, & Goździk, 2010). Frequent assessment of patients' nutritional status is vital before, during, and after transplant. Dietitians are frequently involved in the monitoring of nutrition by assessing weight, as well as caloric and protein intake, and providing patient education on how to maximize both.

Food Safety

Diets should be restricted to reduce the risk of exposure to food-related bacteria, yeasts, molds, viruses, and parasites. Patients should follow food safety precautions until directed by a physician. It typically is recommended that precautions be continued for three months for autologous transplant recipients and until discontinuation of all immunosuppressive drugs for allogeneic transplant recipients (Tomblyn et al., 2009). Patients and caregivers should be instructed in dietary restrictions and appropriate food handling practices beginning before the conditioning regimen. For examples of guidelines and recommendations, see Table 9-3 and Figures 9-3 and 9-4.

Naturopathic medications and herbal supplements should only be prescribed by licensed naturopathic physicians working in conjunction with transplant and infectious disease physicians. During periods of immunosuppression, HSCT recipients should avoid naturopathic medicines that may contain molds (Tomblyn et al., 2009). Patients can be directed to FDA's *Food Safety for People With Cancer* booklet for more detailed information (U.S. Department of Agriculture & U.S. FDA, 2011).

Nutritional Support

In 2009, the American Society for Parenteral and Enteral Nutrition and the European Society for Clinical Nutrition and Metabolism issued guidelines on nutritional support for patients undergoing HSCT (Peric et al., 2018). These guidelines recommend screening for malnutrition and nutritional interventions if patients are unable to maintain their nutritional status on their own. In addition, enteral nutrition is recommended as the first option and is preferred over parenteral nutrition because of the higher risk of side effects, such as central line infections and metabolic complications. Parenteral nutrition should be reserved for patients with severe mucositis (higher than grade 3), ileus, or intractable vomiting.

Water Safety

To avoid possible exposure to *Cryptosporidium* and other waterborne pathogens, HSCT recipients should take precautions regarding water exposure and consumption. Patients should not walk, wade, swim, or play in or drink water from recreational sources such as ponds, rivers, or lakes that may be contaminated with sewage or animal or human wastes (Tomblyn et al., 2009). Water from private or public wells of small communities should not be consumed because of infrequent testing for microbial

Table 9-3. Food Safety to Prevent Foodborne Illnesses

Food Group	Low-Risk Foods to Eat	High-Risk Foods to Avoid
Meat and meat substitutes	Meats, poultry, fish, seafood, or tofu cooked to a safe internal temperature Reheated or cooked hot dogs, sausages, bacon, or bratwurst Canned meat, poultry, fish, or seafood Commercially packaged meats or cold cuts Foods or recipes with cooked eggs or pasteurized eggs Canned, shelf-stable pâtés or meat spreads Roasted nuts, seeds, or commercially packaged nut butters	Raw and undercooked meat, poultry, fish, seafood (including smoked fish, pickled fish, lox, and sushi), and tofu Foods with raw or undercooked unpasteurized eggs (includes over-easy, soft-boiled, or poached cooking styles) All meats and prepared foods from deli counters and sub shops All miso and tempeh products Unpasteurized, refrigerated pâtés and meat spreads Unroasted (raw) nuts, seeds, or nut butters and roasted nuts or seeds in shell
Fruits and vegetables	Well-washed raw or frozen fruits, vegetables, and herbs Cooked, canned, or dried fruits and vegetables Pasteurized juices and frozen juice concentrates Well-washed, cooked sprouts	Unwashed raw fruits, vegetables, or herbs Unpasteurized (often fresh squeezed) fruit and vegetable juice and cider Raw sprouts, such as alfalfa and bean sprouts Salad bar including pre-cut fruit
Dairy products	Pasteurized milk and dairy products Commercially packaged hard cheeses, processed cheeses, cream cheese, and soft cheeses made from pasteurized milk, such as American, mild and medium cheddar, Monterey Jack, mozzarella, Parmesan, and Swiss Pasteurized whipped topping Commercially pasteurized eggnog	Unpasteurized (raw) milk and dairy products Aged, mold-containing, and soft cheeses made from raw milk, such as blue, Brie, Camembert, farmer's cheese, feta, Gorgonzola, Roquefort, queso blanco and fresco, sharp cheddar, or Stilton All cheese from deli counters Cheese containing undercooked vegetables Unrefrigerated cream-filled pastry products
Miscellaneous	Pasteurized honey Cooked yeast Commercially processed, shelf-stable salad dressing with low-risk cheeses and freshly prepared dressing with pasteurized eggs or acceptable cheeses Commercially bottled distilled, spring, and natural water or tap water Dried herbs and spices used in cooked recipes	Raw or unpasteurized honey Raw, uncooked yeast Fresh salad dressing made with raw eggs (often Caesar) or high-risk cheeses All moldy, outdated food products All herbal/botanic products or supplements Well water (unless tested yearly and found to be free of coliforms and *Cryptosporidium*) Unpasteurized beer Salad and soup bars, buffets, bulk bins, sub shops, street vendors, and delicatessens

Note. Based on information from U.S. Department of Agriculture & U.S. Food and Drug Administration, 2011.

Figure 9-3. Food Safety Practices

- Raw poultry, meats, fish, and seafood should be handled on a separate surface (cutting board or countertop) from other food items. Separate cutting boards for poultry, meat, and vegetables should be used.
- All cutting or carving surfaces should be washed with warm water and soap between cutting different food items.
- Uncooked meats should not come into contact with other foods.
- After preparing raw poultry, meats, fish, and seafood and before preparing other foods, food handlers should wash their hands thoroughly in warm, soapy water.
- Cold foods should be stored at temperatures below 40°F (4.4°C); hot foods kept above 140°F (60°C).[a]
- Food handlers should wash their hands in warm, soapy water before handling leftovers.
- Use clean utensils and food preparation surfaces.
- Divide leftovers into small amounts and store in shallow containers for quick cooling.
- Refrigerate leftovers within 2 hours after cooking and discard leftovers kept at room temperature for more than 2 hours.
- Reheat leftovers or partially cooked foods to at least 165°F (73.9°C) throughout before serving.[a]
- Cook meat, fish, casseroles and other foods to temperatures listed in Figure 9-4.
- Bring leftover soups, sauces, and gravies to a rolling boil before serving.
- Shelves, countertops, refrigerators, freezers, utensils, sponges, towels, and other kitchen items should be kept clean.
- All fresh produce should be washed thoroughly under running water before serving.

[a] Internal temperature measured with a thermometer

Note. Based on information from Tomblyn et al., 2009.

pathogens. Water from municipal wells in highly populated areas is safe. In a boil-water advisory, all tap water used for drinking or brushing teeth should be boiled for more than one minute before it is used. Home water filters that remove particles larger than 1 mcm in diameter or filter by reverse osmosis are only safe when used on municipal water sources (Tomblyn et al., 2009). Home water filters are not appropriate or safe for use on water from private or small community public wells. Bottled water can be consumed if it has been processed to remove *Cryptosporidium* by reverse osmosis, distillation, or 1 mcm particulate absolute filtration. Patients should contact the bottler directly. Contact information regarding water bottlers is available from the International Bottled Water Association at www.bottledwater.org (Tomblyn et al., 2009).

Nausea and Vomiting

Nausea and vomiting are common GI symptoms experienced by HSCT recipients. The optimal antiemetic regimen for chemotherapy-induced nausea and vomiting (CINV) in HSCT recipients is unknown and varies in individual transplant settings (Schmitt et al., 2014; Trifilio et al., 2017).

One reason for the lack of antiemetic standardized treatment in this setting is the combination of the numerous chemotherapy regimens that are administered over several days, medication interactions that cause nausea and vomiting, and physiologic factors that cause nausea and vomiting unrelated to CINV (Tendas et al., 2012). Patterns of nausea and vomiting in the HSCT setting are not well described. Delayed nausea and vomiting is reported for days following chemotherapy and continues after discharge. The reason for ongoing nausea and vomiting is multifactorial and related to medication, gastroparesis, and prolonged GI inflammation (Tendas et al., 2012).

Nausea is defined as an unpleasant feeling that occurs in the stomach or the back of the throat. It often occurs in waves and may precede vomiting. *Vomiting* is the expulsion of gastric contents through the mouth. *Retching* is also referred to as dry heaves and involves stomach or esophageal movement without expulsion of gastric contents. Acute nausea and vomiting occur within the first 24 hours, and delayed nausea and vomiting occur after 24 hours and over 4 days. Breakthrough nausea and vomiting occur within five days of chemotherapy administration. Refractory nausea and vomiting do not respond to antiemetic therapy (Kamen et al., 2014; National Cancer Institute, 2018; Navari, 2013).

CINV is associated with serious complications such as electrolyte imbalances, dehydration, anorexia, weight loss, weakness, and more serious complications such as esophageal tears, fractures, aspiration pneumonia, mental status changes, and malnutrition. Moreover, nausea and vomiting can significantly affect patients' quality of life (Clark et al., 2016; Musso et al., 2010; Navari, 2013).

Figure 9-4. Safe Cooking Temperatures for Foods[a]

Beef, Lamb, or Veal
- Ground meats: 160°F (71.2°C)
- Roasts, steaks, chops: 145°F (62.8°C)

Chicken, Duck, or Turkey
- Ground poultry: 165°F (73.9°C)
- Whole, pieces, ground: 165°F (73.9°C)

Pork
- Ham
  - Fresh, raw: 160°F (71.2°C)
  - Fully cooked, USDA inspected: 140°F (60°C)
  - Fully cooked, non-USDA inspected: 165°F (73.9°C)
- Ground pork: 160°F (71.2°C)
- Roasts, steaks, chops: 145°F (62.8°C)

Other Foods
- Sauces, soups, gravy, leftovers: 165°F (73.9°C)
- Casseroles and egg dishes: 160°F (71.2°C)
- Fish and seafood
  - Fish: 145°F (62.8°C)
  - Shrimp, lobster, crab: until opaque
  - Clams, mussels, oysters: until the shells open
- Hot dogs, deli meats: steaming hot or 165°F (73.9°C)

[a] Internal temperature measured with a thermometer

USDA—U.S. Department of Agriculture

Note. Based on information from Tomblyn et al., 2009.

Incidence

Although patients with hematologic malignancies have been treated with HSCT for a number of decades, the incidence of nausea and vomiting for some conditioning regimens remains very high. It is estimated that vomiting occurs in 80%–95% of transplant recipients. Nausea is estimated to occur in approximately 95% of HSCT recipients. Most patients receiving high-dose chemotherapy in the HSCT setting will experience delayed nausea (Schmitt et al., 2014).

Pathophysiology

Nausea and vomiting caused by chemotherapy involve a complex network of neuroanatomic, peripheral centers, neurotransmitters, and receptors. Chemotherapy activates neurotransmitter receptors located in the vomiting center (VC), chemoreceptor trigger zone (CTZ), and GI tract. Vomiting occurs when the VC, located in the medulla, receives stimuli from the cerebral cortex, CTZ, and vagal and pharynx afferent fibers from the GI tract. When this stimulus is received, efferent fibers travel from the VC to the abdominal muscles, salivation center, cranial nerves, and respiratory center, causing vomiting to occur. The nucleus tractus solitarius (NTS) neurons are found in the area postrema in the medulla and have an important role in initiating emesis. The NTS is considered a central site for antiemetics that act in the central nervous system (Janelins et al., 2013; Navari, 2013). Serotonin, dopamine, and substance P are three important neurotransmitters found in the GI tract, CTZ, and VC and mediate the process of emesis.

The main substance found in serotonin is 5-HT$_3$, which mediates the neural signals from the gut to the NTS that increase in acute CINV. Neurokinin-1 (NK$_1$) antagonists prevent substance P from binding to NK$_1$ receptors. NK$_1$ receptors are found along the vagus nerve and the CTZ. These receptors play an active role in delayed CINV. Dopamine antagonists interrupt many CINV pathways and are more likely to decrease chemotherapy-induced vomiting and, to a lesser degree, chemotherapy-induced nausea (Rapoport, 2017). The pathways of nausea and vomiting may not be the same. Each may have different unique pathways; however, more research is needed to determine the exact pathway of each symptom. Other neurotransmitters involved in CINV include histamine, acetylcholine, gamma-aminobutyric acid, and endorphins. The experience of CINV is dependent on the individual's response to the stimuli endured, and the threshold differs for each patient (Janselins et al., 2013).

Assessment

Risk factors should be considered in assessing patients for nausea and vomiting in the HSCT setting. A multicenter prospective study evaluated the patterns of CINV for a total of three cycles. Complete data were obtained for 991 patients in cycle 1, 888 in cycle 2, and 769 in cycle 3.

The key predictor variables for increased CINV included the following: antiemetics that were inconsistent with international guidelines, younger age, prechemotherapy nausea, and a lack of a complete CINV response during previous cycles of therapy (all at p < 0.05). Previously reported risk factors such as history of nausea and vomiting, anxiety, and expectations of nausea were important predictors for some phases of CINV and cycles of therapy but were not consistently correlated across the CINV pathway (Molassiotis et al., 2014).

The emetogenicity of chemotherapy agents is associated with an increased risk of CINV. Chemotherapy is categorized into four groups: highly emetic chemotherapy, risk greater than 90%; moderately emetic chemotherapy, risk 30%–90%; low emetic chemotherapy, risk 10%–30%; and minimal-risk chemotherapy, risk less than 10% (Hesketh et al., 1997). Antiemetic therapy is based on the emetic potential of the prescribed regimen (Navari, 2013). Many HSCT regimens are administered over several days; therefore, appropriate antiemetic therapy should be prescribed each day that chemotherapy is administered (National Comprehensive Cancer Network, 2019). Most HSCT regimens are considered highly emetic, but melphalan used as the preparative agent for multiple myeloma is considered moderately emetic (Schmitt et al., 2014).

Numerous CINV tools exist to measure nausea and vomiting. Some common ones include the Morrow Assessment of Nausea and Emesis, the MASCC nausea assessment tool, the Nausea Questionnaire, and the Common Terminology Criteria for Adverse Events (CTCAE). The Index of Nausea, Vomiting and Retching and the Osoba Nausea and Vomiting Module are tools to measure all nausea, vomiting, and retching. Visual analog scales and numeric rating scales are common tools that also are easy to use. Vomiting is less complicated, as reporting the number of emetic episodes is an objective measurement (Wood, Chapman, & Eilers, 2011).

Assessment of CINV should include additional medications that may contribute to symptoms, such as antibiotics, narcotic analgesics, antihypertensives (e.g., nifedipine), and nonsteroidal anti-inflammatory drugs. Mucositis of the upper GI tract is associated with nausea and vomiting in the transplant setting. Swallowing large quantities of mucus (in patients with severe mucositis) also can produce nausea. Although less common in this population, other conditions that can cause nausea and vomiting include constipation, dehydration, gastroparesis, bowel obstruction, myocardial infarction, pain, viral infections, food sensitivity or food poisoning, and coughing (Glare, Miller, Nikolova, & Tickoo, 2011).

Poorly managed nausea and vomiting can lead to other sequelae such as dehydration, which can affect mobility and safety. The cause of nausea and vomiting should always be investigated and treated aggressively. Appropriate scans and laboratory work should be obtained along with blood work including electrolytes, renal and liver function tests, and a complete blood count. Based on the assessment, a plan of care should be implemented.

Treatment

The treatment of CINV has improved with the addition of the NK_1 inhibitors in the transplant setting, although standardization challenges of CINV remain problematic. Many different conditioning regimens are in use, both with and without total body irradiation. Inherent differences between allogeneic and autologous transplants, pediatric and adult populations, and sequential multiday regimens have contributed to the difficulty in controlling CINV in the HSCT population (Tendas et al., 2012).

Transplants are performed for many types of malignancies and at various disease stages. Given this information, it is difficult to generate one national guideline to fit all types of transplants. Until recently, the recommendation from several national guidelines was to use a 5-HT_3 medication with dexamethasone (Basch, Hesketh, Kris, Prestrud, Temin, & Lyman, 2011; National Comprehensive Cancer Network, 2019). Recent studies have supported the use of an NK_1 inhibitor, specifically fosaprepitant or aprepitant, 5-HT_3, and dexamethasone in the HSCT setting. Two phase 2 and two phase 3 trials support this combination in high-dose BEAM (carmustine, etoposide, cytarabine, melphalan) or high-dose melphalan (Clark et al., 2016; Pielichowski et al., 2011).

In a placebo-controlled phase 3 trial of 179 patients who received a preparative regimen containing high-dose cyclophosphamide, participants were randomized to receive ondansetron and dexamethasone with and without aprepitant (administered daily and for three days after the completion of the preparative regimen). The study reported a reduction in emesis in the aprepitant arm without an increase in toxicity and a complete response of 82%, compared to 66% in the arm not receiving aprepitant (Stiff et al., 2013).

In another phase 3 study, patients with multiple myeloma were randomized to receive either aprepitant (125 mg, followed by 80 mg days 2 and 3), granisetron (days 1–4), and dexamethasone (days 1–4), or granisetron and dexamethasone at the same doses plus placebo (Schmitt et al., 2014). Of the 362 patients evaluated (181 in each arm), 58% of patients in the aprepitant arm reported no nausea or vomiting, compared to 41% in the arm not receiving aprepitant (OR, 1.92; 95% CI [1.23, 3.00]; p = 0.0042) (Schmitt et al., 2014). The absence of major nausea (visual analog scale score > 25 mm) was increased in the aprepitant arm (94%) compared to 88% in the arm not receiving aprepitant (OR, 2.37; 95% CI [1.09, 5.15]; p = 0.026) (Schmitt et al., 2014). Less emesis occurred in the aprepitant arm as well, with 78% reporting no vomiting compared to 65% in the arm not receiving aprepitant (OR, 1.99; 95% CI [1.25, 3.18]; p = 0.0036) (Schmitt et al., 2014).

Based on these findings, MASCC and the European Society for Medical Oncology changed their most recent recommendations for patients receiving high-dose chemotherapy for HSCT. The current recommendations support using the combination of a 5-HT_3 antagonist with dexamethasone and aprepitant (125 mg orally on day 1 and 80 mg on days 2–4) before chemotherapy (Roila et al., 2016).

Based on this information, three main categories of prophylactic antiemetics should be considered: 5-HT_3 antagonists, NK_1 antagonists, and dexamethasone. Figure 9-5 is a list of common 5-HT_3 antagonists and NK_1 antagonists used in the transplant setting. The first-generation 5-HT_3 antagonists are more effective in the acute CINV setting and are equivalent in efficacy and toxicities when the recommended doses are prescribed (Navari, 2013). Over the past several years, 5-HT_3 antagonists have been associated with cardiac arrhythmias. IV dolasetron is no longer commercially available, and IV ondansetron can cause prolonged QT interval and therefore should be used with caution in individuals with cardiac disease.

Figure 9-5. Antiemetic Medications

- 5-HT_3 antagonists
  - Dolasetron: oral
  - Granisetron: oral, IV, transdermal
  - Ondansetron: oral, IV
  - Palonosetron: IV
- NK_1 inhibitors
  - Aprepitant: oral
  - Fosaprepitant: IV

NK_1—neurokinin-1

Note. Based on information from National Comprehensive Cancer Network, 2019.

Delayed Chemotherapy-Induced Nausea and Vomiting

Delayed nausea is a significant problem for HSCT recipients, and breakthrough antiemetic therapy often is needed. Palonosetron is a second-generation 5-HT_3 antagonist with a longer half-life and may have more efficacy in controlling delayed nausea (Navari, 2013). Studies using palonosetron in the HSCT setting have not yielded convincing results. In a randomized, double-blind pilot, palonosetron (for three consecutive days) and dexamethasone (for two consecutive days) were administered to HSCT recipients receiving multiday high-dose melphalan. Although the three-day dosing was well tolerated, only 20% of the patients were emesis free and did not require rescue medication (Giralt et al., 2011).

In a nonrandomized study, 134 patients receiving high-dose chemotherapy and autologous HSCT were administered palonosetron combined with dexamethasone. A second dose of palonosetron and dexamethasone was given for breakthrough CINV. A complete response was reported in 36% of the patients (Musso et al., 2010).

Because delayed nausea in the HSCT setting is difficult to manage, nurses must continually assess for nausea and vomiting and consider using medication from another group of antiemetic medications. These medications include dopamine antagonists, atypical antipsychotics (olanzapine), cannabinoids, and benzodiazepines. Figure 9-6 is a list of breakthrough antiemetic medications.

Over the past few years, olanzapine has been used in the antiemetic prophylaxis setting. The American Society of Clinical Oncology (Basch et al., 2011), MASCC/European Society for Medical Oncology (Roila et al., 2016), and National Comprehensive Cancer Network (2019) now include olanzapine in their guidelines for prophylactic use in highly or moderately emetic chemotherapy. In a randomized, double-blind phase 3 study, the use of olanzapine was compared to placebo (Navari et al., 2016). All patients received aprepitant/fosaprepitant, 5-HT$_3$, and dexamethasone. A total of 380 patients were randomized. Findings showed the olanzapine group had a significantly higher number of patients with no nausea compared to placebo at 24, 25–120, and more than 120 hours. Olanzapine was well tolerated; however, greater sedation was noted on day 2 of the olanzapine group (Navari et al., 2016).

The use of olanzapine has been studied in the HSCT population. A retrospective study compared the use of aprepitant or fosaprepitant to olanzapine for patients receiving high-dose melphalan. Dexamethasone and 5-HT$_3$ medications also were administered to all participants included in the study. The study reported a significant reduction in the olanzapine group compared to the patients who received aprepitant/fosaprepitant in the acute (p < 0.0001) as well as delayed setting (p < 0.004) and reduced the need for rescue medication (p < 0.0046) (Trifilio et al., 2017).

Another retrospective study comparing fosaprepitant to olanzapine found that in 113 patients, the use of breakthrough medication was significantly reduced in the olanzapine arm (p < 0.001) (Nerone, Carlstrom, Weber, & Majhail, 2017). Emesis was similar in each group, and no change was noted in the length of hospital stay. More patients discontinued olanzapine than fosaprepitant because of side effects. Randomized studies using olanzapine in the pretreatment antiemesis HSCT setting are needed to further determine the efficacy of olanzapine. However, given the results of these trials, the use of olanzapine should be considered in the pretreatment setting and as a management strategy for breakthrough CINV.

CINV in the transplant setting remains a significant problem. More research is needed to better understand its pathophysiology and patterns. It is imperative that nurses assess and manage CINV symptoms. Switching to another antiemetic category may be beneficial for patients with poor control. Effective management of CINV will decrease HSCT complications and improve patients' quality of life in this clinical setting.

Diarrhea

Diarrhea is a subjective symptom best defined as an increase in stool frequency that can be quantified but also described as stools that are less formed or loose (Polage, Solnick, & Cohen, 2012; Schiller et al., 2013). An estimated 75%–100% of transplant recipients experience diarrhea (Arango et al., 2006; McQuade, Stojanovska, Abalo, Bornstein, & Nurgali, 2016). Causes can include infection, medications, diet and nutritional supplements, and GVHD (Tuncer, Rana, Milani, Darko, & Al-Homsi, 2012).

Diarrhea is associated with significant complications, including electrolyte imbalances, dehydration, malnutrition, weight loss, perirectal skin breakdown, hemorrhoids, fatigue, and renal failure. Each of these complications can lead to further significant complications. Persistent diarrhea is associated with metabolic acidosis or intestinal inflammation causing thickening and ulceration of the bowel wall. This can lead to a life-threatening bowel obstruction (McQuade et al., 2016; Stein, Voigt, & Jordan, 2010). Uncontrolled diarrhea can lead to infection, prolonged hospitalization, and organ impairment. Fortunately, most complications are avoidable with appropriate interventions. Careful monitoring and replacement of electrolytes is necessary. Symptoms of electrolyte imbalances are muscle cramping, mental status changes, seizures, heart rhythm disturbances, and weakness.

Etiology and Risk Factors

Several chemotherapy agents, particularly busulfan and melphalan, can cause diarrhea by initiating mucosal inflammation (Tuncer et al., 2012). As described elsewhere, the degree of donor–recipient human leukocyte antigen (HLA) incompatibility plays an important role in the devel-

---

Figure 9-6. Breakthrough Antiemetic Medications

- Atypical antipsychotics
  – Olanzapine
- Benzodiazepines
  – Lorazepam
- Cannabinoids
  – Dronabinol
  – Nabilone
- 5-HT$_3$ antagonists
  – Dolasetron
  – Granisetron
  – Ondansetron
- Phenothiazines
  – Prochlorperazine
  – Promethazine
- Steroids
  – Dexamethasone
- Other
  – Haloperidol
  – Metoclopramide
  – Palonosetron
  – Scopolamine

Note. Based on information from National Comprehensive Cancer Network, 2019; Navari, 2013.

opment of GVHD-associated diarrhea. HLA-mismatched donors and unrelated donors increase the risk for developing GVHD (Lorentino et al., 2017). GI GVHD is diarrhea described as secretory diarrhea that produces 1–2 L/day of stool (Malard & Mohty, 2014).

Certain pretransplant viral infections, such as cytomegalovirus, *Herpesviridae*, toxoplasmosis, and hepatitis B and C viruses, should be considered in patients with diarrhea because primary infections, as well as reactivation of certain viruses, can occur (Ullmann et al., 2016). The use of antibiotics is a known risk factor in the development of *Clostridium difficile* infection. Furthermore, the development of early *C. difficile* infection could increase the development of GI GVHD (Alonso et al., 2012).

In a retrospective case-control study describing the epidemiology, timing, and risk factors for *C. difficile* infection, the overall incidence was 9.2%, with 6.5% for autologous patients and 12% for allogeneic patients (Alonso et al., 2012). The median time to diagnosing the infection was 33 days for allogeneic patients. Early *C. difficile* infection was associated with the development of GI GVHD, and GI GVHD was a risk factor for *C. difficile* infection. Other *C. difficile* infection risk factors included chemotherapy prior to HSCT, antibiotic use, and vancomycin-resistant *Enterococcus* colonization (Alonso et al., 2012).

Infection, other than *C. difficile* infection, is another cause of diarrhea in the transplant setting. Neutropenic enterocolitis or typhlitis is a more common complication in the pediatric transplant population. The symptoms of neutropenic enterocolitis include fever, bloody or watery diarrhea, abdominal distension, and right lower quadrant abdominal pain (Chow & Bishop, 2016). Risks associated with neutropenic enterocolitis include high-dose chemotherapy that results in prolonged neutropenia. Abdominal wall integrity is compromised and vulnerable to bacterial invasion, necrosis, or perforation (Cloutier, 2010; del Campo, León, Palacios, Lagana, & Tagarro, 2014). Diagnosis of typhlitis can be delayed because symptoms often begin with vague abdominal cramping and can be confused with other GI symptoms, such as infectious colitis, pseudomembranous colitis, appendicitis, and inflammatory bowel disease (Rodrigues, Dasilva, & Wexner, 2017).

Infectious enterocolitis is common during the pre-engraftment and early post-transplant phases of HSCT. Possible infectious agents include bacteria, fungi, and viruses. Patients often report diarrhea and abdominal pain associated with fever. Thickening of the bowel walls is identified on computed tomography scan (del Campo et al., 2014).

Pathophysiology

Diarrhea is a complicated process, often with measurable damage of the bowel wall. Different pathophysiologic mechanisms are described and vary based on the underlying etiology. Types of diarrhea include secretory, osmotic, inflammatory, and gut dysmotility. When secretory diarrhea occurs, an increase in intestinal secretions of fluid and electrolytes results in decreased absorption (Camilleri, Sellin, & Barrett, 2017). Causes include abnormal mediators, such as enterotoxins (*C. difficile* infection), and *C. difficile* infection should be considered when HSCT recipients present with diarrhea symptoms. A stool specimen should be sent to rule out *C. difficile* infection. GVHD and certain laxatives also can cause secretory diarrhea. In osmotic diarrhea, more water is drawn into the bowel by osmosis. This occurs when certain nonabsorbable laxatives are used (Crombie, Gallagher, & Hall, 2013).

Inflammation of the GI tract causes damage to the intestinal mucosal cells, leading to a loss of fluid and blood and defective absorption of fluid and electrolytes. Chemotherapy is known to cause GI mucosal inflammation resulting in GI damage and degeneration (McQuade et al., 2016). Not all diarrhea is directly related to the transplant process. Other causes associated with inflammatory diarrhea include infectious conditions, such as *Salmonella* and *Shigella* infections, as well as chronic inflammatory conditions, such as ulcerative colitis, Crohn disease, and celiac disease. Abnormal gut motility often experienced in diabetes and hyperthyroidism is another cause of diarrhea. In many of these cases, the volume and weight of the stool are not particularly high, but frequency of defecation is increased (Crombie et al., 2013; Leffler & Lamont, 2015).

Allogeneic HSCT is associated with intense changes in the intestinal microbiota resulting in decreased diversity of bacterial organisms. In a study by Taur et al. (2014), the authors reported that low diversity of bacterial organisms showed an increase in mortality in HSCT recipients. Bacterial microbiota diversity was categorized as low, intermediate, and high. The overall survival of each category in HSCT recipients at three years was 36%, 60%, and 67%, respectively (Taur et al., 2014).

Assessment

Assessment of HSCT recipients experiencing diarrhea is complicated. The pathology, medications, past medical history, and complications associated with the symptoms must be considered. Assessment should begin with the initial report of diarrhea and include the number of episodes, urgency, consistency, and associated symptoms, such as abdominal pain, nausea, vomiting, or bowel incontinence. Pertinent past medical history includes radiation, surgery, travel (particularly outside of the country), and diabetes. The type of transplant (allogeneic vs. autologous), preparative regimen, and timing of symptoms play an important role in narrowing down potential causes (Camilleri et al., 2017). Further documentation of subjective signs and symptoms, such as weakness, fatigue, dizziness, and muscle cramping, should be considered.

Careful attention to physical abnormalities should be recognized. Objective signs and symptoms, such as mental status changes, vital signs (including orthostatics), a decrease in weight, skin turgor, lymphadenopathy, and mucous membrane assessments, should be documented.

Accurate intake and output measurements are imperative. An abdominal examination should include the presence of abdominal pain, distension, and guarding. Laboratory data such as complete blood count with differential and chemistries should be evaluated for abnormalities that may suggest an infectious process, neutropenia, or electrolyte imbalances, as well as renal or hepatic abnormalities. A stool specimen should be sent for bacterial and parasitic organisms. Blood cultures should be considered when patients are febrile or demonstrating signs of sepsis. Reviewing the medication list is vital, and certain medications, such as bowel medications, antibiotics, chemotherapy, immunotherapy, growth factors, and opioids, should be documented (Tuncer et al., 2012).

Radiologic scans (e.g., computed tomography scans and x-rays) may be ordered when ruling out bowel obstruction or colitis or if GI bleeding is present, which is indicative of perforation (Chow & Bishop, 2016). Bacterial, viral, and parasitic infections should be considered in the differential diagnosis (Polage et al., 2012). As previously discussed, *C. difficile* infection is a common bacterial GI infection. Other bacterial infections include *Clostridium perfringens*, *Klebsiella oxytoca*, *Staphylococcus aureus*, and *Bacteroides fragilis* (Polage et al., 2012). Viral infections such as rotavirus and norovirus are commonly identified. Other viruses include adenovirus and cytomegalovirus (Lin & Liu, 2013; Wingard, Hsu, & Hiemenz, 2011). The CTCAE (National Cancer Institute Cancer Therapy Evaluation Program, 2017) is one method used to accurately assess diarrhea in HSCT recipients. Table 9-4 describes CTCAE grading for diarrhea.

Treatment

Treatment should focus on the underlying cause and may involve several management strategies. Volume depletion along with electrolyte imbalances/disturbances is treated with IV infusions. Patients should be encouraged to increase their oral fluid intake whenever possible. Fluids that contain electrolytes (e.g., Pedialyte®, sports drinks) may be beneficial. Dietary intake should be assessed, and patients should be encouraged to adhere to a bland, low-residue diet; eat small, frequent meals; and avoid dairy products

and foods high in fiber and fat (Boyle et al., 2014; Hamdeh et al., 2016; Mayo Clinic, 2018).

If infection is suspected, antibiotics or antiviral medications may be required. When the cause of diarrhea is not infectious, antidiarrheal medications should be used. Different classes of antidiarrheal medications include opioid and opioid-like medications, adrenergic alpha-2 receptor agonists, somatostatin analogs, and bile acid–binding resin drugs. Figure 9-7 includes a categorized summary of antidiarrheal medications. Diarrhea due to suspected or diagnosed GVHD often is treated with steroids. The management of GVHD is discussed in Chapter 7.

Neutropenic patients with diarrhea are at risk for developing perirectal skin breakdown. Although diarrhea often is associated with perirectal skin breakdown, other causes include GVHD, radiation therapy, and chemotherapy. Perirectal skin breakdown is a serious problem, with potential complications including perirectal abscess, fistula, or sepsis (C.-Y. Chen et al., 2013; Solmaz et al., 2016). Common symptoms of perirectal skin breakdown include perirectal discomfort and itching, fever, and bloody or watery stool. It is important to avoid using suppositories in patients with perirectal skin breakdown because of the risk of bacterial migration.

Perirectal skin assessments should take place on a daily basis, and more often if clinically indicated when HSCT recipients are neutropenic with diarrhea. The perirectal area may appear dry or desquamating, and erythema of the area may be present (Dest, 2018). The most important management strategy is to wash the area with warm water after each bowel movement, using water-repellent ointment such as petroleum jelly (Mayo Clinic, 2018).

Summary

The pathophysiology, assessment, and management of HSCT recipients experiencing GI complications are complex. Patients usually have multiple GI complications occurring simultaneously, making assessment and management even more difficult. In most cases, patients experiencing severe oral mucositis will have fluid and electrolyte imbalances, infection, severe pain, and malnutrition. Concur-

Table 9-4. Common Terminology Criteria for Adverse Events Grading of Diarrhea

| Adverse Event | Grade | | | | |
	1	2	3	4	5
Diarrhea	Increase of < 4 stools/day over baseline; mild increase in ostomy output compared to baseline	Increase of 4–6 stools/day over baseline; moderate increase in ostomy output compared to baseline; limiting instrumental ADL	Increase of ≥ 7 stools/day over baseline; hospitalization indicated; severe increase in ostomy output compared to baseline	Life-threatening consequences; urgent interventions indicated	Death

ADL—activity of daily living

Note. From *Common Terminology Criteria for Adverse Events* [v.5.0], by National Cancer Institute Cancer Therapy Evaluation Program, 2017. Retrieved from https://ctep.cancer.gov/protocolDevelopment/electronic_applications/docs/CTCAE_v5_Quick_Reference_8.5x11.pdf.

Figure 9-7. Antidiarrheal Medications

Adrenergic Alpha-2 Receptor Agonists	Bile Acid–Binding Resin Drugs	Opioid and Opioid-Like Receptor Medications	Somatostatin Analogs
• Clonidine	• Cholestyramine • Colestipol	• Codeine • Diphenoxylate • Eluxadoline • Loperamide • Morphine • Opium tincture	• Octreotide

Note. Based on information from Andreyev et al., 2014; Benson et al., 2004; Camilleri et al., 2017; Deng et al., 2017.

rent mucositis of the GI mucosa usually occurs, causing diarrhea that predisposes patients to the development of perineal-rectal skin alterations and GI infection. Following the administration of myeloablative chemotherapy and radiation, patients may experience xerostomia and taste alterations for several months, prolonging nutritional deficiencies. Specialized nursing care, assessments, and management can positively influence patient outcomes and experiences. Nursing research regarding oral hygiene, skin care, nausea, vomiting, pain, and diarrhea management is necessary to identify and implement standards of care that improve patient outcomes.

The authors would like to acknowledge Susan A. Ezzone, MS, RN, CNP, AOCNP®, for her contribution to this chapter that remains unchanged from the previous edition of this book.

References

Al-Dasooqi, N., Sonis, S.T., Bowen, J.M., Bateman, E., Blijlevens, N., Gibson, R.J., ... Lalla, R.V. (2013). Emerging evidence on the pathobiology of mucositis. *Supportive Care in Cancer, 21*, 2075–2083. https://doi.org/10.1007/s00520-013-1810-y

Alonso, C.D., Treadway, S.B., Hanna, D.B., Huff, C.A., Neofytos, D., Carroll, K.C., & Marr, K.A. (2012). Epidemiology and outcomes of *Clostridium difficile* infections in hematopoietic stem cell transplant recipients. *Clinical Infectious Diseases, 54*, 1053–1063. https://doi.org/10.1093/cid/cir1035

Andreyev, J., Ross, P., Donnellan, C., Lennan, E., Leonard, P., Waters, C., ... Ferry, D. (2014). Guidance on the management of diarrhoea during cancer chemotherapy. *Lancet Oncology, 15*(10), e447–e460. https://doi.org/10.1016/S1470-2045(14)70006-3

Arango, J.I., Restrepo, A., Schneider, D.L., Callander, N.S., Ochoa-Bayona, J.L., Restrepo, M.I., Bradshaw, P., ... Freytes, C.O. (2006). Incidence of *Clostridium difficile*-associated diarrhea before and after autologous peripheral blood stem cell transplantation for lymphoma and multiple myeloma. *Bone Marrow Transplantation, 37*, 517–521. https://doi.org/10.1038/sj.bmt.1705269

Basch, E., Hesketh, P.J., Kris, M.G., Prestrud, A.A., Temin, S., & Lyman, G.H. (2011). Antiemetics: American Society of Clinical Oncology clinical practice guideline update. *Journal of Oncology Practice, 7*, 395–398. https://doi.org/10.1200/JOP.2011.000397

Benson, A.B., III, Ajani, J.A., Catalano, R.B., Engelking, C., Kornblau, S.M., Martenson, J.A., ... Wadler, S. (2004). Recommended guidelines for the treatment of cancer treatment-induced diarrhea. *Journal of Clinical Oncology, 22*, 2918–2926. https://doi.org/10.1200/jco.2004.04.132

Bhat, V., Joshi, A., Sarode, R., & Chavan, P. (2015). Cytomegalovirus infection in the bone marrow transplant patient. *World Journal of Transplantation, 5*, 287–291. https://doi.org/10.5500%2Fwjt.v5.i4.287

Botti, S., Liptrott, S.J., Gargiulo, G., & Orlando, L. (2015). Nutritional support in patients undergoing haematopoietic stem cell transplantation: A multicentre survey of the Gruppo Italiano Trapianto Midollo Osseo (GITMO) transplant programmes. *Ecancermedicalscience, 9*, 545. https://doi.org/10.3332/ecancer.2015.545

Bowen, J.M., & Wardill, H.R. (2017). Advances in the understanding and management of mucositis during stem cell transplantation. *Current Opinion in Supportive and Palliative Care, 11*, 341–346. https://doi.org/10.1097/spc.0000000000000310

Boyle, N.M., Podczervinski, S., Jordan, K., Stednick, Z., Butler-Wu, S., McMillen, K., & Pergam, S.A. (2014). Bacterial foodborne infections after hematopoietic cell transplantation. *Biology of Blood and Marrow Transplantation, 11*, 1856–1861. https://doi.org/10.1016/j.bbmt.2014.06.034

Brown, C.G. (2015). Mucositis. In C.G. Brown (Ed.), *A guide to oncology symptom management* (2nd ed., pp. 469–482). Pittsburgh, PA: Oncology Nursing Society.

Camilleri, M., Sellin, J.H., & Barrett, K.E. (2017). Pathophysiology, evaluation, and management of chronic watery diarrhea. *Gastroenterology, 152*, 515–532.e2. https://doi.org/10.1053/j.gastro.2016.10.014

Chaudhry, H.M., Bruce, A.J., Wolf, R.C., Litzow, M.R., Hogan, W.J., Patnaik, M.S., ... Hashmi, S.K. (2016). The incidence and severity of oral mucositis among allogeneic hematopoietic stem cell transplantation patients: A systematic review. *Biology of Blood and Marrow Transplantation, 22*, 605–616. https://doi.org/10.1016/j.bbmt.2015.09.014

Chen, C.-Y., Cheng, A., Huang, S.-Y., Sheng, W.-H., Liu, J.-H., Ko, B.-S., ... Tien, H.-F. (2013). Clinical and microbiological characteristics of perianal infections in adult patients with acute leukemia. *PLOS ONE, 8*, e60624. https://doi.org/10.1371/journal.pone.0060624

Chen, J., Seabrook, J., Fulford, A., & Rajakumar, I. (2017). Icing oral mucositis: Oral cryotherapy in multiple myeloma patients undergoing autologous hematopoietic stem cell transplant. *Journal of Oncology Pharmacy Practice, 23*, 116–120. https://doi.org/10.1177/1078155215620920

Chow, E.J., & Bishop, K.D. (2016). Painless neutropenic enterocolitis in a patient undergoing chemotherapy. *Current Oncology, 23*, e514–e516. https://doi.org/10.3747/co.23.3119

Clark, S.M., Clemmons, A.B., Schaack, L., Garren, J., DeRemer, D.L., & Kota, V.K. (2016). Fosaprepitant for the prevention of nausea and vomiting in patients receiving BEAM or high-dose melphalan before autologous hematopoietic stem cell transplant. *Journal of Oncology Pharmacy Practice, 22*, 416–422. https://doi.org/10.1177/1078155215585190

Cloutier, R.L. (2010). Neutropenic enterocolitis. *Hematology/Oncology Clinics of North America, 24*, 577–584. https://doi.org/10.1016/j.hoc.2010.03.005

Cotogni, P. (2016). Enteral versus parenteral nutrition in cancer patients: Evidences and controversies. *Annals of Palliative Medicine, 5*, 42–49. https://doi.org/10.3978/j.issn.2224-5820.2016.01.05

Crombie, H., Gallagher, R., & Hall, V. (2013). Assessment and management of diarrhoea. *Nursing Times, 109*(30), 22–24.

Daikeler, T., Mauramo, M., Rovó, A., Stern, M., Halter, J., Buser, A., ... Waltimo, T. (2013). Sicca symptoms and their impact on quality of life among very long-term survivors after hematopoietic SCT. *Bone Marrow Transplantation, 48*, 988–993. https://doi.org/10.1038/bmt.2012.260

del Campo, L., León, N.G., Palacios, D.C., Lagana, C., & Tagarro, D. (2014). Abdominal complications following hematopoietic stem cell transplantation. *RadioGraphics, 34*, 396–412. https://doi.org/10.1148/rg.342135046

Deng, C., Deng, B., Jia, L., & Tan, H. (2017). Efficacy of long-acting release octreotide for preventing chemotherapy-induced diarrhoea: Protocol for a systematic review. *BMJ Open, 7*, e014916. https://doi.org/10.1136/bmjopen-2016-014916

de Paula Eduardo, F., Bezinelli, L.M., da Graça Lopes, R.M., Nascimento Sobrinho, J.J., Hamerschlak, N., & Correa, L. (2015). Efficacy of cryotherapy associated with laser therapy for decreasing severity of melphalan-induced oral mucositis during hematological stem-cell transplantation: A prospective clinical study. *Hematological Oncology, 33*, 152–158. https://doi.org/10.1002/hon.2133

Dest, V.M. (2018). Radiation therapy: Toxicities and management. In C.H. Yarbro, D. Wujcik, & B.H. Gobel (Eds.), *Cancer nursing: Principles and practice* (8th ed., pp. 333–374). Burlington, MA: Jones & Bartlett Learning.

Eilers, J.G., Asakura, Y., Blecher, C.S., Burgoon, D., Chiffelle, R., Ciccolini, K., … Valinski, S. (2019, November 26). Symptom interventions: Mucositis. Retrieved from https://www.ons.org/pep/mucositis

Elad, S., Raber-Durlacher, J.E., Brennan, M.T., Saunders, D.P., Mank, A.P., Zadik, Y., … Jensen, S.B. (2015). Basic oral care for hematology–oncology patients and hematopoietic stem cell transplantation recipients: A position paper from the joint task force of the Multinational Association of Supportive Care in Cancer/International Society of Oral Oncology (MASCC/ISOO) and the European Society for Blood and Marrow Transplantation (EBMT). *Supportive Care in Cancer, 23*, 223–236. https://doi.org/10.1007/s00520-014-2378-x

Ferreira, B., da Motta Silveira, F.M., & de Orange, F. (2016). Low-level laser therapy prevents severe oral mucositis in patients submitted to hematopoietic stem cell transplantation: A randomized clinical trial. *Supportive Care in Cancer, 24*, 1035–1042. https://doi.org/10.1007/s00520-015-2881-8

Giralt, S.A., Mangan, K.F., Maziarz, R.T., Bubalo, J.S., Beveridge, R., Hurd, D.D., … Schuster, M.W. (2011). Three palonosetron regimens to prevent CINV in myeloma patients receiving multiple-day high-dose melphalan and hematopoietic stem cell transplantation. *Annals of Oncology, 22*, 939–946. https://doi.org/10.1093/annonc/mdq457

Glare, P., Miller, J., Nikolova, T., & Tickoo, R. (2011). Treating nausea and vomiting in palliative care: A review. *Clinical Interventions in Aging, 6*, 243–259. https://doi.org/10.2147/cia.s13109

Green, S., & Weiss, G.R. (1992). Southwest Oncology Group standard response criteria, endpoint definitions and toxicity criteria. *Investigational New Drugs, 10*, 239–259.

Hamdeh, S., Abdelrahman, A.A.M., Elsallabi, O., Pathak, R., Giri, S., Mosalpuria, K., & Bhatt, V.R. (2016). Clinical approach to diarrheal disorders in allogeneic hematopoietic stem cell transplant recipients. *World Journal of Hematology, 5*, 23–30. https://doi.org/10.5315/wjh.v5.i1.23

Hesketh, P., Kris, M., Grunberg, S., Beck, T., Hainsworth, J., Harker, G., … Lindley, C.M. (1997). Proposal for classifying the acute emetogenicity of cancer chemotherapy. *Journal of Clinical Oncology, 15*, 103–109. https://doi.org/10.1200/jco.1997.15.1.103

Kamen, C., Tejani, M.A., Chandwani, K., Janelsins, M., Peoples, A.R., Roscoe, J.A., & Morrow, G.R. (2014). Anticipatory nausea and vomiting due to chemotherapy. *European Journal of Pharmacology, 722*, 172–179. https://doi.org/10.1016/j.ejphar.2013.09.071

Lalla, R.V., Bowen, J., Barasch, A., Elting, L., Epstein, J., Keefe, D.M., … Mucositis Guidelines Leadership Group of the Multinational Association of Supportive Care in Cancer and International Society of Oral Oncology. (2014). MASCC/ISOO clinical practice guidelines for the management of mucositis secondary to cancer therapy. *Cancer, 120*, 1453–1461. https://doi.org/10.1002/cncr.28592

Leffler, D.A., & Lamont, J.T. (2015). *Clostridium difficile* infection. *New England Journal of Medicine, 317*, 1539–1548. https://doi.org/10.1056/NEJMra1403772

Lemal, R., Cabrespine, A., Pereira, B., Combal, C., Ravinet, A., Hermet, E., … Bouteloup, C. (2015). Could enteral nutrition improve the outcome of patients with haematological malignancies undergoing allogeneic haematopoietic stem cell transplantation? A study protocol for a randomized controlled trial (the NEPHA study). *Trials, 16*, 136. https://doi.org/10.1186/s13063-015-0663-8

Lin, R., & Liu, Q. (2013). Diagnosis and treatment of viral diseases in recipients of allogeneic hematopoietic stem cell transplantation. *Journal of Hematology and Oncology, 6*, 94. https://doi.org/10.1186/1756-8722-6-94

Lorentino, F., Labopin, M., Fleischhauer, K., Ciceri, F., Mueller, C.R., Ruggeri, A., … Mohty, M. (2017). The impact of HLA matching on outcomes of unmanipulated haploidentical HSCT is modulated by GVHD prophylaxis. *Blood Advances, 1*, 669–680. https://doi.org/10.1182/bloodadvances.2017006429

Malard, F., & Mohty, M. (2014). New insight for the diagnosis of gastrointestinal acute graft-versus-host disease. *Mediators of Inflammation, 2014*, 701013. https://doi.org/10.1155/2014/701013

Mayo Clinic. (2018, November). Diarrhea: Cancer-related causes and how to cope. Retrieved from https://www.mayoclinic.org/diseases-conditions/cancer/in-depth/diarrhea/art-20044799

McQuade, R.M., Stojanovska, V., Abalo, R., Bornstein, J.C., & Nurgali, K. (2016). Chemotherapy-induced constipation and diarrhea: Pathophysiology, current and emerging treatments. *Frontiers in Pharmacology, 7*, 414. https://doi.org/10.3389/fphar.2016.00414

Migliorati, C., Hewson, I., Lalla, R.V., Antunes, H.S., Estilo, C.L., Hodgson, B., … Elad, S. (2013). Systematic review of laser and other light therapy for the management of oral mucositis in cancer patients. *Supportive Care in Cancer, 21*, 333–341. https://doi.org/10.1007/s00520-012-1605-6

Molassiotis, A., Aapro, M., Dicato, M., Gascon, P., Novoa, S.A., Isambert, N., … Roila, F. (2014). Evaluation of risk factors predicting chemotherapy-related nausea and vomiting: Results from a European prospective observational study. *Journal of Pain and Symptom Management, 47*, 839–848.e4. https://doi.org/10.1016/j.jpainsymman.2013.06.012

Mozaffari, H.R., Payandeh, M., Ramezani, M., Sadeghi, M., Mahmoudi-ahmadabadi, M., & Sharifi, R. (2017). Efficacy of palifermin on oral mucositis and acute GVHD after hematopoietic stem cell transplantation (HSCT) in hematology malignancy patients: A meta-analysis of trials. *Contemporary Oncology, 21*, 299–305. https://doi.org/10.5114/wo.2017.72400

Musso, M., Scalone, R., Crescimanno, A., Bonanno, V., Polizzi, V., Porretto, F., … Perrone, T. (2010). Palonosetron and dexamethasone for prevention of nausea and vomiting in patients receiving high-dose chemotherapy with auto-SCT. *Bone Marrow Transplantation, 45*, 123–127. https://doi.org/10.1038/bmt.2009.114

National Cancer Institute. (2018). *Nausea and vomiting related to cancer treatment (PDQ®)* [Patient version]. Retrieved from https://www.cancer.gov/about-cancer/treatment/side-effects/nausea/nausea-pdq

National Cancer Institute Cancer Therapy Evaluation Program. (2017). *Common terminology criteria for adverse events* [v.5.0]. Retrieved from https://ctep.cancer.gov/protocolDevelopment/electronic_applications/docs/CTCAE_v5_Quick_Reference_8.5x11.pdf

National Comprehensive Cancer Network. (2019). *NCCN Clinical Practice Guidelines in Oncology (NCCN Guidelines®): Antiemesis* [v.1.2019]. Retrieved from https://www.nccn.org/professionals/physician_gls/pdf/antiemesis.pdf

Navari, R.M. (2013). Management of chemotherapy-induced nausea and vomiting: Focus on newer agents and new uses for older agents. *Drugs, 73*, 249–262. https://doi.org/10.1007/s40265-013-0019-1

Navari, R.M., Qin, R., Ruddy, K.J., Liu, H., Powell, S.F., Bajaj, M., … Loprinzi, C.L. (2016). Olanzapine for the prevention of chemotherapy-induced nausea and vomiting. *New England Journal of Medicine, 375*, 134–142. https://doi.org/10.1056/nejmoa1515725

Nerone, T.A., Carlstrom, K.D., Weber, C., & Majhail, N.S. (2017). Olanzapine for the prevention of chemotherapy-induced nausea and vomiting in autologous hematopoietic cell transplant [Abstract No. 127]. *Biology of Blood and Marrow Transplantation, 23*, S165. https://doi.org/10.1016/j.bbmt.2016.12.148

Pappas, P.G., Kauffman, C.A., Andes, D.R., Clancy, C.J., Marr, K.A., Ostrosky-Zeichner, L., … Sobel, J.D. (2016). Clinical practice guideline for the management of candidiasis: 2016 update by the Infectious Diseases Society of America. *Clinical Infectious Diseases, 62*, e1–e50. https://doi.org/10.1093/cid/civ933

Peric, Z., Botti, S., Stringer, J., Krawczyk, J., van der Werf, S., van Biezen, A., … Basak, G.W. (2018). Variability of nutritional practices in peritransplant period after allogeneic hematopoietic stem cell transplantation: A survey by the Complications and Quality of Life Working Party of the EBMT. *Bone Marrow Transplantation, 53*, 1030–1037. https://doi.org/10.1038/s41409-018-0137-1

Peterson, D.E., Öhrn, K., Bowen, J., Fliedner, M., Lees, J., Loprinzi, C., … Lalla, R.V. (2013). Systematic review of oral cryotherapy for management of oral mucositis caused by cancer therapy. *Supportive Care in Cancer, 21,* 327–332. https://doi.org/10.1007/s00520-012-1562-0

Pielichowski, W., Barzal, J., Gawronski, K., Mlot, B., Oborska, S., Wasko-Grabowska, P., & Rzepecki, P. (2011). A triple-drug combination to prevent nausea and vomiting following BEAM chemotherapy before autologous hematopoietic stem cell transplantation. *Transplantation Proceedings, 43,* 3107–3110. https://doi.org/10.1016/j.transproceed.2011.08.010

Polage, C.R., Solnick, J.V., & Cohen, S.H. (2012). Nosocomial diarrhea: Evaluation and treatment of causes other than *Clostridium difficile. Clinical Infectious Diseases, 55,* 982–989. https://doi.org/10.1093/cid/cis551

Rapoport, B.L. (2017). Delayed chemotherapy-induced nausea and vomiting: Pathogenesis, incidence, and current management. *Frontiers in Pharmacology, 8,* 19. https://doi.org/10.3389/fphar.2017.00019

Rodrigues, F.G., Dasilva, G., & Wexner, S.D. (2017). Neutropenic enterocolitis. *World Journal of Gastroenterology, 23,* 42–47. https://doi.org/10.3748/wjg.v23.i1.42

Roila, F., Molassiotis, A., Herrstedt, J., Aapro, M., Gralla, R.J., Bruera, E., ... van der Wetering, M. (2016). 2016 MASCC and ESMO guideline update for the prevention of chemotherapy- and radiotherapy-induced nausea and vomiting and of nausea and vomiting in advanced cancer patients. *Annals of Oncology, 27*(Suppl. 5), v119–v133. https://doi.org/10.1093/annonc/mdw270

Schiller, L.R., Pardi, D.S., Spiller, R., Semrad, C.E., Surawicz, C.M., Giannella, R.A., ... Sellin, J.H. (2013). Gastro 2013 APDW/WCOG Shanghia Working Party report: Chronic diarrhea: Definition, classification, diagnosis. *Journal of Gastroenterology and Hepatology, 29,* 6–25. https://doi.org/10.1111/jgh.12392

Schmidt, V., Niederwieser, D., Schenk, T., Behre, G., Klink, A., Pfrepper, C., ... Sayer, H.G. (2018). Efficacy and safety of keratinocyte growth factor (palifermin) for prevention of oral mucositis in TBI-based allogeneic hematopoietic stem cell transplantation. *Bone Marrow Transplantation, 53,* 1188–1192. https://doi.org/10.1038/s41409-018-0135-3

Schmitt, T., Goldschmidt, H., Neben, K., Freiberger, A., Hüsing, J., Gronkowski, M., ... Egerer, G. (2014). Aprepitant, granisetron, and dexamethasone for prevention of chemotherapy-induced nausea and vomiting after high-dose melphalan in autologous transplantation for multiple myeloma: Results of a randomized, placebo-controlled phase III trial. *Journal of Clinical Oncology, 32,* 3413–3420. https://doi.org/10.1200/jco.2013.55.0095

Solmaz, S., Korur, A., Gereklioğlu, Ç., Asma, S., Büyükkurt, N., Kasar, M., ... Ozdoğu, H. (2016). Anorectal complications during neutropenic period in patients with hematologic diseases. *Mediterranean Journal of Hematology and Infectious Diseases, 8,* e2016019. https://doi.org/10.4084/mjhid.2016.019

Sonis, S.T. (2004). The pathobiology of mucositis. *Nature Reviews Cancer, 4,* 277–284. https://doi.org/10.1038/nrc1318

Stein, A., Voigt, W., & Jordan, K. (2010). Chemotherapy-induced diarrhea: Pathophysiology, frequency and guideline-based management. *Therapeutic Advances in Medical Oncology, 2,* 51–63. https://doi.org/10.1177/1758834009355164

Stiff, P.J., Fox-Geiman, M.P., Kiley, K., Rychlik, K., Parthasarathy, M., Fletcher-Gonzalez, D., ... Rodriguez, G.T.E. (2013). Prevention of nausea and vomiting associated with stem cell transplant: Results of a prospective, randomized trial of aprepitant used with highly emetogenic preparative regimens. *Biology of Blood and Marrow Transplantation, 19,* 49–55.e1. https://doi.org/10.1016/j.bbmt.2012.07.019

Sung, L., Robinson, P., Treister, N., Baggott, T., Gibson, P., Tissing, W., ... Dupuis, L.L. (2017). Guideline for the prevention of oral and oropharyngeal mucositis in children receiving treatment for cancer or undergoing haematopoietic stem cell transplantation. *BMJ Supportive and Palliative Care, 7,* 7–16. https://doi.org/10.1136/bmjspcare-2014-000804

Taur, Y., Jenq, R.R., Perales, M.-A., Littmann, E.R., Morjaria, S., Ling, L., ... Pamer, E.G. (2014). The effects of intestinal tract bacterial diversity on mortality following allogeneic hematopoietic stem cell transplantation. *Blood, 124,* 1174–1182. https://doi.org/10.1182/blood-2014-02-554725

Tendas, A., Sollazzo, F., Bruno, A., Cupelli, L., Niscola, P., Pignatelli, A.C., ... Arcese, W. (2012). Obstacles to managing chemotherapy-induced nausea and vomiting in high-dose chemotherapy with stem cell transplant. *Supportive Care in Cancer, 20,* 891–892. https://doi.org/10.1007/s00520-012-1411-1

Tomblyn, M., Chiller, T., Einsele, H., Gress, R., Sepkowitz, K., Storek, J., ... Boeckh, M.A. (2009). Guidelines for preventing infectious complications among hematopoietic cell transplantation recipients: A global perspective. *Biology of Blood and Marrow Transplantation, 15,* 1143–1238. https://doi.org/10.1016/j.bbmt.2009.06.019

Trifilio, S., Welles, C., Seeger, K., Mehta, S., Fishman, M., McGowan, K., ... Mehta, J. (2017). Olanzapine reduces chemotherapy-induced nausea and vomiting compared with aprepitant in myeloma patients receiving high-dose melphalan before stem cell transplantation: A retrospective study. *Clinical Lymphoma, Myeloma and Leukemia, 17,* 584–589. https://doi.org/10.1016/j.clml.2017.06.012

Tuncer, H.H., Rana, N., Milani, C., Darko, A., & Al-Homsi, S.A. (2012). Gastrointestinal and hepatic complications of hematopoietic stem cell transplantation. *World Journal of Gastroenterology, 18,* 1851–1860. https://doi.org/10.3748/wjg.v18.i16.1851

Ullmann, A.J., Schmidt-Hieber, M., Bertz, H., Heinz, W.J., Kiehl, M., Krüger, W., ... Maschmeyer, G. (2016). Infectious diseases in allogeneic haematopoietic stem cell transplantation: Prevention and prophylaxis strategy guidelines 2016. *Annals of Hematology, 95,* 1435–1455. https://doi.org/10.1007/s00277-016-2711-1

U.S. Department of Agriculture, & U.S. Food and Drug Administration. (2011, September). *Food safety for people with cancer: A need-to-know guide for those who have been diagnosed with cancer.* Retrieved from https://www.fda.gov/media/83710/download

Vagliano, L., Feraut, C., Gobetto, G., Trunfio, A., Errico, A., Campani, V., ... Dimonte, V. (2011). Incidence and severity of oral mucositis in patients undergoing haematopoietic SCT—Results of a multicentre study. *Bone Marrow Transplantation, 46,* 727–732. https://doi.org/10.1038/bmt.2010.184

Vanhoecke, B., De Ryck, T., Stringer, A., Van de Wiele, T., & Keefe, D. (2015). Microbiota and their role in the pathogenesis of oral mucositis. *Oral Diseases, 21,* 17–30. https://doi.org/10.1111/odi.12224

van Oort, S., Kramer, E., de Groot, J.-W., & Visser, O. (2018). Taste alterations and cancer treatment. *Current Opinion in Supportive and Palliative Care, 12,* 162–167. https://doi.org/10.1097/SPC.0000000000000346

Van Sebille, Z.A., Stansborough, R., Wardill, H.R., Bateman, E., Gibson, R.J., Keefe, D.M. (2015). Management of mucositis during chemotherapy: From pathophysiology to pragmatic therapeutics. *Current Oncology Reports, 17,* 50. https://doi.org/10.1007/s11912-015-0474-9

Wędrychowicz, A., Spodaryk, M., Krasowska-Kwiecień, A., & Goździk, J. (2010). Total parenteral nutrition in children and adolescents treated with high-dose chemotherapy followed by autologous haematopoietic transplants. *British Journal of Nutrition, 103,* 899–906. https://doi.org/10.1017/s000711450999242x

Wingard, J.R., Hsu, J., & Hiemenz, J.W. (2011). Hematopoietic stem cell transplantation: An overview of infection risks and epidemiology. *Infectious Disease Clinics of North America, 25,* 101–116. https://doi.org/10.1016/j.hoc.2010.11.008

Wood, J.M., Chapman, K., & Eilers, J.G. (2011). Tools for assessing nausea, vomiting, and retching: A literature review. *Cancer Nursing, 34,* E14–E24. https://doi.org/10.1097/ncc.0b013e3181e2cd79

World Health Organization. (2017, May 2). Diarrhoeal disease. Retrieved from https://www.who.int/news-room/fact-sheets/detail/diarrhoeal-disease

CHAPTER 10

Hepatorenal and Bladder Complications

Seth Eisenberg, RN, ADN, OCN®, BMTCN®

Introduction

Patients undergoing hematopoietic stem cell transplantation (HSCT) are susceptible to hepatic, renal, and bladder problems. These potentially fatal complications can be related to the preparative regimen, infection, and medications used throughout the transplantation process. Nurses caring for HSCT recipients must have a good understanding of the etiology, appropriate treatment strategies, and specific nursing interventions for these complications.

Hepatic Sinusoidal Obstruction Syndrome

High-dose myeloablative chemoradiation can cause a potentially fatal liver condition known as *hepatic sinusoidal obstruction syndrome* (HSOS), also referred to in the literature as *veno-occlusive disease* or VOD. HSOS can range from mild to severe and can progress to multisystem organ failure. Patients with severe HSOS require almost twice the length of hospitalization, at nearly three times the overall cost (Cao et al., 2017). Nurses play a pivotal role in the management of this toxicity (Botti et al., 2016; Murray, Agreiter, Orlando, & Hutt, 2018). Before discussing HSOS, a brief review of hepatic anatomy and physiology is warranted.

The liver is a highly vascular polyfunctional organ responsible for filtering toxins and removing senescent red blood cells (Barrett, 2014). Distinct areas of the liver known as *portal triads* are divided into smaller functional units referred to as *acini*. Within the acini are narrow sinusoids lined by highly fragile fenestrated endothelial cells (see Figure 10-1). Directly beneath the endothelium is the *space of Disse*, which separates the sinusoid from the hepatocytes. In the absence of pathology, blood flows through the sinusoids to the terminal hepatic venule and finally to the hepatic vein where it reenters venous circulation. The fragility of sinusoidal endothelial cells is due, in part, to the absence of a basement membrane, which is found on other endothelial cells throughout the body (Barrett, 2014). In addition to removing toxins, the liver is solely responsible for producing albumin and clotting proteins and also stores vitamins A, D, E, and K (Barrett, 2014). Therefore, it is not surprising that significant insults to the liver result in disruptions to homeostasis and potential multisystem organ failure.

Pathophysiology

The first cases of HSOS, or VOD, were identified in 1957 as a rare condition resulting from *Senecio* tea poisoning (Bras, Berry, György, & Smith, 1957). Transplant-related VOD was initially reported in 1980 and was thought to be caused by the myeloablative conditioning regimen (Shulman et al., 1980). Autopsies of patients who died of the disease revealed fibrin deposition in the terminal hepatic venules due to hypercoagulation (McDonald, Sharma, Matthews, Shulman, & Thomas, 1984; Shulman et al., 1980). Subsequent studies have shown that damage initially occurs in the sinusoids and that the hypercoagulable state in the venules is coincident rather than causative (DeLeve, Shulman, & McDonald, 2002). For this reason, many authors now commonly use the term *HSOS*.

Drugs metabolized by the cytochrome P450 pathway in the liver rely on glutathione to convert toxic metabolites to nontoxic compounds (Vion, Rautou, Durand, Boulanger, & Valla, 2015). Radiation and drugs such as cyclophosphamide and busulfan are known to deplete glutathione stores, rendering the sinusoids susceptible to damage. Cyclophosphamide in particular is metabolized to acrolein, which is extremely urotoxic (refer to Hemorrhagic Cystitis section) and has a detrimental effect on sinusoidal endothelial cells. Another cyclophosphamide metabolite, phosphoramide mustard, is directly toxic to hepatocytes (Vion et al., 2015). One major challenge in using cyclophosphamide is interpatient variability; patients with the same weight or body surface area can achieve markedly different pharmacokinetic profiles. Unfortunately, dosing based on individual pharmacokinetic data is not commonly used because of practical challenges associated with testing (Hockenberry, Strasser, & McDonald, 2016).

Busulfan has a relatively narrow therapeutic range, and plasma concentration levels greater than 900 ng/ml are associated with hepatotoxicity when used concomitantly with cyclophosphamide (Weil et al., 2017). Total body irradiation greater than 12 Gy, as well as lower doses used in conjunction with cyclophosphamide, can cause HSOS (Hockenberry et al., 2016). Toxic insult from transplant conditioning sets off a chain of physiologic events within the hepatic sinusoids.

It is theorized that injury begins with rounding of the sinusoidal endothelial cells with loss of fenestration

Figure 10-1. Normal Hepatic Sinusoid

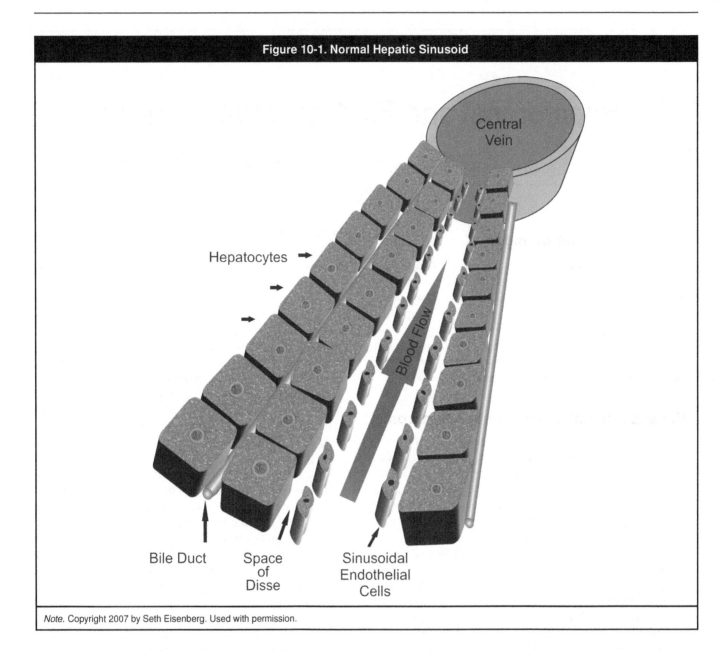

Note. Copyright 2007 by Seth Eisenberg. Used with permission.

(DeLeve et al., 2002). This allows erythrocytes to embolize into the space of Disse, causing subsequent hepatocyte damage (Blix & Husebekk, 2016). The injury results in initial sinusoidal dilation and hemorrhage within the hepatic acinus (Hockenberry et al., 2016). Injured and dead hepatic cells activate the sinusoidal endothelial cells and trigger an immune response, which is further amplified by tumor necrosis factor-alpha (TNF-α), intercellular adhesion molecule-1, vascular adhesion molecule-1, E-selectin, and interleukins IL-1β, IL-6, and IL-8 (Blix & Husebekk, 2016). In addition, stimulation of the sinusoidal endothelial cells produces von Willebrand factor and plasminogen activator inhibitor-1 molecules, which results in platelet activation and initiation of the clotting cascade (Coppell, Brown, & Perry, 2003; Kumar, DeLeve, Kamath, & Tefferi, 2003; Vion et al., 2015; Wadleigh, Ho, Momtaz, & Richardson, 2003).

Matrix metalloproteinase is an enzyme responsible for breaking down cellular components. The generation of matrix metalloproteinase by sinusoidal endothelial cells and the depletion of nitric oxide also contribute to the development of HSOS (DeLeve, Wang, Kanel, et al., 2003; DeLeve, Wang, Tsai, et al., 2003). Lipopolysaccharides from bacteria can worsen sinusoidal endothelial cell damage, as can transplanted allogeneic cluster of differentiation (CD)-positive T cells (Blix & Husebekk, 2016). Bacterial flora is similarly released from the gastrointestinal tract as a result of structural impairment from declining hepatic function adding to a feedback loop (McDonald et al., 1993). The terminal hepatic venules eventually fill with collagen, effectively increasing hepatic pressure and causing hepatic congestion (Ma & Brunt, 2016; see Figure 10-2). Figures 10-3 through 10-5 are hepatic photomicrographs showing a normal hepatic vein, a progres-

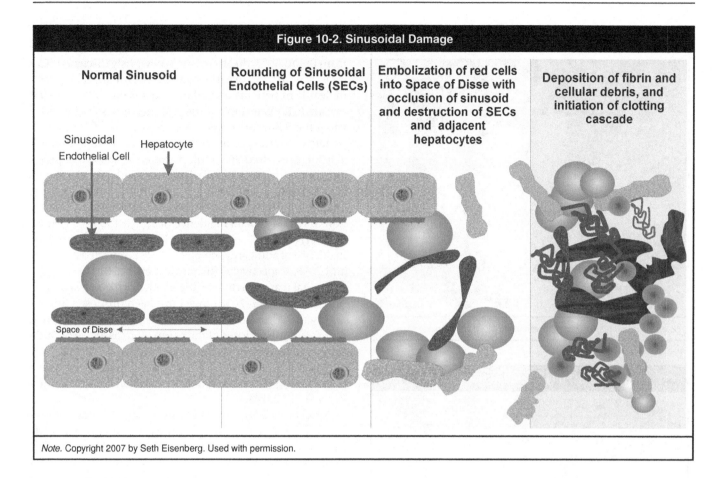

Figure 10-2. Sinusoidal Damage

Normal Sinusoid

Rounding of Sinusoidal Endothelial Cells (SECs)

Embolization of red cells into Space of Disse with occlusion of sinusoid and destruction of SECs and adjacent hepatocytes

Deposition of fibrin and cellular debris, and initiation of clotting cascade

Sinusoidal Endothelial Cell

Hepatocyte

Space of Disse

Note. Copyright 2007 by Seth Eisenberg. Used with permission.

sively narrowing vein, and finally a total occlusion in a patient with HSOS.

Diagnostic Criteria and Diagnosis

Several different criteria for diagnosing HSOS have emerged, beginning with the initial Seattle Criteria, the subsequent Modified Seattle Criteria, and the Baltimore Criteria (Coppell et al., 2010). Although they share general similarities, these differences have negatively affected clinical studies of HSOS: patients who would be diagnosed as having HSOS under one set of criteria would not be diagnosed under the other, significantly influencing reported incidence, effectiveness of interventions, and overall mortality (Coppell et al., 2010; Corbacioglu & Richardson, 2017; Mohty et al., 2016; Skeens et al., 2016). In addition, differences have been observed in the symptoms and clinical course of HSOS in adults as compared to children, a population not specifically described in either the Seattle or Baltimore criteria. The European Society for Blood and Marrow Transplantation (EBMT) has proposed new criteria for HSOS (Mohty et al., 2016). Encompassing much of the Seattle and Baltimore criteria, the EBMT proposal is considerably more detailed and is divided into early and late chronology. Owing to marked differences in pediatric HSOS, new pediatric-specific criteria also have been proposed (Richardson et al., 2018). A comparison of these criteria is represented in Figure 10-6.

A specific laboratory test for the detection of HSOS has not been identified. Elevated liver function tests, although often present, can occur due to a number of other hepatic insults and are therefore nondiagnostic by themselves. Plasminogen activator inhibitor-1 has been identified as a potential marker for HSOS (J.-H. Lee et al., 2002; Pihusch et al.,

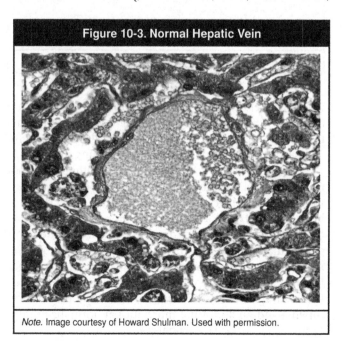

Figure 10-3. Normal Hepatic Vein

Note. Image courtesy of Howard Shulman. Used with permission.

Figure 10-4. Partially Occluded Hepatic Vein

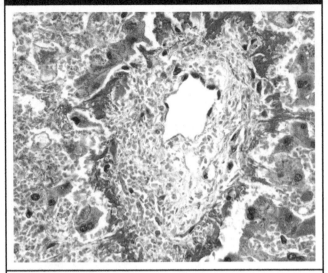

Note. Image courtesy of Dave Myerson. Used with permission.

Figure 10-5. Fully Occluded Hepatic Vein

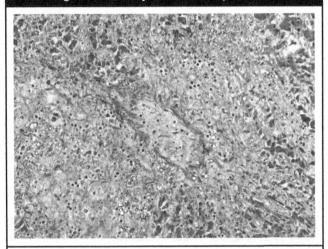

Note. Image courtesy of Dave Myerson. Used with permission.

2005; Salat et al., 1997, 1999), but not all institutions are able to perform the test nor is there agreement on the exact threshold for developing HSOS. Serial levels may be useful in assessing disease progression or confirming diagnosis.

Liver ultrasound may be of some benefit, although it is not useful in early HSOS, and a normal result does not necessarily rule out a positive diagnosis (Bajwa et al., 2017; Hockenberry et al., 2016). Transjugular liver biopsy may be of some benefit, and hepatic venous pressure gradient measurements greater than 10 mm Hg are indicative of HSOS but require platelet counts of at least 50,000/mm³ and normal coagulation studies—limiting their use for patients with marked hepatic impairment who tend to have severe thrombocytopenia and an abnormal international normalized ratio (Bajwa et al., 2017; Hockenberry et al., 2016).

Incidence and Risk Factors

Historical statistics vary widely on the frequency of HSOS, from 0% to 60%, due to reasons previously discussed (Carreras et al., 2011). An early study by McDonald et al. (1984) in Seattle of patients transplanted between 1978 and 1980 revealed HSOS in 21% of the patients. Jones et al. (1987), using the Baltimore criteria, reported a rate of 22% in 235 patients. A retrospective single-center study by Carreras et al. (2011) reviewed 763 adult patients over a 24-year period and found that 13.8% were diagnosed with HSOS using the Seattle Criteria and 8.8% using the Baltimore Criteria (± 1%). Similarly, a review of 135 studies between 1979 and 2010 revealed a mean incidence of 13.7% (95% CI [13.3%, 14.1%]) (Coppell et al., 2010). If EBMT criteria are used, the incidence of adult and pediatric HSOS is reported to be 10% and 20%, respectively (Richardson et al., 2018).

Several reasons as to why the incidence has seemed to stabilize in the 10%–20% range have been proposed, including increased use of reduced-intensity conditioning regimens with lower doses of radiation, increased use of fludarabine, fewer patients with active hepatitis C infections, and better awareness of hepatotoxic drugs in the transplant setting (Corbacioglu & Richardson, 2017; Hockenberry et al., 2016).

Risks factors are either patient specific (associated with the disease status or comorbidities) or transplant specific (attributed to the transplant type or conditioning regimen). In general, HSOS occurs less frequently in autologous transplants compared to allogeneic and is even less common in patients receiving reduced-intensity regimens (Dalle & Giralt, 2016). HSOS is relatively rare in patients receiving nonmyeloablative transplants because fludarabine, which is commonly used for these preparative regimens, is not normally associated with hepatotoxicity (Carreras et al., 2011). Patients with elevated liver function tests or those with GSTM1 null-genotype or heparanase polymorphisms are at an increased risk for developing HSOS (Dalle & Giralt, 2016; Seifert, Wittig, Arndt, & Gruhn, 2015). Pediatric patients transplanted for genetic disorders are at a higher risk than pediatric patients with malignant diseases. When compared with adult patients, in whom late HSOS is considered rare, approximately 20% of pediatric HSOS occurs after day 21 (Richardson et al., 2018). Outside of HSCT, the conjugated monoclonal antibody gemtuzumab ozogamicin (Mylotarg®) can cause HSOS and therefore is a major risk factor for patients proceeding to transplant. A complete list of risk factors is presented in Table 10-1. The Center for International Blood and Marrow Transplant Research has a web-based VOD risk calculator (www.cibmtr.org/ReferenceCenter/Statistical/Tools/Pages/VOD.aspx). Although this free tool is geared toward helping physicians choose the appropriate conditioning regimen based on risk factors, it also is useful for helping nurses gain a better understanding of the complex variables associated with the risk of developing HSOS.

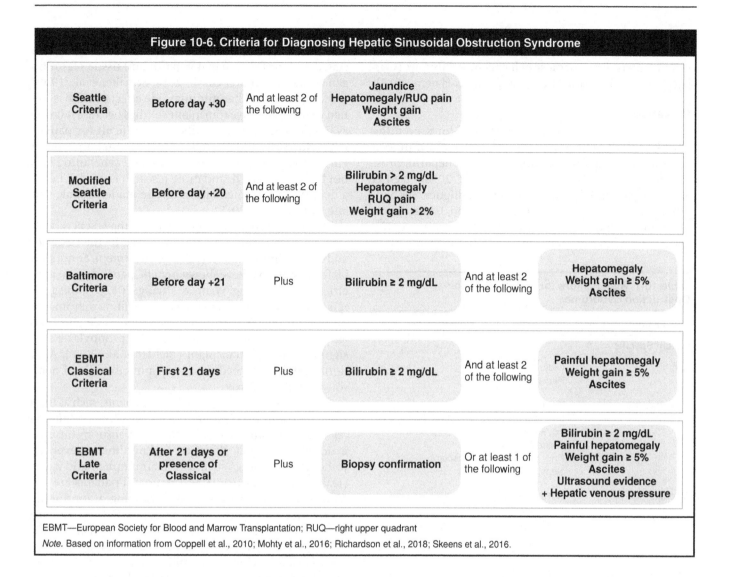

Figure 10-6. Criteria for Diagnosing Hepatic Sinusoidal Obstruction Syndrome

Seattle Criteria	Before day +30	And at least 2 of the following	Jaundice Hepatomegaly/RUQ pain Weight gain Ascites		
Modified Seattle Criteria	Before day +20	And at least 2 of the following	Bilirubin > 2 mg/dL Hepatomegaly RUQ pain Weight gain > 2%		
Baltimore Criteria	Before day +21	Plus	Bilirubin ≥ 2 mg/dL	And at least 2 of the following	Hepatomegaly Weight gain ≥ 5% Ascites
EBMT Classical Criteria	First 21 days	Plus	Bilirubin ≥ 2 mg/dL	And at least 2 of the following	Painful hepatomegaly Weight gain ≥ 5% Ascites
EBMT Late Criteria	After 21 days or presence of Classical	Plus	Biopsy confirmation	Or at least 1 of the following	Bilirubin ≥ 2 mg/dL Painful hepatomegaly Weight gain ≥ 5% Ascites Ultrasound evidence + Hepatic venous pressure

EBMT—European Society for Blood and Marrow Transplantation; RUQ—right upper quadrant

Note. Based on information from Coppell et al., 2010; Mohty et al., 2016; Richardson et al., 2018; Skeens et al., 2016.

Signs and Symptoms

Despite differences in clinical definitions as previously discussed, signs and symptoms of HSOS generally appear during the period immediately after conditioning and before day 30. Late HSOS occurs after day 21 and is included as a separate criterion in the EBMT definition (Corbacioglu & Richardson, 2017; Mohty et al., 2016). Patients typically present with weight gain related to fluid retention, abdominal distension from hepatomegaly or ascites, elevated bilirubin levels with accompanying jaundice, and right upper quadrant pain (Dalle & Giralt, 2016). Importantly, hyperbilirubinemia, historically one of the hallmarks of HSOS, may not be present, as the syndrome has been diagnosed in pediatric patients with normal bilirubin levels (Corbacioglu & Richardson, 2017; Dalle & Giralt, 2016; Myers, Dandoy, El-Bietar, Davies, & Jodele, 2015).

The constellation of signs, symptoms, and abnormal laboratory values attributed to HSOS also can be associated with a number of other conditions that may occur during the same post-transplant time period and must be ruled out before initiating therapy (Eisenberg, 2008). Differen-

tial diagnoses should also include other hepatic pathologies, such as chemical hepatitis from parenteral nutrition or medications, viral hepatitis, congestive heart failure, capillary leak syndrome, sepsis, and fungal liver infections (Dalle & Giralt, 2016; Murray et al., 2018). In particular, careful assessment is required to differentiate between hepatic graft-versus-host disease (GVHD) and late HSOS, both of which occur after engraftment and may have overlapping signs and symptoms (Hockenberry et al., 2016). (Refer to Chapter 7 for information on hepatic GVHD.) A list of differential diagnoses can be found in Table 10-2.

Attempts have been made to classify the severity of HSOS. Bearman first published a classification system using the terms *mild, moderate,* and *severe* based on signs and symptoms and extrapolated the probability of death associated with these categories (Bearman, 1995; Bearman, Anderson, et al., 1993). Recently, a more robust classification system has been proposed, which also takes into account the timeline in which symptoms develop (Mohty et al., 2016). The intent of classifying HSOS is to aid in determining the necessity of aggressive treatment. Mild HSOS in most patients resolves without specific intervention, whereas patients with rapidly developing HSOS require prompt intervention because of higher mortality rates (Corbacioglu & Richardson, 2017; Valla & Cazals-Hatem, 2016).

Prevention

A number of drugs have been studied for preventing HSOS, including antithrombin III, tissue plasminogen activator, fractionated and unfractionated heparin, prostaglandin E, and ursodiol (Dalle & Giralt, 2016; Essell et al., 1998; Imran, Tleyjeh, Zirakzadeh, Rodriguez, & Khan, 2006; Litzow et al., 2002; Song, Seo, Moon, Ghim, & Im, 2006; Tay, Tinmouth, Fergusson, Huebsch, & Allan, 2007). Data have been equivocal for all of these agents, with

severe toxicities associated with prostaglandin E (Bearman, Shen, Hinds, Hill, & McDonald, 1993), and bleeding associated with unfractionated heparin and tissue plasminogen activator (Dalle & Giralt, 2016; Schriber et al., 1999). Although ursodiol has minimal side effects, its use is limited in myeloablative transplant settings because it is only available orally, making adherence difficult for patients with mucositis and altered gastrointestinal absorption. Furthermore, the optimum dosing and scheduling have not been established, and more research is needed before a definitive recommendation can be made (Cheuk, Chiang, Ha, & Chan, 2015).

The most promising drug for preventing HSOS is defibrotide, which is currently only approved by the U.S. Food and Drug Administration (FDA) for treatment. Some studies for prophylaxis have shown benefit, particularly in pediatric patients (Zhang, Wang, & Huang, 2012). At this time, it is unclear which patients would benefit most from defibrotide prophylaxis. Moreover, moderate side effects are associated with the drug, and routine prophylaxis adds significant cost to transplant (Pichler et al., 2017). Additional studies are needed to determine the role of defibrotide for prophylaxis.

Prevention strategies for high-risk patients, such as those with preexisting liver disease, include avoiding conditioning regimens containing cyclophosphamide, ensuring busulfan is dosed by pharmacokinetics, and minimizing exposure to hepatotoxic drugs such as acetaminophen and azoles (Dalle & Giralt, 2016). However, not all patients are candidates for reduced-intensity conditioning or for nonmyeloablative transplants using fludarabine (Hockenberry et al., 2016). When cyclophosphamide is used along with busulfan in patients at higher risk for HSOS, administering busulfan after cyclophosphamide or adding a delay of one to two days after busulfan can potentially help to decrease HSOS. This same reversal strategy can be used for patients receiving busulfan and melphalan by administering melphalan first (Hockenberry et al., 2016).

Treatment

Once HSOS has been presumed or diagnosed, treatment strategies will depend on the severity of the disease and preexisting patient risk factors. The majority of patients (estimated at 70%) will recover with minimal supportive care (Hockenberry et al., 2016). However, it often is difficult to determine which patients will progress versus those in whom the disease will resolve on its own. Despite the challenges in predicting HSOS progression, early treatment has been shown to be beneficial, particularly in the pediatric population (Aziz, Kakadiya, Kush, Weigel, & Lowe, 2018; Mohty et al., 2016; Richardson et al., 2017b).

Defibrotide is the only approved medical treatment for HSOS. Defibrotide was granted FDA approval in 2016 and is administered over two hours at a dosage of 6.25 mg/kg every six hours for at least three weeks. A tremendous amount of information on defibrotide has been amassed

Table 10-1. Risk Factors for Hepatic Sinusoidal Obstruction Syndrome

Risk Factor Category	Risk Factors
Patient Specific	
Age	Older adult Pediatric (< 2 years)
Comorbidities	Karnofsky score < 90 Liver disease (e.g., viral hepatitis, cirrhosis, fibrosis) Osteopetrosis Prior myeloablative transplant Sepsis
Disease	Advanced malignancy Immunodeficiency Leukemia Neuroblastoma Thalassemia
Genetics	C282Y allele GSTM1-null genotype GSMTT1 MTHFR 677CC/1298CC haplotype
Prior medications	Abdominal radiation Acyclovir Gemtuzumab ozogamicin
Transplant Specific	
Conditioning regimen	Busulfan (oral or high dose) Cyclophosphamide Total body irradiation
Donor	Human leukocyte antigen mismatched Unrelated
Drugs used during conditioning	Itraconazole Norethisterone Sirolimus
Transplant type	Allogeneic Autologous Myeloablative

Note. Based on information from Corbacioglu & Richardson, 2017; Dalle & Giralt, 2016; Hockenberry et al., 2016; Mohty et al., 2016; Wallhult & Quinn, 2018.

Table 10-2. Differential Diagnosis for Hepatic Sinusoidal Obstruction Syndrome

Symptom	Also Seen With
Hepatomegaly	Congestive heart failure
	Epstein-Barr virus lymphoproliferative disease
	Fungal infection
	Tumor involvement
Jaundice	Acute graft-versus-host disease
	Biliary infection
	Cholestasis
	Cyclosporine or other drug toxicity
	Hemolysis
	Total parenteral nutrition injury
Rapid weight gain	Acute kidney injury
	Capillary leak syndrome
	Congestive heart failure
	Sepsis syndrome

Note. Based on information from Carreras, 2000; McDonald et al., 1993.

From "Hepatic Sinusoidal Obstruction Syndrome in Patients Undergoing Hematopoietic Stem Cell Transplant," by S. Eisenberg, 2008, *Oncology Nursing Forum, 35*, p. 391. Copyright 2008 by Oncology Nursing Society. Adapted with permission.

over the past two decades. Derived from porcine mucosa, defibrotide has anti-inflammatory, antithrombotic, and anti-ischemic properties, while stimulating the production of endogenous tissue plasminogen activator (Aziz et al., 2018). It is not shown to cause thrombocytopenia or interfere with platelet function but does decrease heparinase activity. The half-life is 1–2 hours, and the area under the curve increases by 50%–60% in patients with renal insufficiency—an important consideration, as patients with HSOS often have concurrent renal compromise (Aziz et al., 2018). The use of a 0.2-micron filter is required for administration.

Although generally well tolerated, defibrotide is contraindicated in patients who are actively bleeding, as the incidence of pulmonary alveolar hemorrhage and epistaxis is increased with administration. Therefore, all medications that can affect coagulation, including heparin and nonsteroidal anti-inflammatory drugs, must be discontinued prior to initiating therapy. Other side effects include diarrhea, hypotension, nausea, and vomiting. Patient and family education for defibrotide should include monitoring for bruising and bleeding, including bloody stools or changes in mentation that could indicate intracerebral hemorrhage (Jazz Pharmaceuticals, 2016).

Gloude et al. (2018) studied the use of defibrotide plus high-dose methylprednisolone (500 mg/m^2 twice daily for three days tapered to 2 mg/kg/day for three days) in 15 pediatric patients. Overall survival was 73%, with a complete response rate of 58% in patients with multisystem organ failure. These results were superior to previously published results, which showed a 54% overall survival rate (Richardson et al., 2017a). Limitations of this study include a very small sample size and lack of randomization. Further stud-

ies will be needed to determine what role, if any, high-dose methylprednisolone has in increasing survival.

Physiologic Effects and Rationale for Nursing Interventions

Although controlled studies are lacking, a number of nursing interventions have been recommended in caring for patients with HSOS (Eisenberg, 2008; Murray et al., 2018; Sosa, 2012). These interventions are based on assessing and managing specific organ systems, which are interrelated; impairment of one system will often affect other systems. Therefore, many nursing interventions are interdependent. Specific nursing interventions can be found in Table 10-3.

Nurses should be able to identify patients who are at risk for developing HSOS prior to conditioning (Wallhult et al., 2017; see Table 10-1) and should understand clinical changes that may assist the transplant team in making a prompt diagnosis (Murray et al., 2018). It also is recommended that nurses accurately monitor and assess patients with early or mild HSOS to discern subtle changes or worsening fluid, respiratory, and mental status. Monitoring laboratory values is an integral part of oncology nursing but is critical in the HSCT setting, where subtle increases in renal or liver function may require immediate notification of the transplant team (Murray et al., 2018). Along with obtaining accurate daily weights with uniform criteria and method (e.g., with or without shoes), abdominal girth measurement is important in monitoring hepatomegaly and ascites (Sosa, 2012). Nursing units should develop a standard method for placement of the measuring tape to ensure accurate repeatability to prevent location-dependent errors (Murray et al., 2018). Another important nursing expectation is understanding the appropriate volume of IV medications, as fluid restrictions dictate minimal volumes whenever possible. Although this normally falls to the pharmacy department, the nurse administering the fluids must be the gatekeeper to ensure each bag of medication is mixed in the lowest volume allowable (Murray et al., 2018).

Changes to the integumentary system can be due to uremia or hyperbilirubinemia. Progressive renal failure leads to increased calcium levels, resulting in pruritis (Chikotas, Gunderman, & Oman, 2006). As circulating levels of bilirubin are unable to be conjugated in the liver and be excreted via normal pathways, bilirubin is instead excreted through other channels, including the eyes, resulting in icteric sclerae; the urine, producing unusually dark orange colored urine; and the skin, where bile acids cause irritation and subsequent itching (Bosonnet, 2003). No standard treatment exists for pruritis related to HSOS. Anecdotal clinical evidence suggests that neither diphenhydramine nor hydroxyzine is effective (Eisenberg, 2008). Newer-generation antihistamines such as cetirizine and loratadine have acceptable side effect profiles but have not been studied in this population. Similarly, drugs such as naltrexone and sertraline, which have been successfully used for treating cholestatic pruritis, and aprepitant, used

Table 10-3. Specific Nursing Interventions for Hepatic Sinusoidal Obstruction Syndrome

Body System	Intervention	Rationale
Renal	Document accurate intake and output.	Evaluate fluid volume status.
	Monitor blood urea nitrogen and creatinine, and report increased values.	Evaluate renal function.
	Administer diuretics as ordered.	Reduce fluid volume excess.
	Avoid concomitant infusion of nephrotoxic medications.	Renal function is preserved.
	Obtain weights twice daily.	Evaluate fluid volume status.
	Monitor cyclosporine A and tacrolimus levels.	Prevent acute kidney injury.
	Coordinate with pharmacy to ensure fluids are concentrated in minimum volumes.	Reduce fluid volume excess.
	Perform abdominal assessment.	Detect ascites.
Hematologic	Monitor platelet count, liver function tests, and coagulation panel.	Assess for risk of bleeding, thrombocytopenia, coagulopathies, and worsening hepatic function.
	Monitor for bleeding associated with defibrotide.	Bleeding is the most common side effect.
	Maintain skin integrity.	Prevent infection and bleeding.
Integumentary	Assess skin color and sclerae.	Assess for jaundice.
	Assess for edema.	Third spacing results in movement of fluid to extravascular compartment.
	Administer topical or oral antipruritic medications.	Decrease itching related to bilirubin or uremia.
	Maintain cool environment.	Decrease itching related to bilirubin or uremia.
	Instruct patients to gently rub skin instead of scratching.	Prevent skin damage.
	Ensure meticulous skin care with skin moisturizers.	Prevent skin damage associated with uremia and/or edema.
	Educate patients and family members to avoid using soap.	Prevent drying of skin.
	Measure abdominal girth daily.	Evaluate for worsening hepatomegaly or ascites.
Neurologic	Assess mental status.	Mental status can worsen due to uremia or hepatic encephalopathy.
	Administer ordered medication for encephalopathy.	Reduce ammonia levels due to accumulation of nitrogenous wastes.
	Maintain safe environment (e.g., use bedrails, assist in ambulation).	Prevent falls.
	Limit use of sedating medications.	Clearance of narcotics and benzodiazepines can be severely delayed, leading to mental status changes or bradypnea/apnea.
Cardiac	Perform postural (orthostatic) vital signs.	Evaluate fluid volume status.
	Elevate feet.	Prevent dependent edema and promote venous circulation.
	Auscultate heart sounds for friction rub or pericardial effusion.	Friction rub or pericardial effusion can occur with acute renal failure.
Respiratory	Assess respiratory rate.	Evaluate for tachypnea related to restricted diaphragm expansion.
	Measure oxygen saturation.	Detect hypoxia.
	Elevate head of bed.	Promote lung expansion.
	Administer oxygen as ordered.	Increase oxygenation.
	Auscultate breath sounds.	Detect fluid overload or other pulmonary insult.
	Assist with paracentesis.	Removal of ascitic fluid can promote diaphragm expansion.
Psychosocial	Allow patients and family time to adjust to changes in physical appearance (e.g., jaundice, edema).	Changes to appearance can be difficult for family members.
	Provide emotional support and facilitate open communication with family regarding rationale for increased assessments, physiologic changes, and need for increased assistance with self-care.	Decline in performance status may require more involvement from family members and/or a change from curative to supportive therapies. Physical changes in the patient's appearance can be difficult for family members.
	Provide support to family for end-of-life issues.	Severe hepatic sinusoidal obstruction syndrome can be fatal.
	Collaborate with interprofessional team.	Management of hepatic sinusoidal obstruction syndrome requires multiple specialties.

Note. Based on information from Eisenberg, 2008; Wallhult et al., 2017; Wallhult & Quinn, 2018.

for drug-induced pruritis, have not been studied in this setting (Pereira, Kremer, Mettang, & Ständer, 2016). General recommendations include using creams and emollients to prevent drying of the skin and avoiding soap, which can potentiate drying. Maintaining a cool environment along with wearing loose-fitting clothing may also help relieve symptoms (Bosonnet, 2003).

Severe HSOS can have a devastating psychosocial effect on patients and family members. Hyperbilirubinemia results in jaundice, producing an unnatural and unnerving change in skin color. Patients also can exhibit profound localized edema or anasarca along with ascites. Such changes in physical appearance can be extremely difficult for family members, and nurses must remain supportive by allowing family members to verbalize their feelings (Eisenberg, 2008; Sosa, 2012).

Damage to the liver can have a major effect on renal and pulmonary function. Albumin is markedly decreased in the presence of HSOS, and hypoalbuminemia results in third spacing due to reduced oncotic pressure, producing ascites and edema. Ascites can impair pulmonary function by impeding expansion of the diaphragm, resulting in hypoventilation and tachypnea, with subsequent carbon dioxide retention and acidosis. Frequent paracentesis may be required, and nurses should be familiar in assisting with the procedure. Oxygen saturation measurements, although useful in ruling out hypoxia, will not indicate carbon dioxide retention or acidosis. In the face of hypoalbuminemia, a prerenal condition results in increasing blood urea nitrogen and serum creatinine. Damaged sinusoidal endothelial cells also cause vasoconstriction within the kidneys, resulting in hypervolemia and eventually oliguria—both of which contribute to potential pulmonary failure (Soubani, 2006). One method of distinguishing prerenal condition from acute kidney injury (discussed later in this chapter) is examination of the blood urea nitrogen/serum creatinine ratio (Tasota & Tate, 2000). While a normal ratio is between 10:1 and 20:1 (e.g., blood urea nitrogen of 18 mg/dl and serum creatinine of 1.8 mg/dl), prerenal ratios are typically 30:1 or greater (Stark, 1994). Albumin should be replaced when serum levels fall below 3 g/dl (Mahadeo et al., 2017).

Decreased intravascular volume—despite an increase in body weight—can result in orthostatic hypotension. Pericardial effusions, friction rub, or tamponade also can occur and require astute nursing assessments (Eisenberg, 2008). Fluid overload has been identified as a risk factor in transplant mortality, irrespective of etiology (Rondón et al., 2017). The use of furosemide is generally avoided because of potential hypovolemia and worsening renal impairment. Spironolactone may be ordered, although adherence may be poor because of concomitant mucositis and nausea. Albumin replacement also may be ordered, although its use is somewhat controversial because without correcting the underlying problem of ascites, the concern exists that albumin leaking into the peritoneal space may, in turn,

result in more osmotic pull. Valid reasons for hydrating patients in the pre- and post-transplant period are based on the need to protect the kidneys from pharmacologic insult and, in the case of cyclophosphamide, to help prevent hemorrhagic cystitis. However, during this same time frame, subclinical changes to renal function along with capillary leak related to conditioning-induced cytokine release predispose patients to fluid overload even before the development of HSOS (Hingorani, 2017; Mahadeo et al., 2017). Therefore, astute attention must be paid to intake and output along with patient weight.

Mental status changes including delirium can be caused by impaired renal function resulting in uremic encephalopathy from hyperbilirubinemia (Chikotas et al., 2006; Saria & Gosselin-Acomb, 2007). Medications that are heavily processed via the liver, such as lorazepam and narcotics, can produce prolonged sedation or confusion in this setting and should be used judiciously (Ovchinsky et al., 2018). Hepatic encephalopathy resulting from ammonia generated by nitrogen by-product degradation can occur, although levels may not be reflective of clinical signs and symptoms (Han & Hyzy, 2006). Lactulose may be used to help lower ammonia levels (Han & Hyzy, 2006), despite lack of efficacy in the transplant setting. Rifaximin, an antibiotic approved for traveler's disease caused by noninvasive strains of *Escherichia coli*, also has been recommended and may have better efficacy than lactulose (Ovchinsky et al., 2018). Ultimately, reversal of neurologic changes associated with elevated ammonia levels requires at least partial resolution of HSOS. Because other concurrent problems, such as infection and intercranial hemorrhage, can produce neurologic changes (Saria & Gosselin-Acomb, 2007), a thorough neurologic assessment is required.

Hepatitis

Between 850,000 and 2.2 million people in the United States are living with the hepatitis B virus (HBV), and an estimated 3.5 million have the hepatitis C virus (HCV) (Centers for Disease Control and Prevention, 2018). HBV and HCV infections in either patients or donors present a challenge for the HSCT team and, in some cases, may require the expertise of a hepatologist.

Hepatitis B

HBV can be seen in the transplant setting in the following situations: occult infection, resolved infection, and chronic infection. Infection can occur in an HBV-naïve patient from a contaminated blood product, although this is extremely rare (Tomblyn et al., 2009).

Serology testing for HBV involves examining specific antigens and antibodies. DNA testing, which may be more precise, can also be performed (Anastasiou et al., 2017). Four serologic markers are commonly used in testing for HBV (Centers for Disease Control and Prevention, 2005):

- HBsAg (hepatitis B surface antigen) indicates the patient is infectious.
- anti-HBs (hepatitis B surface antibody) indicates a normal immune response to HBsAg and also occurs after immunization.
- anti-HBc (total hepatitis B core antibody) appears in acute or prior HBV infection.
- IgM anti-HBc (immunoglobulin M antibody to core antigen) indicates acute infection of six months or less.

Each of these markers has specific clinical implications, described in more detail in Table 10-4.

Patients with resolved infection will test positive for HBc (but will be negative for HBsAg or anti-HBs) and are at risk for reactivation of their disease. Based on HBV testing, patients can be divided into four broad categories influencing their risk for developing a new infection or reactivating the virus during transplant: not infected/susceptible, immune from vaccination, acute infection, and chronic infection (Centers for Disease Control and Prevention, 2005).

Some patients may go on to be inactive carriers, whereas others will have chronic infections (Gentile, Andreoni,

Antonelli, & Sarmati, 2017). Even with treatment, HBV is difficult to eradicate and can remain dormant for many years while patients are asymptomatic (Loomba & Liang, 2017). Because patients aged 30–49 years have the highest rate of HBV infection (Centers for Disease Control and Prevention, 2018), many transplant donors and recipients are potentially affected. Additional information on donor eligibility can be found in Chapters 2 and 5.

The emergence or increase of HBV DNA in patients with active or latent disease is known as *reactivation*, which can occur up to four years after transplant (Anastasiou et al., 2017). Patients with chronic hepatitis or occult infection are at risk for reactivation while undergoing transplant (Gentile et al., 2017; Seto, 2015), with potentially fatal outcomes (Seto et al., 2017). The overall incidence of reactivation in patients previously exposed to HBV varies depending on patient populations but has been reported to be as high as 78% in those who are HBsAg positive (Seto et al., 2017). For patients who are HBsAg negative and HBcAb positive, that number decreases to approximately 50% (Hwang & Lok, 2014). Both the American Society for Transplantation and Cellular Therapy guidelines and those issued by the Foundation for the Accreditation of Cellular Therapy and Joint Accreditation Committee–ISCT and EBMT (FACT-JACIE) recommend all potential HSCT recipients and donors be screened for active and chronic hepatitis during the pretransplant workup (FACT-JACIE, 2018; Tomblyn et al., 2009).

Both the underlying malignancy and medications used for cancer treatment can play a role in determining the level of risk for hepatitis reactivation. Patients with lymphoma and myeloma are considered high risk, although it may be difficult to separate the B-cell–depleting effects of medications used prior to transplant from the underlying diseases (Law et al., 2016). Patients with leukemia are at risk owing to lymphodepleting conditioning regimens and, in particular, prolonged immunosuppressive therapies used for preventing GVHD (Law et al., 2016). Allogeneic HSCT recipients are at risk because the new donor-derived immune system may not contain antibodies to HBV (Anastasiou et al., 2017).

Monoclonal antibodies targeting CD20 (e.g., obinutuzumab, rituximab) carry black box warnings regarding potential HBV reactivation (Genentech, 2017, 2019). In addition to affecting B cells, bortezomib can impair CD4+ T-cell function, an important consideration because cytotoxic T lymphocytes play a major role in viral suppression (Hwang & Lok, 2014; Law et al., 2016). Prednisone, which is often used for treatment of GVHD, is a risk factor when given at dosages greater than 20 mg/day or for longer than four weeks (Law et al., 2016; Perrillo, Gish, & Falck-Ytter, 2015). Both prednisone and cyclosporine A suppress T-cell function, which decreases the production of interleukins that mediate the innate antiviral immune response (Loomba & Liang, 2017). Transplant regimens containing combination fludarabine and rituximab, both

Table 10-4. Hepatitis B Serology

Antigens	Results	Implications
HBsAg anti-HBc anti-HBs	Negative Negative Negative	Patient is susceptible to HBV.
HBsAg anti-HBc anti-HBs	Negative Positive Positive	Patient is immune due to natural infection.
HBsAg anti-HBc anti-HBs	Negative Negative Positive	Patient is immune due to HBV vaccination.
HBsAg anti-HBc IgM anti-HBc anti-HBs	Positive Positive Positive Negative	Patient has acute HBV infection.
HBsAg anti-HBc IgM anti-HBc anti-HBs	Positive Positive Negative Negative	Patient has chronic HBV infection.
HBsAg anti-HBc anti-HBs	Negative Positive Negative	Four possible scenarios: • Patient with resolved HBV infection (most common) • False-positive anti-HBc results • Patient with low-level chronic HBV infection • Patient with resolving acute infection

anti-HBc—total hepatitis B core antibody; anti-HBs—hepatitis B surface antibody; HBsAG—hepatitis B surface antigen; HBV—hepatitis B virus; IgM anti-HBc—immunoglobulin M antibody to hepatitis B core antigen

Note. Adapted from *Interpretation of Hepatitis B Serologic Test Results*, by Centers for Disease Control and Prevention. Retrieved from https://www.cdc.gov/hepatitis/hbv/pdfs/serologicchartv8.pdf.

of which are highly lymphotoxic, have been implicated well (Tomblyn et al., 2009).

Hepatitis C

In contrast to HBV, relatively little has been published on HCV in the HSCT setting. Until recently, standard treatment for nontransplant patients with HCV consisted of a combination of ribavirin and interferon. Concerns regarding the effects of interferon on GVHD exacerbation and potential graft failure have limited its use (Kyvernitakis et al., 2016).

The emergence of newer direct-acting antivirals has provided alternatives to interferon and ribavirin. Although no large-scale studies have been published, one study of 54 HSCT recipients with chronic HCV (78% of which were autologous) examined the efficacy of several combination therapies including interferon, ribavirin, and direct-acting antivirals. Results showed that 85% of patients receiving direct-acting antivirals successfully cleared the virus for a period of at least three months (Kyvernitakis et al., 2016). A list of FDA-approved direct-acting antivirals can be found in Table 10-5 (U.S. FDA, 2018).

In light of limited clinical evidence in the transplant setting, the American Society for Transplantation and Cellular Therapy published preliminary guidelines on HCV in 2015 (Torres et al., 2015). Additional studies are ongoing to determine the optimal therapy and timing of direct-acting antivirals (Kyvernitakis et al., 2016; H.L. Lee et al., 2017). Because transplant patients with HCV are more likely to have thrombocytopenia due to delayed platelet recovery (Murray et al., 2018), they will require additional monitoring as well as patient and family education to prevent bleeding.

Prevention and Treatment

Owing to the complexities of managing HSCT patients with hepatitis, algorithms and guidelines may be useful in determining the optimal treatment course and appropriate medical interventions. Examples of algorithms and guidelines (Fred Hutchinson Cancer Research Center, 2016) for allogeneic donors and patients and for autologous patients are presented in Figures 10-7 through 10-9 and Table 10-6.

Prophylaxis with lamivudine has been used in the past to prevent reactivation. However, resistance has been a problem, and more recent recommendations are to use either entecavir or tenofovir (Di Bisceglie et al., 2015; Sarmati et al., 2017). Entecavir is preferred for all patients with compromised renal function and for any patient undergoing HSCT, as there are no data on tenofovir in the transplant setting. Medication should be started one week prior to conditioning and continued for up to one year after transplant, although disagreement exists regarding precisely when to initiate therapy and the optimal duration (Di Bisceglie et al., 2015; Sarmati et al., 2017).

Nurses caring for patients who have HBV or HCV must understand the general risk factors and monitor liver enzymes and viral load. Daily assessment should include signs and symptoms of worsening hepatic disease as evidenced by ascites, hepatomegaly, jaundice, or mental status changes. Drug interactions between direct-acting antivirals and common transplant medications such as tacrolimus can occur, requiring careful monitoring of drug levels and drug toxicities (Torres et al., 2015).

Although no definitive standard exists for preventing HBV or HCV reactivation after transplant, a number of antiviral medications have been recommended prior to and after transplant, including entecavir, lamivudine, and tenofovir (Murray et al., 2018; Torres et al., 2015). Of these, entecavir appears to have good efficacy (Yoo et al., 2015) and may be preferred because of its ability to overcome lamivudine-associated resistance, although more studies are required (Kimura, Nishikawa, Sakamaki, Mizokami, & Kimura, 2017; Siyahian et al., 2018).

Kidney Injury

Historically referred to as acute renal failure, *acute kidney injury* (AKI) is associated with increased patient mortality, particularly during the first 30 days post-transplant (Ando, 2018). Therefore, prevention requires understanding risk factors and identifying specific patients who may be at a higher risk. Chronic kidney disease in the HSCT setting can be defined as occurring after day 100 post-transplant or the ongoing presence of AKI after that time point (Hingorani, 2016a) and occurs in up to 20% of patients (Troxell, Higgins, & Kambham, 2014).

Table 10-5. Direct-Acting Antiviral Drugs for Hepatitis C

Approval Year	Generic Name	Brand Name	Manufacturer
2016	Sofosbuvir/velpatasvir	Epclusa®	Gilead Sciences
2016	Elbasvir/grazoprevir	Zepatier™	Merck Sharp & Dohme
2015	Ombitasvir/paritaprevir/ritonavir	Technivie™	AbbVie
2014	Ledipasvir/sofosbuvir	Harvoni®	Gilead Sciences
2013	Sofosbuvir	Sovaldi®	Gilead Sciences

Note. Based on information from U.S. Food and Drug Administration, 2018.

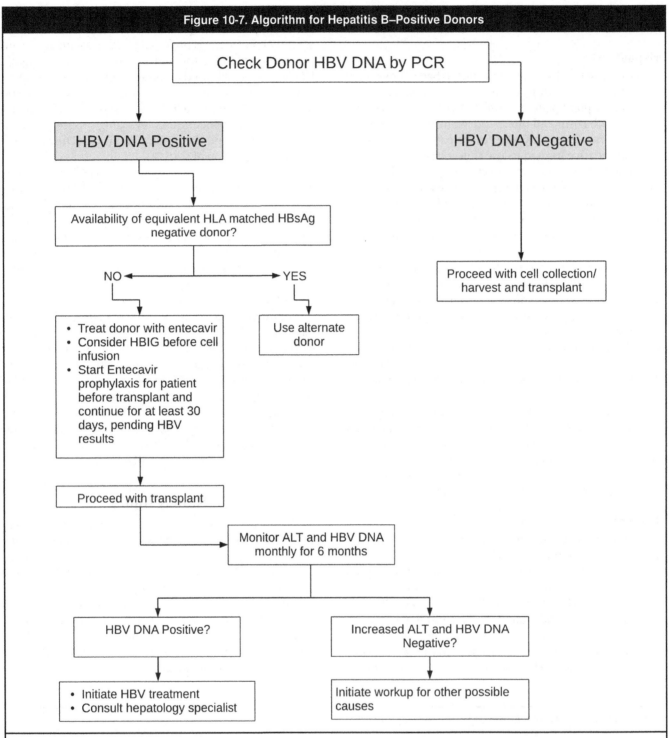

Figure 10-7. Algorithm for Hepatitis B–Positive Donors

Check Donor HBV DNA by PCR

HBV DNA Positive

HBV DNA Negative

Availability of equivalent HLA matched HBsAg negative donor?

NO ← → YES

Proceed with cell collection/harvest and transplant

- Treat donor with entecavir
- Consider HBIG before cell infusion
- Start Entecavir prophylaxis for patient before transplant and continue for at least 30 days, pending HBV results

Use alternate donor

Proceed with transplant

Monitor ALT and HBV DNA monthly for 6 months

HBV DNA Positive?

Increased ALT and HBV DNA Negative?

- Initiate HBV treatment
- Consult hepatology specialist

Initiate workup for other possible causes

ALT—alanine transaminase; HBIG—hepatitis B immunoglobulin; HBsAG—hepatitis B surface antigen; HBV—hepatitis B virus; HLA—human leukocyte antigen; PCR—polymerase chain reaction

Note. From *Blood and Bone Marrow Transplant (BMT)/Immunotherapy (IMTX) Standard Practice Manual (SPM)*, by Fred Hutchinson Cancer Research Center, 2016. *Blood and Bone Marrow Transplant (BMT)/Immunotherapy (IMTX) Standard Practice Manual (SPM)* is a copyrighted work of Fred Hutchinson Cancer Research Center ("Fred Hutch") and the Seattle Cancer Care Alliance ("SCCA") and is being used with permission from Fred Hutch and SCCA.

Disclaimer: These Standard Practice Guidelines are prepared for use only by the personnel of Fred Hutch, Seattle Cancer Care Alliance, and their affiliates. They are made available to others solely for educational purposes. They are not provided as a professional service or as medical advice for specific patients and are not a substitute for professional medical care. If you have, or suspect you may have, a health problem, you should consult a licensed healthcare provider. Fred Hutch and Seattle Cancer Care Alliance expressly disclaim (i) all warranties, express or implied, with respect to these Guidelines and (ii) all liability arising from the use of these Guidelines. These Guidelines are not intended to define the medical standard of care for legal purposes and should not be used in that way. Physicians may deviate from these guidelines if indicated. These Guidelines are not set policies except for the definition of Day "0" which is a policy of Fred Hutch and Seattle Cancer Care Alliance.

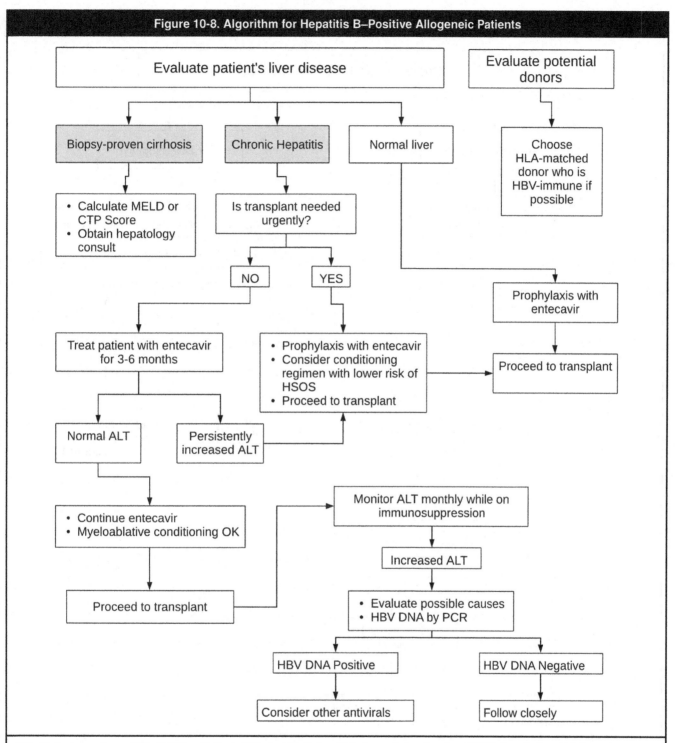

Figure 10-8. Algorithm for Hepatitis B–Positive Allogeneic Patients

Evaluate patient's liver disease

Evaluate potential donors

Biopsy-proven cirrhosis

Chronic Hepatitis

Normal liver

Choose HLA-matched donor who is HBV-immune if possible

- Calculate MELD or CTP Score
- Obtain hepatology consult

Is transplant needed urgently?

NO

YES

Prophylaxis with entecavir

Treat patient with entecavir for 3-6 months

- Prophylaxis with entecavir
- Consider conditioning regimen with lower risk of HSOS
- Proceed to transplant

Proceed to transplant

Normal ALT

Persistently increased ALT

- Continue entecavir
- Myeloablative conditioning OK

Monitor ALT monthly while on immunosuppression

Proceed to transplant

Increased ALT

- Evaluate possible causes
- HBV DNA by PCR

HBV DNA Positive

HBV DNA Negative

Consider other antivirals

Follow closely

ALT—alanine transaminase; CTP—Child-Turcotte-Pugh; HBV—hepatitis B virus; HLA—human leukocyte antigen; HSOS—hepatic sinusoidal obstruction syndrome; MELD—model for end-stage liver disease; PCR—polymerase chain reaction

Note. From *Blood and Bone Marrow Transplant (BMT)/Immunotherapy (IMTX) Standard Practice Manual (SPM)*, by Fred Hutchinson Cancer Research Center, 2016. *Blood and Bone Marrow Transplant (BMT)/Immunotherapy (IMTX) Standard Practice Manual (SPM)* is a copyrighted work of Fred Hutchinson Cancer Research Center ("Fred Hutch") and the Seattle Cancer Care Alliance ("SCCA") and is being used with permission from Fred Hutch and SCCA.

Disclaimer: These Standard Practice Guidelines are prepared for use only by the personnel of Fred Hutch, Seattle Cancer Care Alliance, and their affiliates. They are made available to others solely for educational purposes. They are not provided as a professional service or as medical advice for specific patients and are not a substitute for professional medical care. If you have, or suspect you may have, a health problem, you should consult a licensed healthcare provider. Fred Hutch and Seattle Cancer Care Alliance expressly disclaim (i) all warranties, express or implied, with respect to these Guidelines and (ii) all liability arising from the use of these Guidelines. These Guidelines are not intended to define the medical standard of care for legal purposes and should not be used in that way. Physicians may deviate from these guidelines if indicated. These Guidelines are not set policies except for the definition of Day "0" which is a policy of Fred Hutch and Seattle Cancer Care Alliance.

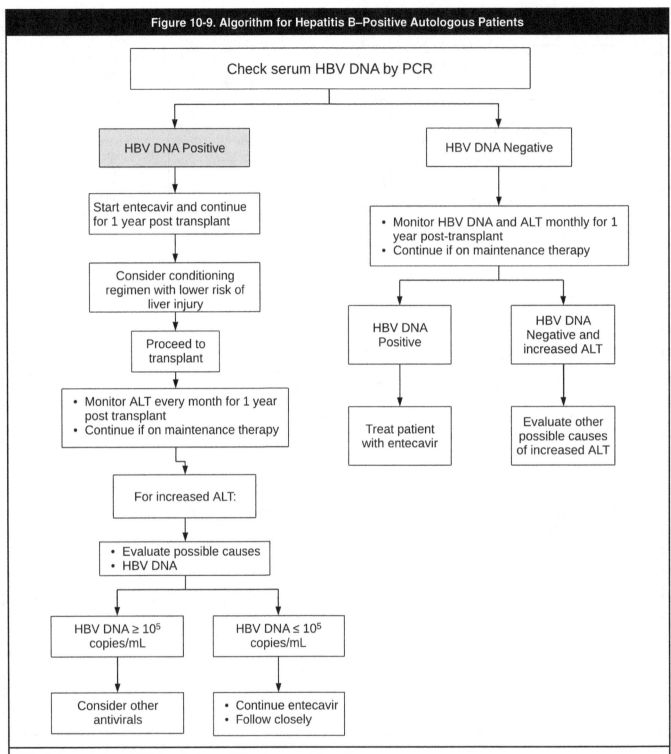

Figure 10-9. Algorithm for Hepatitis B–Positive Autologous Patients

Check serum HBV DNA by PCR

HBV DNA Positive

Start entecavir and continue for 1 year post transplant

Consider conditioning regimen with lower risk of liver injury

Proceed to transplant

- Monitor ALT every month for 1 year post transplant
- Continue if on maintenance therapy

For increased ALT:

- Evaluate possible causes
- HBV DNA

HBV DNA ≥ 10⁵ copies/mL

Consider other antivirals

HBV DNA ≤ 10⁵ copies/mL

- Continue entecavir
- Follow closely

HBV DNA Negative

- Monitor HBV DNA and ALT monthly for 1 year post-transplant
- Continue if on maintenance therapy

HBV DNA Positive

Treat patient with entecavir

HBV DNA Negative and increased ALT

Evaluate other possible causes of increased ALT

ALT—alanine transaminase; HBV—hepatitis B virus; PCR—polymerase chain reaction

Note. From *Blood and Bone Marrow Transplant (BMT)/Immunotherapy (IMTX) Standard Practice Manual (SPM)*, by Fred Hutchinson Cancer Research Center, 2016. *Blood and Bone Marrow Transplant (BMT)/Immunotherapy (IMTX) Standard Practice Manual (SPM)* is a copyrighted work of Fred Hutchinson Cancer Research Center ("Fred Hutch") and the Seattle Cancer Care Alliance ("SCCA") and is being used with permission from Fred Hutch and SCCA.

Disclaimer: These Standard Practice Guidelines are prepared for use only by the personnel of Fred Hutch, Seattle Cancer Care Alliance, and their affiliates. They are made available to others solely for educational purposes. They are not provided as a professional service or as medical advice for specific patients and are not a substitute for professional medical care. If you have, or suspect you may have, a health problem, you should consult a licensed healthcare provider. Fred Hutch and Seattle Cancer Care Alliance expressly disclaim (i) all warranties, express or implied, with respect to these Guidelines and (ii) all liability arising from the use of these Guidelines. These Guidelines are not intended to define the medical standard of care for legal purposes and should not be used in that way. Physicians may deviate from these guidelines if indicated. These Guidelines are not set policies except for the definition of Day "0" which is a policy of Fred Hutch and Seattle Cancer Care Alliance.

Table 10-6. Fred Hutchinson Cancer Research Center Hepatitis Guidelines

Patient Result	Donor Result	Recommendations
HBsAg+	Negative	Refer to Figures 10-7 and 10-8.
anti-HBsAg	Negative	Check for HBV DNA.
anti-HBc	Negative	High risk of post-transplant fulminant hepatic failure exists. Refer to Figures 10-7 and 10-8.
HBV DNA+	Negative	High risk of post-transplant fulminant hepatic failure exists. Refer to Figures 10-7 and 10-8.
Negative	HBsAg+	Donor is infected with HBV and can pass virus to patient. Consider antiviral treatment of donor using entecavir. Refer to Figures 10-7 and 10-8.
Negative	anti-HBsAg	Patient is naturally immune, and no risk to patient exists if donor is HBV DNA negative. Good candidate for infected patient.
Negative	anti-HBc+	No risk to patient exists if donor is HBV DNA negative. However, increased risk of passing virus exists if donor is HBV DNA positive.
Negative	HBV DNA+	Donor will pass virus to patient. Consider antiviral treatment for donor with entecavir. Refer to Figures 10-7 and 10-8.

anti-HBc—total hepatitis B core antibody; anti-HBsAg—hepatitis B surface antigen antibody; HBsAg—hepatitis B surface antigen; HBV—hepatis B virus

Note. Table courtesy of Fred Hutchinson Cancer Research Center.

Disclaimer: These Standard Practice Guidelines are prepared for use only by the personnel of Fred Hutchinson Cancer Research Center, Seattle Cancer Care Alliance, and their affiliates. They are made available to others solely for educational purposes. They are not provided as a professional service or as medical advice for specific patients and are not a substitute for professional medical care. If you have, or suspect you may have, a health problem, you should consult a licensed healthcare provider. Fred Hutchinson Cancer Research Center and Seattle Cancer Care Alliance expressly disclaim (i) all warranties, express or implied, with respect to these Guidelines and (ii) all liability arising from the use of these Guidelines. These Guidelines are not intended to define the medical standard of care for legal purposes and should not be used in that way. Physicians may deviate from these guidelines if indicated. These Guidelines are not set policies except for the definition of Day "0" which is a policy of Fred Hutchinson Cancer Research Center and Seattle Cancer Care Alliance.

Incidence and Risk Factors

Estimates of both acute and chronic kidney injury range from 10% to 73% (Hingorani, 2016b) and are dependent on a number of variables, including patient age, baseline kidney function, diagnosis, and, in particular, type of transplant (Ando, 2018). Different definitions of AKI also contribute to the wide range of reported incidence. While AKI has previously been defined as a doubling of the serum creatinine (da Silva, de Melo Lima, & Secoli, 2014; Hingorani, 2016a), most authors use newer and more precise assessment models. The most commonly cited models for adults are the RIFLE criteria (risk, injury, failure, loss of kidney function, end-stage renal disease) and the AKIN (acute kidney injury) model (Hingorani, 2016b; Krishnappa et al., 2016; Lopes, Jorge, & Neves, 2016). A comparison of these models can be found in Figure 10-10. The RIFLE model is more sensitive than the AKIN model. A variation of the RIFLE model exists for pediatric patients, known as pRIFLE (Kizilbash, Kashtan, Chavers, Cao, & Smith, 2016). Unfortunately, insufficient data exist comparing pRIFLE to AKIN (Koh et al., 2018).

Earlier detection of AKI can result in earlier intervention, and research has identified physiologic diagnostic biomarkers that are more specific than monitoring for increasing serum creatinine and oliguria—both of which tend to occur after kidney damage has already been initiated. Examples of biomarkers include urinary liver-type fatty acid–binding protein, urinary neutrophil gelatinase-associated lipocalin, and IL-18 (Ando, 2018; Lopes et al., 2016). However, testing for these indicators of renal tubule damage is not routinely performed in clinical laboratories, and their role in patient care has yet to be determined.

AKI has a number of different causes and mechanisms, including nephrotoxic medications, sepsis, HSOS, and direct toxicity from infused marrow or DMSO (dimethyl sulfoxide) used for cryopreserved stem cells (Lopes et al., 2016; Sawinski, 2014). A complete list can be found in Figure 10-11. AKI occurs more frequently in adults than children and is more common in patients receiving allogeneic transplants compared to autologous transplants. This is thought to be due to the need for GVHD prophylaxis using calcineurin inhibitors, generation of cytokine-mediated injury from T-cell–mediated inflammation, and generally longer periods of neutropenia, which can contribute to sepsis (Lopes et al., 2016). The risk is lower for patients receiving nonmyeloablative transplants and tends to occur later because of a lower frequency of organ toxicity (Lopes et al., 2016).

The presence of GVHD has been proposed as an independent cause of AKI mediated via inflammatory cytokines as a result of the interaction between donor T cells and the host immune system. Elafin is a protein produced by epithelial cells in response to tissue injury and inflammation in patients with GVHD. One early study demonstrated elevated urinary elafin levels in patients with AKI and chronic kidney disease (Hingorani et al., 2015). Higher levels corresponded to increased risk of death from renal failure.

Figure 10-10. Comparison of RIFLE and AKIN Criteria for Acute Kidney Injury

RIFLE Criteria

R — RISK:
1.5 × baseline serum creatinine or > 25% decrease in GFR. Urine output < 0.5 ml/kg for > 6 hrs.

I — INJURY:
2 × baseline serum creatinine or > 50% decrease in GFR. Urine output < 0.5 ml/kg/hr for > 12 hrs.

F — FAILURE:
3 × baseline serum creatinine, > 75% decrease in GFR, or creatinine > 4 mg/dl with rapid increase of 0.5 mg/dl within 48 hrs. Urine output < 3 ml/kg/hr for > 24 hrs or anuria for > 12 hrs.

L — LOSS:
Dialysis > 4 times per week.

E — END-STAGE RENAL DISEASE:
Complete loss of renal function requiring dialysis > 3 months

AKIN Criteria

STAGE 1 — ≥ 1.5–1.9 × baseline creatinine or ≥ 0.3 mg/dl greater than baseline. Urine output < 0.5 ml/kg/hr for > 6 hrs.

STAGE 2 — > 2–2.9 × baseline creatinine. Urine output < 0.5 ml/kg/hr for > 12 hrs.

STAGE 3 — > 3 × baseline creatinine or creatinine ≥ 4 mg/dl with rapid increase of 0.5 mg/dl within 48 hrs, or need for renal-replacement therapy. Urine output < 0.3 ml/kg/hr ≥ 24 hrs or anuria for > 12 hrs.

GFR—glomerular filtration rate

Note. Based on information from Hingorani, 2016b; Krishnappa et al., 2016; Lopes et al., 2016.

However, further studies are needed to ascertain whether urinary elafin is a reliable marker for AKI and how it could be used in the clinical setting for prevention.

Physiologically, AKI can occur from damage to the renal tubules resulting in acute tubular necrosis, or from vasoconstriction. Fluid shifts and dehydration are common in HSCT recipients and are associated with HSOS, sepsis, diarrhea from conditioning, infection or GVHD, transplantation-associated thrombotic microangiopathy (TMA), and engraftment syndrome (Hingorani, 2017; Lopes et al., 2016). Vasoconstriction of the renal arterials produces a "prerenal" state, leading to a decrease in glomerular filtration rate with subsequent oliguria as the kidneys attempt to compensate (Lopes et al., 2016).

Medications used in transplant often are implicated in the development of acute tubular necrosis (Hahn et al., 2003). These include conditioning chemotherapy, antibiotics, antifungals, antivirals, and drugs to prevent GVHD (Hingorani, 2016a). Nephrotoxic drugs, particularly in the presence of hypovolemia, can potentiate severe AKI (Lopes et al., 2016). Some nephrotoxic medications, including cyclosporine A and tacrolimus, have a narrow therapeutic range and require close monitoring of levels. A low, subtherapeutic level dramatically increases the risk of severe GVHD. High levels increase the risk of AKI in addition to other side effects. A systematic review of nephrotoxicity in adult HSCT recipients reported that cyclosporine A–related AKI occurred in 31% of the qualifying studies (da Silva et al.,

Figure 10-11. Potential Causes of Acute Kidney Injury

Hypovolemia	Systemic Vasodilation	Renal Vasoconstriction	Renal Endothelial Injury	Renal Tubular Injury
• Diarrhea • Excessive diuresis • Vomiting	• Sepsis	• Cyclosporine • Hepatic sinusoidal obstruction syndrome • Hypotension • Tacrolimus	• Acute graft-versus-host disease • Cyclosporine • Tacrolimus • Thrombotic microangiopathy • Total body irradiation	• Acyclovir • Amphotericin • Aminoglycosides • BK nephropathy • Cidofovir • Conditioning chemotherapy • Dimethyl sulfoxide • Entecavir • Foscarnet • Spironolactone • Tumor lysis syndrome • Vancomycin

Note. Based on information from Hahn et al., 2003; Hingorani, 2016b; Krishnappa et al., 2016; Raina et al., 2017; Sawinski, 2014; Zager, 1994.

2014). Nephrotoxicity was also increased when cyclosporine A was administered to patients receiving amphotericin or aminoglycoside antibiotics. The calcineurin inhibitors cause endothelial damage with the subsequent release of complement. Initiation of the complement cascade results in the generation of reactive oxygen species, leading to further tissue damage (Obut, Kasinath, & Abdi, 2016). Prostacyclin, which inhibits clot formation and increases vasodilation, is reduced by both cyclosporine A and tacrolimus (Shayani et al., 2013). The cryopreservative DMSO can be renal toxic by causing hemolysis resulting in the precipitation of heme in the distal nephron, subsequently leading to occlusion (Sawinski, 2014).

Although AKI in the pediatric transplant population is similar to what has been seen in adults, some differences exist. A systematic review focusing solely on pediatric transplant recipients found that 21.7% developed AKI, although different criteria for AKI were used by the authors. Similar to adults, cyclosporine A, amphotericin, and HSOS were implicated as the predominant risk factors, along with the use of foscarnet for cytomegalovirus treatment (Didsbury, Mackie, & Kennedy, 2015). Koh et al. (2018) performed a retrospective single-center study of 1,057 pediatric patients using the AKIN criteria and found that 68% developed AKI by day 100 and 52% within the first month. Older children and those receiving unrelated donor transplants also had a higher risk of developing AKI.

Nursing Management of Acute Kidney Injury

Nurses play an important role in the management of AKI. For patients receiving calcineurin inhibitors, levels must be monitored (da Silva et al., 2014), with pertinent information reported to the transplant team. Outpatients should be instructed on the importance of keeping scheduled laboratory blood draws and to withhold oral calcineurin inhibitors for trough levels. Fluid volume status should be monitored as previously described. Fluid overload, which readily occurs in transplant recipients, can have dire consequences in the presence of oliguria (Hingorani, 2017; Rondón et

al., 2017). Transplant nurses must know which drugs are nephrotoxic and avoid simultaneous administration. This may pose a conundrum for less experienced staff who are accustomed to working with multilumen catheters, particularly when there are many medications to administer within a short time frame. Patients at risk for AKI should be weighed twice daily (if inpatient) and at each outpatient visit (Eisenberg, 2008). Although intake and output are generally not conducted in the outpatient setting, monitoring for insidious progressive weight gain in the face of worsening renal function is prudent.

Transplant-Associated Thrombotic Microangiopathy

First reported in 1981 by Shulman et al., transplant-associated TMA is a complex disease representing two pathologies: hemolytic uremic syndrome and thrombotic thrombocytopenic purpura (Obut et al., 2016). Initially identified as primarily a disease of the kidneys, newer evidence provides insight into a systemic pathology that can affect the gut, lungs, heart, and brain (Jodele et al., 2015). The pathophysiology of TMA is believed to involve platelet aggregation and erythrocyte deposition within the kidneys and vessels, resulting in thrombus formation and ischemia (Hingorani, 2016b; Jodele et al., 2016). Activation of the complement cascade leads to further vascular damage (Obut et al., 2016), along with the recruitment of CD3+, CD8+, and other cytotoxic cells (Hingorani, 2016b). The cytokines TNF-α, IL-6, and IL-8, along with plasminogen activator inhibitor-1, have been implicated in contributing to endothelial damage (Hingorani, 2016b). Platelet consumption occurs along with thrombin formation and fibrin deposition.

Hemolytic uremic syndrome is seen later after transplant compared with thrombotic thrombocytopenic purpura, both of which involve extrarenal sites (Hingorani, 2016b). A diagnosis of TMA is suspected in the presence of unexplained microangiopathic hemolytic anemia, elevated lactic dehydrogenase, and schistocytes in the blood (Jodele et al., 2015). Other post-transplant complications such as regimen-related toxicity and systemic infections contribute to establishing a diagnosis (Shayani et al., 2013). Patients with TMA have higher than normal transfusion demands.

Incidence and Risk Factors

The reported incidence of TMA ranges from 0.5% to 63% (Obut et al., 2016). The wide variation is due to lack of renal biopsies to unequivocally confirm diagnosis, as well as a variety of transplant types and protocols for GVHD prophylaxis. Also, a lack of agreement exists between the Blood and Marrow Transplant Clinical Trials Network and other societies on a definition (Obut et al., 2016). Renal biopsies in the HSCT setting are particularly challenging given the risks associated with a thrombocytopenic population, resulting in delayed diagnosis (Hingorani, 2016b). And because thrombotic thrombocytopenic purpura may be absent in the kidneys but present in other organs such as the gut, an intestinal biopsy may be more beneficial and feasible provided that vascular tissue samples are obtained (Jodele et al., 2016).

Risk factors for TMA include use of calcineurin inhibitors, total body irradiation, grade 2–4 GVHD, transplants from unrelated or haploidentical donors, and BK virus infection (Hingorani, 2016a, 2016b). Conditioning regimens containing busulfan, cyclophosphamide, or fludarabine have also been implicated (Sawinski, 2014). Cyclosporine causes vasoconstriction of the renal arterioles, which appears to be level dependent (Hingorani, 2016b). Shayani et al. (2013) reported on the incidence of TMA in a study of 117 allogeneic patients and found that elevated sirolimus levels or sirolimus used with tacrolimus was a risk factor, although other confounders could not be completely eliminated. In a study of 314 patients, Changsirikulchai et al. (2009) found the use of male donors for female recipients was a risk factor.

Treatment

Early diagnosis of TMA is crucial in having a positive effect on its clinical course, as mortality rates can approach 90% (Sawinski, 2014). Jodele et al. (2016) reported good results with eculizumab, a monoclonal antibody that binds to complement C5. The use of rituximab has also been described (Hingorani, 2016b). Plasmapheresis in nontransplant patients has been used, although the results are equivocal and controlled studies are needed (Sawinski, 2014). Therefore, standardized treatment has yet to be elucidated. Withdrawal of the offending medication may be beneficial but at the expense of exacerbating GVHD—which has been previously described as a risk factor.

Hemorrhagic Cystitis

Initially observed with the administration of cyclophosphamide in 1973 (Cox, 1979; Droller, Saral, & Santos, 1982; Matz & Hsieh, 2017), hemorrhagic cystitis is characterized by edema of the urothelial tissues, ulcers, and necrosis, resulting in hematuria ranging from microscopic to frank blood (Hingorani, 2016b; Takamoto, Sakura, Namera, & Yashiki, 2004). Patients may be asymptomatic but often experience pain and urinary urgency. Hemorrhagic cystitis can be graded using the Common Terminology Criteria for Adverse Events scale as follows: grade 1—microscopic hematuria, grade 2—moderate hematuria, grade 3—gross hematuria with clots, and grade 4—life threatening (National Cancer Institute Cancer Therapy Evaluation Program, 2017). Although mild (grade 1) hemorrhagic cystitis typically resolves without intervention, it can progress, causing severe pain and resulting in urinary obstruction, hydronephrosis with renal failure, and death (Cesaro et al., 2015). Patients often require additional transfusion support and extended hospitalization. Because of its distinct etiologies, hemorrhagic cystitis is classified as *early onset* or *late onset* (Mori et al., 2012).

Early hemorrhagic cystitis is commonly associated with cyclophosphamide administration (Droller et al., 1982; Korkmaz, Topal, & Oter, 2007). After administration, cyclophosphamide is processed by the liver and broken down into its metabolites. One metabolite, aldocyclophosphamide, is further processed into acrolein (McDonald et al., 2003). Acrolein damages the urothelial lining of the bladder via direct inflammatory pyroptotic cellular destruction by increasing reactive oxygen species and the production of nitric oxide (Dobrek & Thor, 2012; Haldar et al., 2016). Cellular protein production is inhibited by both reactive oxygen species and nitric oxide (Matz & Hsieh, 2017). Reactive oxygen species produces nuclear factor kappa beta and activator protein-1, which upregulate the inflammatory cytokine interleukin-1 beta (IL-1β) and TNF-α. Mitogen-activating kinases also are implicated in upregulation of IL-1β (Matz & Hsieh, 2017). Reactive oxygen species are responsible for the inflammatory enzymes nitric oxide synthase and cyclooxygenase-2 (Ribeiro et al., 2012). Autophagy occurs in the muscularis, resulting in destructive ulcerative lesions that expose the vascular bed, ultimately resulting in bleeding (Haldar, Dru, & Bhowmick, 2014; Matz & Hsieh, 2017). Because hemorrhagic cystitis frequently occurs during a period of profound thrombocytopenia in myeloablative transplants, severe hemorrhage is a major concern (Hingorani, 2016b). Figure 10-12 shows the pathophysiology of hemorrhagic cystitis.

Late hemorrhagic cystitis typically is caused by infection with either the BK polyomavirus, JC virus, or adenovirus (Hingorani, 2016b; Peterson et al., 2016). Most cases of late hemorrhagic cystitis in the United States are caused by BK viruses. An estimated 80%–90% of normal healthy adults are infected with these viruses during childhood, although prior viral exposure does not directly correlate with the development of late hemorrhagic cystitis (Mori et al., 2012; Philippe et al., 2016). Several different factors are likely involved, as viruria occurs in approximately 50% of

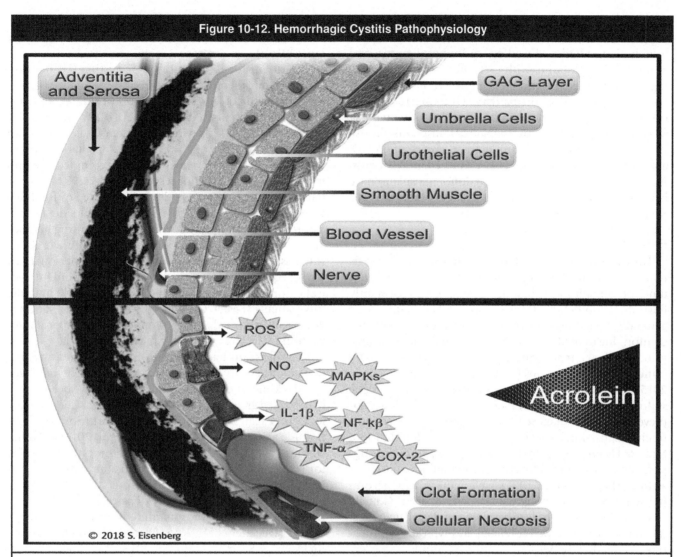

Figure 10-12. Hemorrhagic Cystitis Pathophysiology

Adventitia and Serosa

GAG Layer

Umbrella Cells

Urothelial Cells

Smooth Muscle

Blood Vessel

Nerve

ROS

NO

MAPKs

IL-1β

NF-kβ

TNF-α

COX-2

Acrolein

Clot Formation

Cellular Necrosis

© 2018 S. Eisenberg

Note. Based on information from Dobrek & Thor, 2012; Korkmaz et al., 2007; Matz & Hsieh, 2017; McDonald et al., 2003; Ribeiro et al., 2012. Copyright 2018 by Seth Eisenberg. Used with permission.

HSCT recipients, but the overall incidence is considerably lower (Peterson et al., 2016).

Serum DNA testing for BK virus has not been useful in predicting the development of hemorrhagic cystitis (Dalianis & Ljungman, 2011). Viruria is seen in both autologous and allogeneic transplant recipients, although hemorrhagic cystitis rarely occurs in the former (Peterson et al., 2016). It has been theorized that the BK virus remains dormant until postengraftment and becomes clinically relevant during severe immunosuppression used with allogeneic HSCT (Philippe et al., 2016).

Incidence and Risk Factors

Although reports vary, the incidence of early hemorrhagic cystitis ranges from 6% to 50% (Ribeiro et al., 2012). Late hemorrhagic cystitis occurs in approximately 4%–25% of patients (Dalianis & Ljungman, 2011; Peterson et al., 2016). In a study of 266 adult allogeneic trans-

plant recipients in Japan, 42 (15.8%) developed viral hemorrhagic cystitis (Mori et al., 2012). Of those, 26 were diagnosed with adenovirus and 16 with BK virus. Purging of T cells from the stem cell source was seen as a risk factor for adenovirus hemorrhagic cystitis. The authors noted that unlike in other parts of the world, BK infection is less common in Japan than adenovirus (Mori et al., 2012). A retrospective study of 6,119 pediatric patients revealed an incidence of 1.6% (n = 97). Grade 3 and 4 hemorrhagic cystitis occurred more frequently in patients older than five years old and those whose urine tested positive for BK virus (Riachy et al., 2014). A retrospective study of 1,321 allogeneic patients receiving a variety of conditioning regimens showed an incidence of 16%—the same results as a study done by the institution two decades earlier. The authors concluded that older children and younger adults had an increased risk, along with patients receiving cyclophosphamide (Lunde et al., 2015). Peterson et al. (2016)

reported on a relatively homologous cohort of 73 adult allogeneic transplant recipients receiving combinations of total body irradiation, busulfan, cyclophosphamide, and antithymocyte globulin, with GVHD prophylaxis consisting of mycophenolate and cyclosporine A. BK or JC viruria occurred in 41% of the patients. Of those, 16% developed grade 2 or higher hemorrhagic cystitis. Potential risk factors in adults include myeloablative transplants, the use of busulfan during conditioning, the presence of GVHD, and older age (Laskin et al., 2013). For pediatric patients, male sex and recipients of unrelated donor transplants have been reported to be associated with higher risk (Dalianis & Ljungman, 2011; Hingorani, 2016b).

Prevention

Historically, prophylaxis for early hemorrhagic cystitis relied on continuous bladder irrigation, forcing large volumes of saline into the bladder in an effort to constantly flush the endothelium (Hows et al., 1984). Results were generally mixed and involved considerable patient discomfort due to bladder spasms and the presence of a large urinary catheter. It also carried a significant risk of urinary catheter-related infections (Gonella, di Pasquale, & Palese, 2015; Hingorani, 2016b). Studies using 2-mercaptoethane sulfonate sodium (mesna) had demonstrated efficacy for preventing hemorrhagic cystitis in nontransplant patients receiving ifosfamide (Bryant, Ford, Jarman, & Smith, 1980; Matz & Hsieh, 2017). By the early 1990s, evidence supported the use of mesna for cyclophosphamide in the HSCT setting (Shepherd et al., 1991), paving the way for becoming standard of care along with hyperhydration (Gonella et al., 2015). Mesna binds to acrolein, rendering it an inactive metabolite. It is well tolerated and typically administered immediately before cyclophosphamide and every four hours after for three additional doses. Hyperhydration along with mesna works by diluting the urine and thereby reducing potential acrolein–urothelial interaction (Gonella et al., 2015; Hingorani, 2016b). Mesna use for cyclophosphamide is considered an off-label use, as it is only FDA approved for use with ifosfamide. No approved therapies have been adopted for the prevention of late hemorrhagic cystitis. One anecdotal report (Miller et al., 2011) and one small study have shown benefit of using ciprofloxacin (Leung et al., 2005), but additional controlled studies are needed to determine whether either of these are truly efficacious.

Treatment

The use of mesna for treating cyclophosphamide-induced hemorrhagic cystitis has not been established (Haldar et al., 2014). Continuous bladder irrigation, with or without hydrocortisone, may be indicated in an effort to wash out clots and prevent urethral occlusion. Other substances, such as alum (Westerman, Boorjian, & Linder, 2016), formalin (Ziegelmann, Boorjian, Joyce, Montgomery, & Linder, 2017), and silver nitrate, have also been explored in small

case studies but have potentially significant side effects (Bogris, Johal, Hussein, Duffy, & Mushtaq, 2009; Hingorani, 2016b).

Treatment for late hemorrhagic cystitis has involved both systemic therapy and intravesical installations as previously described. Despite lack of robust studies, antivirals often are used (Hirsch & Pergam, 2016). IV cidofovir has been used for both BK virus and adenovirus (Hingorani, 2016b). In one study of 43 allogeneic transplant recipients with BK hemorrhagic cystitis, 64% had a complete response to cidofovir, 23% did not respond, and 7.7% had a partial resolution. One patient died of unrelated causes (Gilis et al., 2014). Nephrotoxicity is a significant side effect of cidofovir and can result in renal failure requiring hemodialysis. Nurses should also be aware that cidofovir is classified as a hazardous drug, and appropriate personal protective equipment is required for administration. Intravesical cidofovir has had some success, particularly in refractory patients (Foster, Cheng, Nguyen, Krance, & Martinez, 2018; Sakurada et al., 2016). In severe cases, surgical intervention including cystectomy may be required.

Ciprofloxacin has shown promise in decreasing incidence and severity of BK viremia, viruria, and hemorrhagic cystitis (Miller et al., 2011), although there have been reports of increased graft rejection (Zaman, Ettenger, Cheam, Malekzadeh, & Tsai, 2014). The rheumatoid arthritis drug leflunomide also is being studied (Hingorani, 2016b). Animal studies have included IL-11 and keratinocyte growth factor (currently approved for mucositis prevention), which have shown some promise (Ribeiro et al., 2012). Hyperbaric oxygen therapy has been extensively studied for both radiation- and cyclophosphamide-induced hemorrhagic cystitis (Degener et al., 2015; Oscarsson, Arnell, Lodding, Ricksten, & Seeman-Lodding, 2013; Polom et al., 2012; Ribeiro de Oliveira, Carmelo Romão, Gamito Guerreiro, & Matos Lopes, 2015). In the rodent model, hyperbaric oxygen therapy is believed to reduce oxidative stress in irradiated bladder tissue, thereby reducing apoptosis and promoting cellular recovery (Oscarsson et al., 2017). It has not been approved for hemorrhagic cystitis in the United States, and no randomized controlled studies have been performed specifically for cyclophosphamide-induced hemorrhagic cystitis.

Nurses play an important role in the prevention and management of hemorrhagic cystitis and must have a good understanding of the rationale behind hyperhydration and mesna. Because the maximum concentration of acrolein occurs within two to four hours after cyclophosphamide administration and the short half-life of mesna requires repeated administrations at close intervals (Wallhult & Quinn, 2018), ensuring timely administration is critical. Institution-based recommendations may include the administration of IV fluids at least 3 L/m^2/day with accurate intake and output to ensure adequate voiding, as well as specific voiding protocols. Patients should be monitored for potential volume overload, particularly those with underlying cardiopulmonary compromise. Diuretics may be ordered but should be used with caution to prevent unintended volume depletion. Daily or twice-daily weights along with postural vital signs are useful in determining fluid balance. Patients should be monitored for hypertension or hypotension associated with hyperhydration. Maintaining accurate intake and output is also crucial, as cyclophosphamide-induced syndrome of inappropriate antidiarrheic hormone secretion can result in fluid retention (Shepherd et al., 1991). Up to 25% of a dose of cyclophosphamide is excreted unchanged in the urine, requiring appropriate hazardous drug personal protective equipment for nurses and all supportive staff involved with emptying and measuring urine (Eisenberg, 2017; McDonald et al., 2003).

The platelet threshold may be increased to greater than 50,000/mm^3, and plasma or other clotting proteins may need to be given to correct coagulopathy if present (Sawinski, 2014). Complete blood count and platelet counts, renal function (blood urea nitrogen and serum creatinine), and coagulation studies (prothrombin time, partial thromboplastin time, and international normalized ratio) should be monitored. For patients needing a urinary catheter along with continuous bladder irrigation, meticulous catheter care is required. All patients should be monitored for signs and symptoms of urinary tract infections. Pain medication or antispasmodics may be ordered to decrease discomfort.

Summary

HSCT can result in a number of serious complications affecting the liver, kidneys, and bladder. Although some may be preventable, others may occur that require expertise by both medical and nursing personnel. Careful identification of patients at risk and a keen understanding of the physiologic processes are important in providing the best possible outcomes to a vulnerable population.

References

Anastasiou, O.E., Almpani, F., Herrmann, A., Gerken, G., Ditschkowski, M., & Ciesek, S. (2017). HBV reactivation in allogeneic stem cell transplant recipients: Risk factors, outcome, and role of hepatitis B virus mutations. *Hepatology Communications*, 1, 1014–1023. https://doi.org/10.1002/hep4.1118

Ando, M. (2018). An overview of kidney disease following hematopoietic cell transplantation. *Internal Medicine*, 57, 1503–1508. https://doi.org/10.2169/internalmedicine.9838-17

Aziz, M.T., Kakadiya, P.P., Kush, S.M., Weigel, K., & Lowe, D.K. (2018). Defibrotide: An oligonucleotide for sinusoidal obstruction syndrome. *Annals of Pharmacotherapy*, 52, 166–174. https://doi.org/10.1177/1060028017732586

Bajwa, R.P.S., Mahadeo, K.M., Taragin, B.H., Dvorak, C.C., McArthur, J., Jeyapalan, A., ... Woolfrey, A.E. (2017). Consensus report by Pediatric Acute Lung Injury and Sepsis Investigators and Pediatric Blood and Marrow Transplantation Consortium Joint Working Committees: Supportive care guidelines for management of veno-occlusive disease in children and adolescents, part 1: Focus on investigations, prophylaxis, and specific treatment. *Biology of Blood and Marrow Transplantation*, 23, 1817–1825. https://doi.org/10.1016/j.bbmt.2017.07.021

Barrett, K.E. (2014). Functional anatomy of the liver and biliary system. In *Gastrointestinal physiology* (2nd ed.). New York, NY: McGraw-Hill.

Bearman, S.I. (1995). The syndrome of hepatic veno-occlusive disease after marrow transplantation. *Blood*, 85, 3005–3020.

Bearman, S.I., Anderson, G.L., Mori, M., Hinds, M.S., Shulman, H.M., & McDonald, G.B. (1993). Venoocclusive disease of the liver: Development of a model for predicting fatal outcome after marrow transplantation. *Journal of Clinical Oncology*, 11, 1729–1736. https://doi.org/10.1200/jco.1993.11.9.1729

Bearman, S.I., Shen, D.D., Hinds, M.S., Hill, H.A., & McDonald, G.B. (1993). A phase I/II study of prostaglandin E$_1$ for the prevention of hepatic venocclusive disease after bone marrow transplantation. *British Journal of Haematology*, 84, 724–730. https://doi.org/10.1111/j.1365-2141.1993.tb03152.x

Blix, E.S., & Husebekk, A. (2016). Raiders of the lost mark—Endothelial cells and their role in transplantation for hematologic malignancies. *Leukemia and Lymphoma*, 57, 2752–2762. https://doi.org/10.1080/10428194.2016.1201566

Bogris, S.L., Johal, N.S., Hussein, I., Duffy, P.G., & Mushtaq, I. (2009). Is it safe to use aluminum in the treatment of pediatric hemorrhagic cystitis? A case discussion of aluminum intoxication and review of the literature. *Journal of Pediatric Hematology/Oncology*, 31, 285–288. https://doi.org/10.1097/mph.0b013e31819b591c

Bosonnet, L. (2003). Pruritus: Scratching the surface. *European Journal of Cancer Care*, 12, 162–165.

Botti, S., Orlando, L., Gargiulo, G., De Cecco, V., Banfi, M., Duranti, L., ... Bonifazi, F. (2016). Veno-occlusive disease nurse management: Development of a dynamic monitoring tool by the GITMO nursing group. *Ecancermedicalscience*, 10, 661. https://doi.org/10.3332/ecancer.2016.661

Bras, G., Berry, D.M., György, P., & Smith, H.V. (1957). Plants as aetiological factor in veno-occlusive disease of the liver. *Lancet*, 269, 960–962. https://doi.org/10.1016/s0140-6736(57)91283-7

Bryant, B.M., Ford, H.T., Jarman, M., & Smith, I.E. (1980). Prevention of isophosphamide-induced urothelial toxicity with 2-mercaptoethane sulphonate sodium (mesnum) in patients with advanced carcinoma. *Lancet*, 316, 657–659. https://doi.org/10.1016/s0140-6736(80)92703-8

Cao, Z., Villa, K.F., Lipkin, C.B., Robinson, S.B., Nejadnik, B., & Dvorak, C.C. (2017). Burden of illness associated with sinusoidal obstruction syndrome/veno-occlusive disease in patients with hematopoietic stem cell transplantation. *Journal of Medical Economics*, 20, 871–883. https://doi.org/10.1080/13696998.2017.1336623

Carreras, E. (2000). Veno-occlusive disease of the liver after hemopoietic cell transplantation. *European Journal of Haematology*, 64, 281–291.

Carreras, E., Díaz-Beyá, M., Rosiñol, L., Martínez, C., Fernández-Avilés, F., & Rovira, M. (2011). The incidence of veno-occlusive disease following allogeneic hematopoietic stem cell transplantation has diminished and the outcome improved over the last decade. *Biology of Blood and Marrow Transplantation*, 17, 1713–1720. https://doi.org/10.1016/j.bbmt.2011.06.006

Centers for Disease Control and Prevention. (2005). *Interpretation of hepatitis B serologic test results*. Retrieved from https://www.cdc.gov/hbv/pdfs/serologicchartv8.pdf

Centers for Disease Control and Prevention. (2018, April 18). Viral hepatitis. Retrieved from https://www.cdc.gov/hepatitis/statistics/index.htm

Cesaro, S., Tridello, G., Pillon, M., Calore, E., Abate, D., Tumino, M., ... Messina, C. (2015). A prospective study on the predictive value of plasma BK virus-DNA load for hemorrhagic cystitis in pediatric patients after stem cell transplantation. *Journal of the Pediatric Infectious Diseases Society*, 4, 134–142. https://doi.org/10.1093/jpids/piu043

Changsirikulchai, S., Myerson, D., Guthrie, K.A., McDonald, G.B., Alpers, C.E., & Hingorani, S.R. (2009). Renal thrombotic microangiopathy after hematopoietic cell transplant: role of GVHD in pathogenesis. *Clinical Journal of the American Society of Nephrology*, 4, 345–353. https://doi.org/10.2215/cjn.02070508

Cheuk, D.K.L., Chiang, A.K.S., Ha, S.Y., & Chan, G.C.F. (2015). Interventions for prophylaxis of hepatic veno-occlusive disease in people undergoing haematopoietic stem cell transplantation. *Cochrane Database of Systematic Reviews*, 2015(5). https://doi.org/10.1002/14651858.cd009311.pub2

Chikotas, N., Gunderman, A., & Oman, T. (2006). Uremic syndrome and end-stage renal disease: Physical manifestations and beyond. *Journal of the American Academy of Nurse Practitioners, 18,* 195–202. https://doi.org/10.1111/j.1745-7599.2006.00123.x

Coppell, J.A., Brown, S.A., & Perry, D.J. (2003). Veno-occlusive disease: Cytokines, genetics, and haemostasis. *Blood Reviews, 17,* 63–70. https://doi.org/10.1016/s0268-960x(03)00002-x

Coppell, J.A., Richardson, P.G., Soiffer, R., Martin, P.L., Kernan, N.A., Chen, A., ... Niederwieser, D. (2010). Hepatic veno-occlusive disease following stem cell transplantation: Incidence, clinical course, and outcome. *Biology of Blood and Marrow Transplantation, 16,* 157–168. https://doi.org/10.1016/j.bbmt.2009.08.024

Corbacioglu, S., & Richardson, P.G. (2017). Defibrotide for children and adults with hepatic veno-occlusive disease post hematopoietic cell transplantation. *Expert Review of Gastroenterology and Hepatology, 11,* 885–898. https://doi.org/10.1080/17474124.2017.1370372

Cox, P.J. (1979). Cyclophosphamide cystitis—Identification of acrolein as the causative agent. *Biochemical Pharmacology, 28,* 2045–2049. https://doi.org/10.1016/0006-2952(79)90222-3

Dalianis, T., & Ljungman, P. (2011). Full myeloablative conditioning and an unrelated HLA mismatched donor increase the risk for BK virus-positive hemorrhagic cystitis in allogeneic hematopoetic stem cell transplanted patients. *Anticancer Research, 31,* 939–944. Retrieved from http://ar.iiarjournals.org/content/31/3/939.long

Dalle, J.-H., & Giralt, S.A. (2016). Hepatic veno-occlusive disease after hematopoietic stem cell transplantation: Risk factors and stratification, prophylaxis, and treatment. *Biology of Blood and Marrow Transplantation, 22,* 400–409. https://doi.org/10.1016/j.bbmt.2015.09.024

da Silva, J.B., de Melo Lima, M.H., & Secoli, S.R. (2014). Influence of cyclosporine on the occurrence of nephrotoxicity after allogeneic hematopoietic stem cell transplantation: A systematic review. *Revista Brasileira de Hematologia e Hemoterapia, 36,* 363–368. https://doi.org/10.1016/j.bjhh.2014.03.010

Degener, S., Pohle, A., Strelow, H., Mathers, M.J., Zumbé, J., Roth, S., & Brandt, A.S. (2015). Long-term experience of hyperbaric oxygen therapy for refractory radio- or chemotherapy-induced haemorrhagic cystitis. *BMC Urology, 15,* 38. https://doi.org/10.1186/s12894-015-0035-4

DeLeve, L.D., Shulman, H.M., & McDonald, G.B. (2002). Toxic injury to hepatic sinusoids: Sinusoidal obstruction syndrome (veno-occlusive disease). *Seminars in Liver Disease, 22,* 27–42. https://doi.org/10.1055/s-2002-23204

DeLeve, L.D., Wang, X., Kanel, G.C., Ito, Y., Bethea, N.W., McCuskey, M.K., ... McCuskey, R.S. (2003). Decreased hepatic nitric oxide production contributes to the development of rat sinusoidal obstruction syndrome. *Hepatology, 38,* 900–908. https://doi.org/10.1002/hep.1840380416

DeLeve, L.D., Wang, X., Tsai, J., Kanel, G., Strasberg, S., & Tokes, Z.A. (2003). Sinusoidal obstruction syndrome (veno-occlusive disease) in the rat is prevented by matrix metalloproteinase inhibition. *Gastroenterology, 125,* 882–890. https://doi.org/10.1016/s0016-5085(03)01056-4

Di Bisceglie, A.M., Lok, A.S., Martin, P., Terrault, N., Perrillo, R.P., & Hoofnagle, J.H. (2015). Recent US Food and Drug Administration warnings on hepatitis B reactivation with immune-suppressing and anticancer drugs: Just the tip of the iceberg? *Hepatology, 61,* 703–711. https://doi.org/10.1002/hep.27609

Didsbury, M.S., Mackie, F.E., & Kennedy, S.E. (2015). A systematic review of acute kidney injury in pediatric allogeneic hematopoietic stem cell recipients. *Pediatric Transplantation, 19,* 460–470. https://doi.org/10.1111/petr.12483

Dobrek, L., & Thor, P.J. (2012). Bladder urotoxicity pathophysiology induced by the oxazaphosphorine alkylating agents and its chemoprevention. *Advances in Hygiene and Experimental Medicine, 66,* 592–602. https://doi.org/10.5604/17322693.1009703

Droller, M.J., Saral, R., & Santos, G. (1982). Prevention of cyclophosphamide-induced hemorrhagic cystitis. *Urology, 20,* 256–258. https://doi.org/10.1016/0090-4295(82)90633-1

Eisenberg, S. (2008). Hepatic sinusoidal obstruction syndrome in patients undergoing hematopoietic stem cell transplant. *Oncology Nursing Forum, 35,* 385–397. https://doi.org/10.1188/08.ONF.385-397

Eisenberg, S. (2017). Hazardous drugs and USP <800>: Implications for nurses. *Clinical Journal of Oncology Nursing, 21,* 179–187. https://doi.org/10.1188/17.CJON.179-187

Essell, J.H., Schroeder, M.T., Harman, G.S., Halvorson, R., Lew, V., Callander, N., ... Thompson, J.M. (1998). Ursodiol prophylaxis against hepatic complications of allogeneic bone marrow transplantation: A randomized, double-blind, placebo-controlled trial. *Annals of Internal Medicine, 128,* 975–981. https://doi.org/10.7326/0003-4819-128-12_part_1-199806150-00002

Foster, J.H., Cheng, W.S., Nguyen, N.-Y., Krance, R., & Martinez, C. (2018). Intravesicular cidofovir for BK hemorrhagic cystitis in pediatric patients after hematopoietic stem cell transplant. *Pediatric Transplantation, 22,* e13141. https://doi.org/10.1111/petr.13141

Foundation for the Accreditation of Cellular Therapy & Joint Accreditation Committee–ISCT and EBMT. (2018). *FACT-JACIE international standards for hematopoietic cellular therapy product collection, processing, and administration* (7th ed.). Retrieved from https://www.ebmt.org/sites/default/files/2018-06/FACT-JACIE%207th%20Edition%20Standards.pdf

Fred Hutchinson Cancer Research Center. (2016). Hepatitis viruses and hematopoietic cell transplantation. In *Standard practice manual.* Seattle, WA: Author.

Genentech. (2017, November). *Gazyva® (obinutuzumab)* [Package insert]. South San Francisco, CA: Author.

Genentech. (2019, April). *Rituxan® (rituximab)* [Package insert]. South San Francisco, CA: Author.

Gentile, G., Andreoni, M., Antonelli, G., & Sarmati, L. (2017). Screening, monitoring, prevention, prophylaxis and therapy for hepatitis B virus reactivation in patients with haematologic malignancies and patients who underwent haematologic stem cell transplantation: A systematic review. *Clinical Microbiology and Infection, 23,* 916–923. https://doi.org/10.1016/j.cmi.2017.06.024

Gilis, L., Morisset, S., Billaud, G., Ducastelle-Leprêtre, S., Labussière-Wallet, H., Nicolini, F.-E., ... Ader, F. (2014). High burden of BK virus-associated hemorrhagic cystitis in patients undergoing allogeneic hematopoietic stem cell transplantation. *Bone Marrow Transplantation, 49,* 664–670. https://doi.org/10.1038/bmt.2013.235

Gloude, N.J., Jodele, S., Teusink-Cross, A., Grimley, M., Davies, S.M., Lane, A., & Myers, K.C. (2018). Combination of high-dose methylprednisolone and defibrotide for veno-occlusive disease in pediatric hematopoietic stem cell transplant recipients. *Biology of Blood and Marrow Transplantation, 24,* 91–95. https://doi.org/10.1016/j.bbmt.2017.09.007

Gonella, S., di Pasquale, T., & Palese, A. (2015). Preventive measures for cyclophosphamide-related hemorrhagic cystitis in blood and bone marrow transplantation: An Italian multicenter retrospective study [Online exclusive]. *Clinical Journal of Oncology Nursing, 19,* E8–E14. https://doi.org/10.1188/15.CJON.e8-e14

Hahn, T., Rondeau, C., Shaukat, A., Jupudy, V., Miller, A., Alam, A.R., ... McCarthy, P.L., Jr. (2003). Acute renal failure requiring dialysis after allogeneic blood and marrow transplantation identifies very poor prognosis patients. *Bone Marrow Transplantation, 32,* 405–410. https://doi.org/10.1038/sj.bmt.1704144

Haldar, S., Dru, C., & Bhowmick, N.A. (2014). Mechanisms of hemorrhagic cystitis. *American Journal of Clinical and Experimental Urology, 2,* 199–208.

Haldar, S., Dru, C., Mishra, R., Tripathi, M., Duong, F., Angara, B., ... Bhowmick, N.A. (2016). Histone deacetylase inhibitors mediate DNA damage repair in ameliorating hemorrhagic cystitis. *Scientific Reports, 6,* 39257. https://doi.org/10.1038/srep39257

Han, M.K., & Hyzy, R. (2006). Advances in critical care management of hepatic failure and insufficiency. *Critical Care Medicine, 34*(Suppl. 9), S225–S231. https://doi.org/10.1097/01.ccm.0000231882.85350.71

Hingorani, S. (2016a). Kidney and bladder complications of hematopoietic cell transplantation. In S.J. Forman, R.S. Negrin, J.H. Antin, & F.R. Appelbaum (Eds.), *Thomas' hematopoietic cell transplantation: Stem cell transplantation* (5th ed., pp. 1170–1180). https://doi.org/10.1002/9781118416426.ch96

Hingorani, S. (2016b). Renal complications of hematopoietic-cell transplantation. *New England Journal of Medicine, 374,* 2256–2267. https://doi.org/10.1056/NEJMra1404711

Hingorani, S.R. (2017). Fluid: Too much or too little—Transplant mortality may hang in the balance. *Biology of Blood and Marrow Transplantation, 23,* 2020–2022. https://doi.org/10.1016/j.bbmt.2017.10.032

Hingorani, S., Finn, L.S., Pao, E., Lawler, R., Schoch, G., McDonald, G.B., … Gooley, T. (2015). Urinary elafin and kidney injury in hematopoietic cell transplant recipients. *Clinical Journal of the American Society of Nephrology, 10*, 12–20. https://doi.org/10.2215/cjn.01840214

Hirsch, H.H., & Pergam, S.A. (2016). Human adenovirus, polyomavirus, and parvovirus infections in patients undergoing hematopoietic stem cell transplantation. In S.J. Forman, R.S. Negrin, J.H. Antin, & F.R. Appelbaum (Eds.), *Thomas' hematopoietic cell transplantation: Stem cell transplantation* (5th ed., pp. 1129–1139). https://doi.org/10.1002/9781118416426.ch93

Hockenberry, D.M., Strasser, S.I., & McDonald, G.B. (2016). Gastrointestinal and hepatic complications. In S.J. Forman, R.S. Negrin, J.H. Antin, & F.R. Appelbaum (Eds.), *Thomas' hematopoietic cell transplantation: Stem cell transplantation* (5th ed., pp. 1140–1155). https://doi.org/10.1002/9781118416426.ch94

Hows, J.M., Mehta, A., Ward, L., Woods, K., Perez, R., Gordon, M.Y., & Gordon-Smith, E.C. (1984). Comparison of mesna with forced diuresis to prevent cyclophosphamide induced haemorrhagic cystitis in marrow transplantation: A prospective randomised study. *British Journal of Cancer, 50*, 753–756. https://doi.org/10.1038/bjc.1984.252

Hwang, J.P., & Lok, A.S.-F. (2014). Management of patients with hepatitis B who require immunosuppressive therapy. *Nature Reviews Gastroenterology and Hepatology, 11*, 209–219. https://doi.org/10.1038/nrgastro.2013.216

Imran, H., Tleyjeh, I.M., Zirakzadeh, A., Rodriguez, V., & Khan, S.P. (2006). Use of prophylactic anticoagulation and the risk of hepatic veno-occlusive disease in patients undergoing hematopoietic stem cell transplantation: A systematic review and meta-analysis. *Bone Marrow Transplantation, 37*, 677–686. https://doi.org/10.1038/sj.bmt.1705297

Jazz Pharmaceuticals. (2016). *Defitelio® (defibrotide)* [Package insert]. Palo Alto, CA: Author.

Jodele, S., Dandoy, C.E., Myers, K.C., El-Bietar, J., Nelson, A., Wallace, G., & Laskin, B.L. (2016). New approaches in the diagnosis, pathophysiology, and treatment of pediatric hematopoietic stem cell transplantation-associated thrombotic microangiopathy. *Transfusion and Apheresis Science, 54*, 181–190. https://doi.org/10.1016/j.transci.2016.04.007

Jodele, S., Laskin, B.L., Dandoy, C.E., Myers, K.C., El-Bietar, J., Davies, S.M., … Dixon, B.P. (2015). A new paradigm: Diagnosis and management of HSCT-associated thrombotic microangiopathy as multi-system endothelial injury. *Blood Reviews, 29*, 191–204. https://doi.org/10.1016/j.blre.2014.11.001

Jones, R.J., Lee, K.S., Beschorner, W.E., Vogel, V.G., Grochow, L.B., Braine, H.G., … Saral, R. (1987). Venoocclusive disease of the liver following bone marrow transplantation. *Transplantation, 44*, 778–783. https://doi.org/10.1097/00007890-198712000-00011

Kimura, M., Nishikawa, K., Sakamaki, H., Mizokami, M., & Kimura, K. (2017). Reduced therapeutic effect of antiviral drugs in patients with hepatitis B virus reactivation after hematopoietic stem cell transplantation. *Hepatology Research, 48*, 469–478. https://doi.org/10.1111/hepr.13044

Kizilbash, S.J., Kashtan, C.E., Chavers, B.M., Cao, Q., & Smith, A.R. (2016). Acute kidney injury and the risk of mortality in children undergoing hematopoietic stem cell transplantation. *Biology of Blood and Marrow Transplantation, 22*, 1264–1270. https://doi.org/10.1016/j.bbmt.2016.03.014

Koh, K.-N., Sunkara, A., Kang, G., Sooter, A., Mulrooney, D.A., Triplett, B., … Cunningham, L.C. (2018). Acute kidney injury in pediatric patients receiving allogeneic hematopoietic stem cell transplantation: Incidence, risk factors, and outcomes. *Biology of Blood and Marrow Transplantation, 24*, 758–764. https://doi.org/10.1016/j.bbmt.2017.11.021

Korkmaz, A., Topal, T., & Oter, S. (2007). Pathophysiological aspects of cyclophosphamide and ifosfamide induced hemorrhagic cystitis: Implication of reactive oxygen and nitrogen species as well as PARP activation. *Cell Biology and Toxicology, 23*, 303–312. https://doi.org/10.1007/s10565-006-0078-0

Krishnappa, V., Gupta, M., Manu, G., Kwatra, S., Owusu, O.-T., & Raina, R. (2016). Acute kidney injury in hematopoietic stem cell transplantation: A review. *International Journal of Nephrology, 2016*, 5163789. https://doi.org/10.1155/2016/5163789

Kumar, S., DeLeve, L.D., Kamath, P.S., & Tefferi, A. (2003). Hepatic veno-occlusive disease (sinusoidal obstruction syndrome) after hematopoietic stem cell transplantation. *Mayo Clinic Proceedings, 78*, 589–598. https://doi.org/10.4065/78.5.589

Kyvernitakis, A., Mahale, P., Popat, U.R., Jiang, Y., Hosry, J., Champlin, R.E., & Torres, H.A. (2016). Hepatitis C virus infection in patients undergoing hematopoietic cell transplantation in the era of direct-acting antiviral agents. *Biology of Blood and Marrow Transplantation, 22*, 717–722. https://doi.org/10.1016/j.bbmt.2015.12.010

Laskin, B.L., Denburg, M., Furth, S., Diorio, D., Goebel, J., Davies, S.M., & Jodele, S. (2013). BK viremia precedes hemorrhagic cystitis in children undergoing allogeneic hematopoietic stem cell transplantation. *Biology of Blood and Marrow Transplantation, 19*, 1175–1182. https://doi.org/10.1016/j.bbmt.2013.05.002

Law, M.F., Ho, R., Cheung, C.K., Tam, L.H., Ma, K., So, K.C., … Tam, T.H. (2016). Prevention and management of hepatitis B virus reactivation in patients with hematological malignancies treated with anticancer therapy. *World Journal of Gastroenterology, 22*, 6484–6500. https://doi.org/10.3748/wjg.v22.i28.6484

Lee, H.L., Bae, S.H., Jang, B., Hwang, S., Yang, H., Nam, H.C., … Yoon, S.K. (2017). Reactivation of hepatitis C virus and its clinical outcomes in patients treated with systemic chemotherapy or immunosuppressive therapy. *Gut and Liver, 11*, 870–877. https://doi.org/10.5009/gnl16434

Lee, J.H., Lee, K.H., Lee, J.H., Kim, S., Seol, M., Park, C.J., … Lee, J.S. (2002). Plasminogen activator inhibitor-1 is an independent diagnostic marker as well as severity predictor of hepatic veno-occlusive disease after allogeneic bone marrow transplantation in adults conditioned with busulphan and cyclophosphamide. *British Journal of Haematology, 118*, 1087–1094. https://doi.org/10.1046/j.1365-2141.2002.03748.x

Leung, A.Y.H., Chan, M.T.L., Yuen, K.-Y., Cheng, V.C.C., Chan, K.-H., Wong, C.L.P., … Kwong, Y.-L. (2005). Ciprofloxacin decreased polyoma BK virus load in patients who underwent allogeneic hematopoietic stem cell transplantation. *Clinical Infectious Diseases, 40*, 528–537. https://doi.org/10.1086/427291

Litzow, M.R., Repoussis, P.D., Schroeder, G., Schembri-Wismayer, D., Batts, K.P., Anderson, P.M., … Hoagland, H.C. (2002). Veno-occlusive disease of the liver after blood and marrow transplantation: Analysis of pre- and post-transplant risk factors associated with severity and results of therapy with tissue plasminogen activator. *Leukemia and Lymphoma, 43*, 2099–2107. https://doi.org/10.1080/1042819021000032962

Loomba, R., & Liang, T.J. (2017). Hepatitis B reactivation associated with immune suppressive and biological modifier therapies: Current concepts, management strategies, and future directions. *Gastroenterology, 152*, 1297–1309. https://doi.org/10.1053/j.gastro.2017.02.009

Lopes, J.A., Jorge, S., & Neves, M. (2016). Acute kidney injury in HCT: An update. *Bone Marrow Transplantation, 51*, 755–762. https://doi.org/10.1038/bmt.2015.357

Lunde, L.E., Dasaraju, S., Cao, Q., Cohn, C.S., Reding, M., Bejanyan, N., … Ustun, C. (2015). Hemorrhagic cystitis after allogeneic hematopoietic cell transplantation: Risk factors, graft source and survival. *Bone Marrow Transplantation, 50*, 1432–1437. https://doi.org/10.1038/bmt.2015.162

Ma, C., & Brunt, E.M. (2016). Terminal hepatic venule injury in liver biopsies of allogeneic haematopoietic stem cell recipients—A study of 63 cases. *Histopathology, 68*, 996–1003. https://doi.org/10.1111/his.12887

Mahadeo, K.M., McArthur, J., Adams, R.H., Radhi, M., Angelo, J., Jeyapalan, A., … Bajwa, R.P.S. (2017). Consensus report by the Pediatric Acute Lung Injury and Sepsis Investigators and Pediatric Blood and Marrow Transplant Consortium Joint Working Committees on Supportive Care Guidelines for Management of Veno-Occlusive Disease in Children and Adolescents: Part 2—Focus on ascites, fluid and electrolytes, renal, and transfusion issues. *Biology of Blood and Marrow Transplantation, 23*, 2023–2033. https://doi.org/10.1016/j.bbmt.2017.08.014

Matz, E.L., & Hsieh, M.H. (2017). Review of advances in uroprotective agents for cyclophosphamide- and ifosfamide-induced hemorrhagic cystitis. *Urology, 100*, 16–19. https://doi.org/10.1016/j.urology.2016.07.030

McDonald, G.B., Hinds, M.S., Fisher, L.D., Schoch, H.G., Wolford, J.L., Banaji, M., … Clift, R.A. (1993). Veno-occlusive disease of the liver and multiorgan failure after bone marrow transplantation: A cohort study of 355 patients. *Annals of Internal Medicine, 118*, 255–267. https://doi.org/10.7326/0003-4819-118-4-199302150-00003

McDonald, G.B., Sharma, P., Matthews, D.E., Shulman, H.M., & Thomas, E.D. (1984). Venocclusive disease of the liver after bone marrow transplantation: Diagnosis, incidence, and predisposing factors. *Hepatology, 4*, 116–122. https://doi.org/10.1002/hep.1840040121

McDonald, G.B., Slattery, J.T., Bouvier, M.E., Ren, S., Batchelder, A.L., Kalhorn, T.F., ... Gooley, T. (2003). Cyclophosphamide metabolism, liver toxicity, and mortality following hematopoietic stem cell transplantation. *Blood, 101*, 2043–2048. https://doi.org/10.1182/blood-2002-06-1860

Miller, A.N., Glode, A., Hogan, K.R., Schaub, C., Kramer, C., Stuart, R.K., & Costa, L.J. (2011). Efficacy and safety of ciprofloxacin for prophylaxis of polyomavirus BK virus–associated hemorrhagic cystitis in allogeneic hematopoietic stem cell transplantation recipients. *Biology of Blood and Marrow Transplantation, 17*, 1176–1181. https://doi.org/10.1016/j.bbmt.2010.12.700

Mohty, M., Malard, F., Abecassis, M., Aerts, E., Alaskar, A.S., Aljurf, M., ... Carreras, E. (2016). Revised diagnosis and severity criteria for sinusoidal obstruction syndrome/veno-occlusive disease in adult patients: A new classification from the European Society for Blood and Marrow Transplantation. *Bone Marrow Transplantation, 51*, 906–912. https://doi.org/10.1038/bmt.2016.130

Mori, Y., Miyamoto, T., Kato, K., Kamezaki, K., Kuriyama, T., Oku, S., ... Akashi, K. (2012). Different risk factors related to adenovirus- or BK virus-associated hemorrhagic cystitis following allogeneic stem cell transplantation. *Biology of Blood and Marrow Transplantation, 18*, 458–465. https://doi.org/10.1016/j.bbmt.2011.07.025

Murray, J., Agreiter, I., Orlando, L., & Hutt, D. (2018). BMT settings, infection and infection control. In M. Kenyon & A. Babic (Eds.), *The European blood and marrow transplantation textbook for nurses* (pp. 97–134). https://doi.org/10.1007/978-3-319-50026-3_7

Myers, K.C., Dandoy, C., El-Bietar, J., Davies, S.M., & Jodele, S. (2015). Veno-occlusive disease of the liver in the absence of elevation in bilirubin in pediatric patients after hematopoietic stem cell transplantation. *Biology of Blood and Marrow Transplantation, 21*, 379–381. https://doi.org/10.1016/j.bbmt.2014.09.026

National Cancer Institute Cancer Therapy Evaluation Program. (2017). *Common terminology criteria for adverse events* [v.5.0]. Retrieved from https://ctep.cancer.gov/protocolDevelopment/electronic_applications/docs/CTCAE_v5_Quick_Reference_8.5x11.pdf

Obut, F., Kasinath, V., & Abdi, R. (2016). Post-bone marrow transplant thrombotic microangiopathy. *Bone Marrow Transplantation, 51*, 891–897. https://doi.org/10.1038/bmt.2016.61

Oscarsson, N., Arnell, P., Lodding, P., Ricksten, S.-E., & Seeman-Lodding, H. (2013). Hyperbaric oxygen treatment in radiation-induced cystitis and proctitis: A prospective cohort study on patient-perceived quality of recovery. *International Journal of Radiation Oncology, Biology, Physics, 87*, 670–675. https://doi.org/10.1016/j.ijrobp.2013.07.039

Oscarsson, N., Ny, L., Mölne, J., Lind, F., Ricksten, S.-E., Seeman-Lodding, H., & Giglio, D. (2017). Hyperbaric oxygen treatment reverses radiation induced pro-fibrotic and oxidative stress responses in a rat model. *Free Radical Biology and Medicine, 103*, 248–255. https://doi.org/10.1016/j.freeradbiomed.2016.12.036

Ovchinsky, N., Frazier, W., Auletta, J.J., Dvorak, C.C., Ardura, M., Song, E., ... Bajwa, R.P.S. (2018). Consensus report by the Pediatric Acute Lung Injury and Sepsis Investigators and Pediatric Blood and Marrow Transplantation Consortium Joint Working Committees on Supportive Care Guidelines for Management of Veno-Occlusive Disease in Children and Adolescents, Part 3: Focus on cardiorespiratory dysfunction, infections, liver dysfunction, and delirium. *Biology of Blood and Marrow Transplantation, 24*, 207–218. https://doi.org/10.1016/j.bbmt.2017.08.035

Pereira, M.P., Kremer, A.E., Mettang, T., & Ständer, S. (2016). Chronic pruritus in the absence of skin disease: Pathophysiology, diagnosis and treatment. *American Journal of Clinical Dermatology, 17*, 337–348. https://doi.org/10.1007/s40257-016-0198-0

Perrillo, R.P., Gish, R., & Falck-Ytter, Y.T. (2015). American Gastroenterological Association institute technical review on prevention and treatment of hepatitis B virus reactivation during immunosuppressive drug therapy. *Gastroenterology, 148*, 221–244.e223. https://doi.org/10.1053/j.gastro.2014.10.038

Peterson, L., Ostermann, H., Fiegl, M., Tischer, J., Jaeger, G., & Rieger, C.T. (2016). Reactivation of polyomavirus in the genitourinary tract is significantly associated with severe GvHD and oral mucositis following

allogeneic stem cell transplantation. *Infection, 44*, 483–490. https://doi.org/10.1007/s15010-016-0872-4

Philippe, M., Ranchon, F., Gilis, L., Schwiertz, V., Vantard, N., Ader, F., ... Rioufol, C. (2016). Cidofovir in the treatment of BK virus-associated hemorrhagic cystitis after allogeneic hematopoietic stem cell transplantation. *Biology of Blood and Marrow Transplantation, 22*, 723–730. https://doi.org/10.1016/j.bbmt.2015.12.009

Pichler, H., Horner, K., Engstler, G., Poetschger, U., Glogova, E., Karlhuber, S., ... Matthes-Martin, S. (2017). Cost-effectiveness of defibrotide in the prophylaxis of veno-occlusive disease after pediatric allogeneic stem cell transplantation. *Biology of Blood and Marrow Transplantation, 23*, 1128–1133. https://doi.org/10.1016/j.bbmt.2017.03.022

Pihusch, M., Wegner, H., Goehring, P., Salat, C., Pihusch, V., Hiller, E., ... Pihusch, R. (2005). Diagnosis of hepatic veno-occlusive disease by plasminogen activator inhibitor-1 plasma antigen levels: A prospective analysis in 350 allogeneic hematopoietic stem cell recipients. *Transplantation, 80*, 1376–1382. https://doi.org/10.1097/01.tp.0000183288.67746.44

Polom, W., Klejnotowska, A., Matuszewski, M., Sicko, Z., Markuszewski, M., & Krajka, K. (2012). Hyperbaric oxygen therapy (HBOT) in case of hemorrhagic cystitis after radiotherapy. *Central European Journal of Urology, 65*, 200–203. https://doi.org/10.5173/ceju.2012.04.art4

Raina, R., Herrera, N., Krishnappa, V., Sethi, S.K., Deep, A., Kao, W.-M., ... Abu-Arja, R. (2017). Hematopoietic stem cell transplantation and acute kidney injury in children: A comprehensive review. *Pediatric Transplant, 21*(4). https://doi.org/10.1111/petr.12935

Riachy, E., Krauel, L., Rich, B.S., McEvoy, M.P., Honeyman, J.N., Boulad, F., ... La Quaglia, M.P. (2014). Risk factors and predictors of severity score and complications of pediatric hemorrhagic cystitis. *Journal of Urology, 191*, 186–192. https://doi.org/10.1016/j.juro.2013.08.007

Ribeiro, R.A., Lima, R.C.P., Leite, C.A.V.G., Mota, J.M.S.C., Macedo, F.Y.B., Lima, M.V.A., & Brito, G.A.C. (2012). Chemotherapy-induced hemorrhagic cystitis: Pathogenesis, pharmacological approaches and new insights. *Journal of Experimental and Integrative Medicine, 2*, 95–112. https://doi.org/10.5455/jeim.080312.ir.010

Ribeiro de Oliveira, T.M., Carmelo Romão, A.J., Gamito Guerreiro, F.M., & Matos Lopes, T.M. (2015). Hyperbaric oxygen therapy for refractory radiation-induced hemorrhagic cystitis. *International Journal of Urology, 22*, 962–966. https://doi.org/10.1111/iju.12857

Richardson, P.G., Smith, A.R., Triplett, B.M., Kernan, N.A., Grupp, S.A., Antin, J.H., ... Soiffer, R.J. (2017a). Defibrotide for patients with hepatic veno-occlusive disease/sinusoidal obstruction syndrome: Interim results from a treatment IND study. *Biology of Blood and Marrow Transplantation, 23*, 997–1004. https://doi.org/10.1016/j.bbmt.2017.03.008

Richardson, P.G., Smith, A.R., Triplett, B.M., Kernan, N.A., Grupp, S.A., Antin, J.H., ... Soiffer, R.J. (2017b). Earlier defibrotide initiation post-diagnosis of veno-occlusive disease/sinusoidal obstruction syndrome improves day +100 survival following haematopoietic stem cell transplantation. *British Journal of Haematology, 178*, 112–118. https://doi.org/10.1111/bjh.14727

Richardson, P.G., Triplett, B.M., Ho, V.T., Chao, N., Dignan, F.L., Maglio, M., & Mohty, M. (2018). Defibrotide sodium for the treatment of hepatic veno-occlusive disease/sinusoidal obstruction syndrome. *Expert Review of Clinical Pharmacology, 11*, 113–124. https://doi.org/10.1080/17512433.2018.1421943

Rondón, G., Saliba, R.M., Chen, J., Ledesma, C., Alousi, A.M., Oran, B., ... Ciurea, S.O. (2017). Impact of fluid overload as new toxicity category on hematopoietic stem cell transplantation outcomes. *Biology of Blood and Marrow Transplantation, 23*, 2166–2171. https://doi.org/10.1016/j.bbmt.2017.08.021

Sakurada, M., Kondo, T., Umeda, M., Kawabata, H., Yamashita, K., & Takaori-Kondo, A. (2016). Successful treatment with intravesical cidofovir for virus-associated hemorrhagic cystitis after allogeneic hematopoietic stem cell transplantation: A case report and a review of the literature. *Journal of Infection and Chemotherapy, 22*, 495–500. https://doi.org/10.1016/j.jiac.2016.01.013

Salat, C., Holler, E., Kolb, H.J., Pihusch, R., Reinhardt, B., Penovici, M., ... Hiller, E. (1999). The relevance of plasminogen activator inhibitor 1 (PAI-1) as a marker for the diagnosis of hepatic veno-occlusive disease in patients after bone marrow transplantation. *Leukemia and Lymphoma, 33*, 25–32. https://doi.org/10.3109/10428199909093722

Salat, C., Holler, E., Kolb, H.J., Reinhardt, B., Pihusch, R., Wilmanns, W., & Hiller, E. (1997). Plasminogen activator inhibitor-1 confirms the diagnosis of hepatic veno-occlusive disease in patients with hyperbilirubinemia after bone marrow transplantation. *Blood, 89*, 2184–2188. https://doi.org/10.3109/10428199909093722

Saria, M.G., & Gosselin-Acomb, T.K. (2007). Hematopoietic stem cell transplantation: Implications for critical care nurses. *Clinical Journal of Oncology Nursing, 11*, 53–63. https://doi.org/10.1188/07.CJON.53-63

Sarmati, L., Andreoni, M., Antonelli, G., Arcese, W., Bruno, R., Coppola, N., ... Gentile, G. (2017). Recommendations for screening, monitoring, prevention, prophylaxis and therapy of hepatitis B virus reactivation in patients with haematologic malignancies and patients who underwent haematologic stem cell transplantation—A position paper. *Clinical Microbiology and Infection, 23*, 935–940. https://doi.org/10.1016/j.cmi.2017.06.023

Sawinski, D. (2014). The kidney effects of hematopoietic stem cell transplantation. *Advances in Chronic Kidney Disease, 21*, 96–105. https://doi.org/10.1053/j.ackd.2013.08.007

Schriber, J., Milk, B., Shaw, D., Christiansen, N., Baer, M., Slack, J., ... Herzig, G. (1999). Tissue plasminogen activator (tPA) as therapy for hepatotoxicity following bone marrow transplantation. *Bone Marrow Transplantation, 24*, 1311–1314. https://doi.org/10.1038/sj.bmt.1702069

Seifert, C., Wittig, S., Arndt, C., & Gruhn, B. (2015). Heparanase polymorphisms: Influence on incidence of hepatic sinusoidal obstruction syndrome in children undergoing allogeneic hematopoietic stem cell transplantation. *Journal of Cancer Research and Clinical Oncology, 141*, 877–885. https://doi.org/10.1007/s00432-014-1857-2

Seto, W.K. (2015). Hepatitis B virus reactivation during immunosuppressive therapy: Appropriate risk stratification. *World Journal of Hepatology, 7*, 825–830. https://doi.org/10.4254/wjh.v7.i6.825

Seto, W.K., Chan, T.S., Hwang, Y.Y., Wong, D.K., Fung, J., Liu, K.S., ... Yuen, M.F. (2017). Hepatitis B reactivation in occult viral carriers undergoing hematopoietic stem cell transplantation: A prospective study. *Hepatology, 65*, 1451–1461. https://doi.org/10.1002/hep.29022

Shayani, S., Palmer, J., Stiller, T., Liu, X., Thomas, S.H., Khuu, T., ... Nakamura, R. (2013). Thrombotic microangiopathy associated with sirolimus level after allogeneic hematopoietic cell transplantation with tacrolimus/sirolimus-based graft-versus-host disease prophylaxis. *Biology of Blood and Marrow Transplantation, 19*, 298–304. https://doi.org/10.1016/j.bbmt.2012.10.006

Shepherd, J.D., Pringle, L.E., Barnett, M.J., Klingemann, H.G., Reece, D.E., & Phillips, G.L. (1991). Mesna versus hyperhydration for the prevention of cyclophosphamide-induced hemorrhagic cystitis in bone marrow transplantation. *Journal of Clinical Oncology, 9*, 2016–2020. https://doi.org/10.1200/jco.1991.9.11.2016

Shulman, H.M., McDonald, G.B., Matthews, D., Doney, K.C., Kopecky, K.J., Gauvreau, J.M., & Thomas, E.D. (1980). An analysis of hepatic venoocclusive disease and centrilobular hepatic degeneration following bone marrow transplantation. *Gastroenterology, 79*, 1178–1191. https://doi.org/10.1016/0016-5085(80)90911-7

Shulman, H., Striker, G., Deeg, H.J., Kennedy, M., Storb, R., & Thomas, E.D. (1981). Nephrotoxicity of cyclosporin A after allogeneic marrow transplantation—Glomerular thromboses and tubular injury. *New England Journal of Medicine, 305*, 1392–1395. https://doi.org/10.1056/nejm198112033052306

Siyahian, A., Malik, S.U., Mushtaq, A., Howe, C.L., Majeed, A., Zangeneh, T., ... Anwer, F. (2018). Prophylaxis for hepatitis B virus reactivation after allogeneic stem cell transplantation in the era of drug resistance and newer antivirals: A systematic review and meta-analysis. *Biology of Blood and Marrow Transplantation, 24*, 1483–1489. https://doi.org/10.1016/j.bbmt.2018.02.027

Skeens, M.A., McArthur, J., Cheifetz, I.M., Duncan, C., Randolph, A.G., Stanek, J., ... Bajwa, R. (2016). High variability in the reported management of hepatic veno-occlusive disease in children after hematopoietic stem cell transplantation. *Biology of Blood and Marrow Transplantation, 22*, 1823–1828. https://doi.org/10.1016/j.bbmt.2016.07.011

Song, J.S., Seo, J.J., Moon, H.N., Ghim, T., & Im, H.J. (2006). Prophylactic low-dose heparin or prostaglandin E_1 may prevent severe veno-occlusive disease of the liver after allogeneic hematopoietic stem cell transplantation in Korean children. *Journal of Korean Medical Science, 21*, 897–903. https://doi.org/10.3346/jkms.2006.21.5.897

Sosa, E.C. (2012). Veno-occlusive disease in hematopoietic stem cell transplantation recipients. *Clinical Journal of Oncology Nursing, 16*, 507–513. https://doi.org/10.1188/12.CJON.507-513

Soubani, A.O. (2006). Critical care considerations of hematopoietic stem cell transplantation. *Critical Care Medicine, 34*(Suppl. 9), S251–S267. https://doi.org/10.1097/01.ccm.0000231886.80470.b6

Stark, J.L. (1994). Interpreting B.U.N./creatinine levels: It's not as simple as you think. *Nursing, 24*(9), 58–61. https://doi.org/10.1097/00152193-199409000-00025

Takamoto, S., Sakura, N., Namera, A., & Yashiki, M. (2004). Monitoring of urinary acrolein concentration in patients receiving cyclophosphamide and ifosfamide. *Journal of Chromatography B, 806*, 59–63. https://doi.org/10.1016/j.jchromb.2004.02.008

Tasota, F.J., & Tate, J. (2000). Assessing renal function. *Nursing, 30*(5), 20.

Tay, J., Tinmouth, A., Fergusson, D., Huebsch, L., & Allan, D.S. (2007). Systematic review of controlled clinical trials on the use of ursodeoxycholic acid for the prevention of hepatic veno-occlusive disease in hematopoietic stem cell transplantation. *Biology of Blood and Marrow Transplantation, 13*, 206–217. https://doi.org/10.1016/j.bbmt.2006.09.012

Tomblyn, M., Chiller, T., Einsele, H., Gress, R., Sepkowitz, K., Storek, J., ... Boeckh, M.A. (2009). Guidelines for preventing infectious complications among hematopoietic cell transplantation recipients: A global perspective. *Biology of Blood and Marrow Transplantation, 15*, 1143–1238. https://doi.org/10.1016/j.bbmt.2009.06.019

Torres, H.A., Chong, P.P., De Lima, M., Friedman, M.S., Giralt, S., Hammond, S.P., ... Gambarin-Gelwan, M. (2015). Hepatitis C virus infection among hematopoietic cell transplant donors and recipients: American Society for Blood and Marrow Transplantation Task Force recommendations. *Biology of Blood and Marrow Transplantation, 21*, 1870–1882. https://doi.org/10.1016/j.bbmt.2015.07.033

Troxell, M.L., Higgins, J.P., & Kambham, N. (2014). Renal pathology associated with hematopoietic stem cell transplantation. *Advances in Anatomic Pathology, 21*, 330–340. https://doi.org/10.1097/pap.0000000000000034

U.S. Food and Drug Administration. (2018, May 14). Hepatitis B and C treatments. Retrieved from https://www.fda.gov/forpatients/illness/hepatitisbc/ucm408658.htm

Valla, D.-C., & Cazals-Hatem, D. (2016). Sinusoidal obstruction syndrome. *Clinics and Research in Hepatology and Gastroenterology, 40*, 378–385. https://doi.org/10.1016/j.clinre.2016.01.006

Vion, A.-C., Rautou, P.-E., Durand, F., Boulanger, C.M., & Valla, D.C. (2015). Interplay of inflammation and endothelial dysfunction in bone marrow transplantation: Focus on hepatic veno-occlusive disease. *Seminars in Thrombosis and Hemostasis, 41*, 629–643. https://doi.org/10.1055/s-0035-1556728

Wadleigh, M., Ho, V., Momtaz, P., & Richardson, P. (2003). Hepatic veno-occlusive disease: Pathogenesis, diagnosis and treatment. *Current Opinion in Hematology, 10*, 451–462. https://doi.org/10.1097/00062752-200311000-00010

Wallhult, E., Kenyon, M., Liptrott, S., Mank, A., Ní Chonghaile, M., Babic, A., ... Mohty, M. (2017). Management of veno-occlusive disease: The multidisciplinary approach to care. *European Journal of Haematology, 98*, 322–329. https://doi.org/10.1111/ejh.12840

Wallhult, E., & Quinn, B. (2018). Early and acute complications and the principles of HSCT nursing care. In M. Kenyon & A. Babic (Eds.), *The European blood and marrow transplantation textbook for nurses* (pp. 163–195). https://doi.org/10.1007/978-3-319-50026-3_9

Weil, E., Zook, F., Oxencis, C., Canadeo, A., Urmanski, A., Waggoner, M., ... Hari, P. (2017). Evaluation of the pharmacokinetics and efficacy of a busulfan test dose in adult patients undergoing myeloablative hematopoietic cell transplantation. *Biology of Blood and Marrow Transplantation, 23*, 952–957. https://doi.org/10.1016/j.bbmt.2017.02.020

Westerman, M.E., Boorjian, S.A., & Linder, B.J. (2016). Safety and efficacy of intravesical alum for intractable hemorrhagic cystitis: A contemporary evaluation. *International Braz J Urol, 42*, 1144–1149. https://doi.org/10.1590/s1677-5538.ibju.2015.0588

Yoo, J.J., Cho, E.J., Cho, Y.Y., Lee, M., Lee, D.H., Cho, Y., ... Kim, Y.J. (2015). Efficacy of antiviral prophylaxis in HBsAg-negative, anti-HBc positive patients undergoing hematopoietic stem cell transplantation. *Liver International, 35,* 2530–2536. https://doi.org/10.1111/liv.12882

Zager, R.A. (1994). Acute renal failure in the setting of bone marrow transplantation. *Kidney International, 46,* 1443–1458. https://doi.org/10.1038/ki.1994.417

Zaman, R.A., Ettenger, R.B., Cheam, H., Malekzadeh, M.H., & Tsai, E.W. (2014). A novel treatment regimen for BK viremia. *Transplantation, 97,* 1166–1171. https://doi.org/10.1097/01.tp.0000441825.72639.4f

Zhang, L., Wang, Y., & Huang, H. (2012). Defibrotide for the prevention of hepatic veno-occlusive disease after hematopoietic stem cell transplantation: A systematic review. *Clinical Transplantation, 26,* 511–519. https://doi.org/10.1111/j.1399-0012.2012.01604.x

Ziegelmann, M.J., Boorjian, S.A., Joyce, D.D., Montgomery, B.D., & Linder, B.J. (2017). Intravesical formalin for hemorrhagic cystitis: A contemporary cohort. *Canadian Urological Association Journal, 11,* E79–E82. https://doi.org/10.5489/cuaj.4047

CHAPTER 11

Cardiopulmonary Complications

Jennifer M.L. Stephens, MA, PhD, RN, OCN®

Introduction

Research spanning the past decade has confirmed that cardiopulmonary complications remain a significant concern for patients after hematopoietic stem cell transplantation (HSCT). Increased use of HSCT for patients with diverse conditions has increased the incidence of these complications (Chi, Soubani, White, & Miller, 2013). Despite medical and pharmaceutical advancements, intensive care unit (ICU) admission, morbidity, and mortality rates remain high in the post-transplant period for autologous and allogeneic transplants (Chi et al., 2013). According to recent studies of transplant recipients, rates for pulmonary complications remain at 30%–60%, and pulmonary complications are the most common cause of mortality in this patient population (Alsharif et al., 2009; Bertelli et al., 2017; Soubani & Pandya, 2010; Yanik & Kitko, 2013). Cardiac complications, particularly those related to the HSCT conditioning regimen, pose a significant risk for this population as well (Blaes, Konety, & Hurley, 2016).

Lungs that have been exposed to pretransplantation conditioning with chemotherapy and radiation can be particularly vulnerable during the post-transplantation period. Accurate and early diagnosis of complications is critical for improved patient outcomes. Pulmonary complications for HSCT patients can occur in the acute and chronic phases of transplantation. These complications are divided by etiology into two groups: infectious and noninfectious. Because of the nature of conditioning and the myelosuppression that can accompany it, infections from opportunistic bacteria, viruses, and other pathogens are a major concern for autologous and allogeneic transplant recipients. Noninfectious complications include those related to chemotherapy, pulmonary hemorrhage, pulmonary edema, and structural and obstructive disorders, such as acute respiratory distress syndrome (ARDS). Chronic complications are exacerbated by the development of graft-versus-host disease (GVHD) in the lungs and by pulmonary infections, particularly viral infections, such as cytomegalovirus (CMV).

Similarly, cardiac tissue is highly susceptible to the transplantation conditioning regimen of radiation and chemotherapy, such as anthracyclines, which compromise individual cells and the cardiac conduction system. A cardiac comorbidity, such as low ejection fraction, arrhythmias, or hypertension, can substantially increase the risk of complication in the post-transplantation period. Because cardiopulmonary complications are common issues for HSCT patients, it is critical for nurses and other HSCT healthcare providers to have ongoing education in disease etiology, diagnostics, interventions, and contemporary treatments (Blaes et al., 2016; Chi et al., 2013). With each of these complications, early detection and diagnosis with quick treatment initiation is key to improving patient outcomes.

Pulmonary Complications

Recent research confirms that pulmonary complications are the leading cause of post-transplantation morbidity and death in HSCT patients (Chi et al., 2013; Roychowdhury et al., 2005; Yanik & Kitko, 2013; see Figure 11-1). The rate of complications is significantly lower for autologous transplant recipients than for allogeneic transplant recipients. GVHD is typically absent in autologous transplants and subsequently does not require the use of immunosuppressive medications, such as cyclosporine or tacrolimus, and radiation therapy is not always used in the preconditioning regimen (Kotloff, Ahya, & Crawford, 2004). A postmortem study of transplant recipients found that pulmonary complications were generally underdiagnosed, so subclinical infections were often untreated (Sharma et al., 2005). Methods that healthcare professionals can use to improve patient outcomes include raising clinical awareness, improving diagnostic methods and processes, shortening time to medical intervention, and continuing interprofessional research. The spectrum of pulmonary complications for transplant recipients will continue to change, as a result of rapid advances in supportive care, older age of transplant recipients, new antiviral and antifungal agents, and an increased use of prophylactic broad-spectrum antibiotics after transplantation (Sharma et al., 2005). Within the past few years, the increased use of reduced-intensity conditioning regimens has reduced toxicities and mortality in older patient populations (Chi et al., 2013; Clavert et al., 2017). However, the real key to decreasing morbidity and mortality in both adult and pediatric HSCT patient populations remains early identification and subsequent effective diagnostic techniques.

Figure 11-1. Typical Onset of Pulmonary Complications Following Hematopoietic Stem Cell Transplantation

Day 0 to Day 30
- Acute respiratory distress syndrome
- Aspergillosis
- Bacteremias of gastrointestinal origin
- Candidemia (*Candida* sepsis) and candidiasis (general *Candida* infections)
- Chemotherapy-associated pulmonary toxicity
- Diffuse alveolar hemorrhage
- Engraftment syndrome
- Idiopathic pneumonia syndrome
- Infections of central venous catheter origin
- Infections related to conditioning regimen and neutropenia
- Pleural effusion
- Pulmonary edema
- Respiratory viruses (respiratory syncytial virus, parainfluenza, influenza)
- Transfusion-related acute lung injury

Day 31 to Day 100
- Acute respiratory distress syndrome
- Aspergillosis
- Chemotherapy-associated pulmonary toxicity
- Classic opportunistic infections
- Cytomegalovirus
- Diffuse alveolar hemorrhage
- Idiopathic pneumonia syndrome
- *Pneumocystis jirovecii* pneumonia
- Pulmonary sinusoidal obstruction syndrome (due to hepatic sinusoidal obstruction syndrome)
- Respiratory viruses (respiratory syncytial virus, parainfluenza, influenza)
- Toxoplasmosis

Greater Than Day 100
- Acute respiratory distress syndrome
- Aspergillosis
- Bronchiolitis obliterans
- Bronchiolitis obliterans organizing pneumonia
- Chemotherapy-associated pulmonary toxicity
- Cytomegalovirus
- Infections from encapsulated organisms
- *Pneumocystis jirovecii* pneumonia
- Pneumonia
- Post-transplant lymphoproliferative disorder
- Respiratory viruses (respiratory syncytial virus, parainfluenza, influenza)
- Varicella zoster virus

Note. Based on information from Antin & Raley, 2013; Camus & Costabel, 2005; Coomes et al., 2011; Olsen et al., 2019; Soubani & Pandya, 2010.

Diagnostics

Diagnostic techniques for pulmonary disease in patients treated with HSCT are similar to those for other patients. Chest x-ray and thoracic computed tomography (CT) scan remain the most popular and least invasive options. CT scans are particularly useful when compared to two-dimensional x-rays because they can expose acute and chronic changes in the lung parenchyma (Ugai et al., 2015). Respiratory CT scans involve capturing images of cross-sections of lung tissue using special reconstruction during inhalation and exhalation. High-resolution CT scans can view smaller cross-sections (1–5 mm in width), as compared to standard CT scans (5 cm in width). The addition of positron-emission tomography (PET) with CT scans has greatly increased the ability of physicians to create a three-dimensional image of the body (Bomanji, Almuhaideb, & Zumla, 2011). Changes such as nodules, nodules with halo signs, atelectasis, a "glassy" appearance, and other tissue or structural abnormalities will prompt the medical team to consider additional diagnostics (Cornetto et al., 2016). This could include collecting sputum samples, bronchoscopy with or without bronchoalveolar lavage (BAL), open lung biopsy, and needle biopsy (Kaplan, Bashoura, Shannon, Dickey, & Stover, 2011).

Sputum samples can be collected by nurses, physicians, or respiratory therapists according to transplant program protocols. Expectorations in the early morning or after a respiratory procedure can be the easiest for the patient to produce because of the natural accumulation of secretions at these times. Approximately 15 ml of sputum is usually required for adequate laboratory analysis, and this sample should reach the laboratory within a few hours from expectoration (Murray, Doherty, Govan, & Hill, 2010).

Sputum can also be collected during a bronchoscopy, which involves visual examination of the larynx, trachea, and bronchi by a respirologist using a fiber-optic bronchoscope. The bronchoscope—a long, thin tube with video and lighting equipment—is inserted into the nose or mouth and allows for inspection of inflammation, bleeding, and tumors. In some cases, BAL will be performed during the bronchoscopy. BAL involves the flushing of fluid (usually a sterile normal saline solution) into a specific area of the lower respiratory tract and immediately suctioning the fluid through the bronchoscope and into a sterile specimen container. BAL allows for the detection and characterization of several respiratory pathogens, including viral, fungal, and bacterial agents. BAL is considered a major diagnostic mechanism for *Pneumocystis jirovecii* (formerly *Pneumocystis carinii*) (Unnewehr, Friederichs, Bartsch, & Schaaf, 2016).

In some cases, a thoracoscopy may be performed to examine the pleural linings of the lungs. This procedure involves insertion of a device with a video camera and other instruments to identify signs of pulmonary disease, such as inflammation, plaques, and thickening. A brush, needle, and forceps are among the tools at the end of the video-assisted thoracoscope, a slightly longer and more rigid device when compared to the bronchoscope. These tools sit aside a suction catheter in the device and allow for the collection of lung tissue (transbronchial biopsy). This is best utilized in the post-HSCT patient when looking for diffuse interstitial lung diseases (O'Dwyer et al., 2018).

Other diagnostic forms of lung tissue biopsy include open lung biopsy and fine-needle aspiration biopsy. An open lung biopsy is performed in an operating room with the patient under general anesthesia, whereby a surgeon removes a small piece of lung tissue. A chest tube is usually placed to allow accumulating fluid to drain. Open lung biopsy is used to diagnose pulmonary fibrosis, tumors, and infectious processes, as well as noninfectious processes, such as bronchiolitis obliterans and cryptogenic organizing pneumonia.

A fine-needle biopsy is an ultrasound or CT-guided technique in which a very small needle collects cells or fluid from under the skin (or tissue surface). In patients with focal pulmonary lesions, aspergillosis, or pulmonary GVHD, fine-needle aspiration biopsy is considered the first-line diagnostic method (G.-S. Cheng et al., 2016; Gupta et al., 2010).

Despite the highly definitive results, a recent retrospective study of HSCT patients revealed a decrease in the use of the lung biopsy in the post-transplantation phase (G.-S. Cheng et al., 2016). Improvements in radiographic techniques and an increased use of extended-spectrum azoles (e.g., fluconazole, posaconazole, voriconazole) have decreased the need for invasive biopsy testing (G.-S. Cheng et al., 2016).

Pulmonary Infections

Pulmonary infections are the most common cause of post-HSCT morbidity, having been reported in more than one-third of patients and carrying a mortality rate of approximately 20%–32% (Afessa et al., 2012; Cooke, Jannin, & Ho, 2008; Diab et al., 2012; Lucena et al., 2014, 2017). The principal cause of infection is the severe immunocompromised status as a result of the disease process (malignant or nonmalignant), conditioning regimens (myeloablative and nonmyeloablative), and immunosuppressive treatments to prevent and treat GVHD. A study of CT scans by Escuissato et al. (2005) found that viral infections were the most common (51%) in transplant recipients, followed by bacterial infections (23%), fungal infections (19%), and protozoal infections (less than 1%). In 5% of the cases examined, patients had two or more infectious agents concurrently (Escuissato et al., 2005). These infections occurred despite prophylaxis with antibiotics and antivirals, particularly during the initial neutropenic period. A more recent study that examined patient charts retrospectively found that rates of fungal infections were far higher than previously thought, but the study showed decreasing infection rates as antifungal drugs were adopted in prophylactic post-transplantation medication regimens (G.-S. Cheng et al., 2016). Research by Meijer et al. (2004) showed that nonmyeloablative conditioning regimens can reduce the risk of pulmonary infection by more than half. However, more recent research indicates that this type of transplantation conditioning is not always possible or successful (Diab et al., 2012).

Sources of infection can include central venous catheters; innate flora of the mouth, gut, and skin; dormant infections; and infections occurring in the hospital environment with interaction between a patient and staff, family, and friends. Additional research has indicated that stem cells themselves are a potential source of infection, with case reports of vancomycin-resistant *Enterococcus* (VRE) and methicillin-resistant *Staphylococcus aureus* (MRSA) (McCann et al., 2004; Shaw, Boswell, Byrne, Yates, & Russell, 2007). Cases of contaminated stem cell units are rare but do require ongoing monitoring for quality, both in the laboratory and at the bedside (Avenoso et al., 2016; Kozlowska-Skrzypczak et al., 2014).

Unfortunately, research has indicated that the spread of viruses is not prevented by the HEPA filtering systems used on many transplantation units (Ullmann et al., 2016). Viruses and bacteria are smaller than 0.3 mcm, and these HEPA filters can remove particles this size or larger. Traditional safety measures such as consistent handwashing, seasonal vaccination, and quick enactment of respiratory precautions for patients who may be getting sick remain the gold standard for prevention of illness and viral transmission.

Ongoing laboratory research focused on immunology has suggested that following donor cell reconstitution, HSCT patients display impaired immune functioning, particularly in lung tissue (Ogonek et al., 2016). Research has shown that slow T-cell reconstitution may be mostly responsible for harmful infections with latent viruses or fungi, as well as for the occurrence of GVHD and disease relapse. This research also confirmed earlier work by Coomes, Hubbard, and Moore (2011), which proposed that weakened clearance of bacterial and viral pulmonary infections results from changes in immune cell function and cytokine production. Accurate and early diagnosis of infectious complications is crucial to improve patient outcomes, particularly in the case of fungal and viral infections, which are associated with poorer prognoses.

Viral Infections

Awareness of respiratory viruses as a cause of morbidity and mortality after HSCT is increasing (Law & Kumar, 2017; Sim et al., 2018). Viral respiratory tract infections may occur in as many as 3.6%–30% of transplant recipients as determined by viral culture (van Kraaij et al., 2005). The respiratory viruses most commonly identified following transplantation are rhinovirus (strains A, B, and C), respiratory syncytial virus (RSV), human parainfluenza virus (HPIV), and influenza types A and B (Latchford & Shelton, 2003; Saria & Gosselin-Acomb, 2007). Retrospective studies have also identified coronaviruses, including the virus that causes severe acute respiratory syndrome (SARS) and adenovirus as increasingly responsible for viral respiratory tract infections, particularly in patients who have received allogeneic HSCT (Chemaly, Shah, & Boeckh, 2014; Shah, Ghantoji, Mulanovich, Ariza-Heredia, & Chemaly, 2012). In recent years, human metapneumovirus (HMPV) has emerged as a growing concern in the development of quickly progressing pneumonia in post-HSCT populations (Franquet et al., 2005; Shah, Shah, Azzi, El Chaer, & Chemaly, 2016). Human metapneumovirus has also been associated with the development of subsequent bacterial superinfections that are particularly difficult to treat (Ogimi et al., 2019).

Since 2009, concern has increased regarding the H1N1 virus (influenza A subtype) and its successive genetic mutations. According to Ljungman et al. (2011), H1N1 and subsequent new influenza A strains can cause "significant morbidity and even mortality" (p. 1234) in HSCT patients. New molecular testing research by Sim et al. (2018) indicated that rhinoviruses were the most common respiratory viruses infecting HSCT patients. Patients can acquire a respiratory viral infection at any time during the transplantation process. Patients most often acquire viruses from family members, healthcare professionals, or the community. Respiratory viruses infect the epithelium of the upper and lower respiratory tract, resulting in inflammation and possible necrosis. Clinical presentation for viral respiratory tract infections usually includes varying degrees of rhinitis, pharyngitis, malaise, inflammation and irritation of the nasal membranes (coryza), and cough (Peck et al., 2007). Fever can occur in a viral respiratory infection depending on the type of virus and a host of other factors, but research on HSCT patients in the past decade has shown that 13%–85% have at least one febrile episode (Chughtai, Wang, Dung, & Macintyre, 2017; Law & Kumar, 2017). Chest radiographic findings are often nonspecific, and the presence of an associated bacterial infection should be considered (Law & Kumar, 2017).

Respiratory syncytial virus: RSV is classified as a pneumovirus; the usual incubation period is one to four days. RSV is seasonal, with infections typically occurring in winter and spring. Recent studies suggest that up to 12% of HSCT patients develop a respiratory infection caused by RSV (Abbas, Raybould, Sastry, & de la Cruz, 2017). Approximately 50% of these transplant recipients infected with RSV will develop lower tract disease (Avetisyan, Mattsson, Sparrelid, & Ljungman, 2009; Campbell et al., 2015; Neemann & Freifeld, 2015). Rates for contracting and becoming ill from RSV infections are significantly higher in pediatric post-HSCT populations (Anak et al., 2010). Symptoms of RSV infection include rhinorrhea, high fever, cough, and nasal congestion, which can rapidly lead to pneumonia in some patients (Girmenia, Rossolini, & Viscoli, 2017; Seo & Boeckh, 2016). RSV pneumonia has an estimated mortality rate greater than 30% in post-HSCT patients, with higher rates in pediatric populations (Anak et al., 2010; Ljungman, 2014). It should be noted that upper respiratory infection is more irksome than dangerous, as compared to the progression of RSV into the lower respiratory tract. Boeckh (2008) noted that clinical data suggested post-transplantation lymphopenia as an important factor in the transfer of RSV infection from the upper respiratory tract (rhinitis, epiglottitis, laryngitis) to the lower respiratory tract (bronchitis, pneumonia). Combined regions of infection can facilitate potentially fatal complications, particularly regarding comorbidities or development of coinfections.

Parainfluenza: HPIVs belong to the *Paramyxoviridae* family of enveloped RNA viruses. For many decades they were classified into three serotypes: HPIV-1, HPIV-2, and HPIV-3. HPIV-1 and HPIV-3 are the most common, responsible for the majority of respiratory infections, including croup, pneumonia, and bronchiolitis. Recent innovations in the diagnosis and laboratory detection of viral components have revealed additional serotypes HPIV-4 (with subtypes 4a and 4b) and a possible HPIV-5 (J.V. Williams, Piedra, & Englund, 2017). Parainfluenza was first described in the 1950s in an effort to distinguish these viruses from myxoviruses (e.g., influenza), as the *para* indicates they are outside the other class of influenza viruses. HPIV has an incubation period of one to seven days, and approximately 22% of patients experiencing infection will develop pneumonia (McCann et al., 2004). Symptoms of HPIV infection include rhinorrhea, high fever, cough, nasal congestion, and sinusitis (Miller, 2019). Particularly virulent outbreaks of HPIV-3 among post-HSCT patients have resulted in shocking mortality rates, leading researchers to suggest prompt administration of broad-spectrum antimicrobials (Hodson, Kasliwal, Streetly, MacMahon, & Raj, 2011). Currently, no effective treatment strategies are available for HPIV infections in HSCT patients, but research continues with experimental medications that could decrease infection times and complications. DAS181, a sialidase protein given as an inhaler, has shown some promise when used by transplant recipients with HPIV infection (Salvatore et al., 2016).

Influenza: Influenza capable of infecting humans was previously classified into three major types: A, B, and C. Influenza D only affects cattle. Influenza A is divided into subtypes based on the proteins that appear on the viral surface: hemagglutinin (H) and neuraminidase (N). Currently, 18 hemagglutinin subtypes and 11 neuraminidase subtypes have been identified, and the name of the virus indicates which protein subtypes are present (e.g., H1N1, H3N2). Influenza B is divided into two subgroups: B/Yamagata and B/Victoria. Recent pandemics of influenza A, starting with H1N1 (swine flu) in 2008 and 2009, resulted in a variety of paradigm changes around infectious disease transmission and control (Chughtai et al., 2017). The incubation period for influenza averages two days; symptoms include cough, rhinorrhea, and nasal congestion with or without high fever (Miller, 2019). Respiratory involvement with many types of influenza is pronounced and quick, with upper respiratory symptoms moving quickly into the lungs within a matter of hours in immunocompromised patients. High fevers and pneumonia are classic features. For patients who are compromised following transplantation, an influenza infection can be dangerous and potentially fatal. The common influenza vaccination is given to prevent these infections, but it is not active against HPIV.

Other viruses: Several additional viral infections, such as Epstein-Barr virus reactivation with associated pulmonary post-transplantation lymphoproliferative disorder, herpes simplex virus, and varicella zoster virus, can occur in HSCT patients. Despite a lull in activity, a recent resurgence of Epstein-Barr virus has occurred and is responsible for an increasing number of respiratory infections (Piralla et al., 2016).

Prevention and treatment: Continued study into prevention of viral respiratory infections in HSCT patients has resulted in several recommendations, including testing patients for viruses before transplantation and delaying transplantation if a virus is present (Campbell et al., 2015). Because of increasing virulence of these infections, several HSCT programs have added testing for viral infections by polymerase chain reaction when a patient develops an initial neutropenic fever or presents with any new-onset upper respiratory symptoms (Claus, Hodowanec, & Singh, 2015). Standard treatment of respiratory viral pneumonia is supportive care. Aerosolized or oral ribavirin has been increasingly effective in treating and clearing respiratory viruses and simultaneously decreasing mortality (Chemaly, Aitken, Wolfe, Jain, & Boeckh, 2016). However, ribavirin remains one of the only treatments for HSCT patients with viral pneumonia and, despite its high cost, can be administered for situations in which patients have no other option (Chemaly et al., 2016; Shah et al., 2014). Patients who develop respiratory viral pneumonia prior to engraftment have poorer outcomes (Girmenia et al., 2017).

During the respiratory virus season, all HSCT patients are at particular risk for developing infections. Patient and family education are vital in preventing the spread of respiratory viruses (Abbas et al., 2017). Families need to understand the potential implications of sick friends and relatives visiting HSCT patients. Practicing good handwashing technique is the most effective measure for preventing the spread of respiratory viruses. Vaccinating family members and medical staff against influenza may help to control exposure. A study corresponding with the 2008 H1N1 outbreak revealed that cluster of differentiation 8–positive cells increased slightly after vaccination in immunocompromised HSCT patients (Avetisyan, Aschan, Hassan, & Ljungman, 2008). Traditional recommendations suggested that HSCT patients wait six months after transplantation to receive an influenza vaccine. New research, however, suggests that patients receiving the vaccine earlier have greater benefits (Sokol et al., 2017).

Cytomegalovirus

Perhaps the most insidious viral infection in the HSCT population is CMV, which can attack pulmonary tissue, as well as genitourinary and gastrointestinal systems, retina, liver, and central nervous system (Razonable, 2018). CMV infection is defined as isolation of the CMV virus in tissue culture; CMV disease is defined as a symptomatic CMV infection (Ljungman et al., 2006). As a member of the herpesvirus family, CMV is also known as HCMV or human herpesvirus 5. According to some estimates, 40%–80% of adults in the United States and 60%–99% of adults globally test seropositive for the immunoglobulin G antibody

to CMV (Centers for Disease Control and Prevention, 2019; J. Cheng et al., 2009). The Centers for Disease Control and Prevention (2019) reports that one in three children is already infected with CMV by the age of five years. After infection, the virus remains latent in the body and usually only reactivates in the presence of immunosuppression from medications, chemotherapy, cancer, bone marrow diseases (e.g., myelodysplastic syndromes), and infections that compromise the immune system (e.g., HIV) (Centers for Disease Control and Prevention, 2019).

An estimated 10% of HSCT patients will develop a CMV infection (Locatelli, Bertaina, Bertaina, & Merli, 2016). The presence of CMV is widespread in the allogeneic transplant population, with opportunistic infection developing between two and six months after transplantation. Because of the danger of CMV, all patients are and should be screened for CMV immunity as part of the conditioning regimen (George et al., 2010). Those at highest risk for severe post-transplantation CMV infection are CMV-positive patients who receive CMV-seronegative donor cells and those who received T-cell–depleted or umbilical cord blood (UCB) grafts (Ljungman et al., 2003). As a result of the profound immunosuppression required for HSCT, CMV reactivation is a risk (Antin & Raley, 2013). Previous thinking held that all HSCT patients should receive leukocyte-reduced or CMV-seronegative red blood cells and platelets to prevent transfusion-associated infections; however, recent research has supported that CMV unselected blood products do not increase risk of CMV infection in the post-transplantation period (Antin & Raley, 2013; Hall et al., 2015; Peters et al., 2015). In a landmark study, Kekre et al. (2013) found that the presence of CMV in blood products did not adequately predict if the recipient would become CMV positive. The study also found that, even with transfusing CMV-negative blood, HSCT patients still acquired CMV (Kekre et al., 2013). Other risk factors for CMV include ethnicity, socioeconomic status, advanced age, and female sex (Han, 2007; Litjens, van der Wagen, Kuball, & Kwekkeboom, 2018). The highest risk period for developing a CMV infection is days 30–100 after transplantation (acute phase), with higher rates noted in patients with GVHD and delayed T-cell recovery (Ariza-Heredia, Nesher, & Chemaly, 2014). Recent research by Litjens et al. (2018) has suggested that CMV infection may be paradoxically beneficial for patients with acute myeloid leukemia receiving an allogeneic HSCT that used T cell and natural killer cell replete grafts. In only these cases, and not in other hematologic cancers, CMV reactivation is associated with protection from a leukemic relapse (Litjens et al., 2018).

CMV pneumonia is defined as progressive interstitial infiltrates on chest x-ray with concurrent evidence of CMV infection, such as a positive tissue culture (J. Cheng et al., 2009). Symptoms of CMV pneumonia include fever, nonproductive cough, dyspnea, hypoxemia, and diffuse interstitial infiltrates on chest x-ray (Ljungman et al., 2006). CMV pneumonia is usually treated with antivirals, such as ganciclovir or foscarnet (Erard et al., 2015). In some cases, immunoglobulin can be administered to foster an appropriate immune response.

Ganciclovir is an acyclic nucleoside analog of guanine and is a potent inhibitor of CMV replication (Tomblyn et al., 2009). The drug is carcinogenic and teratogenic; therefore, it requires hazardous drug precautions. The healthcare team will carefully monitor the patient's complete blood count and electrolyte profile. As with all cytotoxic medications, pancytopenia is possible, and dosage adjustments may be needed. Ganciclovir is almost entirely renally excreted, so patients must be well hydrated to prevent kidney damage. In some cases of suspected renal failure, ganciclovir dosing may be reduced for patients with renal insufficiency. Serum creatinine and creatinine clearance should be monitored at least weekly (Wilkes & Barton-Burke, 2018).

In the event of severe neutropenia or if the CMV infection fails to respond to the ganciclovir, foscarnet can be administered. Because of its highly nephrotoxic nature and high cost, it is not used as a first-line treatment. Foscarnet causes severe electrolyte imbalances and requires pre- and postadministration hydration with replacement of electrolytes. CMV-specific hyperimmunoglobulin (Cytogam®) continues to be investigated when compared to normal human IV immunoglobulin because of conflicting reports regarding its efficacy (Ariza-Heredia et al., 2014). Improved survival rates have been reported when CMV pneumonia is treated early with Cytogam, but the cost is extraordinary (Ljungman et al., 2006).

CMV surveillance and prophylactic therapy are two standard approaches for preventing infection and decreasing CMV complications after HSCT (Girmenia, 2019). To detect reactivation early, weekly CMV screening for CMV-seropositive patients should commence after transplantation (Antin & Raley, 2013; Tomblyn et al., 2009). Along with screening, the initiation of proactive antiviral prophylaxis over the past decade has reduced the rate of CMV reactivation from a high of 70% to 20%–40% among CMV-seropositive patients who received allogeneic transplant (Ljungman et al., 2006). The most common medications used for CMV prophylaxis are IV ganciclovir or, preferably, oral valganciclovir. However, both medications can cause pancytopenia, which is particularly concerning given the relatively fragile nature of the stem cell graft. Other novel antiviral medications, such as letermovir, seem to be well tolerated with minimal myelotoxicity or nephrotoxicity (Razonable, 2018).

Bacterial Infections

Increased use of prophylactic oral and IV antibiotics has significantly decreased the occurrence of pulmonary infections caused by bacterial agents in HSCT patients (Horton, Haste, & Taplitz, 2018). Additionally, use of nonmyeloablative conditioning has been associated with lower infection rates in several studies (Gjærde, Moser, & Sengeløv, 2017; Meijer et al., 2004). Bacterial infections are found frequently in autologous and allogeneic transplant recipients; however, research suggests that the risk of mortality from bacterial infection is much higher in allogeneic transplant recipients and in those who experience GVHD (Hardak et al., 2016; McCann et al., 2004; Styczynski et al., 2016). Although the reasons for this are not entirely clear, researchers speculate that it could be related to immunosuppression and altered immune responses following an allogeneic transplant (Hardak et al., 2016; Styczynski et al., 2016). Early post-HSCT infections are commonly caused by the patient's own flora that proliferate during the neutropenic period. Other risk factors during this stage include mucosal damage caused by the chemotherapy or radiation therapy conditioning regimen and the presence of a central venous catheter (Abugideiri et al., 2016; Balian, Garcia, & Ward, 2018). Researchers have also found that patients with pretransplantation gut colonization by multidrug-resistant bacteria (e.g., VRE, carbapenem-resistant gram-negative bacteria) are more susceptible to bacterial bloodstream infections (Ferreira et al., 2018). Late post-HSCT infections can be related to the ongoing use of immunosuppressive medications and GVHD. Research by Rieger et al. (2009) did not show any significant difference in bacterial infection rates between related and unrelated matched allogeneic transplant recipients.

Specific organisms common in post-transplantation patients include gram-positive bacteria, such as *Streptococcus* species, MRSA, *Staphylococcus* species, VRE, and *Clostridium difficile* (Engelhard et al., 2009; Freifeld, Zimmer, Zhang, & Meza, 2017; Srinivasan et al., 2013). Pulmonary bacterial infections are most commonly from gram-positive organisms, constituting more than 30% of cases in a recent study using bronchoscopy with BAL alongside classic and molecular polymerase chain reaction detection methods (Aguilar-Guisado et al., 2011; Chi et al., 2014; Freifeld et al., 2017; Wang, Wang, Fan, Tang, & Hu, 2015). Gram-negative bacteria, such as *Legionella* series and *Pseudomonas*, are rarer in post-transplantation respiratory infections, but *Pseudomonas* is increasing in frequency and requires more attention in diagnostics and pharmacology (Hardak et al., 2016; Hofmeister, Czerlanis, Forsythe, & Stiff, 2006). This reflects a parallel increase in nosocomial *Pseudomonas* infections over the past 20 years, and some researchers have speculated that this could be the result of the opportunistic organism's unique ability to thrive in marginal environments (Kossow et al., 2017). In many cases, respiratory complications include acute bronchitis and pneumonia. Polymicrobial pulmonary infections are often more dangerous and harder to treat than monomicrobial infections, with current statistics indicating a 50% mortality rate for HSCT patients who develop a polymicrobial pneumonia (Hardak et al., 2016). In fact, research has shown that a bacterial infection can increase the mortality of fungal or viral infections (Piñana et al., 2018). Treatment includes broad-spectrum and multimodal antibiotics, oxygen therapy, and mechanical ventilation in extreme cases in which the infection has progressed to a critical level.

Preventing bacterial infection begins with education of patients, family members, friends, and staff. Scrupulous handwashing, providing rapid isolation of individuals with highly communicable infections (e.g., MRSA, VRE, *C. difficile*), and restricting sick staff members or visitors from the transplantation unit constitute sound infection control policies (McCann et al., 2004). Nurses are crucial in assessing patients for symptoms of bacterial infection and should perform routine laboratory tests as necessary. Nurses should closely assess and monitor patients for symptoms of progressing respiratory disease, noting decreased breath sounds on auscultation, appearance of a productive cough with colored sputum, and worsening fever. Antibiotics should be initiated as soon as possible. Studies have demonstrated that the commencing of antibiotics as quickly as possible after the onset of a fever can significantly affect length of hospital stay and possible mortality (Perron, Emara, & Ahmed, 2014).

Fungal Infections

Invasive fungal diseases are a major obstacle to patients after HSCT and are a significant cause of pulmonary-related mortality (Ji et al., 2011; Penack et al., 2016). *Aspergillus* is the most common and virulent fungal cause of pneumonia after HSCT (Kosmidis & Denning, 2015). Other fungal respiratory infections in post-HSCT patients, particularly those receiving myeloablative conditioning, include *Malassezia*, zygomycota, and *Candida* species (Kosmidis & Denning, 2015). Over the past decade, a sudden and devastating increase in mucormycosis, a dangerous fungal disease caused by *Mucorales*, has demonstrated an overall mortality rate of about 50% (Danion et al., 2015). Growth in fungal infections has been devastating for many patient populations, but particularly those HSCT patients who are immunocompromised. Several new antifungal medications have demonstrated increased success, showing improved remission rates and thereby decreasing morbidity.

Pulmonary aspergillosis, also known as invasive pulmonary aspergillosis, is a major cause of morbidity and mortality for post-HSCT patients, particularly those who received allogeneic transplants (Samanta & Nguyen, 2017). The incidence varies between regions, with wetter and more humid climates reporting higher rates of fungal infections (Vallabhaneni, Benedict, Derado, & Mody, 2017). Depending on a variety of environmental factors, periodic outbreaks do occur. The mortality rate from *Aspergillus* pneumonia is estimated to be approaching 30%–90% (Bissinger et al., 2005; Jenks & Hoenigl, 2018; Samanta & Nguyen, 2017; Yao & Liao, 2006).

Research into T-cell activity in the past several years has revealed that these cells are a crucial defense mechanism against fungal infections. With the destruction and slow recovery of T cells subsequent to HSCT, voracious fungal spores such as *Aspergillus* have time to multiply rapidly,

overwhelming already weakened immune defenses in the recipient (Tramsen et al., 2009). Risk factors for an HSCT patient to develop aspergillosis include prolonged granulocytopenia, the presence of GVHD, prolonged immunosuppression, human leukocyte antigen (HLA) mismatch, construction near the hospital or a windy external environment, certain foods and plants, and high-dose corticosteroid therapy (Castagnola et al., 2008; Yao & Liao, 2006).

Aspergillosis is primarily contracted by inhalation of *Aspergillus* spores. Teaching should begin early in the transplantation process and include ways to prevent possible exposure, including avoiding areas with high concentrations of dust during the pretransplantation period and avoiding contact with fresh plants, dried plants, or moss. For this reason, most transplantation units are equipped with HEPA filtration systems, which ensure that patients are not exposed to contaminants from outside air. An environmental study at a transplantation unit directly exposed to an active construction site found that the HEPA system was capable of filtering out most, if not all, of the *Aspergillus* spores in the external atmosphere (Nihtinen et al., 2007).

The onset of aspergillosis typically occurs in a bimodal distribution at a median of either 16 days or 96 days after transplantation (Bissinger et al., 2005; Yao & Liao, 2006). The symptoms of *Aspergillus* pneumonia include fever, dyspnea, dry cough, wheezing, pleuritic chest pain, and occasionally, hemoptysis (Yao & Liao, 2006). Although closely resembling other lower respiratory diseases, fungal infection should be suspected in patients who are persistently febrile despite receiving three to five days of broad-spectrum antibiotics. The initial diagnosis can be made via radiography. A chest x-ray will vary from diffuse infiltrates to local infiltrates and cavitating lesions (Yao & Liao, 2006). The CT scan will show a halo surrounding the nodular lesions containing the focal aspergillosis (Patterson et al., 2016; Yao & Liao, 2006). As the disease progresses, these lesions expand to become larger consolidations and cavitary masses. BAL fluid can be useful in diagnosing fungal infections such as aspergillosis, but its use is limited by the minimal amount of mold that can be collected in the drainage and the increased risk of bleeding seen in post-HSCT patients who undergo the procedure (Bissinger et al., 2005; Yao & Liao, 2006).

Aspergillosis is finally diagnosed by tissue culture if the patient can tolerate a transbronchial biopsy and if the *Aspergillus* species is one of the few that can grow in culture (Patterson et al., 2016). A pathologist can usually see the actual fungus on microscopic inspection of the tissue. This visual confirmation coupled with positive serum galactomannan (*Aspergillus* antigen) and halo lesions on a CT scan confirms diagnosis (Patterson et al., 2016). Galactomannan has become a useful method in confirming *Aspergillus* infection in high-risk patients, such as those on steroids or UCB recipients. Some institutions have initiated routine weekly screening in these high-risk groups for the purpose of early detection (Hovi et al., 2007; Nguyen et al., 2011).

Suspected and confirmed fungal infections should be treated empirically. The first-line treatment for infiltrating pulmonary aspergillosis is triazoles, such as fluconazole, itraconazole, isavuconazole, voriconazole, and posaconazole suspension (Lionakis, Lewis, & Kontoyiannis, 2018; Patterson et al., 2016). Voriconazole is highly active against *Aspergillus* species and has replaced amphotericin as a first-line antifungal in many HSCT protocols (Jenks & Hoenigl, 2018; Lortholary et al., 2010; Marr et al., 2009; van de Peppel, Visser, Dekkers, & de Boer, 2018; Wilson, Drew, & Perfect, 2009). Because of concerns related to hepatotoxicity with voriconazole, posaconazole has been replacing voriconazole in some HSCT protocols, but more particularly as pre-HSCT prophylaxis and in salvage regimens (Jenks & Hoenigl, 2018; Kyriakidis, Tragiannidis, Munchen, & Groll, 2017; van de Peppel et al., 2018) Fluconazole and itraconazole are less effective against *Aspergillus* and should be used only when a coinfection with *Candida* is suspected (Yao & Liao, 2006). The literature suggests increased use of posaconazole for aspergillosis in the past few years because of increased efficacy and lower rates of drug resistance (Lionakis et al., 2018). Unfortunately, increased aspergillosis resistance to azoles internationally has created the need to explore additional treatment options (Chowdhary, Sharma, & Meis, 2017; Lionakis et al., 2018).

If a patient is not able to tolerate triazole treatment, the Collaborative Exchange of Antifungal Research (CLEAR) outcome study recommended the use of amphotericin B deoxycholate, or if the patient cannot tolerate this drug, liposomal amphotericin B (AmBisome®) formulations can be used with fewer side effects and lowered renal toxicity rates (Patterson et al., 2016; Yao & Liao, 2006). CLEAR outcomes show a cure rate of 61% for *Aspergillus* lung infections for solid organ transplant populations, with HSCT patients showing slightly decreased rates (Marr et al., 2009; Yao & Liao, 2006). Amphotericin B can be delivered as an IV infusion, and liposomal amphotericin B can be given as an IV infusion or nebulized aerosol (Stone, Bicanic, Salim, & Hope, 2016). Amphotericin B side effects include sudden high fever, severe rigors, and nephrotoxicity. Acute side effects can be reduced and, in many cases, eliminated with premedications, including acetaminophen and diphenhydramine. Serum creatinine and blood urea nitrogen levels should be monitored for signs of renal impairment. Ongoing research in the past decade has expanded the arsenal of treatments for *Aspergillus* infection in the post-HSCT setting beyond azole regimens. Some centers report using an azole–amphotericin combination (Lionakis et al., 2018). More commonly, however, the echinocandin drug class (e.g., caspofungin, anidulafungin, micafungin) is used as prophylaxis during induction chemotherapy, as well as for HSCT in the pre-engraftment period when triazole and polyene antifungals are contraindicated by toxicity or pharmaceutical interactions (Lionakis et al., 2018; Patterson et al., 2016).

In fact, a growing number of organizations are proposing that echinocandins, particularly caspofungin, be used instead of amphotericin B (Tissot et al., 2017). Caspofungin is often used as a first-line therapy for pulmonary invasive fungal infections and shows great efficacy against both *Candida* and *Aspergillus* (Tissot et al., 2017). Micafungin is increasingly used to treat infiltrating pulmonary aspergillosis in combination with an azole, most commonly isavuconazole (Petraitis et al., 2017). This combination has become popular because some species of *Aspergillus*, particularly *A. fumigates*, appear to have mutated against micafungin, so physicians are looking to supplement micafungin or avoid using it altogether (Jiménez-Ortigosa, Moore, Denning, & Perlin, 2017).

When pharmacologic therapies fail, surgical interventions may be an option for patients with invasive chronic pulmonary aspergillosis (Denning et al., 2016). Lung resection, including lobectomies, wedge resectioning, and enucleation, can be an option for a limited number of neutropenic patients. Radical surgical debridement is also an option, particularly if used in conjunction with antifungal medication (Yao & Liao, 2006).

Prophylactic use of antifungals has become standard for HSCT patients, with many post-transplantation regimens including voriconazole (Marr et al., 2009; Patterson et al., 2016). An increase in drug resistance to azoles may be the result of overuse in prophylaxis (Chowdhary et al., 2017). Current research involves the practical growth and transmission of active cytokine-producing anti-*Aspergillus* CD4+ T cells to patients before and after HSCT as a method of combating invasive pulmonary aspergillosis (Beck et al., 2008). A new echinocandin called biafungin (CD101) has demonstrated promising effectiveness against disseminated aspergillosis, but further clinical trials with human participants are needed (Chowdhary et al., 2017; Krishnan et al., 2017; Patterson et al., 2016).

Mucormycosis: Over the past decade, HSCT patients have become increasingly susceptible to developing mucormycosis, a fungal infection caused by *Mucorales*, an order zygomycete fungi. Most cases manifest in the lungs or as rhino-orbito-cerebral infections. They develop more frequently in HSCT patients, as well as those with diabetes mellitus or solid organ transplant recipients (Danion et al., 2015). Mucormycosis and aspergillosis are similar in presentation, and prompt diagnosis by bronchial endoscopy and lung biopsy is necessary to improve outcomes. CT scan of the lungs will show a reversed halo sign, and improvements around diagnosis include a serum blood test for quantitative polymerase chain reaction to detect *Mucorales* DNA (Danion et al., 2015). Current treatment recommendations include liposomal amphotericin in combination with surgery. When mucormycosis brings about neurologic involvement, high-dose liposomal amphotericin with posaconazole as maintenance therapy is recommended (Danion et al., 2015). Echinocandins do not show any activity against *Mucorales*. Mortality from mucormycosis is as high as 90% (Cruz et al., 2016). Strategies to improve treatment options include a push to develop T-cell immunotherapies customized for post-HSCT patients (Cruz et al., 2016).

Pneumocystis Jirovecii Pneumonia

Pneumocystis jirovecii is an opportunistic fungus that can cause a serious pneumonia—*P. jirovecii* pneumonia (PJP)—and fulminant respiratory failure in immunocompromised patients after HSCT (Gea-Banacloche et al., 2009; K.M. Williams et al., 2014). With allogeneic transplant recipients, cases can occur as early as 30 days after transplantation, with major risk factors being lymphopenia and HLA mismatch (K.M. Williams, Ahn, et al., 2016). Definitive diagnosis is made by microbiologic identification, based on positive staining of induced sputum or BAL (Aliouat-Denis et al., 2008; K.M. Williams, Ahn, et al., 2016). This fungus can attach to type I alveolar epithelial cells and proliferate quickly, causing serious pneumonitis (Aliouat-Denis et al., 2008). Symptoms include a dry cough, fever, tachypnea, and escalating dyspnea. Chest x-ray reveals a diffuse interstitial alveolar pneumonia that typically affects the bilateral lower lobes symmetrically. The median time to onset of PJP is two months after transplantation (Tomblyn et al., 2009). A recent retrospective study of autologous and allogeneic recipients showed that PJP, although rare, can occur in a variety of conditions and that GVHD and steroids are risk factors (K.M. Williams et al., 2014).

PJP is generally preventable with prophylactic medications, such as trimethoprim-sulfamethoxazole (TMP-SMX) (Sweiss et al., 2018). Common side effects of TMP-SMX are dermatitis, oral candidiasis, and myelosuppression (K.M. Williams, Ahn, et al., 2016; Yoshida & Ohno, 2004). Prophylaxis should be administered from engraftment for at least six months following transplantation or for as long as the patient is receiving immunosuppressive therapy or has chronic GVHD (Tomblyn et al., 2009). Most centers administer PJP prophylaxis during HSCT conditioning and stop it a few days before transplantation (Cooley et al. 2014; Neumann, Krause, Maschmeyer, Schiel, & von Lilienfeld-Toal, 2013; K.M. Williams, Ahn, et al., 2016). The rationale for this schedule is to reduce PJP burden on patients as they move into increased immunosuppression from conditioning. In addition, prophylactic medications used for PJP can cause further blood count suppression and, thus, contribute to severe pancytopenia, as well as potentially damage transplanted cells (K.M. Williams, Ahn, et al., 2016). Retrospective research suggests continuing PJP prophylaxis for those with GVHD, steroid exposure, or poor immune function can increase survival rates (K.M. Williams et al., 2014).

Alternative agents used for PJP include aerosolized or IV pentamidine, dapsone, atovaquone, clindamycin, and pyrimethamine, but clindamycin and pyrimethamine are no longer commonly used (Crozier, 2011; K.M. Williams, Ahn, et al., 2016). Dapsone has been used in HSCT patients

with sulfonamides allergies. According to a recent study, dapsone for PJP prophylaxis should be started on day +28 at a dosage of 100 mg per day (Abidi, Kozlowski, Ibrahim, & Peres, 2006). Complications from dapsone are very rare but can be severe and include fever, methemoglobinemia, hemolytic anemia, and severe exfoliative dermatitis (Abidi et al., 2006). The primary advantage in using aerosolized pentamidine is that it requires only monthly administration and can be useful for patients who demonstrate poor adherence to oral TMP-SMX or cannot take TMP-SMX or dapsone because of allergies or side effects (Shankar & Nania, 2007; K.M. Williams, Ahn, et al., 2016). However, some researchers have suggested that aerosolized pentamidine be used with caution because of a significant risk of toxic epidermal necrolysis (Watarai, Niiyama, Amoh, & Katsuoka, 2009). A short course of corticosteroids is the gold standard treatment for moderate to severe cases of PJP. Corticosteroids, such as dexamethasone, hydrocortisone, or methylprednisolone, should be initiated within the first 72 hours after diagnosis of PJP to increase efficacy (Shankar & Nania, 2007).

Unspecified Pulmonary Infections

Several pulmonary infections are unspecified in their etiology. These include infection-associated alveolar hemorrhage (IAH) and bronchiolitis obliterans. It should be noted that bronchiolitis obliterans can also occur without the presence of an underlying infection and, for this reason, is discussed in more detail later in this chapter.

The occurrence of IAH in post-transplantation patients has been identified in approximately 4%–6% of this population (Majhail, Parks, Defor, & Weisdorf, 2006). Associated with high mortality rates, IAH can be positively identified one week after an alveolar hemorrhage event in which microorganisms can be isolated in the blood, BAL, or tracheal aspirate (Majhail et al., 2006). Myeloablative conditioning, allogeneic transplant, advanced age, and acute GVHD constitute significant risk factors. IAH is found in higher rates in patients receiving UCB as a donor source, as well as total body irradiation (TBI) during pretransplantation conditioning. The probability of 60-day survival from the onset of hemorrhage was 32%, with slightly increased survivability in patients who received corticosteroids and appropriate medications for the infectious agent (Majhail et al., 2006).

Chemotherapy-Related Pulmonary Toxicity

Damage to the lungs can occur from the administration of chemotherapy as part of a pretransplantation induction or preconditioning regimen (Schwaiblmair et al., 2012). Injury ranges from short-term reversible conditions, such as reactive airway disease, to chronic fibrosis and permanent structural deterioration. Recent studies have estimated that 1%–8% of HSCT patients experience some level of chemotherapy-related pulmonary toxicity (Chernecky, 2009). The increasing use of multimodal and multitargeted therapies over the past decade has amplified patient longevity, concurrently escalating the incidence of pulmonary toxicity.

Chemotherapy-related pulmonary toxicities are divided into acute, undefined, and chronic (Olsen, LeFebvre, & Brassil, 2019). They include interstitial lung disease, alveolar hemorrhage, pleural effusions, pulmonary alveolar proteinosis, and pulmonary sinusoidal obstruction syndrome (SOS). These diseases also occur with radiation treatment and the post-transplantation engraftment process and can be associated with GVHD. It is unclear if pulmonary changes are related exclusively to disease, transplant rejection, chemotherapy, radiation, or a combination of factors. Research on individual chemotherapy agents has yielded specific cases of pulmonary toxicity, but beyond this information, the precise etiology of pulmonary damage can be difficult to ascertain (Olsen et al., 2019; Schwaiblmair et al., 2012). The chemotherapies used in HSCT conditioning have been associated with pulmonary toxicity (see Figure 11-2).

Alkylating Agents

Busulfan is commonly included in preparative regimens for related and unrelated allogeneic transplant. Initially used as a single agent in the 1960s for chronic myeloid leukemia, rare but serious pulmonary complications, known as *busulfan lung*, were observed (Camus & Costabel, 2005; Cho et al., 2007; Smalley & Wall, 1966). Busulfan lung can occur any time from a few months to 10 years after treatment and can be described as a progressive and often fatal pneumonitis (Camus & Costabel, 2005). The onset of pneumonitis is insidious, involving a progressive cough, low-grade fever, and dyspnea. In extreme cases, it progresses to interstitial pulmonary fibrosis, for which no successful treatment is available. Treatment focuses on comfort measures and includes corticosteroids and oxygen therapy. Early detection through baseline pulmonary function tests (PFTs) and chest x-rays for the onset of symptoms remains the cardinal goal.

Cyclophosphamide is another common chemotherapy agent currently integrated in HSCT preparative regimens. Although the incidence of pulmonary toxicity is rare, diffuse alveolar damage can occur within the first 48 days. Studies have failed to show a relationship between toxicity, dose, and duration of administration (Specks, 2019). Recent research has demonstrated an increase in cyclophosphamide-induced lung disease in allogeneic transplant recipients who have received concomitant methotrexate as GVHD prophylaxis (Specks, 2019). Accumulation of the metabolite acrolein causes lipid peroxidation, which can erode the lipid layer in the interstitium of the lungs and cause microvascular damage (Specks, 2019). This, in turn, causes pulmonary edema, alveolar hemorrhage, fibrin deposition, and finally, fibrosis. Research has shown that cyclophosphamide can reduce the diffusion capacity of the lung for carbon monoxide (DLCO), thus making PFT alterations a significant predictor for agent-related

pulmonary toxicity (Hamada et al., 2003). Corticosteroid use at the first signs of pulmonary damage can result in a good response if initiated early in the disease process (Baxter Healthcare Corporation, 2013).

Melphalan is used in pretransplantation conditioning regimens for myeloma, specifically as part of the BEAM regimen (carmustine, etoposide, cytarabine, and melphalan), and for lymphoproliferative disorders in adults. It is the primary conditioning agent in autologous pediatric neuroblastoma protocols. Melphalan-induced pneumonitis is rare and results from epithelial dysplasia that occurs with infusion (Taetle, Dickman, & Feldman, 1978). Corticosteroids can be used to halt pneumonitis at an early stage and to decrease dysplastic damage of late pulmonary toxicity (Aspen Pharmacare Canada, 2019; Camus & Costabel, 2005). Acute hypersensitivity reactions occur in approximately 2.4% of cases when administered before transplantation to patients with myeloma (Aspen Pharmacare Canada, 2019). This type of reaction is dose limit-

---

Figure 11-2. Oncology Medications With Potential Pulmonary Toxicity

- All-trans retinoic acid
- Amphotericin B
- Antithymocyte globulin
- Arsenic trioxide
- Bleomycin
- Bortezomib
- Busulfan
- Carmustine
- Chlorambucil
- Colony-stimulating factors
- Corticosteroids
- Cyclophosphamide
- Cytarabine (cytosine arabinoside)
- Deferoxamine
- Docetaxel
- Doxorubicin
- Erlotinib
- Etoposide
- Fludarabine
- Gefitinib
- Gemcitabine
- Hydroxyurea
- Imatinib
- Interferons (alpha and beta)
- Liposomal amphotericin B
- Lomustine
- Melphalan
- Methotrexate
- Mitomycin-C
- Nitrosoureas
- Paclitaxel
- Procarbazine
- Rituximab
- Thalidomide
- Vinca alkaloids

Note. Based on information from Antin & Raley, 2013; Camus & Costabel, 2005; Olsen et al., 2019; Schwaiblmair et al., 2012.

---

ing for melphalan, and patients should not receive additional IV or oral doses.

Etoposide

The use of etoposide in HSCT conditioning regimens continues to escalate, particularly in patients with lymphoproliferative disorders and those with relapsed acute lymphoblastic leukemia. Most pulmonary reactions are of the hypersensitivity type and include anaphylaxis-like reactions during the initial infusion. Facial and tongue swelling, coughing, diaphoresis, back pain, dyspnea, and syncope have been reported in 0.7%–2% of patients (Bristol-Myers Squibb, 2019; Camus & Costabel, 2005). Treatment is symptomatic with corticosteroids and diphenhydramine.

Carmustine

Carmustine is commonly used to treat lymphoproliferative disorders and in autologous transplantation. Although rare, fatal pulmonary toxicity has been reported in patients receiving a total carmustine dose greater than 1,400 mg/m². Pulmonary fibrosis can occur in patients receiving lower doses at a rate of 1%–10% (Camus & Costabel, 2005; Heritage Pharmaceuticals, 2018). Dosing can be as high as 300–600 mg/m², and pulmonary toxicity can result in the sudden development of severe interstitial pneumonitis. The incidence increases tenfold in patients who have received recent radiation therapy to the mediastinum and who have received concurrent cyclophosphamide therapy (Camus & Costabel, 2005; Cao et al., 2000; Stuart et al., 2001). Risk factors include comorbid lung disease and a history of smoking. Patients with a baseline forced vital capacity and DLCO less than 70% of the predicted value are considered to be at high risk (Heritage Pharmaceuticals, 2018; Olsen et al., 2019).

Cytarabine

Administered as part of the BEAM regimen, cytarabine is also used as an induction chemotherapy agent for a wide variety of hematologic disorders. A "cytarabine syndrome" has been observed 6–12 hours after infusion in patients who have received a high dose (greater than 5 g/m²) (Jirasek & Herrington, 2016; Pfizer, 2018). This syndrome is characterized by sudden respiratory distress that rapidly progresses to pulmonary edema, capillary leak syndrome, and ARDS (Physicians' Desk Reference, 2017). A high-resolution CT scan will show diffuse bilateral patchy infiltrates. Fluid restriction and careful management of fluid balance seems to be the best method to reduce the interstitial fluid (Camus & Costabel, 2005; Forghieri et al., 2007).

Initiating prompt treatment at the first signs of hypersensitivity or toxicity is crucial to increasing positive outcomes. Patients and families should be instructed to notify nurses immediately if dyspnea appears or worsens or if the patient develops a dry cough or experiences rapid deterioration of activity tolerance. Patients should also be monitored closely during their infusions.

Biotherapy-Related Pulmonary Toxicity

The explosion of biotherapies over the past decade has augmented the ability to treat many diseases, including cancer. Patients may receive a biotherapy as part of their initial cancer treatment, as part of their conditioning regimen, or after transplantation. Two particular biotherapies, crizotinib (tyrosine kinase inhibitor) and rituximab (monoclonal antibody) can cause pulmonary toxicity (Schwaiblmair et al., 2012; Shash, Stefanovici, Phillips, & Cuvelier, 2016).

Radiation-Related Pulmonary Toxicity

Radiation therapy used in pretransplantation conditioning and TBI can cause structural damage to delicate lung tissue. The resulting injuries can be acute and chronic. Some conditioning regimens use fractionated TBI, whereby the patient receives divided doses of radiation delivered over three days (Shroff, Marom, Wu, Truong, & Godoy, 2019; Soule et al., 2007). TBI can result in infectious pneumonia and idiopathic pneumonia syndrome (IPS) (Byun et al., 2017). A recent study by Abugideiri et al. (2016) found that TBI dose rate has a significant impact on the development of pulmonary toxicity and IPS.

During the radiation procedure, the patient's lungs and kidneys are shielded to decrease the amount of radiation to these sensitive organs. However, despite these precautions, varying degrees of damage to the epithelial cells of the alveoli and the endothelium of the alveolar capillaries can occur (Ayas et al., 2004; Bledsoe, Nath, & Decker, 2017). Inflammatory responses stimulate the alveoli to release surfactant, which causes increased alveolar wall thickening. Increased capillary permeability causes increased interstitial fluid. This cascading process can result in interstitial lung disease through a process similar to what causes chemotherapy-induced pulmonary toxicity.

The amount of damage to the lung tissue and the resulting diseases are multifactorial, taking into account the amount of radiation administered, use of shielding during the radiation procedure, preexisting pulmonary impairment, chemotherapy used during the conditioning regimen, and previous exposure to pulmonary-toxic agents, such as bleomycin, carmustine, and cyclophosphamide.

Radiation Pneumonitis

Radiation pneumonitis, also known as *interstitial pneumonitis*, can occur after TBI and can be a serious toxicity for allogeneic transplant recipients (Chiang et al., 2016). Initially, patients with acute or sporadic radiation pneumonitis present with a dry, nonproductive cough and diffuse diminished breath sounds. As the pneumonitis progresses, patients can be auscultated with bilateral crackles (rales) representing the openings of alveoli collapsed by increasing interstitial fluid. Pneumonitis can be associated with low-grade fever, tachypnea, cough, and severe fatigue (Bledsoe et al., 2017). As dyspnea progresses and oxygen exchange is increasingly compromised, oxygen therapy and, in some cases, mechanical ventilation will be necessary. Diagnostic methods such as a chest x-ray will reveal interstitial and alveolar infiltrates but only in advanced stages. Laboratory studies will show an increased white blood cell count, presence of C-reactive protein, or increased erythrocyte sedimentation rate (Bledsoe et al., 2017). A chest CT can be useful in diagnosing radiation pneumonitis in its earlier stages, thus facilitating earlier intervention with corticosteroids, antibiotics, antifungals, and antivirals (Bledsoe et al., 2017). Radiation pneumonitis in HSCT patients has been implicated in the development of IPS and bronchiolitis obliterans (Carver et al., 2007).

Radiation Fibrosis

Patients who experience acute radiation pneumonitis have a higher probability of developing radiation fibrosis, a condition that is refractory to treatment (Stubblefield, 2017). Fibrosis occurs when the delicate alveolar membrane is replaced with collagen after continued assault by inflammatory response modulators. Collagen cannot stretch or participate in gas exchange, and the resulting lung tissue is irreversibly incapable of functioning properly. Symptoms of fibrosis are insidious, developing gradually in post-transplantation patients and often mimicking other pulmonary conditions that are more treatable. Mounting dyspnea accompanied by declining exercise tolerance are hallmark symptoms, and over time, patients experience cyanosis, clubbing of the nails, orthopnea, and cor pulmonale. Chest x-ray shows a "ground glass" appearance complemented by hazy pulmonary markings, and a CT scan reveals the damage done to the alveolar tissue (Stubblefield, 2017). Once fibrosis has been diagnosed, medical efforts focus on patient comfort, including the administration of corticosteroids and oxygen therapy; however, no evidence suggests that this treatment halts or reverses the invasive growth of collagen in the alveoli. Patients may be offered a lung transplant, but this is dependent upon individual circumstances and a patient's general health after HSCT (Carver et al., 2007; Shroff et al., 2019).

Noninfectious Pulmonary Complications

Noninfectious complications involving the lungs can occur at any time following HSCT. Examples can include GVHD, which can be a primary complication or can be associated with other conditions, such as eosinophilic pulmonary syndrome (EPS), IPS, noninfectious bronchiolitis obliterans, and cryptogenic organizing pneumonia. According to a recent study by Zhou et al. (2017), IPS and bronchiolitis obliterans are among the most significant causes of post-transplantation mortality. The rates for both increase considerably if patients suffer from a viral infection in the first 100 days after transplantation. Because most noninfectious post-transplantation conditions are associated with GVHD, allogeneic patients in general are at a higher risk.

Graft-Versus-Host Disease

GVHD has gained attention in recent years, corresponding with the increase in allogeneic transplants. The occurrence of acute and chronic GVHD continues to challenge the efficacy of allogeneic transplants, which are being offered to patients who previously would have been excluded because of advanced age, comorbidities, or disease status. GVHD is caused by the donor T cells attacking the host body. Both minor antigens and major histocompatibility antigens are presented to the T cells in the same way that bacterial or viral antigens are presented. In this way, the graft behaves as it would in the presence of an infection and tries to eradicate antigens intrinsic to the host (Paczesny, Hanauer, Sun, & Reddy, 2010). Lymphocytic inflammation and eosinophilic scarring are suggestive of GVHD (Okimoto et al., 2018).

GVHD is classified as acute or chronic (see Figure 11-3). Historically, the distinction between these was based solely on when symptoms appeared: acute GVHD occurring within 100 days after transplantation and chronic occurring later than 100 days. A comprehensive study published in 2005 reclassified acute and chronic GVHD based on clinical manifestations, rather than time after transplantation (Filipovich et al., 2005; Vigorito et al., 2009). Therapy for GVHD is heavily dependent on corticosteroids. Steroids are also the standard of care for GVHD prophylaxis. Additional prophylactic regimens, regardless of stem cell source, include immunosuppressants, such as tacrolimus, cyclosporine, mycophenolate, and sirolimus, with or without methotrexate. Biotherapy agents, including antithymocyte globulin, ruxolitinib, and alemtuzumab, have been used in the past to control GVHD (Koreth & Antin, 2008; Milano, Au, Boeckh, Deeg, & Chien, 2011). A contemporary pilot study on the use of the proteasome inhibitor bortezomib for chronic GVHD showed promising results including increased pulmonary stabilization and decreased toxicity (Jain et al., 2018).

Pulmonary GVHD manifests as a myriad of clinical syndromes for HSCT patients. The interaction between the donor leukocytes in the recipient lung tissue and the

---

Figure 11-3. Taxonomy of Graft-Versus-Host Disease

Acute GVHD
- Day 0–100: Classic acute graft-versus-host disease (GVHD)
- Day > 100: Persistent, recurrent, or late-onset acute GVHD

Overlap Syndrome
- No time limit
- Both acute and chronic GVHD
- Associated with the withdrawal of immunosuppression

Chronic GVHD
- No time limit
- Classic chronic GVHD

Note. Based on information from Antin & Raley, 2013; Filipovich et al., 2005; Rimkus, 2009; Vigorito et al., 2009.

secretion of inflammatory cytokines that follows provides a platform for diffuse tissue injury to occur (Patriarca et al., 2004; Poletti, Costabel, & Semenzato, 2005). Acute disease includes IPS and diffuse alveolar hemorrhage (DAH). Chronic pulmonary GVHD includes EPS and bronchiolitis obliterans. Cryptogenic organizing pneumonia is associated with both acute and chronic GVHD. A retrospective study by Remberger et al. (2016) found that chronic GVHD occurred most commonly in allogeneic transplantation of sibling donor cells. The research showed an increased rate of bronchiolitis obliterans in these patients compared to those who received nonsibling donor cells, a result counterintuitive to long-standing assumptions about the more optimal outcomes using cells from sibling donors.

Eosinophilic Pulmonary Syndrome

Considered part of the clinicopathologic spectrum of pulmonary GVHD, EPS (or eosinophilic lung disease) can develop in patients with active chronic GVHD (Tawfik & Arndt, 2017). In all reported cases, GVHD of the skin preceded pulmonary involvement, which resulted in diffuse bilateral pulmonary infiltrates. Diagnostics revealed peripheral blood eosinophilia, as well as the presence of eosinophils in the small bronchioles. Further evaluation by BAL often reveals an elevated eosinophil count, as well as negative respiratory cultures (Tawfik & Arndt, 2017). For many years, a diagnosis of acute eosinophilic pneumonia was assumed because of similar clinical presentations. However, more recent research suggests a differentiation between EPS and acute eosinophilic pneumonia based on BAL results. In a study by Akhtari, Langston, Waller, and Gal (2009), all patients responded promptly to aggressive systemic corticosteroid therapy, and this result has been replicated in more recent studies (Tawfik & Arndt, 2017). Further research has confirmed that earlier recognition and quick corticosteroid interventions in these patients can significantly improve outcomes when compared to patients who received antibiotic therapy first (Tawfik & Arndt, 2017).

Idiopathic Pneumonia Syndrome

In IPS, patients exhibit classic clinical presentations associated with pneumonia of a noninfectious nature. IPS is an acute lung dysfunction that usually develops around the time of engraftment and neutrophil recovery. The American Thoracic Society (ATS) describes IPS as "an idiopathic syndrome of pneumopathy after HSCT, with evidence of widespread alveolar injury *and* in which infectious etiologies and cardiac dysfunction, acute renal failure, or iatrogenic fluid overload have been excluded" (Panoskaltsis-Mortai et al., 2011, p. 1263). Within the current ATS protocols, IPS is divided into three sites of presumed primary tissue injury: pulmonary parenchyma, vascular endothelium, and airway epithelium (Panoskaltsis-Mortai et al., 2011). The main feature of IPS is diffuse alveolar damage (Tanaka et al., 2016). Several

other pulmonary dysfunctions occurring after HSCT are identified as IPS in the literature, including acute interstitial pneumonitis, ARDS, delayed pulmonary toxicity syndrome, peri-engraftment respiratory distress syndrome, noncardiogenic capillary leak syndrome, DAH, cryptogenic organizing pneumonia, and bronchiolitis obliterans (Panoskaltsis-Mortai et al., 2011). Several of these more common complications are discussed in greater detail in subsequent sections.

IPS is increasingly attributed to transplantation conditioning regimens and usually develops within the first 100 days after allogeneic transplantation (Sano et al., 2014). IPS is associated with significant mortality rates (greater than 50%) despite treatment with systemic corticosteroids and supportive care (Sano et al., 2014; Thompson et al., 2017; Yanik et al., 2014). Etanercept, a tumor necrosis factor–binding protein, is an option used with high-dose corticosteroids in IPS with a later onset (Thompson et al., 2017). Older age, lower pretransplantation performance status, TBI, and HSCT for diseases other than leukemia have all been associated with higher incidence of IPS (Soubani & Pandya, 2010). Allogeneic transplant recipients who took methotrexate for GVHD prophylaxis appear to be at higher risk for IPS (Zhou et al., 2017). A relationship between late IPS (day 30–100) and acute GVHD of the gut has been demonstrated (Zhu et al., 2008). Zhou et al. (2017) also found that patients who developed viral respiratory infections within the first 100 days after transplantation had an increased risk for both IPS and bronchiolitis obliterans. Patients who had human herpesvirus 6 in the first 100 days were at significant risk for developing IPS (Zhou et al., 2017).

IPS is biphasic in nature. The early stage of IPS is characterized by inflammatory cytokines of unknown immunopathogenesis that promote lymphocyte influx into the lungs with minimal fibrosis (Afessa & Peters, 2008). Gradual changes in the lung tissue occur in the presence of continued leukocyte activity and lead to deregulated wound repair mechanisms, resulting in the disintegration of normal alveolar tissue and its replacement with collagen, much in the same manner as occurs with radiation fibrosis (Altmann et al., 2018). In many cases, the deterioration of fragile alveolar tissue presents an environment particularly favorable to attack with such agents as bacteria, viruses (e.g., CMV, human rhinovirus), and *Aspergillus* (Kotloff, Dickey, & Vander Els, 2019).

Patients developing IPS will present with dyspnea, hacking cough, and increasing hypoxemia (Afessa & Peters, 2008; Altmann et al., 2018). Diagnostics such as chest x-ray and CT may detect multilobar pulmonary infiltrates with peribronchial and perivascular cuffing. BAL and subsequent diagnostics for infectious agents are negative. IPS symptoms can sometimes be confused with transfusion-related acute lung injury (TRALI), which occurs during or shortly after a transfusion as a result of preformed anti-HLA antibodies in the transfused product. IPS can appear as fluid overload, cardiac dysfunction, and renal failure, all of which must be excluded before a definitive diagnosis can be made.

The nursing role in managing IPS includes initiating timely interventions, such as oxygen therapy, and prophylactic antibiotics, antivirals, and antifungals, as well as monitoring patient respiratory status frequently (Yanik et al., 2014). High-dose steroids may be efficacious, with dosing as high as 1–2 mg/kg/day for three days and a taper by 50% every three days. Mechanical ventilation may be necessary in the management of IPS. Clinical trials with new agents, such as tumor necrosis factor blockers (e.g., etanercept), have shown disappointing results (Yanik et al., 2014).

Bronchiolitis Obliterans

Bronchiolitis obliterans, also referred to as *bronchiolitis obliterans syndrome*, is an obstructive airway disease associated with chronic GVHD of the lungs (Hakim et al., 2019; Uhlving et al., 2015). Bronchiolitis obliterans has other etiologies, including infectious and noninfectious causes, but in the context of HSCT, it is mostly associated with damage to pulmonary tissue caused by GVHD (Amin et al., 2015). Bronchiolitis obliterans is a critical complication that has the potential to cause enduring pulmonary damage, and it is considered a form of IPS (Lam et al., 2011; Panoskaltsis-Mortai et al., 2011). Onset can occur three months to four years after transplantation and is often associated with patients who have developed other forms of GVHD (Bertelli et al., 2017). Patients who have received cyclosporine and corticosteroids for GVHD treatment or prophylaxis, as well as those with hypogammaglobulinemia or who had TBI in their conditioning regimen are at risk (Bertelli et al., 2017). Unfortunately, bronchiolitis obliterans carries a poor prognosis, particularly those with other forms of chronic GVHD (Amin et al., 2015). Incidence is approximately 5% of allogeneic transplant recipients and 14% of those experiencing chronic extrathoracic GVHD (Barker, Bergeron, Rom, & Hertz, 2014). Another study showed that about 6% of allogeneic HSCT patients will develop bronchiolitis obliterans, with survival of this group at only 13% after five years (K.M. Williams, Chien, Gladwin, & Pavletic, 2009). A study by Zhou et al. (2017) found that CMV infections in the early post-transplantation period (first 100 days) significantly predisposed patients for the development of bronchiolitis obliterans.

An obstructive airway disease, bronchiolitis obliterans involves the narrowing of the lumens in small airways, leading to scarring and impediment and, ultimately, to air trapping (Epler, 2007; Liptzin, DeBoer, Giller, Kroehl, & Weinman, 2018). Symptoms of bronchiolitis obliterans include progressive inspiratory and expiratory wheezing, nonproductive cough, and mounting dyspnea with activity. PFT reveals a severe decrease in the forced expiratory volume in one second (FEV_1) and a normal DLCO (Uhlving et al., 2015; K.M. Williams et al., 2009). Chest x-ray shows hyperinflation of the lungs, diaphragmatic flattening, recurrent pneumothoraces, and focal or diffuse opacities (Epler, 2007). High-resolution CT confirms decreased lung density as evidenced by lobular air trapping with centrilobular nodules and bronchiolectasis (Liptzin et al., 2018). Diagnosis of bronchiolitis obliterans is usually based on clinical presentation, absence of an infectious process, and PFT findings. In some cases, BAL or video-assisted thoracoscopic surgery is used to obtain sufficient deep lung tissue for disease confirmation (Barker et al., 2014). A lung biopsy performed to diagnose bronchiolitis obliterans will show unequivocal dense eosinophilic scarring of the bronchioles, which results in luminal narrowing (Okimoto et al., 2018). A recent retrospective study of patients who underwent lung biopsy for bronchiolitis obliterans confirmed this diagnostic method as the gold standard (Uhlving et al., 2015). This same study also suggested that patients with bronchiolitis obliterans did not necessarily show lower rates of survival than patients without the condition (Uhlving et al., 2015).

As with most other pulmonary complications of HSCT, bronchiolitis obliterans is treated with high-dose corticosteroids—up to 1–2 mg/kg/day for four to six weeks (K.M. Williams, Cheng, et al., 2016). Bronchodilators have been used to decrease inflammation and obstruction of the upper airways, but they provide limited relief (Barisione, Bacigalupo, Crimi, & Brusasco, 2011; Barker et al., 2014). Ongoing studies over the past decade have demonstrated that the use of budesonide/formoterol, an inhaled steroid and long-acting bronchodilator combination, showed significant promise in recovering baseline FEV_1 values for patients with bronchiolitis obliterans (Bergeron et al., 2015).

Other supportive measures used in the treatment of bronchiolitis obliterans include replacement of immunoglobulin G when serum levels decrease to less than 400 mg/dl, as well as administration of azithromycin, which has been used as a treatment for bronchiolitis obliterans with limited success (Lam et al., 2011; K.M. Williams, Cheng, et al., 2016). A novel inhalant including fluticasone, azithromycin, and montelukast has shown good results in treating bronchiolitis obliterans specific to patients who received allogeneic transplant (K.M. Williams, Cheng, et al., 2016). Studies in Europe have focused on donor lymphocyte infusion as a method to diminish the risk of bronchiolitis obliterans in allogeneic HSCT patients (Forslöw, Mattsson, Gustafsson, & Remberger, 2011). In the most extreme cases of severe and treatment-resistant bronchiolitis obliterans in the presence of other factors such as young age and absence of other chronic GVHD manifestations, HSCT patients have received living-donor lobar lung transplants (Okumura et al., 2007). Bilateral sequential lung transplantation has shown better outcomes when compared to only one lung (Gao, Chen, Wei, Wu, & Zhou, 2018).

Cryptogenic Organizing Pneumonia

Cryptogenic organizing pneumonia, formerly referred to as *bronchiolitis obliterans organizing pneumonia*, should not be confused with bronchiolitis obliterans, despite both being obstructive disorders associated with chronic GVHD (Ditschkowski et al., 2007; Jinta et al., 2007; see Table 11-1). Idiopathic bronchiolitis obliterans organizing pneumonia not associated with chronic GVHD is also referred to as *cryptogenic organizing pneumonia* in the medical literature, whereas secondary cryptogenic organizing pneumonia is linked to chronic GVHD (Gea-Banacloche, 2018). Onset involves formation of fibromyxoid connective tissue plugs in the lumens of small distal airways, causing scarring and obstruction that extends into the alveolar ducts and alveoli. As with noninfectious bronchiolitis obliterans and IPS, cultures are negative for infectious agents, and symptoms do not resolve with antibiotics (Ruth-Sahd & White, 2009; Vande Vusse & Madtes, 2017).

As cryptogenic organizing pneumonia progresses, patients develop flu-like symptoms, with complaints of a nonproductive cough, decreased exercise tolerance, and dyspnea (Vande Vusse & Madtes, 2017). Fever, inspiratory wheezing, pleuritic chest pain, hemoptysis, and bilateral crackles can occur as the patient becomes more fatigued and withdrawn (Oymak et al., 2005; Ruth-Sahd & White, 2009). Radiographic diagnostics show bilateral patchy infiltrates with a ground-glass or mosaic appearance, and PFTs have a restrictive pattern with reduced DLCO and lung volumes (Oymak et al., 2005). A definitive diagnosis of cryptogenic organizing pneumonia requires a surgical lung biopsy (Vande Vusse & Madtes, 2017). Despite a treatment course that includes a blend of immunosuppressive agents, including high-dose prednisone, cyclosporine, and mycophenolate, prognosis for HSCT patients with this condition remains poor (Oyan, Koc, Emri, & Kansu, 2006; Ruth-Sahd & White, 2009). The most recent medical recommendations emphasize corticosteroid therapy lasting several months (Vande Vusse & Madtes, 2017). Some researchers have added extracorporeal photopheresis to the cryptogenic organizing pneumonia treatment protocol. In a case study, extracorporeal photopheresis achieved notable clinical response, as evidenced by improved pulmonary function and DLCO, but the patient did not regain pretransplantation lung capacity (Oyan et al., 2006).

Cardiovascular Considerations

Diffuse Alveolar Damage and Diffuse Alveolar Hemorrhage

Diffuse alveolar damage specifically refers to systemic and widespread damage of the pulmonary small vessels from a variety of noninfective factors after transplantation. If the damage to these vessels continues, DAH syndrome develops, leading to blood collection within the alveoli. As these crucial structures are overwhelmed and collapse, the exchange of oxygen and carbon dioxide is disrupted. Depending on the speed of the hemorrhage, which itself is based on underlying conditions such as blood coagulability and platelet availability, DAH can cause rapid deterioration and is the hallmark of ARDS (MacLaren & Stringer, 2007). For this reason, DAH is considered an oncologic emergency (Escuissato, Warszawiak, & Marchiori, 2015). According to recent studies, DAH develops in approximately 5% of autologous and allogeneic transplant recipients (Afessa, Tefferi, Litzow, & Peters, 2002; Soubani & Pandya, 2010). Concurrently, DAH has been found in more than 10% of transplant recipients at autopsy (Lewis, DeFor, & Weisdorf, 2000; Sharma et al., 2005). The development of DAH is often fatal—not from the hemorrhage itself but from the underlying damage to lung tissue (Wanko, Broadwater, Folz, & Chao, 2006). Allogeneic transplants seem to carry a higher risk of DAH when compared to autologous transplants, particularly in pediatric populations (Kaur et al., 2018). As a result, ongoing research highlights the need for increased assessment and early intervention in the management of DAH.

The unknown and multifactorial etiology of diffuse alveolar damage and DAH makes these complications difficult to predict. Research in the past decade has shown that older age, allogeneic transplant, myeloablative conditioning, and severe acute GVHD significantly increase the risk of

Table 11-1. Characteristics of Cryptogenic Organizing Pneumonia Versus Bronchiolitis Obliterans Syndrome

Diagnostic	Cryptogenic Organizing Pneumonia	Bronchiolitis Obliterans Syndrome
Pathology	Granulation tissue plugs in small airway lumens; granulation tissue extends into alveolar ducts and alveoli	Granulation tissue plugs in small airway lumens
Chest x-ray	Bilateral patchy infiltrates with a ground-glass or mosaic appearance	Normal or hyperinflation with diaphragmatic flattening, pneumothoraces, focal opacities
Pulmonary function	Severely reduced DLCO, reduced FEV_1	Normal DLCO, severely reduced FEV_1
Lung auscultation	Inspiratory wheezing, bilateral crackles	Progressive inspiratory and expiratory wheezing
Other symptoms	Flu-like symptoms, nonproductive cough, fever, pleuritic chest pain, hemoptysis, fatigue	Nonproductive cough, dyspnea with activity

DLCO—diffusion capacity of the lung for carbon monoxide; FEV_1—forced expiratory volume in one second

Note. Based on information from Epler, 2007; Feinstein et al., 2015; Huisman et al., 2006; Oyan et al., 2006; Oymak et al., 2005; Ruth-Sahd & White, 2009; Soubani & Pandya, 2010; K.M. Williams et al., 2009.

DAH (Majhail et al., 2006; Sharma et al., 2005). Children who receive transplants for Hurler syndrome also have an increased risk of DAH. Figure 11-4 lists the various medications associated with DAH. Both diffuse alveolar damage and DAH are associated with the first 30 days after transplantation, but recent postmortem studies have shown the presence of undiagnosed diffuse alveolar damage in 33% of patients past 100 days (Roychowdhury et al., 2005). Similarly, patients who develop DAH in the first 30 days after transplantation have a 32% mortality rate when compared to patients with a late hemorrhage (Afessa et al., 2002). Symptoms first appear as sudden hypoxemia, dyspnea, nonproductive cough, wheezing, and occasionally a low-grade fever. As the hemorrhage process progresses, patients show progressive hemoptysis and worsening hypoxemia (Escuissato et al., 2015; Majhail et al., 2006). Immediate diagnostics should include chest x-ray, which will indicate diffuse pulmonary infiltrates. A bronchoscopy, when safely indicated, will show increasing amounts of bloody lavage, but no damage to the airway structures will be visible. BAL fluid staining will show hemosiderin-laden macrophages, a hallmark sign of DAH (Patel et al., 2010).

First-line treatment for DAH has traditionally been high-dose corticosteroids, usually methylprednisolone (IV 250–1,000 mg/day in adults and IV 2–5 mg/kg/day in children) (Rathi et al., 2015; Wanko et al., 2006). The rationale behind this treatment is that DAH may represent a nonspecific inflammatory response to an unidentified initial insult. HSCT patients showed a 16% probability of 60-day survival from the onset of hemorrhage, and patients receiving high-dose corticosteroids had a 26% survival rate for this same period (Majhail et al., 2006). A more recent study by Rathi et al. (2015) demonstrated a mortality rate of 85% by day 100 after transplantation for patients who developed DAH. The addition of aminocaproic acid to the methylprednisolone regimen in recent years has shown conservative improvements in rates of mortality and median transplantation survival without significant side effects (Rathi et al., 2015). Additional treatment for DAH includes addressing coagulation issues and administering platelet transfusions for thrombocytopenia, treating associated renal fail-

ure, and providing supportive oxygen management. Consultation with pulmonology, as well as the ICU team, can offer improved survival if DAH continues to progress. In more critical cases, patients will require mechanical ventilation (Majhail et al., 2006). Long-term survivors treated with HSCT who experience DAH often return to normal lung function (Lewis et al., 2000; Soubani & Pandya, 2010).

Pulmonary Embolism and Venous Thromboembolism

A venous thromboembolism (VTE) is characterized by blood clots that form in the deeper veins of the groin, arms, or legs. These thrombi can lodge themselves within the delicate vascular structure of the lungs and become pulmonary embolisms. As with any medical treatment, the risk of pulmonary embolism, although rare in transplant recipients, exists because of the potential for thrombocytopenia with associated coagulation and liver dysfunction. This should be monitored with each nursing assessment (Kaur et al., 2018). A pulmonary embolism is an occlusion of a portion of the vascular bed in the lung tissue, causing ischemia and, in severe cases, infarction. An embolus in the case of an HSCT patient could include a thrombus, tissue fragments, lipids, or an air bubble infused through the central venous catheter (Sharma et al., 2005). In the case of a patient receiving bone marrow, poorly filtered bone marrow can result in emboli made of fat or bone spicules (Chaturvedi et al., 2016). Risk of pulmonary embolism can also increase after conditioning with radiation and chemotherapy (Heidrich, Konau, & Hesse, 2009). Increasing use of lenalidomide in patients with multiple myeloma has resulted in higher rates of thromboembolism and deep vein thrombosis after autologous transplantation (Chaturvedi et al., 2016). Immobility and a lack of physical conditioning can lead to deep vein thrombosis in HSCT patients (Chaturvedi et al., 2016). An allogeneic transplant recipient who develops GVHD carries a higher risk of developing a pulmonary embolism (Chaturvedi et al., 2016; Kekre et al., 2017; Zahid et al., 2016). Kekre et al. (2017) speculated that autologous transplant recipients are at decreased risk for pulmonary embolism because of the lower rate of GVHD and hepatic SOS compared to allogeneic transplant recipients. A systematic review placed the risk for VTE in HSCT patients at 1%–20% (Hashmi et al., 2015).

The possibility of a pulmonary embolism in the immediate post-transplantation period is often overlooked because of the lack of platelets and possible dysfunction in the coagulation pathway due to liver involvement. As in non-HSCT cases, a pulmonary embolism causes varying degrees of sudden unilateral or referred chest pain, anxiety, tachypnea, tachycardia, hypoxia, pulmonary edema, atelectasis, and hypotension. Chest x-ray can show opacity over the emboli field; however, definitive diagnosis of a pulmonary embolism is through a spiral CT scan, which displays venous circulation in the lungs and pulmonary lesions. Treatment typically involves anticoagulants, which

---

Figure 11-4. Select Medications Associated With Diffuse Alveolar Hemorrhage

- Amiodarone
- Bleomycin
- Infliximab
- Lenalidomide
- Methotrexate
- Montelukast
- Nitrofurantoin
- Phenytoin
- Propylthiouracil
- Warfarin

Note. Based on information from Mogili et al., 2009; Sakai et al., 2011; Schwaiblmair et al., 2012; Sharma et al., 2005.

---

can be difficult to manage in the post-transplantation population (Chaturvedi et al., 2016). Some programs still adhere to heparin infusions as a prophylaxis for SOS, a practice that can decrease the risk for pulmonary embolism (Ibrahim et al., 2005).

Pleural Effusion

Pleural effusion is defined as an accumulation of fluid in the pleural space as the result of malignant or nonmalignant factors (Brashers & Huether, 2016). In HSCT patients, pleural effusion can occur in the first few weeks after transplantation and is most associated with fluid overload (Lee, Modi, Jang, Uberti, & Kim, 2017). The pleural space is a gap between the visceral pleura, which envelops the lung, and the parietal pleura, which is attached to the thoracic cavity. The space typically contains 5–15 ml of serous fluid, which serves the dual purposes of allowing the lungs to expand and to glide easily in the thoracic cavity (Abinun & Cavet, 2007; Brashers & Huether, 2016). This pleural fluid is produced by the intercostal arteries, flows through the pleural space, and is reabsorbed into the lymphatic system. Larger quantities of fluid can accumulate in the pleural space when the rate of production exceeds the rate of reabsorption. Pleural effusion, a profound increase in pleural fluid, occurs when the production of fluid is increased or when fluid reabsorption is prevented (Shidham & Atkinson, 2007).

Pleural effusions in HSCT patients can be caused by ascites secondary to hepatic SOS, vascular leak secondary to GVHD, hypoproteinemia, congestive heart failure (CHF), pulmonary emboli, pneumonia, lung infections, and pericardial effusion (Modi et al., 2016). A relationship between pleural effusion and GVHD has been uncovered in recent research whereby allogeneic patients exhibit a higher risk for GVHD complications after developing a pleural effusion and vice versa (Lee et al., 2017). Another retrospective study placed the risk for developing pleural effusion within the first year after HSCT at 9.9% (Modi et al., 2016). Additional risk factors for pleural effusion include previous chest irradiation, methotrexate, cyclophosphamide, and malignancies such as lymphomas and leukemias (Cooke & Yanik, 2016). Symptoms of pleural effusion include shortness of breath, tachypnea, nonproductive cough, chest pain, and fever. Chest x-ray reveals blunting of the costophrenic angle and fluid accumulation, and chest CT scan further confirms the quality of the effusion (Cooke & Yanik, 2016; Modi et al., 2016). A thoracentesis is often necessary to determine the cause of the pleural effusion. The pleural fluid should be sent to the laboratory to be cultured and tested for cytology (Shidham & Atkinson, 2007).

Treatment is aimed at eliminating the cause, removing the fluid, and obliterating the pleural space so that fluid has no place to collect. Asymptomatic patients may be managed by diuresis or no treatment at all (Cooke & Yanik, 2016). The fluid can be removed by thoracentesis, but recurrent effusions may require chest tube placement. Eliminating the excess fluid in the pleural space is achieved through pleurodesis (Shidham & Atkinson, 2007). Pleurodesis involves instillation of chemicals into the pleural space, resulting in fibrotic lesions that cause the visceral pleura and parietal pleura to stick together. This procedure is generally not a first-line treatment and is reserved for patients with recurrent effusions. Most effusions in the transplantation setting do not require pleurodesis or even chest tube placement. If effusions require a chest tube, it is usually with a flexible tube (often called a "pigtail") to allow drainage. Pleurodesis is commonly performed for malignant pleural effusions. The most common agents used in pleurodesis are talc, bleomycin, and doxycycline. Chest tubes often are inserted at the bedside on the unit in stable patients; however, the unique erythrocytopenia and thrombocytopenia in transplant recipients may require preparatory transfusions and necessitate advanced monitoring equipment (Gilbert et al., 2015; Modi et al., 2016). HSCT nurses may need an educational update on chest tube management, which includes positioning the patient to prevent the tube from kinking, "milking" the tubing as ordered, avoiding dependent loops when positioning the chest drainage system, and increasing patient activity as tolerated. All these measures are aimed at promoting chest tube drainage. Patients with pleural effusions often are most comfortable sitting upright and may require analgesia or sedation. Prognosis varies and depends on the cause of the pleural effusion and whether it can be managed effectively.

Transfusion-Related Acute Lung Injury

TRALI is another variation of IPS (Vande Vusse et al., 2014). Frequent transfusions in post-transplantation patients as a result of chemotherapy, radiation, and disease processes present an increased risk for TRALI (Corash, Lin, Sherman, & Eiden, 2011; Vande Vusse et al., 2014). Whole blood, red blood cells, platelets, plasma, immunoglobulins, and stem cells can produce noncardiac pulmonary edema. The resulting acute lung injury is caused by the complement-mediated binding of donor antileukocyte, antineutrophil, or anti-HLA antibodies with the recipient leukocytes (Camus & Costabel, 2005; Kopko & Popovsky, 2004). Studies have shown an increased risk of TRALI for patients with recent or concurrent infection and sepsis, as well as those receiving granulocyte–colony-stimulating factor (Camus & Costabel, 2005; Tanaka et al., 2016). Some evidence suggests that platelet transfusions are associated with higher incidents of IPS, specifically of TRALI (Vande Vusse et al., 2014).

Symptoms of TRALI include profound and abrupt respiratory failure with dyspnea, tachypnea, cyanosis, hypotension, and frothy sputum. Patients can develop a fever with associated chills and rigors. Usually, these symptoms develop up to six hours after a transfusion. For post-HSCT patients, TRALI can be found in the early period (before 30 days), when the administration of supportive blood products, along with granulocyte–colony-stimulating factor, is most common. Because of the large number of transfusions that patients can receive, diagnosing TRALI can be difficult. A chest x-ray will show "whiteout" of the lungs, indicating pulmonary edema or infection (Kleinman et al., 2004).

Medical management of TRALI includes careful fluid management, oxygen therapy, and in cases of ARDS, mechanical ventilation (Toy et al., 2005). Corticosteroids remain a popular treatment, but their role in decreasing noncardiac pulmonary edema is unproven (Camus & Costabel, 2005; Gajic et al., 2007). Diuretics may exacerbate hypotension because of noncardiac pulmonary edema and third-spacing of fluids. Diuretics must be given with caution and only in patients with documented fluid overload or in left ventricular failure (Popovsky, 2004).

Pulmonary Hypertension Due to Sinusoidal Obstruction Syndrome

Pulmonary SOS, formerly referred to as pulmonary veno-occlusive disease, is a rare complication of HSCT and is often a subcategory of cardiovascular pressure–related conditions called pulmonary arterial hypertension (Harch, Whitford, & McLean, 2009; Soubani & Pandya, 2010; Vion, Rautou, Durand, Boulanger, & Valla, 2015). SOS, explained in more detail in Chapter 8, can result in pulmonary hypertension (Corbacioglu et al., 2018; Harch et al., 2009).

Patients experiencing pulmonary hypertension present with dyspnea, decreased activity tolerance, and increasing oxygenation requirements. Many have a baseline reduced partial pressure of arterial oxygen (PaO_2). PFTs are normal, and evidence does not indicate an underlying infection (Dalle & Giralt, 2016; Montani et al., 2008). Chest x-ray reveals increased interstitial bronchovascular markings, enlarged proximal pulmonary arteries, and, in some cases, scattered pleural effusions (Montani et al., 2008). CT scans reveal nodular and ground-glass opacities. Angiography can be used to exclude thrombi. Right-sided cardiac catheterization to monitor pulmonary artery pressure can be used to confirm pulmonary hypertension independent of emboli, but potentially dangerous issues arise in the HSCT population because of thrombocytopenia and hemorrhaging concerns (Antin & Raley, 2013; Dalle & Giralt, 2016). Treatment of SOS is difficult because the condition has a poor response to the usual vasodilators with nitric oxide, immunosuppressants, and anticoagulant therapies (Dalle & Giralt, 2016).

Treatment for pulmonary SOS is directly dependent on treating hepatic SOS but with modifications necessary based on clinical presentation and comorbidities. Maintenance of baseline weight and restriction of extracellular fluids are goals to avoid fluid overload. The use of defibrotide and ursodeoxycholic acid can be treatment or prophylactic options (Dalle & Giralt, 2016). Defibrotide is a sodium salt of complex single-stranded oligodeoxyribonucleotides derived from porcine intestinal mucosa DNA, and it is the only drug approved by the U.S. Food and Drug Adminis-

tration for adult and pediatric SOS. The use of anticoagulant, antithrombin, or unfractionated heparin is not recommended in the HSCT population because of the significant risk for hemorrhaging (Dalle & Giralt, 2016). Despite recent advancements in diagnosing SOS earlier in HSCT patients, mortality rates remain high (Dalle & Giralt, 2016; Mohty et al., 2015).

Acute Respiratory Distress Syndrome

ARDS, also known as respiratory distress syndrome, has infectious and noninfectious etiologies. ARDS is defined as a clinical syndrome of acute lung injury that occurs in adults or children for a variety of situations and diseases (Mackay & Al-Haddad, 2009). ARDS typically has an acute onset that rapidly moves to respiratory failure requiring mechanical ventilation (Seong et al., 2020; Yadav et al., 2016). For this reason, timely and accurate medical intervention is crucial for patient survival. One study has demonstrated the incidence of ARDS in 15.6% of allogeneic transplant recipients and 2.7% in autologous transplant recipients (Yadav et al., 2016).

In HSCT patients, the most common causes of ARDS are sepsis, frequent transfusions, and pneumonia, but research has indicated that neutrophilia is a major risk factor in the early post-transplantation period (Azoulay, 2009; Yadav et al., 2016). Respiratory deterioration during neutropenia has been shown to be pivotal in the pathophysiology of ARDS. Complex interactions between resident macrophages and migrated neutrophils in the lung interstitium promote the secretion of proinflammatory cytokines (Azoulay, 2009).

The development of ARDS is characterized by three distinct stages: acute, subacute, and chronic. The acute or exudative phase is characterized by the rapid onset of respiratory failure and hypoxemia that do not respond to supplemental oxygen. In the medical literature, this is referred to as *acute lung injury* to describe lung tissue that has suffered external or internal assault and is progressively deteriorating (Mackay & Al-Haddad, 2009). The acute phase can last up to seven days, during which leakage of protein-rich fluid in the alveoli, activated neutrophils, and blood trigger endothelial and epithelial injury. The subacute or proliferative phase occurs from day 5 onward, characterized by worsening hypoxemia, reduced lung compliance, and early interstitial fibrosis. Disruption of capillary function causes microvascular thrombi to form. Chest x-ray shows linear opacities with evolving fibrosis. CT scan shows diffuse interstitial opacities and bullae. Pathology reveals fibrosis, acute and chronic inflammatory cells, and partial resolution of the pulmonary edema. Some patients have clinical improvement during this stage as the body proliferates type 2 alveolar cells to replace those that have been damaged beyond repair. Other patients progress after day 14 into the chronic or fibrotic phase of ARDS, whereby pulmonary fibrosis increases and overtakes much of the compliant alveoli tissue. The resulting loss of normal lung structure leads to poor lung compliance and increased dead space. Clinically, patients in this stage have a significantly reduced capacity to exhale carbon dioxide. In some patients, prognosis improves as the body creates new structures to fulfill oxygenation requirements. In other patients, ARDS leads to respiratory failure (Djamel, Julien, Florence, Chetaille, & Jean-Louis, 2011; Finan & Pastores, 2018).

Treatment of ARDS involves supportive care and treatment of the underlying cause (Finan & Pastores, 2018; Wheeler & Berard, 2007). Appropriate treatment of any underlying infection is critical. Patients receiving prolonged mechanical ventilation may require enteral or parenteral feedings. It is important to maintain intravascular volume to maintain adequate systemic perfusion. However, excessive fluids will contribute to pulmonary edema, and vasopressors may be needed for adequate organ perfusion. Mechanical ventilation often is necessary, with high tidal volumes remaining the treatment standard despite the risk of further lung injury (Finan & Pastores, 2018; Gattinoni & Caironi, 2008). The mortality from ARDS is 40%–60%, and the majority of deaths are the result of sepsis or multiorgan failure, rather than respiratory failure (Leaver & Evans, 2007; Yadav et al., 2016). In patients who survive, lung function can return to nearly normal within 6–12 months, but in severe cases and in patients requiring prolonged mechanical ventilation, permanent pulmonary damage can affect quality of life (Gattinoni & Caironi, 2008).

Novel Pulmonary Diagnoses

With increased interest and research in pulmonary toxicity occurring after autologous and allogeneic HSCT, new diagnoses based on nuanced understandings are inevitable. For example, a new disease with unknown etiology called pleuroparenchymal fibroelastosis (PPFE) has been described in recent literature as a complex and serious late-onset complication of HSCT (Rosenbaum et al., 2015; Shioya et al., 2018). Research by Okimoto et al. (2018) discounted a relationship between PPFE and GVHD or bronchiolitis obliterans. PPFE occurs in less than 0.3% of patients receiving HSCT, but it is associated with a high mortality rate (Okimoto et al., 2018). Lung tissue examination obtained from biopsy reveals fibroelastosis with pleural thickening. Persistent pneumothorax is a vexing problem. PPFE's most problematic characteristic is that, unlike in bronchiolitis obliterans and chronic GVHD, immunosuppressive and anti-inflammatory therapies are totally ineffective (Okimoto et al., 2018).

A possibly related disease of the lungs in post-HSCT patients has been identified as acute fibrinous organizing pneumonia (AFOP). Currently, AFOP is considered part of a nonspecific dysregulated response to lung injury that can occur with alveolar damage and cryptogenic organizing pneumonia (Vande Vusse & Madtes, 2017). AFOP is characterized by fibrin balls, which are patchy aggregates of intra-alveolar fibrin, and inflamed alveolar walls infiltrated by neutrophils. Corticosteroids are the treatment of choice, but patients may also receive mycophenolate mofetil dual therapy (Vande Vusse & Madtes, 2017).

Nursing Care of Pulmonary Complications

All patients undergoing HSCT are at risk for pulmonary complications. Bedside nurses are the most likely to observe subtle changes in a patient's condition, and for this reason, it is critical that nursing staff working with the HSCT population are highly trained in oncology and critical care interventions (Wallhult & Quinn, 2018). Prompt reporting of symptoms can ensure proper and timely medical intervention and facilitate improved patient outcomes. This has been found particularly true in identifying GVHD, with clinical nurses at the forefront of identifying and reporting suspicious symptoms to the healthcare team (Mattson, 2007). Nurses play a central role in patient and family education regarding the course of treatment, complications, and other key pieces of the HSCT process, including central line care. By educating patients on what to expect after transplantation with regard to troubling symptoms, nurses ensure patient participation in early identification of developing complications and improved HSCT outcomes.

The most critical aspect of evaluating HSCT patients for pulmonary complications is obtaining baseline PFTs and an admission chest x-ray (Olsen et al., 2019). Some programs perform PFTs as part of the workup to obtain a baseline before conditioning, in addition to a comprehensive patient history and physical. When assessing for pulmonary complications in a post-transplantation patient, frequent and careful nursing assessment of laboratory tests and weight changes, with a focus on the cardiopulmonary systems, is customary. A thorough assessment can assist the nursing staff in detecting changes indicative of developing complications. Vital signs, including the rate and quality of respirations, and oximetry should be performed per program protocols, usually every four hours and more frequently for patients at risk for pulmonary insufficiency. Taking a patient's temperature every four hours or as necessary is another critical element of monitoring, as most post-HSCT complications are infectious in nature.

In the post-transplantation period, it is important to encourage patients to pace their activities with their level of ability (Wallhult & Quinn, 2018). Coughing and deep-breathing exercises accompanying the regular use of an incentive spirometer constitute critical methods to open deep alveolar tissue and encourage pulmonary hygiene on patients prone to fatigue and malaise and those whose blood counts are very low. Patients with stabilized hemoglobin levels who exhibit platelet recovery either through engraftment or transfusions can be encouraged to engage in greater activity levels. However, movements straining large muscle groups, such as using a stationary bike or treadmill, must be reserved for patients with even higher hemoglobin and platelet counts. Working closely with a physiotherapist and occupational therapist, nurses facilitate an interprofessional care plan that encourages respiratory well-being, physical safety, and improved mental and emotional health.

If patients develop pulmonary complications, nurses must work closely with physicians, pharmacists, and other team members in creating a plan of care. Anxiolytic agents, oxygen therapy, and complementary and alternative medicine modalities, such as guided imagery, can be used as auxiliary treatments to help patients who are experiencing shortness of breath and dyspnea. In all cases, the development of pulmonary complications necessitates quick interventions and diagnostics including chest radiography, cultures, and laboratory tests, such as arterial gases, so that treatment decisions can be made. In some cases, a patient's respiratory condition may deteriorate rapidly, requiring consultation with the center's rapid response team or critical care outreach team. This team should be notified per facility protocol, but usually when an HSCT nurse thinks that patient status has deteriorated to a point that ICU admission may be necessary. Respiratory complications constitute the majority of reasons for ICU admissions, with mechanical ventilation necessary in approximately 30% of these patients (Foucar & Galvin, 2017; Moreau et al., 2014). Pulmonary clinical symptoms that would necessitate further medical intervention include tachypnea, oxygen desaturation requiring increasing oxygen supplementation, sudden and severe chest pain, sudden increase in frank hemoptysis, and a condition unresponsive to corticosteroid and antihistamine administration.

The outcomes for HSCT patients transferred to the ICU are poor, especially if they require mechanical ventilation (Saria & Gosselin-Acomb, 2007). Transfer to the ICU is a frightening experience for patients and families. Transfer frequently involves getting to know new nursing and medical staff. Ongoing involvement and support from the transplantation team is critical. HSCT clinicians vary greatly in their opinions about what constitutes the appropriate level of care for these patients. However, it is not unusual for HSCT patients to receive measures such as mechanical ventilation, Swan-Ganz catheter placement, dialysis, and medications to support blood pressure. Nurses play an important role in supporting and educating families during this difficult time. If withdrawal of life support is discussed, the nursing perspective is critical for family support. Because of the lack of proven therapeutic interventions to manage and improve transplant-related pulmonary complications, dilemmas arise both in the transplantation unit and in the ICU regarding diagnostic procedures for comorbidities, the course of treatment, and the perception of patient survivability (Saria & Gosselin-Acomb, 2007).

Discharge of HSCT patients from inpatient wards or day clinics has become an important topic in recent years. With increasing numbers of patients receiving transplants and improvements in mortality rates associated with these procedures, issues of post-HSCT survivorship demand increasing attention from nurses. Regarding long-term HSCT-related pulmonary complications, patients should be carefully educated on the signs and symptoms of pulmonary complications and instructed to report these symptoms immediately to their healthcare providers. Patients should particularly be aware of signs of chronic GVHD, as well as the potential to develop late-onset pulmonary complications (Shapiro, 2016).

Cardiac Complications

Cardiac complications in HSCT patients are extremely rare but carry high mortality rates (Shinohara et al., 2016). Post-HSCT cardiac complications predominantly include arrhythmias, myocardial infarction (MI), and CHF. Other problems include pericardial effusions with tamponade, cardiomyopathy, hypertensive crisis, and possibly GVHD of the heart. In some cases, preexisting cardiac conditions lead to complications for transplant recipients (Hildebrandt et al., 2013). Long-term survivors treated with HSCT seem particularly vulnerable to developing late-onset cardiovascular disease secondary to their transplantation experience (Rovó & Tichelli, 2012).

A study by Qazilbash et al. (2009) showed that the presence of at least one of seven cardiac risk factors was associated with a significant increase in cardiac complications following allogeneic HSCT: history of smoking, hypertension, hyperlipidemia, coronary artery disease, arrhythmia, prior MI, and CHF. For this reason, baseline cardiac function studies are often mandatory before conditioning begins. The suggested pre-HSCT safe minimal left ventricular ejection fraction is more than 50% (Qazilbash et al., 2009; Sucak et al., 2008). Reduced-intensity conditioning may decrease the incidence of cardiac complications in older adults or debilitated patients who do not have optimal cardiac functioning. In these cases, however, mortality can be as high as 40% because of dangerous arrhythmias, MI, and CHF (Chow et al., 2011; Peres et al., 2010). Treatment with antineoplastic agents and radiation can cause or complicate cardiac disease, as can infectious processes and GVHD.

Chemotherapy- and Radiation-Induced Cardiotoxicity

The cardiac tissue is delicate yet resilient, in that it can withstand a number of pre- and post-transplantation assaults. However, antineoplastic conditioning regimens and TBI can cause temporary or permanent cardiac damage (Poręba et al., 2016). Chemotherapy-induced cardiotoxicity is potentially life threatening and, therefore, necessitates discontinuation or dosing reductions (Poręba et al., 2016). Figure 11-5 lists common chemotherapy agents that can cause cardiotoxicity, and Figure 11-6 lists several biotherapy agents that have demonstrated cardiopulmonary toxicity. Overall, it can be difficult to determine whether post-transplantation cardiac complications are related to the conditioning regimen, but specific factors are well documented as causing cardiotoxic-

Figure 11-5. Chemotherapy Agents Potentially Toxic to the Heart

- Busulfan
- Carmustine
- Cisplatin
- Clofarabine
- Cyclophosphamide
- Cytarabine
- Dacarbazine
- Daunorubicin
- Daunorubicin liposomal
- Doxorubicin
- Doxorubicin liposomal
- Epirubicin
- Etoposide
- 5-Fluorouracil
- Idarubicin
- Ifosfamide
- Mitoxantrone
- Paclitaxel

Note. Based on information from Antin & Raley, 2013; Camus & Costabel, 2005; Di Lisi et al., 2016; Olsen et al., 2019; Rimkus, 2009; Yeh et al., 2009.

Figure 11-6. Biotherapy Agents Potentially Toxic to the Heart

- Alemtuzumab
- Bevacizumab
- Cetuximab
- Crizotinib
- Imatinib
- Interferons (alpha and beta)
- Ipilimumab
- Rituximab
- Trastuzumab
- Tumor necrosis factor-alpha blockers

Note. Based on information from Asnani, 2018; Olsen et al., 2019; Schwaiblmair et al., 2012; Shash et al., 2016.

ity. Studies in the past decade have implicated preexisting high blood glucose as a predisposing factor for increased risk of cardiotoxic results from chemotherapy (Brunello, Kapoor, & Extermann, 2011). Cardiotoxicity is usually measured using serum values of troponin 1 and brain natriuretic peptide, as both are indicators of tissue damage and decreased ventricular function (Poręba et al., 2016). Assessment of cardiac function by serial echocardiography or radionuclide angiography (also known as a multigated acquisition or radionuclide ventriculogram) is an effective way to monitor patient outcomes and improve morbidity (Chia, Chiang, Snyder, & Dowling, 2018; Pfeffer, Tziros, & Katz, 2009). Immediate corrective medications include diuretics to manage fluid balance and digitalis to control potentially hazardous tachycardias (Pallera & Schwartzberg, 2004). Angiotensin-converting enzyme (ACE) inhibitors, angiotensin II receptor blockers, and carvedilol are pharmacologic interventions to minimize

cardiotoxic effects (Di Lisi et al., 2016). Patients are also encouraged to make lifestyle modifications to decrease stress on cardiac tissue (Rotz et al., 2017). Anthracyclines and the alkylating agents cyclophosphamide and busulfan are responsible for most cases of cardiotoxicity in HSCT patients. Cyclophosphamide-induced cardiotoxicity can occur in HSCT patients independent of baseline cardiac function (Ishida et al., 2016; Olsen et al., 2019; Wilkes & Barton-Burke, 2018). High doses of cyclophosphamide, particularly in conjunction with TBI, can induce acute or chronic myopericarditis that has been associated with a fatal pericardial tamponade, hemorrhagic myocardial necrosis, or pulseless electrical activity based on an effect on left ventricular function (Morandi, Ruffini, Benvenuto, Raimondi, & Fosser, 2005; Poręba et al., 2016). Milder toxicities lead to CHF and myocardial edema (Baxter Healthcare Corporation, 2013). Patients developing cyclophosphamide cardiotoxicity will present with shortness of breath, pleuritic chest pain and orthopnea, cough, fever, and tachycardia that occurs 1–10 days following administration (Curigliano, Mayer, Burstein, Winer, & Goldhirsch, 2010; Shapiro, 2016). Some patients, particularly children and women, may complain of abdominal pain and vomiting. Anthracycline-induced cardiomyopathy from daunorubicin or doxorubicin is similar to cyclophosphamide toxicity (Olsen et al., 2019). Symptoms often are insidious and include signs of fluid overload such as weight gain, peripheral edema, tachycardia, dyspnea, orthopnea, and adventitious break sounds such as rales. No specific therapy exists for chemotherapy-induced cardiotoxicity, and patients are treated symptomatically. Biotherapy agents, such as alemtuzumab and imatinib, can also have cardiotoxic effects (Kebriaei et al., 2012; Olsen et al., 2019).

Radiation can also cause cardiotoxicity when used in the HSCT conditioning, particularly for those allogeneic transplant recipients who undergo TBI. Radiation therapy can cause injury to the myocardium, pericardium, valvular apparatus, and coronary vasculature. The tissue damage can occur anywhere from the epicardial to the microvascular level (Herrmann et al., 2014). Estimates of radiation-induced cardiotoxicity in the post-transplantation period vary greatly, but the literature seems to suggest an occurrence rate of 10%–35% (Carver et al., 2007; Majhail et al., 2014). Radiation to the mediastinum has been implicated as a major cause of cardiomyopathy, as pericardial thickening resulting from radiation exposure leads to thickening of the cardiac tissue (Felicetti, Fortunati, & Brignardello, 2018; Herrmann et al., 2014). Acute and chronic pericarditis are frequent complications that can occur for patients who receive radiation to the chest greater than 35 grays (Herrmann et al., 2014). Changes to the myocardium can also result in diffuse interstitial fibrosis, as well as thickening of the arterioles and capillaries. Current research suggests that the deterioration of the endothelial cells with associated microhemorrhaging can lead to extravasation of albumin. This can cause amyloid formation and progress to a form of restrictive cardiomyopathy that can lead to sudden death (Herrmann et al., 2014). Combination anthracyclines and TBI has demonstrated high rates of altered cardiac function and valve disease (Herrmann et al., 2014; van Leeuwen-Segarceanu et al., 2011).

Arrhythmias

An arrhythmia is characterized as an alteration in the heart rhythm or heart rate caused by abnormal electrical activity. Arrhythmias are the most common cardiac complication of autologous or allogeneic HSCT (Herrmann et al., 2014). The heartbeats may be tachycardic, bradycardic, irregular, or regular. The clinical significance of arrhythmias in HSCT patients can vary and largely depends on symptom manifestation (Tonorezos et al., 2015). Several studies have shown that arrhythmias develop in as many as 9%–27% of HSCT patients and often begin immediately after or within a few days of transplantation (Blaes et al., 2016; Peres et al., 2010). Symptoms of less severe arrhythmias include stable sinus rhythm with occasional missed or extra beats auscultated, with rates within normal parameters of 60–100 beats per minute for adults. Patients with minor arrhythmias may feel slight palpitations or fluttering in the sternum but will not complain of chest pain or dyspnea. Vital signs will otherwise be stable, as will pulse oximetry. A retrospective study examining a decade of HSCT patient data revealed that post-transplantation arrhythmias are associated with high rates of mortality within the first year (Tonorezos et al., 2015).

Severe arrhythmias are characterized by the presence of palpitations; anxiety; chest discomfort; dyspnea; mental status changes; a weak, thready pulse; abnormal heart sounds; or hypotension (Hidalgo et al., 2004). Arrhythmias are diagnosed by a 12-lead electrocardiogram (ECG), which will show the rate, regularity, and pattern of the heart rhythm. HSCT patients are at increased risk for supraventricular tachyarrhythmias, occurring a few days to two weeks after transplantation (Blaes et al., 2016; Herrmann et al., 2014). This potentially fatal arrhythmia first begins as an atrial flutter or fibrillation or a narrow-complex tachycardia, persisting for an average of 72 hours. It has been suggested that increased age, cardiac comorbidity, high-dose anthracycline conditioning, low ejection fraction, and lymphoma diagnosis increase HSCT patients' risk of developing potentially dangerous arrhythmias (Peres et al., 2010; Singla et al., 2013).

Treatment is based on the specific arrhythmia diagnosed and the patient's tolerance to the treatment. Agents used in transplantation that can cause arrhythmias include cisplatin, etoposide, ifosfamide, and cyclophosphamide (Tonorezos et al., 2015; see Figure 11-5). DMSO (dimethyl sulfoxide) and voriconazole have been well documented as causes of arrhythmia (Alkan et al., 2004). Post-transplantation medications such as amphotericin B, liposomal amphotericin, and corticosteroids used in GVHD treatment can change electrical activity in cardiac muscles (El-Cheikh et al., 2007). In many cases, if arrhythmias are progressively worsening and the patient becomes symptomatic, aggressive medical therapy along with electrical cardioversion can be used to restore sinus rhythm and hemodynamic stability (Hidalgo et al., 2004).

Inflammation of the Heart: Endocarditis and Pericarditis

Inflammation of the cardiac tissue can lead to sudden death or chronic heart insufficiency. Pericarditis occurs when the pericardium tissue layer of the heart becomes agitated and inflamed. The pericardium is the sac layer around the heart that holds the pericardial fluid. In the case of HSCT, pericarditis has been recently associated with peri-engraftment (Shinohara et al., 2016). Endocarditis occurs when the endocardium, including valves, interventricular septum, and chordae tendineae, and the mural endocardium become inflamed. The etiology of this inflammation can include a mass of platelets or fibrin (vegetation) and is known as marantic, or nonbacterial, thrombotic endocarditis. Infective endocarditis is the more common complication seen in post-transplantation patients (Kuruvilla et al., 2004). Among the most frequently reported causative organisms are *Candida albicans*, *Aspergillus*, *Pseudomonas*, *Clostridium*, *Streptococcus*, and *Staphylococcus* (Kuruvilla et al., 2004). Bacterial infections of the heart usually seed from the gastrointestinal tract but can be associated with indwelling central venous catheters, immunosuppression in allogeneic transplant recipients, and the disruption of skin and mucosa during antineoplastic and radiation conditioning with GVHD, allowing bacteria to enter the bloodstream. Bacteremia predisposes the HSCT patient to valvular disease. Valvular vegetations can break off and become emboli (Kuruvilla et al., 2004). *Aspergillus* is associated with endocarditis and pericarditis secondary to extrapulmonary spread.

Diagnosing cardiac infections is difficult because the symptoms are nonspecific: fever, cough, and new-onset heart murmur (American Heart Association, 2017; Kuruvilla et al., 2004). Additional clinical findings that may indicate cardiac involvement include heart sound changes, ECG changes, or symptoms of CHF. A cardinal sign of infective endocarditis is persistently positive blood cultures (Kuruvilla et al., 2004). Chest x-ray is nonspecific but may reveal increased heart size or pulmonary edema. Echocardiogram may reveal valvular vegetations and decreased ventricular function. Treatment should include quick initiation of broad-spectrum antibiotics. Antifungal treatment with caspofungin, low-dose amphotericin B, fluconazole, or voriconazole may be considered if a neutropenic patient remains febrile after several days of antibiotic therapy, with special attention paid to the culture results and engraftment status (Pappas et al., 2016). Fluids should be carefully managed, and administration of diuretics, digitalis, and nitroglycerin may be indicated.

Cardiomyopathy

Cardiomyopathy is defined as damage and deterioration of the myocardium (Bush & Griffin-Sobel, 2004). This can cause a variety of conditions depending on the area of the heart that is affected or changed. Cyclophosphamide can cause an acute myocardial hemorrhage as a result of endothelial capillary damage (Baxter Healthcare Corporation, 2013; Blaes et al., 2016; Morandi et al., 2005). A pretransplantation left ventricular ejection fraction of less than 50% increases the risk for cardiotoxicity and, thus, increases the risk of weakened heart tissue (Morandi et al., 2005). Radiation to the mediastinum is a well-known causative agent of cardiomyopathy. The pathology involves pericardial thickening that eventually leads to fibrosis and malfunction of the cardiac tissue, as fibrotic tissue is akinetic (Hensley et al., 2009).

Cardiomyopathy is associated with CHF, particularly if the damaged tissue prevents the ventricles from working correctly (Rimkus, 2009). Clinical manifestations resemble any form of heart disease and can include mild to severe chest pain, peripheral edema, pulmonary edema as evidenced by rales and a moist cough, dyspnea, and decreased activity tolerance. ECG can show signs of left ventricular hypertrophy as the heart tries to compensate, observed as flat or inverted T waves and low-voltage QRS complexes. A bundle branch block, particularly of the left side, can also be identified. Chest x-ray shows evidence of pulmonary edema or cardiomegaly associated with CHF (Kawano et al., 2015). Patients who develop cardiomyopathy have an increased risk of arrhythmia and sudden cardiac death because of inherent changes to the electrical conduction pathways resulting from a change in tissue mass or structure. Serum electrolytes, troponin, and brain natriuretic peptide should be tested regularly to determine if cardiac tissue ischemia is present (Rotz et al., 2017). Right heart pressures can be monitored by a pulmonary arterial balloon catheter system (Swan-Ganz catheter). Medications for patients with CHF from cardiomyopathy include ACE inhibitors, beta-blockers, and antiarrhythmics. Strict hemodynamic management for post-transplantation advanced cardiomyopathy should take place in the ICU.

Pericardial Effusion and Cardiac Tamponade

A pericardial effusion is a serious complication for patients who have received an HSCT, and recent studies suggest poor outcomes (Chen et al., 2016; Cox, Punn, Weiskopf, Pinsky, & Kharbanda, 2017). A pericardial effusion can occur as a complication to any antineoplastic therapy, but it is mostly associated with cyclophosphamide. Pericardial effusion is an abnormal accumulation of fluid in the pericardial cavity or space, an area that normally contains 15–50 ml of serous fluid, which lubricates the visceral and parietal layers of the pericardium (Ren & Lilly, 2011). Typical pericardial fluid is thought to be ultrafiltrate from the plasma and is released into the pericardial space by the visceral pericardium. Although total protein levels are low, pericardial fluid has a high concentration of albumin because of its low molecular weight. Fluid production in this space can increase for many reasons, but in the HSCT setting, it can be the result of exudative fluid secondary to inflammatory, infectious, malignant, or autoimmune processes. Pericarditis and any injury to the pericardium from chemotherapy or radiation can also trigger increased pericardial fluid production (Ren & Lilly, 2011). A recent study estimated rates of late-onset pericardial effusion in allogeneic HSCT patients at approximately 3% and attributed risk to age older than 50 years and chronic GVHD (Liu et al., 2015).

Cardiac tamponade develops when the pericardial sac fills with excess fluid, restricting the ventricles from filling properly and leading to low stroke volume. As fluid accumulates in the pericardial space, right ventricular filling is impaired and may even cause collapse of the right ventricle during diastole. This results in increased venous pressure, systemic venous congestion, and symptoms of right heart failure, such as distended jugular veins, edema, and hepatomegaly. As a result, less blood is delivered to the lungs, and left ventricle and cardiac output is reduced. Ineffective circulation that lacks both volume and pressure for gas exchange causes a rapid deterioration of a patient's cardiovascular status and necessitates immediate intervention (Dandoy et al., 2017; Ren & Lilly, 2011).

According to a study of pediatric HSCT patients, rates of pericardial effusion average 4.4% when cardiac function is normal prior to transplantation (Rhodes et al., 2005). Allogeneic transplants are associated with increased risk of pericardial effusions with tamponade complications because of the higher incidence of acute and chronic GVHD. Post-HSCT high-dose cyclophosphamide is an additional risk factor for pericardial effusion development (Liu et al., 2015). Innovative research by Lev et al. (2010) has implicated cardiac GVHD as a major post-transplantation obstacle. According to their research, premature B cells have been found in pericardial effusions, indicating an isolated GVHD symptom.

Clinical manifestations of pericardial effusion are dependent on the rate and volume of fluid accumulating in the pericardial sac. Rapid accumulation may cause elevated intrapericardial pressures leading to chest pain and discomfort, syncope, tachycardia, tachypnea, palpitations, hiccoughs, cough, and dyspnea (Holler, 2008; Pfeiffer et al., 2017). Widened pulse pressure can be accompanied by the classic Beck triad of pericardial tamponade including hypotension, muffled heart sounds, and jugular vein distension. Pulsus paradoxus, in which the systolic blood pressure falls more than 10 mm Hg with inspiration, signals failing cardiac output. As with pericarditis, a pericardial friction rub may be heard on the left lower sternal border during expiration. With the patient positioned upright and leaning forward, a high-pitched, scratching and grating sound can be heard near the tricuspid valve of the heart, signifying a change of pressure and constitution in the pericardial sac

(Ren & Lilly, 2011). The Ewart sign—dullness to percussion beneath the angle of the left scapula—indicates compression of the left lung by increasing volume of pericardial fluid (Holler, 2008).

Chest radiography may reveal a "water bottle" configuration of the cardiac silhouette. An echocardiogram may show the position and size of the pericardial effusion. The heart may present with a diastolic indentation or a collapsed right ventricle. Monitoring also includes laboratory values of electrolytes for renal function and cardiac enzymes, such as troponin and creatine kinase levels. Minimal troponin elevation in pericardial effusion indicates the involvement of the epicardium in the inflammatory process affecting fluid production, and an angiogram will confirm an effusion as the etiology. Supportive care is adequate if the patient is asymptomatic. In many cases, a cardiologist may choose to perform a fluoroscopic aspiration of the pericardial fluid to determine if it is infectious or malignant. In extreme conditions of threatening tamponade, pericardiocentesis or a pericardial window may be necessary (Ren & Lilly, 2011).

Nursing interventions for pericardial infusions include frequent monitoring of vital signs, close monitoring of intake and output, telemetry, oxygen administration, assessment for pulsus paradoxus, and administration of corrective medications, including beta-blockers, ACE inhibitors, calcium channel blockers, diuretics, and corticosteroids (Dandoy et al., 2017; Norkin et al., 2011; Rimkus, 2009). Special attention must be given to allogeneic transplant recipients receiving methotrexate as part of a GVHD prophylaxis regimen, because the drug easily crosses into the pericardial fluid and can cause extensive damage to the surrounding tissue (Koreth & Antin, 2008). Prognosis often depends on the prompt recognition and treatment of the underlying cause and effective management of symptoms. A cardiac tamponade is an emergency, and an affected patient typically requires timely transfer to the ICU. Malignant cardiac tamponade is typically fatal (Deaver, 2008; Holler, 2008; Ren & Lilly, 2011).

Hypertensive Crisis

Hypertensive crisis is an HSCT complication seen in patients with underlying hypertension, usually diagnosed well before the transplantation conditioning regimen begins (Antin & Raley, 2013; Dandoy, Hirsch, Chima, Davies, & Jodele, 2013). Hypertension can be a frequent toxicity for patients with GVHD and for those on long-term steroid therapy. Other risk factors include the administration of calcineurin inhibitors (e.g., cyclosporine, tacrolimus) used as GVHD prophylaxis and treatment (Hendriks, Blijlevens, Schattenberg, Burger, & Donnelly, 2006).

Patients present with gradual or sudden increases in mean arterial pressure (Najima et al., 2009). Hypertension can be defined as a systolic blood pressure above 140 mm Hg and a diastolic blood pressure above 90 mm Hg (Touzot et al., 2010). Symptoms include headache, blurred vision,

arrhythmias, or the sensation of pounding in the chest, neck, or ears. Post-transplantation patients with thrombocytopenia may experience increased ecchymosis, petechiae, and scleral hemorrhaging and are at risk for internal bleeding because of a decreased ability to quickly coagulate ruptures. Posterior encephalopathy and cortical blindness may be experienced if the IV pressure rises and if the hypertensive episode is complicated by GVHD or hepatic SOS (Najima et al., 2009).

Treatment of a hypertensive crisis can be challenging. It usually begins with identifying underlying causes, such as renal disease or pulmonary complications (Farge & Gluckman, 2011; Glezerman et al., 2010). Conditions or disorders that could be contributing to a hypertensive crisis, such as electrolyte imbalances, should be explored, particularly if a patient has shown sudden changes in blood pressure readings (Guinan, Hewett, Domaney, & Margossian, 2011). In some cases, acute renal failure secondary to transplantation complications may be responsible for a hypertensive crisis (Kang et al., 2012). Medications such as tacrolimus and cyclophosphamide can precipitate hypertensive events, and patients with preexisting hypertension may be particularly susceptible (Yanagisawa et al., 2011). Treatment can include administration of antihypertensive medications, such as diuretics, beta-blockers (e.g., metoprolol), calcium channel blockers (e.g., amlodipine), and angiotensin II receptor antagonists (e.g., candesartan) or ACE inhibitors (e.g., captopril). Patients with severe high blood pressure and elevated mean arterial pressure should be monitored frequently for changes in neurologic or cardiovascular function (Jodele et al., 2012). The risk of cerebral hemorrhage, for example, is particularly high for post-HSCT patients who still exhibit thrombocytopenia (Dandoy et al., 2013).

Graft-Versus-Host Disease of the Heart

The literature contains a few reported cases of GVHD of the cardiac tissue following HSCT (New et al., 2002; Rackley et al., 2005; Roberts et al., 2006). In most of these cases, preexisting cardiac complications, such as CHF, may have served as a significant risk factor, but this is not supported by the clinical evidence (Coghlan, Handler, & Kottaridis, 2007). Some researchers have speculated that specific conditioning regimens, such as combination busulfan and cyclophosphamide, can cause changes in cardiac tissue (Al-Hashmi, Hassan, Sadeghi, Rozell, & Hassan, 2011). GVHD of the heart is extremely rare and is associated with higher mortality rates. Manifesting as chronic and unexplained bradycardia associated with coronary disease, many researchers have postulated that GVHD of the heart often results in a stricture of vessels, which can precede complete heart block or sudden death (Morley-Smith, Cowie, & Vazir, 2013). As most of the clinical reports are from pediatric HSCT cases (Roberts et al., 2006), authors such as Coghlan et al. (2007) have questioned whether cases in adult HSCT populations are underreported. More recent research has focused on whether GVHD can actually occur in cardiac tissue, recognizing that cardiomyopathy associated with chronic GVHD may be a more appropriate diagnosis (Kawano et al., 2015).

Nursing Care of Cardiac Complications

The potential for cardiotoxicity should be recognized before the commencement of the HSCT preparative regimen, whether for autologous or allogeneic recipients. Identifying and responding to cardiac events in the HSCT patient population requires a team effort (Dandoy et al., 2017). Nurses must be aware of the chemotherapy and radiation conditioning schedule their patients received, including a strong theoretical understanding of potential side effects and complications affecting cardiac function. Baseline ECG and ejection fraction measurements constitute foundational observations required before transplantation to determine comorbidity and estimate potential toxicity risks. For example, it is important for the nurse to facilitate a 12-lead ECG before administering cyclophosphamide and again within 48 hours of the final dose according to institutional protocol. With variations in practice among geographical areas, healthcare systems, and nursing units, such procedures may or may not be part of a recognized protocol. Vigilance and continual self-education regarding current research and evidence-based practice are mandatory for HSCT nursing practice.

Nursing assessments are critical in detecting cardiac problems; vital signs, including apical rhythm regularity and quality, blood pressure, and oximetry, should be measured at least every four hours (Ford, Wickline, & Heye, 2016). If possible, HSCT nurses should become trained in rudimentary reading of 12-lead ECGs and be able to detect and identify fundamental heart sound discrepancies, including diastolic and systolic murmurs, ventricular gallop, and pericardial friction rubs. Distinguishing between variations of pulse sensations in the radial pulse when compared to the apical pulse can help nurses determine if a patient is having atrial fibrillation or flutter versus a tachycardic sinus rhythm.

Blood cultures, which could potentially detect infectious vegetations, should be drawn daily for febrile patients. Positive results should be immediately reported to the physician so that antibiotic therapy can be quickly initiated, or current regimens can be modified. Troponin, creatine kinase, and brain natriuretic peptide levels can provide information regarding cardiac function by revealing tissue damage and the subsequent release of chemicals into the vascular system (Brashers, 2016; Bush & Griffin-Sobel, 2004). Additionally, attentive monitoring of electrolytes, including calcium, sodium, magnesium, and potassium, can assist in diagnosing potential aggravating factors for arrhythmias and pericardial effusions. Cardiology consultations can be helpful in managing these patients.

The discharge of patients affected by cardiac complications following HSCT will require careful education and attention to detail by the nursing staff and other healthcare providers. Issues of survivorship after HSCT are becoming critical for oncology nurses caring for these patients in both acute care and outpatient settings (Shapiro, 2016). As more patients are receiving transplants, more will be surviving with the potential for short- or long-term multiorgan complications. Working closely with patients encompasses educating them about personal cardiac risk factors and encouraging regular checkups with their healthcare providers. Most importantly, nurses should educate patients and the support team on important signs and symptoms that may signal a cardiac problem.

Summary

Despite recent advancements in anticipating, detecting, and treating potentially life-threatening complications following HSCT, cardiopulmonary disorders continue to be the most common conditions seen in this patient population. It is important for transplantation nurses to be aware of these complications and to be able to recognize the signs and symptoms as early as possible. Informed and ongoing nursing assessments must occur at all stages of the transplantation process to ensure patient safety through timely interventions if problems arise. Early detection, intervention, and treatment of cardiopulmonary complications can lead to improved patient outcomes and higher quality of care.

References

Abbas, S., Raybould, J.E., Sastry, S., & de la Cruz, O. (2017). Respiratory viruses in transplant recipients: More than just a cold. Clinical syndromes and infection prevention principles. *International Journal of Infectious Diseases, 62,* 86–93. https://doi.org/10.1016/j.ijid.2017.07.011

Abidi, M.H., Kozlowski, J.R., Ibrahim, R.B., & Peres, E. (2006). The sulfone syndrome secondary to dapsone prophylaxis in a patient undergoing unrelated hematopoietic stem cell transplantation. *Hematological Oncology, 24,* 164–165. https://doi.org/10.1002/hon.780

Abinun, M., & Cavet, J. (2007). Gastrointestinal, respiratory and renal/urogenital complications of HSCT. In A.J. Cant, A. Galloway, & G. Jackson (Eds.), *Practical hematopoietic stem cell transplantation* (pp. 126–132). https://doi.org/10.1002/9780470988763.ch11

Abugideiri, M., Nanda, R.H., Butker, C., Zhang, C., Kim, S., Chiang, K.-Y., … Esiashvili, N. (2016). Factors influencing pulmonary toxicity in children undergoing allogeneic hematopoietic stem cell transplantation in the setting of total body irradiation-based myeloablative conditioning. *International Journal of Radiation Oncology, Biology, Physics, 94,* 349–359. https://doi.org/10.1016/j.ijrobp.2015.10.054

Afessa, B., Abdulai, R.M., Kremers, W.K., Hogan, W.J., Litzow, M.R., & Peters, S.G. (2012). Risk factors and outcome of pulmonary complications after autologous hematopoietic stem cell transplant. *Chest, 141,* 442–450. https://doi.org/10.1378/chest.10-2889

Afessa, B., & Peters, S. (2008). Noninfectious pneumonitis after blood and marrow transplant. *Current Opinion in Oncology, 20,* 227–233. https://doi.org/10.1097/cco.0b013e3282f50ff5

Afessa, B., Tefferi, A., Litzow, M.R., & Peters, S.G. (2002). Outcome of diffuse alveolar hemorrhage in hematopoietic stem cell transplant recipients. *American Journal of Respiratory and Critical Care Medicine, 166,* 1364–1368. https://doi.org/10.1164/rccm.200208-792oc

Aguilar-Guisado, M., Jiménez-Jambrina, M., Espigado, I., Rovira, M., Martino, R., Oriol, A., … Cisneros, J.M. (2011). Pneumonia in allogeneic stem cell transplantation recipients: A multicenter prospective study. *Clinical Transplantation, 25,* E629–E638. https://doi.org/10.1111/j.1399-0012.2011.01495.x

Akhtari, M., Langston, A.A., Waller, E.K., & Gal, A.A. (2009). Eosinophilic pulmonary syndrome as a manifestation of GVHD following hematopoietic stem cell transplantation in three patients. *Bone Marrow Transplantation, 43,* 155–158. https://doi.org/10.1038/bmt.2008.302

Al-Hashmi, S., Hassan, Z., Sadeghi, B., Rozell, B., & Hassan, M. (2011). Dynamics of early histopathological changes in GVHD after busulphan/cyclophosphamide conditioning regimen. *International Journal of Clinical and Experimental Pathology, 4,* 596–605.

Aliouat-Denis, C.-M., Chabé, M., Demanche, C., Aliouat, E.M., Viscogliosi, E., Guillot, J., … Dei-Cas, E. (2008). *Pneumocystis* species, co-evolution and pathogenic power. *Infection, Genetics and Evolution, 8,* 708–726. https://doi.org/10.1016/j.meegid.2008.05.001

Alkan, Y., Haefeli, W.E., Burhenne, J., Stein, J., Yaniv, I., & Shalit, I. (2004). Voriconazole-induced QT interval prolongation and ventricular tachycardia: A non–concentration-dependent adverse effect. *Clinical Infectious Diseases, 39,* e49–e52. https://doi.org/10.1086/423275

Alsharif, M., Cameron, S.E.H., Young, J.-A.H., Savik, K., Henriksen, J.C., Gulbahce, H.E., & Pambuccian, S.E. (2009). Time trends in fungal infections as a cause of death in hematopoietic stem cell transplant recipients: An autopsy study. *American Journal of Clinical Pathology, 132,* 746–755. https://doi.org/10.1309/ajcpv9dc4hgpankr

Altmann, T., Slack, J., Slatter, M.A., O'Brien, C., Cant, A., Thomas, M., … Gennery, A.R. (2018). Endothelial cell damage in idiopathic pneumonia syndrome. *Bone Marrow Transplantation, 53,* 515–518. https://doi.org/10.1038/s41409-017-0042-z

American Heart Association. (2017, March 31). Heart valves and infective endocarditis. Retrieved from http://www.heart.org/en/health-topics/heart-valve-problems-and-disease/heart-valve-problems-and-causes/heart-valves-and-infective-endocarditis

Amin, E.N., Phillips, G.S., Elder, P., Jaglowski, S., Devine, S.M., & Wood, K.L. (2015). Health-related quality of life in patients who develop bronchiolitis obliterans syndrome following allo-SCT. *Bone Marrow Transplantation, 50,* 289–295. https://doi.org/10.1038/bmt.2014.264

Anak, S., Atay, D., Unuvar, A., Garipardic, M., Agaoglu, L., Ozturk, G., … Devecioglu, O. (2010). Respiratory syncytial virus infection outbreak among pediatric patients with oncologic diseases and/or BMT. *Pediatric Pulmonology, 45,* 307–311. https://doi.org/10.1002/ppul.21184

Antin, J.H., & Raley, D.Y. (2013). *Manual of stem cell and bone marrow transplantation* (2nd ed.). https://doi.org/10.1017/CBO9781139507080

Ariza-Heredia, E.J., Nesher, L., & Chemaly, R.F. (2014). Cytomegalovirus diseases after hematopoietic stem cell transplantation: A mini-review. *Cancer Letters, 342,* 1–8. https://doi.org/10.1016/j.canlet.2013.09.004

Asnani, A. (2018). Cardiotoxicity of immunotherapy: Incidence, diagnosis, and management. *Current Oncology Reports, 20,* 44. https://doi.org/10.1007/s11912-018-0690-1

Aspen Pharmacare Canada. (2019, February). *Alkeran® (melphalan)* [Package insert]. Ontario, Canada: Author.

Avenoso, D., Bradshaw, A., Innes, A., de la Fuente, J., Olavarria, E., Apperley, J.F., & Pavlů, J. (2016). Microbial contamination of haematopoietic stem cell products: A single centre experience [Abstract]. *Blood, 128,* 5741. https://doi.org/10.1182/blood.V128.22.5741.5741

Avetisyan, G., Aschan, J., Hassan, M., & Ljungman, P. (2008). Evaluation of immune responses to seasonal influenza vaccination in healthy volunteers and in patients after stem cell transplantation. *Transplantation, 86,* 257–263. https://doi.org/10.1097/tp.0b013e3181772a75

Avetisyan, G., Mattsson, J., Sparrelid, E., & Ljungman, P. (2009). Respiratory syncytial virus infection in recipients of allogeneic stem-cell transplantation: A retrospective study of the incidence, clinical features, and outcome. *Transplantation, 88,* 1222–1226. https://doi.org/10.1097/TP.0b013e3181bb477e

Ayas, M., Al-Jefri, A., Al-Mahr, M., Rifai, S., Moussa, E., Karaoui, M., … El-Solh, H. (2004). Allogeneic stem cell transplantation in patients with Fanconi's anemia and myelodysplasia or leukemia utilizing low-dose cyclophosphamide and total body irradiation. *Bone Marrow Transplantation, 33,* 15–17. https://doi.org/10.1038/sj.bmt.1704340

Azoulay, É. (2009). Pulmonary infiltrates in patients with malignancies: Why and how neutropenia influences clinical reason-

ing. *European Respiratory Journal, 33,* 6–8. https://doi.org/10.1183/09031936.00164208

Balian, C., Garcia, M., & Ward, J. (2018). A retrospective analysis of bloodstream infections in pediatric allogeneic stem cell transplant recipients: The role of central venous catheters and mucosal barrier injury. *Journal of Pediatric Oncology Nursing, 35,* 210–217. https://doi.org/10.1177/1043454218762706

Barisione, G., Bacigalupo, A., Crimi, E., & Brusasco, V. (2011). Acute bronchodilator responsiveness in bronchiolitis obliterans syndrome following hematopoietic stem cell transplantation. *Chest, 139,* 633–639. https://doi.org/10.1378/chest.10-1442

Barker, A.F., Bergeron, A., Rom, W.N., & Hertz, M.I. (2014). Obliterative bronchiolitis. *New England Journal of Medicine, 370,* 1820–1828. https://doi.org/10.1056/nejmra1204664

Baxter Healthcare Corporation. (2013). *Cyclophosphamide* [Package insert]. Deerfield, IL: Author.

Beck, O., Koehl, U., Tramsen, L., Mousset, S., Latgé, J.P., Müller, K., … Lehrnbecher, T. (2008). Enumeration of functionally active anti-*Aspergillus* T-cells in human peripheral blood. *Journal of Immunological Methods, 335,* 41–45. https://doi.org/10.1016/j.jim.2008.02.014

Bergeron, A., Chevret, S., Chagnon, K., Godet, C., Bergot, E., de Latour, R.P., … Tazi, A. (2015). Budesonide/formoterol for bronchiolitis obliterans after hematopoietic stem cell transplantation. *American Journal of Respiratory and Critical Care Medicine, 191,* 1242–1249. https://doi.org/10.1164/rccm.201410-1818oc

Bertelli, L., Cazzato, S., Belotti, T., Prete, A., Ricci, G., & Pession, A. (2017). Prevalence, risk factors, and outcomes of bronchiolitis obliterans after allogeneic hematopoietic stem cell transplantation. *Pediatric Allergy, Immunology, and Pulmonology, 30,* 113–115. https://doi.org/10.1089/ped.2017.0754

Bissinger, A.L., Einsele, H., Hamprecht, K., Schumacher, U., Kandolf, R., Loeffler, J., … Hebart, H. (2005). Infectious pulmonary complications after stem cell transplantation or chemotherapy: Diagnostic yield of bronchoalveolar lavage. *Diagnostic Microbiology and Infectious Disease, 52,* 275–280. https://doi.org/10.1016/j.diagmicrobio.2005.03.005

Blaes, A., Konety, S., & Hurley, P. (2016). Cardiovascular complications of hematopoietic stem cell transplantation. *Current Treatment Options in Cardiovascular Medicine, 18,* 25. https://doi.org/10.1007/s11936-016-0447-9

Bledsoe, T.J., Nath, S.K., & Decker, R.H. (2017). Radiation pneumonitis. *Clinics in Chest Medicine, 38,* 201–208. https://doi.org/10.1016/j.ccm.2016.12.004

Boeckh, M. (2008). The challenge of respiratory virus infections in hematopoietic cell transplant recipients. *British Journal of Haematology, 143,* 455–467. https://doi.org/10.1111/j.1365-2141.2008.07295.x

Bomanji, J., Almuhaideb, A., & Zumla, A. (2011). Combined PET and x-ray computed tomography imaging in pulmonary infections and inflammation. *Current Opinion in Pulmonary Medicine, 17,* 197–205. https://doi.org/10.1097/mcp.0b013e328344db8a

Brashers, V.L. (2016). Alterations in cardiovascular function. In S. Huether & K. McCance (Eds.), *Understanding pathophysiology* (6th ed., pp. 598–651). St. Louis, MO: Elsevier.

Brashers, V.L., & Huether, S.E. (2016). Alterations in pulmonary function. In S. Huether & K. McCance (Eds.), *Understanding pathophysiology* (6th ed., pp. 687–713). St. Louis, MO: Elsevier.

Bristol-Myers Squibb. (2019, May). *Etopophos® (etoposide phosphate)* [Package insert]. Princeton, NJ: Author.

Brunello, A., Kapoor, R., & Extermann, M. (2011). Hyperglycemia during chemotherapy for hematologic and solid tumors is correlated with increased toxicity. *American Journal of Clinical Oncology, 34,* 292–296. https://doi.org/10.1097/coc.0b013e3181e1d0c0

Bush, N.J., & Griffin-Sobel, J.P. (2004). Chemotherapy-induced cardiomyopathy. *Oncology Nursing Forum, 31,* 185–187. https://doi.org/10.1188/04.ONF.185-187

Byun, H.K., Yoon, H.I., Cho, J., Kim, H.J., Min, Y.H., Lyu, C.J., … Suh, C.-O. (2017). Factors associated with pulmonary toxicity after myeloablative conditioning using fractionated total body irradiation. *Radiation Oncology Journal, 35,* 257–267. https://doi.org/10.3857/roj.2017.00290

Campbell, A.P., Guthrie, K.A., Englund, J.A., Farney, R.M., Minerich, E.L., Kuypers, J., … Boeckh, M. (2015). Clinical outcomes associated with respiratory virus detection before allogeneic hematopoietic stem cell transplant. *Clinical Infectious Diseases, 61,* 192–202. https://doi.org/10.1093/cid/civ272

Camus, P., & Costabel, U. (2005). Drug-induced respiratory disease in patients with hematological diseases. *Seminars in Respiratory and Critical Care Medicine, 26,* 458–481. https://doi.org/10.1055/s-2005-922030

Cao, T.M., Negrin, R.S., Stockerl-Goldstein, K.E., Johnston, L.J., Shizuru, J.A., Taylor, T.L., … Hu, W.W. (2000). Pulmonary toxicity syndrome in breast cancer patients undergoing BCNU-containing high-dose chemotherapy and autologous hematopoietic cell transplantation. *Biology of Blood and Marrow Transplantation, 6,* 387–394. https://doi.org/10.1016/s1083-8791(00)70015-2

Carver, J.R., Shapiro, C.L., Ng, A., Jacobs, L., Schwartz, C., Virgo, K.S., … Vaughn, D.J. (2007). American Society of Clinical Oncology clinical evidence review on the ongoing care of adult cancer survivors: Cardiac and pulmonary late effects. *Journal of Clinical Oncology, 25,* 3991–4008. https://doi.org/10.1200/jco.2007.10.9777

Castagnola, E., Faraci, M., Moroni, C., Bandettini, R., Granata, C., Caruso, S., … Viscoli, C. (2008). Invasive mycoses in children receiving hemopoietic SCT. *Bone Marrow Transplantation, 41*(Suppl. 2), S107–S111. https://doi.org/10.1038/bmt.2008.67

Centers for Disease Control and Prevention. (2019, June 17). About cytomegalovirus (CMV). Retrieved from https://www.cdc.gov/cmv/overview.html

Chaturvedi, S., Neff, A., Nagler, A., Savani, U., Mohty, M., & Savanti, B.N. (2016). Venous thromboembolism in hematopoietic stem cell transplant recipients. *Bone Marrow Transplantation, 51,* 473–478. https://www.nature.com/articles/bmt2015308

Chemaly, R.F., Aitken, S.L., Wolfe, C.R., Jain, R., & Boeckh, M.J. (2016). Aerosolized ribavirin: The most expensive drug for pneumonia. *Transplant Infectious Disease, 18,* 634–636. https://doi.org/10.1111/tid.12551

Chemaly, R.F., Shah, D.P., & Boeckh, M.J. (2014). Management of respiratory viral infections in hematopoietic cell transplant recipients and patients with hematologic malignancies. *Clinical Infectious Diseases, 59*(Suppl. 5), S344–S351. https://doi.org/10.1093/cid/ciu623

Chen, X., Zou, Q., Yin, J., Wang, C., Xu, J., Wei, J., & Zhang, Y. (2016). Pericardial effusion post transplantation predicts inferior overall survival following allo-hematopoietic stem cell transplant. *Bone Marrow Transplantation, 51,* 303–306. https://doi.org/10.1038/bmt.2015.227

Cheng, G.-S., Stednick, Z.J., Madtes, D.K., Boeckh, M., McDonald, G.B., & Pergam, S.A. (2016). Decline in the use of surgical biopsy for diagnosis of pulmonary disease in hematopoietic cell transplantation recipients in an era of improved diagnostics and empirical therapy. *Biology of Blood and Marrow Transplantation, 22,* 2243–2249. https://doi.org/10.1016/j.bbmt.2016.08.023

Cheng, J., Ke, Q., Jin, Z., Wang, H., Kocher, O., Morgan, J.P., … Crumpacker, C.S. (2009). Cytomegalovirus infection causes an increase of arterial blood pressure. *PLOS Pathogens, 5,* e1000427. https://doi.org/10.1371/journal.ppat.1000427

Chernecky, C.C. (2009). Pulmonary fibrosis. In C.C. Chernecky & K. Murphy-Ende (Eds.), *Acute care oncology nursing* (2nd ed., pp. 442–454). St. Louis, MO: Elsevier Saunders.

Chi, A.K., Soubani, A.O., White, A.C., & Miller, K.B. (2013). An update on pulmonary complications of hematopoietic stem cell transplantation. *Chest, 144,* 1913–1922. https://doi.org/10.1378/chest.12-1708

Chia, P.L., Chiang, K., Snyder, R., & Dowling, A. (2018). The utility of routine pre-chemotherapy screening with cardiac gated blood pool scan for patients at low risk of anthracycline toxicity. *Journal of Oncology Pharmacy Practice, 24,* 264–271. https://doi.org/10.1177/1078155217697487

Chiang, Y., Tsai, C.-H., Kuo, S.-H., Liu, C.-Y., Yao, M., Li, C.-C., … Chen, Y.-H. (2016). Reduced incidence of interstitial pneumonitis after allogeneic hematopoietic stem cell transplantation using a modified technique of total body irradiation. *Scientific Reports, 6,* 36730. https://doi.org/10.1038/srep36730

Cho, Y.-H., Lim, H.-A., Lee, M.H., Kim, I., Lee, J.S., Park, S.Y., … Yoon, S.-S. (2007). Pharmacokinetics and tolerability of intravenous busulfan in hematopoietic stem cell transplantation. *Clinical Transplantation, 21,* 417–422. https://doi.org/10.1111/j.1399-0012.2007.00664.x

Chow, E.J., Mueller, B.A., Baker, K.S., Cushing-Haugen, K.L., Flowers, M.E.D., Martin, P.J., … Lee, S.J. (2011). Cardiovascular hospitaliza-

tions and mortality among recipients of hematopoietic stem cell transplantation. *Annals of Internal Medicine, 155,* 21–32. https://doi.org/10.7326/0003-4819-155-1-201107050-00004

Chowdhary, A., Sharma, C., & Meis, J.F. (2017). Azole-resistant aspergillosis: Epidemiology, molecular mechanisms, and treatment. *Journal of Infectious Diseases, 216*(Suppl. 3), S436–S444. https://doi.org/10.1093/infdis/jix210

Chughtai, A.A., Wang, Q., Dung, T.C., & Macintyre, C.R. (2017). The presence of fever in adults with influenza and other viral respiratory infections. *Epidemiology and Infection, 145,* 148–155. https://doi.org/10.1017/s0950268816002181

Claus, J.A., Hodowanec, A.C., & Singh, K. (2015). Poor positive predictive value of influenza-like illness criteria in adult transplant patients: A case for multiplex respiratory virus PCR testing. *Clinical Transplantation, 29,* 938–943. https://doi.org/10.1111/ctr.12600

Clavert, A., Peric, Z., Brissot, E., Malard, F., Guillaume, T., Delaunay, J., … Chevallier, P. (2017). Late complications and quality of life after reduced-intensity conditioning allogeneic stem cell transplantation. *Biology of Blood and Marrow Transplantation, 23,* 140–146. https://doi.org/10.1016/j.bbmt.2016.10.011

Coghlan, J.G., Handler, C.E., & Kottaridis, P.D. (2007). Cardiac assessment of patients for haematopoietic stem cell transplantation. *Best Practice and Research Clinical Haematology, 20,* 247–263. https://doi.org/10.1016/j.beha.2006.09.005

Cooke, K.R., Jannin, A., & Ho, V. (2008). The contribution of endothelial activation and injury to end-organ toxicity following allogeneic hematopoietic stem cell transplantation. *Biology of Blood and Marrow Transplantation, 14*(Suppl. 1), 23–32. https://doi.org/10.1016/j.bbmt.2007.10.008

Cooke, K.R., & Yanik, G.A. (2016). Lung injury following hematopoietic cell transplantation. In S.J. Forman, R.S. Negrin, J.H. Antin, & F.R. Appelbaum (Eds.), *Thomas' hematopoietic cell transplantation: Stem cell transplantation* (5th ed., pp. 1156–1169). https://doi.org/10.1002/9781118416426.ch95

Cooley, L., Dendle, C., Wolf, J., Teh, B.W., Chen, S.C., Boutlis, C., & Thursky, K.A. (2014). Consensus guidelines for diagnosis, prophylaxis and management of *Pneumocystis jirovecii* pneumonia in patients with haematological and solid malignancies, 2014. *Internal Medicine, 44,* 1350–1363. https://doi.org/10.1111/imj.12599

Coomes, S.M., Hubbard, L.L.N., & Moore, B.B. (2011). Impaired pulmonary immunity post-bone marrow transplant. *Immunologic Research, 50,* 78–86. https://doi.org/10.1007/s12026-010-8200-z

Corash, L., Lin, J.S., Sherman, C.D., & Eiden, J. (2011). Determination of acute lung injury after repeated platelet transfusions. *Blood, 117,* 1014–1020. https://doi.org/10.1182/blood-2010-06-293399

Corbacioglu, S., Carreras, E., Ansari, M., Balduzzi, A., Cesaro, S., Dalle, J.-H., … Bader, P. (2018). Diagnosis and severity criteria for sinusoidal obstruction syndrome/veno-occlusive disease in pediatric patients: A new classification from the European Society for Blood and Marrow Transplantation. *Bone Marrow Transplantation, 53,* 138–145. https://doi.org/10.1038/bmt.2017.161

Cornetto, M.A., Chevret, S., Abbes, S., de Margerie-Mellon, C., Hussenet, C., Sicre de Fontbrune, F., … Bergeron, A. (2016). Early lung computed tomography scan after allogeneic hematopoietic stem cell transplantation. *Biology of Blood and Marrow Transplantation, 22,* 1511–1516. https://doi.org/10.1016/j.bbmt.2016.05.009

Cox, K., Punn, R., Weiskopf, E., Pinsky, B.A., & Kharbanda, S. (2017). Pericardial effusion following hematopoietic cell transplantation in children and young adults is associated with increased risk of mortality. *Biology of Blood and Marrow Transplantation, 23,* 1165–1169. https://doi.org/10.1016/j.bbmt.2017.03.028

Crozier, F. (2011). *Pneumocystis carinii* pneumonia prophylaxis: Current therapies and recommendations. *Journal of Pediatric Oncology Nursing, 28,* 179–184. https://doi.org/10.1177/1043454211408101

Cruz, C.R,Y., Castillo, P., Wright, K., Albert, N.D., Bose, S., Hazrat, Y., … Bollard, C.M. (2016). Developing an adoptive T-cell therapy for mucormycosis in high-risk patients after HSCT. *Biology of Blood and Marrow Transplantation, 22*(Suppl. 3), S161–S162. https://doi.org/10.1016/j.bbmt.2015.11.520

Curigliano, G., Mayer, E.L., Burstein, H.J., Winer, E.P., & Goldhirsch, A. (2010). Cardiac toxicity from systemic cancer therapy: A comprehensive review. *Progress in Cardiovascular Diseases, 53,* 94–104. https://doi.org/10.1016/j.pcad.2010.05.006

Dalle, J.-H., & Giralt, S.A. (2016). Hepatic veno-occlusive disease after hematopoietic stem cell transplantation: Risk factors and stratification, prophylaxis, and treatment. *Biology of Blood and Marrow Transplantation, 22,* 400–409. https://doi.org/10.1016/j.bbmt.2015.09.024

Dandoy, C.E., Hirsch, R., Chima, R., Davies, S.M., & Jodele, S. (2013). Pulmonary hypertension after hematopoietic stem cell transplantation. *Biology of Blood and Marrow Transplantation, 19,* 1546–1556. https://doi.org/10.1016/j.bbmt.2013.07.017

Dandoy, C.E., Jodele, S., Paff, Z., Hirsch, R., Ryan, T.D., Jefferies, J.L., ... Chima, R.S. (2017). Team-based approach to identify cardiac toxicity in critically ill hematopoietic stem cell transplant recipients. *Pediatric Blood and Cancer, 64,* e26513. https://doi.org/10.1002/pbc.26513

Danion, F., Aguilar, C., Catherinot, E., Alanio, A., DeWolf, S., Lortholary, O., & Lanternier, F. (2015). Mucormycosis: New developments into a persistently devastating infection. *Seminars in Respiratory and Critical Care Medicine, 36,* 692–705. https://doi.org/10.1055/s-0035-1562896

Deaver, D. (2008). The development of pericarditis following peripheral blood stem cell transplantation: A case report. *Clinical Journal of Oncology Nursing, 12,* 201–205. https://doi.org/10.1188/08.cjon.201-205

Denning, D.W., Cadranel, J., Beigelman-Aubry, C., Ader, F., Chakrabarti, A., Blot, S., ... Lange, C. (2016). Chronic pulmonary aspergillosis: Rationale and clinical guidelines for diagnosis and management. *European Respiratory Journal, 47,* 45–68. https://doi.org/10.1183/13993003.00583-2015

Diab, K.J., Yu, Z., Wood, K.L., Shmalo, J.A., Sheski, F.D., Farber, M.O., ... Nelson, R.P., Jr. (2012). Comparison of pulmonary complications after nonmyeloablative and conventional allogeneic hematopoietic cell transplant. *Biology of Blood and Marrow Transplantation, 18,* 1827–1834. https://doi.org/10.1016/j.bbmt.2012.06.013

Di Lisi, D., Leggio, G., Vitale, G., Arrotti, S., Iacona, R., Inciardi, R.M., ... Novo, S. (2016). Chemotherapy cardiotoxicity: Cardioprotective drugs and early identification of cardiac dysfunction. *Journal of Cardiovascular Medicine, 17,* 270–275. https://doi.org/10.2459/jcm.0000000000000232

Ditschkowski, M., Elmaagacli, A.H., Trenschel, R., Peceny, R., Koldehoff, M., Schulte, C., & Beelen, D.W. (2007). T-cell depletion prevents from *bronchiolitis obliterans* and bronchiolitis obliterans with organizing pneumonia after allogeneic hematopoietic stem cell transplantation with related donors. *Haematologica, 92,* 558–561. https://doi.org/10.3324/haematol.10710

Djamel, M., Julien, T., Florence, E., Chetaille, B., & Jean-Louis, B. (2011). Acute respiratory distress syndrome (ARDS) in neutropenic patients. In É. Azoulay (Ed.), *Pulmonary involvement in patients with hematological malignancies* (pp. 477–490). https://doi.org/10.1007/978-3-642-15742-4_36

El-Cheikh, J., Faucher, C., Fürst, S., Duran, S., Berger, P., Vey, N., ... Mohty, M. (2007). High-dose weekly liposomal amphotericin B antifungal prophylaxis following reduced-intensity conditioning allogeneic stem cell transplantation. *Bone Marrow Transplantation, 39,* 301–306. https://doi.org/10.1038/sj.bmt.1705592

Engelhard, D., Akova, M., Boeckh, M.J., Freifeld, A., Sepkowitz, K., Viscoli, C., ... Radd, I. (2009). Bacterial infection prevention after hematopoietic cell transplantation. *Bone Marrow Transplantation, 44,* 467–470. https://doi.org/10.1038/bmt.2009.257

Epler, G.R. (2007). Constrictive bronchiolitis obliterans: The fibrotic airway disorder. *Expert Review of Respiratory Medicine, 1,* 139–147. https://doi.org/10.1586/17476348.1.1.139

Erard, V., Guthrie, K.A., Seo, S., Smith, J., Huang, M., Chien, J., ... Boeckh, M. (2015). Reduced mortality of cytomegalovirus pneumonia after hematopoietic cell transplantation due to antiviral therapy and changes in transplantation practices. *Clinical Infectious Diseases, 61,* 31–39. https://doi.org/10.1093/cid/civ215

Escuissato, D.L., Gasparetto, E.L., Marchiori, E., de Melo Rocha, G., Inoue, C., Pasquini, R., & Müller, N.L. (2005). Pulmonary infections after bone marrow transplantation: High-resolution CT findings in 111 patients. *American Journal of Roentgenology, 185,* 608–615. https://doi.org/10.2214/ajr.185.3.01850608

Escuissato, D.L., Warszawiak, D., & Marchiori, E. (2015). Differential diagnosis of diffuse alveolar haemorrhage in immunocompromised patients. *Current Opinion in Infectious Diseases, 28,* 337–342. https://doi.org/10.1097/qco.0000000000000181

Farge, D., & Gluckman, E. (2011). Autologous HSCT in systemic sclerosis: A step forward. *Lancet, 378,* 460–462. https://doi.org/10.1016/s0140-6736(11)61100-8

Feinstein, M.B., DeSouza, S.A., Moreira, A.L., Stover, D.E., Heelan, R.T., Iyriboz, T.A., ... Travis, W.D. (2015). A comparison of the pathological, clinical and radiographical, features of cryptogenic organising pneumonia, acute fibrinous and organising pneumonia and granulomatous organising pneumonia. *Journal of Clinical Pathology, 68,* 441–447. https://doi.org/10.1136/jclinpath-2014-202626

Felicetti, F., Fortunati, N., & Brignardello, E. (2018). Cancer survivors: An expanding population with an increased cardiometabolic risk. *Diabetes Research and Clinical Practice, 143,* 432–442. https://doi.org/10.1016/j.diabres.2018.02.016

Ferreira, A.M., Moreira, F., Guimaraes, T., Spadão, F., Ramos, J.F., Batista, M.V., ... Rocha, V. (2018). Epidemiology, risk factors and outcomes of multi-drug-resistant bloodstream infections in haematopoietic stem cell transplant recipients: Importance of previous gut colonization. *Journal of Hospital Infection, 100,* 83–91. https://doi.org/10.1016/j.jhin.2018.03.004

Filipovich, A.H., Weisdorf, D., Pavletic, S., Socie, G., Wingard, J.R., Lee, S.J., ... Flowers, M.E.D. (2005). National Institutes of Health consensus Development Project on Criteria for Clinical Trials in Chronic Graft-Versus-Host Disease: I. Diagnosis and Staging Working Group report. *Biology of Blood and Marrow Transplantation, 11,* 945–956. https://doi.org/10.1016/j.bbmt.2005.09.004

Finan, M., & Pastores, S.M. (2018). Acute respiratory failure after hematopoietic stem cell transplantation. In A.M. Esquinas, S.E. Pravinkumar, & A.O. Soubani (Eds.), *Mechanical ventilation in critically ill cancer patients* (pp. 347–354). https://doi.org/10.1007/978-3-319-49256-8_34

Ford, R.C., Wickline, M.M., & Heye, D. (2016). Nursing role in hematopoietic stem cell transplantation. In S.J. Forman, R.S. Negrin, J.H. Antin, & F.R. Appelbaum (Eds.), *Thomas' hematopoietic cell transplantation: Stem cell transplantation* (5th ed., pp. 362–372). https://doi.org/10.1002/9781118416426.ch30

Forghieri, F., Luppi, M., Morselli, M., Potenza, L., Volzone, F., Riva, G., ... Torelli, G. (2007). Cytarabine-related lung infiltrates on high resolution computerized tomography: A possible complication with benign outcome in leukemic patients. *Haematologica, 92,* e85–e90. https://doi.org/10.3324/haematol.11697

Forslöw, U., Mattsson, J., Gustafsson, T., & Remberger, M. (2011). Donor lymphocyte infusion may reduce the incidence of bronchiolitis obliterans after allogeneic stem cell transplantation. *Biology of Blood and Marrow Transplantation, 17,* 1214–1221. https://doi.org/10.1016/j.bbmt.2010.12.701

Foucar, C., & Galvin, J.P. (2017). Prognostic factors of patients undergoing an allogeneic stem cell transplant admitted to an intensive care unit [Abstract]. *Blood, 130*(Suppl. 1), 5476. https://doi.org/10.1097/01.rct.0000157087.14838.4c

Franquet, T., Rodríguez, S., Martino, R., Salinas, T., Giménez, A., & Hidalgo, A. (2005). Human metapneumovirus infection in hematopoietic stem cell transplant recipients: High-resolution computed tomography findings. *Journal of Computer Assisted Tomography, 29,* 223–227. https://doi.org/10.1097/01.rct.0000157087.14838.4c

Freifeld, A., Zimmer, A., Zhang, Y., & Meza, J. (2017). Bloodstream infection survey in high-risk oncology patients (BISHOP): Preliminary report [Abstract]. *Blood, 130*(Suppl. 1), 2284. https://doi.org/10.1182/blood.V130.Suppl_1.2284.2284

Gajic, O., Rana, R., Winters, J.L., Yilmaz, M., Mendez, J.L., Rickman, O.B., ... Moore, S.B. (2007). Transfusion-related acute lung injury in the critically ill: Prospective nested case-control study. *American Journal of Respiratory and Critical Care Medicine, 176,* 886–891. https://doi.org/10.1164/rccm.200702-271oc

Gao, F., Chen, J., Wei, D., Wu, B., & Zhou, M. (2018). Lung transplantation for bronchiolitis obliterans syndrome after allogenic hematopoietic stem cell transplantation. *Frontiers of Medicine, 12,* 224–228. https://doi.org/10.1007/s11684-017-0538-3

Gattinoni, L., & Caironi, P. (2008). Refining ventilatory treatment for acute lung injury and acute respiratory distress syndrome. *JAMA, 299,* 691–693. https://doi.org/10.1001/jama.299.6.691

Gea-Banacloche, J. (2018). Pulmonary infectious complications after hematopoietic stem cell transplantation: A practical guide to clinicians. *Current Opinion in Organ Transplantation, 23,* 375–380. https://doi.org/10.1097/mot.0000000000000549

Gea-Banacloche, J., Masur, H., Arns da Cuhna, C., Chiller, T., Kirchoff, L., Shaw, P., ... Cordonnier, C. (2009). Regionally limited or rare infections: Prevention after hematopoietic cell transplantation. *Bone Marrow Transplantation, 44,* 489–494. https://doi.org/10.1038/bmt.2009.260

George, B., Pati, N., Gilroy, N., Ratnamohan, M., Huang, G., Kerridge, I., ... Bradstock, K. (2010). Pre-transplant cytomegalovirus (CMV) serostatus remains the most important determinant of CMV reactivation after allogeneic hematopoietic stem cell transplantation in the era of surveillance and preemptive therapy. *Transplant Infectious Disease, 12,* 322–329. https://doi.org/10.1111/j.1399-3062.2010.00504.x

Gilbert, C.R., Lee, H.J., Skalski, J.H., Maldonado, F., Wahidi, M., Choi, P.J., ... Yarmus, L. (2015). The use of indwelling tunneled pleural catheters for recurrent pleural effusions in patients with hematologic malignancies: A multicenter study. *Chest, 148,* 752–758. https://doi.org/10.1378/chest.14-3119

Girmenia, C. (2019). Advances in CMV infection prevention and treatment after allo-HSCT. *Advances in Cell and Gene Therapy, 2,* e53. https://doi.org/10.1002/acg2.53

Girmenia, C., Rossolini, G.M., & Viscoli, C. (2017). Prevention and treatment of infection. In S.A. Abulatib & P. Hari (Eds.), *Clinical manual of blood and bone marrow transplantation* (pp. 348–358). https://doi.org/10.1002/9781119095491.ch39

Gjærde, L.I., Moser, C., & Sengeløv, H. (2017). Epidemiology of bloodstream infections after myeloablative and non-myeloablative allogeneic hematopoietic stem cell transplantation: A single-center cohort study. *Transplant Infectious Disease, 19,* e12730. https://doi.org/10.1111/tid.12730

Glezerman, I.G., Jhaveri, K.D., Watson, T.H., Edwards, A.M., Papadopoulos, E.B., Young, J.W., ... Jakubowski, A.A. (2010). Chronic kidney disease, thrombotic microangiopathy, and hypertension following T cell-depleted hematopoietic stem cell transplantation. *Biology of Blood and Marrow Transplantation, 16,* 976–984. https://doi.org/10.1016/j.bbmt.2010.02.006

Guinan, E.C., Hewett, E.K., Domaney, N.M., & Margossian, R. (2011). Outcome of hematopoietic stem cell transplant in children with congenital heart disease. *Pediatric Transplantation, 15,* 75–80. https://doi.org/10.1111/j.1399-3046.2010.01317.x

Gupta, S., Sultenfuss, M., Romaguera, J.E., Ensor, J., Krishnamurthy, S., Wallace, M.J., ... Hicks, M.E. (2010). CT-guided percutaneous lung biopsies in patients with haematologic malignancies and undiagnosed pulmonary lesions. *Hematological Oncology, 28,* 75–81. https://doi.org/10.1002/hon.923

Hakim, A., Cooke, K.R., Pavletic, S.Z., Khalid, M., Williams, K.M., & Hashmi, S.K. (2019). Diagnosis and treatment of bronchiolitis obliterans syndrome accessible universally. *Bone Marrow Transplantation, 54,* 383–392. https://doi.org/10.1038/s41409-018-0266-6

Hall, S., Danby, R., Osman, H., Peniket, A., Rocha, V., Craddock, C., ... Chaganti, S. (2015). Transfusion in CMV seronegative T-depleted allogeneic stem cell transplant recipients with CMV-unselected blood components results in zero CMV transmissions in the era of universal leukocyte reduction: A UK dual centre experience. *Transfusion Medicine, 25,* 418–423. https://doi.org/10.1111/tme.12219

Hamada, K., Nagai, S., Kitaichi, M., Jin, G., Shigematsu, M., Nagao, T., ... Mishima, M. (2003). Cyclophosphamide-induced late-onset lung disease. *Internal Medicine, 42,* 82–87. https://doi.org/10.2169/internalmedicine.42.82

Han, X.Y. (2007). Epidemiologic analysis of reactivated cytomegalovirus antigenemia in patients with cancer. *Journal of Clinical Microbiology, 45,* 1126–1132. https://doi.org/10.1128/jcm.01670-06

Harch, S., Whitford, H., & McLean, C. (2009). Failure of medical therapy in pulmonary arterial hypertension: Is there an alternative diagnosis? *Chest, 135,* 1462–1469. https://doi.org/10.1378/chest.08-2006

Hardak, E., Avivi, I., Berkun, L., Raz-Pasteur, A., Lavi, N., Geffen, Y., ... Oren, I. (2016). Polymicrobial pulmonary infection in patients with hematological malignancies: Prevalence, co-pathogens, course and outcome. *Infection, 44,* 491–497. https://doi.org/10.1007/s15010-016-0873-3

Hashmi, S., Khorana, A., Hogan, W., Gastineau, D.A., Patnaik, M., Prokop, L., ... Litzow, M.R. (2015). Venous thromboembolism is hematopoietic stem cell transplant patients—A meta-analysis and systemic review [Abstract No. 63]. *Biology of Blood and Marrow Transplantation, 21*(Suppl.), S74–S75. https://doi.org/10.1016/j.bbmt.2014.11.083

Heidrich, H., Konau, E., & Hesse, P. (2009). Asymptomatic venous thrombosis in cancer patients—A problem often overlooked. Results of a retrospective and prospective study. *Vasa, 38,* 160–166. https://doi.org/10.1024/0301-1526.38.2.160

Hendriks, M.P., Blijlevens, N.M.A., Schattenberg, A.V.M.B., Burger, D.M., & Donnelly, J.P. (2006). Cyclosporine short infusion and C$_2$ monitoring in haematopoietic stem cell transplant recipients. *Bone Marrow Transplantation, 38,* 521–525. https://doi.org/10.1038/sj.bmt.1705481

Hensley, M.L., Hagerty, K.L., Kewalramani, T., Green, D.M., Meropol, N.J., Wasserman, T.H., ... Schuchter, L.M. (2009). American Society of Clinical Oncology 2008 clinical practice guideline update: Use of chemotherapy and radiation therapy protectants. *Journal of Clinical Oncology, 27,* 127–145. https://doi.org/10.1200/jco.2008.17.2627

Heritage Pharmaceuticals. (2018, October). *BICNU (carmustine)* [Package insert]. East Brunswick, NJ: Author.

Herrmann, J., Lerman, A., Sandhu, N.P., Villarraga, H.R., Mulvagh, S.L., & Kohli, M. (2014). Evaluation and management of patients with heart disease and cancer: Cardio-oncology. *Mayo Clinic Proceedings, 89,* 1287–1306. https://doi.org/10.1016/j.mayocp.2014.05.013

Hidalgo, J.D., Krone, R., Rich, M.W., Blum, K., Adkins, D., Fan, M.-Y., ... Khoury, H. (2004). Supraventricular tachyarrhythmias after hematopoietic stem cell transplantation: Incidence, risk factors and outcomes. *Bone Marrow Transplantation, 34,* 615–619. https://doi.org/10.1038/sj.bmt.1704623

Hildebrandt, G.C., Munker, R., Duffner, U., Wolff, D., Stadler, M., Dietrich-Ntoukas, T., ... Atkinson, K. (2013). Organ-related and miscellaneous complications. In R. Munker, G.C. Hildebrandt, H.M. Lazarus, & K. Atkinson (Eds.), *The BMT data book* (3rd ed., pp. 348–410). https://doi.org/10.1017/cbo9781139519205.028

Hodson, A., Kasliwal, M., Streetly, M., MacMahon, E., & Raj, K. (2011). A parainfluenza-3 outbreak in a SCT unit: Sepsis with multi-organ failure and multiple co-pathogens are associated with increased mortality. *Bone Marrow Transplantation, 46,* 1545–1550. https://doi.org/10.1038/bmt.2010.347

Hofmeister, C.C., Czerlanis, C., Forsythe, S., & Stiff, P.J. (2006). Retrospective utility of bronchoscopy after hematopoietic stem cell transplant. *Bone Marrow Transplantation, 38,* 693–698. https://doi.org/10.1038/sj.bmt.1705505

Holler, T. (2008). *Cardiology essentials.* Sudbury, MA: Jones & Bartlett Learning.

Horton, L.E., Haste, N.M., & Taplitz, R.A. (2018). Rethinking antimicrobial prophylaxis in the transplant patient in the world of emerging resistant organisms—Where are we today? *Current Hematologic Malignancy Reports, 13,* 59–67. https://doi.org/10.1007/s11899-018-0435-0

Hovi, L., Saxen, H., Saarinen-Pihkala, U.M., Vettenranta, K., Meri, T., & Richardson, M. (2007). Prevention and monitoring of invasive fungal infections in pediatric patients with cancer and hematologic disorders. *Pediatric Blood and Cancer, 48,* 28–34. https://doi.org/10.1002/pbc.20717

Huisman, C., van der Straaten, H.M., Canninga-van Dijk, M.R., Fijnheer, R., & Verdonck, L.F. (2006). Pulmonary complications after T-cell-depleted allogeneic stem cell transplantation: Low incidence and strong association with acute graft-versus-host disease. *Bone Marrow Transplantation, 38,* 561–566. https://doi.org/10.1038/sj.bmt.1705484

Ibrahim, R.B., Peres, E., Dansey, R., Abidi, M.H., Abella, E.M., Gumma, M.M., ... Klein, J. (2005). Safety of low-dose low-molecular-weight-heparins in thrombocytopenic stem cell transplantation patients: A case series and review of the literature. *Bone Marrow Transplantation, 35,* 1071–1077. https://doi.org/10.1038/sj.bmt.1704952

Ishida, S., Doki, N., Shingai, N., Yoshioka, K., Kakihana, K., Sakamaki, H., & Ohashi, K. (2016). The clinical features of fatal cyclophosphamide-induced cardiotoxicity in a conditioning regimen for allogeneic hematopoietic stem cell transplantation (allo-HSCT). *Annals of Hematology, 95,* 1145–1150. https://doi.org/10.1007/s00277-016-2654-6

Jain, M., Budinger, G., Jovanovic, B., Dematte, J., Duffey, S., & Mehta, J. (2018). Bortezomib is safe in and stabilizes pulmonary function in patients with allo-HSCT-associated pulmonary CGVHD. *Bone Marrow Transplantation, 53*, 1124–1130. https://doi.org/10.1038/s41409-018-0134-4

Jenks, J.D., & Hoenigl, M. (2018). Treatment of aspergillosis. *Journal of Fungi, 4*, 98–117. https://doi.org/10.3390/jof4030098

Ji, Y., Xu, L.-P., Liu, D.-H., Chen, Y.-H., Han, W., Zhang, X.-H., … Huang, X.-J. (2011). Positive results of serum galactomannan assays and pulmonary computed tomography predict the higher response rate of empirical antifungal therapy in patients undergoing allogeneic hematopoietic stem cell transplantation. *Biology of Blood and Marrow Transplantation, 17*, 759–764. https://doi.org/10.1016/j.bbmt.2010.11.002

Jiménez-Ortigosa, C., Moore, C., Denning, D.W., & Perlin, D.S. (2017). Emergence of echinocandin resistance due to a point mutation in the *fks1* gene of *Aspergillus fumigatus* in a patient with chronic pulmonary aspergillosis. *Antimicrobial Agents and Chemotherapy, 61*, e01277-17. https://doi.org/10.1128/aac.01277-17

Jinta, M., Ohashi, K., Ohta, T., Ieki, R., Abe, K., Kamata, N., … Sakamaki, H. (2007). Clinical features of allogeneic hematopoietic stem cell transplantation-associated organizing pneumonia. *Bone Marrow Transplantation, 40*, 465–472. https://doi.org/10.1038/sj.bmt.1705768

Jirasek, M.A., & Herrington, J.D. (2016). Cytarabine syndrome despite corticosteroid premedication in an adult undergoing induction treatment for acute myelogenous leukemia. *Journal of Oncology Pharmacy Practice, 22*, 795–800. https://doi.org/10.1177/1078155215607090

Jodele, S., Chima, R., Hor, K., Witte, D., Laskin, B.L., Goebel, J., … Davies, S.M. (2012). Pulmonary hypertension (PH) in patients with hematopoietic stem cell transplant-associated thrombotic microangiopathy (TMA) [Abstract]. *Biology of Blood and Marrow Transplantation, 18*(Suppl. 2), S232. https://doi.org/10.1016/j.bbmt.2011.12.088

Kang, S.H., Park, H.S., Sun, I.O., Choi, S.R., Chung, B.H., Choi, B.S., … Park, C.W. (2012). Changes in renal function in long-term survivors of allogeneic hematopoietic stem-cell transplantation: Single-center experience. *Clinical Nephrology, 77*, 225–230. https://doi.org/10.5414/cn107280

Kaplan, R., Bashoura, L., Shannon, V.R., Dickey, B.F., & Stover, D.E. (2011). Noninfectious lung infiltrates that may be confused with pneumonia in the cancer patient. In A. Safdar (Ed.), *Principles and practice of cancer infectious diseases* (pp. 153–165). https://doi.org/10.1007/978-1-60761-644-3_13

Kaur, D., Ashrani, A.A., Pruthi, R., Khan, S.P., Bailey, K., & Rodriguez, V. (2018). Thrombotic and hemorrhagic complications in children and young adult recipients of hematopoietic stem cell transplant (HSCT). *Thrombosis Research, 167*, 44–49. https://doi.org/10.1016/j.thromres.2018.04.023

Kawano, H., Tanaka, H., Yamashita, T., Hirata, K.-I., Ishii, S., Suzuki, T., … Katayama, Y. (2015). Very late-onset reversible cardiomyopathy in patients with chronic GvHD. *Bone Marrow Transplantation, 50*, 870–872. https://doi.org/10.1038/bmt.2015.40

Kebriaei, P., Saliba, R., Rondon, G., Chiattone, A., Luthra, R., Anderlini, P., … Champlin, R. (2012). Long-term follow-up of allogeneic hematopoietic stem cell transplantation for patients with Philadelphia chromosome-positive acute lymphoblastic leukemia: Impact of tyrosine kinase inhibitors on treatment outcomes. *Biology of Blood and Marrow Transplantation, 18*, 584–592. https://doi.org/10.1016/j.bbmt.2011.08.011

Kekre, N., Kim, H.T., Ho, V.T., Cutler, C., Armand, P., Nikiforow, S., … Koreth, J. (2017). Venous thromboembolism is associated with graft-*versus*-host disease and increased non-relapse mortality after allogeneic hematopoietic stem cell transplantation. *Haematologica, 102*, 1185–1191. https://doi.org/10.3324/haematol.2017.164012

Kekre, N., Tokessy, M., Mallick, R., McDiarmid, S., Huebsch, L., Bredeson, C., … Sheppard, D. (2013). Is cytomegalovirus testing of blood products still needed for hematopoietic stem cell transplant recipients in the era of universal leukoreduction? *Biology of Blood and Marrow Transplantation, 19*, 1719–1724. https://doi.org/10.1016/j.bbmt.2013.09.013

Kleinman, S., Caulfield, T., Chan, P., Davenport, R., McFarland, J., McPhedran, S., … Slinger, P. (2004). Toward an understanding of transfusion-related acute lung injury: Statement of a consensus panel. *Transfusion, 44*, 1774–1789. https://doi.org/10.1111/j.0041-1132.2004.04347.x

Kopko, P.M., & Popovsky, M.A. (2004). Pulmonary injury from transfusion-related acute lung injury. *Clinics in Chest Medicine, 25*, 105–113. https://doi.org/10.1016/s0272-5231(03)00135-7

Koreth, J., & Antin, J.H. (2008). Current and future approaches for control of graft-versus-host disease. *Expert Review of Hematology, 1*, 111–128. https://doi.org/10.1586/17474086.1.1.111

Kosmidis, C., & Denning, D.W. (2015). Republished: The clinical spectrum of pulmonary aspergillosis. *Postgraduate Medical Journal, 91*, 403–410. https://doi.org/10.1136/postgradmedj-2014-206291rep

Kossow, A., Kampmeier, S., Willems, S., Berdel, W.E., Groll, A.H., Burckhardt, B., … Stelljes, M. (2017). Control of multidrug-resistant *Pseudomonas aeruginosa* in allogeneic hematopoietic stem cell transplant recipients by a novel bundle including remodeling of sanitary and water supply systems. *Clinical Infectious Diseases, 65*, 935–942. https://doi.org/10.1093/cid/cix465

Kotloff, R.M., Ahya, V.N., & Crawford, S.W. (2004). Pulmonary complications of solid organ and hematopoietic stem cell transplantation. *American Journal of Respiratory and Critical Care Medicine, 170*, 22–48. https://doi.org/10.1164/rccm.200309-1322so

Kotloff, R.M., Dickey, B.F., & Vander Els, N. (2019). Respiratory tract diseases that may be mistaken for infection. In A. Safdar (Ed.), *Principles and practice of transplant infectious diseases* (pp. 351–364). https://doi.org/10.1007/978-1-4939-9034-4_21

Kozlowska-Skrzypczak, M., Bembnista, E., Kubiak, A., Matuszak, P., Schneider, A., & Komarnicki, M. (2014). Microbial contamination of peripheral blood and bone marrow hematopoietic cell products and environmental contamination in a stem cell bank: A single-center report. *Transplantation Proceedings, 46*, 2873–2876. https://doi.org/10.1016/j.transproceed.2014.09.002

Krishnan, B.R., James, K.D., Polowy, K., Bryant, B.J., Vaidya, A., Smith, S., & Laudeman, C.P. (2017). CD101, a novel echinocandin with exceptional stability properties and enhanced aqueous solubility. *Journal of Antibiotics, 70*, 130–135. https://doi.org/10.1038/ja.2016.89

Kuruvilla, J., Forrest, D.L., Lavoie, J.C., Nantel, S.H., Shepherd, J.D., Song, K.W., … Nevill, T.J. (2004). Characteristics and outcome of patients developing endocarditis following hematopoietic stem cell transplantation. *Bone Marrow Transplantation, 34*, 969–973. https://doi.org/10.1038/sj.bmt.1704655

Kyriakidis, I., Tragiannidis, A., Munchen, S., & Groll, A.H. (2017). Clinical hepatotoxicity associated with antifungal agents. *Expert Opinion on Drug Safety, 16*, 149–165. https://doi.org/10.1080/14740338.2017.1270264

Lam, D.C.L., Lam, B., Wong, M.K.Y., Lu, C., Au, W.Y., Tse, E.W.C., … Lie, A.K.W. (2011). Effects of azithromycin in bronchiolitis obliterans syndrome after hematopoietic SCT—A randomized double-blinded placebo-controlled study. *Bone Marrow Transplantation, 46*, 1551–1556. https://doi.org/10.1038/bmt.2011.1

Latchford, T., & Shelton, B.K. (2003). Respiratory syncytial virus in blood and marrow transplant recipients. *Clinical Journal of Oncology Nursing, 7*, 418–422. https://doi.org/10.1188/03.CJON.418-422

Law, N., & Kumar, D. (2017). Post-transplant viral respiratory infections in the older patient: Epidemiology, diagnosis, and management. *Drugs and Aging, 34*, 743–754. https://doi.org/10.1007/s40266-017-0491-5

Leaver, S.K., & Evans, T.W. (2007). Acute respiratory distress syndrome. *BMJ, 335*, 389–394. https://doi.org/10.1136/bmj.39293.624699.ad

Lee, J., Modi, D., Jang, H., Uberti, J.P., & Kim, S. (2017). Multistate models on pleural effusion after allogeneic hematopoietic stem cell transplantation. *Open Access Medical Statistics, 7*, 15–26. https://doi.org/10.2147/oams.s125465

Lev, A., Amariglio, N., Spirer, Z., Katz, U., Bielorai, B., Rechavi, G., & Somech, R. (2010). Specific self-antigen-driven immune response in pericardial effusion as an isolated GVHD manifestation. *Bone Marrow Transplantation, 45*, 1084–1087. https://doi.org/10.1038/bmt.2009.314

Lewis, I., DeFor, T., & Weisdorf, D.J. (2000). Increasing incidence of diffuse alveolar hemorrhage following allogeneic bone marrow transplantation: Cryptic etiology and uncertain therapy. *Bone Marrow Transplantation, 26*, 539–543. https://doi.org/10.1038/sj.bmt.1702546

Lionakis, M.S., Lewis, R.E., & Kontoyiannis, D.P. (2018). Breakthrough invasive mold infections in the hematology patient: Current concepts and future directions. *Clinical Infectious Disease, 67*, 1621–1630. https://doi.org/10.1093/cid/ciy473

Liptzin, D.R., DeBoer, E.M., Giller, R.H., Kroehl, M.E., & Weinman, J.P. (2018). Evaluating for bronchiolitis obliterans with low-attenuation computed tomography three-dimensional reconstructions. *American Journal of Respiratory and Critical Care Medicine, 197*, 814–815. https://doi.org/10.1164/rccm.201707-1340im

Litjens, N.H.R., van der Wagen, L., Kuball, J., & Kwekkeboom, J. (2018). Potential beneficial effects of cytomegalovirus infection after transplantation. *Frontiers in Immunology, 9*, 389. https://doi.org/10.3389/fimmu.2018.00389

Liu, Y.-C., Chien, S.-H., Fan, N.-W., Hu, M.-H., Gau, J.-P., Liu, C.-J., ... Tzeng, C.-H. (2015). Risk factors for pericardial effusion in adult patients receiving allogeneic haematopoietic stem cell transplantation. *British Journal of Haematology, 169*, 737–745. https://doi.org/10.1111/bjh.13357

Ljungman, P. (2014). Respiratory syncytial virus in hematopoietic cell transplant recipients: Factors determining progression to lower respiratory tract disease. *Journal of Infectious Diseases, 209*, 1151–1152. https://doi.org/10.1093/infdis/jit833

Ljungman, P., Brand, R., Einsele, H., Frassoni, F., Niederwieser, D., & Cordonnier, C. (2003). Donor CMV serologic status and outcome of CMV-seropositive recipients after unrelated donor stem cell transplantation: An EBMT megafile analysis. *Blood, 102*, 4255–4260. https://doi.org/10.1182/blood-2002-10-3263

Ljungman, P., de la Camara, R., Perez-Bercoff, L., Abecasis, M., Nieto Campuzano, J.B., Cannata-Ortiz, M.J., ... Engelhard, D. (2011). Outcome of pandemic H1N1 infections in hematopoietic stem cell transplant recipients. *Haematologica, 96*, 1231–1235. https://doi.org/10.3324/haematol.2011.041913

Ljungman, P., Perez-Bercoff, L., Jonsson, J., Avetisyan, G., Sparrelid, E., Aschan, J., ... Ringden, O. (2006). Risk factors for the development of cytomegalovirus disease after allogeneic stem cell transplantation. *Haematologica, 91*, 78–83. Retrieved from http://www.haematologica.org/content/91/1/78.long

Locatelli, F., Bertaina, A., Bertaina, V., & Merli, P. (2016). Cytomegalovirus in hematopoietic stem cell transplant recipients—Management of infection. *Expert Review of Hematology, 9*, 1093–1105. https://doi.org/10.1080/17474086.2016.1242406

Lortholary, O., Obenga, G., Biswas, P., Caillot, D., Chachaty, E., Bienvenu, A.-L., ... Troke, P. (2010). International retrospective analysis of 73 cases of invasive fusariosis treated with voriconazole. *Antimicrobial Agents and Chemotherapy, 54*, 4446–4450. https://doi.org/10.1128/aac.00286-10

Lucena, C.M., Rovira, M., Gabarrús, A., Filella, X., Martínez, C., Domingo, R., ... Agustí, C. (2017). The clinical value of biomarkers in respiratory complications in hematopoietic SCT. *Bone Marrow Transplantation, 52*, 415–422. https://doi.org/10.1038/bmt.2016.280

Lucena, C.M., Torres, A., Rovira, M., Marcos, M.A., de la Bellacasa, J.P., Sánchez, M., ... Agustí, C. (2014). Pulmonary complications in hematopoietic SCT: A prospective study. *Bone Marrow Transplantation, 49*, 1293–1299. https://doi.org/10.1038/bmt.2014.151

Mackay, A., & Al-Haddad, M. (2009). Acute lung injury and acute respiratory distress syndrome. *Continuing Education in Anesthesia, Critical Care and Pain, 9*, 152–156. https://doi.org/10.1093/bjaceaccp/mkp028

MacLaren, R., & Stringer, K.A. (2007). Emerging role of anticoagulants and fibrinolytics in the treatment of acute respiratory distress syndrome. *Pharmacotherapy, 27*, 860–873. https://doi.org/10.1592/phco.27.6.860

Majhail, N.S., Parks, K., Defor, T.E., & Weisdorf, D.J. (2006). Diffuse alveolar hemorrhage and infection-associated alveolar hemorrhage following hematopoietic stem cell transplantation: Related and high-risk clinical syndromes. *Biology of Blood and Marrow Transplantation, 12*, 1038–1046. https://doi.org/10.1016/j.bbmt.2006.06.002

Majhail, N.S., Rizzo, J.D., Lee, S.J., Aljurf, M., Atsuta, Y., Bonfim, C., ... Tichelli, A. (2014). Recommended screening and preventive practices for long-term survivors after hematopoietic cell transplantation. *Hematology/Oncology and Stem Cell Therapy, 5*, 1–30. https://doi.org/10.5144/1658-3876.2012.1

Marr, K.A., Bow, E., Chiller, T., Maschmeyer, G., Ribaud, P., Segal, B., ... Nucci, M. (2009). Fungal infection prevention after hematopoietic cell transplantation. *Bone Marrow Transplantation, 44*, 483–487. https://doi.org/10.1038/bmt.2009.259

Mattson, M.R. (2007). Graft-versus-host disease: Review and nursing implications. *Clinical Journal of Oncology Nursing, 11*, 325–328. https://doi.org/10.1188/07.cjon.325-328

McCann, S., Byrne, J.L., Rovira, M., Shaw, P., Ribaud, P., Sica, S., ... Cordonnier, C. (2004). Outbreaks of infectious diseases in stem cell transplant units: A silent cause of death for patients and transplant programmes. *Bone Marrow Transplantation, 33*, 519–529. https://doi.org/10.1038/sj.bmt.1704380

Meijer, E., Dekker, A.W., Lokhorst, H.M., Petersen, E.J., Nieuwenhuis, H.K., & Verdonck, L.F. (2004). Low incidence of infectious complications after nonmyeloablative compared with myeloablative allogeneic stem cell transplantation. *Transplant Infectious Disease, 6*, 171–178. https://doi.org/10.1111/j.1399-3062.2004.00075.x

Milano, F., Au, M.A., Boeckh, M.J., Deeg, H.J., & Chien, J.W. (2011). Evaluation of the impact of antithymocyte globulin on lung function at 1 year after allogeneic stem cell transplantation. *Biology of Blood and Marrow Transplantation, 17*, 703–709. https://doi.org/10.1016/j.bbmt.2010.08.012

Miller, S. (2019). Paramyxoviruses and rubella virus. In S. Riedel, S.A. Morse, T. Mietzner, & S. Miller (Eds.), *Jawetz, Melnick, and Adelberg's medical microbiology* (28th ed., pp. 595–616). New York, NY: McGraw-Hill Education.

Modi, D., Jang, H., Kim, S., Deol, A., Ayash, L., Bhutani, D., ... Uberti, J.P. (2016). Incidence, etiology, and outcome of pleural effusions in allogeneic hematopoietic stem cell transplantation. *American Journal of Hematology, 91*, E341–E347. https://doi.org/10.1002/ajh.24435

Mogili, S., Krishnamurthy, M., Alkhoury, Z.A., & Lyons, J.J. (2009). Warfarin induced intra alveolar hemorrhage: A case report. *Internet Journal of Internal Medicine, 8*(2), 1–3. Retrieved from http://ispub.com/IJIM/8/2/9419

Mohty, M., Malard, F., Abecassis, M., Aerts, E., Alaskar, A.S., Aljurf, M., ... Carreras, E. (2015). Sinusoidal obstruction syndrome/veno-occlusive disease: Current situation and perspectives—A position statement from the European Society for Blood and Marrow Transplantation (EBMT). *Bone Marrow Transplantation, 50*, 781–789. https://doi.org/10.1038/bmt.2015.52

Montani, D., Achouh, L., Dorfmüller, P., Le Pavec, J., Sztrymf, B., Tchérakian, C., ... Humbert, M. (2008). Pulmonary veno-occlusive disease: Clinical, functional, radiologic, and hemodynamic characteristics and outcome of 24 cases confirmed by histology. *Medicine, 87*, 220–233. https://doi.org/10.1097/md.0b013e31818193bb

Morandi, P., Ruffini, P.A., Benvenuto, G.M., Raimondi, R., & Fosser, V. (2005). Cardiac toxicity of high-dose chemotherapy. *Bone Marrow Transplantation, 35*, 323–334. https://doi.org/10.1038/sj.bmt.1704763

Moreau, A.-S., Seguin, A., Lemiale, V., Yakoub-Agha, I., Girardie, P., Robriquet, L., ... Jourdain, M. (2014). Survival and prognostic factors of allogeneic hematopoietic stem cell transplant recipients admitted to intensive care unit. *Leukemia and Lymphoma, 55*, 1417–1420. https://doi.org/10.3109/10428194.2013.836602

Morley-Smith, A.C., Cowie, M.R., & Vazir, A. (2013). Pericardial constriction attributable to graft-versus-host disease: Importance of early immunosuppression. *Circulation: Heart Failure, 6*, e59–e61. https://doi.org/10.1161/circheartfailure.113.000462

Murray, M.P., Doherty, C.J., Govan, J.R.W., & Hill, A.T. (2010). Do processing time and storage of sputum influence quantitative bacteriology in bronchiectasis? *Journal of Medical Microbiology, 59*, 829–833. https://doi.org/10.1099/jmm.0.016683-0

Najima, Y., Ohashi, K., Miyazawa, M., Nakano, M., Kobayashi, T., Yamashita, T., ... Sakamaki, H. (2009). Intracranial hemorrhage following allogeneic hematopoietic stem cell transplantation. *American Journal of Hematology, 84*, 298–301. https://doi.org/10.1002/ajh.21382

Neemann, K., & Freifeld, A. (2015). Respiratory syncytial virus in hematopoietic stem cell transplantation and solid-organ transplantation. *Current Infectious Disease Reports, 17*, 38. https://doi.org/10.1007/s11908-015-0490-9

Neumann, S., Krause, S.W., Maschmeyer, G., Schiel, X., & von Lilienfeld-Toal, M. (2013). Primary prophylaxis of bacterial infections and *Pneumocystis jirovecii* pneumonia in patients with hematological malignancies and solid tumors: Guidelines of the Infectious Diseases Working Party (AGIHO) of the German Society of Hematology and Oncology (DGHO). *Annals of Hematology, 92*, 433–442. https://doi.org/10.1007/s00277-013-1698-0

New, J.Y., Li, B., Koh, W.P., Ng, H.K., Tan, S.Y., Yap, E.H., ... Hu, H.Z. (2002). T cell infiltration and chemokine expression: Relevance to the disease localization in murine graft-versus-host disease. *Bone Marrow Transplantation, 29*, 979–986. https://doi.org/10.1038/sj.bmt.1703563

Nguyen, M.H., Leather, H., Clancy, C.J., Cline, C., Jantz, M.A., Kulkarni, V., ... Wingard, J.R. (2011). Galactomannan testing in bronchoalveolar lavage fluid facilitates the diagnosis of invasive pulmonary aspergillosis in patients with hematologic malignancies and stem cell transplant recipients. *Biology of Blood and Marrow Transplantation, 17*, 1043–1050. https://doi.org/10.1016/j.bbmt.2010.11.013

Nihtinen, A., Anttila, V.-J., Richardson, M., Meri, T., Volin, L., & Ruutu, T. (2007). The utility of intensified environmental surveillance for pathogenic moulds in a stem cell transplantation ward during construction work to monitor the efficacy of HEPA filtration. *Bone Marrow Transplantation, 40*, 457–460. https://doi.org/10.1038/sj.bmt.1705749

Norkin, M., Ratanatharathorn, V., Ayash, L., Abidi, M.H., Al-Kadhimi, Z., Lum, L.G., & Uberti, J.P. (2011). Large pericardial effusion as a complication in adults undergoing SCT. *Bone Marrow Transplantation, 46*, 1353–1356. https://doi.org/10.1038/bmt.2010.297

O'Dwyer, D.N., Duvall, A.S., Xia, M., Hoffman, T.C., Bloye, K.S., Bulte, C.A., ... Yanik, G.A. (2018). Transbronchial biopsy in the management of pulmonary complications of hematopoietic stem cell transplantation. *Bone Marrow Transplantation, 53*, 193–198. https://doi.org/10.1038/bmt.2017.238

Ogimi, C., Xie, H., Campbell, A.P., Waghmare, A., Kuypers, J.M., Jerome, K.R., ... Boeckh, M.J. (2019). Human metapneumovirus or influenza A upper respiratory tract infection associated with increased risk of bacterial superinfection in allogeneic hematopoietic cell transplant recipients. *Biology of Blood and Marrow Transplantation, 25*(Suppl. 3), S350–S351. https://doi.org/10.1016/j.bbmt.2018.12.568

Ogonek, J., Juric, M.K., Ghimire, S., Varanasi, P.R., Holler, E., Greinix, H., & Weissinger, E. (2016). Immune reconstitution after allogeneic hematopoietic stem cell transplantation. *Frontiers in Immunology, 7*, 507. https://doi.org/10.3389/fimmu.2016.00507

Okimoto, T., Tsubata, Y., Hamaguchi, M., Sutani, A., Hamaguchi, S., & Isobe, T. (2018). Pleuroparenchymal fibroelastosis after haematopoietic stem cell transplantation without graft-versus-host disease findings. *Respirology Case Reports, 6*, e000298. https://doi.org/10.1002/rcr2.298

Okumura, H., Ohtake, S., Ontachi, Y., Ozaki, J., Shimadoi, S., Waseda, Y., ... Nakao, S. (2007). Living-donor lobar lung transplantation for broncho-bronchiolitis obliterans after allogeneic hematopoietic stem cell transplantation: Does bronchiolitis obliterans recur in transplanted lungs? *International Journal of Hematology, 86*, 369–373. https://doi.org/10.1532/ijh97.07045

Olsen, M.M., LeFebvre, K.B., & Brassil, K.J. (Eds.). (2019). *Chemotherapy and immunotherapy guidelines and recommendations for practice.* Pittsburgh, PA: Oncology Nursing Society.

Oyan, B., Koc, Y., Emri, S., & Kansu, E. (2006). Improvement of chronic pulmonary graft-vs-host disease manifesting as bronchiolitis obliterans organizing pneumonia following extracorporeal photopheresis. *Medical Oncology, 23*, 125–129. https://doi.org/10.1385/mo:23:1:125

Oymak, F.S., Demirbaş, H.M., Mavili, E., Akgun, H., Gulmez, I., Demir, R., & Ozesmi, M. (2005). Bronchiolitis obliterans organizing pneumonia: Clinical and roentgenological features in 26 cases. *Respiration, 72*, 254–262. https://doi.org/10.1159/000085366

Paczesny, S., Hanauer, D., Sun, Y., & Reddy, P. (2010). New perspectives on the biology of acute GVHD. *Bone Marrow Transplantation, 45*, 1–11. https://doi.org/10.1038/bmt.2009.328

Pallera, A.M., & Schwartzberg, L.S. (2004). Managing the toxicity of hematopoietic stem cell transplant. *Journal of Supportive Oncology, 2*, 223–237.

Pappas, P.G., Kauffman, C.A., Andes, D.R., Clancy, C.J., Marr, K.A., Ostrosky-Zeichner, L., ... Sobel, J.D. (2016). Clinical practice guideline for the management of candidiasis: 2016 update by the Infectious Diseases Society of America. *Clinical Infectious Diseases, 62*, e1–e50. https://doi.org/10.1093/cid/civ933

Patel, A.V., Hahn, T., Bogner, P.N., Loud, P.A., Brown, K., Paplham, P., ... McCarthy, P.L. (2010). Fatal diffuse alveolar hemorrhage associated with sirolimus after allogeneic hematopoietic cell transplantation. *Bone Marrow Transplantation, 45*, 1363–1364. https://doi.org/10.1038/bmt.2009.339

Patriarca, F., Skert, C., Sperotto, A., Damiani, D., Cerno, M., Geromin, A., ... Fanin, R. (2004). Incidence, outcome, and risk factors of late-onset noninfectious pulmonary complications after unrelated donor stem cell transplantation. *Bone Marrow Transplantation, 33*, 751–758. https://doi.org/10.1038/sj.bmt.1704426

Patterson, T.F., Thompson, G.R., III, Denning, D.W., Fishman, J.A., Hadley, S., Herbrecht, R., ... Bennett, J.E. (2016). Practice guidelines for the diagnosis and management of aspergillosis: 2016 update by the Infectious Diseases Society of America. *Clinical Infectious Diseases, 63*, e1–e60. https://doi.org/10.1093/cid/ciw326

Peck, A.J., Englund, J.A., Kuypers, J., Guthrie, K.A., Corey, L., Morrow, R., ... Boeckh, M. (2007). Respiratory virus infection among hematopoietic cell transplant recipients: Evidence for asymptomatic parainfluenza virus infection. *Blood, 110*, 1681–1688. https://doi.org/10.1182/blood-2006-12-060343

Penack, O., Tridello, G., Hoek, J., Socié, G., Blaise, D., Passweg, J., ... Cesaro, S. (2016). Influence of pre-existing invasive aspergillosis on allo-HSCT outcome: A retrospective EBMT analysis by the Infectious Diseases and Acute Leukemia Working Parties. *Bone Marrow Transplantation, 51*, 418–423. https://doi.org/10.1038/bmt.2015.237

Peres, E., Levine, J.E., Khaled, Y.A., Ibrahim, R.B., Braun, T.M., Krijanovski, O.I., ... Abidi, M.H. (2010). Cardiac complications in patients undergoing a reduced-intensity conditioning hematopoietic stem cell transplantation. *Bone Marrow Transplantation, 45*, 149–152. https://doi.org/10.1182/blood.V126.23.2346.2346

Perron, T., Emara, M., & Ahmed, S. (2014). Time to antibiotics and outcomes in cancer patients with febrile neutropenia. *BMC Health Services Research, 14*, 162. https://doi.org/10.1186/1472-6963-14-162

Peters, J., Elliott, J., Bloor, A., Dennis, M., Murray, J., Cavet, J., ... Kulkarni, S. (2015). Use of CMV unselected blood products does not increase the risk of CMV reactivation in patients undergoing hematopoetic stem cell transplant (HSCT). *Blood, 126*, 2346. Retrieved from http://www.bloodjournal.org/content/126/23/2346

Petraitis, V., Petraitiene, R., McCarthy, M.W., Kovanda, L.L., Zaw, M.H., Hussain, K., ... Walsh, T.J. (2017). Combination therapy with isavuconazole and micafungin for treatment of experimental invasive pulmonary aspergillosis. *Antimicrobial Agents and Chemotherapy, 61*, 1–12. https://doi.org/10.1128/aac.00305-17

Pfeffer, B., Tziros, C., & Katz, R.J. (2009). Current concepts of anthracycline cardiotoxicity: Pathogenesis, diagnosis, and prevention. *British Journal of Cardiology, 16*, 85–89.

Pfeiffer, T.M., Rotz, S.J., Ryan, T.D., Hirsch, R., Taylor, M., Chima, R., ... Dandoy, C. (2017). Pericardial effusion requiring surgical intervention after stem cell transplantation: A case series. *Bone Marrow Transplantation, 52*, 630–633. https://doi.org/10.1038/bmt.2016.331

Pfizer. (2018). *Cytarabine* [Package insert]. New York, NY: Author.

Physicians' Desk Reference. (2017). *PDR nurse's drug handbook* (2017 ed.). Montvale, NJ: Author.

Piñana, J.L., Gómez, M.D., Pérez, A., Madrid, S., Balaguer-Roselló, A., Giménez, E., ... Navarro, D. (2018). Community-acquired respiratory virus lower respiratory tract disease in allogeneic stem cell transplantation recipient: Risk factors and mortality from pulmonary virus-bacterial mixed infections. *Transplant Infectious Disease, 20*, e12926. https://doi.org/10.1111/tid.12926

Piralla, A., Gagliardone, C., Girello, A., Premoli, M., Campanini, G., Decembrino, N., ... Baldanti, F. (2016). The impact of viral respiratory infections in the first year post-transplant period of pediatric hematopoietic stem cell transplant (HSCT) recipients. *Journal of Clinical Virology, 82*(Suppl.), S98–S99. https://doi.org/10.1016/j.jcv.2016.08.196

Poletti, V., Costabel, U., & Semenzato, G. (2005). Pulmonary complications in patients with hematological disorders: Pathobiological bases and practical approach. *Seminars in Respiratory and Critical Care Medicine, 26*, 439–444. https://doi.org/10.1055/s-2005-922028

Popovsky, M.A. (2004). Transfusion and the lung: Circulatory overload and acute lung injury. *Vox Sanguinis, 87*(Suppl. 2), 62–65. https://doi.org/10.1111/j.1741-6892.2004.00453.x

Poręba, M., Gać, P., Usnarska-Zubkiewicz, L., Pilecki, W., Kuliczkowski, K., Mazur, G., ... Poręba, R. (2016). Echocardiographic evaluation of the early cardiotoxic effect of hematopoietic stem cell transplantation in patients with hematologic malignancies. *Leukemia and Lymphoma, 57*, 2119–2125. https://doi.org/10.3109/10428194.2015.1122782

Qazilbash, M.H., Amjad, A.I., Qureshi, S., Qureshi, S.R., Saliba, R.M., Khan, Z.U., … Champlin, R.E. (2009). Outcome of allogeneic hematopoietic stem cell transplantation in patients with low left ventricular ejection fraction. *Biology of Blood and Marrow Transplantation, 15*, 1265–1270. https://doi.org/10.1016/j.bbmt.2009.06.001

Rackley, C., Schultz, K.R., Goldman, F.D., Chan, K.W., Serrano, A., Hulse, J.E., & Gilman, A.L. (2005). Cardiac manifestations of graft-versus-host disease. *Biology of Blood and Marrow Transplantation, 11*, 773–780. https://doi.org/10.1016/j.bbmt.2005.07.002

Rathi, N.K., Tanner, A.R., Dinh, A., Dong, W., Feng, L., Ensor, J., … Nates, J.L. (2015). Low-, medium- and high-dose steroids with or without aminocaproic acid in adult hematopoietic SCT patients with diffuse alveolar hemorrhage. *Bone Marrow Transplantation, 50*, 420–426. https://doi.org/10.1038/bmt.2014.287

Razonable, R.R. (2018). Role of letermovir for prevention of cytomegalovirus infection after allogeneic haematopoietic stem cell transplantation. *Current Opinion in Infectious Diseases, 31*, 286–291. https://doi.org/10.1097/qco.0000000000000459

Remberger, M., Afram, G., Sundin, M., Uhlin, M., LeBlanc, K., Björklund, A., … Ljungman, P. (2016). High incidence of severe chronic GvHD after HSCT with sibling donors. A single center analysis. *Bone Marrow Transplantation, 51*, 1518–1521. https://doi.org/10.1038/bmt.2016.159

Ren, Y., & Lilly, L.S. (2011). Diseases of the pericardium. In L.S. Lilly (Ed.), *Pathophysiology of heart disease: A collaborative project of medical students and faculty* (5th ed., pp. 324–338). Philadelphia, PA: Lippincott Williams & Wilkins.

Rhodes, M., Lautz, T., Kavanaugh-Mchugh, A., Manes, B., Calder, C., Koyama, T., … Frangoul, H.J. (2005). Pericardial effusion and cardiac tamponade in pediatric stem cell transplant recipients. *Bone Marrow Transplantation, 36*, 139–144. https://doi.org/10.1038/sj.bmt.1705023

Rieger, C.T., Rieger, H., Kolb, H., Peterson, L., Huppmann, S., Fiegl, M., & Ostermann, H. (2009). Infectious complications after allogeneic stem cell transplantation: Incidence in matched-related and matched-unrelated transplant settings. *Transplant Infectious Disease, 11*, 220–226. https://doi.org/10.1111/j.1399-3062.2009.00379.x

Rimkus, C. (2009). Acute complications of stem cell transplant. *Seminars in Oncology Nursing, 25*, 129–138. https://doi.org/10.1016/j.soncn.2009.03.007

Roberts, S.S., Leeborg, N., Loriaux, M., Johnson, F.L., Huang, M.-L., Stenzel, P., … Godder, K.T. (2006). Acute graft-versus-host disease of the heart. *Pediatric Blood and Cancer, 47*, 624–628. https://doi.org/10.1002/pbc.20621

Rosenbaum, J.N., Butt, Y.M., Johnson, K.A., Meyer, K., Batra, K., Kanne, J.P., & Torrealba, J.R. (2015). Pleuroparenchymal fibroelastosis: A pattern of chronic lung injury. *Human Pathology, 46*, 137–146. https://doi.org/10.1016/j.humpath.2014.10.007

Rotz, S.J., Ryan, T.D., Hlavaty, J., George, S.A., El-Bietar, J., & Dandoy, C.E. (2017). Cardiotoxicity and cardiomyopathy in children and young adult survivors of hematopoietic stem cell transplant. *Pediatric Blood and Cancer, 64*, e26600. https://doi.org/10.1002/pbc.26600

Rovó, A., & Tichelli, A. (2012). Cardiovascular complications in long-term survivors after allogeneic hematopoietic stem cell transplantation. *Seminars in Hematology, 49*, 25–34. https://doi.org/10.1053/j.seminhematol.2011.10.001

Roychowdhury, M., Pambuccian, S.E., Aslan, D.L., Jessurun, J., Rose, A.G., Manivel, J.C., & Gulbahce, H.E. (2005). Pulmonary complications after bone marrow transplantation: An autopsy study from a large transplantation center. *Archives of Pathology and Laboratory Medicine, 129*, 366–371. Retrieved from https://www.archivesofpathology.org/doi/10.1043/1543-2165(2005)129%3C366:PCABMT%3E2.0.CO;2

Ruth-Sahd, L.A., & White, K.A. (2009). Bronchiolitis obliterans organizing pneumonia. *Dimensions of Critical Care Nursing, 28*, 204–208. https://doi.org/10.1097/dcc.0b013e3181ac49ce

Sakai, M., Kubota, T., Kuwayama, Y., Ikezoe, T., & Yokoyama, A. (2011). Diffuse alveolar hemorrhage associated with lenalidomide. *International Journal of Hematology, 93*, 830–831. https://doi.org/10.1007/s12185-011-0871-2

Salvatore, M., Satlin, M.J., Jacobs, S.E., Jenkins, S.G., Schuetz, A.N., Moss, R.B., … Soave, R. (2016). DAS181 for treatment of parainfluenza virus infections in hematopoietic stem cell transplant recipients at a single center. *Biology of Blood and Marrow Transplantation, 22*, 965–970. https://doi.org/10.1016/j.bbmt.2016.02.011

Samanta, P., & Nguyen, M.H. (2017). Pathogenesis of invasive pulmonary aspergillosis in transplant recipients. *Current Fungal Infection Reports, 11*, 148–157. https://doi.org/10.1007/s12281-017-0278-5

Sano, H., Kobayashi, R., Iguchi, A., Suzuki, D., Kishimoto, K., Yasuda, K., & Kobayashi, K. (2014). Risk factor analysis of idiopathic pneumonia syndrome after allogeneic hematopoietic SCT in children. *Bone Marrow Transplantation, 49*, 38–41. https://doi.org/10.1038/bmt.2013.123

Saria, M.G., & Gosselin-Acomb, T.K. (2007). Hematopoietic stem cell transplantation: Implications for critical care nurses. *Clinical Journal of Oncology Nursing, 11*, 53–63. https://doi.org/10.1188/07.cjon.53-63

Schwaiblmair, M., Behr, W., Haeckel, T., Märkl, B., Foerg, W., & Berghaus, T. (2012). Drug induced interstitial lung disease. *Open Respiratory Medicine Journal, 6*, 63–74. https://doi.org/10.2174/1874306401206010063

Seo, S., & Boeckh, M. (2016). Respiratory viruses after hematopoietic cell transplantation. In S.J. Forman, R.S. Negrin, J.H. Antin, & F.R. Appelbaum (Eds.), *Thomas' hematopoietic cell transplantation: Stem cell transplantation* (5th ed., pp. 1112–1125). https://doi.org/10.1002/9781118416426.ch91

Seong, G.M., Lee, Y., Hong, S.-B., Lim, C.-M., Koh, Y., & Huh, J.W. (2020). Prognosis of acute respiratory distress syndrome in patients with hematological malignancies. *Journal of Intensive Care Medicine, 35*, 364–370. https://doi.org/10.1177/0885066617753566

Shah, D.P., Ghantoji, S.S., Ariza-Heredia, E.J., Shah, J.N., El Taoum, K.K., Shah, P.K., … Chemaly, R.F. (2014). Immunodeficiency scoring index to predict poor outcomes in hematopoietic cell transplant recipients with RSV infections. *Blood, 123*, 3263–3268. https://doi.org/10.1182/blood-2013-12-541359

Shah, D.P., Ghantoji, S.S., Mulanovich, V.E., Ariza-Heredia, E.J., & Chemaly, R.F. (2012). Management of respiratory viral infections in hematopoietic cell transplant recipients. *American Journal of Blood Research, 2*, 203–218.

Shah, D.P., Shah, P.K., Azzi, J.M., El Chaer, F., & Chemaly, R.F. (2016). Human metapneumovirus infections in hematopoietic cell transplant recipients and hematologic malignancy patients: A systematic review. *Cancer Letters, 379*, 100–106. https://doi.org/10.1016/j.canlet.2016.05.035

Shankar, S.M., & Nania, J.J. (2007). Management of *Pneumocystis jiroveci* pneumonia in children receiving chemotherapy. *Pediatric Drugs, 9*, 301–309. https://doi.org/10.2165/00148581-200709050-00003

Shapiro, T.W. (2016). Nursing implications of blood and bone marrow transplantation. In J. Iatano (Ed.), *Core curriculum for oncology nursing* (5th ed., pp. 212–225). St Louis, MO: Elsevier.

Sharma, S., Nadrous, H.F., Peters, S.G., Tefferi, A., Litzow, M.R., Aubry, M.-C., & Afessa, B. (2005). Complications in adult blood and marrow transplant recipients. *Chest, 128*, 1385–1392. https://doi.org/10.1378/chest.128.3.1385

Shash, H., Stefanovici, C., Phillips, S., & Cuvelier, G.E. (2016). Aggressive metastatic inflammatory myofibroblastic tumor after allogeneic stem cell transplant with fatal pulmonary toxicity from crizotinib. *Journal of Pediatric Hematology/Oncology, 38*, 642–645. https://doi.org/10.1097/mph.0000000000000594

Shaw, B.E., Boswell, T., Byrne, J.L., Yates, C., & Russell, N.H. (2007). Clinical impact of MRSA in a stem cell transplant unit: Analysis before, during and after an MRSA outbreak. *Bone Marrow Transplantation, 39*, 623–629. https://doi.org/10.1038/sj.bmt.1705654

Shidham, V., & Atkinson, B. (2007). *Cytopathologic diagnosis of serous fluids*. St. Louis, MO: Elsevier Saunders.

Shinohara, A., Honda, A., Nukina, A., Takaoka, K., Tsukamoto, A., Hangai, S., … Kurokawa, M. (2016). Acute pericarditis before engraftment in hematopoietic stem cell transplantation. *Bone Marrow Transplantation, 51*, 459–461. https://doi.org/10.1038/bmt.2015.282

Shioya, M., Otsuka, M., Yamada, G., Umeda, Y., Ikeda, K., Nishikiori, H., … Takahashi, H. (2018). Poorer prognosis of idiopathic pleuroparenchymal fibroelastosis compared with idiopathic pulmonary fibrosis in advanced stage. *Canadian Respiratory Journal, 2018*, 1–7. https://doi.org/10.1155/2018/6043053

Shroff, G.S., Marom, E.M., Wu, C.C., Truong, M.T., & Godoy, M.C.B. (2019). Imaging of pneumonias and other thoracic complications after hematopoietic stem cell transplantation. *Current Problems in Diagnostic Radiology, 48*, 393–401. https://doi.org/10.1067/j.cpradiol.2018.07.006

Sim, S.A., Leung, V.K.Y., Ritchie, D., Slavin, M.A., Sullivan, S.G., & Teh, B.W. (2018). Viral respiratory tract infections in allogeneic hematopoietic stem cell transplantation recipients in the era of molecular testing. *Biology of Blood and Marrow Transplantation, 24*, 1490–1496. https://doi.org/10.1016/j.bbmt.2018.03.004

Singla, A., Hogan, W.J., Ansell, S.M., Buadi, F.K., Dingli, D., Dispenzieri, A., … Kumar, S.K. (2013). Incidence of supraventricular arrhythmias during autologous peripheral blood stem cell transplantation. *Biology of Blood and Marrow Transplantation, 19*, 1233–1237. https://doi .org/10.1016/j.bbmt.2013.05.019

Smalley, R.V., & Wall, R.L. (1966). Two cases of busulfan toxicity. *Annals of Internal Medicine, 64*, 154–164. https://doi.org/10.7326/0003-4819 -64-1-154

Sokol, K.A., Kim-Schulze, S., Robins, H., Obermoser, G., Blankenship, D., Qi, J., … Merad, M. (2017). Timing of influenza vaccine response in patients that receive autologous hematopoietic cell transplantation [Abstract]. *Biology of Blood and Marrow Transplantation, 23*(Suppl. 3), S143–S144. https://doi.org/10.1016/j.bbmt.2016.12.266

Soubani, A.O., & Pandya, C.M. (2010). The spectrum of noninfectious pulmonary complications following hematopoietic stem cell transplantation. *Hematology/Oncology and Stem Cell Therapy, 3*, 143–157. https://doi.org/10.1016/s1658-3876(10)50025-6

Soule, B.P., Simone, N.L., Savani, B.N., Ning, B., Albert, P.S., Barrett, A.J., & Singh, A.K. (2007). Pulmonary function following total body irradiation (with or without lung shielding) and allogeneic peripheral blood stem cell transplant. *Bone Marrow Transplantation, 40*, 573–578. https://doi.org/10.1038/sj.bmt.1705771

Specks, U. (2019). Cyclophosphamide pulmonary toxicity. In H. Hollingsworth & D.M.F. Savarese (Eds.), *UpToDate*. Retrieved October 22, 2019, from https://www.uptodate.com/contents/cyclophosphamide -pulmonary-toxicity

Srinivasan, A., Wang, C., Srivastava, D.K., Burnette, K., Shenep, J.L., Leung, W., & Hayden, R.T. (2013). Timeline, epidemiology, and risk factors for bacterial, fungal, and viral infections in children and adolescents after allogeneic hematopoietic stem cell transplantation. *Biology of Blood and Marrow Transplantation, 19*, 94–101. https://doi.org/10.1016 /j.bbmt.2012.08.012

Stone, N.R.H., Bicanic, T., Salim, R., & Hope, W. (2016). Liposomal amphotericin B (*AmBisome*®): A review of the pharmacokinetics, pharmacodynamics, clinical experience and future directions. *Drugs, 76*, 485–500. https://doi.org/10.1007/s40265-016-0538-7

Stuart, M.J., Chao, N.S., Horning, S.J., Wong, R.M., Negrin, R.S., Johnston, L.J., … Stockerl-Goldstein, K.E. (2001). Efficacy and toxicity of a CCNU-containing high-dose chemotherapy regimen followed by autologous hematopoietic cell transplantation in relapsed or refractory Hodgkin's disease. *Biology of Blood and Marrow Transplantation, 7*, 552–560. https://doi.org/10.1016/s1083-8791(01)70015-8

Stubblefield, M.D. (2017). Clinical evaluation and management of radiation fibrosis syndrome. *Physical Medicine and Rehabilitation Clinics of North America, 28*, 89–100. https://doi.org/10.1016/j.pmr.2016.08.003

Styczynski, J., Czyzewski, K., Wysocki, M., Gryniewicz-Kwiatkowska, O., Kolodziejczyk-Gietka, A., Salamonowicz, M., … Gil, L. (2016). Increased risk of infections and infection-related mortality in children undergoing haematopoietic stem cell transplantation compared to conventional anticancer therapy: A multicentre nationwide study. *Clinical Microbiology and Infection, 22*, 179.e1–179.e10. https://doi.org /10.1016/j.cmi.2015.10.017

Sucak, G.T., Ozkurt, Z.N., Akı, Z., Yağci, M., Çengel, A., & Haznedar, R. (2008). Cardiac systolic function in patients receiving hematopoetic stem cell transplantation: Risk factors for posttransplantation cardiac toxicity. *Transplantation Proceedings, 40*, 1586–1590. https://doi.org/10 .1016/j.transproceed.2007.11.077

Sweiss, K., Anderson, J., Wirth, S., Oh, A., Quigley, J.G., Khan, I., … Patel, P. (2018). A prospective study of intravenous pentamidine for PJP prophylaxis in adult patients undergoing intensive chemotherapy or hematopoietic stem cell transplant. *Bone Marrow Transplantation, 53*, 300–306. https://doi.org/10.1038/s41409-017-0024-1

Taetle, R., Dickman, P.S., & Feldman, P.S. (1978). Pulmonary histopathologic changes associated with melphalan therapy. *Cancer, 42*, 1239–

1245. https://doi.org/10.1002/1097-0142(197809)42:3<1239::aid -cncr2820420332>3.0.co;2-i

Tanaka, N., Kunihiro, Y., Kobayashi, T., Yujiri, T., Kido, S., Ueda, K., & Matsunaga, N. (2016). High-resolution CT findings of idiopathic pneumonia syndrome after haematopoietic stem cell transplantation: Based on the updated concept of idiopathic pneumonia syndrome by the American Thoracic Society in 2011. *Clinical Radiology, 71*, 953–959. https://doi.org/10.1016/j.crad.2016.06.109

Tawfik, P., & Arndt, P. (2017). The rare complication and diagnostic challenges of pulmonary eosinophilia in graft versus host disease patients after hematopoietic stem cell transplantation. *Lung, 195*, 805–811. https://doi.org/10.1007/s00408-017-0060-z

Thompson, J., Yin, Z., D'Souza, A., Fenske, T., Hamadani, M., Hari, P., … Drobyski, W.R. (2017). Etanercept and corticosteroid therapy for the treatment of late-onset idiopathic pneumonia syndrome. *Biology of Blood and Marrow Transplantation, 23*, 1955–1960. https://doi.org/10 .1016/j.bbmt.2017.07.019

Tissot, F., Agrawal, S., Pagano, L., Petrikkos, G., Groll, A.H., Skiada, A., … Herbrecht, R. (2017). ECIL-6 guidelines for the treatment of invasive candidiasis, aspergillosis and mucormycosis in leukemia and hematopoietic stem cell transplant patients. *Haematologica, 102*, 433–444. https://doi.org/10.3324/haematol.2016.152900

Tomblyn, M., Chiller, T., Einsele, H., Gress, R., Sepkowitz, K., Storek, J., … Boeckh, M.J. (2009). Guidelines for preventing infectious complications among hematopoietic cell transplantation recipients: A global perspective. *Biology of Blood and Marrow Transplantation, 15*, 1143–1238. https://doi.org/10.1016/j.bbmt.2009.06.019

Tonorezos, E.S., Stillwell, E.E., Calloway, J.J., Glew, T., Wessler, J.D., Rebolledo, B.J., … Schaffer, W.L. (2015). Arrhythmias in the setting of hematopoietic cell transplants. *Bone Marrow Transplantation, 50*, 1212–1216. https://doi.org/10.1038/bmt.2015.127

Touzot, M., Elie, C., van Massenhove, J., Maillard, N., Buzyn, A., & Fakhouri, F. (2010). Long-term renal function after allogenic haematopoietic stem cell transplantation in adult patients: A single-centre study. *Nephrology Dialysis Transplantation, 25*, 624–627. https://doi.org/10 .1093/ndt/gfp529

Toy, P., Popovsky, M.A., Abraham, E., Ambruso, D.R., Holness, L.G., Kopko, P.M., … Stroncek, D. (2005). Transfusion-related acute lung injury: Definition and review. *Critical Care Medicine, 33*, 721–726. https://doi .org/10.1097/01.ccm.0000159849.94750.51

Tramsen, L., Koehl, U., Tonn, T., Latgé, J.-P., Schuster, F.R., Borkhardt, A., … Lehrnbecher, T. (2009). Clinical-scale generation of human anti-*Aspergillus* T cells for adoptive immunotherapy. *Bone Marrow Transplantation, 43*, 13–19. https://doi.org/10.1038/bmt.2008.271

Ugai, T., Hamamoto, K., Kimura, S.-I., Akahoshi, Y., Nakano, H., Harada, N., … Kanda, Y. (2015). A retrospective analysis of computed tomography findings in patients with pulmonary complications after allogeneic hematopoietic stem cell transplantation. *European Journal of Radiology, 84*, 2663–2670. https://doi.org/10.1016/j.ejrad.2015.08 .020

Uhlving, H.H., Andersen, C.B., Christensen, I.J., Gormsen, M., Pedersen, K.D., Buchvald, F., … Müller, K.G. (2015). Biopsy-verified bronchiolitis obliterans and other noninfectious lung pathologies after allogeneic hematopoietic stem cell transplantation. *Biology of Blood and Marrow Transplantation, 21*, 531–538. https://doi.org/10.1016/j.bbmt .2014.12.004

Ullmann, A.J., Schmidt-Hieber, M., Bertz, H., Heinz, W.J., Kiehl, M., Krüger, W., … Maschmeyer, G. (2016). Infectious diseases in allogeneic haematopoietic stem cell transplantation: Prevention and prophylaxis strategy guidelines 2016. *Annals of Hematology, 95*, 1435–1455. https://doi .org/10.1007/s00277-016-2711-1

Unnewehr, M., Friederichs, H., Bartsch, P., & Schaaf, B. (2016). High diagnostic value of a new real-time pneumocystis PCR from bronchoalveolar lavage in a real-life clinical setting. *Respiration, 92*, 144–149. https://doi.org/10.1159/000448626

Vallabhaneni, S., Benedict, K., Derado, G., & Mody, R.K. (2017). Trends in hospitalizations related to invasive aspergillosis and mucormycosis in the United States, 2000–2013. *Open Forum Infectious Diseases, 4*, ofw268. https://doi.org/10.1093/ofid/ofw268

van de Peppel, R.J., Visser, L.G., Dekkers, O.M., & de Boer, M.G.J. (2018). The burden of invasive aspergillosis in patients with haematological malignancy: A meta-analysis and systematic review. *Journal of Infection, 76*, 550–562. https://doi.org/10.1016/j.jinf.2018.02.012

Vande Vusse, L.K., & Madtes, D.K. (2017). Early onset noninfectious pulmonary syndromes after hematopoietic cell transplantation. *Clinics in Chest Medicine, 38*, 233–248. https://doi.org/10.1016/j.ccm.2016.12.007

Vande Vusse, L.K., Madtes, D.K., Guthrie, K.A., Gernsheimer, T.B., Curtis, J.R., & Watkins, T.R. (2014). The association between red blood cell and platelet transfusion and subsequently developing idiopathic pneumonia syndrome after hematopoietic stem cell transplantation. *Transfusion, 54*, 1071–1080. https://doi.org/10.1111/trf.12396

van Kraaij, M.G.J., van Elden, L.J.R., van Loon, A.M., Hendriksen, K.A.W., Laterveer, L., Dekker, A.W., & Nijhuis, M. (2005). Frequent detection of respiratory viruses in adult recipients of stem cell transplants with the use of real-time polymerase chain reaction, compared with viral culture. *Clinical Infectious Diseases, 40*, 662–669. https://doi.org/10.1086/427801

van Leeuwen-Segarceanu, E.M., Bos, W.-J.W., Dorresteijn, L.D.A., Rensing, B.J.W.M., van der Heyden, J.A.S., Vogels, O.J.M., & Biesma, D.H. (2011). Screening Hodgkin lymphoma survivors for radiotherapy induced cardiovascular disease. *Cancer Treatment Reviews, 37*, 391–403. https://doi.org/10.1016/j.ctrv.2010.12.004

Vigorito, A.C., Campregher, P.V., Storer, B.E., Carpenter, P.A., Moravec, C.K., Kiem, H.-P., ... Flowers, M.E.D. (2009). Evaluation of the NIH consensus criteria for classification of late acute and chronic GVHD. *Blood, 114*, 702–708. https://doi.org/10.1182/blood-2009-03-208983

Vion, A.-C., Rautou, P.-E., Durand, F., Boulanger, C.M., & Valla, D.C. (2015). Interplay of inflammation and endothelial dysfunction in bone marrow transplantation: Focus on hepatic veno-occlusive disease. *Seminars in Thrombosis and Hemostasis, 41*, 629–643. https://doi.org/10.1055/s-0035-1556728

Wallhult, E., & Quinn, B. (2018). Early and acute complications and the principles of HSCT nursing care. In M. Kenyon & A. Babic (Eds.), *The European blood and marrow transplantation textbook for nurses* (pp. 163–195). https://doi.org/10.1007/978-3-319-50026-3_9

Wang, L., Wang, Y., Fan, X., Tang, W., & Hu, J. (2015). Prevalence of resistant gram-negative bacilli in bloodstream infection in febrile neutropenia patients undergoing hematopoietic stem cell transplantation: A single center retrospective cohort study. *Medicine, 94*, e1931. https://doi.org/10.1097/md.0000000000001931

Wanko, S.O., Broadwater, G., Folz, R.J., & Chao, N.J. (2006). Diffuse alveolar hemorrhage: Retrospective review of clinical outcome in allogeneic transplant recipients treated with aminocaproic acid. *Biology of Blood and Marrow Transplantation, 12*, 949–953. https://doi.org/10.1016/j.bbmt.2006.05.012

Watarai, A., Niiyama, S., Amoh, Y., & Katsuoka, K. (2009). Toxic epidermal necrolysis caused by aerosolized pentamidine. *American Journal of Medicine, 122*, e1–e2. https://doi.org/10.1016/j.amjmed.2008.08.022

Wheeler, A.P., & Berard, G.R. (2007). Acute lung injury and the acute respiratory distress syndrome: A clinical review. *Lancet, 369*, 1553–1564. https://doi.org/10.1016/s0140-6736(07)60604-7

Wilkes, G.M., & Barton-Burke, M. (2018). *2018 oncology nursing drug handbook*. Burlington, MA: Jones & Bartlett Learning.

Williams, J.V., Piedra, P.A., & Englund, J.A. (2017). Respiratory syncytial virus, human metapneumovirus, and parainfluenza viruses. In D.D. Richman, R.J. Whitley, & F.G. Hayden (Eds.), *Clinical virology* (4th ed., pp. 873–900). https://doi.org/10.1128/9781555819439.ch37

Williams, K.M., Agwu, A.G., Chen, M., Ahn, K.W., Szabolcs, P., Boeckh, M.J., ... Tomblyn, M.R. (2014). CIBMTR retrospective analysis reveals incidence, mortality, and timing of pneumocystis jiroveci pneumonia (PCP) after hematopoietic stem cell transplantation (HSCT). *Biology of Blood and Marrow Transplantation, 20*(Suppl. 2), S94. https://doi.org/10.1016/j.bbmt.2013.12.123

Williams, K.M., Ahn, K.W., Chen, M., Aljurf, M.D., Agwu, A.L., Chen, A.R., ... Riches, M.R. (2016). The incidence, mortality and timing of *Pneumocystis jiroveci* pneumonia after hematopoietic cell transplantation: A CIBMTR analysis. *Bone Marrow Transplantation, 51*, 573–580. https://doi.org/10.1038/bmt.2015.316

Williams, K.M., Cheng, G.-S., Pusic, I., Jagasia, M., Burns, L., Ho, V.T., ... Lee, S.J. (2016). Fluticasone, azithromycin, and montelukast treatment for new-onset bronchiolitis obliterans syndrome after hematopoietic cell transplantation. *Biology of Blood and Marrow Transplantation, 22*, 710–716. https://doi.org/10.1016/j.bbmt.2015.10.009

Williams, K.M., Chien, J.W., Gladwin, M.T., & Pavletic, S.Z. (2009). Bronchiolitis obliterans after allogeneic hematopoietic stem cell transplantation. *JAMA, 302*, 306–314. https://doi.org/10.1001/jama.2009.1018

Wilson, D.T., Drew, R.H., & Perfect, J.R. (2009). Antifungal therapy for invasive fungal diseases in allogeneic stem cell transplant recipients: An update. *Mycopathologia, 168*, 313–327. https://doi.org/10.1007/s11046-009-9193-9

Yadav, H., Nolan, M.E., Bohman, J.K., Cartin-Ceba, R., Peters, S.G., Hogan, W.J., ... Kor, D.J. (2016). Epidemiology of acute respiratory distress syndrome following hematopoietic stem cell transplantation. *Critical Care Medicine, 44*, 1082–1090. https://doi.org/10.1097/ccm.0000000000001617

Yanagisawa, R., Katsuyama, Y., Shigemura, T., Saito, S., Tanaka, M., Nakazawa, Y., ... Koike, K. (2011). Engraftment syndrome, but not acute GVHD, younger age, CYP3A5 or MDR1 polymorphisms, increases tacrolimus clearance in pediatric hematopoietic SCT. *Bone Marrow Transplantation, 46*, 90–97. https://doi.org/10.1038/bmt.2010.64

Yanik, G.A., Horowitz, M.M., Weisdorf, D.J., Logan, B.R., Ho, V.T., Soiffer, R.J., ... Cooke, K.R. (2014). Randomized, double-blind, placebo-controlled trial of soluble tumor necrosis factor receptor: Enbrel (etanercept) for the treatment of idiopathic pneumonia syndrome after allogeneic stem cell transplantation: Blood and Marrow Transplant Clinical Trials Network protocol. *Biology of Blood and Marrow Transplantation, 20*, 858–864. https://doi.org/10.1016/j.bbmt.2014.02.026

Yanik, G., & Kitko, C. (2013). Management of noninfectious lung injury following hematopoietic cell transplantation. *Current Opinion in Oncology, 25*, 187–194. https://doi.org/10.1097/cco.0b013e32835dc8a5

Yao, Z., & Liao, W. (2006). Fungal respiratory disease. *Current Opinion in Pulmonary Medicine, 12*, 222–227. https://doi.org/10.1097/01.mcp.0000219272.57933.01

Yeh, E.T.H., Tong, A.T., Lenihan, D.J., Yusuf, S.W., Swafford, J., Champion, C., ... Ewer, M.S. (2004). Cardiovascular complications of cancer therapy: Diagnosis, pathogenesis, and management. *Circulation, 109*, 3122–3131. https://doi.org/10.1161/01.cir.0000133187.74800.b9

Yoshida, M., & Ohno, R. (2004). Antimicrobial prophylaxis in febrile neutropenia. *Clinical Infectious Diseases, 39*(Suppl. 1), S65–S67. https://doi.org/10.1086/383058

Zahid, M.F., Murad, M.H., Litzow, M.R., Hogan, W.J., Patnaik, M.S., Khorana, A., ... Hashmi, S.K. (2016). Venous thromboembolism following hematopoietic stem cell transplantation—A systematic review and meta-analysis. *Annals of Hematology, 95*, 1457–1464. https://doi.org/10.1007/s00277-016-2673-3

Zhou, X., Trulik, K., Chadwick, M.M., Hoffman, T., Bulte, C., Bloye, K., ... Yanik, G.A. (2017). Early post-transplant viral infections and the incidence of acute and chronic noninfectious pulmonary complications following hematopoietic stem cell transplantation (HSCT). *Biology of Blood and Marrow Transplantation, 23*(Suppl.), 1–2. https://doi.org/10.1016/j.bbmt.2016.12.069

Zhu, K.-E., Hu, J.-Y., Zhang, T., Chen, J., Zhong, J., & Lu, Y.-H. (2008). Incidence, risks, and outcome of idiopathic pneumonia syndrome early after allogeneic hematopoietic stem cell transplantation. *European Journal of Haematology, 81*, 461–466. https://doi.org/10.1111/j.1600-0609.2008.01149.x

CHAPTER 12

Neurologic Complications

Jean A. Ridgeway, DNP, MSN, APN, AOCN®, Rebecca Pape, MSN, APN, FNP-C, and Keriann Kordas, MSN, APN

Introduction

According to the Worldwide Network for Blood and Marrow Transplantation and the World Health Organization, more than one million hematopoietic stem cell transplantations (HSCTs) have been performed worldwide to date (Gratwohl et al., 2015; World Health Organization, n.d.). As the number of HSCT recipients continues to grow, a corresponding increase in toxicities can be anticipated. Neurologic complications after HSCT are an uncommon but serious cause of treatment-related mortality. It has been reported that neurotoxicities after HSCT can vary widely in incidence (3%–44%) and severity, ranging from mild, transient disorders to serious clinical illness or death (Barba et al., 2009; Bhatt et al., 2015; Dowling et al., 2018; Maffini et al., 2017; Siegal et al., 2007). Chimeric antigen receptor (CAR) T-cell therapy, discussed elsewhere in this book, has also emerged as a viable treatment option for some cancers. CAR T-cell therapy is a new and developing strategy aimed at treating cancers by engineering a patient's own immune system to attack and eradicate cancer cells. At the time of this writing, the most common diseases treated with CAR T-cell therapy are relapsed or refractory B-cell malignancies (some types of acute lymphoblastic leukemia and lymphomas), but clinical trials and investigations into utilizing CAR T cells for other malignancies remain underway. Unlike HSCT, neurotoxicities of CAR T-cell therapies are common.

The causes of neurologic complications after HSCT are numerous and include infectious pathogens, neurotoxic medications, metabolic encephalopathy, cerebrovascular disease, and immune-mediated toxicities (Table 12-1). Neurologic complications can occur at any time during the HSCT treatment trajectory. In a study of 191 allogeneic HSCT recipients, the nonrelapse mortality at one year was 42% in patients with central nervous system (CNS) complications, compared to 20% in patients without CNS involvement (Barba et al., 2009; Dhar, 2018). The majority of neurologic complications occur in the early post-transplant period, but recipients remain at risk for opportunistic infections and other nervous system disorders for many years (Dhar, 2018). Dowling et al. (2018) performed a retrospective study of 263 consecutive patients undergoing allogeneic HSCT for hematologic malignancies to determine the

incidence, risk factors, and clinical impact of neurotoxicities in the first five years after transplantation. They examined the incidence of CNS infection, intracranial hemorrhage, ischemic stroke, metabolic encephalopathy, posterior reversal encephalopathy syndrome (PRES), seizure, and peripheral neuropathy. In their series, 50 patients experienced 63 neurotoxicities: 37 early (before day +100), 21 late (day +101 to 2 years), and 5 very late (2–5 years after HSCT) (Dowling et al., 2018). Cumulatively, the one-year incidence for all neurotoxicities was 15.6%, and the five-year incidence was 19.2% (Dowling et al., 2018).

With wide variability in incidence and severity, clinicians must understand the significance of neurologic com-

Table 12-1. Categories of Hematopoietic Stem Cell Transplantation Neurologic Complications

Category	Causative Agent
Drug-related	Calcineurin inhibitors Methotrexate Cytotoxic agents Monoclonal antibodies Antibiotics
Metabolic	Hepatic encephalopathy Uremic encephalopathy
Infectious	Bacteria Viruses Fungi Protozoa
Cerebrovascular	Hemorrhage Ischemic stroke
Immune-mediated	Myositis Myasthenia gravis Demyelinating diseases CNS cGVHD CRS

cGVHD—chronic graft-versus-host disease; CNS—central nervous system; CRS—cytokine release syndrome

Note. From "Neurologic Complications After Allogeneic Hematopoietic Stem Cell Transplantation," by E. Maffini, M. Festuccia, L. Brunello, M. Boccadoro, L. Giaccone, and B. Bruno, 2017, *Biology of Blood and Marrow Transplantation, 23*, p. 389. Copyright 2017 by American Society for Blood and Marrow Transplantation. Retrieved from https://doi.org/10.1016/j.bbmt.2016.12.632. Licensed under CC BY-NC-ND 4.0 (https://creativecommons.org/licenses/by-nc-nd/4.0).

plications related to commonly used drugs and treatments, infections, and numerous other causes. Early identification of these complications and their treatment is also essential.

Neurotoxicities of Common Agents

Busulfan

Busulfan is a common component of many conditioning regimens for HSCT and has been associated with seizure activity, but the exact mechanism of this toxicity is unclear. Busulfan is lipophilic, so it can cross the blood–brain barrier and enter the cerebrospinal fluid (CSF) at the same ratio found in plasma. This can lead to continuous exposure of the brain to the parent drug or accumulation of metabolites to produce seizures despite prophylaxis with phenytoin (Hassan, Ehrsson, & Ljungman, 1996).

Neurotoxicity with high-dose busulfan (e.g., 3.2–4 mg/kg/day IV for 1–4 days) can result in generalized tonic-clonic seizures (Eberly, Anderson, Bubalo, & McCune, 2008). In addition, busulfan area under the concentration-time curve greater than 1,500 micromolar per minute increases the risk of developing neurotoxicity (Ciurea & Andersson, 2009). Seizures can occur during administration and up to 24 hours after administration (Grigg, Shepherd, & Phillips, 1989; S. Mathew, Harnicar, Adel, & Papadopoulos, 2011). Other neurologic side effects seen with busulfan use include reversible encephalopathy with confusion, somnolence, and decreased alertness; myoclonus; headache; and hallucinations (Rosenfeld & Pruitt, 2006).

Anticonvulsive prophylaxis decreases the rate of busulfan-induced seizures to 0%–5.5% (Grigg et al., 1989). However, the estimated incidence of neurotoxicity is approximately 10% in the absence of adequate pharmacologic prophylaxis (Maffini et al., 2017). Ideally, prophylaxis should be loaded to therapeutic levels within 8 hours before the start of busulfan, then continued until 25 hours after the final dose (Diaz-Carrasco et al., 2013). Current practice recommends using an agent that can be loaded rapidly prior to busulfan administration and does not add to toxicity, alter the pharmacokinetics, or impede donor cell engraftment. Drugs that have been studied in adults include phenytoin, levetiracetam, and benzodiazepines (see Table 12-2).

Ifosfamide

Ifosfamide is an alkylating agent that is commonly used in the treatment of a variety of solid and hematologic malignancies.

Ifosfamide-induced encephalopathy, a dose-dependent neurotoxicity, is a serious potential complication (Richards, Marshall, & McQuary, 2011). As with busulfan, ifosfamide and its metabolites also cross the blood–brain barrier. The incidence of encephalopathy is approximately 5%–60% (Richards et al., 2011). Onset of symptoms usually occurs in the first 24 hours of exposure but can be delayed up to 146 hours after the start of the infusion (Richards et al.,

2011). Ifosfamide is a prodrug that requires activation in the liver by the cytochrome P450 enzymatic system. Thus, concomitant use of drugs that inhibit this system may increase neurotoxicity. Renal insufficiency can alter excretion of ifosfamide. It is thought that the accumulation of the metabolite chloroacetaldehyde may be responsible because elevated levels have been found in patients who develop neurotoxicities. Other factors that may predispose a patient to develop neurotoxicity include older age, female sex, cisplatin-induced renal insufficiency, hypoalbuminemia, and pelvic structural abnormalities (e.g., urinary obstruction). The most common neurotoxicity seen with ifosfamide use is encephalopathy that reveals altered sensorium ranging from mild confusion to coma (Richards et al., 2011). Other symptoms may include sleepiness, disorientation, agitation, drowsiness, hallucinations, psychosis, amnesia, epileptic episodes, and extrapyramidal symptoms (Cavaliere & Schiff, 2006; Richards et al., 2011). This type of encephalopathy is more common with initial exposure to the drug and is usually less frequent or intense with subsequent treatments (Richards et al., 2011; Rieger, Fiegl, Tischer, Ostermann, & Schiel, 2004).

Symptoms are usually self-limited and resolve within hours or days of discontinuation of the drug. Irreversible mental status changes have been reported in children. Long-term sequelae, such as emotional instability, apathy, short-term memory problems, and mental focus problems, have also been reported (Cain & Bender, 1995; Kerbusch et al., 2001). Serious long-term sequelae are rare, but brain damage, coma, and death have occurred (David & Picus, 2005; Richards et al., 2011).

Fludarabine

Fludarabine is one of the main components in reduced-intensity or nonmyeloablative conditioning regimens for HSCT (Annaloro et al., 2015).

Fludarabine can induce significant dose-related neurotoxicity consisting of cortical blindness, altered mental status, and generalized seizures. Beitinjaneh, McKinney, Cao, and Weisdorf (2011) described a retrospective study of 1,596 patients, in which 39 (2.4%) were reported to have fludarabine-related neurotoxicity with different manifestations, including PRES, acute toxic leukoencephalopathy, and other leukoencephalopathy syndromes. Fludarabine-induced acute toxic leukoencephalopathy commonly presents as confusion, somnolence, seizure, severe persisting headache, and blurred vision. Prognosis is poor, with decreased median time of survival (Beitinjaneh et al., 2011). The median overall survival for patients with fludarabine-associated encephalopathy was 169 days. Patients with acute toxic leukoencephalopathy had a median overall survival of 66 days, and those with PRES survived a median of 208 days (Beitinjaneh et al., 2011).

When fludarabine was administered at daily doses in excess of 100 mg/m² for five to seven days in various phase I/II studies, fludarabine-related neurotoxicity was reported in

Table 12-2. Busulfan Seizure Prophylaxis

Drug	Study Design	Dose	Efficacy	Side Effects	Drug Interactions
Clonazepam	Retrospective, descriptive (N = 33)	12 hrs prior to busulfan, 1 mg IV every 8 hrs, continued until 24 hrs after final busulfan dose	100%	Sedation	None
Diazepam	Prospective randomized cohort compared with phenytoin (N = 8)	Day of busulfan; 5 mg PO QID for 4 days	100%	Sedation	None
Levetiracetam	Retrospective comparison to phenytoin (N = 32)	24 hrs prior to busulfan, 500 mg PO BID, continue until 24 hrs after final busulfan dose	100%	Liver enzyme elevation	None
Lorazepam	Prospective cohort compared to retrospective control of phenytoin (N = 49)	Evening prior to busulfan, 0.5 mg PO every 6 hrs, continued until 24 hrs after final busulfan dose	Not reported	Sedation, rash	None
Phenytoin	Prospective (N = 50)	24 hrs prior to busulfan, 18 mg/kg/day load dose in divided doses, then 300 mg PO daily until 24 hrs after final busulfan dose	100%	Rash, mild liver enzyme elevation	Busulfan, voriconazole, posaconazole, dexamethasone

BID—twice a day; hrs—hours; PO—by mouth; QID—four times a day

Note. Based on information from Grigg et al., 1989; Hassan et al., 1993.

30%–40% of patients (Annaloro et al., 2015). Potential risk factors include age greater than 60 years, prior CNS treatment, or prior HSCT with fludarabine conditioning. Renal impairment can cause elevated fludarabine concentrations in the CNS (Long-Boyle et al., 2011). The onset of neurotoxicity occurs approximately two months after receiving fludarabine and develops progressively over four weeks with increasing severity (Beitinjaneh et al., 2011). Albeit uncommon, toxicity can be seen several weeks after administration (Beitinjaneh et al., 2011; M.S. Lee, McKinney, Brace, & SantaCruz, 2010). The combination of fludarabine and busulfan for reduced-intensity conditioning has not been shown to increase the risk of neurologic complications (de Lima et al., 2004). Beitinjaneh et al. (2011) described acute toxic leukoencephalopathy as a possible clinical and imaging counterpart of fludarabine neurotoxicity. The most common clinical features of acute toxic leukoencephalopathy include cognitive impairment associated with visual and sensitive defects. The clinical outcome was frequently, but not always, irreversible and progressive, with a magnetic resonance imaging (MRI) pattern characterized by the presence of bilateral signal alteration in the deep white matter, which is distinct from PRES (Beitinjaneh et al., 2011).

Cytarabine

High-dose cytarabine (e.g., ≥ 2 g/m^2) is frequently used for induction therapy with acute myeloid leukemia and in some preparative regimens.

Cerebellar toxicity is the most common neurologic complication of high-dose cytarabine. Documented risk factors for neurotoxicities include increased age (older than 55 years), renal insufficiency, and repeated exposure (Cavaliere

& Schiff, 2006; Schiller & Lee, 1997). A cerebellar syndrome can be observed within hours of administration and presents as ataxia of gait and limbs (Cavaliere & Schiff, 2006). Other neurologic changes usually develop gradually, typically observed several days after the initiation of therapy, and include confusion, somnolence, ataxia, dysarthria, and sometimes seizures and coma (Macdonald, 1991). These toxicities usually resolve within two weeks after therapy is stopped. Rapid infusion may cause an abrupt onset of these symptoms. Long-term neurologic effects can occur and include cerebellar toxicity manifested by ataxia and slapping gait. Computed tomography (CT) scan and MRI may reveal cerebellar atrophy (de Magalhaes-Silverman & Hammert, 2000; Macdonald, 1991). The cause of this toxicity is unclear, but reports have suggested that a loss of Purkinje cells in the cerebellum and apoptosis of neurons may be to blame (Cavaliere & Schiff, 2006; Courtney & Coffey, 1999).

Signs and symptoms of cerebellar toxicity should be assessed prior to administering each dose of cytarabine. Brown (2010) described a standardized approach to completing an assessment for cerebellar toxicity that included checking for nystagmus, orientation, body tremors, and changes in speech pattern or handwriting. Other tests include rapid alternating hand movements, point-to-point testing, observation of gait, and Romberg test. If signs of cerebellar toxicity are present, subsequent doses of cytarabine should be held (Brown, 2010).

Methotrexate

Because the dose of methotrexate used in the post-HSCT setting for graft-versus-host disease (GVHD) prophylaxis is much lower compared to the high doses used outside a transplant setting, it is less likely to cause neurotoxicity. Occasional minor neurotoxicities associated with methotrexate include headaches, dizziness, and very rarely, seizures (Maffini et al., 2017). Leukoencephalopathy, most frequently associated with high-dose methotrexate, has been reported following use of low-dose oral methotrexate (Maffini et al., 2017).

Carmustine

Carmustine is often used in the autologous HSCT setting and is known to cross the blood–brain barrier. Mild toxicities include headaches, facial flushing, and paresthesias (Maffini et al., 2017). Acute encephalopathy (delirium), dementia (chronic encephalopathy), and seizures can also occur (Magge & DeAngelis, 2015). Carmustine has been associated with optic disc and retinal microvasculopathy, resulting in varying degrees of vision loss and, in high doses, irreversible severe encephalopathy (R.M. Mathew & Rosenfeld, 2007).

Total Body Irradiation

Many HSCT preparatory regimens use total body irradiation (TBI) and cranial radiation prior to transplant. Factors that influence the development of radiation-associated neurologic complications include radiation dosage and fractionation, as well as younger age (Shih, 2019).

Toxicities resulting from this therapy are classified as acute, early-delayed, and late sequelae (Shih, 2019). Acute complications occur within two weeks of radiation therapy and abate over two months. Fatigue, headaches, nausea and vomiting, anorexia, hearing loss, parotitis, and worsening of preexisting neurologic issues are cited as acute neurotoxicities (Shih, 2019). The most severe, but least common, acute reaction to TBI and cranial radiation is encephalopathy. Early-delayed side effects occur within six months after radiation therapy and most commonly involve persistent fatigue (Shih, 2019). Late adverse effects of radiation occur beyond six months following treatment and involve cognitive deficits, stroke, and neuroendocrine dysfunction (Shih, 2019).

Dimethyl Sulfoxide

Dimethyl sulfoxide (DMSO) is a solvent used to protect cryopreserved stem cells. DMSO may also be used in the setting of an allogeneic transplant if logistics of donor collection prohibit an infusion of freshly collected cells or if the infusion is delayed. Reported neurotoxicities include headache, migraine, cerebral infarction, seizure, encephalopathy, transient global amnesia, and coma (Júnior et al., 2008; Marcacci et al., 2009). Most examples of neurotoxicities are from isolated, anecdotal case reports. The variation of symptoms within these reports makes it difficult to determine one unifying or single pathogenic hypothesis for the etiology (Marcacci et al., 2009). The severity of neurotoxicities may be related to the volume of DMSO infused and the rate of infusion (Rowley, 2016). The maximum recommended dose to be infused at one time is 1 g/kg, or

10 ml/kg or 10% (Júnior et al., 2008). If the anticipated dose is greater than 1 g/kg, it is recommended to divide the cell infusion into two or three separate infusions that occur over several hours or days. The stem cells may also be washed to remove DMSO if an infusion reaction occurs.

Marcacci et al. (2009) reported that animal models have suggested that DMSO may affect the vascular system, causing prolonged vasoconstriction; therefore, it may cause cerebrovascular ischemia. MRI changes have been reported in patients with DMSO-related neurotoxicity (Bauwens et al., 2005).

Otrock et al. (2008) reported on a case of transient global amnesia associated with infusion of DMSO cryopreserved stem cells that manifested as acute onset of disorientation to place and time, retrograde amnesia, and perseveration (asking the same questions repeatedly). As with other DMSO-related neurotoxicity, the mechanism of transient global amnesia is not well understood. It is thought to be secondary to pathologic changes that affect the mediobasal temporal region of the brain, hippocampus, and parahippocampus, which can be seen on MRI.

According to Mueller et al. (2007), a history of preexisting cerebral disease is not associated with DMSO-related neurotoxicity. In a study of 51 patients receiving stem cells cryopreserved with DMSO, eight of whom had a preexisting cerebral disease, only one of the 51 total patients had reported neurotoxicity (a generalized tonic seizure during stem cell reinfusion). The authors did not observe any neurotoxicity in those patients with preexisting cerebral disease (Mueller et al., 2007).

Neurotoxicities of Infectious Diseases

The use of potent and effective immunosuppressive regimens has prolonged the survival and reduced the risk of graft rejection for HSCT recipients. However, use of these drugs along with prolonged post-transplant survival can result in a higher risk of opportunistic infections (Dhar, 2018). Maschke et al. (1999) reported a study of 655 patients who had undergone allogeneic, syngeneic, or autologous HSCT. All CNS infections occurred in allogeneic HSCT recipients, with a 4% incidence. *Toxoplasma* and *Aspergillus* were the most common pathogens. Overall, mortality in patients with opportunistic CNS infections was 67% (Maschke et al., 1999). A CNS infection should always be suspected if the patient has new neurologic signs, fever, or a systemic infection, particularly pulmonary (R.M. Mathew & Rosenfeld, 2007; Pruitt et al., 2013). Factors influencing susceptibility include disruption of the blood–brain barrier, such as past treatment with TBI. CT, MRI, and CSF evaluation should be included when any neurologic abnormality is found.

Viral

Herpes Simplex Virus Type 1

Herpes simplex virus type 1 (HSV-1) infections can occur in HSCT recipients, although dissemination to the

CNS is uncommon (Maffini et al., 2017). HSV encephalitis is a rare, serious complication affecting 1 in 250,000–500,000 patients, with reported mortality ranging 4%–28% and approximately 15%–38% of survivors returning to their baseline level of functioning (Tan, McArthur, Venkatesan, & Nath., 2012). Herpesviruses and John Cunningham (JC) virus are commonly latent in the brain or cell ganglia (Dhar, 2018). These can reactivate in periods of immunosuppression, causing herpes zoster encephalitis (at times without skin lesions), or in the case of JC virus, progressive multifocal leukoencephalopathy (PML) (Dhar, 2018). Tan et al. (2012) conducted a retrospective review of HSV encephalitis, comparing HSV-1 encephalitis manifestations of immunocompetent patients against immunocompromised patients. The outcomes for the immunocompromised group were worse compared to the immunocompetent group. The mortality rate was nearly six times higher in the immunocompromised group (35.7% vs. 6.7%) (Tan et al., 2012). The time from onset of symptoms to time of death was shorter for the immunocompromised group compared to the immunocompetent group (17.6 ± 2 days vs. 30 days) (Tan et al., 2012). Incidence and survival data for immunocompromised patients is currently lacking; however, Tan et al. (2012) hypothesized survival to be grim, with a rapid course of HSV progression and increased morbidity and mortality for immunocompromised patients.

Patients may experience nonspecific symptoms, such as headache, complex partial seizures, fever with or without nuchal rigidity, and limbic features in their presentation of HSV encephalitis (Benninger & Steiner, 2018). Immunocompromised patients are likely to experience fewer prodromal symptoms and focal deficits compared to immunocompetent patients; brain involvement may be more extensive and may include the brain stem, cerebellum, and other atypical regions. Patients may not have an expected increase of cells in the CSF (Tracy & Mowzoon, 2006). For the diagnosis of HSV encephalitis, it is recommended to obtain both a CSF sample and a brain MRI. Additionally, if patients have been symptomatic for 24 hours to 10 days, a CSF sample for polymerase chain reaction (PCR) for HSV-1 should be obtained (Tracy & Mowzoon, 2006). HSV PCR of CSF is a highly sensitive diagnostic technique (Maffini et al., 2017). If a patient has been symptomatic for 10 days or longer, the IgM antibody count from CSF for HSV-1 should be obtained as well (Pruitt, 2012).

Treatment for HSV encephalitis consists of high-dose acyclovir (Maffini et al., 2017). It may take more time for the PCR to return a positive result, especially for patients who have received prior brain irradiation due to low white blood cell CSF count or polymorphonuclear cell predominance (Tan et al., 2012). If HSV encephalitis is suspected and brain MRI reveals temporal lobe involvement, it is recommended to begin empiric acyclovir 10–12 mg/kg IV every 8 hours (Styczynski et al., 2009; Tomblyn et al., 2009). Acyclovir treatment is to be continued for 14–21 days. Foscarnet is the treatment of choice for HSV resistant to acyclovir. If a patient is unable to receive foscarnet, treatment with cidofovir should be considered (Styczynski et al., 2009; Tomblyn et al., 2009).

Human Herpesvirus 6

Human herpesvirus 6 (HHV-6)–associated encephalitis in the HSCT population is reported to have an incidence of 4%, with the median time to initial symptoms being 18–21 days (range 6–145 days) (Bhanushali et al., 2013; Sakai et al., 2011). HHV-6 is increasingly recognized as a cause of limbic encephalitis, especially after HSCT (Shimazu, Kondo, Ishikawa, Yamashita, & Takaori-Kondo, 2013). Patients may present with headaches, altered mental status, amnesia, and seizures (Bhanushali et al., 2013; Sakai et al., 2011). HHV-6 poses the greatest threat to the CNS when compared to other herpesviruses. After exposure during childhood, it lies dormant and reactivates during periods of immunosuppression, attacking cluster of differentiation (CD) 4 lymphocytes, suggesting hematogenous spread (Sakai et al., 2011; Seeley et al., 2007). The term *post-transplant acute limbic encephalitis*, or PALE, was coined to describe the syndrome of amnesia with limbic abnormalities on MRI associated with HHV-6 (Seeley et al., 2007). In a retrospective analysis, Shimazu et al. (2013) examined the influence of symptomatic HHV-6 reactivation and HHV-6 encephalitis on overall survival of 140 consecutive adult allogeneic HSCT recipients who were treated at Kyoto University Hospital between January 2005 and September 2009. Using multivariate logistic models, the survival analysis identified a high risk of disease (p = 0.021) and HHV-6 encephalitis (p = 0.003) as independent risk factors for poor overall survival (Shimazu et al., 2013). Although HHV-6 encephalitis was associated with a poor prognosis, the prognosis of cases with symptomatic HHV-6 reactivation without HHV-6 encephalitis was identical to that of cases without symptomatic HHV-6 reactivation (Shimazu et al., 2013).

MRI of the brain for patients who have HHV-6 may be normal, but the most common imaging pattern is fluid-attenuated inversion recovery (FLAIR) hyperintensity in the early phase involving the mesial temporal lobes, with subsequent hippocampal atrophy (Pruitt, 2012; Tracy & Mowzoon, 2006). Maffini et al. (2017) reported that ganciclovir and foscarnet are common treatments for HHV-6, although their efficacy does not appear to be optimal. Given the rapidly progressive onset of neurologic symptoms, prompt initiation of antiviral therapy is mandatory (Maffini et al., 2017; Pruitt, 2012).

Varicella Zoster Virus

Varicella zoster virus (VZV) reactivation can occur in the HSCT setting; however, the disease usually is restricted to a specific dermatomal distribution or the viscera and responds well to antiviral therapy. Reactivation rate is reported to be as high as 40% in allogeneic HSCT and

25% in autologous HSCT (Rosenfeld & Pruitt, 2006). Painful peripheral neuropathy has been associated with VZV.

John Cunningham Virus

PML is a rare demyelinating disorder of the CNS caused by the JC virus. A DNA polyomavirus, JC virus has been found to cause PML more commonly in patients with prolonged immunosuppression. Potent lymphotoxic drugs, such as rituximab and fludarabine, and the protease inhibitor bortezomib are associated with the development of PML. Patients present with slowly progressing focal deficits with visual changes, subacute dementia, and sometimes brain stem syndrome. A decrease in immunosuppression may cause regression both clinically and radiographically; however, there are no known treatment options for PML at this time. PML is generally considered to be fatal if it occurs (R.M. Mathew & Rosenfeld, 2007; Raajasekar, Ayyapan, Khan, Mantzaris, & Janakiram, 2013; Rosenfeld & Pruitt, 2006).

Cytomegalovirus

Cytomegalovirus (CMV) encephalitis after allogeneic HSCT is a late-onset disease with a median time of onset of 210 days. It has CT or MRI changes suggestive of encephalitis in the absence of other sites of CMV disease (Reddy, Winston, Territo, & Schiller, 2010). CMV can cause encephalitis, which may be associated with CNS mass lesions, ascending polyradiculitis or polyradiculomyelitis, polyneuropathy, and rarely, vasculopathy with stroke (Marra, 2018). Reddy et al. (2010) reviewed 11 cases of CMV encephalitis and found the development of CMV CNS disease was associated with risk factors such as T-cell depletion, antithymocyte globulin, and umbilical cord blood transplantation, which cause severe and protracted T-cell immunodeficiency (8 of 11 cases); a history of recurrent CMV viremia treated with multiple courses of preemptive ganciclovir or foscarnet therapy (11 of 11 cases); and ganciclovir-resistant CMV infection (11 of 11 cases). Despite therapy with a combination of antiviral drugs (ganciclovir, foscarnet, and cidofovir), mortality was high (10 of 11 cases). Given this, extended prophylaxis with current or novel antiviral drugs and strategies to enhance CMV immunity need to be considered in high-risk patients (Reddy et al., 2010).

Clinical manifestations of CMV encephalitis can be progressive encephalopathy or dementia (Marra, 2018). Diagnosis of CMV encephalitis includes obtaining CSF for CMV PCR (Benninger & Steiner, 2018). PCR has 95% sensitivity and 99% specificity. PCR reports are routinely available in less than 24 hours. If CMV is suspected, empiric antiviral treatment can be initiated early in the clinical course. Benninger and Steiner (2018) recommended a typical minimum extraction volume of CSF of 100–300 mcl for diagnostic testing. If brain MRI is obtained, it may show hyperintense signals in the basal ganglia and nonspecific white matter abnormalities (Denier et al., 2006; Tunkel et al., 2008).

No standard therapy exists for the treatment of CMV encephalitis. A retrospective review of published literature recommends considering combination of ganciclovir (5 mg/kg IV every 12 hours) and foscarnet (60 mg/kg IV every 8 hours or 90 mg/kg IV every 12 hours) for three weeks, followed by maintenance therapy (Raffi, Taburet, Ghaleh, Huart, & Singlas, 1993; Tunkel et al., 2008). Cidofovir therapy is not recommended, as its ability to penetrate the blood–brain barrier has not been well studied (Ljungman et al., 1998). Current data does not support the addition of immune globulin for the treatment of CMV disease other than pneumonia; thus, it is not recommended (Ljungman et al., 1998).

Fungal

Mucorales

Mucormycosis is the most common non-*Aspergillus* fungal infection among transplant recipients (Parize, Rammaert, & Lortholary, 2012). Mucormycosis refers to a group of potentially lethal opportunistic mycoses that occur in immunocompromised or diabetic patients. Infections are caused by *Mucorales*, ubiquitous filamentous fungi with broad, thin-walled, sparsely septate, and ribbon-like hyphae (Lanternier et al., 2012). The predominant source of these fungi is soil containing organic matter in a state of decay, such as leaves, compost and vegetable matter, or rotting wood (M. Richardson, 2009). Immunocompetent people do not need added protection from mucormycosis; however, HSCT recipients require prophylaxis with azole antifungals to prevent infection. Current incidence and epidemiologic data in 10 European and American studies ranged 0.1%–2%, with the highest rates observed among patients with GVHD (Lanternier et al., 2012). Lanternier et al. (2012) reported a cumulative 12-month incidence of 0.29% among HSCT recipients in the United States, and incidence was higher in transplants from human leukocyte antigen-matched unrelated donors. Patients most at risk for acquiring mucormycotic encephalopathy are those who have received T-cell-depletion chemotherapy, those with profound neutropenia for more than 21 days, those treated with corticosteroids dosed at 1 mg/kg/day, and those with uncontrolled hyperglycemia (Kontoyiannis & Lewis, 2011).

During infection, the hyphae invade blood vessels, causing tissue infarction and necrosis (Lanternier et al., 2012). In the past two decades, mucormycosis has emerged as an important invasive fungal infection in solid-organ transplant and HSCT recipients, in whom it often has an aggressive clinical course and substantial mortality rates (Lanternier et al., 2012). Inhaled mucormycotic spores travel through the bloodstream to the brain (Pruitt, 2012). Patients present with seizures, cranial nerve dysfunction, and embolic cerebrovascular accident (Pruitt, 2012). Symptoms can have a more subtle presentation in the form of headaches or vision changes. Identification, biopsy, and culture of specific infected sites is critical to correctly diagnosing mucormycotic encephalitis (Pruitt, 2012). Antifungal agents alone are inadequate treatment; surgical excision of infectious tissue is also necessary (Pruitt, 2012). Improvement of immune and metabolic factors should be routinely considered by administering tapering steroids and immunosuppressive agents when feasible and by controlling hyperglycemia (Lanternier et al., 2012). Liposomal amphotericin B offers the best cerebral tissue penetration for pharmacologic management (Schwartz et al., 2005). Most experts suggest administering liposomal amphotericin B at a starting dose of 5 mg/kg/day, which can be escalated to 10 mg/kg/day if needed to control the infection (Lanternier et al., 2012).

Aspergillus

In patients with invasive aspergillosis and acute leukemia or those treated with allogeneic HSCT, CNS aspergillosis has an incidence of 14%–42% (Schwartz et al., 2005). Reportedly, localized pulmonary aspergillosis has the lowest rate of mortality, but disseminated or CNS aspergillosis has nearly a 100% mortality rate (Schwartz et al., 2005). Poor penetration of antifungal drugs into the CNS has historically contributed to the grim prognosis (Schwartz et al., 2005). HSCT recipients are treated with azoles as a means of prophylaxis against aspergillosis. The main risk factor that predisposes patients to infection is prolonged severe neutropenia (neutrophil count less than 500/mm³ for 10 days or more) (Zunt & Baldwin, 2012). Infection occurs when inhaled spores travel from the sinuses to the bloodstream (Pruitt, 2012). Presentation of illness can be subtle and include headaches and visual change but can also present more severely as cranial neuropathies or embolic stroke (Pruitt, 2012).

MRI of the brain may show infarction, hemorrhagic lesions, hyperintense foci, or ring-enhancing lesions (Kourkoumpetis, Fuchs, Coleman, Desalermos, & Mylonakis, 2012; Pruitt, 2012; Zunt & Baldwin, 2012). However, definitive diagnosis is best determined through biopsy of infectious lesions. Several new agents to treat aspergillosis have come into clinical use. Systemic voriconazole is first-line treatment followed by the lipid formulations of amphotericin, itraconazole, or posaconazole (Walsh et al., 2008; Zunt & Baldwin, 2012). Voriconazole has excellent penetration into the CNS and is the treatment of choice for patients with CNS aspergillosis. Schwartz et al. (2005) reported improved outcomes in CNS aspergillosis using voriconazole treatment in a retrospective chart review of 81 HSCT recipients who were treated with voriconazole for definite (n = 48) or probable (n = 33) CNS aspergillosis. Complete and partial responses were recorded as 35%, with 22% of HSCT recipients surviving a median of 203 days (Schwartz et al., 2005). Cases of treatment resistance have been reported, and patients have shown progression of neurologic deficits while receiving first-line therapy. Such cases necessitate the use of salvage therapy with voriconazole with caspofungin, as well as surgical debridement of infectious lesions (Walsh et al., 2008; Zunt & Baldwin, 2012).

Parasitic

Although parasitic infectious complications rarely occur among HSCT recipients, the consequences involving the neurologic system are frequently fatal (Miyagi et al., 2015). Encephalopathy from parasites in HSCT recipients is most frequently caused by the protozoa *Toxoplasma gondii*. Exposure to meat infected with the cysts of *T. gondii* can transmit infection to humans, especially undercooked pork, lamb, venison, or other game (Centers for Disease Control and Prevention, 2018). *T. gondii* replicates most rapidly in the gastrointestinal tract of felines, making their feces or soil contaminated with their feces an alternate source of infection. Mueller-Mang, Mang, Kalhs, and Thurnher (2006) stated that between 1992 and 2006, only 100 cases of toxoplasmic encephalitis were confirmed, with another 22 reported cases since then.

The patients most at risk are those with positive *Toxoplasma* PCR prior to transplant or those who are PCR negative but whose donor is PCR positive (Martino et al., 2000). Other risk factors include lack of prophylaxis, insufficient CD4 lymphocyte count, and GVHD. Preventive treatment includes trimethoprim-sulfamethoxazole. Diagnosing toxoplasmic encephalitis can be challenging because of the generalized presentation of symptoms, including fevers, headaches, disorientation, and impairment in speech and balance (Miyagi et al., 2015). Patients presenting with such symptoms should prompt CT and MRI scans and *Toxoplasma* PCR testing. Imaging frequently shows an abundance of ring-enhancing lesions. In a case report review by Miyagi et al. (2015), two allogeneic HSCT recipients diagnosed by PCR were treated with pyrimethamine and sulfadiazine. Both patients survived and were free of neurologic sequelae as late as 400 days following onset of encephalopathy (Miyagi et al., 2015). The obvious limitation of this report is the small scale, and neither case yields further information about length of treatment.

Bacterial

Bacterial infections have not been shown to be a significant burden of neurologic complications and CNS infection in HSCT recipients (Barba et al., 2009; Bhatt et al., 2015). Bacterial CNS infections usually occur concomitantly with systemic infection and neutropenia (Maffini et al., 2017). They can present as either meningitis or brain abscess. A brain abscess is a rare but severe CNS complication. Teive et al. (2008) reported a retrospective study in Brazil of 1,000 HSCT recipients, finding a 3% incidence of bacterial meningitis and a 1% incidence of brain abscess. Meningitis commonly has sensorium alteration, but classical meningeal signs may be mild or absent, owing to impaired inflammatory response (Maffini et al., 2017). Acute bacterial meningitis is one of the most severe acute inflammatory diseases of the CNS, leading to severe morbidity and death (Benninger & Steiner, 2018).

CSF culture is the gold standard for the diagnosis of bacterial meningitis. The results of CSF cultures are positive in 70%–85% of patients who have not received prior antimicrobial therapy, but cultures may take up to 48 hours for organism identification (Benninger & Steiner, 2018). Appropriate treatment with antibiotics is recommended.

Other Causes of Neurologic Complications

Encephalopathy

Various forms of encephalopathy occur as complications of HSCT, including metabolic encephalopathy, hepatic encephalopathy secondary to hepatic sinusoidal obstruction syndrome (veno-occlusive disease), and leukoencephalopathy. It is unclear what the exact incidence of encephalopathy is following transplant; however, a mortality rate of 84% has been reported (Fichet et al., 2009; Kansu, 2012).

Specifically, hepatic encephalopathy has a survival rate of less than 50% by one year following HSCT and less than 25% after three years following HSCT (Fichet et al., 2009; Kansu, 2012). Female sex, recipients of abdominal radiation, high-dose busulfan and cyclophosphamide, and previous hepatic disease are classified as risk factors. Patients may present with cognitive changes and lethargy. After exclusion of all other sources of mental status changes, the offending factors in hepatic encephalopathy are typically hepatic sinusoidal obstruction syndrome and GVHD. Plasma exchange and management of acute electrolyte imbalances are part of treatment (Blei & Córdoba, 2001; Myers, Lawrence, Marsh, Davies, & Jodele, 2013). Similar to management of patients with hepatic failure, restricted dietary intake of protein and lactulose administration for reduction of serum ammonia levels are imperative.

Leukoencephalopathy has a variety of causative factors, including HHV-6 and JC virus, as well as various chemotherapy agents. PML predominantly effects the cerebellum or cerebral hemispheres but can also involve the brain stem (Pruitt, 2012). Patients present with hemiparesis, dysphasia, vision changes, and although atypically, seizures (Aksamit, 2012; Berger, 2007; de Lima et al., 2006). Diagnosis is confirmed with MRI, which reveals supratentorial white matter lesions. First-line treatment is removing immunosuppression along with pharmacologic therapy, including mirtazapine, interleukin-2, and cidofovir (Focosi et al., 2010; Owczarczyk, Hilker, Brunn, Hallek, & Rubbert, 2007; Verma et al., 2007).

Cerebrovascular Disease

Hemorrhagic or thrombotic complications are potentially lethal events for HSCT recipients (Maffini et al., 2017). Colosimo et al. (2000) reported a low incidence of 2.6% of subdural hematomas in a retrospective analysis of 657 patients who received autologous or allogeneic HSCT, and they were not associated with an increased patient mortality. Refractoriness to platelet transfusions was correlated with an increased risk of bleeding (Graus et al., 1996). Other factors, such as arterial hypertension, fibrinogen serum level, and grade III–IV acute GVHD have also been shown to play roles in cerebrovascular hemorrhagic events (Zhang et al., 2013). In a retrospective study of 351 patients who underwent allogeneic HSCT between 2002 and 2011 at the University of Nebraska Medical Center, a 24% incidence of stroke or transient ischemic attack was reported (Bhatt et al., 2015). None of the patients who developed stroke had a history of cerebrovascular disease (Bhatt et al., 2015). Najima et al. (2009) reported intraparenchymal hemorrhage incidence of 1.1%–2.4% after transplant with a median onset time after transplant of 122 days with high mortality.

The clinical picture of hemorrhagic or thrombotic complications can be characterized by headache and worsening sensorium without lateralizing signs. Diagnosis can at times be challenging in sedated patients and patients with encephalopathy (Maffini et al., 2017). CT scans generally show a hyperdense signal of blood at least 12 hours before MRI (Maffini et al., 2017). Neurosurgery, if clinically possible, especially in those patients who present with progressive neurologic deterioration or voluminous lesions, is recommended (Barba et al., 2009).

Posterior Reversible Encephalopathy Syndrome

PRES is a disorder that can occur after allogeneic HSCT. It is characterized by neurologic symptoms (e.g., headache, seizure, encephalopathy, visual disturbances) in the setting of high blood pressure, renal impairment, and immunosuppressive medications (Fugate & Rabinstein, 2015). The incidence of PRES following an allogeneic HSCT is 1.1%–20% (Chen et al., 2016). As suggested in the name, PRES is generally reversible, with most patients making a full recovery (Fugate & Rabinstein, 2015).

The pathophysiology of PRES is largely unknown, but it is thought to be a combination of hyperperfusion and endothelial damage. A sudden and significant rise in blood pressure can lead to hyperperfusion and subsequent breakdown of the blood–brain barrier. However, it should be noted that 15%–20% of patients with PRES are normotensive or hypotensive (Fugate & Rabinstein, 2015). It is also hypothesized that cytokines released during an inflammatory response may also contribute to PRES. Cytokines, such as tumor necrosis factor-alpha and interleukin-1, allow endothelial cells to secrete vasoactive factors, which, in turn, increase vascular permeability leading to interstitial brain edema (Fugate & Rabinstein, 2015).

Immunosuppressive medications, such as tacrolimus and cyclosporine, are known risk factors for PRES. Studies have shown that these medications can damage the cell membrane and, in the case of cyclosporine, induce apoptosis in the capillary endothelial cells of the brain. These cellular changes can then lead to increased permeability of the blood–brain barrier (Chen et al., 2016). Patients can develop PRES secondary to immunosuppressive medications, even after several months and despite normal or therapeutic drug levels (Fugate & Rabinstein, 2015).

Diagnosis of PRES is made by assessment of clinical symptoms in combination with specific findings on brain MRI. Common clinical manifestations include headache, seizure, encephalopathy (confusion, stupor), decreased visual acuity, visual field deficits, hallucinations, and cortical blindness (Fugate & Rabinstein, 2015). Dysarthria, ataxia, paresis, and sensory deficits are less common (Chen et al., 2016). An MRI of the brain will generally reveal vasogenic edema in both hemispheres of the parieto-occipital region, as well as subcortical white matter changes (Fugate & Rabinstein, 2015).

Treatment of PRES involves discontinuing or reducing the offending agent (Chen et al., 2016). Schmidt et al. (2016) suggested that tacrolimus or cyclosporine can be safely discontinued, and other immunosuppressive medications can be used as GVHD prophylaxis (steroids, mycophenolate mofetil, or sirolimus). Hypertension should be carefully managed with a goal of decreasing the blood pressure by 25% within a few hours, while avoiding large fluctuations in the blood pressure (Fugate & Rabinstein, 2015).

Immune Effector Cell–Associated Neurologic Syndrome

CAR T-cell therapy has been associated with significant toxicities including cytokine release syndrome (CRS) and neurotoxicity, otherwise known as immune effector cell–associated neurotoxicity syndrome (ICANS) (D.W. Lee et al., 2019). CAR T cell–related encephalopathy syndrome can be grouped within ICANS. The overall incidence of neurotoxicity varies across clinical trials, with an average of 13%–63% in patients with acute lymphoblastic leukemia and 7%–31% in those with non-Hodgkin lymphoma (Gauthier & Turtle, 2018). One study that examined the incidence of neurotoxicity in 133 adult patients across disease populations showed that 40% of patients had one or more neurologic adverse events within 28 days of CAR T-cell infusion (Gust et al., 2017). Of the patients that developed a neurologic adverse event, 91% also had CRS (Gust et al., 2017). Neurotoxicity was observed more frequently in younger patients, those with high tumor burden, those with B-cell acute lymphoblastic leukemia, and those with a preexisting neurologic comorbidity (Gust et al., 2017).

The onset of ICANS can happen in two phases. The first occurs concurrently with CRS (high fevers, hypotension), typically within five days following CAR T-cell infusion. The second phase occurs after that five-day period, when the CRS symptoms have begun to resolve. Symptoms of neurotoxicity last for two to four days on average but can be present for a few hours to a few weeks (Neelapu et al., 2018).

The pathophysiology of CAR T-cell–related neurotoxicity is not fully understood, but it is thought to involve a breakdown in the blood–brain barrier, allowing cytokines to enter the CNS. One study found that neurotoxicity after CAR T-cell therapy is associated with early onset of high serum concentrations of cytokines and vascular dysfunction (Gust et al., 2017). The authors noted that patients with grade 3 or higher neurologic adverse events often have evidence of systemic capillary leak (weigh gain, low serum albumin, and low serum protein), and those with severe neurotoxicity exhibited disseminated intravascular coagulation. The severity of neurotoxicity directly correlated with higher serum levels of C-reactive protein, ferritin, and cytokines (interleukin-6, interferon-gamma, tumor necrosis factor-alpha) (Gust et al., 2017). Gust et al. (2017) believe this evidence of endothelial activation and systemic capillary leak can lead to disruption of the blood–brain barrier. This breakdown in the blood–brain barrier then allows for cytokines and even CAR T cells to move into the CSF.

ICANS can present as a variety of neurologic symptoms, including delirium, headache, loss of consciousness, impaired attention, aphasia, agitation, tremor, and impaired handwriting. More severe symptoms include seizure, ataxia, incontinence, increased intracranial pressure, papilledema, and cerebral edema (Gust et al., 2017; Neelapu et al., 2018). Careful nursing assessment of a patient's mental status is key to grading and treatment of these symptoms. D.W. Lee et al. (2019) have proposed an assessment tool known as the immune effector cell–associated encephalopathy (ICE) score. This tool can be easily adopted and provides an objective score that can assist in grading ICANS, thus driving treatment. The tool assigns one point each to the following: ability to name the hospital and city (1 point each), ability to identify the month and year (1 point each), ability to name three objects (1 point for each object), ability to write a standard sentence, ability to follow a command, and ability to count backward from 100 by 10s. A total score of 10 on the ICE indicates normal cognitive function. A score of 7–9 indicates grade 1 ICANS; 3–6 indicates grade 2 ICANS; and 0–2 indicates grade 3 ICANS (see Table 12-3).

As one can infer by the grading criteria, patients with suspected ICANS should undergo a thorough neurologic workup, including CT and MRI of the brain, electroencephalograph, lumbar puncture, and eye examination. In most cases, the CT and MRI scans will be normal and are used as a means of excluding other possible causes of neurologic events. Gust et al. (2017) noted acute abnormalities on MRI scans in 7 of 23 patients. Four of these patients had severe neurotoxicity that was fatal. These MRI changes included indications of vasogenic edema, leptomeningeal enhancement, and multifocal microhemorrhages.

According to Neelapu et al. (2018), management is driven by the overall grade of neurotoxicity. Throughout all grades, the neurology team should be consulted to assist with fundoscopic examinations for papilledema and to assist in interpretation of diagnostic testing. Grade 1 toxicity management includes close monitoring and supportive care, such as aspiration precautions, fall precautions, and withholding oral medications and nutrition. Grade 2 and higher neurotoxicity may be managed with steroids (dexa-

Table 12-3. Grading of Immune Effector Cell–Associated Neurotoxicity Syndrome

Grade	ICE Score	Additional Symptoms
1	7–9	None
2	3–6	None
3	0–2	Awakens to touch Electroencephalograph with partial or nonconvulsive seizures Focal or generalized seizure Focal edema on neuroimaging
4	Unarousable, unable to participate in ICE assessment	Coma New motor weakness Generalized convulsive or nonconvulsive seizures, status epilepticus Papilledema Diffuse cerebral edema on imaging Decerebrate or decorticate posturing Cushing triad

ICE—immune effector cell–associated encephalopathy

Note. Based on information from D.W. Lee et al., 2019.

methasone 10 mg IV every 6 hours or methylprednisolone 1 mg/kg every 12 hours). Patients with grade 2 or higher neurotoxicity may require transfer to the intensive care unit for closer monitoring or mechanical ventilation if they are no longer able to protect their airways.

Calcineurin Inhibitor–Induced Neurotoxicity

Calcineurin inhibitors work by binding to immunophilins to form a complex that inhibits calcineurin (Dhar, 2018). This results in inhibition of calcium-dependent signaling pathways that release interleukin-2 and activate T cells. Their neurotoxicity may also be mediated through their effects on calcineurin, a critical regulator of neuronal function and excitability (Gijtenbeek, van den Bent, & Vecht, 1999). Neurotoxic effects are more frequent with elevated serum level but can occur at therapeutic serum concentrations as well (Maffini et al., 2017).

Calcineurin inhibitor toxicity may present with a myriad of symptoms. Minor complaints can include headache, paresthesia, and tremor. Moderate neuropsychiatric disturbances include insomnia, anxiety, agitation, and seizures—mainly single and generalized, sometimes with transient postseizure deficits, such as cortical blindness or behavioral abnormalities. Severe symptoms include decreased responsiveness and pyramidal motor weakness (Dhar, 2018; Maffini et al., 2017). These symptoms may occur in isolation or precede the development of more overt delirium with hallucinations and delusions that may culminate in seizures and persistent encephalopathy if not detected (Syed, Couriel, Frame, & Srinivasan, 2016). The radiographic corre-

late of calcineurin inhibitor toxicity is PRES in many cases (Syed et al., 2016).

Grotz et al. (2001) described a rare pain syndrome involving the feet and legs—calcineurin inhibitor–induced pain syndrome. Although the exact pathophysiology remains unclear, it is thought to represent a variant of reflex sympathetic dystrophy, as it can be accompanied by signs of limb (and bone marrow) edema, albeit with fewer trophic changes or vasomotor instability. Pain can be debilitating, but often resolves with reduction in drug dose. Unfortunately, there is no standard therapy, but anecdotal reports suggest it may be amenable to calcium channel–blocking medications (Prommer, 2012).

Cyclosporine

Cyclosporine was the first calcineurin inhibitor introduced in the HSCT setting and often is used for GVHD prophylaxis. Neurotoxicity from cyclosporine can occur early or late in the HSCT course. Acute, early onset is associated with high peak levels of cyclosporine, which occurs most often during initiation of therapy but can also occur when changing route of administration (IV to oral) or the dose. Late neurotoxicity occurs in patients on chronic, long-term immunosuppression whose trough levels of cyclosporine are within therapeutic range. Risk factors are low cholesterol, as it facilitates higher unbound circulating drug levels to diffuse into the brain; hypomagnesemia; hypertension; fluid overload; damage to the vascular endothelium; and breakdown of the blood–brain barrier from chemotherapy or radiation (Gijtenbeek et al., 1999; Openshaw & Chen, 2016). Concomitant therapy with CYP3A inhibitors or inducers and concomitant therapy with methylprednisolone may also increase the risk (Serkova, Christians, & Benet, 2004). The likelihood of developing cyclosporine-induced neurotoxicity may depend on underlying disease.

Cyclosporine toxicity is reversible in early stages; thus, early diagnosis is imperative. Failure to intervene early can result in irreversible toxicity with a potentially fatal outcome. Cyclosporine neurotoxicity is confirmed by MRI, which is more sensitive than CT. Electroencephalography is a sensitive test for identifying cerebral dysfunction but lacks specificity (Syed et al., 2016).

Treatment of cyclosporine neurotoxicity depends on the severity of the symptoms. For mild symptoms, such as tremor, dose reduction is not always required (Gijtenbeek et al., 1999). For most patients with significant symptoms, discontinuation or dose reduction should be considered (Syed et al., 2016).

Tacrolimus

Tacrolimus, another calcineurin inhibitor, may also cause neurotoxicity. In a retrospective study evaluating tacrolimus and cyclosporine in 87 HSCT recipients, the investigators showed no significant differences in neurotoxicity between the drugs in the first 100 days after transplantation. Seizures were noted in 5 of the 87 patients, and altered mental status occurred in the presence of significant metabolic abnormalities and infection (Syed et al., 2016). Appignani et al. (1996) reported rates of tacrolimus neurotoxicity at 5%–30%. Syed et al. (2016) reported a decreased incidence rate because current clinical practice targets lower trough levels. The pathogenesis of tacrolimus-induced neurotoxicity is unclear; and several hypotheses exist. As with cyclosporine, early diagnosis is critical for reversing CNS toxicity (Mammoser, 2012).

Risk factors for neurotoxicity are similar to those of cyclosporine. Patients may experience a range of symptoms that can be mild or severe when presenting with neurotoxicity. Mild symptoms, occurring in 40%–60% of patients, include visual disturbances, headache, agitation, paresthesias, and tremor (Openshaw & Chen, 2016). Severe symptoms, found in 5%–8% of patients, include seizure, cortical blindness, encephalopathy, and coma (Dhar, 2018). Tacrolimus neurotoxicity can occur acutely—immediately after HSCT as a result of supratherapeutic blood levels—or it can occur late after HSCT when tacrolimus levels are therapeutic. Diagnosis is confirmed by MRI (Dhar, 2018; Syed et al., 2016). Treatment is dependent on the time frame of neurotoxicity as it relates to HSCT; discontinuation or decrease in dose leads to symptom resolution (Dhar, 2018).

Neurocognitive Dysfunction

Neurocognitive dysfunction, including symptoms such as memory impairment, impaired concentration, and difficulty in performing multiple tasks simultaneously, has been recognized as a common complication in patients with cancer (Askins & Moore, 2008; Meyers, 2000). Neurocognitive function refers to the activities of the brain that generate the complex behaviors of day-to-day life (Kelly et al., 2018). Although several brain structures may be involved in generating these behaviors, unique neurocognitive functions can be described most comprehensively by evaluating eight domains (Scott, Ostermeyer, & Shah, 2016; see Table 12-4). Neurocognitive dysfunction describes a negative change in neurocognitive function that is independent of normal aging and may affect activities of daily living, including social interactions, complex behaviors, and occupational or academic functioning; this change may have a profound effect on quality of life (Scott et al., 2016). Patients presenting for treatment of hematologic cancers may be at increased risk for neurocognitive dysfunction before HSCT. Neurocognitive dysfunction can significantly affect the early and late post-HSCT course, and it has emerged as a major cause for post-transplant morbidity and mortality. In adult transplant recipients, an incidence of neurocognitive dysfunction of up to 60% has been documented at 22–82 months after HSCT (Harder et al., 2002; Sostak et al., 2003). A recent survey performed in a heterogeneous group of more than 400 HSCT recipients and caregivers by a patient advocacy group (BMT InfoNet; www.bmtinfonet.org) showed that finding

information about neurocognitive dysfunction was the top concern for patients and second most important concern for caregivers (Kelly et al., 2018). Neurocognitive dysfunction is associated with pretransplant chemotherapy, physical deconditioning, TBI in conditioning, immunosuppressive therapies, length of hospital stay, infections, GVHD, and fatigue (Root et al., 2018).

Although neurocognitive dysfunction is a serious cause of morbidity after HSCT, little is known about this phenomenon. The Center for International Blood and Marrow Transplant Research and the European Society for Blood and Marrow Transplantation collaborated to close this knowledge gap and created an expert review of neurocognitive dysfunction after HSCT. This review defined what constitutes a neurocognitive dysfunction, characterized its risk factors and sequelae, described tools and methods to assess neurocognitive dysfunction, and discussed possible interventions (Kelly et al., 2018).

Subjective and objective measures have been used to assess neurocognitive function in the HSCT setting. However, no standard recommendations exist for the timing or types of measures to assess neurocognitive function in adults or children (Kelly et al., 2018). Many unique age range–specific evaluations are available to test neurocognitive domains. The tests are common in the published literature and address the domains most affected by neurocognitive dysfunction. All commonly used neurocognitive tests are standardized measures that are psychometrically validated and widely available in multiple languages. In the current transplant literature, it has been reported that a variety of screening tools to assess neurocognitive function of adults are available. However, their use is controversial, and the National Comprehensive Cancer Network does not recommend neurocognitive dysfunction screening tools in patients with cancer, including HSCT recipients (Denlinger et al., 2014). Kelly et al. (2018) speculated that this recommendation is the result of screening tools being developed for patients with dementia, so they may not detect the subtle neurocognitive dysfunction found in HSCT recipients. Kelly et al. (2018) proposed that future research should focus on the development of a standardized risk factor profile for patients who may be at risk of poor neurocognitive functioning after HSCT.

Kelly et al. (2018) also acknowledged that several significant gaps exist in the research on neurocognitive dysfunction and urged for future research focusing on specific populations, including children and older adults, to delineate neurocognitive dysfunction and to define potential risk and protective factors for patients with neurocognitive dysfunction.

Potential cognitive dysfunction or frank impairment may affect treatment decision making or the ability to recall and follow post-HSCT treatment plan recommendations, which may affect medication and treatment adherence after discharge and, thus, overall survival. Clarification of potential pre-HSCT neurocognitive dysfunction is an important goal

Table 12-4. Domains of Neurocognitive Function in Adults and Children

Domain	Alternative Names	Subdomains	Characteristics
Attention and concentration	• Attention	• Arousal • Focused attention • Divided attention • Vigilance or sustained attention	Alertness sufficient to the completion of tasks. Ability to focus and sustain attention throughout tasks (distractibility). Aspects of attention include the level of alertness or arousal of an individual, which is maintained by the reticular activating system.
Perceptual processing	• Sensory-perceptual • Sensory-motor • Visuospatial and constructional processing	• Agnosia • Visual-spatial cognition	Object recognition. Ability to recognize where objects are located in space. The ventromedial occipital parietal tract aids in the identification of objects, whereas the dorsolateral occipital parietal pathway serves to determine their location in space.
Learning and working memory	• Visual learning and memory	• Verbal • Visual • Working memory • Short- and long-term recall recognition	Learning is the capacity to store and recall new information. Working member is used to describe the capacity to hold, process, and manipulate information.
Abstract thinking and executive function	• Executive function	• Initiation and planning • Cognitive flexibility • Self-regulation	Ability to reason beyond given information to arrive at an interpretation or understand, or a course of action consistent with goals. Many executive functions are served by the frontal lobes.
Language		• Reception • Repetition • Self-expression	Ability to use written or spoken communication to understand or convey information.
Information processing speed			Ability to rapidly process simple and complex information. Information processing speed is a measure of the efficiency of cognitive function and is necessary for motor function.
Motor functions	• Motor speed and strength • Fine motor	• Speed • Dexterity • Coordination	Ability to perform tasks rapidly, precisely and in a smooth, coordinated way
Emotions	• Inhibition • Mood, thought content, personality, and behavior • Motivation/symptom validity	• Behavioral • Perceptual	Ability to suppress actions that interfere with goal driven behavior

Note. From "Neurocognitive Dysfunction in Hematopoietic Cell Transplant Recipients: Expert Review From the Late Effects and Quality of Life Working Committee of the Center for International Blood and Marrow Transplant Research and Complications and Quality of Life Working Party of the European Society for Blood and Marrow Transplantation," by D.L. Kelly, D. Buchbinder, R.F. Duarte, J.J. Auletta, N. Bhatt, M. Byrne, … B.E. Shaw, 2018, *Biology of Blood and Marrow Transplantation, 24,* p. 230. Copyright 2017 by American Society for Blood and Marrow Transplantation. Retrieved from https://doi.org/10.1016/j.bbmt.2017.09.004. Licensed under CC BY-NC-ND 4.0 (https://creativecommons.org/licenses/by-nc-nd/4.0).

to guide treatment planning. Enlisting caregivers for compensatory support and cognitive rehabilitation can enhance postdischarge monitoring (Root et al., 2018).

Long-Term Neurotoxicities

Peripheral Neuropathy

Peripheral neuropathy is a form of neurologic impairment that can occur at any time during a malignant disease course and is best characterized by a change in sensation (Fairman & Bilotti, 2013). The pathophysiology of peripheral neuropathy is not well understood. Tariman, Love, McCullagh, and Sandifer (2008) reported that for patients with multiple myeloma, sensory changes of peripheral neuropathy become progressive and often followed a glove-and-stocking pattern of hypesthesia and dysesthesia in the hands, fingers, legs, toes, or feet. Severe muscle weakness and gait ataxia may also occur (Wick, Hertenstein, & Platten, 2016). Recognizing and evaluating peripheral neuropathy can be challenging because of its diverse presentations.

Understanding and diagnosing peripheral neuropathy involves obtaining a thorough patient history, conducting a neurologic examination, possibly placing a referral to a neurologist for confirming tests with electromyography and nerve conduction studies. Unfortunately, the use of neuroimaging and electrodiagnostic evaluation is debatable for most patients with suspected neuropathy (Doughty & Seyedsadjadi, 2018). Providers should obtain a history that includes the type of symptoms present and the pace of their progress. Table 12-5 lists common signs and symptoms seen in patients with peripheral neuropathy.

Peripheral neuropathy can be a symptom of multiple myeloma or related to the use of medications for treatment, such as lenalidomide or bortezomib. These agents are commonly used before a transplant and are being studied as part of post-transplant maintenance. A high incidence of peripheral neuropathy was demonstrated in several early trials using IV bortezomib (Harousseau et al., 2006; Jagannath et al., 2009; P. Richardson et al., 2008). Most studies have reported an incidence of mild to moderate peripheral neuropathy up to 80% by the end of standard multiple myeloma treatment prior to transplant, and approximately 10%–20% of patients needed to discontinue treatment because of peripheral neuropathy (Dimopoulos et al., 2011; Jagannath et al., 2009; P. Richardson et al., 2008). The incidence of peripheral neuropathy with bortezomib is substantially decreased when administered subcutaneously, rather than by IV push.

Sensory peripheral neuropathy can result from treatment with chemotherapy agents, such as bortezomib, lenalidomide, and vincristine. Specifically, bortezomib-induced peripheral neuropathy typically develops within the first four months of treatment, and lenalidomide-induced peripheral neuropathy develops within the first six months. If detected early, symptoms can be reversed to some degree with dose reductions or discontinuation. Unfortunately, complete resolution of peripheral neuropathy is rare (Argyriou, Iconomou, & Kalofonos, 2008; P. Richardson et al., 2008). Supportive treatments include ion channel blockers, such as gabapentin, and the antidepressant duloxetine for dysesthesia (Wick et al., 2016). Evidence from a phase 3 study suggests that symptomatic treatment with duloxetine may be effective for painful chemotherapy-induced neuropathy (Smith et al., 2013). No other phase 3 data affirm the use of supportive medications for peripheral neuropathy.

Graft-Versus-Host Disease

The manifestations of GVHD in the CNS are less clearly delineated by comparison to the peripheral nervous system (Openshaw & Chen, 2016). Chronic CNS GVHD is best described as a diagnosis of exclusion. According to Openshaw and Chen (2016), the presence of neurologic abnormalities by examination, apparent abnormalities on MRI, abnormalities in CSF, and chronic GVHD of other organ systems are collectively indicative of CNS GVHD. Changes to large and medium neurologic vasculature have been attributed to chronic GVHD, and symptomatology ranges from headaches to seizures and cerebrovascular accident (Grauer et al., 2010). When neurologic symptoms are concurrent with chronic GVHD of other organ systems, treatment should involve immunosuppressive therapy with steroids (Grauer et al., 2010).

Peripheral Nervous System Toxicities

Myositis

Myositis is considered a peripheral nervous system disorder. Patients may present 3–70 months following HSCT (Openshaw & Chen, 2016). No clear risk factors are associated with the development of myositis, but it is most often associated with chronic GVHD (Grauer et al., 2010). Symptomatology includes proximal muscle weakness, either moderate or severe, and dysphasia (Openshaw & Chen, 2016).

A serum creatinine kinase level of 5–50 times above normal correlates with diagnosis of myositis. Lactate dehydrogenase and transaminases may also be above normal (Grauer et al., 2010). Myositis is treated with steroids; however, improvement in symptoms can take days or up to six weeks (Albayda & Christopher-Stine, 2012; Grauer et al., 2010). Alternative agents for treatment include etanercept, rituximab, IV immunoglobulin, methotrexate, and cyclosporine.

Myopathy

Corticosteroid therapy at doses equivalent to 30 mg daily of prednisolone presents a risk for developing steroid-induced myopathy. Proximal muscles (e.g., quad-

Table 12-5. Types of Peripheral Neuropathy and Examination Findings

Type	Examination Findings
Distal symmetric polyneuropathy	Length-dependent: diffuse involvement, affects distal segments first Symptoms occurring below the knees prior to affecting fingers Often caused by diabetes
Hereditary neuropathies	Distal calf atrophy, hammertoes, pes cavus Motor deficits worse than or equal to sensory deficits Diffuse areflexia
Mononeuropathy	Symptoms restricted to distribution of single nerve, myotome, or dermatome Asymmetric reflexes
Mononeuropathy multiplex	Occurrence of several concurrent mononeuropathies Vasculitic etiology
Myelopathy	Disease affecting spinal cord Hyperreflexia, spasticity, sensory deficits occurring in the trunk
Radiculopathy	Degenerative disease affecting cervical or lumbosacral spine Asymmetric reflexes Lower back pain, pain radiating to legs, bladder/bowel dysfunction

Note. Based on information from Doughty & Sevedsadjadi, 2018.

riceps) are the most frequently affected. Myopathy has no prominent diagnostic features; symptoms improve with tapering and discontinuation of steroids (Albayda & Christopher-Stine, 2012).

Guillain-Barré Syndrome

Guillain-Barré syndrome is understood to be an immune dysfunction that leads to the destruction of myelin or axons of peripheral nerves. Onset is rapid and progressive beginning with ascending motor weakness and leading to paralysis (Hughes & Cornblath, 2005). The autonomic nervous system is also involved, leading to respiratory, cardiac, and digestive dysfunction, as well as urinary retention. Guillain-Barré syndrome is rare, but it has been reported in allogeneic and autologous HSCT recipients. It occurs most frequently within three months of HSCT but can develop as early as two weeks and as late as 15 months (Bulsara, Baron, Tuttle-Newhall, Clavien, & Morgenlander, 2001; Wen et al., 1997). Risk for Guillain-Barré syndrome pertaining specifically to HSCT recipients may be attributed to impaired humoral immunity and presence of GVHD. Pathogenic workup is extensive and should include coxsackie virus, Epstein-Barr virus, CMV, hepatitis C virus, *Chlamydophila pneumoniae, Mycoplasma pneumoniae, Campylobacter jejuni*, and VZV (Grauer et al., 2010). CSF analysis reveals elevated protein. Plasma exchange and treatment of the underlying infectious agent are most effective for recovery (Albayda & Christopher-Stine, 2012; Grauer et al., 2010). Rituximab with IV immunoglobulin are also considered appropriate therapy.

Myasthenia Gravis

Myasthenia gravis is an autoimmune disorder in which antibodies attack acetylcholine receptors causing dysfunction at the neuromuscular junction. The result is skeletal muscle weakness, facial muscle weakness, ptosis and visual disturbance, joint pain, shortness of breath, and dysphagia (Bolger et al., 1986; Dowell, Moots, & Stein, 1999).

Less than 1% of HSCT recipients reportedly develop myasthenia gravis, and it occurs most frequently 22–60 months after transplant (Tse et al., 1999). Decreased amplitude in muscle potential following repetitive nerve stimulation is diagnostic. Blood tests for muscle-specific tyrosine kinase antibodies and acetylcholine receptor antibodies may be used in diagnosis, but patients with myasthenia gravis may be seronegative (Rezania et al., 2012). Six months of treatment with cholinesterase inhibitors and steroids are first-line treatment for myasthenia gravis. Second-line agents include azathioprine, cyclosporine, mycophenolate mofetil, tacrolimus, methotrexate, or rituximab (Díaz-Manera, García, & Illa, 2012).

Summary

Neurologic complications for patients undergoing HSCT are important clinical issues, and the etiology is multifactorial. HSCT recipients are at a high risk for these complications. Neurologic complications can arise from the primary disease being treated with HSCT or as a consequence of immunosuppressive treatment, infection, or hemorrhage that may develop following transplant. The occurrence of a neurologic complication is an independent risk factor for increased mortality and a surrogate marker of poor prognosis and increased nonrelapse mortality (Bhatt et al., 2015). Overall, prompt diagnosis and immediate treatment intervention may improve the prognosis and outcome of a neurologic complication and are essential in preventing long-term neurologic disabilities. The toxic effects of medications used in conditioning and immunosuppressive agents account for most of these complications in the early post-transplantation period.

Oncology nurses play a key role in recognizing neurologic changes of the patients. Communication with the transplant team can aid in the successful outcomes and management of neurotoxicities in HSCT recipients. Patient and family education on neurotoxicity promotes self-care, which can allow patients to take control of the side effects by reporting uncommon but potentially frightening toxicities. Prompt interruption or discontinuation of therapy and dose delays or reductions may be necessary to manage certain toxicities.

For the patients undergoing CAR T-cell therapy, neurotoxicities are expected and common. Nursing plays an important role in the care and management of patients with CAR T-cell–related encephalopathy syndrome. Careful and thorough neurologic examinations are key to noting the early signs and symptoms of CAR T-cell–related encephalopathy syndrome, which can be subtle. Nurses can complete CARTOX assessments at a minimum of every shift and as often as neurologic changes are noted. Options for CAR T-cell therapy are increasing, so oncology nurses must remain current with this evolving treatment environment. Oncology nurses need to continuously monitor CAR T cell–recipients' neurologic status for CAR T-cell–related encephalopathy syndrome. Nurses should build a routine evaluation of toxicities and create a standard assessment to care for this unique group of patients.

References

Aksamit, A.J., Jr. (2012). Progressive multifocal leukoencephalopathy. *Continuum, 18*, 1374–1391. https://doi.org/10.1212/01.CON.0000423852.70641.de

Albayda, J., & Christopher-Stine, L. (2012). Novel approaches in the treatment of myositis and myopathies. *Therapeutic Advances in Musculoskeletal Disease, 4*, 369–377. https://doi.org/10.1177/1759720x12447705

Annaloro, C., Costa, A., Fracchiolla, N.S., Mometto, G., Artuso, S., Saporiti, G., … Cortelezzi, A. (2015). Severe fludarabine neurotoxicity after reduced intensity conditioning regimen to allogeneic hematopoietic stem cell transplantation: A case report. *Clinical Case Reports, 3*, 650–655. https://doi.org/10.1002/ccr3.308

Appignani, B.A., Bhadelia, R.A., Blacklow, S.C., Wang, A.K., Roland, S.F., & Freeñman, R.B., Jr. (1996). Neuroimaging findings in patients on immunosuppressive therapy: Experience with tacrolimus toxicity. *American Journal of Roentgenology, 166*, 683–688. https://doi.org/10.2214/ajr.166.3.8623651

Argyriou, A.A., Iconomou, G., & Kalofonos, H.P. (2008). Bortezomib-induced peripheral neuropathy in multiple myeloma: A comprehensive review of the literature. *Blood, 112*, 1593–1599. https://doi.org/10.1182/blood-2008-04-149385

Askins, M.A., & Moore, B.D., III. (2008). Preventing neurocognitive late effects in childhood cancer survivors. *Journal of Child Neurology, 23*, 1160–1171. https://doi.org/10.1177/0883073808321065

Barba, P., Piñana, J.L., Valcárcel, D., Querol, L., Martino, R., Sureda, A., … Sierra, J. (2009). Early and late neurological complications after reduced-intensity conditioning allogeneic stem cell transplantation. *Biology of Blood and Marrow Transplantation, 15*, 1439–1446. https://doi.org/10.1016/j.bbmt.2009.07.013

Bauwens, D., Hantson, P., Laterre, P.-F., Michaux, L., Latinne, D., De Tourtchaninoff, M., … Hernalsteen, D. (2005). Recurrent seizure and sustained encephalopathy associated with dimethylsulfoxide-preserved stem cell infusion. *Leukemia and Lymphoma, 46*, 1671–1674. https://doi.org/10.1080/10428190500235611

Beitinjaneh, A., McKinney, A.M., Cao, Q., & Weisdorf, D.J. (2011). Toxic leukoencephalopathy following fludarabine-associated hematopoietic cell transplantation. *Biology of Blood and Marrow Transplantation, 17*, 300–308. https://doi.org/10.1016/j.bbmt.2010.04.003

Benninger, F., & Steiner, I. (2018). CSF in acute and chronic infectious disease. In F. Deisenhammer, C.E. Teunissen, & H. Tumani (Eds.), *Handbook of clinical neurology: Vol. 146. Cerebrospinal fluid in neurologic disorders* (pp. 187–206). https://doi.org/10.1016/b978-0-12-804279-3.00012-5

Berger, J.R. (2007). Progressive multifocal leukoencephalopathy. *Current Neurology and Neuroscience Reports, 7*, 461–469. https://doi.org/10.1007/s11910-007-0072-9

Bhanushali, M.J., Kranick, S.M., Freeman, A.F., Cuellar-Rodriguez, J.M., Battiwalla, M., Gea-Banacloche, J.C., … Nath, A. (2013). Human herpes 6 virus encephalitis complicating allogeneic hematopoietic stem cell transplantation. *Neurology, 80*, 1494–1500. https://doi.org/10.1212/wnl.0b013e31828cf8a2

Bhatt, V.R., Balasetti, V., Jasem, J.A., Giri, S., Armitage, J.O., Loberiza, F.R., Jr., … Akhtari, M. (2015). Central nervous system complications and outcomes after allogeneic hematopoietic stem cell transplantation. *Clinical Lymphoma, Myeloma and Leukemia, 15*, 606–611. https://doi.org/10.1016/j.clml.2015.06.004

Blei, A.T., & Córdoba, J. (2001). Hepatic encephalopathy. *American Journal of Gastroenterology, 96*, 1968–1976. Retrieved from https://journals.lww.com/ajg/Citation/2001/07000/Hepatic_Encephalopathy.9.aspx

Bolger, G.B., Sullivan, K.M., Spence, A.M., Appelbaum, F.R., Johnston, R., Sanders, J.E., … Storb, R. (1986). Myasthenia gravis after allogeneic bone marrow transplantation: Relationship to chronic graft-versus-host disease. *Neurology, 36*, 1087–1091. https://doi.org/10.1212/WNL.36.8.1087

Brown, C. (2010). Cerebellar assessment for patients receiving high-dose cytarabine: A standardized approach to nursing assessment and documentation. *Clinical Journal of Oncology Nursing, 14*, 371–373. https://doi.org/10.1188/10.cjon.371-373

Bulsara, K., Baron, P., Tuttle-Newhall, J., Clavien, P.-A., & Morgenlander, J. (2001). Guillain-Barre syndrome in organ and bone marrow transplant patients. *Transplantation, 71*, 1169–1172. https://doi.org/10.1097/00007890-200104270-00026

Cain, J.W., & Bender, C.M. (1995). Ifosfamide-induced neurotoxicity: Associated symptoms and nursing implications. *Oncology Nursing Forum, 22*, 659–666.

Cavaliere, R., & Schiff, D. (2006). Neurologic toxicities of cancer therapies. *Current Neurology and Neuroscience Reports, 6*, 218–226. https://doi.org/10.1007/s11910-006-0009-8

Centers for Disease Control and Prevention. (2018, September 28). Toxoplasmosis frequently asked questions (FAQs). Retrieved from http://www.cdc.gov/parasites/toxoplasmosis/gen_info/faqs.html

Chen, S., Hu, J., Xu, L., Brandon, D., Yu, J., & Zhang, J. (2016). Posterior reversible encephalopathy syndrome after transplantation: A review. *Molecular Neurobiology, 53*, 6897–6909. https://doi.org/10.1007/s12035-015-9560-0

Ciurea, S.O., & Andersson, B.S. (2009). Busulfan in hematopoietic stem cell transplantation. *Biology of Blood and Marrow Transplantation, 15*, 523–536. https://doi.org/10.1016/j.bbmt.2008.12.489

Colosimo, M., McCarthy, N., Jayasinghe, R., Morton, J., Taylor, K., & Durrant, S. (2000). Diagnosis and management of subdural haematoma complicating bone marrow transplantation. *Bone Marrow Transplantation, 25*, 549–552. https://doi.org/10.1038/sj.bmt.1702166

Courtney, M.J., & Coffey, E.T. (1999). The mechanism of ara-C-induced apoptosis of differentiating cerebellar granule neurons. *European Journal of Neuroscience, 11*, 1073–1084. https://doi.org/10.1046/j.1460-9568.1999.00520.x

David, K.A., & Picus, J. (2005). Evaluating risk factors for the development of ifosfamide encephalopathy. *American Journal of Clinical Oncology, 28*, 277–280. https://doi.org/10.1097/01.coc.0000158439.02724.5a

de Lima, M., Couriel, D., Thall, P.F., Wang, X., Madden, T., Jones, R., … Andersson, B.S. (2004). Once-daily intravenous busulfan and fludarabine: Clinical and pharmacokinetic results of a myeloablative, reduced-toxicity conditioning regimen for allogeneic stem cell transplantation in AML and MDS. *Blood, 104*, 857–864. https://doi.org/10.1182/blood-2004-02-0414

de Magalhaes-Silverman, M., & Hammert, L. (2000). Neurologic complications. In E. Ball, J. Lister, & P. Law (Eds.), *Hematopoietic stem cell therapy* (pp. 578–588). New York, NY: Churchill Livingstone.

Denier, C., Bourhis, J.-H., Lacroix, C., Koscielny, S., Bosq, J., Sigal, R., … Adams, D. (2006). Spectrum and prognosis of neurologic complications after hematopoietic transplantation. *Neurology, 67*, 1990–1997. https://doi.org/10.1212/01.wnl.0000247038.43228.17

Denlinger, C.S., Ligibel, J.A., Are, M., Baker, K.S., Demark-Wahnefried, W., Friedman, D.L., … Freedman-Cass, D.A. (2014). Survivorship: Cognitive function, version 1.2014. *Journal of the National Comprehensive Cancer Network, 12*, 976–986. https://doi.org/10.6004/jnccn.2014.0094

Dhar, R. (2018). Neurologic complications of transplantation. *Neurocritical Care, 28*, 4–11. https://doi.org/10.1007/s12028-017-0387-6

Diaz-Carrasco, S.M., Olmos, R., Blanquer, M., Velasco, J., Sánchez-Salinas, A., & Moraleda, J.M. (2013). Clonazepam for seizure prophylaxis in adult patients treated with high dose busulfan. *International Journal of Clinical Pharmacology, 35*, 339–343. https://doi.org/10.1007/s11096-013-9768-x

Díaz-Manera, J., García, R.R., & Illa, I. (2012). Treatment strategies for myasthenia gravis: An update. *Expert Opinion on Pharmacotherapy, 13*, 1873–1883. https://doi.org/10.1517/14656566.2012.705831

Dimopoulos, M.A., Mateos, M.-V., Richardson, P.G., Schlag, R., Khuageva, N.K., Shpilberg, O., … San Miguel, J.F. (2001). Risk factors for, and reversibility of, peripheral neuropathy associated with bortezomib-melphalan-prednisone in newly diagnosed patients with multiple myeloma: Subanalysis of the phase 3 VISTA study. *European Journal of Haematology, 86*, 23–31. https://doi.org/10.1111/j.1600-0609.2010.01533.x

Doughty, C.T., & Seyedsadjadi, R. (2018). Approach to peripheral neuropathy for the primary care clinician. *American Journal of Medicine, 131*, 1010–1016. https://doi.org/10.1016/j.amjmed.2017.12.042

Dowell, J.E., Moots, P.L., & Stein, R.S. (1999). Myasthenia gravis after allogeneic bone marrow transplantation for lymphoblastic lymphoma. *Bone Marrow Transplantation, 24*, 1359–1361. https://doi.org/10.1038/sj.bmt.1702067

Dowling, M.R., Li, S., Dey, B.R., McAfee, S.L., Hock, H.R., Spitzer, T.R., … Ballen, K.K. (2018). Neurologic complications after allogeneic hematopoietic stem cell transplantation: Risk factors and impact. *Bone Marrow Transplantation, 53*, 199–206. https://doi.org/10.1038/bmt.2017.239

Eberly, A.L., Anderson, G.D., Bubalo, J.S., & McCune, J.S. (2008). Optimal prevention of seizures induced by high-dose busulfan. *Pharmacotherapy, 28*, 1502–1510. https://doi.org/10.1592/phco.28.12.1502

Fichet, J., Mercier, E., Genée, O., Garot, D., Legras, A., Dequin, P.-F., & Perrotin, D. (2009). Prognosis and 1-year mortality of intensive care unit patients with severe hepatic encephalopathy. *Journal of Critical Care, 24*, 364–370. https://doi.org/10.1016/j.jcrc.2009.01.008

Focosi, D., Marco, T., Kast, R.E., Maggi, F., Ceccherini-Nelli, L., & Petrini, M. (2010). Progressive multifocal leukoencephalopathy: What's new? *Neuroscientist, 16*, 308–323. https://doi.org/10.1177/1073858409356594

Fugate, J.E., & Rabinstein, A.A. (2015). Posterior reversible encephalopathy syndrome: Clinical and radiological manifestations, pathophysiology, and outstanding questions. *Lancet Neurology, 14*, 914–925. https://doi.org/10.1016/s1474-4422(15)00111-8

Gauthier, J., & Turtle, C.J. (2018). Insights into cytokine release syndrome and neurotoxicity after CD19-specific CAR T-cell therapy. *Current Research in Translational Medicine, 66*, 50–52. https://doi.org/10.1016/j.retram.2018.03.003

Gijtenbeek, J.M.M., van den Bent, M.J., & Vecht, C.J. (1999). Cyclosporine neurotoxicity: A review. *Journal of Neurology, 246*, 339–346. https://doi.org/10.1007/s004150050360

Gratwohl, A., Pasquine, M.C., Aljurf, M., Atsuta, Y., Baldomero, H., Foeken, L., ... Niederwieser, D. (2015). One million haemopoietic stem-cell transplants: A retrospective observational study. *Lancet Haematology, 2*, e91–e100. https://doi.org/10.1016/s2352-3026(15)00028-9

Grauer, O., Wolff, D., Bertz, H., Greinix, H., Kühl, J.-S., Lawitschka, A., ... Kleiter, I. (2010). Neurologic manifestations of chronic graft-versus-host disease after allogeneic haematopoietic stem cell transplantation: Report from the Consensus Conference on Clinical Practice in chronic graft-versus-host disease. *Brain, 133*, 2852–2865. https://doi.org/10.1093/brain/awq245

Graus, F., Saiz, A., Sierra, J., Arbaiza, D., Rovira, M., Carreras, E., ... Rozman, C. (1996). Neurologic complications of autologous and allogeneic bone marrow transplantation in patients with leukemia: A comparative study. *Neurology, 46*, 1004–1009. https://doi.org/10.1212/wnl.46.4.1004

Grigg, A.P., Shepherd, J.D., & Phillips, G.L. (1989). Busulfan and phenytoin [Letter to the editor]. *Annals of Internal Medicine, 111*, 1049–1050. https://doi.org/10.7326/0003-4819-111-12-1049_2

Grotz, W.H., Breitenfeldt, M.K., Braune, S.W., Allmann, K.-H., Krause, T.M., Schollmeyer, P.J., & Rump, J.A. (2001). Calcineurin-inhibitor induced pain syndrome (CIPS): A severe disabling complication after organ transplantation. *Transplant International, 14*, 16–23. https://doi.org/10.1007/s001470000285

Gust, J., Hay, K.A., Hanafi, L.-A., Li, D., Myerson, D., Gonzalez-Cuyar, L.F., ... Turtle, C.J. (2017). Endothelial activation and blood–brain barrier disruption in neurotoxicity after adoptive immunotherapy with CD19 CAR-T cells. *Cancer Discovery, 7*, 1404–1419. https://doi.org/10.1158/2159-8290.cd-17-0698

Harder, H., Cornelissen, J.J., Van Gool, A.R., Duivenvoorden, H.J., Eijkenboom, W.M.H., & van den Bent, M.J. (2002). Cognitive functioning and quality of life in long-term adult survivors of bone marrow transplantation. *Cancer, 95*, 183–192. https://doi.org/10.1002/cncr.10627

Harousseau, J.-L., Attal, M., Leleu, X., Troncy, J., Pegourie, B., Stoppa, A.M., ... Avet-Loiseau, H. (2006). Bortezomib plus dexamethasone as induction treatment prior to autologous stem cell transplantation in patients with newly diagnosed multiple myeloma: Results of an IFM phase II study. *Haematalogica, 91*, 1498–1505. Retrieved from http://www.haematologica.org/content/91/11/1498

Hassan, M., Ehrsson, H.E., & Ljungman, P. (1996). Aspects concerning busulfan pharmacokinetics and bioavailability. *Leukemia and Lymphoma, 22*, 395–407. https://doi.org/10.3109/10428199609054777

Hassan, M., Öberg, G., Björkholm, M., Wallin, I., & Lindgren, M. (1993). Influence of prophylactic anticonvulsant therapy of high-dose busulphan kinetics. *Cancer Chemotherapy and Pharmacology, 33*, 181–186. https://doi.org/10.1007/bf00686213

Hughes, R.A.C., & Cornblath, D.R. (2005). Guillain-Barré syndrome. *Lancet, 366*, 1653–1666. https://doi.org/10.1016/s0140-6736(05)67665-9

Jagannath, S., Durie, B.G.M., Wolf, J.L., Camacho, E.S., Irwin, D., Lutzky, J., ... Vescio, R. (2009). Extended follow-up of a phase 2 trial of bortezomib alone and in combination with dexamethasone for the frontline treatment of multiple myeloma. *British Journal of Haematology, 146*, 619–626. https://doi.org/10.1111/j.1365-2141.2009.07803.x

Júnior, A.M., Arrais, C.A., Saboya, R., Velasques, R.D., Junqueira, P.L., & Dulley, F.L. (2008). Neurotoxicity associated with dimethylsulfoxide-preserved hematopoietic progenitor cell infusion. *Bone Marrow Transplantation, 41*, 95–96. https://doi.org/10.1038/sj.bmt.1705883

Kansu, E. (2012). Thrombosis in stem cell transplantation. *Hematology, 17*(Suppl. 1), s159–s162. https://doi.org/10.1179/102453312X13336169156735

Kelly, D.L., Buchbinder, D., Duarte, R.F., Auletta, J.J., Bhatt, N., Byrne, M., ... Shaw, B.E. (2018). Neurocognitive dysfunction in hematopoietic cell transplant recipients: Expert review from the Late Effects and Quality of Life Working Committee of the Center for International Blood and Marrow Transplant Research and Complications and Quality of Life Working Party of the European Society for Blood and Marrow Transplantation. *Biology of Blood and Marrow Transplantation, 24*, 228–241. https://doi.org/10.1016/j.bbmt.2017.09.004

Kerbusch, T., de Kraker, J., Keizer, H.J., van Putten, J.W.G., Groen, H.J.M., Jansen, R.L.H., ... Beijnen, J.H. (2001). Clinical pharmacokinetics and pharmacodynamics of ifosfamide and its metabolites. *Clinical Pharmacokinetics, 40*, 41–62. https://doi.org/10.2165/00003088-200140010-00004

Kontoyiannis, D.P., & Lewis, R.E. (2011). How I treat mucormycosis. *Blood, 118*, 1216–1224. https://doi.org/10.1182/blood-2011-03-316430

Kourkoumpetis, T.K., Fuchs, B.B., Coleman, J.J., Desalermos, A., & Mylonakis, E. (2012). Polymerase chain reaction–based assays for the diagnosis of invasive fungal infections. *Clinical Infectious Diseases, 54*, 1322–1331. http://doi.org/10.1093/cid/cis132

Lanternier, F., Sun, H.-Y., Ribaud, P., Singh, N., Kontoyiannis, D.P., & Lortholary, O. (2012). Mucormycosis in organ and stem cell transplant recipients. *Clinical Infectious Diseases, 54*, 1–8. https://doi.org/10.1093/cid/cis195

Lee, D.W., Santomasso, B.D., Locke, F.L., Ghobadi, A., Turtle, C.J., Brudno, J.N., ... Neelapu, S.S. (2019). ASTCT consensus grading for cytokine release syndrome and neurologic toxicity associated with immune effector cells. *Biology of Blood and Marrow Transplantation, 25*, 625–638. https://doi.org/10.1016/j.bbmt.2018.12.758

Lee, M.S., McKinney, A.M., Brace, J.R., & SantaCruz, K. (2010). Clinical and imaging features of fludarabine neurotoxicity. *Journal of Neuro-Ophthalmology, 30*, 37–41. https://doi.org/10.1097/wno.0b013e3181ce8087

Ljungman, P., Cordonnier, C., Einsele, H., Bender-Götze, C., Bosi, A., Dekker, A., ... Veil, D. (1998). Use of intravenous immune globulin in addition to antiviral therapy in the treatment of CMV gastrointestinal disease in allogeneic bone marrow transplant patients: A report from the European Group for Blood and Marrow Transplantation (EBMT). *Bone Marrow Transplantation, 21*, 473–476. https://doi.org/10.1038/sj.bmt.1701113

Long-Boyle, J.R., Green, K.G., Brunstein, C.G., Cao, Q., Rogosheske, J., Weisdorf, D.J., ... Jacobson, P.A. (2011). High fludarabine exposure and relationship with treatment-related mortality after nonmyeloablative hematopoietic cell transplantation. *Bone Marrow Transplantation, 46*, 20–26. https://doi.org/10.1038/bmt.2010.53

Macdonald, D.R. (1991). Neurologic complications of chemotherapy. *Neurologic Clinics, 9*, 955–967. https://doi.org/10.1016/s0733-8619(18)30259-7

Maffini, E., Festuccia, M., Brunello, L., Boccadoro, M., Giaccone, L., & Bruno, B. (2017). Neurologic complications after allogeneic hematopoietic stem cell transplantation. *Biology of Blood and Marrow Transplantation, 23*, 388–397. https://doi.org/10.1016/j.bbmt.2016.12.632

Magge, R.S., & DeAngelis, L.M. (2015). The double-edged sword: Neurotoxicity of chemotherapy. *Blood Reviews, 29*, 93–100. https://doi.org/10.1016/j.blre.2014.09.012

Mammoser, A. (2012). Calcineurin inhibitor encephalopathy. *Seminars in Neurology, 23*, 517–524. https://doi.org/10.1055/s-0033-1334471

Marcacci, G., Corazzelli, G., Becchimanzi, C., Arcamone, M., Capobianco, G., Russo, F., ... Pinto, A. (2009). DMSO-associated encephalopathy during autologous peripheral stem cell infusion: A predisposing role of preconditioning exposure to CNS-penetrating agents? *Bone Marrow Transplantation, 44*, 133–135. https://doi.org/10.1038/bmt.2008.442

Marra, C.M. (2018). Other central nervous system infections: Cytomegalovirus, *Mycobacterium tuberculosis*, and *Treponema pallidum*. In B.J. Brew (Ed.), *Handbook of clinical neurology: Vol. 152. The neurology of HIV infection* (pp. 151–166). https://doi.org/10.1016/b978-0-444-63849-6.00012-8

Martino, R., Maertens, J., Bretagne, S., Rovira, M., Deconinck, E., Ullmann, A.J., ... Cordonnier, C. (2000). Toxoplasmosis after hematopoietic stem cell transplantation. *Clinical Infectious Diseases, 31*, 1188–1194. https://doi.org/10.1086/317471

Maschke, M., Dietrich, U., Prumbaum, M., Kastrup, O., Turowski, B., Schaefer, U.W., & Diener, H.C. (1999). Opportunistic CNS infection after bone marrow transplantation. *Bone Marrow Transplantation, 23*, 1167–1176. https://doi.org/10.1038/sj.bmt.1701782

Mathew, R.M., & Rosenfeld, M.R. (2007). Neurologic complications of bone marrow and stem-cell transplantation in patients with cancer. *Current Treatment Options in Neurology, 9*, 308–314. https://doi.org/10.1007/s11940-007-0016-3

Mathew, S., Harnicar, S., Adel, N., & Papadopoulos, E. (2011). Retrospective comparison of phenytoin and levetiracetam as seizure prophylaxis with high dose busulfan during allogeneic stem cell transplant [Abstract]. *Biology of Blood and Marrow Transplantation, 17*(Suppl. 2), S353. https://doi.org/10.1016/j.bbmt.2010.12.595

Meyers, C.A. (2000). Neurocognitive dysfunction in cancer patients. *Oncology, 14*, 75–79.

Miyagi, T., Itonaga, H., Aosai, F., Taguchi, J., Norose, K., Mochizuki, K., … Miyazaki, Y. (2015). Successful treatment of toxoplasmic encephalitis diagnosed early by polymerase chain reaction after allogeneic hematopoietic stem cell transplantation: Two case reports and review of literature. *Transplant Infectious Disease, 17*, 593–598. https://doi.org/10.1111/tid.12401

Mueller, L.P., Theurich, S., Christopeit, M., Grothe, W., Muetherig, A., Weber, T., … Behre, G. (2007). Neurotoxicity upon infusion of dimethylsulfoxide-cryopreserved peripheral blood stem cells in patients with and without pre-existing cerebral disease. *European Journal of Haematology, 78*, 527–531. https://doi.org/10.1111/j.1600-0609.2007.00851.x

Mueller-Mang, C., Mang, T.G., Kalhs, P., & Thurnher, M.M. (2006). Imagining characteristics of toxoplasmosis encephalitis after bone marrow transplantation: Report of two cases and review of the literature. *Neuroradiology, 48*, 84–89. https://doi.org/10.1007/s00234-005-0018-3

Myers, K.C., Lawrence, J., Marsh, R.A., Davies, S.M., & Jodele, S. (2013). High-dose methylprednisolone for veno-occlusive disease of the liver in pediatric hematopoietic stem cell transplantation recipients. *Biology of Blood and Marrow Transplantation, 19*, 500–503. https://doi.org/10.1016/j.bbmt.2012.11.011

Najima, Y., Ohashi, K., Miyazawa, M., Nakano, M., Kobayashi, T., Yamashita, T., … Sakamaki, H. (2009). Intracranial hemorrhage following allogeneic hematopoietic stem cell transplantation. *American Journal of Hematology, 84*, 298–301. https://doi.org/10.1002/ajh.21382

Neelapu, S.S., Tummala, S., Kebriaei, P., Wierda, W., Gutierrez, C., Locke, F.L., … Shpall, E.J. (2018). Chimeric antigen receptor T-cell therapy—Assessment and management of toxicities. *Nature Reviews Clinical Oncology, 15*, 47–62. https://doi.org/10.1038/nrclinonc.2017.148

Openshaw, H., & Chen, B.T. (2016). Neurologic complications of hematopoietic cell transplantation. In S.J. Forman, R.S. Negrin, J.H. Antin, & F.R. Appelbaum (Eds.), *Thomas' hematopoietic cell transplantation: Stem cell transplantation* (5th ed., pp. 1287–1296). https://doi.org/10.1002/9781118416426.ch105

Otrock, Z.K., Beydoun, A., Barada, W.M., Masrouleh, R., Hourani, R., & Bazarbachi, A. (2008). Transient global amnesia associated with the infusion of DMSO-cryopreserved autologous peripheral blood stem cells. *Haematologica, 93*, e36–e37. https://doi.org/10.3324/haematol.12249

Owczarczyk, K., Hilker, R., Brunn, A., Hallek, M., & Rubbert, A. (2007). Progressive multifocal leucoencephalopathy in a patient with sarcoidosis—Successful treatment with cidofovir and mirtazapine. *Rheumatology, 46*, 888–890. https://doi.org/10.1093/rheumatology/kem049

Parize, P., Rammaert, B., & Lortholary, O. (2012). Emerging invasive fungal diseases in transplantation. *Current Infectious Disease Reports, 14*, 668–675. https://doi.org/10.1007/s11908-012-0296-y

Prommer, E. (2012). Calcineurin-inhibitor pain syndrome. *Clinical Journal of Pain, 28*, 556–559. https://doi.org/10.1097/ajp.0b013e31823a67f1

Pruitt, A.A. (2012). CNS infections in patients with cancer. *Continuum, 18*, 384–405. https://doi.org/10.1212/01.CON.0000413665.80915.c4

Raajasekar, A.K.A., Ayyapan, S., Khan, H., Mantzaris, I., & Janakiram, M. (2016). Progressive multifocal leukoencephalopathy associated with hematopoietic stem cell transplant (HSCT) has better prognosis than PML associated with monoclonal antibodies or chemotherapy in hematological malignancies: Analysis of a case series [Abstract]. *Biology of Blood and Marrow Transplantation, 22*(Suppl. 3), S153–S154. https://doi.org/10.1016/j.bbmt.2015.11.505

Raffi, F., Taburet, A.M., Ghaleh, B., Huart, A., & Singlas, E. (1993). Penetration of foscarnet into cerebrospinal fluid of AIDS patients. *Antimicrobial Agents and Chemotherapy, 37*, 1777–1780. https://doi.org/10.1128/aac.37.9.1777

Reddy, S.M., Winston, D.J., Territo, M.C., & Schiller, G.J. (2010). CMV central nervous system disease in stem-cell transplant recipients: An increasing complication of drug-resistant CMV infection and protracted immunodeficiency. *Bone Marrow Transplantation, 45*, 979–984. https://doi.org/10.1038/bmt.2010.35

Rezania, K., Soliven, B., Baron, J., Lin, H., Penumalli, V., & van Besien, K. (2012). Myasthenia gravis, an autoimmune manifestation of lymphoma and lymphoproliferative disorders: Case reports and review of literature. *Leukemia and Lymphoma, 53*, 371–380. https://doi.org/10.3109/10428194.2011.615426

Richards, A., Marshall, H., & McQuary, A. (2011). Evaluation of methylene blue, thiamine, and/or albumin in the prevention of ifosfamide-related neurotoxicity. *Journal of Oncology Pharmacy Practice, 17*, 372–380. https://doi.org/10.1177/1078155210385159

Richardson, M. (2009). The ecology of the zygomycetes and its impact on environmental exposure. *Clinical Microbiology and Infection, 15*(Suppl. 5), 2–9. https://doi.org/10.1111/j.1469-0691.2009.02972.x

Richardson, P., Lonial, S., Jakubowiak, A.J., Jagannath, S., Raje, N., Avigan, D., … Anderson, K.C. (2008). Lenalidomide, bortezomib, and dexamethasone in patients with newly diagnosed multiple myeloma: Encouraging efficacy in high risk groups with updated results of a phase I/II study [Abstract]. *Blood, 112*, 92. https://doi.org/10.1182/blood.V112.11.92.92

Rieger, C., Fiegl, M., Tischer, J., Ostermann, H., & Schiel, X. (2004). Incidence and severity of ifosfamide-induced encephalopathy. *Anti-Cancer Drugs, 15*, 347–350. https://doi.org/10.1097/00001813-200404000-00006

Root, J.C., Rocha-Cadman, X., Kasven-Gonzalez, N., Campbell, C., Maloy, M., Flynn, J., … Jakubowski, A.A. (2018). Pre-transplant cognitive dysfunction in hematologic cancers, predictors and associated outcomes [Abstract]. *Biology of Blood and Marrow Transplantation, 24*(Suppl. 3), S308. https://doi.org/10.1016/j.bbmt.2017.12.354

Rosenfeld, M.R., & Pruitt, A. (2006). Neurologic complications of bone marrow, stem cell, and organ transplantation in patients with cancer. *Seminars in Oncology, 33*, 352–361. https://doi.org/10.1053/j.seminoncol.2006.03.003

Rowley, S.D. (2016). Cryopreservation of hematopoietic cells. In S.J. Forman, R.S. Negrin, J.H. Antin, & F.R. Appelbaum (Eds.), *Thomas' hematopoietic cell transplantation: Stem cell transplantation* (5th ed., pp. 469–479). https://doi.org/10.1002/9781118416426.ch42

Sakai, R., Kanamori, H., Motohashi, K., Yamamoto, W., Matsuura, S., Fujita, A., … Fujisawa, S. (2011). Long-term outcome of human herpesvirus-6 encephalitis after allogeneic stem cell transplantation. *Biology of Blood and Marrow Transplantation, 17*, 1389–1394. https://doi.org/10.1016/j.bbmt.2011.01.014

Schiller, G., & Lee, M. (1997). Long-term outcome of high-dose cytarabine-based consolidation chemotherapy for older patients with acute myelogenous leukemia. *Leukemia and Lymphoma, 25*, 111–119. https://doi.org/10.3109/10428199709042501

Schmidt, V., Prell, T., Treschl, A., Klink, A., Hochhaus, A., & Sayer, H.G. (2016). Clinical management of posterior reversible encephalopathy syndrome after allogeneic hematopoietic stem cell transplantation: A case series and review of the literature. *Acta Haematologica, 135*, 1–10. https://doi.org/10.1159/000430489

Schwartz, S., Ruhnke, M., Ribaud, P., Corey, L., Driscoll, T., Cornely, O.A., … Thiel, E. (2005). Improved outcome in central nervous system aspergillosis, using voriconazole treatment. *Blood, 106*, 2641–2645. https://doi.org/10.1182/blood-2005-02-0733

Scott, J.G., Ostermeyer, B., & Shah, A.A. (2016). Neuropsychological assessment in neurocognitive disorders. *Psychiatric Annals, 46*, 118–126. https://doi.org/10.3928/00485713-20151229-01

Seeley, W.W., Marty, F.M., Holmes, T.M., Upchurch, K., Soiffer, R.J., Antin, J.H., … Broomfield, E.B. (2007). Post-transplant acute limbic encephalitis: Clinical features and relationship to HHV6. *Neurology, 69*, 156–165. https://doi.org/10.1212/01.wnl.0000265591.10200.d7

Serkova, N.J., Christians, U., & Benet, L.Z. (2004). Biochemical mechanisms of cyclosporine neurotoxicity. *Molecular Interventions, 4*, 97–107.

Shih, H.A. (2019). Acute complications of cranial radiation. In A.F. Eichler (Ed.), *UpToDate*. Retrieved September 16, 2019, from https://www.uptodate.com/contents/acute-complications-of-cranial-irradiation

Shimazu, Y., Kondo, T., Ishikawa, T., Yamashita, K., & Takaori-Kondo, A. (2013). Human herpesvirus-6 encephalitis during hematopoietic stem cell transplantation leads to poor prognosis. *Transplant Infectious Disease, 15,* 195–201. https://doi.org/10.1111/tid.12049

Siegal, D., Keller, A., Xu, W., Bhuta, S., Kim, D.H., Kuruvilla, J., ... Gupta, V. (2007). Central nervous system complications after allogeneic hematopoietic stem cell transplantation: Incidence, manifestations, and clinical significance. *Biology of Blood and Marrow Transplantation, 13,* 1369–1379. https://doi.org/10.1016/j.bbmt.2007.07.013

Smith, E.M.L., Pang, H., Cirrincione, C., Fleishman, S., Paskett, E.D., Ahles, T., ... Shapiro, C.L. (2013). Effect of duloxetine on pain, function, and quality of life among patients with chemotherapy-induced painful peripheral neuropathy: A randomized clinical trial. *JAMA, 309,* 1359–1367. https://doi.org/10.1001/jama.2013.2813

Sostak, P., Padovan, C.S., Yousry, T.A., Ledderose, G., Kolb, H.-J., & Straube, A. (2003). Prospective evaluation of neurological complications after allogeneic bone marrow transplantation. *Neurology, 60,* 842–848. https://doi.org/10.1212/01.wnl.0000046522.38465.79

Styczynski, J., Reusser, P., Einsele, H., de la Camara, R., Cordonnier, C., Ward, K.N., ... Engelhard, D. (2009). Management of HSV, VZV and EBV infections in patients with hematological malignancies and after SCT: Guidelines from the Second European Conference on Infections in Leukemia. *Bone Marrow Transplantation, 43,* 757–770. https://doi.org/10.1038/bmt.2008.386

Syed, F.I., Couriel, D.R., Frame, D., & Srinivasan, A. (2016). Central nervous system complications of hematopoietic stem cell transplant. *Hematology/Oncology Clinics of North America, 30,* 887–898. https://doi.org/10.1016/j.hoc.2016.03.009

Tan, I.L., McArthur, J.C., Venkatesan, A., & Nath, A. (2012). Atypical manifestations and poor outcome of herpes simplex encephalitis in the immunocompromised. *Neurology, 79,* 2125–2132. https://doi.org/10.1212/wnl.0b013e3182752ceb

Tariman, J.D., Love, G., McCullagh, E., & Sandifer, S. (2008). Peripheral neuropathy associated with novel therapies in patients with multiple myeloma: Consensus statement of the IMF Nurse Leadership Board. *Clinical Journal of Oncology Nursing, 12,* 29–35. https://doi.org/10.1188/08.cjon.s1.29-35

Teive, H.A.G., Funke, V., Bitencourt, M.A., de Oliveira, M.M., Bonfim, C., Zanis-Neto, J., ... Pasquini, R. (2008). Neurological complications of hematopoietic stem cell transplantation (HSCT): A retrospective study in a HSCT center in Brazil. *Arquivos de Neuro-Psiquiatria, 66,* 685–690. https://doi.org/10.1590/s0004-282x2008000500014

Tomblyn, M., Chiller, T., Einsele, H., Gress, R., Sepkowitz, K., Storek, J., ... Boeckh, M.A. (2009). Guidelines for preventing infectious complications among hematopoietic cell transplantation recipients: A global perspective. *Biology of Blood and Marrow Transplantation, 15,* 1143–1238. https://doi.org/10.1016/j.bbmt.2009.06.019

Tracy, J.A., & Mowzoon, N. (2006). In N. Mowzoon, & K.D. Fleming (Eds.), *Neurology board review: An illustrated study guide* (pp. 601–615). https://doi.org/10.1201/b14430

Tse, S., Saunders, E.F., Silverman, E., Vajsar, J., Becker, L., & Meaney, B. (1999). Myasthenia gravis and polymyositis as manifestations of chronic graft-versus-host disease. *Bone Marrow Transplantation, 23,* 397–399. https://doi.org/10.1038/sj.bmt.1701575

Tunkel, A.R., Glaser, C.A., Bloch, K.C., Sejvar, J.J., Marra, C.M., Roos, K.L., ... Whitley, R.J. (2008). The management of encephalitis: Clinical practice guidelines by the Infectious Diseases Society of America. *Clinical Infectious Diseases, 47,* 303–327. https://doi.org/10.1086/589747

Verma, S., Cikurel, K., Koralnik, I.J., Morgello, S., Cunningham-Rundles, C., Weinstein, Z.R., ... Simpson, D.M. (2007). Mirtazipine in progressive multifocal leukoencephalopathy associated with polycythemia vera. *Journal of Infectious Diseases, 196,* 709–711. https://doi.org/10.1086/520514

Walsh, T.J., Anaissie, E.J., Denning, D.W., Herbrecht, R., Kontoyiannis, D.P., Marr, K.A., ... Patterson, T.F. (2008). Treatment of aspergillosis: Clinical practice guidelines of the Infectious Diseases Society of America. *Clinical Infectious Disease, 46,* 327–360. https://doi.org/10.1086/525258

Wen, P.Y., Alyea, E.P., Simon, D., Herbst, R.S., Soiffer, R.J., & Antin, J.H. (1997). Guillian-Barré syndrome following allogeneic bone marrow transplantation. *Neurology, 49,* 1711–1714. https://doi.org/10.1212/wnl.49.6.1711

Wick, W., Hertenstein, A., & Platten, M. (2016). Neurological sequelae of cancer immunotherapies and targeted therapies. *Lancet Oncology, 17,* e529–e541. https://doi.org/10.1016/s1470-2045(16)30571-x

World Health Organization. (n.d.). Transplantation: GKT1 activity and practices. Retrieved from http://www.who.int/transplantation/gkt/statistics/en

Zhang, X., Han, W., Chen, Y., Chen, H., Liu, D., Xu, L., ... Huang, X. (2013). Intracranial hemorrhage and mortality in 1461 patients after allogeneic hematopoietic stem cell transplantation for 6-year follow-up: Study of 44 cases [Abstract]. *Blood, 122,* 3322. https://doi.org/10.1182/blood.V122.21.3322.3322

Zunt, J., & Baldwin, K.J. (2012). Chronic and subacute meningitis. *Continuum, 18,* 1290–1318. https://doi.org/10.1212/01.CON.0000423848.17276.21

CHAPTER 13

Relapse and Subsequent Malignancies

Suni Dawn Elgar, MPH, BSN, RN, OCN®, and Mihkaila Maurine Wickline, MN, RN, AOCN®, BMTCN®

Introduction

Hematopoietic stem cell transplantation (HSCT) is a curative treatment modality for many malignant and nonmalignant conditions. For some disorders, HSCT is used to control or delay the progression of the malignancy but is not curative in intent. HSCT may not adequately treat the disease, resulting in either disease persistence or relapse after initial response. A defined standard for relapse management does not currently exist. For patients whom HSCT initially fails, they may proceed to palliative support or additional treatment, either with a relapse regimen, donor lymphocyte infusion (DLI), subsequent transplant, or experimental therapy, including immunotherapy. Even after successful HSCT, subsequent malignancies can occur. As the risk of relapse declines over time, the risk for development of second malignancies continues to rise. With patients facing multiple post-HSCT challenges, it is necessary for nurses to understand these issues and their implications for nursing.

Relapse After Hematopoietic Stem Cell Transplantation

Autologous Transplantation

Since 2010, the total number of autologous HSCTs performed in the United States has been increasing at a faster rate than allogeneic HSCTs (D'Souza & Fretham, 2018). According to the Center for International Blood and Marrow Transplant Research, multiple myeloma (MM), non-Hodgkin lymphoma, and Hodgkin lymphoma accounted for more than 60% of all HSCTs performed in 2017 (D'Souza & Fretham, 2018). For patients with certain malignant diseases who have relapsed after conventional chemotherapy treatments, autologous HSCT can be curative. However, relapse or recurrence of primary disease after autologous HSCT remains the most common cause of death in this population, representing 71% of post-transplant deaths from 2015 to 2016 (D'Souza & Fretham, 2018).

Several approaches have been proposed to reduce the rate of relapse following autologous HSCT. Identifying potential candidates and scheduling transplantation earlier may decrease resistance to therapies while decreasing exposure of stem cells to multiple therapies. Patients with chemosensitive MM who have sustained complete response have the most favorable outcomes following autologous HSCT (Lehners et al., 2018). Improved and intensified preparative regimens increase the likelihood that high-dose chemotherapy will eradicate the malignancy during transplant, with every attempt made to achieve minimal residual disease before stem cells are collected.

Oncologists rely more and more on post-transplant consolidation and maintenance therapy to induce durable remissions. The often-held differentiation between consolidation and maintenance therapy is that consolidation therapy is administered acutely after autologous HSCT for a finite duration with the goal of achieving a deeper disease response, ideally to a state of minimal residual disease. Maintenance therapy is usually less intensive and administered over a longer period of time, often until disease progression (Krishnan & Giralt, 2016). The subtleties can be blurred, and the terms are at times used interchangeably. For some generally incurable diseases, such as mantle cell lymphoma and MM, the main purpose of autologous HSCT is to extend the duration of remission and delay relapse (Le Gouill et al., 2017; Lehners et al., 2018). Maintenance therapy can then be instituted while balancing disease control and quality of life (Gay et al., 2018). Likewise, Le Gouill et al. (2017) showed that in mantle cell lymphoma, a three-year course of maintenance rituximab after autologous transplant was superior to receiving no maintenance therapy, prolonging event-free survival, progression-free survival, and overall survival. Current maintenance options and future medications currently being studied may continue to improve the survival of patients after autologous transplant (see Table 13-1).

Worldwide, HSCT is most commonly used to treat MM, and the number of individuals transplanted continues to increase each year (D'Souza & Fretham, 2018). Fortunately, MM treatment has achieved a major improvement in median survival after diagnosis over the past two decades. Previously, patients with MM requiring therapy experienced a median survival with chemotherapy alone of three years after diagnosis (Sengsayadeth, Malard, Savani, Garderet, & Mohty, 2017). By 2016, MM treatment with autologous HSCT alone had a median survival of seven years (Sengsayadeth et al., 2017). With time and additional therapy,

Table 13-1. Maintenance Therapy After Autologous Hematopoietic Stem Cell Transplantation

Class of Therapy	Treatment Modality	Toxicities	Nursing Implications
Hodgkin Lymphoma			
Standard of care: antibody–drug conjugate	Brentuximab	Neutropenia Sensory and motor neuropathy	Efficacy in patients with prior brentuximab exposure not known Fall precautions Financial toxicity Risk of infectious complications
Future advances	Anti–PD-1 monoclonal antibody (immune checkpoint inhibitor)	Typically well tolerated Adrenal insufficiency	Financial toxicity
Mantle Cell Lymphoma			
Standard of care: anti-CD20 monoclonal antibodies	Rituximab	Cytopenia and neutropenia Immune reconstitution and hypogammaglobulinemia	Efficacy of post-transplant revaccination Myeloid growth factor support Periodic IV immunoglobulin support Risk of infectious complications
Future advances	Bruton tyrosine kinase inhibitor Combination treatments Immunomodulatory agents Proteasome inhibitors Radioimmunotherapy	Cardiovascular issues Cytopenia Edema Gastrointestinal symptoms Musculoskeletal symptoms Peripheral neuropathy Thromboembolic events	Financial toxicity May require large time commitment (if IV administration only) Not widely available
Multiple Myeloma			
Standard of care: immunomodulatory agents	Lenalidomide • Less toxic profile; has replaced thalidomide as standard of care • Standard-risk disease	Dermatologic toxicity Hematologic adverse events (neutropenia) SPM Venous thromboembolism	Antithrombotic therapy Discussion of SPM prior to initiating therapy Monitoring for SPM
	Thalidomide (standard-risk disease)	Peripheral neuropathy Subsequent malignancies Venous thromboembolic events	Fall precautions Long-term use minimized due to significant dose-limiting toxicity
Standard of care: proteasome inhibitors	Bortezomib • Intermediate- to high-risk disease • Renal impairment)	Peripheral neuropathy	Fall precautions Lower risk of neurotoxicity with subcutaneous administration versus IV Only available for IV and subcutaneous administration
Future advances	Histone deacetylase inhibitors Immunotherapy Monoclonal antibodies Next-generation proteasome inhibitors	Asthenia Cardiopulmonary complications Diarrhea Infusion reactions Peripheral neuropathy Thrombocytopenia Tumor lysis syndrome	Fall precautions Financial toxicity May have proven efficacy as treatment; more studies needed to understand use as maintenance therapy May require large time commitment (if IV administration only)

PD-1—programmed cell death protein 1; SPM—secondary primary malignancy

Note. Based on information from Chim et al., 2018; Gay et al., 2018; Hari et al., 2017; Jethava et al., 2017; Kumar et al., 2008; Le Gouill et al., 2017; Lehners et al., 2018; Rajkumar, 2016; Sengsayadeth et al., 2017; Yan et al., 2017.

relapsed or progressive MM becomes more resistant as a result of additional genetic alterations, leading to progressively shorter durations of response to therapy (Chim et al. 2018; Rajkumar, 2016). In the absence of a highly curative therapy, long-term disease control for MM is the most important part of disease management. Multiple factors, including aggressive nature of the relapse, types of therapy used for prior treatment, and the number of previous ther-

apies, can complicate determination of treatment at relapse (Rajkumar, 2016).

Patients with MM who have relapsed after an initial autologous HSCT may receive either a second autologous transplant or an allogeneic transplant. Htut et al. (2018) found superior survival after relapse in patients who received an allogeneic transplant after an autologous transplant compared to patients who received a second autologous transplant. However, the utility of allogeneic HSCT after relapse following an initial autologous HSCT remains controversial and warrants additional study because of inconsistent survival benefits. For patients with MM, allogeneic transplant may be most beneficial in those with a poor prognosis and high-risk cytogenetics or those who relapse within the first year after autologous transplant (Chim et al., 2018). Historical post–autologous HSCT treatment for patients with Hodgkin lymphoma included a second autologous HSCT or salvage chemotherapy followed by consolidation with allogeneic HSCT. Recent data suggest that some newer drugs may be valuable treatment options, and allogeneic HSCT could be reserved for younger, fit patients who have responsive disease (Jethava, Murthy, & Hamadani, 2017).

Allogeneic Transplantation

According to the Center for International Blood and Marrow Transplant Research, in 2017, 72% of allogeneic HSCTs were performed to treat acute leukemias and myelodysplastic syndrome (MDS) (D'Souza & Fretham, 2018). Disease status at the time of transplant and the donor type were the major predictors of post-transplant survival. At 100 days or more after allogeneic HSCT, primary disease accounted for 57% of deaths in human leukocyte antigen (HLA)-matched sibling donor transplants and 48% of deaths in unrelated transplants (D'Souza & Fretham, 2018). When relapse occurs, disease has not been completely eradicated in the patient. In general, early post–allogeneic HSCT relapse leads to poor outcomes with only 10%–20% of patients surviving more than two years after relapse; later relapse is associated with longer survival (Weisdorf, 2016). For patients with advanced myeloid malignancies or aggressive lymphoid malignancies, stage and remission status are among the strongest predictors for relapse following allogeneic HSCT. Therefore, it is imperative that patients begin the transplantation process at the earliest possible stage, as soon as remission has been achieved (Gyurkocza & Sandmaier, 2014). Transplant centers continue to push the upper age limit of transplant eligibility. However, because older age is associated with an increase in comorbidities, many may not be eligible for high-dose conditioning regimens. Reduced-intensity conditioning regimens offer a potential cure but with the tradeoff of a higher relapse rate (Sorror et al., 2011).

High-dose chemotherapy and radiation therapy followed by allogeneic HSCT can successfully cure many hematologic malignancies and nonmalignant disorders in adults and children. The advantage gained from allogeneic HSCT in malignant diseases when compared to autologous transplant is the antineoplastic effect of the donor graft. Myeloablative allogeneic HSCT relies not only on the conditioning therapy to control disease initially but has the added benefit of the graft-versus-tumor (GVT) effect, which provides disease surveillance after transplant. The GVT effect, a powerful adoptive immunotherapy reaction, is generated from donor T cells and natural killer cells, as well as ancillary involvement of B cells, dendritic cells, and minor histocompatibility antigens (Singh & McGuirk, 2016). Donor cells react against residual host tumor and impart a cytotoxic effect. Sorror et al. (2011) noted that most post-HSCT relapses in malignant diseases occur during the first year when the full effects of GVT have yet to become fully established. Attempts to enhance the GVT effect after allogeneic HSCT have had mixed success, as they have been complicated by graft-versus-host disease (GVHD), which is also mediated by T cells (see Chapter 7). Acute GVHD has not been shown to be associated with GVT. However, chronic GVHD has been shown to have a protective effect and is associated with fewer incidences of late relapse in patients with chronic myeloid leukemia (CML) but not in patients with acute myeloid leukemia (AML), acute lymphoblastic leukemia, or MDS (Boyiadzis et al., 2015). Because CML proliferates at a slower pace than acute leukemia, the GVT effect may become well established in time to react against the disease. Scientists continue to research the safest, most efficacious strategies to increase the GVT effect while minimizing the detrimental effects of GVHD.

Treatment of relapsed disease following allogeneic transplantation continues to evolve. Although controversial, one approach in patients without evidence of GVHD is to rapidly reduce or withdraw immunosuppression in an attempt to trigger a GVT effect. It is important to ensure that GVHD is not present, as treating relapse in the presence of GVHD proves to be a clinically complicated situation. Despite some reports supporting withdrawal of immunosuppression leading to positive outcomes, its efficacy in AML and MDS is unlikely (Champlin, 2016).

Another attempt to capitalize on the GVT effect is DLI after chemotherapy or as a stand-alone infusion. Multiple DLIs may be given for a single incidence of relapse. DLI from related, unrelated, and haploidentical donors has been shown to be efficacious (Zeidan et al., 2014). Important predictors of success are the underlying disease, donor type, time to relapse after transplant, and the extent of relapse at the time of DLI. Response to DLI may be durable or temporary with relapse occurring later. DLI is limited to use in patients without current active GVHD. The development of severe or life-threatening GVHD is a risk of immunosuppression withdrawal and DLI. Additionally, DLI can cause transient bone marrow aplasia, which may lead to infectious complications. Marrow aplasia can result when the donor lymphocytes destroy the host's functioning hematopoietic cells.

DLI has shown promising results for patients with CML in the chronic phase, with remission rates of 70%–80% (Martin & Shlomchik, 2016). Unfortunately, this approach is less effective in patients with CML in blast crisis or patients with MM, myelodysplasias, lymphomas, and acute leukemias (Chalandon et al., 2014; Dickinson et al., 2017; Martin & Shlomchik, 2016; Miyamoto et al., 2017; Singh & McGuirk, 2016; see Figure 13-1). In order to capitalize on the GVT effect, researchers continue to study dif-

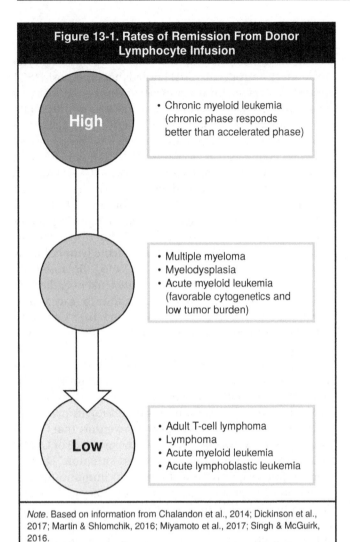

Figure 13-1. Rates of Remission From Donor Lymphocyte Infusion

High
- Chronic myeloid leukemia (chronic phase responds better than accelerated phase)

- Multiple myeloma
- Myelodysplasia
- Acute myeloid leukemia (favorable cytogenetics and low tumor burden)

Low
- Adult T-cell lymphoma
- Lymphoma
- Acute myeloid leukemia
- Acute lymphoblastic leukemia

Note. Based on information from Chalandon et al., 2014; Dickinson et al., 2017; Martin & Shlomchik, 2016; Miyamoto et al., 2017; Singh & McGuirk, 2016.

ferent ways to increase the effect without increasing GVHD. Recently, prophylactic or preemptive DLI has been given to patients with minimal residual disease after HSCT, with or without the addition of hypomethylating agents (Dickinson et al., 2017). A potential future improvement on current DLI is to engineer it to be less toxic while simultaneously increasing the antitumor activity through the addition of immune checkpoint inhibition (Warren & Deeg, 2013). The possibility presented by suicide gene therapy to quickly reverse unwanted GVHD could allow for safe administration of post-transplant engineered DLI that experiences rapid cell death when the suicide gene is activated (Singh & McGuirk, 2016). Clinical trials, which are active in this arena, may hold the key to maximizing GVT effect while minimizing GVHD.

The role of maintenance therapy after allogeneic HSCT is an evolving area in relapse prevention. The utility of tyrosine kinase inhibitors (TKIs) after allogenic HSCT for Philadelphia chromosome–positive acute lymphoblastic leukemia to improve response rates and survival has been understood for years. Post-HSCT disease-free survival using TKIs

has increased from 41% to 58% (Lussana et al., 2016). Second-generation TKIs may build on that success by deepening responses and increasing cure rates (Wieduwilt, 2018).

As discussed in Chapter 16, emerging interventions that attempt to harness the powerful therapeutic benefits of the donor's immune system to eliminate residual host tumor have been promising in some leukemias and lymphomas (Singh & McGuirk, 2016). Antitumor immunity–enhancing interventions, such as genetically modified T-cell receptors and chimeric antigen receptors will likely have the largest positive impact on outcomes of allogeneic HSCT (Warren & Deeg, 2013).

A second myeloablative or reduced-intensity HSCT following allogeneic HSCT carries a significant risk of treatment-related mortality. Notably, risk factors associated with poor outcome after a second allogeneic HSCT include relapse less than 7.5 months after the first HSCT, presence of disease at the time of second HSCT, and chemoresistant disease (Schmid et al., 2018; Weisdorf, 2016). Nonrelapse mortality after myeloablative conditioning complicates a second HSCT with the potential for organ damage. Thus, consideration for reduced-intensity regimens should be weighed (Vrhovac et al., 2016). Pediatric patients who proceed to a second HSCT have better outcomes than those who receive salvage therapy alone (Bajwa et al., 2013). Interestingly, no difference in the incidence of relapse, nonrelapse mortality, overall survival, or relapse-free survival has been observed when using the same donor for both allogeneic HSCTs versus enlisting a different donor for the second transplant (Weisdorf, 2016). Poon et al. (2013) noted that although long-term survival after a second HSCT is limited, it remains a treatment option that can provide more time to administer additional options to prevent relapse. Well-designed clinical trials are needed to understand which patients will benefit from a second allogeneic HSCT without a prohibitive increase in nonrelapse mortality.

Patients with relapsed disease following HSCT who are ineligible for clinical trials may choose not to receive any further therapy. As treatment goals change, supportive and palliative care options should be revisited to best support patients and families through end-of-life care. Nurses can bolster families by providing information so that informed decisions regarding end-of-life care can be made in a timely manner.

Patients for whom HSCT is a cure will continue to follow-up with the oncology team to monitor for late treatment toxicities, along with periodic long-term follow-up for transplant-related toxicities at the transplant center. Periodic restaging, including physical assessment, blood tests, scans, and bone marrow studies, will be necessary to evaluate patients for engraftment, relapse, or subsequent malignancies. Transplant recipients should also receive routine health maintenance and health promotion education. Post-transplant follow-up care is discussed in greater detail in Chapter 14.

Nursing Implications

The path followed by patients treated with HSCT and their families can be challenging even in the best of circumstances. It can be even more burdensome when the outcome is not as hoped. Post-HSCT care must include stringent monitoring of disease status and, if relapse is detected, early intervention. HSCT nurses who understand the significant potential for post-HSCT relapse can be instrumental advocates for the patients they support.

HSCT comes with a host of complex physical and psychosocial challenges, many of which can be supported through early palliative care interventions, such as goal clarification, symptom management, and advanced care planning, to improve quality of life (Tierney, Passaglia, & Jenkins, 2014). Button, Gavin, and Keogh (2014) cited the need for early integration of palliative care for HSCT recipients through nurse-led education sessions, advanced care planning, and nurse-initiated referral to palliative care services. Nurses in the inpatient, outpatient ambulatory, and community settings spend a considerable amount of time as patient advocates, listening to patient and family concerns, aiding in interpretation of clinical discussions, and providing education on outcomes and next steps. Nurses will continue to support patients and families as patients prepare for postrelapse care, ensuring that a patient's individual goals are clearly understood by the entire care team (Ford, Wickline, & Heye, 2016).

Fear of cancer recurrence/progression (FCR) is a complex phenomenon reported by many post-treatment cancer survivors, and it can affect their physical and mental health (Simard, Savard, & Ivers, 2010). FCR in the post-treatment general oncology setting has been studied for years, and studies have shown that certain psychosocial interventions, although not universally beneficial, may help alleviate FCR in this population (Chen et al., 2018). FCR in the HSCT setting has not been well studied and is an area that requires additional research. In a cohort of patients with hematologic cancer treated with allogeneic HSCT, Sarkar et al. (2014) found that 23%–36% of patients had high levels of FCR, which had a significant influence on health-related quality of life. Levels of FCR declined over time, notably at two time points: 100 days and 12 months post-HSCT (Sarkar et al., 2014). Hefner et al. (2014) identified that younger HSCT recipients experience a significantly higher level of FCR than their older counterparts, suggesting that they require additional scrutiny and guidance. Psychological screenings beginning in the pretreatment evaluation phase of HSCT could help identify patients who may benefit from early interventions for psychological symptom management (Hoodin, Zhao, Carey, Levine, & Kitko, 2013; Sarkar et al., 2014). Research has elucidated the limited attention paid to FCR in the HSCT setting. Additional research is needed in this area to better understand the phenomenon and to find interventions for patients who experience FCR.

In 2017, more than half of all autologous HSCT recipients and 31% of allogeneic HSCT recipients were over the age of 60 years, with an increasing trend of HSCT being performed on patients older than 70 years (D'Souza & Fretham, 2018). Nurses can offer pivotal education surrounding common HSCT complications that create challenges for older patients, including weakness, dehydration, and medication side effects. Older patients have higher rates of comorbidities, which may complicate their opportunities for postrelapse treatment. In a retrospective study on the impact of age and comorbidities on outcomes of patients with relapsed or refractory MM, those patients with both cardiovascular disease and renal insufficiency faced the highest risk of progression to death compared to individuals with only one comorbidity or no comorbidities (Hari et al., 2018). Practitioners may be more resistant to offer high-intensity or newer regimen options to this group of patients, as they are underrepresented in clinical trials because of exclusion criteria. Medinger, Lengerke, and Passweg (2016) suggested that the grading of an older patient's fitness, vulnerability, and frailty should be assessed using standard geriatric assessment tools, as opposed to using chronologic age, when selecting safe and appropriate therapy. Comorbidities associated with aging are not the only factors that may complicate treatment after HSCT. Additional questions, such as how to appropriately dose for obese patients without compromising disease control, will continue to need clarification (Shultes, Arp, Stockerl-Goldstein, Trinkaus, & DeFrates, 2018). Nurses can ensure that patients and families understand not only the disease-specific risks of relapse but also the risks associated with underlying comorbidities, frailty, or aging.

As treatment options for post-HSCT relapse continue to grow in number, nurses will play a pivotal role in aiding patients and families to fully understand the potential toxicities associated with newer treatments. Some post-HSCT relapse therapies have the potential to cause subsequent GVHD. Nurses will be instrumental in up-front and continued patient education about signs and symptoms associated with acute and chronic GVHD. The financial toll of a serious illness can be quite profound, and the prolonged treatment that HSCT necessitates may become financially toxic for patients and their families. Nurses can collaborate with the healthcare team, including social workers and clinical pharmacists, to help patients find alternative sources of funding for high-cost medications and treatments that may be prescribed in the post-HSCT relapse setting.

Nurses who work in HSCT-dedicated clinical settings play an important role in providing hand-off communication as patients transition out of active transplant care to other sites. Information about patient and family goals, educational needs, and financial barriers to continue post-HSCT disease monitoring and medications must be adequately communicated to nurses in community settings. As the post-HSCT patient population continues to grow, nurses in the community setting will need to familiarize themselves with post-HSCT monitoring for relapse, symptom management, and long-term complications. Additionally, understanding the complexities of evaluation of physical and psychological sequelae of HSCT is imperative for all nurses who care for HSCT recipients.

Subsequent Malignancies After Hematopoietic Stem Cell Transplantation

Subsequent malignancies are a known complication of conventional chemotherapy and radiation. Additionally, subsequent malignancies following HSCT have long been reported. Not all subsequent malignancies, however, are thought to be the result of treatment exposures for the primary cancer, but they may reflect a shared etiology with host characteristics and environmental exposures. The nomenclature change from *secondary malignancy* to *subsequent malignancy* better reflects both the potential for the diagnosis of more than one cancer after a primary cancer diagnosis, and accounting for the potential of noncausality from HSCT treatment exposures (M. Flowers, personal communication, March 26, 2018). HSCT recipients who are alive at two years after transplant have an 85% chance of living 10 years or longer (Chang, Armenian, & Dellinger, 2018). Projections suggest that the number of HSCT survivors in the United States could reach 500,000 by 2030 (Hashmi, Carpenter, Khera, Tichelli, & Savani, 2015). With the increase in long-term survival comes the increased risk for new cancers in this population, estimated to be the cause of up to 10% of all late deaths in HSCT recipients (Adhikari, Sharma, & Bhatt, 2015). Pediatric transplant recipients are especially at risk, as their lifetime risk of any subsequent malignancy has been reported to be up to 45 times higher. This risk is inversely correlated with age (Baker et al., 2003).

Subsequent malignancies are classified into three discrete categories: post-transplant lymphoproliferative disorder (PTLD), therapy-related MDS and AML, and subsequent solid malignancies. Each have distinct features, risk factors, and prognoses. Table 13-2 highlights the features of these three categories of malignancies following HSCT.

Post-Transplant Lymphoproliferative Disorder

PTLD is an aggressive, rare, and potentially fatal proliferation of lymphoid cells of donor origin, usually occurring within the first four months after allogeneic HSCT (Baker et al., 2003; Danylesko & Shimoni, 2018; Styczynski et al., 2013). PTLD is caused by the opportunistic expansion of Epstein-Barr virus (EBV)-transformed donor B cells in a host with suppressed T-cell function. The incidence varies with the number of risk factors, and reported incidence ranges from less than 1% to approximately 10%, with the largest studies putting the incidence at 1.4%–3.22%. This disorder is strongly influenced by T-cell depletion of the graft (in vivo or ex vivo) and antithymocyte globulin use, as well as unrelated or mismatched grafts, presence of acute or chronic GVHD, older age of recipient, and multiple transplants. Late PTLD that occurs following the first year after

transplant and PTLD after autologous transplant are rare (Danylesko & Shimoni, 2018).

Although PTLD once carried significant mortality, early detection of EBV load in at-risk patients and rituximab therapy have improved survival rates significantly over the past two decades from a one-year overall survival of 25% to a three-year overall survival of 47.3% (Baker et al., 2003; Styczynski et al., 2013). In patients who do not respond to rituximab therapy, outcomes remain poor with a median survival of 33 days (Fox et al., 2014). Risk factors for poor survival are age older than 30 years, extranodal involvement, presence of acute GVHD grade II or higher, and inability to reduce immunosuppression. Pediatric patients tend to have superior survival advantage compared to adults (Styczynski et al., 2013). In addition to rituximab, other therapies include withdrawal of immunosuppression if GVHD allows, EBV-specific cytotoxic T lymphocytes, DLI, or variations on classic lymphoma chemotherapy regimens (Fox et al., 2014; Styczynski et al., 2013).

For allogeneic HSCT recipients at risk for the development of PTLD, sequential blood samples should be obtained for measurement of EBV load by quantitative polymerase chain reaction–based assays for at least the first six months after allogeneic HSCT (Landgren et al., 2009). The doubling time for EBV is estimated to be approximately two to three days, so serial testing that reveals rising EBV loads will need to be repeated frequently. When the threshold is met, rapid intervention is warranted as treatment is more efficacious in patients without mass lesions (Danylesko & Shimoni, 2018; Styczynski et al., 2013).

For patients at risk for PTLD, nurses play a role in coordination of blood draws and monitoring, as well as patient education and guidance. This role expands to administration of therapies and supportive care with diagnosis of PTLD.

Myelodysplastic Syndrome and Acute Myeloid Leukemia

According to the World Health Organization, therapy-related MDS and AML are distinctly separate from other types of MDS and AML and characterized by certain mutations, unfavorable karyotypes, and poor prognosis (Berger et al., 2018). These malignancies occur in 0.8%–6.3% of recipients of autologous HSCT and develop with a median latency period of 2.5 years. The relative risk of developing hematologic malignancies is reported as high as 300-fold over an age-matched healthy population (Baker et al., 2003; Danylesko & Shimoni, 2018). The pathogenesis of therapy-related MDS/AML after autologous transplant is thought to be caused by genetic damage to stem cells from cytotoxic treatment. It is postulated that this may be potentiated by the transplant process itself with damage caused during cell mobilization, collection, and storage, as well as conditioning with chemotherapy and radiation (Bhatia, 2013). The stress of engraftment and regeneration of the marrow on the precursor cells may also be potentiat-

Table 13-2. Subsequent Malignancies After Hematopoietic Stem Cell Transplantation[a]

Malignancy	Timing	Plateau	Risk Factors	Incidence	Excess Risk (Standardized Incidence Ratio[b])
Solid	Median 4.2 years after HSCT	No plateau	Autologous or allogeneic HSCT Age < 10 years at time of HSCT Total body irradiation > 1,200 cGy Smoking history	3.8%–8.8% at 20 years	2.8
Therapy-related MDS/AML	Median 3 years after HSCT	Plateau at 10 years Greatly reduced risk after 10 years	Autologous HSCT Pre-HSCT diagnosis of multiple myeloma, non-Hodgkin lymphoma, or Hodgkin lymphoma Exposure to alkylating agents, topoisomerase inhibitors, or radiation prior to HSCT Older age at time of HSCT Total body irradiation	0.8%–6.3% at 20 years	300
PLTD	Median 2–4 months after HSCT	Plateau at 10 years	Allogeneic HSCT Age < 10 years at time of HSCT EBV proliferation after HSCT Intensive immunosuppression Mismatched related donor Pre-HSCT diagnosis of immune deficiency Antithymocyte globulin use any time during HSCT process T-cell depletion Unrelated donor Multiple HSCTs Graft-versus-host disease EBV sero-mismatch	1.4%–3.22% at 20 years	54.3

[a] Excludes nonmelanoma skin cancers

[b] The ratio of observed cancer cases in an HSCT cohort to expected cancer cases in the general population of a similar age and gender

AML—acute myeloid leukemia; cGy—centigray; EBV—Epstein-Barr virus; HSCT—hematopoietic stem cell transplantation; MDS—myelodysplastic syndrome; PTLD—post-transplant lymphoproliferative disorder

Note. Based on information from Adhikari et al., 2015; Baker et al., 2003; Berger et al., 2018; Bhatia, 2013; Danylesko & Shimoni, 2018; Dyer et al., 2016; Vaxman et al., 2015.

ing factor (Bhatia, 2013). Evidence also suggests that therapy administered prior to the transplant can cause cytogenetic abnormalities and dysplastic changes that can affect the development of therapy-related MDS/AML. Age older than 35 years at time of transplant also appears to affect the risk of developing these diseases (Baker et al., 2003; Danylesko & Shimoni, 2018). HSCT recipients who were mobilized with etoposide; those who received a dose greater than 10 Gy for a total body irradiation–based conditioning regimen; those who were exposed to alkylating agents or topoisomerase II inhibitors; those who received peripheral blood stem cells, instead of bone marrow, as a cell source; and those who received a transplant for a lymphoproliferative disease are also at risk (Baker et al., 2003; Danylesko & Shimoni, 2018; Vaxman et al., 2015). Therapy-related MDS and AML are rare after allogeneic HSCT (Baker et al., 2003; Bhatia, 2013; Vaxman et al., 2015), and this is postulated to be caused by the lack of exposure of donor progenitor cells to chemotherapy (Danylesko & Shimoni, 2018). The conditioning regimen BEAM (carmustine, etoposide, cytarabine, melphalan) has been shown to have low leukemogenic potential (Danylesko & Shimoni, 2018).

When treated with conventional therapy, therapy-related MDS/AML after autologous HSCT has a uniformly dismal prognosis, with a median survival of six months (Bhatia, 2013). Because of the poor response to conventional chemotherapy, allogeneic transplant for therapy-related MDS/AML has been explored with better outcomes. A predictive model of survival after allogeneic transplant has been developed based on four risk factors: age older than 35 years, poor-risk cytogenetics, therapy-related AML not in remission or advanced therapy-related MDS, and a donor other than an HLA-identical sibling or well-matched unrelated donor (Bhatia, 2013). Five-year survival rates range from 4% (all risk factors) to 50% (no risk factors) (Bhatia, 2013). Overall, relapse after allogeneic transplant is lowest in patients who receive a busulfan and cyclophosphamide conditioning regimen and cells from an unrelated donor (Bhatia, 2013).

Emerging science using highly sensitive probes has enabled the identification of clonal hematopoiesis of indeterminate potential (CHIP) in healthy individuals has shown to slightly increase the risk of developing a hematologic malignancy. A recent study showed that 70% of the autologous transplant recipients who eventually developed therapy-related MDS/AML had the presence of CHIP before transplant (Berger et al., 2018). In the future, the early detection of premalignant mutations and close monitoring over time may predict the development of therapy-related MDS/AML and guide early detection and intervention. Currently, best practice for monitoring for therapy-related MDS/AML involves monitoring peripheral blood counts over time with further testing when aberrant cell regeneration, such as prolonged low counts, is noted (Berger et al., 2018).

For patients at risk for therapy-related MDS/AML, the role of nurses includes coordination of outpatient blood draws and monitoring, as well as patient education and guidance. When a patient is diagnosed with therapy-related MDS/AML, the nursing role expands to education, psychosocial support, treatment coordination, and possibly preparation for a second transplant. Given the poor prognosis, nurses may also serve as advocates for palliative care involvement and for medical decision making with patient and family goals and priorities in mind. For the patient who has already been through an autologous transplant, facing a second transplant with an allogeneic donor presents challenges for the patient and family that expert HSCT nursing care can help them meet.

Solid Malignancies

Subsequent solid malignancies have been described after autologous and allogeneic HSCT. The risk is greater among those who have survived longer than five years after transplantation, with a reported incidence of up to 8.8% at 20 years after transplant (Adhikari et al., 2015). In children receiving a transplantation at age 10 years or younger, studies have reported a 33-fold to 55-fold higher risk of developing a subsequent solid malignancy in their lifetime than age-matched peers (Baker et al., 2003; Rizzo et al., 2009). Nearly every type of solid tumor has been reported in HSCT recipients, but those that occur most commonly are melanoma and nonmelanoma skin cancers and cancers of the oral cavity, thyroid, breast, esophagus, brain, liver, bone, lung, soft tissue, and female reproductive tract (Danylesko & Shimoni, 2018; see Table 13-3). No plateau of risk exists with solid tumors after transplant; the risk continues to rise with a longer survival.

The two strongest risk factors for nonsquamous cell solid malignancies are younger age at time of transplant (especially for pediatric patients but also for young adults) and total body irradiation. The radiation exposure is thought to induce breaks in the DNA, causing mutations, deletions, translocations, and genomic instability that may play a role in tumor development (Danylesko & Shimoni, 2018). For squamous cell carcinomas of the oral cavity and skin, chronic GVHD is a strong risk factor. Other risk factors are length of immunosuppression therapy and male sex (Rizzo et al., 2009). Oncogenic viruses that may proliferate with prolonged immunosuppression may also play a role in the development of subsequent cancers (Danylesko & Shimoni, 2018). Additionally, host-related factors, such as genetic predisposition to cancer and health-related behaviors (e.g., smoking, obesity, excess alcohol intake, sun exposure) are thought to contribute to cancer development in HSCT recipients (Adhikari et al., 2015).

Reduced-intensity (nonmyeloablative) regimens, which use little or no total body irradiation, had been hypothesized to confer less risk of subsequent cancers, but the limited literature exploring cancers after reduced-intensity regimens does not support the hypothesis. Studies have shown a higher risk of solid cancers in certain sites (lip, tonsil, oropharynx, bone, soft tissue, vulva, melanoma) after reduced-intensity transplant regimens compared to the general population risk, and some have shown that the risk is comparable to that of myeloablative regimens (Adhikari et al., 2015). Fludarabine, a drug commonly used in reduced-intensity regimens, has been implicated in inhibiting DNA repair following DNA damage and may be one of the reasons that the risk of subsequent cancers after reduced-intensity regimens remains as high as the risk in myeloablative regimens (Danylesko & Shimoni, 2018). More studies need to evaluate subsequent cancers after reduced-intensity transplants (Adhikari et al., 2015).

Subsequent solid malignancies should be treated with the best available therapy for that tumor, unless compelling evidence demonstrates that the patient will not be able to tolerate that therapy (Bhatia & Bhatia, 2009). Patients with operable or nonmetastatic disease on diagnosis can often be cured (Danylesko & Shimoni, 2018). Survival following a subsequent solid tumor has been reported to be 44% at five years (Baker et al., 2003), although the subsequent cancer is the cause of death in 63%–86% of patients who develop this complication. Overall, survival tends to be best for patients with thyroid, breast, and skin cancers and worst for patients with central nervous system, lung, or liver cancers (Danylesko & Shimoni, 2018).

For patients at high risk for developing subsequent solid malignancies, close monitoring and reporting of suspicious signs and symptoms is essential. Nurses should also recommend that patients closely adhere to cancer screenings. When a solid tumor is diagnosed, patients and families may reach out to their transplant center for advice, recalling the transplant team's expertise in curing the primary cancer. HSCT nurses can provide psychosocial support and education and direct patients to a specialist with expertise in treating their subsequent malignancies.

Prevention and Screening

When possible, the transplant regimen can be selected to offset the risk of development of subsequent cancers in HSCT recipients. Limited interventions are available for preventing a subsequent malignancy after the transplant has occurred. Many of the risks for cancer development are inherent to the transplant process, and treating the patient's primary diagnosis with a goal to cure the life-threatening disease is the priority. To manage the risk of subsequent malignancies, the long-term follow-up team

Table 13-3. Nonmelanoma Skin Cancers After Hematopoietic Stem Cell Transplantation

Cancer Type	Timing	Plateau	Risk Factors	Incidence	Excess Risk as Hazard Ratio[a]
Basal cell carcinoma	Median 7.9 years after HSCT	No plateau	Age < 10 years at time of HSCT Attained age Caucasian race Chronic graft-versus-host disease Diagnosis of actinic keratosis Pre-HSCT diagnosis of malignancy Total body irradiation, especially unfractionated or doses ≥ 1,400 cGy	6.5% at 20 years	3.1
Squamous cell carcinoma	Median 6.3 years after HSCT	No plateau	Acute graft-versus-host disease Age < 10 years at time of HSCT Chronic graft-versus-host-disease Diagnosis of actinic keratosis Longer time on immunosuppression Male sex Pre-HSCT diagnosis of malignancy	3.4% at 20 years	18.3

[a] How often a cancer is diagnosed in an HSCT cohort compared to a background cohort of age- and gender-matched controls

cGy—centigray; HSCT—hematopoietic stem cell transplantation

Note. Based on information from Curtis et al., 2005; Inamoto et al., 2015; Leisenring et al., 2006; Omland et al., 2016.

can recognize the risk associated with chronic GVHD treatment and select the least immunosuppressive agents to control the signs and symptoms of GVHD. Closely monitoring patients with the goal of tapering immunosuppressive therapy at the first opportunity can also manage risk of subsequent cancers.

Other than these efforts made by the transplant team, most preventive efforts fall to the patient to reduce risk by maintaining a healthy lifestyle. Survivors should follow a healthy diet that is high in whole grains, fruits, and vegetables; incorporate physical activity into their routines; and maintain a healthy weight. Survivors should avoid all tobacco products and passive tobacco exposure and follow safe practices to avoid unprotected ultraviolet exposure. Other interventions include avoiding excessive alcohol intake and needless computed tomography scans to reduce radiation exposure (Adhikari et al., 2015; Danylesko & Shimoni, 2018; Majhail et al., 2012). Female survivors who need hormone-replacement therapy should use progesterone-estrogen preparations because estrogen alone may increase the risk of endometrial cancers (Inamoto et al., 2015). Survivors aged 9–26 years should receive a human papillomavirus (HPV) vaccination series, as this oncogenic virus can be more active in immunocompromised people. In addition, more than 90% of all cervical cancers and at least 60% of all vulvovaginal cancers are related to HPV (Chang et al., 2018). HPV vaccination is typically given one year after transplant (Inamoto et al., 2015).

Screening for subsequent cancers tends to be site specific, but general principles exist. These general principles rely on patients being aware of their increased risk; performing self-examinations of the skin, oral cavity, and breasts or testes; and reporting suspicious signs and symptoms promptly. Evaluation by a dentist every 6–12 months

is recommended to screen for oral cancer, and an annual visit to a medical provider for appropriate cancer screenings is also recommended. HSCT recipients need to minimally follow the cancer screening guidance for the general population, although selected sites may require increased monitoring (Danylesko & Shimoni, 2018).

Female survivors should be screened via mammography and breast magnetic resonance imaging starting at age 25 years or 8 years after total body irradiation or chest radiation—whichever occurs later but no later than age 40 years. Clinical breast examination should take place annually in addition to self-examinations. Women also need an annual Pap test and HPV DNA test to screen for cervical cancer (Adhikari et al., 2015; Danylesko & Shimoni, 2018; Inamoto et al., 2015; Majhail et al., 2012). There are no specific screening recommendations for male survivors; they are encouraged to follow guidelines for the general population for prostate and testicular cancer screening (Inamoto et al., 2015).

Survivors who have persistent oral GVHD, have been on immunosuppressive therapy for more than two years, have a history of oral field radiation, were younger than 10 years old at time of transplant, or are male should be evaluated for oral cancers every six months. Survivors with lower risk need screening at least every 12 months. Changes in the oral mucosa due to GVHD can make a diagnosis of oral cancer difficult because GVHD may mimic cancers and cancers may mimic oral GVHD. It is important that patients see a dentist who understands their cancer history and who takes an aggressive approach to early detection and treatment of oral cancers (Danylesko & Shimoni, 2018; Haverman et al., 2014; Inamoto et al., 2015).

In addition to self-examinations, all survivors need to have a full body, naked skin examination annually by a provider trained to detect skin cancers. If a survivor notes a new skin lesion, it needs to be reported immediately for further evaluation and biopsy. A handheld dermatoscope can be a helpful diagnostic tool (Adhikari et al., 2015; Danylesko & Shimoni, 2018; Inamoto et al., 2015). All survivors should be screened annually for thyroid cancer with a physical examination and a thyroid ultrasound ordered if a suspicious nodule is detected on palpation. A fine-needle aspiration should be utilized for diagnosis with any nodule larger than 5 mm (Adhikari et al., 2015; Inamoto et al., 2015). Survivors with persistent gastroesophageal reflux disease or new dysphagia should have an upper gastrointestinal endoscopy, and an endoscopic screening may be considered in survivors with prolonged chronic GVHD requiring immunosuppressive therapy. A liver ultrasound every six months should be considered for survivors with hepatitis B infection or with a history of cirrhosis (Inamoto et al., 2015).

Two studies, one with 441 Australian HSCT recipients (Dyer et al., 2016) and the other with 1,549 American HSCT recipients (Khera et al., 2011), examined adherence to cancer screening following transplantation and provided insight into understanding the factors that influence adherence. Both studies were similar with respect to survivor age at the time of survey and at the time of transplant, as well as gender. In the self-reported Australian study, 24% indicated at least one cancer following HSCT (Dyer et al., 2016). Overall, the adherence rates for cancer screenings varied widely based on nationality and tended to be lower in the Australian group. Dyer et al. (2016) reported that 52.3% of patients had a dermatologic assessment after transplant, compared to 61% in the study by Khera et al. (2011). Dyer et al. (2016) reported that 53.3% of female patients had a mammogram within the preceding two years; Khera et al. (2011) reported that 90% of female patients had mammograms. Many factors were identified by these studies for lower adherence to cancer screenings (see Figure 13-2). Nurses can intervene on the modifiable factors to increase the number of survivors that are getting the important

screenings. Early detection of subsequent cancers can lead to better outcomes (Dyer et al., 2016; Khera et al., 2011).

Nursing Implications

Currently, no published papers describe the fear of a subsequent malignancy after HSCT as a phenomenon or discuss evidence-based interventions for this problem. This is a clear opportunity for future nursing or interdisciplinary research. In the absence of evidence, the risk of subsequent malignancy can be a target for nursing interventions, such as anticipatory guidance, education, and psychosocial support. HSCT nurses need to teach patients and families the importance of close monitoring and early reporting of suspicious signs and symptoms prior to discharge from the transplant program. Nurses can also use educational interventions, counseling, and motivational interviewing to help survivors make healthy lifestyle choices and adhere to recommended screenings. When needed, nurses can play an important role in exploring and mitigating barriers to assist patients in accessing preventive activities (e.g., smoking cessation, dietary interventions) and screening (e.g., Pap tests, mammograms) that are important for prevention and early detection of cancers. When a new cancer is diagnosed, nurses can support HSCT recipients through psychosocial interventions, as well as anticipatory guidance and education around preparing for further treatment or palliative care. Nurses are also important as partners in research that explores methods to improve adherence to screening and early detection, as well as in the evaluation of directed therapies at subsequent cancers after transplant. Nurses who work in dedicated long-term follow-up or HSCT survivorship roles are at the forefront of working with HSCT recipients and play an important role in identifying nursing interventions to support patients and their families, as well as their local healthcare providers, when a subsequent cancer is diagnosed.

Summary

The HSCT community has long known of the risk of relapse and subsequent malignancies after transplant. These problems remain two of the biggest challenges to morbidity and mortality after transplant. Future research efforts are needed to continue to refine available maintenance therapy protocols after transplant to reduce the risk of relapse, improve methods of early detection of relapse, and discover the best methods to treat relapse. Researchers must also continue investigating the factors that influence subsequent malignancy development in HSCT recipients so that clinicians can modify the risk factors at the time of transplant when possible. Researchers need to explore methods for increasing adherence to screening for subsequent malignancies after transplant to find cancers early and study treatments and outcomes in patients who develop malignancies after transplant to better serve future patients. Systematic, prospective follow-up, vigilant screening processes,

---

Figure 13-2. Risk Factors for Nonadherence to Recommended Cancer Screenings

- Autologous transplantation
- Concerns about medical cost (less common in Australian cohort, who have access to free screenings)
- Time since transplant > 15 years
- Non-Caucasian race
- Male sex
- Lower physical functioning
- No chronic graft-versus-host disease
- Age < 40
- Self-reported lack of knowledge about needed screenings
- Self-reported lack of time
- Belief that screening is unnecessary
- Current provider not advocating for screenings

Note. Based on information from Dyer et al., 2016; Khera et al., 2011.

and well-maintained survivorship clinics and databases are necessities to effective patient care and should be included in the infrastructure of individual transplant centers and networks (Lowe, Bhatia, & Somlo, 2007). Nurses play important roles in all of these areas of caring for HSCT recipients who experience late effects.

References

Adhikari, J., Sharma, P., & Bhatt, V.R. (2015). Risk of secondary solid malignancies after allogeneic hematopoietic stem cell transplantation and preventive strategies. *Future Oncology, 11*, 3175–3185. https://doi.org/10.2217/fon.15.252

Bajwa, R., Schechter, T., Soni, S., Gassas, A., Doyle, J., Sisler, I., ... Frangoul, H. (2013). Outcome of children who experience disease relapse following allogeneic hematopoietic SCT for hematologic malignancies. *Bone Marrow Transplantation, 48*, 661–665. https://doi.org/10.1038/bmt.2012.209

Baker, K.S., DeFor, T.E., Burns, L.J., Ramsay, N.K.C., Neglia, J.P., & Robison, L.L. (2003). New malignancies after blood or marrow stem-cell transplantation in children and adults: Incidence and risk factors. *Journal of Clinical Oncology, 21*, 1352–1358. https://doi.org/10.1200/jco.2003.05.108

Berger, G., Kroeze, L.I., Koorenhof-Scheele, T.N., de Graaf, A.O., Yoshida, K., Ueno, H., ... Jansen, J.H. (2018). Early detection and evolution of preleukemic clones in therapy-related myeloid neoplasms following autologous SCT. *Blood, 131*, 1846–1857. https://doi.org/10.1182/blood-2017-09-805879

Bhatia, S. (2013). Therapy-related myelodysplasia and acute myeloid leukemia. *Seminars in Oncology, 40*, 666–675. https://doi.org/10.1053/j.seminoncol.2013.09.013

Bhatia, S., & Bhatia, R. (2009). Secondary malignancies after hematopoietic cell transplantation. In F.R. Appelbaum, S.J. Forman, R.S. Negrin, & K.G. Blume (Eds.), *Thomas' hematopoietic cell transplantation: Stem cell transplantation* (4th ed., pp. 1638–1652). https://doi.org/10.1002/9781444303537.ch106

Boyiadzis, M., Arora, M., Klein, J.P., Hassebroek, A., Hemmer, M., Urbano-Ispizua, A., ... Pavletic, S.Z. (2015). Impact of chronic graft-versus-host disease on late relapse and survival on 7,489 patients after myeloablative allogeneic hematopoietic cell transplantation for leukemia. *Clinical Cancer Research, 21*, 2020–2028. https://doi.org/10.1158/1078-0432.ccr-14-0586

Button, E.B., Gavin, N.C., & Keogh, S.J. (2014). Exploring palliative care provision for recipients of allogeneic hematopoietic stem cell transplantation who relapsed. *Oncology Nursing Forum, 41*, 370–381. https://doi.org/10.1188/14.onf.370-381

Chalandon, Y., Passweg, J.R., Guglielmi, C., Iacobelli, S., Apperley, J., Schaap, N.P.M., ... Olavarria, E. (2014). Early administration of donor lymphocyte infusions upon molecular relapse after allogeneic hematopoietic stem cell transplantation for chronic myeloid leukemia: A study by the Chronic Malignancies Working Party of the EBMT. *Haematologica, 99*, 1492–1498. https://doi.org/10.3324/haematol.2013.100198

Champlin, R. (2016). Relapse of hematologic malignancy after allogeneic hematopoietic transplantation. In S.J. Forman, R.S. Negrin, J.H. Antin, & F.R. Appelbaum (Eds.), *Thomas' hematopoietic cell transplantation: Stem cell transplantation* (5th ed., pp. 836–841). https://doi.org/10.1002/9781118416426.ch70

Chang, H.A., Armenian, S.H., & Dellinger, T.H. (2018). Secondary neoplasms of the female lower genital tract after hematopoietic cell transplantation. *Journal of the National Comprehensive Cancer Network, 16*, 211–218. https://doi.org/10.6004/jnccn.2018.7005

Chen, D., Sun, W., Liu, N., Wang, J., Zhao, J., Zhang, Y., ... Zhang, W. (2018). Fear of cancer recurrence: A systematic review of randomized, controlled trials. *Oncology Nursing Forum, 45*, 703–712. https://doi.org/10.1188/18.onf.703-712

Chim, C.S., Kumar, S.K., Orlowski, R.Z., Cook, G., Richardson, P.G., Gertz, M.A., ... Anderson, K.C. (2018). Management of relapsed and refractory multiple myeloma: Novel agents, antibodies, immunotherapies and beyond. *Leukemia, 32*, 252–262. https://doi.org/10.1038/leu.2017.329

Curtis, R.E., Metayer, C., Rizzo, J.D., Socié, G., Sobocinski, K.A., Flowers, M.E.D., ... Deeg, H.J. (2005). Impact of chronic GVHD therapy on the development of squamous-cell cancers after hematopoietic stem-cell transplantation: An international case-control study. *Blood, 105*, 3802–3811. https://doi.org/10.1182/blood-2004-09-3411

Danylesko, I., & Shimoni, A. (2018). Second malignancies after hematopoietic stem cell transplantation. *Current Treatment Options in Oncology, 19*, 9. https://doi.org/10.1007/s11864-018-0528-y

Dickinson, A.M., Norden, J., Li, S., Hromadnikova, I., Schmid, C., Schmetzer, H., & Jochem-Kolb, H. (2017). Graft-versus-leukemia effect following hematopoietic stem cell transplantation for leukemia. *Frontiers in Immunology, 8*, 496. https://doi.org/10.3389/fimmu.2017.00496

D'Souza, A., & Fretham, C. (2018). *Current uses and outcomes of hematopoietic cell transplantation (HCT): 2018 summary slides.* Retrieved from https://www.cibmtr.org/ReferenceCenter/SlidesReports/SummarySlides/_layouts/15/WopiFrame.aspx?sourcedoc=/ReferenceCenter/SlidesReports/SummarySlides/Documents/2018%20Summary%20Slides%20-%20final%20-%20for%20web%20posting.pptx&action=default

Dyer, G., Larsen, S.R., Gilroy, N., Brice, L., Greenwood, M., Hertzberg, M., ... Kerridge, I. (2016). Adherence to cancer screening guidelines in Australian survivors of allogeneic blood and marrow transplantation (BMT). *Cancer Medicine, 5*, 1702–1716. https://doi.org/10.1002/cam4.729

Ford, R.C., Wickline, M.M., & Heye, D. (2016). Nursing role in hematopoietic cell transplantation. In S.J. Forman, R.S. Negrin, J.H. Antin, & F.R. Appelbaum (Eds.), *Thomas' hematopoietic cell transplantation: Stem cell transplantation* (5th ed., pp. 362–373). https://doi.org/10.1002/9781118416426.ch30

Fox, C.P., Burns, D., Parker, A.N., Peggs, K.S., Harvey, C.M., Natarajan, S., ... Chaganti, S. (2014). EBV-associated post-transplant lymphoproliferative disorder following *in vivo* T-cell-depleted allogeneic transplantation: Clinical features, viral load correlates and prognostic factors in the rituximab era. *Bone Marrow Transplantation, 49*, 280–286. https://doi.org/10.1038/bmt.2013.170

Gay, F., Engelhardt, M., Terpos, E., Wäsch, R., Giaccone, L., Auner, H.W., ... Sonneveld, P. (2018). From transplant to novel cellular therapies in multiple myeloma: European Myeloma Network guidelines and future perspectives. *Haematologica, 103*, 197–211. https://doi.org/10.3324/haematol.2017.174573

Gyurkocza, B., & Sandmaier, B.M. (2014). Conditioning regimens for hematopoietic cell transplantation: One size does not fit all. *Blood, 124*, 344–353. https://doi.org/10.1182/blood-2014-02-514778

Hari, P., Mateos, M.-V., Abonour, R., Knop, S., Bensinger, W., Ludwig, H., ... Goldschmidt, H. (2017). Efficacy and safety of carfilzomib regimens in multiple myeloma patients relapsing after autologous stem cell transplant: ASPIRE and ENDEAVOR outcomes. *Leukemia, 31*, 2630–2641. https://doi.org/10.1038/leu.2017.122

Hari, P., Romanus, D., Luptakova, K., Blazer, M., Yong, C., Raju, A., ... Morrison, V.A. (2018). The impact of age and comorbidities on practice patterns and outcomes in patients with relapsed/refractory multiple myeloma in the era of novel therapies. *Journal of Geriatric Oncology, 9*, 138–144. https://doi.org/10.1016/j.jgo.2017.09.007

Hashmi, S., Carpenter, P., Khera, N., Tichelli, A., & Savani, B.N. (2015). Lost in transition: The essential need for long-term follow-up clinic for blood and marrow transplantation survivors. *Biology of Blood and Marrow Transplantation, 21*, 225–232. https://doi.org/10.1016/j.bbmt.2014.06.035

Haverman, T.M., Raber-Durlacher, J.E., Rademacher, W.M.H., Vokurka, S., Epstein, J.B., Huisman, C., ... Rozema, F.R. (2014). Oral complications in hematopoietic stem cell recipients: The role of inflammation. *Mediators of Inflammation, 2014*, 378281. https://doi.org/10.1155/2014/378281

Hefner, J., Kapp, M., Drebinger, K., Dannenmann, A., Einsele, H., Grigoleit, G.-U., ... Mielke, S. (2014). High prevalence of distress in patients after allogeneic hematopoietic SCT: Fear of progression is associated with a younger age. *Bone Marrow Transplantation, 49*, 581–584. https://doi.org/10.1038/bmt.2013.228

Hoodin, F., Zhao, L., Carey, J., Levine, J.E., & Kitko, C. (2013). Impact of psychological screening on routine outpatient care of hematopoietic cell transplantation survivors. *Biology of Blood and Marrow Transplantation, 19*, 1493–1497. https://doi.org/10.1016/j.bbmt.2013.07.019

Htut, M., D'Souza, A., Krishnan, A., Bruno, B., Zhang, M.-J., Fei, M., … Hari, P. (2018). Autologous/allogeneic hematopoietic cell transplantation versus tandem autologous transplantation for multiple myeloma: Comparison of long-term postrelapse survival. *Biology of Blood and Marrow Transplantation, 24*, 478–485. https://doi.org/10.1016/j.bbmt .2017.10.024

Inamoto, Y., Shah, N.N., Savani, B.N., Shaw, B.E., Abraham, A.A., Ahmed, I.A., … Majhail, N.S. (2015). Secondary solid cancer screening following hematopoietic cell transplantation. *Bone Marrow Transplantation, 50*, 1013–1023. https://doi.org/10.1038/bmt.2015.63

Jethava, Y., Murthy, G.S.G., & Hamadani, M. (2017). Relapse of Hodgkin lymphoma after autologous transplantation: Time to rethink treatment? *Hematology/Oncology and Stem Cell Therapy, 10*, 47–56. https://doi.org/10.1016/j.hemonc.2016.12.002

Khera, N., Chow, E.J., Leisenring, W.M., Syrjala, K.L., Baker, K.S., Flowers, M.E.D., … Lee, S.J. (2011). Factors associated with adherence to preventive care practices among hematopoietic cell transplantation survivors. *Biology of Blood and Marrow Transplantation, 17*, 995–1003. https://doi .org/10.1016/j.bbmt.2010.10.023

Krishnan, A., & Giralt, S.A. (2016). Hematopoietic cell transplantation for multiple myeloma. In S.J. Forman, R.S. Negrin, J.H. Antin, & F.R. Appelbaum (Eds.), *Thomas' hematopoietic cell transplantation: Stem cell transplantation* (5th ed., pp. 625–635). https://doi.org/10.1002 /9781118416426.ch55

Kumar, S.K., Rajkumar, S.V., Dispenzieri, A., Lacy, M.Q., Hayman, S.R., Buadi, F.K., … Gertz, M.A. (2008). Improved survival in multiple myeloma and the impact of novel therapies. *Blood, 111*, 2516–2520. https://doi.org/10.1182/blood-2007-10-116129

Landgren, O., Gilbert, E.S., Rizzo, J.D., Socié, G., Banks, P.M., Sobocinski, K.A., … Curtis, R.E. (2009). Risk factors for lymphoproliferative disorders after allogeneic hematopoietic cell transplantation. *Blood, 113*, 4992–5001. https://doi.org/10.1182/blood-2008-09-178046

Le Gouill, S., Thieblemont, C., Oberic, L., Moreau, A., Bouabdallah, K., Dartigeas, C., … Hermine, O. (2017). Rituximab after autologous stem-cell transplantation in mantle-cell lymphoma. *New England Journal of Medicine, 377*, 1250–1260. https://doi.org/10.1056 /nejmoa1701769

Lehners, N., Becker, N., Benner, A., Pritsch, M., Löpprich, M., Mai, E.K., … Raab, M.-S. (2018). Analysis of long-term survival in multiple myeloma after first-line autologous stem cell transplantation: Impact of clinical risk factors and sustained response. *Cancer Medicine, 7*, 307–316. https://doi.org/10.1002/cam4.1283

Leisenring, W., Friedman, D.L., Flowers, M.E.D., Schwartz, J.L., & Deeg, H.J. (2006). Nonmelanoma skin and mucosal cancers after hematopoietic cell transplantation. *Journal of Clinical Oncology, 24*, 1119–1126. https://doi.org/10.1200/jco.2005.02.7052

Lowe, T., Bhatia, S., & Somlo, G. (2007). Second malignancies after allogeneic hematopoietic cell transplantation. *Biology of Blood and Marrow Transplantation, 13*, 1121–1134. https://doi.org/10.1016/j.bbmt .2007.07.002

Lussana, F., Intermesoli, T., Gianni, F., Boschini, C., Masciulli, A., Spinelli, O., … Rambaldi, A. (2016). Achieving molecular remission before allogeneic stem cell transplantation in adult patients with Philadelphia chromosome–positive acute lymphoblastic leukemia: Impact on relapse and long-term outcome. *Biology of Blood and Marrow Transplantation, 22*, 1983–1987. https://doi.org/10.1016/j.bbmt.2016.07.021

Majhail, N.S., Rizzo, J.D., Lee, S.J., Aljurf, M., Atsuta, Y., Bonfim, C., … Tichelli, A. (2012). Recommended screening and preventive practices for long-term survivors after hematopoietic cell transplantation. *Biology of Blood and Marrow Transplantation, 18*, 348–371. https://doi.org /10.1016/j.bbmt.2011.12.519

Martin, P.J., & Shlomchik, W.D. (2016). Overview of hematopoietic cell transplantation immunology. In S.J. Forman, R.S. Negrin, J.H. Antin, & F.R. Appelbaum (Eds.), *Thomas' hematopoietic cell transplantation: Stem cell transplantation* (5th ed., pp. 96–111). https://doi.org/10.1002 /9781118416426.ch9

Medinger, M., Lengerke, C., & Passweg, J. (2016). Novel therapeutic options in acute myeloid leukemia. *Leukemia Research Reports, 6*, 39–49. https:// doi.org/10.1016/j.lrr.2016.09.001

Miyamoto, T., Fukuda, T., Nakashima, M., Henzan, T., Kusakabe, S., Kobayashi, N., … Mori, S.-I. (2017). Donor lymphocyte infusion for relapsed hematological malignancies after unrelated allogeneic bone marrow transplantation facilitated by the Japan Marrow Donor Program. *Biology of Blood and Marrow Transplantation, 23*, 938–944. https:// doi.org/10.1016/j.bbmt.2017.02.012

Omland, S.H., Gniadecki, R., Hædersdal, M., Helweg-Larsen, J., & Omland, L.H. (2016). Skin cancer risk in hematopoietic stem-cell transplant recipients compared with background population and renal transplant recipients: A population-based cohort study. *JAMA Dermatology, 152*, 177–183. https://doi.org/10.1001/jamadermatol.2015 .3902

Poon, L.M., Bassett, R., Jr., Rondon, G., Hamdi, A., Qazilbash, M., Hosing, C., … Kebriaei, P. (2013). Outcomes of second allogeneic hematopoietic stem cell transplantation for patients with acute lymphoblastic leukemia. *Bone Marrow Transplantation, 48*, 666–670. https:// doi.org/10.1038/bmt.2012.195

Rajkumar, S.V. (2016). Multiple myeloma: 2016 update on diagnosis, risk-stratification, and management. *American Journal of Hematology, 91*, 719–734. https://doi.org/10.1002/ajh.24402

Rizzo, J.D., Curtis, R.E., Socié, G., Sobocinski, K.A., Gilbert, E., Landgren, O., … Deeg, H.J. (2009). Solid cancers after allogeneic hematopoietic cell transplantation. *Blood, 113*, 1175–1183. https://doi.org/10.1182 /blood-2008-05-158782

Sarkar, S., Scherwath, A., Schirmer, L., Schulz-Kindermann, F., Neumann, K., Kruse, M., … Mehnert, A. (2014). Fear of recurrence and its impact on quality of life in patients with hematological cancers in the course of allogeneic hematopoietic SCT. *Bone Marrow Transplantation, 49*, 1217–1222. https://doi.org/10.1038/bmt.2014.139

Schmid, C., de Wreede, L.C., van Biezen, A., Finke, J., Ehninger, G., Ganser, A., … Kröger, N. (2018). Outcome after relapse of myelodysplastic syndrome and secondary acute myeloid leukemia following allogeneic stem cell transplantation: A retrospective registry analysis on 698 patients by the Chronic Malignancies Working Party of the European Society of Blood and Marrow Transplantation. *Haematologica, 103*, 237–245. https://doi.org/10.3324/haematol.2017.168716

Sengsayadeth, S., Malard, F., Savani, B.N., Garderet, L., & Mohty, M. (2017). Posttransplant maintenance therapy in multiple myeloma: The changing landscape. *Blood Cancer Journal, 7*, e545. https://doi.org /10.1038/bcj.2017.23

Shultes, K.C., Arp, C., Stockerl-Goldstein, K., Trinkaus, K., & DeFrates, S. (2018). Impact of dose-adjusted melphalan in obese patients undergoing autologous stem cell transplantation. *Biology of Blood and Marrow Transplantation, 24*, 687–693. https://doi.org/10.1016/j.bbmt .2017.11.041

Simard, S., Savard, J., & Ivers, H. (2010). Fear of cancer recurrence: Specific profiles and nature of intrusive thoughts. *Journal of Cancer Survivorship, 4*, 361–371. https://doi.org/10.1007/s11764-010-0136-8

Singh, A.K., & McGuirk, J.P. (2016). Allogeneic stem cell transplantation: A historical and scientific overview. *Cancer Research, 76*, 6445–6451. https://doi.org/10.1158/0008-5472.can-16-1311

Sorror, M.L., Sandmaier, B.M., Storer, B.E., Franke, G.N., Laport, G.G., Chauncey, T.R., … Storb, R. (2011). Long-term outcomes among older patients following nonmyeloablative conditioning and allogeneic hematopoietic cell transplantation for advanced hematologic malignancies. *JAMA, 306*, 1874–1883. https://doi.org/10.1001/jama .2011.1558

Styczynski, J., Gil, L., Tridello, G., Ljungman, P., Donnelly, J.P., van der Velden, W., … Cesaro, S. (2013). Response to rituximab-based therapy and risk factor analysis in Epstein Barr Virus–related lymphoproliferative disorder after hematopoietic stem cell transplant in children and adults: A study from the Infectious Diseases Working Party of the European Group for Blood and Marrow Transplantation. *Clinical Infectious Diseases, 57*, 794–802. https:// doi.org/10.1093/cid/cit391

Tierney, D.K., Passaglia, J., & Jenkins, P. (2014). Palliative care of hematopoietic cell transplant recipients and families. *Seminars in Oncology Nursing, 30*, 253–261. https://doi.org/10.1016/j.soncn.2014.08.007

Vaxman, I., Ram, R., Gafter-Gvili, A., Vidal, L., Yeshurun, M., Lahav, M., & Shpilberg, O. (2015). Secondary malignancies following high dose therapy and autologous hematopoietic cell transplantation–Systematic review and meta-analysis. *Bone Marrow Transplantation, 50*, 706–714. https://doi.org/10.1038/bmt.2014.325

Vrhovac, R., Labopin, M., Ciceri, F., Finke, J., Holler, E., Tischer, J., … Mohty, M. (2016). Second reduced intensity conditioning allogeneic transplant as a rescue strategy for acute leukaemia patients who relapse after an initial RIC allogeneic transplantation: Analysis of risk factors and treatment outcomes. *Bone Marrow Transplantation, 51,* 186–193. https://doi.org/10.1038/bmt.2015.221

Warren, E.H., & Deeg, H.J. (2013). Dissecting graft-versus-leukemia from graft-versus-host-disease using novel strategies. *Tissue Antigens, 81,* 183–193. https://doi.org/10.1111/tan.12090

Weisdorf, D. (2016). The role of second transplants for leukemia. *Best Practice and Research Clinical Haematology, 29,* 359–364. https://doi.org/10.1016/j.beha.2016.10.011

Wieduwilt, M.J. (2018). In the era of BCR-ABL1 inhibitors, are we closing the survival gap between allogeneic hematopoietic cell transplanta-tion and chemotherapy for Philadelphia chromosome-positive acute lymphoblastic leukemia in first complete remission? *Biology of Blood and Marrow Transplantation, 24,* 637–638. https://doi.org/10.1016/j.bbmt.2018.02.011

Yan, F., Gopal, A.K., & Graf, S.A. (2017). Targeted drugs as maintenance therapy after autologous stem cell transplantation in patients with mantle cell lymphoma. *Pharmaceuticals, 10,* 28. https://doi.org/10.3390/ph10010028

Zeidan, A.M., Forde, P.M., Symons, H., Chen, A., Smith, B.D., Pratz, K., … Bolaños-Meade, J. (2014). HLA-haploidentical donor lymphocyte infusions for patients with relapsed hematologic malignancies after related HLA-haploidentical bone marrow transplantation. *Biology of Blood and Marrow Transplantation, 20,* 314–318. https://doi.org/10.1016/j.bbmt.2013.11.020

CHAPTER 14

Late Effects and Survivorship Care

Lisa A. Pinner, RN, MSN, CNS, CPON®, BMTCN®, and D. Kathryn Tierney, RN, BMTCN®, PhD

Introduction

The number of successful hematopoietic stem cell transplantations (HSCTs) being performed each year is increasing, and it is estimated that by 2030, the number of survivors treated with HSCT in the United States will exceed 500,000 (Majhail et al., 2013). Numerous factors have led to an increase in the utilization of HSCT, including improved outcomes, decreased early transplant-related mortality, expanding indications, use of alternative donors, improved supportive care, and older age of eligibility (Gooley et al., 2010; Hahn et al., 2013; Hashmi, Carpenter, Khera, Tichelli, & Savani, 2015). The enlarging population of HSCT survivors is an accomplishment to celebrate but brings new challenges to understand and address late effects.

In 2015, the National Cancer Institute and National Heart, Lung, and Blood Institute convened a panel of HSCT experts across multiple disciplines, HSCT survivors, and advocates to develop research priorities and establish best practices to improve the health of survivors (Battiwalla et al., 2017). This 12-month initiative focused on patient-centered outcomes, immune dysregulation and pathobiology, cardiovascular disease and risk factors, subsequent neoplasms, healthcare delivery, research methodology, and study design (Battiwalla et al., 2017). The cumulative insults from the underlying disease, comorbidities, lifestyle factors, genetic susceptibilities, therapy antecedent to transplant, preparative regimen, and prevention and treatment of HSCT complications contribute to late effects. It is estimated that, compared to the general population, HSCT survivors more than two years after transplant have a tenfold greater risk for premature death (Bhatia et al., 2007). Compared to siblings, HSCT survivors are 3.5 times more likely to develop severe chronic health conditions, and the cumulative incidence of life-threatening and severe chronic health conditions is estimated to be greater than 40% (Sun et al., 2010, 2013). Understanding of the incidence, risk factors, pathophysiology, prevention, and treatment of late effects continues to evolve (Battiwalla et al., 2017). Risk factors for and presentation of late effects may be different in HSCT survivors compared to the general population (Bhatia, Armenian, & Landier, 2017).

Health-related quality of life (HRQOL) impairments, infections, organ-specific toxicities, and subsequent neoplasms in pediatric and adult survivors are common late effects. With a goal of minimizing morbidity and mortality, preventive measures and monitoring strategies are essential. However, it is important to note that clinical trials evaluating screening and preventive practices specific to HSCT survivors are lacking (Bhatia et al., 2017). It must also be acknowledged that as the field of transplantation changes, new challenges for HSCT survivors may emerge. It is vital for nurses in this field to also understand survivorship care, the importance of educating HSCT survivors on taking a lead role in their health monitoring and maintenance, and the burdens faced by the HSCT caregiver.

Survivorship Care

The goal of survivorship care is to minimize morbidity and mortality from late effects of treatment and improve the health and HRQOL of HSCT survivors. Follow-up care, including examinations and testing, is targeted not only at assessing for recurrence of the underlying disease but also health maintenance and early detection of late effects. Lifelong monitoring for HSCT survivors is essential because many complications will develop years after transplantation. The need for lifelong monitoring is especially true for pediatric survivors, who are at risk for late effects for a longer period of time. Consideration of each survivor's unique risk factors and individualization of screening practices are essential (Tichelli & Rovó, 2015).

Discharge from an HSCT center has the potential for fragmentation of care, as the number of healthcare providers increases significantly. The expanded healthcare team includes the referring physician (e.g., oncologist, hematologist), primary care provider (PCP), medical specialists (e.g., dentist, gynecologist, ophthalmologist), and HSCT team. As the age of HSCT recipients has increased, the role of the PCP has become even more vital to address common comorbidities, such as diabetes and hypertension. For pediatric survivors, it is critical to be in the care of a PCP who can manage routine health care and the unique challenges facing these survivors as they mature from children to adults.

Frequent communication between the expanded healthcare team can reduce fragmentation. Letters, emails, and phone calls are some options for coordinating care. A brief yet comprehensive review of post-HSCT complications and recommended monitoring sent to the referring oncologist or hematologist and PCP can serve as a reference guide. Table 14-1 reviews common late effects of HSCT, risk factors, and recommended screenings (Majhail et al., 2012). Many HSCT survivors have been enrolled in a clinical trial, and coordinating care with the oncologist or hematologist and PCP can ensure that required assessments and testing are completed so that outcome data for the clinical trial are complete. Survivorship care plans are a useful tool to facilitate communication and care coordination (Bevans et al., 2017; Hashmi et al., 2015). Each clinic visit should include a comprehensive care summary and review of the follow-up plan to be shared with all providers and the survivor.

Existing and emerging technologies may offer opportunities to change care delivery models and improve care. Examples include joint clinic visits with the HSCT provider and PCP, video conferencing, and utilization of electronic health record systems to send health maintenance reminders. The National Marrow Donor Program (NMDP) publishes a comprehensive guide to long-term follow-up for HSCT survivors on its website (https://bethematch.org/patients-and-families). To address the special needs of pediatric survivors, the Children's Oncology Group offers a survivorship guide on its website (www.survivorshipguidelines.org). The American Society for Transplantation and Cellular Therapy and NMDP have also developed computer applications for healthcare providers that include survivorship practice guidelines.

Developing survivorship clinics may minimize fragmentation of care, facilitate completion of study assessments, allow for collection of outcome data, coordinate the complex needs of survivors, and provide the infrastructure for research to better understand and characterize late effects. Many models of survivorship care are available, but the ability to deliver comprehensive care by experts to HSCT survivors is the key to their success (Hashmi et al., 2015; Tichelli & Rovó, 2015). Models for survivorship clinics include an HSCT long-term follow-up clinic, a cancer survivorship clinic that includes HSCT survivors, or a combined chronic graft-versus-host disease (GVHD) and HSCT survivorship clinic (Hashmi et al., 2015). One group of investigators explored the use of an Internet-based survivorship program known as INSPIRE (Syrjala et al., 2011). The INSPIRE program contained three main intervention sections: boosting health, restoring energy, and renewing outlook. Two additional sections were also included: getting connected, which facilitated communication between participants and study coordinators, and tips and tools, which provided additional resources. The investigators concluded that an Internet-based survivorship program providing resources for HSCT survivors is feasible and a useful adjunct to clinical care.

An educated HSCT survivor is essential to reduce the morbidity and mortality of late effects. Education for the HSCT survivor should include long-term health risks, such as subsequent neoplasms, chronic GVHD, infectious com-plications and risks, medication administration and side effects, reportable signs and symptoms, and recommended follow-up care. An application that covers these topics and provides alerts for scheduling follow-up appointments, suggested interventions to minimize symptoms and improve HRQOL, and links to online resources may be a powerful tool for enabling HSCT survivors to take a lead role in their health care. Areas of future research include motivation of HSCT survivors to engage in healthy lifestyles, adherence to medication schedules, and recommended screening guidelines.

Late Infectious Complications

The primary risk factor for late infectious complications—defined as occurring at 100 days or more after transplantation—is delayed recovery of the immune system, which is generally slower in allogeneic transplants than autologous transplants. Variables affecting immune reconstitution include age-associated thymic involution, thymic damage from the conditioning regimen, GVHD, immunosuppressive medications, graft manipulation (particularly T-cell depletion), umbilical cord blood grafts, and the degree of histocompatibility (Bosch, Khan, & Storek, 2012; Dudakov, Perales, & van den Brink, 2016; Rizzo et al., 2006; Tomblyn et al., 2009; Welniak, Blazar, & Murphy, 2007). These variables will delay immune reconstitution for years (Tomblyn et al., 2009). Two measures of immune recovery to guide the healthcare provider in determining how long to continue prophylactic measures are CD4+ counts and the CD4/CD8 ratio (Majhail et al., 2012). Measuring antigen-specific antibodies following infection or vaccination is a means of assessing recovery of humoral immunity (Tomblyn et al., 2009).

Opportunistic bacterial, fungal, and viral infections pose a risk for immunocompromised HSCT survivors (Tomblyn et al., 2009). In two recent reports of relapse-free survivors, infections remained a significant risk for late mortality (Atsuta et al., 2016; Solh et al., 2018).

Administration of IV immunoglobulin (IVIG) as a means of providing passive immunity in HSCT survivors with a low IgG level (less than 400 mg/dl) is a practice followed at some centers (Tomblyn et al., 2009). This practice is controversial because of the high costs of IVIG and lack of proven efficacy.

Bacterial Infections

Late bacterial infections are more common in allogeneic than autologous HSCT survivors. In general, survivors with chronic GVHD remain vulnerable to potentially life-threatening infections from encapsulated bacteria, including *Streptococcus pneumoniae*, *Haemophilus influenzae*, and *Neisseria meningitidis* (Majhail et al., 2012). One center reported seven cases of *S. pneumoniae* per 1,000 transplants over a 17-year period and a mortality rate of 13% (Youssef et al., 2007). It is important to note that 69% of survi-

Table 14-1. Summary Recommendations for Screening and Prevention of Late Complications in Long-Term Hematopoietic Cell Transplantation Survivors

Tissue/Organs	Late Complication	General Risk Factors	Monitoring Tests	Monitoring Tests and Preventive Measures in All HCT Recipients	Monitoring Tests and Preventive Measures in Special Populations
Immune system	• Infections	• Donor source • HLA disparity • T cell depletion • GVHD • Prolonged immuno-suppression • Venous access devices	• CMV antigen or PCR in patients at high risk for CMV reactivation	• PJP prophylaxis for initial 6 months after HCT • Immunizations posttransplantation according to published guidelines • Administration of antibiotics for endocarditis prophylaxis according to American Heart Association guidelines	• Patients with cGVHD: Antimicrobial prophylaxis targeting encapsulated organisms and PJP for the duration of immunosuppressive therapy • Patients with cGVHD: Screening for CMV reactivation should be based on risk factors, including intensity of immunosuppression.
Ocular	• Cataracts • Sicca syndrome • Microvascular reti-nopathy	• TBI/radiation expo-sure to head and neck • Corticosteroids • GVHD	• Ophthalmologic exam	• Routine clinical evaluation at 6 months and 1 year after HCT and at least yearly thereafter • Ophthalmologic examination with measure-ment of visual acuity and fundus examina-tion at 1 year after HCT, subsequent evalu-ations based on findings and risk factors • Prompt ophthalmologic examination in patients with visual symptoms	• Patients with cGVHD: Routine clinical evaluation, and if indicated, ophthalmologic examination more frequently
Oral	• Sicca syndrome • Caries	• GVHD • TBI/radiation expo-sure to head and neck	• Dental assessment	• Education about preventive oral health practices • Clinical oral assessment at 6 months and 1 year after HCT and at least yearly thereafter with particular attention to intraoral malig-nancy evaluation • Dental assessment at 1 year after HCT and then at least yearly thereafter	• Pediatric recipients: Yearly assess-ment of teeth development • Patients with cGVHD: Consider more frequent oral and dental assessments with particular attention to intraoral malignancy evaluation
Respiratory	• Idiopathic pneumonia syndrome • Bronchiolitis obliterans syndrome • Cryptogenic organiz-ing pneumonia • Sinopulmonary infec-tions	• TBI/radiation expo-sure to chest • GVHD • Infectious agents • Allogeneic HCT • Busulfan exposure	• PFTs • Radiologic studies (eg, chest x-ray, CT scan)	• Routine clinical evaluation at 6 months and 1 year after HCT and at least yearly thereafter • Assessment of tobacco use and counselling against smoking • PFTs and focused radiologic assessment for allogeneic HCT recipients with symp-toms or signs of lung compromise	• Patients with cGVHD: Some experts recommend earlier and more frequent clinical evaluation and PFTs

(Continued on next page)

Table 14-1. Summary Recommendations for Screening and Prevention of Late Complications in Long-Term Hematopoietic Cell Transplantation Survivors *(Continued)*

Tissue/Organs	Late Complication	General Risk Factors	Monitoring Tests	Monitoring Tests and Preventive Measures in All HCT Recipients	Monitoring Tests and Preventive Measures in Special Populations
Cardiac and vascular	• Cardiomyopathy • Congestive heart failure • Arrhythmias • Valvular anomaly • Coronary artery disease • Cerebrovascular disease • Peripheral arterial disease	• Anthracycline exposure • TBI/radiation to neck or chest • Older age at HCT • Allogeneic HCT • Cardiovascular risk factors before/after HCT • Chronic kidney disease • Metabolic syndrome	• Cumulative dose of anthracyclines • Echocardiogram with ventricular function, ECG in patients at risk and in symptomatic patients • Fasting lipid profile (including HDL-C, LDL-C and triglycerides) • Fasting blood sugar	• Routine clinical assessment of cardiovascular risk factors as per general health maintenance at 1 year and at least yearly thereafter • Education and counseling on "heart-healthy" lifestyle (regular exercise, healthy weight, no smoking, dietary counseling) • Early treatment of cardiovascular risk factors such as diabetes, hypertension, and dyslipidemia • Administration of antibiotics for endocarditis prophylaxis according to American Heart Association guidelines	
Liver	• GVHD • Hepatitis B • Hepatitis C • Iron overload	• Cumulative transfusion exposure • Risk factors for viral hepatitis transmission	• LFTs • Liver biopsy • Serum ferritin • Imaging for iron overload (MRI or SQUID)	• LFTs every 3–6 months in the first year, then individualized, but at least yearly thereafter • Monitor viral load by PCR for patients with known hepatitis B or C, with liver and infectious disease specialist consultation • Consider lifer biopsy at 8–10 years after HCT to assess cirrhosis in patients with chronic HCV infection • Serum ferritin at 1 year after HCT in patients who have received RBC transfusions; consider liver biopsy or imaging study for abnormal results based on magnitude of elevation and clinical context; subsequent monitoring is suggested for patients with elevated LFTs, continued RBC transfusions, or presence of HCV infection	
Renal and genitourinary	• Chronic kidney disease • Bladder dysfunction • Urinary tract infections	• TBI • Drug exposure (eg, calcineurin inhibitors, amphotericin, aminoglycosides) • CMV • Hemorrhagic cystitis	• Urine protein • Serum creatinine • BUN	• Blood pressure assessment at every clinic visit, with aggressive hypertension management • Assess renal function with BUN, creatinine and urine protein at 6 months, 1 year and at least yearly thereafter • Consider further workup (kidney biopsy or renal ultrasound) for further workup of renal dysfunction as clinically indicated	

(Continued on next page)

Table 14-1. Summary Recommendations for Screening and Prevention of Late Complications in Long-Term Hematopoietic Cell Transplantation Survivors (Continued)

Tissue/Organs	Late Complication	General Risk Factors	Monitoring Tests	Monitoring Tests and Preventive Measures in All HCT Recipients	Monitoring Tests and Preventive Measures in Special Populations
Muscle and connective tissue	• Myopathy • Fasciitis/scleroderma • Polymyositis	• Corticosteroids • GVHD	• Evaluate ability to stand from a sitting position • Clinical evaluation of joint range of motion	• Follow general population guidelines for physical activity • Frequent clinical evaluation for myopathy in patients on corticosteroids	• Patients with cGVHD: Physical therapy consultation in patients with prolonged corticosteroids exposure, fasciitis or scleroderma • Patients with cGVHD: Frequent clinical evaluation by manual muscle tests or by assessing ability to go from sitting to standing position for patients on prolonged corticosteroids
Skeletal	• Osteopenia/osteoporosis • Avascular necrosis	• Inactivity • TBI • Corticosteroids • GVHD • Hypogonadism • Allogeneic HCT	• Dual photon densitometry • MRI to evaluate patients with joint symptoms	• Dual photon densitometry at 1 year for adult women, all allogeneic HCT recipients and patients who are at high risk for bone loss; subsequent testing determined by defects or to assess response to therapy • Physical activity, vitamin D, and calcium supplementation to prevent loss of bone density	• Patients with cGVHD: Consider dual photon densitometry at an earlier date in patients with prolonged corticosteroid or calcineurin inhibitor exposure.
Nervous system	• Leukoencephalopathy • Late infections • Neuropsychological and cognitive defects • Calcineurin neurotoxicity • Peripheral neuropathy	• TBI/radiation exposure to the head • GVHD • Exposure to fludarabine • Intrathecal chemotherapy		• Clinical evaluation for symptoms and signs of neurologic dysfunction at 1 year and yearly thereafter • Diagnostic testing (eg, radiographs, nerve conduction studies) for those with symptoms or signs	• Pediatric recipients: Annual assessment for cognitive development milestones
Endocrine	• Hypothyroidism • Hypoadrenalism • Hypogonadism • Growth retardation	• TBI/radiation exposure (eg, head and neck, CNS) • Corticosteroids • Young age at HCT • Chemotherapy exposure	• Thyroid function tests • FSH, LH, testosterone • Growth velocity in children	• Thyroid function testing yearly post-HCT, or if relevant symptoms develop • Clinical and endocrinologic gonadal assessment for postpubertal women at 1 year, subsequent follow-up based on menopausal status • Gonadal function in men, including FSH, LH, and testosterone, should be assessed as warranted by symptoms	• Pediatric recipients: clinical and endocrine and gonadal assessment for prepubertal boys and girls within year of transplantation, with further follow-up as determined in consultation with a pediatric endocrinologist • Pediatric recipients: Monitor growth velocity in children annually; assessment of thyroid and growth hormone function if clinically indicated • Patients with cGVHD: Slow terminal tapering of corticosteroids for those with prolonged exposure • Patients with cGVHD: Consider stress doses of corticosteroids during acute illness for patients who have received chronic corticosteroids

(Continued on next page)

Table 14-1. Summary Recommendations for Screening and Prevention of Late Complications in Long-Term Hematopoietic Cell Transplantation Survivors *(Continued)*

Tissue/Organs	Late Complication	General Risk Factors	Monitoring Tests	Monitoring Tests and Preventive Measures in All HCT Recipients	Monitoring Tests and Preventive Measures in Special Populations
Mucocutaneous	• Cutaneous sclerosis • Genital GVHD	• GVHD • TBI/radiation exposure to the pelvis	• Pelvic exam	• Counsel patients to perform routine self-exam of skin and avoid excessive exposure to sunlight without adequate protection • Annual gynecologic exam in woman to detect early involvement of vaginal mucosa by GVHD	• Patients with cGVHD and TBI recipients: Consider more frequent gynecologic evaluation based on clinical symptoms
Second cancers	• Solid tumors • Hematologic malignancies • PTLD	• GVHD • TBI/radiation exposure • T cell depletion • Exposure to alkylating agents or etoposide	• Mammogram • Screening for colon cancer (eg, colonoscopy, sigmoidoscopy, fecal occult blood testing) • Pap smear	• Counsel patients about risks of secondary malignancies annually and encourage them to perform self-exam (eg, skin, testicles/genitalia) • Council patients to avoid high risk behaviors (eg, smoking) • Follow general population recommendations for cancer screening	• Patients with cGVHD: Clinical and dental evaluation with particular attention toward oral and pharyngeal cancer • TBI and chest irradiation recipients: Screening mammography in women starting at age 25 or 8 years after radiation exposure, whichever occurs later but no later than age 40
Psychosocial and sexual	• Depression • Anxiety • Fatigue • Sexual dysfunction	• Prior psychiatric morbidity • Hypogonadism	• Psychological evaluation	• Clinical assessment throughout recovery period, at 6 months, 1 year, and annually thereafter, with mental health professional counseling recommended for those with recognized deficits • Encouragement of robust support networks • Regularly assess level of spousal/caregiver psychological adjustment and family functioning • Query adults about sexual function at 6 months, 1 year, and at least annually thereafter	
Fertility	• Infertility	• TBI/radiation exposure • Chemotherapy exposure	• FSH, LH levels	• Consider referral to appropriate specialists for patients who are contemplating a pregnancy or are having difficulty conceiving • Counsel sexually active patients in reproductive age group about birth control post-HCT	
General Health				• Recommended screening as per general population	

BUN—blood urea nitrogen; cGVHD—chronic graft-versus-host disease; CMV—cytomegalovirus; CNS—central nervous system; CT—computed tomography; ECG—electrocardiogram; FSH—follicle-stimulating hormone; GVHD—graft-versus-host disease; HCT—hematopoietic cell transplantation; HCV—hepatitis C virus; HDL-C—high-density lipoprotein cholesterol; HLA—human leukocyte antigen; LDL-C—low-density lipoprotein cholesterol; LFT—liver function test; LH—luteinizing hormone; MRI—magnetic resonance imaging; PCR—polymerase chain reaction; PFT—pulmonary function test; PJP—*Pneumocystis jirovecii* pneumonia; PTLD—post-transplant lymphoproliferative disorders; RBC—red blood cell; SQUID—superconducting quantum interference device; TBI—total body irradiation

Note. From "Recommended Screening and Preventive Practices for Long-Term Survivors After Hematopoietic Cell Transplantation," by N.S. Majhail, J.D. Rizzo, S.J. Lee, M. Aljurf, Y. Astuta, C. Bonfim, … A. Tichelli, 2012, *Biology of Blood and Marrow Transplantation, 18,* pp. 350–352. Copyright 2012 by Elsevier. Retrieved from https://doi.org/10.1016/j.bbmt.2011.12.519. Licensed under CC BY-NC-ND 4.0 (https://creativecommons.org/licenses/by-nc-nd/4.0).

vors who developed *S. pneumoniae* infections did not have chronic GVHD. A second report also showed that four of five fatal cases of bacterial infections occurred in allogeneic transplant recipients without chronic GVHD (Bjorklund et al., 2007). Splenectomy and functional asplenia are additional risk factors for infection. Prophylaxis against encapsulated bacterial infections in an allogeneic transplant recipient with chronic GVHD is recommended until the resolution of GVHD and discontinuation of immunosuppressive agents (Majhail et al., 2012). Bacterial prophylaxis should be guided by local antibiotic resistance patterns (Tomblyn et al., 2009).

Fungal Infections

Invasive fungal infections following allogeneic HSCT carry up to a 51% mortality rate (Kontoyiannis et al., 2010; Vehreschild et al., 2010). Invasive fungal infections in autologous transplant recipients are infrequent once mucositis and neutropenia have resolved (Tomblyn et al., 2009). Selection of appropriate antifungal prophylaxis should be guided by local fungal epidemiology, risk factors, knowledge of antifungal agents, and awareness of emerging fungal pathogens (Fleming et al., 2014; Marr, 2008). Risk stratification is a useful means of determining which HSCT survivors should be considered for antifungal prophylaxis. Prophylaxis should be considered for survivors at high risk, including those with chronic GVHD and those receiving corticosteroids (Bjorklund et al., 2007; Pagano et al., 2011). Other risk factors for late invasive fungal infections include umbilical cord blood or unrelated donor grafts, iron overload, cytomegalovirus (CMV) infection, and acute and chronic GVHD (Girmenia et al., 2014; Pagano et al., 2011).

Classes of antifungal agents include the polyenes (amphotericin B, lipid-based amphotericin, aerosolized amphotericin), echinocandins (caspofungin, anidulafungin, micafungin), and azoles (fluconazole, itraconazole, voriconazole, posaconazole) (Marr, 2008). Selection and optimal use of these agents must involve knowledge of antifungal coverage, drug interactions, and toxicity profile (Chau et al., 2014).

Self-care strategies for HSCT survivors to reduce the risk of invasive fungal infection due to *Candida* species include protecting the integrity of the skin and mucosal barriers. Strategies to reduce the risk of invasive fungal infections due to *Aspergillus* species include avoiding construction sites and direct contact with soil, as well as use of an N95 particulate filter mask (Fleming et al., 2014). Healthcare providers should educate HSCT survivors on the increased risk of photosensitivity and skin carcinomas associated with receiving immunosuppressive therapy and voriconazole prophylaxis for longer than one year (Clancy & Nguyen, 2011).

Pneumocystis jirovecii, formerly classified as *Pneumocystis carinii*, is a fungus once thought to be a protozoal organism that can cause life-threatening pneumonia in susceptible individuals. Effective prophylaxis can be achieved with trimethoprim-sulfamethoxazole administered for three to six months after autologous HSCT and continuing for three months after completion of immunosuppressive therapy in allogeneic HSCT survivors (Majhail et al., 2012; Tomblyn et al., 2009). Alternative prophylactic agents include dapsone, atovaquone, or pentamidine (IV or aerosolized) for survivors who have an allergy or intolerance to trimethoprim-sulfamethoxazole.

Viral Infections

CMV is a latent herpes virus that contributes to morbidity and mortality in HSCT survivors. Late CMV infection and disease occurred in 31% and 6%, respectively, of 269 allogeneic HSCT survivors in one report (Özdemir et al., 2007). In this study, risk factors for late CMV infection (more than 100 days after HSCT) included more than two early episodes of CMV infection, diagnosis of a lymphoid malignancy, unrelated or mismatched related donor grafts, seropositive recipients with a seronegative donor, donors aged 26–45 years, prior acute GVHD, lymphopenia at day 100, and the development of chronic GVHD (Özdemir et al., 2007). A recent review of studies from 1995 to 2017 to identify and classify risk factors for CMV infection disease concluded that the major risk factors for CMV disease included seropositive recipients with seronegative donors, GVHD, and unrelated or mismatched donors (Dziedzic, Sadowska-Krawczenko, & Styczynski, 2017). Late CMV disease most commonly presents as pneumonia or gastrointestinal disease. Manifestations of CMV pneumonia include fever, nonproductive cough, hypoxia, and chest x-ray abnormalities (Ljungman, Hakki, & Boeckh, 2010). Although the risk is low, CMV pneumonia should be included in the differential diagnosis of an autologous transplant recipient who presents with constitutional symptoms, hypoxia, and abnormal chest x-ray findings.

A longer duration of CMV monitoring is necessary, as prophylactic and preemptive treatment with ganciclovir has resulted in an increase in late CMV infection (Asano-Mori et al., 2008; Özdemir et al., 2007). Monitoring for late CMV infection with CMV antigen or CMV polymerase chain reaction (PCR) testing is recommended for allogeneic transplant recipients at high risk for late CMV disease (Boeckh et al., 2003). Two strategies are used for the prevention of late CMV disease: preemptive therapy based on monitoring CMV infection or prophylaxis to treat every survivor at risk. An advantage of preemptive therapy is that only those with evidence of infection are exposed to the toxicities of the antiviral therapy; however, it requires the capability to perform diagnostic testing and to quickly initiate antiviral therapy (Tomblyn et al., 2009). Letermovir, one of the newest pharmacologic agents for prevention of CMV infection, received U.S. Food and Drug Administration (FDA) approval in November 2017. Ganciclovir can be used for both preemptive therapy and treatment of CMV disease (Boeckh, Murphy, & Peggs, 2015). CMV of the gastrointestinal tract is generally treated with antiviral therapy alone, but for CMV pneumonia, some recommend the addition of IVIG (Boeckh, 2011). However, a recent report showed no benefit with the addition of IVIG for the treatment of CMV pneumonia (Erard et al., 2015). Foscarnet is an alternative choice for ganciclovir-resistant CMV, and cidofovir is an option for ganciclovir-induced cytopenias (Erard et al., 2015; Kotton et al., 2013). Newer approaches include adoptive therapy with CMV-specific T cells or natural killer cells and the development of a CMV vaccine (Boeckh et al., 2015; Melenhorst et al., 2010; Peggs et al., 2009; Schleiss, 2016).

A second latent herpes virus associated with morbidity and mortality in HSCT survivors is varicella zoster virus (VZV). The majority of cases of zoster or shingles are the result of viral reactivation; however, approximately 5% of survivors will develop a primary infection in the first year following HSCT with the rate of primary infection higher in pediatric survivors (Ho & Arvin, 2016). Autologous and allogeneic transplant recipients have a similar risk of developing VZV disease. Varicella, the primary infection, manifests with fever, malaise, and disseminated vesicular rash (Ho & Arvin, 2016). In contrast, with VZV reactivation (herpes zoster), the rash typically presents with a specific dermatomal distribution and is often proceeded by paresthesia (Ho & Arvin, 2016). VZV reactivation generally occurs at 2–10 months after transplant, with a median onset of five months (Ho & Arvin, 2016). Complications of VZV infection include postherpetic neuralgia, scarring, and dissemination. Acyclovir and valaciclovir are effective as prophylaxis, and acyclovir is effective as treatment of primary and recurrent VZV infections (Ho & Arvin, 2016; Milano et al., 2010). Both allogeneic and autologous transplant recipients should receive prophylaxis for the first year following transplantation, and it should be continued beyond one year in allogeneic transplant recipients with chronic GVHD (Majhail et al., 2012). HSCT survivor education should include signs and symptoms of VZV infection, rationale for prophylaxis, and review of acyclovir administration and side effects. For survivors who are VZV seronegative, education should include signs and symptoms of primary infection and the importance of avoiding contact with anyone with VZV infection. Vaccination of healthcare providers and family members who do not have a history of varicella infection or are VZV seronegative is an additional prevention strategy (Tomblyn et al., 2009).

Respiratory viral infections, including influenza, parainfluenza, rhinovirus, respiratory syncytial virus, adenovirus, and human metapneumovirus, pose a serious risk for immunocompromised HSCT survivors, with mortality for lower respiratory tract infection of 28%–36% (Chemaly et al., 2006; D'Angelo et al., 2016; Ljungman et al., 2001). Risk factors for respiratory viral infections include high corticosteroid doses, bacterial or viral coinfections, and lymphopenia. Risk factors for progression to lower respiratory tract infection include alternative donors, chronic GVHD, neutropenia, lymphopenia, and age older than 65 years (Martino et al., 2005; Paulsen & Danziger-Isakov, 2017). The diagnosis of respiratory viral infections is made with PCR testing of swabs of the nasopharynx or oropharynx and bronchoalveolar lavage (Husain et al., 2011; Paulsen & Danziger-Isakov, 2017). Prevention of respiratory viral infections in a hospital setting includes respiratory or contact precautions, rigorous hand hygiene, and screening of visitors and staff (Garcia et al., 1997; Kassis et al., 2010). Meticulous handwashing and avoiding contact with infected individuals are essential measures to reduce the risk of respiratory viral infections. Given the high mortality of these infections in immunocompromised survivors, education of patients and caregivers cannot be overemphasized. Treatment options for respiratory viral infections is limited, and efficacy of available therapies has not been adequately studied.

Spread of respiratory syncytial virus is seasonal, beginning in late fall and lasting through spring. The incidence is less than 2% in autologous transplant recipients and 17% in allogeneic transplant recipients (Chemaly, Shah, & Boeckh, 2014; Renaud & Campbell, 2011). Prompt initiation of therapy can reduce the development of respiratory syncytial virus pneumonia from nearly 60% to less than 20% (Chemaly et al., 2006). Treatment may include ribavirin (aerosolized, IV, or oral), IVIG, and respiratory syncytial virus–specific IVIG, but the efficacy of and evidence for these therapies are not supported by placebo-controlled clinical trials (Boeckh et al., 2007; Paulsen & Danziger-Isakov, 2017; Small et al., 2002).

Influenza infection typically occurs in the winter through early spring. An inactivated vaccine is widely available and is strongly recommended for HSCT survivors, household members, and healthcare professionals (Paulsen & Danziger-Isakov, 2017). The neuraminidase inhibitors may be used for prevention and treatment of influenza (Paulsen & Danziger-Isakov, 2017).

Four distinct serotypes of parainfluenza have activity throughout the year, including the summer months (Paulsen & Danziger-Isakov, 2017). Of the four serotypes of parainfluenza, serotype 3 is the most common (Seo & Boeckh, 2016). In one report, the incidence of parainfluenza was 1.3% in autologous transplant recipients and 5.5% in allogeneic transplant recipients (Chemaly et al., 2012). In this analysis, 30% had lower respiratory tract infection at presentation, with a mortality rate of 17% (Chemaly et al., 2012).

In immunocompromised HSCT survivors, adenovirus may present as asymptomatic viremia or disseminated disease and may occur from reactivation or primary infection (Paulsen & Danziger-Isakov, 2017). Presentation may include hemorrhagic cystitis, hepatitis, central nervous system disease, and pneumonia (Hirsch & Pergam, 2016). Disseminated infection and lower respiratory tract infection are associated with a mortality rate ranging 50%–100% (Hubmann et al., 2016; Lion et al., 2003; Robin et al., 2007). No therapy for adenovirus has been approved by FDA, and the most common antiviral agents used, ribavirin and cidofovir, have not been evaluated in randomized clinical trials (Hirsch & Pergam, 2016).

Human metapneumovirus belongs to the same paramyxovirus family as respiratory syncytial virus and parainfluenza (Paulsen & Danziger-Isakov, 2017). In a systematic review of human metapneumovirus, the incidence in HSCT survivors was reported to be 4% in children and 7% in adults (Renaud et al., 2013; Shah, Shah, Azzi, El Chaer, & Chemaly, 2016). Progression to lower respiratory tract infection carries a mortality rate approaching 30% (Shah et al., 2016). No therapy for human metapneumovirus has been approved by FDA (Paulsen & Danziger-Isakov, 2017).

Vaccinations

It is recommended that HSCT survivors be revaccinated against preventable illnesses, and consensus guidelines for vaccination in this population have been published (Ljungman et al., 2009; Tomblyn et al., 2009). NMDP offers an application that includes a vaccination schedule for influenza (inactivated); polio (inactivated); meningococcal conjugate; recombinant hepatitis B; measles, mumps, and rubella (live); pneumococcal conjugate; *H. influenzae* conjugate; and tetanus, diphtheria, and acellular pertussis. With the exception of live virus vaccines, vaccinations should not be delayed in HSCT survivors with chronic GVHD, as it has been demonstrated that these individuals can respond to vaccination (Majhail et al., 2012). Measuring pre- and postvaccination antibody levels may guide the clinician in evaluating the need for booster immunizations (Majhail et al., 2012).

Organ-Specific Toxicities

Endocrine Complications

Endocrine complications can result from therapy prior to, during, and after HSCT, including chemotherapy, radiation, and treatment for chronic GVHD (Cohen et al., 2008). Endocrine problems include hypothyroidism, growth disturbances, and gonadal dysfunction (Cohen et al., 2008). In pediatric survivors, the incidence of endocrine complications is 65%, and the incidence will likely increase as survivors age (Shalitin et al., 2018).

Subclinical compensated hypothyroidism occurs in 7%–15% of survivors in the first year after HSCT and is characterized by elevated thyroid-stimulating hormone and normal serum free thyroxine levels (Berger et al., 2005; Cohen et al., 2008; Majhail et al., 2012; Rizzo et al., 2006). The incidence of overt hypothyroidism varies with the preparative regimen, with a 50% risk associated with total body irradiation (TBI), decreasing to 15% with fractionated TBI and 11% with busulfan and cyclophosphamide regimens (Majhail et al., 2012). The greatest risk is in survivors treated for Hodgkin lymphoma (Sanders et al., 2009). The thyroid may be more susceptible to the effects of radiation during childhood, especially children younger than 10 years (Wei & Albanese, 2014). Once thyroid replacement is initiated, thyroid assessment should be repeated every six weeks

until stable dosing is achieved, followed by testing every six months (Majhail et al., 2012).

Growth failure in children treated with HSCT ranges 20%–80% and results in short stature, defined as two standard deviations below the mean for age (Dvorak et al., 2011; Jackson, Mostoufi-Moab, Hill-Kayser, Balamuth, & Arkader, 2018). Factors that can influence growth failure include deficiencies in growth hormone, prolonged corticosteroid use, hypothyroidism, radiation, gonadal failure, and improper nutrition (Wei & Albanese, 2014). Cranial radiation may damage the hypothalamus, resulting in growth hormone–releasing hormone deficiency (Wei & Albanese, 2014). Endocrinology specialists should closely follow pediatric survivors to ensure that they reach growth and developmental milestones. The response to growth hormone replacement is effective for most childhood survivors; however, most children will not reach full spinal height because of radiation therapy damage to the vertebral epiphysis (Wei & Albanese, 2014).

Multiple variables affect the risk of hypogonadism, including age, therapy antecedent to HSCT, dose intensity of the conditioning regimen, TBI, and the type of chemotherapy, with alkylating agents being particularly toxic to gonadal tissue. Infertility was once presumed to occur in nearly all survivors following myeloablative conditioning regimens; longer follow-up indicates variable rates of infertility, particularly in male survivors (Rovó et al., 2006). In addition to the risk of infertility, children treated are also at risk for delayed or arrested puberty and postpubertal gonadal insufficiency (Chow et al., 2013; Felicetti et al., 2011; Kenney et al., 2012; Steffens et al., 2008).

Elevated levels of follicle-stimulating hormone in men are associated with impaired or absent spermatogenesis (Rovó et al., 2006). One study found that in 39 men tested, 28% had spermatozoa detected in semen, but the sperm analysis was not normal (Rovó et al., 2006). The investigators reported that younger age at the time of HSCT and a longer time interval since HSCT were identified as variables associated with recovery of spermatogenesis. In one report, azoospermia was detected in 81% of men who received TBI and in 46% of men who did not receive TBI (Rovó et al., 2013). Chronic GVHD has also been reported to negatively impact male fertility (Rovó et al., 2006). Testosterone levels generally remain normal; however, men who report problems with sexual functioning may need more extensive hormonal testing and referral to an endocrinologist or urologist (Majhail et al., 2012; Rovó et al., 2006). Prepubescent males should be screened for testicular function by assessing Tanner stages of development, testicular volume, and sperm counts (Cohen et al., 2008; van Dorp et al., 2012).

Women and girls undergoing HSCT are at a significant risk of hypogonadism and infertility, especially those treated with TBI and alkylating agents (Majhail et al., 2012; Rovó et al., 2006). Nearly all women older than 25 years of age treated with myeloablative HSCT experience premature ovarian failure with associated infertility and early menopause. Prepubescent females have a better chance of ovarian recovery and reaching spontaneous menarche, but premature menopause remains common. In the setting of raising follicle-stimulating hormone levels or an absence of signs of puberty based on the Tanner scale, hormone replacement should be started by 12–13 years of age (Wei & Albanese, 2014). Female survivors with premature ovarian failure should be referred to a gynecologist to thoroughly evaluate the risks and benefits of hormone replacement therapy.

Hepatic Complications

The primary reasons for late hepatic complications include hepatotoxic medications, chronic hepatitis B and C infection, chronic GVHD, and iron overload (McDonald, 2010). The incidence of hepatic complications due to iron overload is reported as 75%, and the incidence due to chronic GVHD is 54% (Sucak et al., 2008). Hepatitis B virus is associated with mild to moderate liver dysfunction, whereas chronic hepatitis C virus can lead to cirrhosis in 11% and 24% of survivors at 15 and 20 years, respectively (Majhail et al., 2012). Hepatitis C antiviral therapy should be initiated after consultation with a hepatologist (Hockenbery, Strasser, & McDonald, 2016).

Recipients of autologous and allogeneic HSCT may develop iron overload, which is primarily related to transfusions of red blood cells prior to and during transplantation. Those patients with an underlying diagnosis of thalassemia or hemoglobinopathies are at a particularly high risk of developing iron overload (Majhail et al., 2012). Diagnosis is based on ferritin levels, magnetic resonance imaging, superconducting quantum interference device (SQUID) testing, and liver biopsy (Majhail et al., 2012). Survivors with iron overload are at risk for hepatic dysfunction, as well as other organ dysfunctions, including cardiac, pituitary, and pancreatic (McDonald, 2006). Initiation of therapy is based on the degree of iron overload and liver dysfunction. Therapy may include phlebotomy and chelation therapy.

Monitoring for liver dysfunction includes liver function tests every three to six months for the first year after HSCT, then annually (Majhail et al., 2012). PCR testing for viral load (hepatitis B and C) and ferritin levels should be assessed regularly for those at risk (Majhail et al., 2012). Survivors with iron overload or other evidence of liver dysfunction should avoid vitamin supplementation that includes iron, minimize hepatotoxic medications when possible, and limit alcohol intake (Majhail et al., 2012).

Metabolic Syndrome and Cardiovascular Disease

Metabolic syndrome occurs in an estimated 34%–49% of adult HSCT survivors (Annaloro et al., 2008; Majhail, Flowers, et al., 2009; McMillen, Schmidt, Storer, & Bar, 2014; Oudin et al., 2015). One cross-sectional study of allogeneic HSCT survivors found that the incidence of metabolic syndrome was 2.2 times higher in HSCT survivors compared to an aged- and gender-matched control group (Majhail,

Flowers, et al., 2009). This study also reported that 56% of survivors had elevated blood pressure and 58% had elevated triglycerides compared to the control group (Majhail, Flowers, et al., 2009). The impact of metabolic syndrome on the risk of cardiovascular disease in HSCT survivors is unknown, but in the general population, metabolic syndrome is associated with diabetes mellitus, cardiovascular disease, and an increase in all-cause mortality (Alberti et al., 2009; DeFilipp et al., 2016; Isomaa et al., 2001; Shin et al., 2013). Key clinical measures used in evaluating metabolic syndrome include abdominal obesity and elevated waist circumference, hypertension, reduced high-density lipoprotein cholesterol, elevated triglycerides, and elevated fasting glucose (Alberti et al., 2009). HSCT survivors are at risk for metabolic syndrome as a result of changes in body composition, dyslipidemia, hypertension, diabetes mellitus and insulin resistance, male hypogonadism, premature ovarian failure, and hypothyroidism (Baker et al., 2007; DeFilipp et al., 2016; Majhail, Challa, Mulrooney, Baker, & Burns, 2009).

In a large study of allogeneic HSCT survivors, the risk of premature death due to cardiovascular disease was 2.3 times higher when compared to the general population (Bhatia et al., 2007). Cardiovascular disease includes arterial disease, coronary artery disease, and cardiac disease (Armenian & Chow, 2014). Risk factors for the development of arterial disease include allogeneic HSCT, older age at the time of HSCT, GVHD, TBI, dyslipidemia, diabetes, obesity, and hypertension (Armenian & Chow, 2014; Armenian et al., 2012). Risk factors for cardiac disease include autologous HSCT, female sex, hypertension, diabetes, cardiotoxic chemotherapy, and chest radiation (Armenian & Chow, 2014). Assessment of risk factors for cardiovascular disease and metabolic syndrome should begin one year after HSCT and be repeated annually (Majhail et al., 2012). Recognizing the individual risk factors for cardiovascular disease in HSCT survivors should guide healthcare providers to initiate screening and therapy earlier than what is recommended for the general population (Armenian & Chow, 2014). In the absence of clinical trials focused on management of cardiovascular disease in HSCT survivors, management of hypertension, diabetes, and dyslipidemia should be based on current evidence-based practice guidelines for the general population.

Education of HSCT survivors involves reviewing cardiovascular disease risk factors and encouraging a healthy lifestyle, including eating a primarily plant-based diet high in fruits and vegetables; avoiding smoking; maintaining a healthy weight; limiting alcohol consumption; and exercising regularly.

Musculoskeletal Complications

Myopathy is common among HSCT survivors and is associated with functional impairments (Majhail et al., 2012). Prolonged use of corticosteroids is a major risk factor for the development of myopathy. HSCT survivors may experience a cycle of fatigue, decreased activity levels, and progressive muscle weakness, and this debilitating constellation of symptoms can negatively affect HRQOL. It may be difficult to distinguish myositis due to chronic GVHD and steroid-induced myopathy (Majhail et al., 2012).

Exercise and increased physical activity should be encouraged, although it is recognized that research is needed to understand motivational factors and strategies to improve adherence to exercise guidelines. Survivors should be informed of the risk of muscle atrophy and counseled to engage in routine exercise to mitigate further atrophy and as a strategy to decrease fatigue. Referral to a physical therapist is recommended for those with myopathy.

Late skeletal complications include avascular necrosis and loss of bone mineral density (BMD) (McClune, Majhail, & Flowers, 2012). A decrease in BMD, both osteoporosis and osteopenia, has been reported in more than 45% of allogeneic HSCT survivors within the first two years following transplant (Yao et al., 2008). Loss of BMD may place an HSCT survivor at increased risk of fractures. In the first year after transplantation, all skeletal sites lose BMD (Pundole, Barbo, Lin, Champlin, & Lu, 2015). Recovery of BMD is first noted in the lumbar spine followed by a long recovery period (up to 10 years) in the femur (Pundole et al., 2015). In one study of 7,620 survivors, the incidence of fracture was 11% and 5% in autologous and allogeneic transplant recipients, respectively (Pundole et al., 2015). Compared to an age- and gender-matched control group, the risk of fracture in female HSCT survivors was eight times higher, and the risk for male survivors was seven to nine times higher (Pundole et al., 2015). In this study, risk factors for fracture included age over 50 years, autologous HSCT, diagnosis of multiple myeloma, and transplant for a solid tumor. Both corticosteroids and prolonged use of calcineurin inhibitors contribute to loss of BMD in allogeneic transplant recipients (McClune et al., 2012).

Pediatric survivors are at risk for short stature, slipped capital femoral epiphysis, and development of benign osteochondromas and malignant bone tumors (Gawade et al., 2014; Liu, Tsai, & Huang, 2004; Sanders, 2008). Treatment with fractionated TBI places children at risk for short stature, defined as two standard deviations below the mean for age and includes both standing and sitting height (Jackson et al., 2018; Vrooman et al., 2017). Both growth hormone deficiency and diffuse physeal damage place the pediatric survivor at risk for impaired growth (Jackson et al., 2018; Pekic & Popovic, 2014; Sanders et al., 2005). Pediatric survivors should be regularly assessed for attainment of growth and developmental milestones. Bone age radiograph and laboratory testing of the hypothalamic-pituitary axis should be considered in survivors with severe impaired growth (Hammell, Bunin, Edgar, & Jaramillo, 2013).

Strategies to improve or maintain bone health include physical activity, adequate intake of calcium and vitamin D, consideration of bisphosphonate therapy, and hormone replacement therapy in female survivors. A baseline dual energy x-ray densitometry should be obtained before HSCT,

and screening should begin six months after HSCT (Pundole et al., 2015).

Avascular necrosis is the result of decreased blood flow to the bones and results in ischemic bone damage (Faraci, Békássy, De Fazio, Tichelli, & Dini, 2008). The incidence of avascular necrosis ranges 4%–19% (Majhail et al., 2012). All bones are at risk for avascular necrosis, but the femur is the most common site (Faraci et al., 2008; Jackson et al., 2018; Majhail et al., 2012). Factors that contribute to the development of avascular necrosis include risk factors for BMD loss and TBI (Jackson et al., 2018; Majhail et al., 2012). Joint pain is a common presenting symptom and should be evaluated with magnetic resonance imaging (Faraci et al., 2008; Majhail et al., 2012). Prevention of avascular necrosis includes engaging in regular weight-bearing physical activity, and treatment involves non-weight-bearing activities to rest the affected bone and joint replacement (Faraci et al., 2008).

Neurocognitive and Neurologic Complications

Neurocognitive dysfunction has been reported in 11%–60% of adult HSCT survivors (Harder et al., 2002; Harder, Duivenvoorden, van Gool, Cornelissen, & van den Bent, 2006; Sostak et al., 2003). Risk factors include TBI, pre-HSCT high-dose chemotherapy, immunosuppressive medications for the prevention and treatment of GVHD, and infections (Buchbinder et al., 2018; Harder et al., 2006). Table 14-2 summarizes neurocognitive dysfunction associated with HSCT (Buchbinder et al., 2018). To accurately evaluate the impact of HSCT on neurocognitive function, assessment should be performed before transplantation, with serial assessments afterward. Multiple domains of neurocognitive function need to be evaluated to accurately diagnose dysfunction, and a wide variety of assessment tools are available (Buchbinder et al., 2018). In a study of 171 HSCT survivors three years after HSCT, the most common neurocognitive dysfunction reported was difficulty with concentration (Bevans et al., 2014). Another study of 25 survivors found that one-fourth experienced changes on multiple cognitive domains, including intelligence and complex tasks, attention and executive function, and psychomotor functions and speed (Harder et al., 2002; Harder et al., 2006). Intervention strategies may include job retraining, cognitive rehabilitation, and pharmacologic interventions. Reducing risk factors when possible, such as utilizing preparative regimens that do not involve TBI, may prevent neurocognitive dysfunction (Buchbinder et al., 2018).

Pediatric HSCT survivors are at risk for developing neurocognitive deficits and developmental delays (Faraci et al., 2008; Rizzo et al., 2006). Neurocognitive changes are more common in children who receive a transplant at developmentally vulnerable ages, especially those treated at younger than three years old (Faraci et al., 2008). Neurologic complications vary in intensity. Signs of neurologic complications include changes in mentation, problems with memory and attention span, impaired speech, and impaired motor and sensory function (Buchbinder et al., 2018; Mulcahy Levy et al., 2013). Data are not conclusive on the risk of alterations in IQ in pediatric HSCT survivors (Buchbinder et al., 2018). Regardless, even if pediatric survivors do not show decreases in IQ, they can experience executive function deficits, such as decreased attention span, processing, response, and visual-motor integration skills (Buchbinder et al., 2018; Nathan et al., 2007; Perkins et al., 2007). Approximately 40% of children treated with HSCT for sickle cell disease have experienced silent

Table 14-2. Risk Factors for Neurocognitive Dysfunction and Manifestations

Risk Factor	Manifestations
Conditioning Regimen	
Total body irradiation	Headache, fatigue
Busulfan	Reversible encephalopathy with some somnolence, confusion, decreased alertness, myoclonus, hallucinations; seizures
Carboplatin	Ototoxicity in patients with neuroblastoma
Carmustine	Variable degrees of optic disc and retinal microvasculopathy with variable degrees of visual loss
Cytarabine arabinoside	Pancerebellar syndrome +/– diffuse encephalopathy with lethargy, confusion, and seizures
Etoposide	Confusion, somnolence and seizures, which resolve spontaneously
Fludarabine	Neurological decline, blindness, leukoencephalopathy
Ifosfamide	Encephalopathy with lethargy, confusion and seizures in 10–40% of patients. Visual or auditory hallucinations, myoclonus or muscle rigidity have been reported, which is often self-limited, but there are reports of progressing to coma
Thiotepa	Chronic encephalopathy with progressive declines in cognitive and behavioral function and memory loss
Immunosuppressive therapy	
Cyclosporine A	TMA, PRES
Tacrolimus	
Sirolimus	
Steroids	Psychosis, myopathy
ATG	Neurotoxicity, seizures
Cyclophosphamide	Neurotoxicity
Methotrexate	Leukoencephalopathy
Central nervous system infections	
HHV6	Encephalitis, AMS
HSV	Meningoencephalitis, seizures
VZV	Encephalitis, post-herpetic neuralgias, zoster ophthalmicus
JC	Encephalitis, AMS
EBV	Post-transplant lymphoproliferative disease
CMV	Vision loss, CMV retinitis, meningoencephalitis
Toxoplasma gondii	Mild to severe encephalopathy

AMS—altered mental status; ATG—antithymocyte globulin; CMV—cytomegalovirus; EBV—Epstein-Barr virus; HHV6—human herpesvirus 6; HSV—herpes simplex virus; JC—John Cunningham virus; PRES—posterior reversible encephalopathy syndrome; TMA—thrombotic microangiopathy; VZV—varicella zoster virus

Note. From "Neurocognitive Dysfunction in Hematopoietic Cell Transplant Recipients: Expert Review From the Late Effects and Quality of Life Working Committee of the CIBMTR and Complications and Quality of Life Working Party of the EBMT," by D. Buchbinder, D.L. Kelly, R.F. Duarte, J.J. Auletta, N. Bhatt, M. Byrne, ... B.E. Shaw, 2018, *Bone Marrow Transplantation, 53,* p. 541. Copyright 2018 by Springer. Reprinted with permission.

cerebral infarcts, which increase the risk of neurocognitive dysfunction (DeBaun et al., 2012; Shenoy et al., 2017). These children need frequent assessment of neurocognitive function and may need additional education interventions (Shenoy et al., 2017).

Central nervous system complications include infection, calcineurin-induced neurotoxicity, GVHD, and leukoencephalopathy (Majhail et al., 2012). Peripheral nervous system complications include peripheral neuropathies and ototoxicity (Faraci et al., 2008; Majhail et al., 2012). Risk factors for neurologic impairments include prolonged exposure to calcineurin inhibitors, TBI, cranial radiation, and intrathecal therapy (Faraci et al., 2008; Majhail et al., 2012).

Assessment for neurologic changes should be initiated one year after HSCT and repeated annually (Majhail et al., 2012). Executive function and IQ testing in pediatric survivors should begin one year after HSCT and be repeated every one to two years to assess learning needs. Testing is especially important during transitional years, such as junior high to high school and high school to college (Nathan et al., 2007). The Children's Oncology Group provides guidelines for identification of, advocacy for, and interventions for neurocognitive dysfunction in pediatric survivors (Nathan et al., 2007). Survivors may face a multitude of cognitive and psychosocial challenges as they enter or return to school. Federal laws mandate that education be provided to all children and outline provisions to ensure children obtain the assistance they require. The Individuals With Disabilities Act requires school districts to identify children with special education needs and to develop an individual education plan to address the identified needs (American Psychological Association, n.d.). The Rehabilitation Act of 1973 requires schools and universities with federal funding to provide reasonable accommodations to students with perceived impairments, including childhood cancer survivors (U.S. Department of Education, 2020). Although these laws exist to aid survivors, families may need assistance in navigating the school systems to ensure access to available services.

Ocular Complications

Late ocular complications after HSCT include cataracts, keratoconjunctivitis sicca, and ischemic microvascular retinopathy (Majhail et al., 2012). In a study of 248 HSCT survivors, cataracts were reported by 38%, which was significantly higher than a sibling comparison group (Baker et al., 2004). TBI, prolonged use of corticosteroids, allogeneic transplant, and older age are risk factors for the development of cataracts (Buchsel, 2009; Majhail et al., 2012). Surgery for cataracts involves removing the clouded lens and replacing it with a clear artificial lens.

Keratoconjunctivitis sicca occurs in approximately 20% of HSCT survivors within 15 years and occurs twice as frequently in those affected by chronic GVHD (Jensen et al., 2010; Rizzo et al., 2006). Symptoms of keratoconjunctivitis include pain, burning, irritation, blurred vision, photophobia, sensation of a foreign body, and excess tearing (Kamoi et al., 2007; Majhail et al., 2012; Motolese et al., 2007). Management of keratoconjunctivitis includes the use of topical lubricants, artificial tears, occlusion of the tear duct, occlusive scleral lens contacts, and autologous serum in addition to ongoing therapy for chronic GVHD. Topical corticosteroids should be used with caution in the presence of ocular viral or bacterial infections (Majhail et al., 2012).

Risk factors for ischemic microvascular retinopathy include TBI and cyclosporine for GVHD prophylaxis (Majhail et al., 2012). Signs and symptoms include cotton-wool spots observed on funduscopic examination and optic-disc edema. Effective therapy includes the reduction or withdrawal of immunosuppressive therapy (Majhail et al., 2012).

HSCT survivor education regarding late ocular complications should include reportable signs and symptoms to ensure timely reporting and early intervention. Preventive self-care strategies include using sunglasses when outdoors and generally avoiding contact lenses to reduce the risk of abrasion. Routine ophthalmologic examinations should begin at six months after transplant, then at 12 months, and yearly thereafter. More frequent ophthalmologic examinations are required in survivors with ocular complications (Majhail et al., 2012; Motolese et al., 2007).

Oral Complications

Reported by 44% of HSCT survivors in one study (Hull, Kerridge, & Schifter, 2012), xerostomia is a common complication that can occur in the absence of chronic GVHD. Xerostomia increases the risk of dental caries, tooth decay, infections, sleep disturbances, and difficulty with speaking, swallowing and chewing (Jensen et al., 2010; Majhail et al., 2012). Fluoride gel or rinses may reduce the risk of caries and facilitate remineralization of teeth (Epstein, Raber-Drulacher, Wilkins, Chavarria, & Myint, 2009). Xerostomia may increase oral sensitivities and place survivors at risk for nutritional deficits. Additionally, taste alterations (hypogeusia and ageusia) have been reported—by 20% of HSCT survivors in one study—and may further contribute to impaired nutritional intake and compromised nutritional status (Epstein et al., 2009). Sialagogues (e.g., pilocarpine) can be used in adults to increase salivary secretions (Effinger et al., 2014; Majhail et al., 2012). Acupuncture and artificial saliva substitutes may provide some relief (Effinger et al., 2014). Chewing gum or sugarless candy may improve mastication of food and improve nutritional intake (Epstein et al., 2009; Majhail et al., 2012).

Pediatric HSCT survivors are at risk for alterations in tooth development, including hypodontia, microdontia, root malformation, and enamel hypoplasia (Cubukcu, Sevinir, & Ercan, 2012). Survivors treated before 12 years of age can experience disruptions in the genetic signaling of tooth development (Cubukcu et al., 2012). Pediatric survivors at highest risk of oral complications include those who received a transplant before the age of five years, high doses of alkylating agents, and fractionated TBI.

Survivor education should include a review of oral complications, signs and symptoms, the need for meticulous oral hygiene to prevent infections, and frequency of dental evaluations. Additional teaching points include avoidance of tobacco products, beverages with high sugar content, and intraoral piercing (Majhail et al., 2012). HSCT survivors should learn to conduct a thorough inspection of the oral cavity. A dietary consult for recommendations on strategies to decrease xerostomia and mitigate taste alterations may improve nutritional intake. Frequent dental examinations may be required and should begin six months after HSCT (Majhail et al., 2012). Ideally, the HSCT program should have access to a dentist familiar with the unique oral complications of HSCT survivors (van der Pas-van Voskuilen et al., 2009).

Pulmonary Complications

Pulmonary complications that typically develop within the first two years following allogeneic HSCT include bronchiolitis obliterans, cryptogenic organizing pneumonia (also referred to as *bronchiolitis obliterans organizing pneumonia*), and idiopathic pneumonia syndrome (IPS) (Yoshihara, Yanik, Cooke, & Mineishi, 2007). Pediatric HSCT survivors have a ninefold increased risk of dying of respiratory complications (Armstrong et al., 2009). Pulmonary complications following autologous HSCT are rare after three months (Tichelli, Rovó, & Gratwohl, 2008). Risk factors include prior infections, exposure to pulmonary-toxic chemotherapy antecedent to and during HSCT, exposure to radiation, and immune-mediated lung injury such as chronic GVHD.

Bronchiolitis obliterans is a nonspecific inflammatory injury of the small airways characterized by an obstructive pattern that progresses to peribronchiolar fibrosis (Tichelli et al., 2008). Pathologically, bronchiolitis obliterans is a fixed airflow obstruction (Santo Tomas et al., 2005). It is a life-threatening complication that typically develops in the first two years but can develop as late as four to five years after transplantation (Santo Tomas et al., 2005). Symptoms include dry cough, wheezing, and progressive dyspnea (Tichelli et al., 2008). In a report summarizing multiple studies, the incidence of bronchiolitis obliterans in HSCT survivors was 8.3%, but this percentage varies widely (Afessa, Litzow, & Tefferi, 2001; Tichelli et al., 2008). The incidence of bronchiolitis obliterans is approximately 6% in allogeneic HSCT survivors without chronic GVHD and increases to 14% in those with chronic GVHD (Au, Au, & Chien, 2011; Dudek & Mahaseth, 2006). The development of bronchiolitis obliterans carries a poor prognosis, especially if associated with chronic GVHD, and a 10-year mortality rate of 40% (Chien et al., 2003). In a report using registry data of 6,275 allogeneic HSCT survivors, contributing causes for the development of bronchiolitis obliterans included GVHD, a prior episode of interstitial pneumonia, male recipient with a female donor, more than 14 months from diagnosis to transplant, a peripheral blood stem cell graft, and busulfan-containing regimens (Rizzo et al., 2006; Santo Tomas et al., 2005; Tichelli et al., 2008). Diagnosis of bronchiolitis obliterans can be made using pulmonary function testing, high-resolution computed tomography, and lung biopsy (Bacigalupo, Chien, Barisione, & Pavletic, 2012; Filipovich et al., 2005). Treatment strategies include systemic immunosuppressive therapy, inhaled corticosteroids, or cyclosporine and azithromycin (Bacigalupo et al., 2012; Hildebrandt et al., 2011).

Cryptogenic organizing pneumonia is rare, reported in approximately 2% of allogeneic HSCT survivors, and typically occurs in the first year (Tichelli et al., 2008). Presentation resembles an interstitial pneumonia with an acute onset of a dry cough, fever, and dyspnea (Tichelli et al., 2008). The diagnostic workup may include pulmonary function testing, chest x-ray, bronchoscopy with bronchoalveolar lavage, and lung biopsy (Tichelli et al., 2008). Treatment of cryptogenic organizing pneumonia includes systemic and inhaled corticosteroids and treatment of any identified infections (Tichelli et al., 2008).

IPS usually presents within the first 120 days after HSCT but may occur as a late complication (Majhail et al., 2012). In a study of 1,100 HSCT survivors, 81 individuals developed IPS, with an incidence of 8.4% after myeloablative conditioning and 2.2% after nonmyeloablative conditioning (Fukuda et al., 2003). In this study, risk factors for the development of IPS included myeloablative conditioning, age older than 40 years, acute GVHD, TBI, and a diagnosis of acute myeloid leukemia (AML) or myelodysplastic syndrome (MDS). The study reported an overall survival after diagnosis of IPS of 23% at day 100 and 17% at one year (Fukuda et al., 2003).

Survivorship education on pulmonary complications should include strategies for infection risk reduction, lifelong abstinence from smoking, and avoidance of environmental factors that increase the risk of lung damage. A screening history and physical examination should begin at six months, and in those with chronic GVHD, screening may include pulmonary function tests (Majhail et al., 2012).

Renal Complications

In HSCT survivors, chronic kidney disease may progress to end-stage renal disease (Tichelli et al., 2008). Risk factors for the development of chronic kidney disease include receiving nephrotoxic medications, especially antimicrobial agents and calcineurin inhibitors, before, during, and after transplantation. In a retrospective study of 266 HSCT survivors, the cumulative incidence of chronic kidney disease was 20% at 5 years and 27% at 10 years, which is twice the rate seen in the general population (Kersting, Hené, Koomans, & Verdonck, 2007). Of the 61 survivors who developed chronic kidney disease, the mean time of onset was 2.6 years, with a range of 6 months to 12 years (Kersting et al., 2007). Pretransplantation risk factors for developing chronic kidney disease included female sex, older age, lower glomerular filtration rate, and higher serum creatinine. The study identified hypertension as the only post-transplantation risk factor. The development of chronic kidney disease did not impact overall survival for this group (Kersting et al., 2007). Screening for chronic kidney disease includes tests of renal function and urine protein analysis (Tichelli et al., 2008).

Relapse and Subsequent Malignancies

For those who survive the immediate risks of HSCT, the most significant threat to survival is relapse of the primary malignancy. The risk of relapse is highest in the first two to four years following transplantation (Majhail, 2017). Multiple variables impact the risk of relapse, including underlying disease, cytogenetic abnormalities, response to therapy before HSCT, remission status at the time of transplantation, intensity of the preparative regimen, and degree of donor–recipient histocompatibility (Majhail, 2008). Outcome data submitted by transplant centers to the Center for International Blood and Marrow Transplant Research are analyzed annually and published on its website (www. cibmtr.org/Pages/index.aspx).

For survivors 10 years or more after allogeneic HSCT, the risk of death from subsequent neoplasms ranges 5%–12% (Wingard et al., 2011). Compared to the general population, autologous HSCT survivors have a 12-fold higher risk of death from subsequent neoplasms (Bhatia et al., 2005). Subsequent neoplasms fall into three broad categories: post-transplant lymphoproliferative disorder (PTLD), hematologic malignancies (MDS, AML), and solid tumors (Majhail et al., 2012).

PTLD most often occurs in the first year following allogeneic HSCT (Landgren et al., 2009). In a report of nearly 27,000 HSCT survivors, risk factors for developing PTLD include T-cell depletion, antithymocyte globulin administration, unrelated or mismatched donors, age older than 50 years at transplantation, and acute and chronic GVHD (Landgren et al., 2009; Majhail, 2011). HSCT survivors at risk for PTLD should be screened for Epstein-Barr virus reactivation with consideration for early therapy (Landgren et al., 2009; Majhail, 2011).

In one review of secondary MDS or AML following autologous HSCT, risk factors included older age, TBI, use of peripheral blood stem cells, and large cumulative doses of alkylating agents (Pedersen-Bjergaard, Andersen, & Christiansen, 2000). The incidence of secondary MDS or AML after autologous HSCT varies widely between studies, with a range of 1.3%–24.3% (Kollmannsberger et al., 1998; Pedersen-Bjergaard, Pedersen, Myhre, & Geisler, 1997). In some cases, the development of MDS or AML occurred within the first year following autologous HSCT (Pedersen-Bjergaard et al., 2000).

Allogeneic HSCT survivors have twice the incidence of solid tumors compared to age-matched controls, and the risk increases with time from transplantation (Majhail et al., 2011; Ringdén et al., 2014; Rizzo et al., 2009). The incidence of solid tumors after allogeneic HSCT is 1%–2% at 10 years and 3%–5% at 20 years (Majhail et al., 2011; Ringdén et al., 2014; Rizzo et al., 2009). Significant risk factors for developing solid malignancies after allogeneic HSCT include TBI and chronic GVHD (Socié & Rizzo, 2012). The types of solid tumors reported include oral, brain and central nervous system, thyroid, bone, soft tissue, and skin cancers (Rizzo et al., 2009).

Established screening guidelines published by the American Society for Transplantation and Cellular Therapy and NMDP for subsequent malignancies are available to guide healthcare providers as downloadable applications. Lifelong surveillance is required, as the risk of subsequent neoplasms increases with time.

HSCT survivors need education not only on the risk of subsequent malignancies but also on healthy lifestyles, prevention strategies, and self-examinations of the skin, breasts, oral cavity, and testes. Healthy lifestyle choices include weight management, exercise, healthy diet, stress reduction, sun protection, moderate use of alcohol, smoking cessation, safe sex, and avoidance of illicit substances.

Health-Related Quality of Life

HRQOL is a subjective multidimensional construct that commonly includes physical, psychological, and social dimensions. The majority of HSCT survivors report good to excellent HRQOL (Bevans et al., 2006; Bush, Donaldson, Haberman, Dacanay, & Sullivan, 2000; Pidala, Anasetti, & Jim, 2009; Syrjala et al., 2004; Wettergren, Sprangers, Björkholm, & Langius-Eklöf, 2008). Findings indicate that overall HRQOL improves for the majority by one year after transplantation, but full recovery may take up to five years (Pidala et al., 2009; Syrjala et al., 2004; Syrjala, Martin, & Lee, 2012). Common impairments in the physical domain include fatigue, sleep disturbances, musculoskeletal pain, sexual dysfunction, and decreased physical functioning (Andrykowski et al., 2005; Hjermstad et al., 2004; Jim et al., 2014; Li et al., 2015; Syrjala et al., 2004; Syrjala, Langer, Abrams, Storer, & Martin, 2005). Chronic GVHD is cited in many studies as exerting a negative impact on HRQOL (Fraser et al., 2006; Lee et al., 2006; Worel et al., 2002). Emotional distress is reported in 22%–43% of HSCT survivors, but evidence is also suggestive of positive psychological and interpersonal growth (Andrykowski et al., 2005; Jeon, Yoo, Kim, & Lee, 2015; Rusiewicz et al., 2008; Sun et al., 2011).

Caregivers

Informal caregivers, typically spouses, parents, adult children, or friends, are essential members of the HSCT team and, unlike professional caregivers, have a personal relationship with the survivors. Caregiver responsibilities include assisting with activities of daily living and medications, preparing meals, managing finances, facilitating transportation, being an advocate, and showing physical and emotional support (Beattie & Lebel, 2011). Caregivers are usually well prepared for the initial months of caregiving, but when the demands extend for years after transplantation, caregivers are at risk for developing physical and psychosocial health problems. A growing body of literature has documented the burdens of caregiving and its physical and emotional demands (Bevans & Sternberg, 2012; Bevans et al., 2016; Laudenslager et al., 2015). Caregivers report sleep impairments, fatigue, social isolation, depression, anxiety, and decreased marital satisfaction (Bishop et al., 2007). Healthcare providers may help mitigate the burdens of caregiving by counseling caregivers to stay connected with family and friends, attend to their own physical and emotional health needs, provide resources, and encourage engagement in stress management strategies such as exercise and meditation.

Summary

Late effects of HSCT affect the health and HRQOL of many survivors and are significant causes of premature death. The cumulative insults to organ systems from the primary malignancy, comorbidities, lifestyle factors, genetic susceptibilities, therapy antecedent to transplantation, preparative regimens, and prevention and treatment of HSCT complications contribute to late effects. The National Cancer Institute and National Heart, Lung, and Blood Institute late effects initiative has highlighted the need for further research on patient-centered outcomes, immune dysregulation and pathobiology, cardiovascular disease and risk factors, and subsequent neoplasms. As risk factors are identified and the pathobiology of late effects evolves, HSCT healthcare professionals will be in a better position to mitigate the impact of late effects and prevent premature death. Despite the burden of late effects, most HSCT survivors report good to excellent HRQOL.

The goal of survivorship care is to minimize morbidity and mortality from late effects and improve the health and HRQOL of HSCT survivors. HSCT nurses play a key role in survivorship care by providing education on late effects, healthy lifestyles, and recommended screening. HSCT survivors, as integral members of the healthcare team, need to be active participants in their care by acquiring the necessary knowledge and skills to make informed decisions regarding their health and well-being.

Future research efforts should include a focus on understanding the educational needs of HSCT survivors and caregivers, motivation for adherence to medication administration, and recommended screening and interventions to improve the HRQOL of survivors and caregivers.

References

Afessa, B., Litzow, M.R., & Tefferi, A. (2001). *Bronchiolitis obliterans* and other late onset non-infectious pulmonary complications in hematopoietic stem cell transplantation. *Bone Marrow Transplantation, 28,* 425–434. https://doi.org/10.1038/sj.bmt.1703142

Alberti, K.G.M.M., Eckel, R.H., Grundy, S.M., Zimmet, P.Z., Cleeman, J.I., Donato, K.A., … Smith, S.C., Jr. (2009). Harmonizing the metabolic syndrome: A joint interim statement of the International Diabetes Federation Task Force on Epidemiology and Prevention; National Heart, Lung, and Blood Institute; American Heart Association; World Heart Federation; International Atherosclerosis Society; and International Association for the Study of Obesity. *Circulation, 120,* 1640–1645. https://doi.org/10.1161/circulationaha.109.192644

American Psychological Association. (n.d.). Individuals with Disability Education Act (IDEA). Retrieved from https://www.apa.org/advocacy/education/idea/index

Andrykowski, M.A., Bishop, M.M., Hahn, E.A., Cella, D.F., Beaumont, J.L., Brady, M.J., … Wingard, J.R. (2005). Long-term health-related quality of life, growth, and spiritual well-being after hematopoietic stem-cell transplantation. *Journal of Clinical Oncology, 23,* 599–608. https://doi.org/10.1200/jco.2005.03.189

Annaloro, C., Usardi, P., Airaghi, L., Giunta, V., Forti, S., Orsatti, A., … Lambertenghi Deliliers, G. (2008). Prevalence of metabolic syndrome in long-term survivors of hematopoietic stem cell transplantation. *Bone Marrow Transplantation, 41,* 797–804. https://doi.org/10.1038/sj.bmt.1705972

Armenian, S.H., & Chow, E.J. (2014). Cardiovascular disease in survivors of hematopoietic cell transplantation. *Cancer, 120,* 469–479. https://doi.org/10.1002/cncr.28444

Armenian, S.H., Sun, C.-L., Vase, T., Ness, K.K., Blum, E., Francisco, L., … Bhatia, S. (2012). Cardiovascular risk factors in hematopoietic cell transplantation survivors: role in development of subsequent cardiovascular disease. *Blood, 120,* 4505–4512. https://doi.org/10.1182/blood-2012-06-437178

Armstrong, G.T., Liu, Q., Yasui, Y., Neglia, J.P., Leisenring, W., Robison, L.L., & Mertens, A.C. (2009). Late mortality among 5-year survivors of childhood cancer: A summary from the Childhood Cancer Survivor Study. *Journal of Clinical Oncology, 27,* 2328–2338. https://doi.org/10.1200/jco.2008.21.1425

Asano-Mori, Y., Kanda, Y., Oshima, K., Kako, S., Shinohara, A., Nakasone, H., … Kurokawa, M. (2008). Clinical features of late cytomegalovirus infection after hematopoietic stem cell transplantation. *International Journal of Hematology, 87,* 310–318. https://doi.org/10.1007/s12185-008-0051-1

Atsuta, Y., Hirakawa, A., Nakasone, H., Kurosawa, S., Oshima, K., Sakai, R., … Yamashita, T. (2016). Late mortality and causes of death among long-term survivors after allogeneic stem cell transplantation. *Biology of Blood and Marrow Transplantation, 22,* 1702–1709. https://doi.org/10.1016/j.bbmt.2016.05.019

Au, B.K.C., Au, M.A., & Chien, J.W. (2011). Bronchiolitis obliterans syndrome epidemiology after allogeneic hematopoietic cell transplantation. *Biology of Blood and Marrow Transplantation, 17,* 1072–1078. https://doi.org/10.1016/j.bbmt.2010.11.018

Bacigalupo, A., Chien, J., Barisione, G., & Pavletic, S. (2012). Late pulmonary complications after allogeneic hematopoietic stem cell transplantation: Diagnosis, monitoring, prevention, and treatment. *Seminars in Hematology, 49,* 15–24. https://doi.org/10.1053/j.seminhematol.2011.10.005

Baker, K.S., Gurney, J.G., Ness, K.K., Bhatia, R., Forman, S.J., Francisco, L., … Bhatia, S. (2004). Late effects in survivors of chronic myeloid leukemia treated with hematopoietic cell transplantation: Results from the Bone Marrow Transplant Survivor Study. *Blood, 104,* 1898–1906. https://doi.org/10.1182/blood-2004-03-1010

Baker, K.S., Ness, K.K., Steinberger, J., Carter, A., Francisco, L., Burns, L.J., … Bhatia, S. (2007). Diabetes, hypertension, and cardiovascular events in survivors of hematopoietic cell transplantation: A report from the Bone Marrow Transplantation Survivor Study. *Blood, 109,* 1765–1772. https://doi.org/10.1182/blood-2006-05-022335

Battiwalla, M., Hashmi, S., Majhail, N., Pavletic, S., Savani, B.N., & Shelburne, N. (2017). National Institutes of Health Hematopoietic Cell Transplantation Late Effects Initiative: Developing recommendations to improve survivorship and long-term outcomes. *Biology of Blood and Marrow Transplantation, 23,* 6–9. https://doi.org/10.1016/j.bbmt.2016.10.020

Beattie, S., & Lebel, S. (2011). The experience of caregivers of hematological cancer patients undergoing a hematopoietic stem cell transplant: A comprehensive literature review. *Psycho-Oncology, 20,* 1137–1150. https://doi.org/10.1002/pon.1962

Berger, C., Le-Gallo, B., Donadieu, J., Richard, O., Devergie, A., Galambrun, C., ... Stephan, J.L. (2005). Late thyroid toxicity in 153 long-term survivors of allogeneic bone marrow transplantation for acute lymphoblastic leukaemia. *Bone Marrow Transplantation, 35,* 991–995. https://doi.org/10.1038/sj.bmt.1704945

Bevans, M.F., El-Jawahri, A., Tierney, D.K., Wiener, L., Wood, W.A., Hoodin, F., ... Syrjala, K.L. (2017). National Institutes of Health Hematopoietic Cell Transplantation Late Effects Initiative: The Patient-Centered Outcomes Working Group report. *Biology of Blood and Marrow Transplantation, 23,* 538–551. https://doi.org/10.1016/j.bbmt.2016.09.011

Bevans, M.F., Marden, S., Leidy, N.K., Soeken, K., Cusack, G., Rivera, P., ... Barrett, A.J. (2006). Health-related quality of life in patients receiving reduced-intensity conditioning allogeneic hematopoietic stem cell transplantation. *Bone Marrow Transplantation, 38,* 101–109. https://doi.org/10.1038/sj.bmt.1705406

Bevans, M.F., Mitchell, S.A., Barrett, J.A., Bishop, M.R., Childs, R., Fowler, D., ... Yang, L. (2014). Symptom distress predicts long-term health and well-being in allogeneic stem cell transplantation survivors. *Biology of Blood and Marrow Transplantation, 20,* 387–395. https://doi.org/10.1016/j.bbmt.2013.12.001

Bevans, M.F., Ross, A., Wehrlen, L., Klagholz, S.D., Yang, L., Childs, R., ... Pacak, K. (2016). Documenting stress in caregivers of transplantation patients: Initial evidence of HPA dysregulation. *Stress, 19,* 175–184. https://doi.org/10.3109/10253890.2016.1146670

Bevans, M.F., & Sternberg, E.M. (2012). Caregiving burden, stress, and health effects among family caregivers of adult cancer patients. *JAMA, 307,* 398–403. https://doi.org/10.1001/jama.2012.29

Bhatia, S., Armenian, S.H., & Landier, W. (2017). How I monitor long-term and late effects after blood or marrow transplantation. *Blood, 130,* 1302–1314. https://doi.org/10.1182/blood-2017-03-725671

Bhatia, S., Francisco, L., Carter, A., Sun, C.-L., Baker, K.S., Gurney, J.G., ... Weisdorf, D.J. (2007). Late mortality after allogeneic hematopoietic cell transplantation and functional status of long-term survivors: Report from the Bone Marrow Transplant Survivor Study. *Blood, 110,* 3784–3792. https://doi.org/10.1182/blood-2007-03-082933

Bhatia, S., Robison, L.L., Francisco, L., Carter, A., Liu, Y., Grant, M., ... Forman, S.J. (2005). Late mortality in survivors of autologous hematopoietic-cell transplantation: Report from the Bone Marrow Transplant Survivor Study. *Blood, 105,* 4215–4222. https://doi.org/10.1182/blood-2005-01-0035

Bishop, M.M., Beaumont, J.L., Hahn, E.A., Cella, D., Andrykowski, M.A., Brady, M.J., ... Wingard, J.R. (2007). Late effects of cancer and hematopoietic stem-cell transplantation on spouses or partners compared with survivors and survivor-matched controls. *Journal of Clinical Oncology, 25,* 1403–1411. https://doi.org/10.1200/jco.2006.07.5705

Bjorklund, A., Aschan, J., Labopin, M., Remberger, M., Ringden, O., Winiarski, J., & Ljungman, P. (2007). Risk factors for fatal infectious complications developing late after allogeneic stem cell transplantation. *Bone Marrow Transplantation, 40,* 1055–1062. https://doi.org/10.1038/sj.bmt.1705856

Boeckh, M. (2011). Complications, diagnosis, management, and prevention of CMV infections: Current and future. *Hematology: American Society of Hematology Education Program Book, 2011,* 305–309. https://doi.org/10.1182/asheducation-2011.1.305

Boeckh, M., Englund, J., Li, Y., Miller, C., Cross, A., Fernandez, H., ... Whitley, R. (2007). Randomized controlled multicenter trial of aerosolized ribavirin for respiratory syncytial virus upper respiratory tract infection in hematopoietic cell transplant recipients. *Clinical Infectious Diseases, 44,* 245–249. https://doi.org/10.1086/509930

Boeckh, M., Leisenring, W., Riddell, S.R., Bowden, R.A., Huang, M.-L., Myerson, D., ... Corey, L. (2003). Late cytomegalovirus disease and mortality in recipients of allogeneic hematopoietic stem cell transplants: Importance of viral load and T-cell immunity. *Blood, 101,* 407–414. https://doi.org/10.1182/blood-2002-03-0993

Boeckh, M., Murphy, W.J., & Peggs, K.S. (2015). Recent advances in cytomegalovirus: An update on pharmacologic and cellular thera-

pies. *Biology of Blood and Marrow Transplantation, 21,* 24–29. https://doi.org/10.1016/j.bbmt.2014.11.002

Bosch, M., Khan, F.M., & Storek, J. (2012). Immune reconstitution after hematopoietic cell transplantation. *Current Opinion in Hematology, 19,* 324–335. https://doi.org/10.1097/moh.0b013e328353bc7d

Buchbinder, D., Kelly, D.L., Duarte, R.F., Auletta, J.J., Bhatt, N., Byrne, M., ... Shaw, B.E. (2018). Neurocognitive dysfunction in hematopoietic cell transplant recipients: Expert review from the Late Effects and Quality of Life Working Committee of the CIBMTR and Complications and Quality of Life Working Party of the EBMT. *Bone Marrow Transplantation, 53,* 535–555. https://doi.org/10.1038/s41409-017-0055-7

Buchsel, P.C. (2009). Survivorship issues in hematopoietic stem cell transplantation. *Seminars in Oncology Nursing, 25,* 159–169. https://doi.org/10.1016/j.soncn.2009.03.003

Bush, N.E., Donaldson, G.W., Haberman, M.H., Dacanay, R., & Sullivan, K.M. (2000). Conditional and unconditional estimation of multidimensional quality of life after hematopoietic stem cell transplantation: A longitudinal follow-up of 415 patients. *Biology of Blood and Marrow Transplantation, 6,* 576–591. https://doi.org/10.1016/s1083-8791(00)70067-x

Chau, M.M., Kong, D.C.M., van Hal, S.J., Urbancic, K., Trubiano, J.A., Cassumbhoy, M., ... Worth, L.J. (2014). Consensus guidelines for optimising antifungal drug delivery and monitoring to avoid toxicity and improve outcomes in patients with haematological malignancy, 2014. *Internal Medicine Journal, 44,* 1364–1388. https://doi.org/10.1111/imj.12600

Chemaly, R.F., Ghosh, S., Bodey, G.P., Rohatgi, N., Safdar, A., Keating, M.J., ... Raad, I.I. (2006). Respiratory viral infections in adults with hematologic malignancies and human stem cell transplantation recipients: A retrospective study at a major cancer center. *Medicine, 85,* 278–287. https://doi.org/10.1097/01.md.0000232560.22098.4e

Chemaly, R.F., Hanmod, S.S., Rathod, D.B., Ghantoji, S.S., Jiang, Y., Doshi, A., ... Champlin, R. (2012). The characteristics and outcomes of parainfluenza virus infections in 200 patients with leukemia or recipients of hematopoietic stem cell transplantation. *Blood, 119,* 2738–2745. https://doi.org/10.1182/blood-2011-08-371112

Chemaly, R.F., Shah, D.P., & Boeckh, M.J. (2014). Management of respiratory viral infections in hematopoietic cell transplant recipients and patients with hematologic malignancies. *Clinical Infectious Diseases, 59*(Suppl. 5), S344–S351. https://doi.org/10.1093/cid/ciu623

Chien, J.W., Martin, P.J., Gooley, T.A., Flowers, M.E., Heckbert, S.R., Nichols, W.G., & Clark, J.G. (2003). Airflow obstruction after myeloablative allogeneic hematopoietic stem cell transplantation. *American Journal of Respiratory and Critical Care Medicine, 168,* 208–214. https://doi.org/10.1164/rccm.200212-1468oc

Chow, E.J., Liu, W., Srivastava, K., Leisenring, W.M., Hayashi, R.J., Sklar, C.A., ... Baker, K.S. (2013). Differential effects of radiotherapy on growth and endocrine function among acute leukemia survivors: A childhood cancer survivor study report. *Pediatric Blood and Cancer, 60,* 110–115. https://doi.org/10.1002/pbc.24198

Clancy, C.J., & Nguyen, M.H. (2011). Long-term voriconazole and skin cancer: Is there cause for concern? *Current Infectious Disease Reports, 13,* 536–543. https://doi.org/10.1007/s11908-011-0220-x

Cohen, A., Békássy, A.N., Gaiero, A., Faraci, M., Zecca, S., Tichelli, A., & Dini, G. (2008). Endocrinological late complications after hematopoietic SCT in children. *Bone Marrow Transplantation, 41*(Suppl. 2), S43–S48. https://doi.org/10.1038/bmt.2008.54

Cubukcu, C.E., Sevinir, B., & Ercan, İ. (2012). Disturbed dental development of permanent teeth in children with solid tumors and lymphomas. *Pediatric Blood and Cancer, 58,* 80–84. https://doi.org/10.1002/pbc.22902

D'Angelo, C.R., Kocherginsky, M., Pisano, J., Bishop, M.R., Godley, L.A., Kline, J., ... Artz, A.S. (2016). Incidence and predictors of respiratory viral infections by multiplex PCR in allogeneic hematopoietic cell transplant recipients 50 years and older including geriatric assessment. *Leukemia and Lymphoma, 57,* 1807–1813. https://doi.org/10.3109/10428194.2015.1113279

DeBaun, M.R., Armstrong, F.D., McKinstry, R.C., Ware, R.E., Vichinsky, E., & Kirkham, F.J. (2012). Silent cerebral infarcts: A review on a prevalent and progressive cause of neurologic injury in sickle cell anemia. *Blood, 119,* 4587–4596. https://doi.org/10.1182/blood-2011-02-272682

DeFilipp, Z., Duarte, R.F., Snowden, J.A., Majhail, N.S., Greenfield, D.M., Miranda, J.L., ... Shaw, B.E. (2016). Metabolic syndrome and cardiovascular disease after hematopoietic cell transplantation: Screening and preventive practice recommendations from the CIBMTR and EBMT. *Biology of Blood and Marrow Transplantation, 22,* 1493–1503. https://doi.org/10.1016/j.bbmt.2016.05.007

Dudakov, J.A., Perales, M.-A., & van den Brink, M.R.M. (2016). Immune reconstitution following hematopoietic cell transplantation. In S.J. Forman, R.S. Negrin, J.H. Antin, & F.R. Appelbaum (Eds.), *Thomas' hematopoietic cell transplantation: Stem cell transplantation* (5th ed., pp. 160–165). https://doi.org/10.1002/9781118416426.ch15

Dudek, A.Z., & Mahaseth, H. (2006). Hematopoietic stem cell transplant–related airflow obstruction. *Current Opinion in Oncology, 18,* 115–119. https://doi.org/10.1097/01.cco.0000208782.61452.08

Dvorak, C.C., Gracia, C.R., Sanders, J.E., Cheng, E.Y., Baker, K.S., Pulsipher, M.A., & Petryk, A. (2011). NCI, NHLBI/PBMTC first international conference on late effects after pediatric hematopoietic cell transplantation: Endocrine challenges—Thyroid dysfunction, growth impairment, bone health, and reproductive risks. *Biology of Blood and Marrow Transplantation, 17,* 1725–1738. https://doi.org/10.1016/j.bbmt.2011.10.006

Dziedzic, M., Sadowska-Krawczenko, I., & Styczynski, J. (2017). Risk factors for cytomegalovirus infection after allogeneic hematopoietic cell transplantation in malignancies: Proposal for classification. *Anticancer Research, 37,* 6551–6556. https://doi.org/10.21873/anticanres.12111

Effinger, K.E., Migliorati, C.A., Hudson, M.M., McMullen, K.P., Kaste, S.C., Ruble, K., ... Castellino, S.M. (2014). Oral and dental late effects in survivors of childhood cancer: A Children's Oncology Group report. *Supportive Care in Cancer, 22,* 2009–2019. https://doi.org/10.1007/s00520-014-2260-x

Epstein, J.B., Raber-Drulacher, J.E., Wilkins, A., Chavarria, M.-G., & Myint, H. (2009). Advances in hematologic stem cell transplant: An update for oral health care providers. *Oral Surgery, Oral Medicine, Oral Pathology, Oral Radiology, and Endodontology, 107,* 301–312. https://doi.org/10.1016/j.tripleo.2008.12.006

Erard, V., Guthrie, K.A., Seo, S., Smith, J., Huang, M., Chien, J., ... Boeckh, M. (2015). Reduced mortality of cytomegalovirus pneumonia after hematopoietic cell transplantation due to antiviral therapy and changes in transplantation practices. *Clinical Infectious Diseases, 61,* 31–39. https://doi.org/10.1093/cid/civ215

Faraci, M., Békássy, A.N., De Fazio, V., Tichelli, A., & Dini, G. (2008). Non-endocrine late complications in children after allogeneic haematopoietic SCT. *Bone Marrow Transplantation, 41*(Suppl. 2), S49–S57. https://doi.org/10.1038/bmt.2008.55

Felicetti, F., Manicone, R., Corrias, A., Manieri, C., Biasin, E., Bini, I., ... Brignardello, E. (2011). Endocrine late effects after total body irradiation in patients who received hematopoietic cell transplantation during childhood: A retrospective study from a single institution. *Journal of Cancer Research and Clinical Oncology, 137,* 1343–1348. https://doi.org/10.1007/s00432-011-1004-2

Filipovich, A.H., Weisdorf, D., Pavletic, S., Socie, G., Wingard, J.R., Lee, S.J., ... Flowers, M.E.D. (2005). National Institutes of Health consensus development project on criteria for clinical trials in chronic graft-versus-host disease: I. Diagnosis and Staging Working Group report. *Biology of Blood and Marrow Transplantation, 11,* 945–956. https://doi.org/10.1016/j.bbmt.2005.09.004

Fleming, S., Yannakou, C.K., Haeusler, G.M., Clark, J., Grigg, A., Heath, C.H., ... Slavin, M.A. (2014). Consensus guidelines for antifungal prophylaxis in haematological malignancy and haemopoietic stem cell transplantation, 2014. *Internal Medicine Journal, 44,* 1283–1297. https://doi.org/10.1111/imj.12595

Fraser, C.J., Bhatia, S., Ness, K., Carter, A., Francisco, L., Arora, M., ... Baker, K.S. (2006). Impact of chronic graft-versus-host disease on the health status of hematopoietic cell transplantation survivors: A report from the Bone Marrow Transplant Survivor Study. *Blood, 108,* 2867–2873. https://doi.org/10.1182/blood-2006-02-003954

Fukuda, T., Hackman, R.C., Guthrie, K.A., Sandmaier, B.M., Boeckh, M., Maris, M.B., ... Madtes, D.K. (2003). Risks and outcomes of idiopathic pneumonia syndrome after nonmyeloablative and conventional conditioning regimens for allogeneic hematopoietic stem cell transplantation. *Blood, 102,* 2777–2785. https://doi.org/10.1182/blood-2003-05-1597

Garcia, R., Raad, I., Abi-Said, D., Bodey, G., Champlin, R., Tarrand, J., ... Whimbey, E. (1997). Nosocomial respiratory syncytial virus infections: Prevention and control in bone marrow transplant patients. *Infection Control and Hospital Epidemiology, 18,* 412–416. https://doi.org/10.2307/30141248

Gawade, P.L., Hudson, M.M., Kaste, S.C., Neglia, J.P., Wasilewski-Masker, K., Constine, L.S., ... Ness, K.K. (2014). A systematic review of selected musculoskeletal late effects in survivors of childhood cancer. *Current Pediatric Reviews, 10,* 249–262. https://doi.org/10.2174/1573400510666141114223827

Girmenia, C., Raiola, A.M., Piciocchi, A., Algarotti, A., Stanzani, M., Cudillo, L., ... Locasciulli, A. (2014). Incidence and outcome of invasive fungal diseases after allogeneic stem cell transplantation: A prospective study of the Gruppo Italiano Trapianto Midollo Osseo (GITMO). *Biology of Blood and Marrow Transplantation, 20,* 872–880. https://doi.org/10.1016/j.bbmt.2014.03.004

Gooley, T.A., Chien, J.W., Pergam, S.A., Hingorani, S., Sorror, M.L., Boeckh, M., ... McDonald, G.B. (2010). Reduced mortality after allogeneic hematopoietic-cell transplantation. *New England Journal of Medicine, 363,* 2091–2101. https://doi.org/10.1056/NEJMoa1004383

Hahn, T., McCarthy, P.L., Jr., Hassebroek, A., Bredeson, C., Gajewski, J.L., Hale, G.A., ... Majhail, N.S. (2013). Significant improvement in survival after allogeneic hematopoietic cell transplantation during a period of significantly increased use, older recipient age, and use of unrelated donors. *Journal of Clinical Oncology, 31,* 2437–2449. https://doi.org/10.1200/jco.2012.46.6193

Hammell, M.T.K., Bunin, N., Edgar, J.C., & Jaramillo, D. (2013). Paraphyseal changes on bone-age studies predict risk of delayed radiation-associated skeletal complications following total body irradiation. *Pediatric Radiology, 43,* 1152–1158. https://doi.org/10.1007/s00247-013-2669-2

Harder, H., Cornelissen, J.J., Van Gool, A.R., Duivenvoorden, H.J., Eijkenboom, W.M.H., & van den Bent, M.J. (2002). Cognitive functioning and quality of life in long-term adult survivors of bone marrow transplantation. *Cancer, 95,* 183–192. https://doi.org/10.1002/cncr.10627

Harder, H., Duivenvoorden, H.J., van Gool, A.R., Cornelissen, J.J., & van den Bent, M.J. (2006). Neurocognitive functions and quality of life in haematological patients receiving haematopoietic stem cell grafts: A one-year follow-up pilot study. *Journal of Clinical and Experimental Neuropsychology, 28,* 283–293. https://doi.org/10.1080/13803390490918147

Hashmi, S., Carpenter, P., Khera, N., Tichelli, A., & Savani, B.N. (2015). Lost in transition: The essential need for long-term follow-up clinic for blood and marrow transplantation survivors. *Biology of Blood and Marrow Transplantation, 21,* 225–232. https://doi.org/10.1016/j.bbmt.2014.06.035

Hildebrandt, G.C., Fazekas, T., Lawitschka, A., Bertz, H., Greinix, H., Halter, J., ... Wolff, D. (2011). Diagnosis and treatment of pulmonary chronic GVHD: Report from the Consensus Conference on Clinical Practice in Chronic GVHD. *Bone Marrow Transplantation, 46,* 1283–1295. https://doi.org/10.1038/bmt.2011.35

Hirsch, H., & Pergam, S.A. (2016). Human adenovirus, polyomavirus, and parvovirus infections in patients undergoing hematopoietic stem cell transplantation. In S.J. Forman, R.S. Negrin, J.H. Antin, & F.R. Appelbaum (Eds.), *Thomas' hematopoietic cell transplantation: Stem cell transplantation* (5th ed., pp. 1129–1139). https://doi.org/10.1002/9781118416426.ch93

Hjermstad, M.J., Knobel, H., Brinch, L., Fayers, P.M., Loge, J.H., Holte, H., & Kaasa, S. (2004). A prospective study of health-related quality of life, fatigue, anxiety and depression 3–5 years after stem cell transplantation. *Bone Marrow Transplantation, 34,* 257–266. https://doi.org/10.1038/sj.bmt.1704561

Ho, D.Y., & Arvin, A.M. (2016). Varicella zoster virus infections. In S.J. Forman, R.S. Negrin, J.H. Antin, & F.R. Appelbaum (Eds.), *Thomas' hematopoietic cell transplantation: Stem cell transplantation* (5th ed., pp. 1085–1104). https://doi.org/10.1002/9781118416426.ch89

Hockenbery, D.M., Strasser, S.I., & McDonald, G.B. (2016). Gastrointestinal and hepatic complications. In S.J. Forman, R.S. Negrin, J.H. Antin, & F.R. Appelbaum (Eds.), *Thomas' hematopoietic cell transplantation: Stem cell transplantation* (5th ed., pp. 1140–1155). https://doi.org/10.1002/9781118416426.ch94

Hubmann, M., Fritsch, S., Zoellner, A.-K., Prevalsek, D., Engel, N., Bücklein, V., ... Tischer, J. (2016). Occurrence, risk factors and outcome of adenovirus infection in adult recipients of allogeneic hematopoietic stem cell transplantation. *Journal of Clinical Virology, 82*, 33–40. https://doi.org/10.1016/j.jcv.2016.07.002

Hull, K.M., Kerridge, I., & Schifter, M. (2012). Long-term oral complications of allogeneic haematopoietic SCT. *Bone Marrow Transplantation, 47*, 265–270. https://doi.org/10.1038/bmt.2011.63

Husain, S., Mooney, M.L., Danziger-Isakov, L., Mattner, F., Singh, N., Avery, R., ... Hannan, M. (2011). A 2010 working formulation for the standardization of definitions of infections in cardiothoracic transplant recipients. *Journal of Heart and Lung Transplantation, 30*, 361–374. https://doi.org/10.1016/j.healun.2011.01.701

Isomaa, B., Almgren, P., Tuomi, T., Forsén, B., Lahti, K., Nissén, M., ... Groop, L. (2001). Cardiovascular morbidity and mortality associated with the metabolic syndrome. *Diabetes Care, 24*, 683–689. https://doi.org/10.2337/diacare.24.4.683

Jackson, T.J., Mostoufi-Moab, S., Hill-Kayser, C., Balamuth, N.J., & Arkader, A. (2018). Musculoskeletal complications following total body irradiation in hematopoietic stem cell transplant patients. *Pediatric Blood and Cancer, 65*, e26905. https://doi.org/10.1002/pbc.26905

Jensen, S.B., Pedersen, A.M.L., Vissink, A., Andersen, E., Brown, C.G., Davies, A.N., ... Brennan, M.T. (2010). A systematic review of salivary gland hypofunction and xerostomia induced by cancer therapies: Prevalence, severity and impact on quality of life. *Supportive Care in Cancer, 18*, 1039–1060. https://doi.org/10.1007/s00520-010-0827-8

Jeon, M., Yoo, I.Y., Kim, S., & Lee, J. (2015). Post-traumatic growth in survivors of allogeneic hematopoietic stem cell transplantation. *Psycho-Oncology, 24*, 871–877. https://doi.org/10.1002/pon.3724

Jim, H.S.L., Evans, B., Jeong, J.M., Gonzalez, B.D., Johnston, L., Nelson, A.M., ... Palesh, O. (2014). Sleep disruption in hematopoietic cell transplantation recipients: Prevalence, severity, and clinical management. *Biology of Blood and Marrow Transplantation, 20*, 1465–1484. https://doi.org/10.1016/j.bbmt.2014.04.010

Kamoi, M., Ogawa, Y., Dogru, M., Uchino, M., Kawashima, M., Goto, E., ... Tsubota, K. (2007). Spontaneous lacrimal punctal occlusion associated with ocular chronic graft-versus-host disease. *Current Eye Research, 32*, 837–842. https://doi.org/10.1080/02713680701586409

Kassis, C., Champlin, R.E., Hachem, R.Y., Hosing, C., Tarrand, J.J., Perego, C.A., ... Chemaly, R.F. (2010). Detection and control of a nosocomial respiratory syncytial virus outbreak in a stem cell transplantation unit: The role of palivizumab. *Biology of Blood and Marrow Transplantation, 16*, 1265–1271. https://doi.org/10.1016/j.bbmt.2010.03.011

Kenney, L.B., Cohen, L.E., Shnorhavorian, M., Metzger, M.L., Lockart, B., Hijiya, N., ... Meacham, L. (2012). Male reproductive health after childhood, adolescent, and young adult cancers: A report from the Children's Oncology Group. *Journal of Clinical Oncology, 30*, 3408–3416. https://doi.org/10.1200/jco.2011.38.6938

Kersting, S., Hené, R.J., Koomans, H.A., & Verdonck, L.F. (2007). Chronic kidney disease after myeloablative allogeneic hematopoietic stem cell transplantation. *Biology of Blood and Marrow Transplantation, 13*, 1169–1175. https://doi.org/10.1016/j.bbmt.2007.06.008

Kollmannsberger, C., Beyer, J., Droz, J.P., Harstrick, A., Hartmann, J.T., Biron, P., ... Bokemeyer, C. (1998). Secondary leukemia following high cumulative doses of etoposide in patients treated for advanced germ cell tumors. *Journal of Clinical Oncology, 16*, 3386–3391. https://doi.org/10.1200/jco.1998.16.10.3386

Kontoyiannis, D.P., Marr, K.A., Park, B.J., Alexander, B.D., Anaissie, E.J., Walsh, T.J., ... Pappas, P.G. (2010). Prospective surveillance for invasive fungal infections in hematopoietic stem cell transplant recipients, 2001–2006: Overview of the Transplant-Associated Infection Surveillance Network (TRANSNET) Database. *Clinical Infectious Diseases, 50*, 1091–1100. https://doi.org/10.1086/651263

Kotton, C.N., Kumar, D., Caliendo, A.M., Åsberg, A., Chou, S., Danziger-Isakov, L., & Atul, H. (2013). Updated International Consensus Guidelines on the Management of Cytomegalovirus in Solid-Organ Transplantation. *Transplantation, 96*, 333–360. https://doi.org/10.1097/tp.0b013e31829df29d

Landgren, O., Gilbert, E.S., Rizzo, J.D., Socié, G., Banks, P.M., Sobocinski, K.A., ... Curtis, R.E. (2009). Risk factors for lymphoproliferative disorders after allogeneic hematopoietic cell transplantation. *Blood, 113*, 4992–5001. https://doi.org/10.1182/blood-2008-09-178046

Laudenslager, M.L., Simoneau, T.L., Kilbourn, K., Natvig, C., Philips, S., Spradley, J., ... Mikulich-Gilbertson, S.K. (2015). A randomized control trial of a psychosocial intervention for caregivers of allogeneic hematopoietic stem cell transplant patients: Effects on distress. *Bone Marrow Transplantation, 50*, 1110–1118. https://doi.org/10.1038/bmt.2015.104

Lee, S.J., Kim, H.T., Ho, V.T., Cutler, C., Alyea, E.P., Soiffer, R.J., & Antin, J.H. (2006). Quality of life associated with acute and chronic graft-versus-host disease. *Bone Marrow Transplantation, 38*, 305–310. https://doi.org/10.1038/sj.bmt.1705434

Li, Z., Mewawalla, P., Stratton, P., Yong, A.S.M., Shaw, B.E., Hashmi, S., ... Rovó, A. (2015). Sexual health in hematopoietic stem cell transplant recipients. *Cancer, 121*, 4124–4131. https://doi.org/10.1002/cncr.29675

Lion, T., Baumgartinger, R., Watzinger, F., Matthes-Martin, S., Suda, M., Preuner, S., ... Gadner, H. (2003). Molecular monitoring of adenovirus in peripheral blood after allogeneic bone marrow transplantation permits early diagnosis of disseminated disease. *Blood, 102*, 1114–1120. https://doi.org/10.1182/blood-2002-07-2152

Liu, S.-C., Tsai, C.-C., & Huang, C.-H. (2004). Atypical slipped capital femoral epiphysis after radiotherapy and chemotherapy. *Clinical Orthopaedics and Related Research, 426*, 212–218. https://doi.org/10.1097/01.blo.0000136655.51838.84

Ljungman, P., Cordonnier, C., Einsele, H., Englund, J., Machado, C.M., Storek, J., & Small, T. (2009). Vaccination of hematopoietic cell transplant recipients. *Bone Marrow Transplantation, 44*, 521–526. https://doi.org/10.1038/bmt.2009.263

Ljungman, P., Hakki, M., & Boeckh, M. (2010). Cytomegalovirus in hematopoietic stem cell transplant recipients. *Infectious Disease Clinics of North America, 24*, 319–337. https://doi.org/10.1016/j.idc.2010.01.008

Ljungman, P., Ward, K.N., Crooks, B.N.A., Parker, A., Martino, R., Shaw, P.J., ... Cordonnier, C. (2001). Respiratory virus infections after stem cell transplantation: A prospective study from the Infectious Diseases Working Party of the European Group for Blood and Marrow Transplantation. *Bone Marrow Transplantation, 28*, 479–484. https://doi.org/10.1038/sj.bmt.1703139

Majhail, N.S. (2008). Old and new cancers after hematopoietic-cell transplantation. *Hematology: American Society of Hematology Education Program Book, 2008*, 142–149. https://doi.org/10.1182/asheducation-2008.1.142

Majhail, N.S. (2011). Secondary cancers following allogeneic haematopoietic cell transplantation in adults. *British Journal of Haematology, 154*, 301–310. https://doi.org/10.1111/j.1365-2141.2011.08756.x

Majhail, N.S. (2017). Long-term complications after hematopoietic cell transplantation. *Hematology/Oncology and Stem Cell Therapy, 10*, 220–227. https://doi.org/10.1016/j.hemonc.2017.05.009

Majhail, N.S., Brazauskas, R., Rizzo, J.D., Sobecks, R.M., Wang, Z., Horowitz, M.M., ... Socie, G. (2011). Secondary solid cancers after allogeneic hematopoietic cell transplantation using busulfan-cyclophosphamide conditioning. *Blood, 117*, 316–322. https://doi.org/10.1182/blood-2010-07-294629

Majhail, N.S., Challa, T.R., Mulrooney, D.A., Baker, K.S., & Burns, L.J. (2009). Hypertension and diabetes mellitus in adult and pediatric survivors of allogeneic hematopoietic cell transplantation. *Biology of Blood and Marrow Transplantation, 15*, 1100–1107. https://doi.org/10.1016/j.bbmt.2009.05.010

Majhail, N.S., Flowers, M.E., Ness, K.K., Jagasia, M., Carpenter, P.A., Arora, M., ... Burns, L.J. (2009). High prevalence of metabolic syndrome after allogeneic hematopoietic cell transplantation. *Bone Marrow Transplantation, 43*, 49–54. https://doi.org/10.1038/bmt.2008.263

Majhail, N.S., Rizzo, J.D., Lee, S.J., Aljurf, M., Atsuta, Y., Bonfim, C., ... Tichelli, A. (2012). Recommended screening and preventive practices for long-term survivors after hematopoietic cell transplantation. *Biology of Blood and Marrow Transplantation, 18*, 348–371. https://doi.org/10.1016/j.bbmt.2011.12.519

Majhail, N.S., Tao, L., Bredeson, C., Davies, S., Dehn, J., Gajewski, J.L., ... Kuntz, K.M. (2013). Prevalence of hematopoietic cell transplant survivors in the United States. *Biology of Blood and Marrow Transplantation, 19*, 1498–1501. https://doi.org/10.1016/j.bbmt.2013.07.020

Marr, K.A. (2008). Primary antifungal prophylaxis in hematopoietic stem cell transplant recipients: Clinical implications of recent studies. *Current *Opinion in Infectious Diseases, 21,* 409–414. https://doi.org/10.1097/qco.0b013e328307c7d9

Martino, R., Porras, R.P., Rabella, N., Williams, J.V., Rámila, E., Margall, N., … Sierra, J. (2005). Prospective study of the incidence, clinical features, and outcome of symptomatic upper and lower respiratory tract infections by respiratory viruses in adult recipients of hematopoietic stem cell transplants for hematologic malignancies. *Biology of Blood and Marrow Transplantation, 11,* 781–796. https://doi.org/10.1016/j.bbmt.2005.07.007

McClune, B., Majhail, N.S., & Flowers, M.E.D. (2012). Bone loss and avascular necrosis of bone after hematopoietic cell transplantation. *Seminars in Hematology, 49,* 59–65. https://doi.org/10.1053/j.seminhematol.2011.10.007

McDonald, G.B. (2006). Review article: Management of hepatic disease following haematopoietic cell transplant. *Alimentary Pharmacology and Therapeutics, 24,* 441–452. https://doi.org/10.1111/j.1365-2036.2006.03001.x

McDonald, G.B. (2010). Hepatobiliary complications of hematopoietic cell transplantation, 40 years on. *Hepatology, 51,* 1450–1460. https://doi.org/10.1002/hep.23533

McMillen, K.K., Schmidt, E.M., Storer, B.E., & Bar, M. (2014). Metabolic syndrome appears early after hematopoietic cell transplantation. *Metabolic Syndrome and Related Disorders, 12,* 367–371. https://doi.org/10.1089/met.2014.0051

Melenhorst, J.J., Leen, A.M., Bollard, C.M., Quigley, M.F., Price, D.A., Rooney, C.M., … Heslop, H.E. (2010). Allogeneic virus-specific T cells with HLA alloreactivity do not produce GVHD in human subjects. *Blood, 116,* 4700–4702. https://doi.org/10.1182/blood-2010-06-289991

Milano, F., Campbell, A.P., Guthrie, K.A., Kuypers, J., Englund, J.A., Corey, L., & Boeckh, M. (2010). Human rhinovirus and coronavirus detection among allogeneic hematopoietic stem cell transplantation recipients. *Blood, 115,* 2088–2094. https://doi.org/10.1182/blood-2009-09-244152

Motolese, E., Rubegni, P., Poggiali, S., Motolese, P.A., Marotta, G., Russo, L., … Fimiani, M. (2007). Ocular manifestations of chronic graft-versus-host disease in patients treated with extracorporeal photochemotherapy. *European Journal of Ophthalmology, 17,* 961–969. https://doi.org/10.1177/112067210701700615

Mulcahy Levy, J.M., Tello, T., Giller, R., Wilkening, G., Quinones, R., Keating, A.K., & Liu, A.K. (2013). Late effects of total body irradiation and hematopoietic stem cell transplant in children under 3 years of age. *Pediatric Blood and Cancer, 60,* 700–704. https://doi.org/10.1002/pbc.24252

Nathan, P.C., Patel, S.K., Dilley, K., Goldsby, R., Harvey, J., Jacobsen, C., … Armstrong, F.D. (2007). Guidelines for identification of, advocacy for, and intervention in neurocognitive problems in survivors of childhood cancer: A report from the Children's Oncology Group. *Archives of Pediatrics and Adolescent Medicine, 161,* 798–806. https://doi.org/10.1001/archpedi.161.8.798

Oudin, C., Auquier, P., Bertrand, Y., Contet, A., Kanold, J., Sirvent, N., … Michel, G. (2015). Metabolic syndrome in adults who received hematopoietic stem cell transplantation for acute childhood leukemia: An LEA study. *Bone Marrow Transplantation, 50,* 1438–1444. https://doi.org/10.1038/bmt.2015.167

Özdemir, E., Saliba, R.M., Champlin, R.E., Couriel, D.R., Giralt, S.A., de Lima, M., … Komanduri, K.V. (2007). Risk factors associated with late cytomegalovirus reactivation after allogeneic stem cell transplantation for hematological malignancies. *Bone Marrow Transplantation, 40,* 125–136. https://doi.org/10.1038/sj.bmt.1705699

Pagano, L., Akova, M., Dimopoulos, G., Herbrecht, R., Drgona, L., & Blijlevens, N. (2011). Risk assessment and prognostic factors for mould-related diseases in immunocompromised patients. *Journal of Antimicrobial Chemotherapy, 66*(Suppl. 1), i5–i14. https://doi.org/10.1093/jac/dkq437

Paulsen, G.C., & Danziger-Isakov, L. (2017). Respiratory viral infections in solid organ and hematopoietic stem cell transplantation. *Clinics in Chest Medicine, 38,* 707–726. https://doi.org/10.1016/j.ccm.2017.07.012

Pedersen-Bjergaard, J., Andersen, M.K., & Christiansen, D.H. (2000). Therapy-related acute myeloid leukemia and myelodysplasia after high-dose chemotherapy and autologous stem cell transplantation. *Blood, 95,* 3273–3279.

Pedersen-Bjergaard, J., Pedersen, M., Myhre, J., & Geisler, C. (1997). High risk of therapy-related leukemia after BEAM chemotherapy and autologous stem cell transplantation for previously treated lymphomas is mainly related to primary chemotherapy and not to the BEAM-transplantation procedure. *Leukemia, 11,* 1654–1660. https://doi.org/10.1038/sj.leu.2400809

Peggs, K.S., Verfuerth, S., Pizzey, A., Chow, S.-L.C., Thomson, K., & Mackinnon, S. (2009). Cytomegalovirus-specific T cell immunotherapy promotes restoration of durable functional antiviral immunity following allogeneic stem cell transplantation. *Clinical Infectious Diseases, 49,* 1851–1860. https://doi.org/10.1086/648422

Pekic, S., & Popovic, V. (2014). Alternative causes of hypopituitarism: Traumatic brain injury, cranial irradiation, and infections. In E. Fliers, M. Korbonits, & J.A. Romijn (Eds.), *Handbook of Clinical Neurology: Vol. 124* (pp. 271–290). https://doi.org/10.1016/b978-0-444-59602-4.00018-6

Perkins, J.L., Kunin-Batson, A.S., Youngren, N.M., Ness, K.K., Ulrich, K.J., Hansen, M.J., … Baker, K.S. (2007). Long-term follow-up of children who underwent hematopoeitic cell transplant (HCT) for AML or ALL at less than 3 years of age. *Pediatric Blood and Cancer, 49,* 958–963. https://doi.org/10.1002/pbc.21207

Pidala, J., Anasetti, C., & Jim, H. (2009). Quality of life after allogeneic hematopoietic cell transplantation. *Blood, 114,* 7–19. https://doi.org/10.1182/blood-2008-10-182592

Pundole, X.N., Barbo, A.G., Lin, H., Champlin, R.E., & Lu, H. (2015). Increased incidence of fractures in recipients of hematopoietic stem-cell transplantation. *Journal of Clinical Oncology, 33,* 1364–1370. https://doi.org/10.1200/jco.2014.57.8195

Renaud, C., & Campbell, A.P. (2011). Changing epidemiology of respiratory viral infections in hematopoietic cell transplant recipients and solid organ transplant recipients. *Current Opinion in Infectious Diseases, 24,* 333–343. https://doi.org/10.1097/qco.0b013e3283480440

Renaud, C., Xie, H., Seo, S., Kuypers, J., Cent, A., Corey, L., … Englund, J.A. (2013). Mortality rates of human metapneumovirus and respiratory syncytial virus lower respiratory tract infections in hematopoietic cell transplantation recipients. *Biology of Blood and Marrow Transplantation, 19,* 1220–1226. https://doi.org/10.1016/j.bbmt.2013.05.005

Ringdén, O., Brazauskas, R., Wang, Z., Ahmed, I., Atsuta, Y., Buchbinder, D., … Majhail, N.S. (2014). Second solid cancers after allogeneic hematopoietic cell transplantation using reduced-intensity conditioning. *Biology of Blood and Marrow Transplantation, 20,* 1777–1784. https://doi.org/10.1016/j.bbmt.2014.07.009

Rizzo, J.D., Curtis, R.E., Socié, G., Sobocinski, K.A., Gilbert, E., Landgren, O., … Deeg, H.J. (2009). Solid cancers after allogeneic hematopoietic cell transplantation. *Blood, 113,* 1175–1183. https://doi.org/10.1182/blood-2008-05-158782

Rizzo, J.D., Wingard, J.R., Tichelli, A., Lee, S.J., Van Lint, M.T., Burns, L.J., … Socié, G. (2006). Recommended screening and preventive practices for long-term survivors after hematopoietic cell transplantation: Joint recommendations of the European Group for Blood and Marrow Transplantation, the Center for International Blood and Marrow Transplant Research, and the American Society of Blood and Marrow Transplantation. *Biology of Blood and Marrow Transplantation, 12,* 138–151. https://doi.org/10.1016/j.bbmt.2005.09.012

Robin, M., Marque-Juillet, S., Scieux, C., Peffault de Latour, R., Ferry, C., Rocha, V., … Socié, G. (2007). Disseminated adenovirus infections after allogeneic hematopoietic stem cell transplantation: Incidence, risk factors and outcome. *Haematologica, 92,* 1254–1257. https://doi.org/10.3324/haematol.11279

Rovó, A., Aljurf, M., Chiodi, S., Spinelli, S., Salooja, N., Sucak, G., … Tichelli, A. (2013). Ongoing graft-*versus*-host disease is a risk factor for azoospermia after allogeneic hematopoietic stem cell transplantation: A survey of the Late Effects Working Party of the European Group for Blood and Marrow Transplantation. *Haematologica, 98,* 339–345. https://doi.org/10.3324/haematol.2012.071944

Rovó, A., Tichelli, A., Passweg, J.R., Heim, D., Meyer-Monard, S., Holzgreve, W., … De Geyter, C. (2006). Spermatogenesis in long-term survivors after allogeneic hematopoietic stem cell transplantation is associated with age, time interval since transplantation, and apparently absence of chronic GvHD. *Blood, 108,* 1100–1105. https://doi.org/10.1182/blood-2006-01-0176

Rusiewicz, A., DuHamel, K.N., Burkhalter, J., Ostroff, J., Winkel, G., Scigliano, E., … Redd, W. (2008). Psychological distress in long-term survivors of hematopoietic stem cell transplantation. *Psycho-Oncology, 17,* 329–337. https://doi.org/10.1002/pon.1221

Sanders, J.E. (2008). Growth and development after hematopoietic cell transplant in children. *Bone Marrow Transplantation, 41,* 223–227. https://doi.org/10.1038/sj.bmt.1705875

Sanders, J.E., Guthrie, K.A., Hoffmeister, P.A., Woolfrey, A.E., Carpenter, P.A., & Appelbaum, F.R. (2005). Final adult height of patients who received hematopoietic cell transplantation in childhood. *Blood, 105,* 1348–1354. https://doi.org/10.1182/blood-2004-07-2528

Sanders, J.E., Hoffmeister, P.A., Woolfrey, A.E., Carpenter, P.A., Storer, B.E., Storb, R.F., & Appelbaum, F.R. (2009). Thyroid function following hematopoietic cell transplantation in children: 30 years' experience. *Blood, 113,* 306–308. https://doi.org/10.1182/blood-2008-08-173005

Santo Tomas, L.H., Loberiza, F.R., Jr., Klein, J.P., Layde, P.M., Lipchik, R.J., Rizzo, J.D., … Horowitz, M.M. (2005). Risk factors for bronchiolitis obliterans in allogeneic hematopoietic stem-cell transplantation for leukemia. *Chest, 128,* 153–161. https://doi.org/10.1378/chest.128.1.153

Schleiss, M.R. (2016). Cytomegalovirus vaccines under clinical development. *Journal of Virus Eradication, 2,* 198–207.

Seo, S., & Boeckh, M. (2016). Respiratory viruses after hematopoietic cell transplantation. In S.J. Forman, R.S. Negrin, J.H. Antin, & F.R. Appelbaum (Eds.), *Thomas' hematopoietic cell transplantation: Stem cell transplantation* (5th ed., pp. 1112–1121). https://doi.org/10.1002/9781118416426.ch91

Shah, D.P., Shah, P.K., Azzi, J.M., El Chaer, F., & Chemaly, R.F. (2016). Human metapneumovirus infections in hematopoietic cell transplant recipients and hematologic malignancy patients: A systematic review. *Cancer Letters, 379,* 100–106. https://doi.org/10.1016/j.canlet.2016.05.035

Shalitin, S., Pertman, L., Yackobovitch-Gavan, M., Yaniv, I., Lebenthal, Y., Phillip, M., & Stein, J. (2018). Endocrine and metabolic disturbances in survivors of hematopoietic stem cell transplantation in childhood and adolescence. *Hormone Research in Paediatrics, 89,* 108–121. https://doi.org/10.1159/000486034

Shenoy, S., Angelucci, E., Arnold, S.D., Baker, K.S., Bhatia, M., Bresters, D., … Walters, M.C. (2017). Current results and future research priorities in late effects after hematopoietic stem cell transplantation for children with sickle cell disease and thalassemia: A consensus statement from the Second Pediatric Blood and Marrow Transplant Consortium International Conference on Late Effects after Pediatric Hematopoietic Stem Cell Transplantation. *Biology of Blood and Marrow Transplantation, 23,* 552–561. https://doi.org/10.1016/j.bbmt.2017.01.009

Shin, J.-A., Lee, J.-H., Lim, S.-Y., Ha, H.-S., Kwon, H.-S., Park, Y.-M., … Son, H.-Y. (2013). Metabolic syndrome as a predictor of type 2 diabetes, and its clinical interpretations and usefulness. *Journal of Diabetes Investigation, 4,* 334–343. https://doi.org/10.1111/jdi.12075

Small, T.N., Casson, A., Malak, S.F., Boulad, F., Kiehn, T.E., Stiles, J., … Sepkowitz, K.A. (2002). Respiratory syncytial virus infection following hematopoietic stem cell transplantation. *Bone Marrow Transplantation, 29,* 321–327. https://doi.org/10.1038/sj.bmt.1703365

Socié, G., & Rizzo, J.D. (2012). Second solid tumors: Screening and management guidelines in long-term survivors after allogeneic stem cell transplantation. *Seminars in Hematology, 49,* 4–9. https://doi.org/10.1053/j.seminhematol.2011.10.013

Solh, M.M., Bashey, A., Solomon, S.R., Morris, L.E., Zhang, X., Brown, S., & Holland, H.K. (2018). Long term survival among patients who are disease free at 1-year post allogeneic hematopoietic cell transplantation: A single center analysis of 389 consecutive patients. *Bone Marrow Transplantation, 53,* 576–583. https://doi.org/10.1038/s41409-017-0076-2

Sostak, P., Padovan, C.S., Yousry, T.A., Ledderose, G., Kolb, H.-J., & Straube, A. (2003). Prospective evaluation of neurological complications after allogeneic bone marrow transplantation. *Neurology, 60,* 842–848. https://doi.org/10.1212/01.wnl.0000046522.38465.79

Steffens, M., Beauloye, V., Brichard, B., Robert, A., Alexopoulou, O., Vermylen, C., & Maiter, D. (2008). Endocrine and metabolic disorders in young adult survivors of childhood acute lymphoblastic leukaemia (ALL) or non-Hodgkin lymphoma (NHL). *Clinical Endocrinology, 69,* 819–827. https://doi.org/10.1111/j.1365-2265.2008.03283.x

Sucak, G.T., Yegin, Z.A., Özkurt, Z.N., Akı, Ş.Z., Karakan, T., & Akyol, G. (2008). The role of liver biopsy in the workup of liver dysfunction late after SCT: Is the role of iron overload underestimated? *Bone Marrow Transplantation, 42,* 461–467. https://doi.org/10.1038/bmt.2008.193

Sun, C.-L., Francisco, L., Baker, K.S., Weisdorf, D.J., Forman, S.J., & Bhatia, S. (2011). Adverse psychological outcomes in long-term survivors of hematopoietic cell transplantation: A report from the Bone Marrow Transplant Survivor Study (BMTSS). *Blood, 118,* 4723–4731. https://doi.org/10.1182/blood-2011-04-348730

Sun, C.-L., Francisco, L., Kawashima, T., Leisenring, W., Robison, L.L., Baker, K.S., … Bhatia, S. (2010). Prevalence and predictors of chronic health conditions after hematopoietic cell transplantation: A report from the Bone Marrow Transplant Survivor Study. *Blood, 116,* 3129–3139; quiz 3377. https://doi.org/10.1182/blood-2009-06-229369

Sun, C.-L., Kersey, J.H., Francisco, L., Armenian, S.H., Baker, K.S., Weisdorf, D.J., … Bhatia, S. (2013). Burden of morbidity in 10+ year survivors of hematopoietic cell transplantation: Report from the Bone Marrow Transplantation Survivor Study. *Biology of Blood and Marrow Transplantation, 19,* 1073–1080. https://doi.org/10.1016/j.bbmt.2013.04.002

Syrjala, K.L., Langer, S.L., Abrams, J.R., Storer, B.E., & Martin, P.J. (2005). Late effects of hematopoietic cell transplantation among 10-year adult survivors compared with case-matched controls. *Journal of Clinical Oncology, 23,* 6596–6606. https://doi.org/10.1200/jco.2005.12.674

Syrjala, K.L., Langer, S.L., Abrams, J.R., Storer, B., Sanders, J.E., Flowers, M.E.D., & Martin, P.J. (2004). Recovery and long-term function after hematopoietic cell transplantation for leukemia or lymphoma. *JAMA, 291,* 2335–2343. https://doi.org/10.1001/jama.291.19.2335

Syrjala, K.L., Martin, P.J., & Lee, S.J. (2012). Delivering care to long-term adult survivors of hematopoietic cell transplantation. *Journal of Clinical Oncology, 30,* 3746–3751. https://doi.org/10.1200/jco.2012.42.3038

Syrjala, K.L., Stover, A.C., Yi, J.C., Artherholt, S.B., Romano, E.M., Schoch, G., … Flowers, M.E.D. (2011). Development and implementation of an Internet-based survivorship care program for cancer survivors treated with hematopoietic stem cell transplantation. *Journal of Cancer Survivorship, 5,* 292–304. https://doi.org/10.1007/s11764-011-0182-x

Tichelli, A., & Rovó, A. (2015). Survivorship after allogeneic transplantation—Management recommendations for the primary care provider. *Current Hematologic Malignancy Reports, 10,* 35–44. https://doi.org/10.1007/s11899-014-0243-0

Tichelli, A., Rovó, A., & Gratwohl, A. (2008). Late pulmonary, cardiovascular, and renal complications after hematopoietic stem cell transplantation and recommended screening practices. *Hematology: American Society of Hematology Education Program Book, 2008,* 125–133. https://doi.org/10.1182/asheducation-2008.1.125

Tomblyn, M., Chiller, T., Einsele, H., Gress, R., Sepkowitz, K., Storek, J., … Boeckh, M.A. (2009). Guidelines for preventing infectious complications among hematopoietic cell transplantation recipients: A global perspective. *Biology of Blood and Marrow Transplantation, 15,* 1143–1238. https://doi.org/10.1016/j.bbmt.2009.06.019

U.S. Department of Education. (2020, January 10). Protecting students with disabilities. Retrieved from https://www2.ed.gov/about/offices/list/ocr/504faq.html

van der Pas-van Voskuilen, I.G.M., Veerkamp, J.S.J., Raber-Durlacher, J.E., Bresters, D., van Wijk, A.J., Barasch, A., … Gortzak, R.A.T. (2009). Long-term adverse effects of hematopoietic stem cell transplantation on dental development in children. *Supportive Care in Cancer, 17,* 1169–1175. https://doi.org/10.1007/s00520-008-0567-1

van Dorp, W., van Beek, R.D., Laven, J.S.E., Pieters, R., de Muinck Keizer-Schrama, S.M.P.F., & van den Heuvel-Eibrink, M.M. (2012). Long-term endocrine side effects of childhood Hodgkin's lymphoma treatment: A review. *Human Reproduction Update, 18,* 12–28. https://doi.org/10.1093/humupd/dmr038

Vehreschild, J.J., Rüping, M.J.G.T., Wisplinghoff, H., Farowski, F., Steinbach, A., Sims, R., … Cornely, O.A. (2010). Clinical effectiveness of posaconazole prophylaxis in patients with acute myelogenous leukaemia (AML): A 6-year experience of the Cologne AML cohort. *Journal of Antimicrobial Chemotherapy, 65,* 1466–1471. https://doi.org/10.1093/jac/dkq121

Vrooman, L.M., Millard, H.R., Brazauskas, R., Majhail, N.S., Battiwalla, M., Flowers, M.E., … Duncan, C. (2017). Survival and late effects after allogeneic hematopoietic cell transplantation for hematologic malignancy at less than three years of age. *Biology of Blood and Marrow Transplantation, 23*, 1327–1334. https://doi.org/10.1016/j.bbmt.2017.04.017

Wei, C., & Albanese, A. (2014). Endocrine disorders in childhood cancer survivors treated with haemopoietic stem cell transplantation. *Children, 1*, 48–62. https://doi.org/10.3390/children1010048

Welniak, L.A., Blazar, B.R., & Murphy, W.J. (2007). Immunobiology of allogeneic hematopoietic stem cell transplantation. *Annual Review of Immunology, 25*, 139–170. https://doi.org/10.1146/annurev.immunol.25.022106.141606

Wettergren, L., Sprangers, M., Björkholm, M., & Langius-Eklöf, A. (2008). Quality of life before and one year following stem cell transplantation using an individualized and a standardized instrument. *Psycho-Oncology, 17*, 338–346. https://doi.org/10.1002/pon.1240

Wingard, J.R., Majhail, N.S., Brazauskas, R., Wang, Z., Sobocinski, K.A., Jacobsohn, D., … Socié, G. (2011). Long-term survival and late deaths after allogeneic hematopoietic cell transplantation. *Journal of Clinical Oncology, 29*, 2230–2239. https://doi.org/10.1200/jco.2010.33.7212

Worel, N., Biener, D., Kalhs, P., Mitterbauer, M., Keil, F., Schulenburg, A., … Greinix, H.T. (2002). Long-term outcome and quality of life of patients who are alive and in complete remission more than two years after allogeneic and syngeneic stem cell transplantation. *Bone Marrow Transplantation, 30*, 619–626. https://doi.org/10.1038/sj.bmt.1703677

Yao, S., McCarthy, P.L., Dunford, L.M., Roy, D.M., Brown, K., Paplham, P., … Hahn, T. (2008). High prevalence of early-onset osteopenia/osteoporosis after allogeneic stem cell transplantation and improvement after bisphosphonate therapy. *Bone Marrow Transplantation, 41*, 393–398. https://doi.org/10.1038/sj.bmt.1705918

Yoshihara, S., Yanik, G., Cooke, K.R., & Mineishi, S. (2007). Bronchiolitis obliterans syndrome (BOS), bronchiolitis obliterans organizing pneumonia (BOOP), and other late-onset noninfectious pulmonary complications following allogeneic hematopoietic stem cell transplantation. *Biology of Blood and Marrow Transplantation, 13*, 749–759. https://doi.org/10.1016/j.bbmt.2007.05.001

Youssef, S., Rodriguez, G., Rolston, K.V., Champlin, R.E., Raad, I.I., & Safdar, A. (2007). *Streptococcus pneumoniae* infections in 47 hematopoietic stem cell transplantation recipients: Clinical characteristics of infections and vaccine-breakthrough infections, 1989–2005. *Medicine, 86*, 69–77. https://doi.org/10.1097/md.0b013e31803eb176

CHAPTER 15

Ethical Considerations

Joyce L. Neumann, PhD, APRN, AOCN®, BMTCN®

Introduction

Hematopoietic stem cell transplantation (HSCT) nurses encounter numerous clinical situations that may challenge their technical skills and intellect, as well as their beliefs, values, and principles. Nurses have a professional responsibility and obligation to advocate for patients during all phases of the treatment experience (American Nurses Association, 2015). Nurses must come to terms with competing ethical principles presented by differences in resource allocation, religious beliefs, societal mores, and the research aspect of the treatment regimen. HSCT nursing is unique because the patients in this setting frequently present with life-threatening illnesses for which standard therapy has failed or has a low probability of controlling the refractory disease. Increased uncertainty about treatment outcomes can contribute to difficulty for patients and caregivers in making the decision to undergo therapy, as well as at critical points along the treatment course. As such, it is necessary for nurses to understand the ethical and legal dilemmas related to treatment options, the outcome of treatment, and end-of-life care that challenge HSCT nurses and their patients.

In 2019, the Oncology Nursing Society (ONS) published *Oncology Nursing: Scope and Standards of Practice* (Lubejko & Wilson, 2019). Included in this publication is a standard of ethics, which states that an oncology nurse's decisions and actions on behalf of clients are determined using ethical principles. It encourages oncology nurses to examine their own philosophical, spiritual, and personal beliefs; discuss ethical issues with colleagues; address advance directives and advance care planning with patients and families; act as patient advocates; maintain a sensitivity to patients' cultural diversity; protect patient autonomy, dignity, and rights; and seek resources to examine issues and formulate ethical decisions. In addition, oncology nurses are encouraged to self-assess their cultural competence as it relates to life-and-death decision making, alert patient and families to potential ethical issues specific for their clinical situation, maintain patient confidentiality and privacy, deliver nondiscriminatory care, and initiate ethics consultations to assist in solving ethical dilemmas when appropriate (Lubejko & Wilson, 2019).

Figures 15-1 and 15-2 provide a brief review of ethical principles relevant in current U.S. society that may influence decision making in certain clinical situations. It is impor-

tant to remember that these ethical principles do not stand alone. Different clinicians will have varied opinions; therefore, policies are frequently necessary to promote consistency in practice.

Figure 15-1. Bioethical Principles

- Beneficence: Clinicians act to benefit or help people.
- Nonmaleficence: Clinicians must act in a way to prevent or avoid harm to people (do no harm).
- Sanctity of life: Human life is held in high regard and respect.
- Justice: Professionals have a duty to act with fairness and to give every individual what is owed.
- Personal autonomy: Competent individuals or their surrogates have a right to decide for or against treatment.
- Benefit–burden: Only medical treatments that provide more benefit than burden are ethically mandated.

Note. Based on information from Beauchamp & Childress, 2012.

Figure 15-2. Ethical Considerations in Clinical Situations

- Norms of family life: Familial relationships give rise to moral responsibility. Clinicians expect families to act in the best interest of the person.
- Relationship between clinician and patient: Clinicians have a fiduciary responsibility to care for patients. This relationship requires mutual trust, and the patient must be treated as a whole person.
- Professional integrity of clinicians: Clinicians have no responsibility to offer treatment that is not medically indicated.
- Cost-effectiveness and justice: In a system with limited resources, allocation needs to be prioritized for the most appropriate use. Clinicians must be stewards of resources.
- Cultural or religious variations: Differences in beliefs or cultural norms may create disparity in values and principles.

Note. Based on information from Jonsen et al., 2015.

Transplantation as a Treatment Option: Beneficence and Nonmaleficence

Many factors must be considered when cancer treatment decisions are made. When little or no chance of cure or control exists, offering treatments to patients can contradict the ethical principles of beneficence and nonmaleficence (Caocci et al., 2011; see Table 15-1). Some centers have written or unwritten rules relating prognosis, comorbidity, and availability of social support to the appropriateness of offering HSCT. For example, therapies may not be offered if the chance of cure or appreciably controlling disease is less than 5%–10%. Yet other clinicians might consider that all treatment options should be offered and administered if the patient knows the survival outcome data and consents to treatment. With new "right to try" laws in most states and at the federal level, this may include experimental treatments that have not received U.S. Food and Drug Administration approval (Carrieri, Peccatori, & Boniolo, 2018). When clinicians take this position unanimously, it may conflict with what others consider to be best medical practice. Additionally, consideration must be given to resource allocation and cultural differences of patients from varying ethnic backgrounds and international patients who are seeking state-of-the-art care at larger medical centers where HSCT is offered.

As a culture, Americans have been grappling with resource allocation as it relates to healthcare costs and access. This can become more challenging when the proposed treatment is unproven but promising or a last-chance therapy, as is the case with some HSCT and cellular therapy research protocols. The Patient Protection and Affordable Care Act (2010) has made provisions for this with the establishment of the nonprofit Patient-Centered Outcomes Research Institute to identify research priorities and support comparative effectiveness research (Kaiser Family Foundation, 2013). In recent years, the research related to immunotherapy and cellular therapy has increased the legal and ethical debate. Issues related to insurance coverage and the high cost of new therapies have mobilized citizen action groups (e.g., Patients for Affordable Drugs) and professional groups to participate in the debate (Prasad, De Jesús, & Mailankody, 2017).

Table 15-1. Ethical Issues Related to Patient or Donor Selection

Potential Issue	Ethical or Moral Dilemma
Hematopoietic stem cell transplantation patient with relapse or less-than-optimal condition (high comorbidity)	Benefit vs. burden Nonmaleficence
No reliable caregiver or housing	Nonmaleficence
Nonadherence to prescribed medication, scheduled appointments, or recommendations of hematopoietic stem cell transplantation program	Patient autonomy vs. nonmaleficence vs. provider integrity
Current use or abuse of illicit drugs, tobacco, or alcohol	Patient autonomy vs. do no harm Justice—use of limited resources
Vulnerable donor cleared by recipient provider	Conflict of interest, autonomy of donor, coercive influence

Legal decisions related to resource allocation versus the principle of justice attained public attention through landmark cases, such as that of Colby Howard of Oregon in the mid-1980s. Colby, a seven-year-old boy with leukemia, needed a bone marrow transplant. Initially, Oregon Medicaid agreed to fund the procedure, which was to be performed in the neighboring state of Washington. Before the transplant process was started, the Oregon legislature voted to discontinue funding of solid organ and bone marrow transplantation, which was expected to benefit only 34 people over a two-year period. The $2.8 million was reallocated to fund prenatal and pediatric care for 1,500 low-income mothers and children. Colby died waiting for the funds needed for the transplant (Pence, 2004; Wiener, 1992). The competing ethical principles or considerations that lawmakers were faced with in making their decision were justice (i.e., Colby was entitled to what was promised) and benefit versus burden (i.e., the greater good for the most people).

When considering aggressive therapies, such as HSCT, as treatment options, evidence demonstrates that many factors will affect outcomes (Bayraktar et al., 2017; Khera et al., 2017; Patel et al., 2018; Shaw et al., 2018; Shouval et al., 2018). The aftercare of the patient requires adherence to medications, clinic visits to monitor blood counts and perform physical examinations, and adherence to guidelines for self-care activities. Many HSCT programs require a patient to have a caregiver available 24 hours a day. Some centers have developed an algorithm for patients who meet the medical eligibility for transplantation but have special needs or situations that may put them at risk for harm (nonmaleficence) with the prescribed therapy. Ideally, these issues should be addressed and resolved before the patient begins therapy, whether inpatient or outpatient. The goal is to provide a means of success in the cure or control of the patient's disease. Clinicians have a responsibility to be good stewards of available resources and create criteria with guidelines for judicious use of therapies, especially those that are extremely costly, such as HSCT and cellular therapy.

Frequently, a research nurse or clinical nurse ascertains that the patient understands the prescribed therapy. It is imperative that the patient understands that alternative treatment options exist, even though the goal of cure may not be achievable. If patients are enrolling in a clinical trial, it is important that they know if their physician is the principal investigator of the study and, therefore, may have a vested interest in the study. In recent years, knowledge of alternative therapies and potential conflicts of interest have been added to most informed consent documents (Little et al., 2008).

Members of the nursing staff may have difficulty accepting the aggressive nature of HSCT. New nurses on a transplantation staff need to understand the research program's goals and acknowledge that the patient accepts the experimental nature of a treatment with uncertain outcomes.

Nurses may have the perception of being caught in the middle of competing goals of the medical team and the patient and family. It takes skill and a strong advocacy role on the nurse's part to ensure that mutual goals are understood.

To achieve unity in care and goals, it may be helpful for HSCT team members to agree on certain basic assumptions and ethical considerations, which may include the following:

- Care providers have an obligation to provide potential life-saving treatment (beneficence).
- Numerous factors, in addition to medical eligibility, will influence outcomes and patient safety (nonmaleficence).
- Success is dependent on a team of professionals who are empowered to make decisions.
- A patient's verbal commitment should be demonstrated with actions (e.g., adherence with appointments, tests, and treatments).
- Individuals (patients) do not change coping styles during a high-stress situation, such as during HSCT treatment.

HSCT healthcare providers will want to provide resources to decrease dependence on maladaptive coping skills or a psychiatric diagnosis that may have negative health-related outcomes for patients. Concern is raised when patients refuse psychosocial assessments and interventions (Foster et al., 2009). Evidence supports the correlation between depression and overall survival in allogeneic HSCT patients (El-Jawahri et al., 2017; Grulke, Larbig, Kächele, & Bailer, 2008; Pillay, Lee, Katona, Burney, & Avery, 2014; Sun et al., 2011).

Other variables that may influence a clinician's decisions related to treatment include patient age, toxicities, and cost of treatment. In the past, HSCT was a treatment modality for younger patients, but nonmyeloablative transplants and reduced-intensity conditioning regimens allow this therapy to be offered to older patients with responsive and less aggressive diseases. Although reduced-intensity conditioning is associated with less toxicity than conventional regimens, complications related to comorbid conditions of older patients can make management equally complex and costly (Preussler et al., 2017). In addition, post-transplantation complications, such as graft-versus-host disease, can be more devastating and have a longer recovery time in older patients. Several centers are exploring prehabilitation or enhanced recovery programs that offer older patients or those with the potential for increased deconditioning a method to mitigate the debilitating effects of HSCT (Hacker, Peters, Patel, & Rondelli, 2018; Sullivan & Caguioa, 2018). An interprofessional approach includes evaluation before admission by the rehabilitation team (physical therapist, occupational therapist, and physician), gerontology, clinical nutrition, and clinical pharmacy. In some centers, patients will receive education about the program by advanced practice providers and nursing coordinators. During hospitalization and after discharge, nursing, physical and occupational therapy, and nutrition support teams will follow-up with patients (Szewczyk et al., 2019).

Informed Consent: Autonomous Decision

Telling the truth (veracity) regarding HSCT and a patient's prognosis can pose a great concern for clinicians. Frequently, in an attempt to "protect" a patient, families will request an alteration to the truth so that their loved one will not give up hope or decide to stop treatment. If the patient is very young, older, or of an ethnic background following a different decision-making model (e.g., paternalistic), a patient surrogate may serve as the decision maker or spokesperson. The use of a professional interpreter is required if a patient speaks a different language than providers. If possible, the consent form should be written in a patient's native language (Sheldon & Hilaire, 2016). The interpreter can assist in the acquisition of culturally sensitive information that could influence the decision-making process. A clinician requires cultural awareness to meet the challenge of ensuring that a patient's wishes or interests are understood and protected.

A patient's physical and psychosocial condition must be considered in selecting the most appropriate treatment or clinical trial. The concepts of informed consent and informed decision making are important issues at this point. The purpose of informed consent is to protect human rights through an ongoing process of providing a patient or surrogate with information related to the treatment plan, medications, side effects, complications, risks, costs, benefits, and rights (Ermete, 2016; Lesko, Dermatis, Penman, & Holland, 2006; Raj, Choi, Gurtekin, & Platt, 2018). Informed consent does not end with signing a document; rather, it extends throughout the patient's treatment (Ermete, 2016). As the clinical situation changes, a patient or surrogate can make appropriate decisions for specific events.

A patient's awareness of all potential side effects is crucial to informed consent. Clinicians may have differing opinions on whether to tell patients about side effects that they may occur infrequently. Acute (potentially life-threatening) side effects are most often discussed, and long-term effects are less frequently mentioned (Ramirez et al., 2009). As more quality-of-life research involving HSCT is conducted, clinicians can provide more information on morbidity (e.g., neurocognitive dysfunction) to patients and families so they can make more informed decisions (Bevans et al., 2014; Buchbinder et al., 2018; Jim et al., 2014). It is important to present unbiased information when educating patients treated with HSCT on the side effects that are most likely to occur, providing additional detail when requested.

In research protocols, a written informed consent document provides information and obtains the patient's permission to provide treatment that is considered experimental. The patient should receive a copy of the signed document. The written consent also serves to document and register the patient on a protocol. Providing an informed consent for standard therapies (rather than research protocols) is a suggested practice but not one uniformly exercised. By having the patient sign consent, the clinician is demonstrating an increased sense of responsibility to have the patient understand the treatment plan (Kunneman & Montori, 2017).

In the case of a minor undergoing HSCT, most institutions have a policy in place and an assent clause in the informed consent document that a parent or legal guardian signs. Assent is obtained from minors who are younger than 18 years old and have the mental comprehension equivalent to a child older than 7 years (American Academy of Pediatrics Committee on Bioethics, 2016; Lesko et al., 2006). Courts have recognized an adolescent may possess the cognitive ability, maturity of judgment, and moral authority in situations to independently make decisions about their health care, and many states have the mature minor doctrine, which permits adolescents to make these decisions (American Academy of Pediatrics Committee on Bioethics, 2016).

Patient Education: Preparing for Treatment Outcomes

Knowledge about treatment outcomes and expectations will not only assist the patient in making an autonomous decision about pursuing HSCT but also increase self-efficacy, decrease distress, and increase satisfaction (Burns et al., 2018). Patient, caregiver, and family education and support has been identified as a major area of interest in setting future patient-centered outcomes research (Burns et al., 2018). The nurse, as a primary patient advocate, provides detailed information of what the patient can expect during the therapy and aftercare to help prevent potential ethical issues (see Table 15-2). Some HSCT centers provide a care contract or agreement—a document that specifically

Table 15-2. Ethical Issues Related to Patient Preparation for All Possible Outcomes

Potential Issue	Ethical or Moral Dilemma
Advance care planning, advance directives	Autonomy, surrogate decision making
Continual patient education	Shared decision making, autonomy
Cultural difference—request by family not to discuss negative aspects	Veracity, patient autonomy
Explanation of potential negative outcomes—physical and psychological burdens after treatment	Veracity, uncertainty, therapeutic misconception
Informed consent—understanding risks and choices	Autonomy
Self-care and caregiver responsibility	Autonomy, informed decision making

outlines what is expected of the patient and caregiver and what they can expect of the healthcare facility and providers. This is especially helpful if clinicians are concerned about a patient's or caregiver's level of understanding, commitment, or adherence to HSCT program guidelines. Ensuring that a patient knows about these non-negotiable care requirements may help to prevent issues as treatment progresses. Facilitating patient-centered care and maintaining patients' sense of control over aspects of their care are equally important (Jim et al., 2014; Khera et al., 2017).

Asking patients to identify their most important concern or issue and to communicate this to all providers through the plan of care may help to eliminate misunderstandings, individualize care, and inform patients that the team is willing to address their personal needs. For some patients, receiving information about their blood counts daily is most important. For others, it is knowing about premedication for blood products or that every effort will be made to ensure that they get four uninterrupted hours of sleep in the hospital. Communicating a patient's individual requests to all care providers may help to lessen patient distress, possible conflict, and potential ethical dilemmas, such as autonomy versus beneficence.

Occasionally, a patient wants to know little or nothing of the details of a treatment, whereas others may request that only positive information be given. These types of patient preferences present some ethical challenges, as it is the healthcare provider's responsibility to inform the patient of undesirable conditions or complications. One suggested way to deal with these issues is to have the patient identify a family member who can act as a surrogate and assist in the information-sharing and decision-making processes.

To increase the patient's knowledge of planned therapy, an HSCT nurse can assist the patient in formulating questions and provide additional information concerning the long-term consequences of treatment. When discussing the treatment plan, the patient may have questions or concerns regarding fertility issues, plans to return to work or "normal" life, the plan for complications, and end-of-life care (Jim et al., 2014). These questions and concerns should be addressed before treatment begins.

When conducting phase 1 clinical trials, the clinician must ensure that patients understand that the treatment may have little or no direct benefit to them and that the goal of the trial is to define the maximum tolerated dose of therapy (Anderson & Kimmelman, 2010). Studies suggest that even after being informed that a protocol is a phase 1 study, patients often believe they will personally gain a clinical benefit from participation (Ermete, 2016; Kvale, Woodby, & Williams, 2010). This has been referred to as *therapeutic misconception*. With the advent of targeted therapies and immunotherapies in the field, understanding the goal of therapy has become more important. Uncertain benefit of expensive novel therapies that are in the early stages of research and development can make it more challenging to assist desperate patients to make well-informed decisions and prepare for all possible outcomes (Hey & Kesselheim, 2016; Jecker, Wightman, Rosenberg, & Diekema, 2017; Jones & Campbell, 2016; Ogba et al., 2018). The Internet gives patients the opportunity to explore treatment options, such as standard therapies, as well as experimental and unproven treatments. Practitioners need to be able to explain these options to patients in such a way that they understand that not all options are suitable or appropriate for their conditions.

Donor Issues

Healthcare professionals have an ethical responsibility to inform healthy donors of the risks associated with stem cell donation via bone marrow harvest or apheresis procedures. The risks to a young, healthy donor are minimal for either procedure. However, as HSCT has become more available to older adult patients, the donors may also be older and have multiple comorbid conditions. These factors may increase the risks for donors.

Special consideration is required when the donor is a child or minor (American Academy of Pediatrics Committee on Bioethics, 2010, 2016). If the treatment has a low chance of success, the risks to the healthy donor may be the primary factor in the decision not to proceed (Bitan et al., 2016). Parents may become desperate to find treatment options for their ill child and may coerce a healthy sibling to donate. Donors' rights must be protected through program or institutional policies that provide a mechanism to ensure voluntary, confidential, and safe practices when harvesting stem cells, whether through apheresis or bone marrow procurement.

The American Academy of Pediatrics and the World Marrow Donor Association recommend that a minor donor be appointed an independent advocate and undergo extensive psychosocial and developmental assessment by a child psychologist (American Academy of Pediatrics Committee on Bioethics, 2010; Stegenga et al., 2018). The emotional dilemmas may be profound because of the ages of the patient and donor, as well as the need for immediacy of decision making in some clinical situations. In the case of a child donor, separate healthcare teams are usually assigned for the patient and donor to eliminate the possibility of competing interests. When obtaining informed consent for a minor donor, most centers will obtain consent or assent from the donor, as well as the parents or guardians, if possible (American Academy of Pediatrics Committee on Bioethics, 2010). In the case of a very young or incompetent minor donor, a formal ethics consult may be standard practice during the consenting process. In the extreme but infrequent case of dissension of the minor donor, it is recommended that further discussion should occur with the involvement of the donor advocate, child mental health professional, and ethics consultants (American Academy of Pediatrics Committee on Bioethics, 2010). The preparative regimen for the recipient is held until this issue is resolved. Regardless of the donor's age, if any concerns develop regarding donor rights or interests, a formal ethics consult should be initiated by any member of the healthcare team.

Caring for international patients coming from countries where systems and ethics are different from those in the United States may pose other problems. In countries where laws are less stringent than in the United States, donors may be solicited by unauthorized review of hospital records or offered incentives. In these situations when care is provided in the United States, an institutional ethics committee and administrative review board may be involved to ensure donors' rights are protected (van Walraven et al., 2018).

In the case of an unrelated donor, national and international bone marrow registries have set up strict guidelines to protect donor and recipient rights and confidentiality (van Walraven et al., 2018). Assessment of the donor is performed for possible increased risk factors related to general anesthesia in bone marrow harvest or increased fluid and electrolyte shifts in an apheresis procedure. Personnel at the center where donation takes place manage concerns about potential withdrawal of consent by the donor after the transplant recipient's conditioning regimen has been started by validating the level of commitment of the donor and having the donor sign a letter of intent. Selection of a date for the donation may be somewhat complicated and sometimes is inflexible. Specific information (e.g., donor name and address) is provided to the patient and donor after a year and only if both parties agree (National Marrow Donor Program, 2018).

Outcomes of Disease and Treatment: Undesirable Consequences

Most cancer therapies are aimed at cure, but with advanced disease, the goal of therapy may be control of disease or palliation. Issues that may pose ethical dilemmas during the treatment or aftercare for HSCT patients include advance directives, do-not-resuscitate (DNR) orders, and discontinuation of medically inappropriate care (futility) (see Table 15-3). Individual states and institutions may have differing regulations related to each of these issues. In addition, other factors such as ethnicity, religion, coping style, and socioeconomic status may have a profound effect on patient and family wishes and responses to issues at the end of life (Smith et al., 2008). For example, low socioeconomic status was associated with increased mortality (Patel et al., 2018).

Advance Care Planning

In 1990, U.S. Congress enacted the Patient Self-Determination Act, which mandates that patients must be informed of their rights to accept or refuse treatments, including resuscitative measures, in accordance with state laws or statutes (Jezewski & Finnell, 1998). The term *advance directive* usually refers to three separate documents: living

Table 15-3. Ethical Issues Related to Life-Threatening Complications and End of Life

Potential Issue	Ethical or Moral Dilemma
Cultural difference—end-of-life care, after-death care	Patient/surrogate–provider communication and agreement
Decision to end life-sustaining treatment	Shared decision making, autonomy
Do-not-resuscitate order	Patient/surrogate–provider communication and agreement
Goal of care (transition of curative to comfort)	Level of appropriate medical care
Goals of care	Shared decision making, veracity, autonomy
Offering life-sustaining treatment with little chance of success	Veracity, patient–provider communication
Symptoms adequately managed (palliative care consult)	Level of responsiveness vs. symptom control
Treatment uncertainty, offering unproven treatment	Patient–provider communication

will, medical power of attorney, and DNR order. The social work or clinical ethics department usually assists patients and families in completing the advance directive forms and answers their questions. Historically, people who do not wish to be kept alive by artificial means if their medical condition is considered irreversible have a living will. For example, in Texas, an irreversible condition may be defined as

A condition, injury, or illness:
(A) that may be treated but is never cured or eliminated;
(B) that leaves a person unable to care for or make decisions for the person's own self; and
(C) that, without life-sustaining treatment provided in accordance with the prevailing standard of medical care, is fatal. (Advance Directives Act, 1999, § 166.002[9])

An additional statement was added to the living will document in several states, through support from the National Right to Life Committee; individuals can indicate that they want all life support measures to be maintained despite having a terminal or irreversible condition. The additional statements in the Texas living will document read, "I request that I be kept alive in this terminal condition using available life-sustaining treatment," and "I request that I be kept alive in this irreversible condition using available life-sustaining treatment" (Texas Health and Human Services Commission, 2015, p. 1). It should be noted that these statements do not apply to hospice care. Although this may give more choices to the individ-

ual completing the document, it is more challenging to the healthcare provider. To some, this reflects the principle of autonomy to the extreme and has the potential to create a barrier to clinicians exercising what would be viewed as appropriate medical practice. For example, CPR may not be indicated in a terminally ill patient treated with HSCT in multisystem failure. The importance for autonomy in decision making, especially at the end of life, is a core value in Western culture but may be complex and unpredictable for nurses caring for culturally diverse groups of patients (Sheldon & Hilaire, 2016). Except for Oregon, Montana, Washington, Vermont, and California, current advance directive documents and state laws do not include the choice of hastening death for patients whose wishes may include ending their lives if their condition is intolerable (Svenson, 2010). Nursing professional organizations, such as the American Nurses Association, ONS, and the Hospice and Palliative Nurses Association, also support the nurses' right to refuse to be part of such actions resulting in euthanasia, assisted suicide, and aid in dying (Haddad, 2016).

Review of advance directive documents can ideally create a forum for preemptive discussions, especially when the patient is about to undergo treatment regimens with a high risk for complications that may necessitate transfer to an intensive care unit (ICU) and intubation (Cappell et al., 2018). In a study by Needle and Smith (2016) involving adolescents and young adults undergoing HSCT, although the percentage of patients with advance directives was relatively small (23%), those with advance directives expressing preference for life-sustaining treatment were more likely to receive CPR than those without. Advance directive documents are an important part of the advance care planning process. Advance care planning has broader implications in helping to identify more than the care provided at the end of life; it also focuses on how patients want to live and their wishes in various circumstances. Advance care planning in HSCT patients has been examined as a factor influencing treatment outcomes (Cappell et al., 2018; Ganti et al., 2007; Needle & Smith, 2016), and these studies suggest it should be investigated further. The communication skills of clinicians are essential when presenting information related to diagnosis and treatment options to patients and families. Improved communication skills with compassionate and clear messages will naturally lead to decreased conflict and fewer ethical dilemmas (Sheldon & Hilaire, 2016). Figure 15-3 provides an example of an advance care planning document to be given as part of patient education before treatment begins.

Do-Not-Resuscitate Orders

The choice to use a DNR order is a medical decision based on the judgment of the patient's physician that the use of extraordinary measures (e.g., CPR, defibrillation, emergency medications, intubation) in irreversible conditions will not change the outcome for the patient who has

Figure 15-3. Advance Care Planning Before Stem Cell Transplantation

An important part of the stem cell transplant process is advance care planning—talking about your goals, values and wishes in terms of your health care. This will help prepare you and your caregivers before, during and after your treatment, which can be difficult and confusing at times.

Advance Directives

Advance directive is one way for you to make your wishes known about medical treatment before you need such care. Advance directives include medical power of attorney, living will and Out-of-Hospital Do Not Resuscitate Order (DNR). Although it is difficult and sometimes scary to think about situations or problems that could happen, it is important to learn about your medical treatment before you need such care.

Talking or thinking about it does not mean it is going to happen. If you have questions, please talk to your social work counselor, or call the Department of Social Work at 713-792-6195.

Stem Cell Transplant

Stem cell transplant is an aggressive treatment that comes with the risk of serious problems. Some can be life-threatening. Most likely, you have already read or talked with your doctor about some of these risks. Every patient we treat is different. Throughout your treatment, your health care team will discuss your medical condition with you and your family. This includes plans and options to treat problems as they occur.

Here are some of the risks or problems that may occur during treatment and how your health care team might address them:

Disease Relapse

Your disease may come back within one to two months after having a transplant. If that happens, your health care team will discuss other treatment options with specialists who treat your type of cancer. These options may include other types of chemotherapy or new drugs being evaluated for the treatment of the disease.

If you had a donor transplant, we may decrease or stop the immunosuppressive drugs. In most cases, this is tacrolimus or steroids. This allows the donor's immune system to "fight" your disease, also called graft versus tumor effect. Your doctor may also ask your donor to donate cells again (donor lymphocyte infusion).

If we stop the drugs or if we give you a boost of donor cells, you could develop graft versus host disease (GVHD). If you develop GVHD from your initial transplant, your health care team may not be able to stop the drugs or give you more donor cells because it will make the GVHD worse.

Graft Failure

Your blood counts may take two or more weeks to recover. This depends on the type of stem cells you received. Although rare, sometimes blood counts may not recover because the new graft or stem cells do not take hold in the bone marrow. Or, if the counts do recover, they stay very low for a long time. If this happens, we try to get more stem cells from your donor or use stem cells that were frozen and stored, if available. Also, blood products (platelets and red blood cells) and antibiotics are given to help your own cells do their job. With graft failure, there is a high risk for serious or life-threatening infections and bleeding.

Infection

After transplant, the immune system must rebuild itself, which takes many months. This means that stem cell transplant patients have an increased risk of infection for several years after the transplant.

Anti-bacterial, anti-viral and anti-fungal medicines are given at the start of the transplant to prevent infections. Yet, many patients often still develop a fever and infection that require going back to the hospital for treatment. Different IV antibiotics are used to fight the infection. Sometimes, bacterial, fungal or viral infections that are resistant to treatment may occur. Patients with an active fungal infection or a recent history of fungal infections are at high risk for those infections to become active again. Fungal and viral infections both require long-term treatment that can take weeks or months to control. Viral infections can also be resistant to treatment. A simple infection can be life threatening for a stem cell transplant patient.

Graft-Versus-Host Disease

After transplant, the immune system recovers using the stem cells (the graft) from the donor. The new immune system may recognize you (the host) as being different. So, instead of protecting your body, the graft reacts as though the body is "foreign" and attacks the body, causing GVHD signs and symptoms.

There are two types of GVHD: **acute and chronic**. Acute GVHD usually starts within three months after transplant. Chronic GVHD usually starts three months or more after the transplant. But, the type of GVHD may be better determined based on the current symptoms and which organs are affected. GVHD can affect the eyes, throat/esophagus, mouth, lips, skin, hair, nails, GI (gastrointestinal) system, lungs, joints/muscles and vagina.

Treatment depends on how much of the body is involved and the severity of the GVHD. Many of the treatments include steroid medicines. If GVHD does not respond to the steroids, this is called steroid refractory GVHD. Other immunosuppressive drugs are then used to treat the GVHD, but the risk of infection also increases as these drugs are added. If the patient does not respond to any of the treatments, the overall chance of survival is very low.

(Continued on next page)

Respiratory and Multiple Organ Failure
- Pneumonia is a common problem that can occur after transplant. Some types of pneumonias, such fungal and viral, are more serious than others. In some cases, an infection may not respond to even the best therapy, and this can be life-threatening.
- Bleeding into the lungs is another problem that can happen with an infection. It is extremely serious because it can make it very difficult for the lungs to work properly and requires the use of a breathing machine (ventilator).
- Some patients may require small amounts of oxygen while on the stem cell transplant floor. If more oxygen is needed quickly or at higher amounts, the health care team will consider placing a tube in the airway and the use of a breathing machine. If this happens, care is provided in the intensive care unit.
- Intubation (a tube in the airway) and the use of a breathing machine may be needed to support you while you wait for treatment to work. Your health care team will explain and discuss intubation and the breathing machine with you. Even if you have a living will, your health care team will review your options with you because your condition may improve with aggressive support. But, some patients may not respond despite all forms of therapy. Your doctors will discuss specific matters and concerns with you if this should happen.
- Multiple organ failure can occur if a patient has a serious infection or problem. If organs do not work properly, this can be a severe, life-threatening situation. Multiple organ failure can include the kidneys, lungs, liver, heart, brain and/or the blood system. Each organ system is vital for the body to work properly.

Treatment Goal
The goal with a stem cell transplant is to cure or control your disease. Our approach is to hope for the best, but prepare for all possible events. This includes the chance of not getting better. A stem cell transplant is a high-risk treatment. Sometimes, it does not always cure or control the disease.

It is important that you and your family prepare for the chance of serious medical problems that might occur. Take time to discuss your thoughts and values about life support, such as breathing machines and kidney dialysis. This will help your family and the medical team make the right treatment decision based on your wishes.

This is why you are strongly encouraged to have a living will and a medical power of attorney stating your wishes before treatment begins. Our general approach is to use all available treatments, including life support, if there is a chance for recovery. If a situation occurs and recovery is not possible, heroic measures like a breathing machine, cardiac resuscitation or invasive procedures will not be used.

Treatment Considerations
Communication is important. Your doctors will always keep you and your family informed about your condition and recovery. Our aim is to provide the best treatment based on your medical condition and support your full recovery. Despite the best possible treatment, some patients do not get better, making recovery and survival unlikely. If this happens, your health care team may change your treatment goal and focus on maintaining your comfort, quality of life and end-of-life care.

These matters will be discussed with you in detail. If you are unable to talk about these matters with us, your health care team will work with your family or the person with medical power of attorney to make decisions.

Once the decision has been made to focus on comfort and quality of life, your health care team will not perform any new life-sustaining or heroic measures or invasive procedures. Your comfort, dignity and helping you and your family cope during this difficult time will be our main goal.

If you have any questions or concerns, please talk with your doctor or other health care team members.

no reasonable hope for recovery. It is never advocated that the physician does this unilaterally, nor should the physician put the burden of the DNR decision on the patient or family exclusively. Frequently, disparity exists in the definitions and meaning of DNR among patients, providers, and families, which can lead to conflict in the consent process (Sheldon & Hilaire, 2016). Patients and families might assume that they need to sign a document before the DNR order can be written, and in a few states, this is the case. Some states have statutes mandating that adult patients (or their designee) give verbal or written consent before a physician writes the DNR order (Health Care Facility Do-Not-Resuscitate Orders, 2018; Sulmasy et al., 2006). Physicians or patients and families may have the perception and concern that the quality of nursing care will be less in the setting of a DNR order. Some may believe that by writing a DNR order, the patient will lose all hope and give up. Literature has supported the use of the verbiage *allow natural death* (AND) instead of DNR to increase the likelihood of patient and surrogate decision maker endorsement of the order (Venneman, Narnor-Harris, Perish, & Hamilton, 2008).

Some institutions have created an order set in which the physician has various treatment options to choose from, including cardiac defibrillation, vasoactive drugs, antiarrhythmic drugs, cardiac pacemaker, tracheostomy, chemotherapy, antibiotics, dialysis, blood products, hyperalimentation, tube feeding, IV fluids, oxygen, and tests. These order sets also specify that patient comfort always takes priority. Establishing the specific goal of care is paramount in deciding which of these measures are to be provided or withheld.

Knowledge of HSCT patient trends is critical in making sound judgments about which conditions may be considered irreversible. Studies suggest that specific variables have been shown to influence the mortality of patients with cancer admitted to the ICU. CPR within 24 hours prior to admission, intubation, intracranial mass, allogeneic HSCT, recurrence of disease, poor baseline performance status, prothrombin time longer than 15 seconds, albumin less than 2.5 g/dl, bilirubin greater than 2 mg/dl, blood urea nitrogen greater than 50 mg/dl, and the number of hospital days prior to ICU admission increase mortality in the ICU (Gilli, Remberger, Hjelmqvist, Ringden, & Mattsson, 2010; Johnston et al., 2018; Lin et al., 2019; Shaw et al., 2018; Shouval et al., 2018). The development of a prognostic index specific for allogeneic HSCT patients who require ICU management has been helpful in predicting mortality and is more accurate than other instruments (Bayraktar et al., 2017). As critical care medicine has made advances, recent studies support improved outcomes for HSCT patients who are admitted to the ICU.

Discontinuation of Medically Inappropriate Care

At times, measures are instituted when it is not clear whether a patient's condition is reversible. When it becomes apparent that a patient has little or no chance of recovery, the decision may be made to discontinue life-sustaining measures and switch to measures with the goal of a peaceful death with dignity. This may be difficult for families, and they may liken it to euthanasia. Many factors must be considered when having this discussion, such as individual preferences, religious beliefs, and cultural traditions. For example, Muslims may believe that withholding or withdrawing life-sustaining measures would be totally unacceptable under any circumstances (Searight & Gafford, 2005; Sheldon & Hilaire, 2016). Institutions and hospitals, especially those with religious affiliations, may hold the ethical principle of the sanctity of life in the highest regard. This may lead to conflict with what practitioners might consider an appropriate medical decision regarding termination of life-sustaining treatment. With the exception of aggressive relapsed disease, the transplant medical team frequently has difficulty discontinuing aggressive therapy for complications of transplantation (Ganti et al., 2007). Decision making and practices related to stopping or withholding treatment for HSCT patients with life-threatening organ failure or relapse disease should be addressed before treatment begins (Johnston et al., 2018; Lin et al., 2019). The authors concluded that greater attention should be paid to these topics during pretransplantation counseling, including the identification of treatment limits (Johnston et al., 2018; Lin et al., 2019).

When families and clinicians disagree on medical care, an ethics consult is usually called. Some states have enacted laws that support institutional policy, if available, for determination of medically inappropriate interventions (Advance Directives Act, 1999). This policy usually involves a review process that includes clinical experts not directly involved in the case, members of the ethics committee, the patient's family, the medical team, and a representative from the hospital administration. If the decision is made to terminate life support, a designated waiting period will be established so that the patient and family can find another care facility that will continue to provide the level of care requested. During this process, provisions usually are in place to maintain the same level of life-sustaining care, and an agreement (within the institution's physician group) is made that no other physician will take over the case, thereby risking a change in the goal and plan of care as decided by the committee. If the family decides not to move the patient to another facility, life-sustaining measures will be discontinued, and comfort measures will be continued until the patient dies.

Summary

HSCT nurses encounter many ethical issues in their role as patient advocates. Studies are currently trying to quantify the issues nurses face in practice (Neumann et al., 2018). Oncology nurses who face unresolved ethical issues in their practice often experience moral distress (Cohen & Erickson, 2006; Ferrell, 2006; Neumann et al., 2018). Nurses working in research centers where phase 1 trials take place may face additional ethical challenges because of the unpredictable results of these studies and the possibility of severe side effects and complications as new therapies are being developed (Chang, 2008; Ermete, 2016). Nurses' knowledge of advance directive documents, the Patient Self-Determination Act, and state law is inconsistent, so it is necessary for nurses to familiarize themselves with laws and policies related to advance directives (Jezewski & Feng, 2007). Nurses are encouraged to become involved in their institution's ethics committee and in writing policies that can help to define practice and lessen potential conflicts. Measures to support nurses in the role of caregiver and patient advocate should be examined (Bowman, 2018; Vaclavik, Staffileno, & Carlson, 2018). For example, the University of Texas MD Anderson Cancer Center initiated monthly nursing ethics rounds on an inpatient HSCT unit that included the nursing staff, assistant nurse manager, HSCT advanced practice registered nurse, and a member of the institutional ethics committee.

Nurses have a responsibility to know their state's current regulations, as well as the policies of their institutions, related to ethical issues. Finally, to truly advocate for patients, it is imperative to know the goal of care and to challenge inconsistencies if they arise between the patient's understanding of that goal and the medical plan of care.

References

Advance Directives Act, Texas Health & Safety Code Ann. §§166.001 et seq. (1999). Retrieved from http://www.statutes.legis.state.tx.us/Docs /HS/htm/HS.166.htm

American Academy of Pediatrics Committee on Bioethics. (2010). Policy statement—Children as hematopoietic stem cell donors. *Pediatrics, 125*, 392–404. https://doi.org/10.1542/peds.2009-3078

American Academy of Pediatrics Committee on Bioethics. (2016). Informed consent in decision-making in pediatric practice. *Pediatrics, 138*, e20161484. https://doi.org/10.1542/peds.2016-1484

American Nurses Association. (2015). *Code of ethics for nurses with interpretive statements.* Retrieved from https://www.nursingworld.org/practice-policy/nursing-excellence/ethics/code-of-ethics-for-nurses/coe-view-only

Anderson, J.A., & Kimmelman, J. (2010). Extending clinical equipoise to phase 1 trials involving patients: Unresolved problems. *Kennedy Institute of Ethics Journal, 20*, 75–98. https://doi.org/10.1353/ken.0.0307

Bayraktar, U.D., Milton, D.R., Shpall, E.J., Rondon, G., Price, K.J., Champlin, R.E., & Nates, J.L. (2017). Prognostic index for critically ill allogeneic transplantation patients. *Biology of Blood and Marrow Transplantation, 23*, 991–996. https://doi.org/10.1016/j.bbmt.2017.03.003

Beauchamp, T.L., & Childress, J.F. (2012). *Principles of biomedical ethics* (7th ed.). New York, NY: Oxford University Press.

Bevans, M.F., Mitchell, S.A., Barrett, J.A., Bishop, M.R., Childs, R., Fowler, D., … Yang, L. (2014). Symptom distress predicts long-term health and well-being in allogeneic stem cell transplantation survivors. *Biology of Blood and Marrow Transplantation, 20*, 387–395. https://doi.org/10.1016/j.bbmt.2013.12.001

Bitan, M., van Walraven, S.M., Worel, N., Ball, L.M., Styczynski, J., Torrabadella, M., … Pulsipher, M.A. (2016). Determination of eligibility in related pediatric hematopoietic cell donors: Ethical and clinical consideration. Recommendation from a working group of the Worldwide Network for Blood and Marrow Transplantation Association. *Biology of Blood and Marrow Transplantation, 22*, 96–103. https://doi.org/10.1016/j.bbmt.2015.08.017

Bowman, P. (2018, May 22). How to have ethical discussions in your practice. Retrieved from https://voice.ons.org/news-and-views/how-to-have-ethical-discussions-in-your-practice

Buchbinder, D., Kelly, D.L., Duarte, R.F., Auletta, J.J., Bhatt, N., Byrne, M., … Shaw, B.E. (2018). Neurocognitive dysfunction in heamatopoietic cell transplant recipients: Expert review from the Late Effects and Quality of Life Working Committee of the CIBMTR and Complications and Quality of Life Working Party of the EBMT. *Bone Marrow Transplantation, 53*, 535–555. https://doi.org/10.1038/s41409-017-0055-7

Burns, L.J., Abbetti, B., Arnold, S.D., Bender, J., Doughtie, S., El-Jawahiri, A., … Denzen, E.M. (2018). Engaging patients in setting a patient-centered outcomes research agenda in hematopoietic cell transplantation. *Biology of Blood and Marrow Transplantation, 24*, 1111–1118. https://doi.org/10.1016/j.bbmt.2018.01.029

Caocci, G., La Nasa, G., d'Aloja, E., Vacca, A., Piras, E., Pintor, M., … Pisu, S. (2011). Ethical issues of unrelated hematopoietic stem cell transplantation in adult thalassemia patients. *BMC Medical Ethics, 12*, 4. https://doi.org/10.1186/1472-6939-12-4

Cappell, K., Sundaram, V., Park, A., Shiraz, P., Gupta, R., Jenkins, P., … Muffly, L. (2018). Advance directive utilization is associated with less aggressive end-of-life care in patients undergoing allogeneic hematopoietic cell transplantation. *Biology of Blood and Marrow Transplantation, 24*, 1035–1040. https://doi.org/10.1016/j.bbmt.2018.01.014

Carrieri, D., Peccatori, F.A., & Boniolo, G. (2018). The ethical plausibility of the 'Right to Try' laws. *Critical Reviews in Oncology/Hematology, 122*, 64–71. https://doi.org/10.1016/j.critrevonc.2017.12.014

Chang, A. (2008). An exploratory survey of nurses' perceptions of phase I clinical trials in pediatric oncology. *Journal of Pediatric Oncology Nursing, 25*, 14–23. https://doi.org/10.1177/1043454207311742

Cohen, J.S., & Erickson, J.M. (2006). Ethical dilemmas and moral distress in oncology nursing practice. *Clinical Journal of Oncology Nursing, 10*, 775–780. https://doi.org/10.1188/06.cjon.775-780

El-Jawahri, A., Chen, Y.-B., Brazauskas, R., He, N., Lee, S.J., Knight, J.M., … Saber, W. (2017). Impact of pre-transplant depression on outcomes of allogeneic and autologous hematopoietic stem cell transplantation. *Cancer, 123*, 1828–1838. https://doi.org/10.1002/cncr.30546

Ermete, R. (2016). Medical research and clinical trials. In J.M. Erickson & K. Payne (Eds.), *Ethics in oncology nursing* (pp. 21–39). Pittsburgh, PA: Oncology Nursing Society.

Ferrell, B.R. (2006). Understanding the moral distress of nurses witnessing medically futile care. *Oncology Nursing Forum, 33*, 922–930. https://doi.org/10.1188/06.onf.922-930

Foster, L.W., McLellan, L., Rybicki, L., Dabney, J., Visnosky, M., & Bolwell, B. (2009). Utility of the psychosocial assessment of candidates for transplantation (PACT) scale in allogeneic BMT. *Bone Marrow Transplantation, 44*, 375–380. https://doi.org/10.1038/bmt.2009.37

Ganti, A.K., Lee, S.J., Vose, J.M., Devetten, M.P., Bociek, R.G., Armitage, J.O., … Loberiza, F.R., Jr. (2007). Outcomes after hematopoietic stem-cell transplantation for hematologic malignancies in patients with or without advance care planning. *Journal of Clinical Oncology, 25*, 5643–5648. https://doi.org/10.1200/jco.2007.11.1914

Gilli, K., Remberger, M., Hjelmqvist, H., Ringden, O., & Mattsson, J. (2010). Sequential organ failure assessment predicts the outcome of SCT recipients admitted to intensive care unit. *Bone Marrow Transplantation, 45*, 682–688. https://doi.org/10.1038/bmt.2009.220

Grulke, N., Larbig, W., Kächele, H., & Bailer, H. (2008). Pre-transplant depression as risk factor for survival of patients undergoing allogeneic haematopoietic stem cell transplantation. *Psycho-Oncology, 17*, 480–487. https://doi.org/10.1002/pon.1261

Hacker, E., Peters, T., Patel, P., & Rondelli, D. (2018). Steps to enhance early recovery after hematopoietic stem cell transplantation: Lessons learned from a physical activity feasibility study. *Clinical Nurse Specialist, 32*, 152–162. https://doi.org/10.1097/nur.0000000000000374

Haddad, A.M. (2016). Principles of ethics. In J.M. Erickson & K. Payne (Eds.), *Ethics in oncology nursing* (pp. 1–20). Pittsburgh, PA: Oncology Nursing Society.

Health Care Facility Do-Not-Resuscitate Orders, Tex. Health & Safety Code Ann. § 166.201 et seq. (2018). Retrieved from https://statutes.capitol.texas.gov/Docs/HS/htm/HS.166.htm

Hey, S.P., & Kesselheim, A.S. (2016). The FDA, Juno Therapeutics, and the ethical imperative of transparency. *BMJ, 354*, i4435. https://doi.org/10.1136/bmj.i4435

Jecker, N.S., Wightman, A.G., Rosenberg, A.R., & Diekema, D.S. (2017). From protection to entitlement: Selecting research subjects for early phase clinical trials involving breakthrough therapies. *Journal of Medical Ethics, 43*, 391–400. https://doi.org/10.1136/medethics-2016-103868

Jezewski, M.A., & Feng, J.-Y. (2007). Emergency nurses' knowledge, attitudes, and experiential survey on advance directives. *Applied Nursing Research, 20*, 132–139. https://doi.org/10.1016/j.apnr.2006.05.003

Jezewski, M.A., & Finnell, D.S. (1998). The meaning of DNR status: Oncology nurses' experiences with patients and families. *Cancer Nursing, 21*, 212–221. https://doi.org/10.1097/00002820-199806000-00009

Jim, H.S.L., Quinn, G.P., Gwede, C.K., Cases, M.G., Barata, A., Cessna, J., … Pidala, J. (2014). Patient education in allogeneic hematopoietic cell transplant: What patients wish they had known about quality of life. *Bone Marrow Transplantation, 49*, 299–303. https://doi.org/10.1038/bmt.2013.158

Johnston, E.E., Muffly, L., Alvarez, E., Saynina, O., Sanders, L.M., Bhatia, S., & Chamberlain, L.J. (2018). End-of-life care intensity in patients undergoing allogeneic hematopoietic cell transplantation: A population-level analysis. *Journal of Clinical Oncology, 36*, 3023–3030. https://doi.org/10.1200/jco.2018.78.0957

Jones, R.A., & Campbell, C. (2016). Treatment decision making. In J. Erickson & K. Payne (Eds.), *Ethics in oncology nursing* (pp. 41–58). Pittsburgh, PA: Oncology Nursing Society.

Jonsen, A.R., Siegler, M., & Winslade, W.J. (2015). *Clinical ethics: A practical approach to ethical decisions in clinical medicine* (8th ed.). New York, NY: McGraw-Hill Medical.

Kaiser Family Foundation. (2013, April 25). Summary of the Affordable Care Act (Publication No. 8061-02). Retrieved from https://www.kff.org/health-reform/fact-sheet/summary-of-the-affordable-care-act

Khera, N., Martin, P., Edsall, K., Bonagura, A., Burns, L.J., Juckett, M., … Majhail, N.S. (2017). Patient-centered care coordination in hematopoietic cell transplantation. *Blood Advances, 1*, 1617–1627. https://doi.org/10.1182/bloodadvances.2017008789

Kunneman, M., & Montori, V.M. (2017). When patient-centered care is worth doing well: Informed consent or shared decision-making. *BMJ Quality and Safety, 26*, 522–524. https://doi.org/10.1136/bmjqs-2016-005969

Kvale, E.A., Woodby, L., & Williams, B.R. (2010). The experience of older patients with cancer in phase 1 clinical trials: A qualitative case series. *American Journal of Hospice and Palliative Care, 27*, 474–481. https://doi.org/10.1177/1049909110365072

Lesko, L.M., Dermatis, H., Penman, D., & Holland, J.C. (2006). Patients', parents', and oncologists' perceptions of informed consent for bone marrow transplantation. *Medical and Pediatric Oncology, 17*, 181–187. https://doi.org/10.1002/mpo.2950170303

Lin, R.J., Elko, T.A., Perales, M.-A., Alexander, K., Jakubowski, A.A., Devlin, S.M., … Nelson, J.E. (2019). End-of-life care for older AML patients relapsing after allogeneic stem cell transplant at a dedicated cancer center. *Bone Marrow Transplantation, 54*, 700–706. https://doi.org/10.1038/s41409-018-0311-5

Little, M., Jordens, C.F.C., McGrath, C., Montgomery, K., Lipworth, W., & Kerridge, I. (2008). Informed consent and medical ordeal: A qualitative study. *Internal Medicine Journal, 38*, 624–628. https://doi.org/10.1111/j.1445-5994.2008.01700.x

Lubejko, B.G., & Wilson, B.J. (2019). *Oncology nursing: Scope and standards of practice.* Pittsburgh, PA: Oncology Nursing Society.

National Marrow Donor Program. (2018). *National Marrow Donor Program®/Be The Match® 24th edition standards and glossary.* Retrieved from https://bethematch.org/workarea/downloadasset.aspx?id=10093

Needle, J., & Smith, A.R. (2016). The impact of advance directives on end-of-life care for adolescents and young adults undergoing hematopoietic stem cell transplant. *Journal of Palliative Medicine, 19*, 300–305. https://doi.org/10.1089/jpm.2015.0327

Neumann, J.L., Mau, L.-W., Virani, S., Denzen, E.M., Boyle, D.A., Boyle, N.J., … Burns, L.J. (2018). Burnout, moral distress, work–life balance, and career satisfaction among hematopoietic cell transplantation professionals. *Biology of Blood and Marrow Transplantation, 24*, 849–860. https://doi.org/10.1016/j.bbmt.2017.11.015

Ogba, N., Arwood, N.M., Bartlett, N.L., Bloom, M., Brown, P., Brown, C., … Rosen, S.T. (2018). Chimeric antigen receptor T-cell therapy. *Journal of the National Comprehensive Cancer Network, 16*, 1092–1106. https://doi.org/10.6004/jnccn.2018.0073

Patel, S.S., Rybicki, L.A., Corrigan, D., Bolwell, B., Dean, R., Liu, H., … Hamilton, B.K. (2018). Prognostic factors for morality among day +100 survivors after allogeneic cell transplantation. *Biology of Blood and Marrow Transplantation, 24*, 1029–1034. https://doi.org/10.1016/j.bbmt.2018.01.016

Patient Protection and Affordable Care Act, Pub. L. No. 111-148, 124 Stat. 119 (2010).

Pence, G.E. (2004). *Classic cases in medical ethics: Accounts of cases that have shaped medical ethics, with philosophical, legal, and historical backgrounds* (4th ed.). Boston, MA: McGraw-Hill.

Pillay, B., Lee, S.J., Katona, L., Burney, S., & Avery, S. (2014). Psychosocial factors predicting survival after allogeneic stem cell transplant. *Supportive Care in Cancer, 22*, 2547–2555. https://doi.org/10.1007/s00520-014-2239-7

Prasad, V., De Jesús, K., & Mailankody, S. (2017). The high price of anticancer drugs: Origins, implications, barriers, solutions. *Nature Reviews Clinical Oncology, 14*, 381–390. https://doi.org/10.1038/nrclinonc.2017.31

Preussler, J.M., Meyer, C.L., Mau, L.-W., Najhail, N.S., Denzen, E.M., Edsall, K.C., … Vanness, D.J. (2017). Healthcare costs and utilization for patients age 50 to 64 years with acute myeloid leukemia treated with chemotherapy or with chemotherapy and allogeneic hematopoietic cell transplantation. *Biology of Blood and Marrow Transplantation, 23*, 1021–1028. https://doi.org/10.1016/j.bbmt.2017.02.017

Raj, M., Choi, S.W., Gurtekin, T.S., & Platt, J. (2018). Improving the informed consent process in hematopoietic cell transplantation: Patient, caregiver, and provider perspectives. *Biology of Blood and Marrow Transplantation, 24*, 156–162. https://doi.org/10.1016/j.bbmt.2017.08.037

Ramirez, L.Y., Huestis, S.E., Yap, T.Y., Zyzanski, S., Drotar, D., & Kodish, E. (2009). Potential chemotherapy side effects: What do oncologists tell parents? *Pediatric Blood and Cancer, 52*, 497–502. https://doi.org/10.1002/pbc.21835

Searight, H.R., & Gafford, J. (2005). Cultural diversity at the end of life: Issues and guidelines for family physicians. *American Family Physician, 71*, 515–522. Retrieved from https://www.aafp.org/afp/2005/0201/p515.html

Shaw, B.E., Logan, B.R., Spellman, S.R., Marsh, S.G.E., Robinson, J., Pidala, J., … Lee, S.J. (2018). Development of an unrelated donor selection score predictive of survival after HCT: Donor age matters most. *Biology of Blood and Marrow Transplantation, 24*, 1049–1056. https://doi.org/10.1016/j.bbmt.2018.02.006

Sheldon, L.K., & Hilaire, D.M. (2016). Communication and ethics. In J.M. Erickson & K. Payne (Eds.), *Ethics in oncology nursing* (pp. 101–122). Pittsburgh, PA: Oncology Nursing Society.

Shouval, R., de Jong, C.N., Fein, J., Broers, A.E.C., Danylesko, I., Shimoni, A., … Cornelissen, J.J. (2018). Baseline renal function and albumin are powerful predictors for allogeneic transplantation-related mortality. *Biology of Blood and Marrow Transplantation, 24*, 1685–1691. https://doi.org/10.1016/j.bbmt.2018.05.005

Smith, A.K., McCarthy, E.P., Paulk, E., Balboni, T.A., Maciejewski, P.K., Block, S.D., & Prigerson, H.G. (2008). Racial and ethnic differences in advance care planning among patients with cancer: Impact of terminal illness acknowledgment, religiousness, and treatment preferences. *Journal of Clinical Oncology, 26*, 4131–4137. https://doi.org/10.1200/jco.2007.14.8452

Stegenga, K., Pentz, R.D., Alderfer, M.A., Pelletier, W., Fairclough, D., & Hinds, P.S. (2018). Child and parent access to transplant information and involvement in treatment decision making. *Western Journal of Nursing Research, 41*, 576–591. https://doi.org/10.1177/0193945918770440

Sullivan, H.B., & Caguioa, N., (2018). Preparing the frontline: Nursing education for enhanced recovery in stem cell transplant, an interdisciplinary program targeting improved outcomes in patients 65+ years old receiving allogeneic transplant [Abstract]. *Biology of Blood and Marrow Transplantation, 24*(Suppl. 3), S455–S456. https://doi.org/10.1016/j.bbmt.2017.12.755

Sulmasy, D.P., Sood, J.R., Texiera, K., McAuley, R.L., McGugins, J., & Ury, W.A. (2006). A prospective trial of a new policy eliminating signed consent for do not resuscitate orders. *Journal of General Internal Medicine, 21*, 1261–1268. https://doi.org/10.1111/j.1525-1497.2006.00612.x

Sun, C.-L., Francisco, L., Baker, K.S., Weisdorf, D.J., Forman, S.J., & Bhatia, S. (2011). Adverse psychological outcomes in long-term survivors of hematopoietic cell transplantation: A report from the Bone Marrow Transplant Survivor Study (BMTSS). *Blood, 118*, 4723–4731. https://doi.org/10.1182/blood-2011-04-348730

Svenson, A.G. (2010). Montana's courting of physician aid in dying. Could Des Moines follow suit? *Politics and the Life Sciences, 29*(2), 2–16. https://doi.org/10.2990/29_2_2

Szewczyk, N., Neumann, J.L., Kruse, B., Pang, L., Ngo-Huang, A., Ferguson, J., … & Popat, U.R. (2019). Experience with applying and improving feasibility of an enhanced recovery model for allogenic stem cell transplant patients aged 65 and older [Abstract]. *Biology of Blood and Marrow Transplantation, 25*(Suppl. 3), S432. https://doi.org/10.1016/j.bbmt.2018.12.497

Texas Health and Human Services Commission. (2015). *Directive to physicians and family or surrogates.* Retrieved from https://hhs.texas.gov/sites/default/files/documents/laws-regulations/forms/LivingWill/LivingWill.pdf

Vaclavik, E.A., Staffileno, B.A., & Carlson, E. (2018). Moral distress: Using mindfulness-based stress reduction interventions to decrease nurse perceptions of distress. *Clinical Journal of Oncology Nursing, 22*, 326–332. https://doi.org/10.1188/18.cjon.326-332

van Walraven, S.M., Egeland, T., Borrill, V., Nicoloso-de Faveri, G., Rall, G., & Szer, J. (2018). Addressing ethical and procedural principles for unrelated allogeneic hematopoietic progenitor cell donation in a changing medical environment. *Biology of Blood and Marrow Transplantation, 24*, 887–894. https://doi.org/10.1016/j.bbmt.2018.01.018

Venneman, S.S., Narnor-Harris, P., Perish, M., & Hamilton, M. (2008). "Allow natural death" versus "do not resuscitate": Three words that can change a life. *Journal of Medical Ethics, 34*, 2–6. https://doi.org/10.1136/jme.2006.018317

Wiener, J.M. (1992). Oregon's plan for health care rationing: Bold initiative or terrible mistake? *The Brookings Review, 10*, 26–31. https://doi.org/10.2307/20080268

Emerging Cellular Therapies: Chimeric Antigen Receptor T Cells

Theresa Latchford, RN, MS, BMTCN®, AOCNS®, and D. Kathryn Tierney, RN, BMTCN®, PhD

Introduction

Immunotherapy is considered the fourth pillar of cancer therapy after surgery, radiation, and chemotherapy (McCune, 2018). Immense strides have been made in recent years to harness the power of the immune system to treat cancer. The recent U.S. Food and Drug Administration (FDA) approval of chimeric antigen receptor (CAR) T-cell therapy has generated a great deal of enthusiasm for the treatment of acute lymphoblastic leukemia (ALL) and non-Hodgkin lymphoma (NHL) that are refractory to other therapies. The major focus of this chapter is the cancer immunotherapy treatment option of CAR T-cell therapy, including mechanism of action, manufacturing process, pioneering studies leading to FDA approval, infrastructure to develop and administer CAR T-cell therapy, management of toxicities, staff education, financial concerns, and future directions.

Overview of the Immune System and Immunotherapy

The immune system maintains homeostasis by protecting the host from microorganisms and foreign tissue. Cells are identified by specific markers on the cell surface called cluster of differentiation (CD) markers. Cellular immunity is principally orchestrated by a variety of T lymphocytes, including cytotoxic T cells, helper T cells, natural killer T cells, and memory T cells—each having a specific function. T lymphocytes function by recognizing a specific antigen on a cell surface. After recognizing the antigen, a cascade of events occurs, resulting in the proliferation of T lymphocytes and a coordinated attack on cells carrying that specific antigen. B lymphocytes are the key cells involved in humoral immunity. B lymphocytes secrete antibodies, such as immunoglobulin (Ig) G, A, M, D, and E. Each antibody has a specific function. Similar to T lymphocytes, B lymphocytes also respond to a specific antigen on a cell's surface. Recognition of the antigen then stimulates B lymphocytes to secrete antibodies to eliminate all cells with that specific antigen. Both cellular and humoral immunity play a key role in protecting the host from microorganisms, foreign tissue, and cancer.

Cancer cells evade detection by the immune system in several ways. The antigens on the surface of cancer cells may appear similar to antigens on healthy cells, so the immune system does not recognize the cell as abnormal and target it for destruction. As cancer progresses, multiple mutations can occur that change the antigens expressed on the cell surface, again allowing the cancer cells to evade detection by the immune system. A goal of cancer research has been to find antigens that are unique to cancer cells and not found on healthy cells. Therapies can then be developed to target that specific antigen and spare healthy cells. Cancer immunotherapy is an emerging field with that goal in mind.

Cancer immunotherapy consists of four major categories: monoclonal antibodies, checkpoint inhibitors, oncolytic viral therapies, and CAR T-cell therapy (Bayer et al., 2017). FDA has approved numerous monoclonal antibodies for cancer treatment. For example, rituximab is a common monoclonal antibody therapy that targets a specific antigen (CD20) found on healthy B lymphocytes in addition to malignant B lymphocytes in the majority of B-cell NHL cases (Zhang, Medeiros, & Young, 2018). Rituximab was first approved in 1997 for the treatment of B-cell NHL. Checkpoint inhibitors are a class of drugs that target immune checkpoint pathways that enable the cancer to evade the immune system. Immune checkpoints are regulators of the immune system that inhibit or stimulate its actions. FDA has approved multiple checkpoint inhibitors for cancer treatment, including ipilimumab for melanoma; nivolumab for non-small cell lung cancer, melanoma, renal cell carcinoma, and Hodgkin lymphoma; and pembrolizumab for non-small cell lung cancer, melanoma, and squamous cell carcinoma of the head and neck. Each of these drugs targets a different immune system checkpoint, including cytotoxic T lymphocyte–associated proteins, programmed cell death protein 1 (PD-1) and programmed cell death-ligand 1 (PD-L1). The majority of oncolytic viral therapies are under investigation with the exception of talimogene laherparepvec, which is an FDA-approved intralesional injection using a modified herpes simplex type 1 virus to treat metastatic melanoma (Bayer et al., 2017). It is unknown specifically how viral targeted therapy kills the cancer cells. Talimogene laherparepvec is injected into the tumor, and as the virus replicates, it stimulates the immune system to produce granulocyte macrophage–colony-stimulating factor to cause cell death and an antitumor response.

CARs, the fourth type of immunotherapy, are genetically engineered receptors and a form of targeted therapy using T cells. T cells have long been recognized as contributing to curing hematologic malignancies, known as graft-versus-tumor benefit of allogeneic transplantation. T cells that are equipped with CAR are one of the most recent advances in immunotherapy. Currently, the available CAR T-cell products target the CD19 antigen found on B-cell malignancies. An advantage of CAR T-cell therapy against CD19 is that CD19 is expressed at all stages of B-cell maturation with the exception of plasma cells (Chavez & Locke, 2017). CD19 is expressed in most B-cell malignancies, such as chronic lymphocytic leukemia, B-cell NHL, and B-cell ALL, which makes these malignancies ideal targets for CAR T-cell therapy. CD19 is also expressed on healthy B cells resulting in B-cell hypoplasia after these therapies. Sufficient data support the notion that depletion of healthy B cells following chemotherapy and monoclonal antibody therapies, such as rituximab, is tolerated (Chavez & Locke, 2018). According to Elahi, Khosh, Tahmasebi, and Esmaeilzadeh (2018), development of CAR T cells against other targets including CD5, CD13, CD20, CD22, and B-cell maturation antigen (BCMA)/transmembrane activator and CAML interactor (TACI), found in other hematologic malignancies, including multiple myeloma, is under investigation. BCMA is a tumor necrosis factor that helps plasma cells survive. Similar to CD19 on healthy and malignant B cells, BCMA is expressed on healthy plasma cells and multiple myeloma cells, and it is the main target for many promising anti-BCMA CAR T-cell therapies in phase 1 and 2 clinical trials for myeloma (Adaniya, Cohen, & Garfall, 2019). The use of CAR T cells for the treatment of solid cancers is also an emerging field. Identification of surface-expressed tumor targets unique to cancer is a major challenge in expanding the use of CAR T-cell therapy. For example, epidermal growth factor receptor variant III and ephrin receptor A2 in glioblastoma, GD2 in neuroblastoma and sarcoma, and alpha fetoprotein in hepatocellular carcinoma are being investigated as targets of CAR T-cell therapy for the treatment of solid tumors (Elahi et al., 2018).

Other immune effector cells are being used for the treatment of cancer or are under investigation. Immune effector cell therapies include natural killer cells with or without ex vivo activation; cytotoxic T lymphocytes expanded ex vivo against viral or tumor peptides to target infection or malignancy; regulatory cells with or without genetic modification to induce tolerance; and dendritic cells loaded with peptides or genetically engineered to express cytokines to enhance immune system recognition (Maus & Nikiforow, 2017). CAR T-cell therapy is an emerging cancer immunotherapy that is rapidly changing treatment options and oncology clinical practice.

Building a Chimeric Antigen Receptor T Cell

CAR T cells are genetically modified autologous T cells. These modified T cells recognize a specific target on the surface of a cancer cell and destroy the cell. The manufacture of CAR T cells has multiple steps. First, peripheral mononuclear cells are collected by leukapheresis and sent to a manufacturing facility for stimulation and activation of the T cells. Some manufacturing begins with enrichment of the mononuclear cells for specific T-cell subsets, including CD4 and CD8 cells. The enriched cells are then stimulated with a bead conjugated with human anti-CD3 and anti-CD28 monoclonal antibodies (Vormittag, Gunn, Ghorashian, & Veraitch, 2018). The activated T-cells are then transduced with a viral vector encoding the CAR. The viral vectors most commonly used for CAR T-cell therapy are retroviral or lentiviral vectors. These viral vectors encode the receptor, which is integrated into the DNA of the T cell, allowing for CAR expression. The transduced T cells are then cultured for several days in the presence of growth-promoting cytokines (interleukin [IL]-2, IL-7, or IL-15) prior to the final formulation (Elahi et al., 2018). The viral vector and the final T-cell product undergo extensive biosafety testing to ensure that the infused product is sterile and free of unwanted agents, including the replication-competent virus. Currently, the most common and efficient method to deliver genetic modifications into T cells is via viral vectors; however, work to develop nonviral vector strategies to introduce genetic modifications into T cells, such as messenger RNA, transposons, and DNA plasmid, are underway (Elahi et al., 2018). Transfection of the CAR genes into the cell and expansion can take two weeks or more (Elahi et al., 2018). Efforts to improve the efficacy of the manufacturing process are ongoing, with a focus on reducing overall production time, as well as improving methodologies for genetic modification of T cells.

Mechanism of Action

Four components make up a CAR, including the extracellular binding domain, which provides the tumor antigen specificity and is referred to as the *single-chain variable fragment* (ScFv) (Ghobadi, 2018). The extracellular ScFv attaches and binds to the target tumor antigen. The hinge or spacer connects the ScFv to the transmembrane domain and provides flexibility for the extracellular domain (Elahi et al., 2018; Whilding & Maher, 2015). Based on the number and type of intracellular signaling domains, CARs are designated as first, second, or third generation (Elahi et al., 2018; Ghobadi, 2018; Whilding & Maher, 2015; Zhang et al., 2018). A first-generation CAR has only a CD3-zeta (CD247) signaling domain. Second-generation CARs, in addition to CD3-zeta signaling, typically have a second signaling domain, either CD28 or 4-1BB (CD137). Third-generation CARs contain a combination of three signaling domains

(Ghobadi, 2018; Zhang et al., 2018). When the CAR T cell encounters antigen, the T cell is activated through the signal transduction domain. T-cell expansion and direct cell cytotoxicity occur (Heyman & Yang, 2018). The specific activation and costimulation increases cytokine production, resulting in proliferation and activation of CAR T cells (Neelapu, Tummala, Kebriaei, Wierda, Gutierrez, et al., 2018; Salter, Pont, & Riddell, 2018).

First-generation CAR T cells yielded important insights and experience, but they lacked efficacy and long-term persistence (Maude, 2017). Second-generation CAR T cells have improved cell expansion and persistence (Zhang et al., 2018). This generation of T cells, which includes the CD28 costimulatory domain, had both a rapid expansion and low persistence in the blood, whereas 4-1BB CAR T cells exhibited slower initial expansion but appeared to persist longer without exhibiting exhaustion (Perica, Curran, Brentjens, & Giralt, 2018; Whilding & Maher, 2015). Long-term outcomes of the different costimulatory domains need further evaluation. The third generation of CAR T cells combine three costimulatory domains, such as CD28, CD27, 4-1BB (CD137), inducible T-cell costimulator (ICOS; CD278) or OX40 (CD134), in addition to CD3-zeta (Zhang et al., 2018). It is thought that the presence of three costimulatory domains will improve clinical outcomes (Zhang et al., 2018). Engineering CAR T cells with multiple costimulatory domains carries the risk of an increase in the release of life-threatening cytokines resulting from signaling activation of the CAR T cells when they encounter antigen. New technologies to control CAR expansion and activation are being developed, which could be considered fourth-generation CAR T cells (Zhang et al., 2018). One fourth-generation CAR T-cell therapy under investigation is T cells redirected for universal cytokine-mediated killing (TRUCKs). TRUCKs, or "armored" CAR T cells, increase the activation of the CAR T cells, induce cytokine release, and attract innate immune cells for cancer destruction (Elahi et al., 2018; Zhang et al., 2018). Figure 16-1 provides a comparison of the different CD19-directed CAR T cell constructs. A variety of CAR constructs are actively being investigated with the goal of reducing toxicity and improving the efficacy of cancer immunotherapies. While research of CAR T-cell therapies continues to develop and improve, as of May 2018, FDA has approved two CAR T-cell therapies for commercial use. At the time of this writing, several CAR T-cell therapies are at various stages of the clinical trial process: ZUMA-7 is active (Kite Pharma, 2019a); KarMMa-3 (Novick, 2019) and BELINDA (Novartis Pharmaceuticals, 2019a) are recruiting participants; and OBERON (Novartis Pharmaceuticals, 2019b) will soon begin recruiting.

Pivotal Trials

Several clinical trials led to the approval of axicabtagene ciloleucel and tisagenlecleucel for various hematologic malignancies.

ZUMA-1, a multicenter phase 2 trial of axicabtagene ciloleucel by Kite Pharma, included 111 participants with diffuse large B-cell lymphoma (DLBCL), primary mediastinal B-cell lymphoma, or transformed follicular lymphoma who received axicabtagene ciloleucel (Locke, Neelapu, Bartlett, Siddiqi, et al., 2017; Neelapu et al., 2017). Axicabtagene ciloleucel is genetically modified to have ScFv with a CD3-zeta extracellular domain and a CD28 intracellular costimulatory domain that signals and initiates T-cell activation against CD19 found on certain malignant cells (Neelapu et al., 2017). All participants had refractory NHL. The study defined *refractory* as progressive or stable disease as the best response to most recent chemotherapy or disease progression within one year of autologous hematopoietic stem cell transplantation (HSCT). The median participant age was 58 years, with a range of 23–76 years. Most of the patients had stage III or IV disease, and 77% of participants had disease that was shown to be resistant to two or more lines of therapy. Disease relapse occurred in 21% of participants after autologous transplantation; 69% received at least three lines of previous therapies; and 26% had a history of primary refractory disease.

Following leukapheresis at the treatment center, the collected cells were sent to the pharmaceutical company for manufacturing. The median time from leukapheresis to the return of the cells was 17 days, with a 99% manufacturing success rate for 110 of the 111 participants. To prepare the participants, low doses of lymphodepleting chemotherapy were administered. No bridging chemotherapy was administered for disease management after leukapheresis and prior to lymphodepleting chemotherapy (Neelapu et al., 2017). The lymphodepleting chemotherapy included cyclophosphamide at 500 mg/m^2 and fludarabine at 30 mg/m^2 on days –5, –4, and –3 prior to receiving the genetically modified autologous CAR T cells. In this study, of the 111 participants enrolled, axicabtagene ciloleucel was infused into 101 patients. The infused CAR T-cell dose was 2×10^6/kg and given as a one-time infusion (Neelapu et al., 2017).

The study used the incidence of adverse events as one outcome measure. Cytokine release syndrome (CRS) was graded using the Lee criteria (Lee et al., 2014). Individual symptoms of CRS and neurologic events were graded using the National Cancer Institute Common Terminology Criteria for Adverse Events (CTCAE). Of the 101 participants who received infusion, 95% experienced a grade 3 or higher adverse event (Neelapu et al., 2017). Including all grades of adverse events, the most common were pyrexia (85%), neutropenia (84%), anemia (66%), and hypotension (59%). CRS occurred in 94 (93%) of the participants, with 13% experiencing grade 3 or higher (Neelapu et al., 2017). The median time from infusion to the onset of CRS was two days (range 1–12 days), and the median duration of CRS was seven days (range 2–58 days) (Kite Pharma, 2019b). Neurologic events were also common,

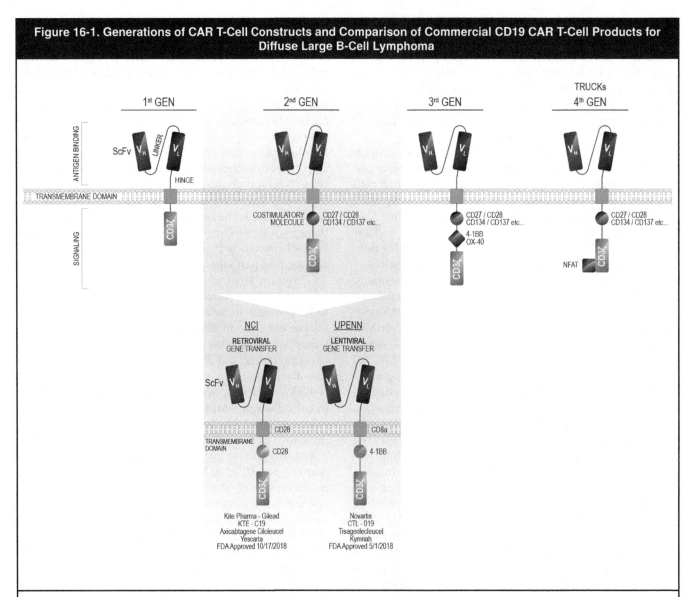

CAR—chimeric antigen receptor; CD—cluster of differentiation; FDA—U.S. Food and Drug Administration; NCI—National Cancer Institute; NFAT—nuclear factor of activated T cells; ScFv—single-chain variable fragment; TRUCKs—T cells redirected for universal cytokine-mediated killing; UPENN—University of Pennsylvania

Note. Image designed by Chris Filart.

occuring in 64% of participants, with 28% experiencing grade 3 or higher (Neelapu et al., 2017). Encephalopathy, occurred in 34% of participants; headache (5%), tremor (29%), confusion (29%), aphasia (18%), somnolence (15%), and agitation (9%) were also reported (Neelapu et al., 2017). Word finding or dysphagia, attention or calculation defects, and difficulty completing complex commands (e.g., handwriting) were frequently observed. The median time to onset of neurologic events was four days (range 1–43 days), and median duration was 17 days (Kite Pharma, 2019b). Toxicity management of neurologic events and CRS included administration of tocilizumab to 43% and glucocorticoids to 27% of the participants (Neelapu et al., 2017). Tocilizumab and steroids were not found to negatively affect the overall response

rates. A positron-emission tomography–computed tomography scan on day 28 post–CAR T-cell infusion showed an objective response rate of 82%, with 54% obtaining a complete remission and 28% achieving a partial remission (Neelapu et al., 2017). With a median follow-up at 15 months, 40% of participants remained in complete remission, and overall survival at 18 months was 52% (Neelapu et al., 2017). In a two-year follow-up of ZUMA-1 by an independent review committee, the ongoing complete response was 35% of patients, with a median duration of complete response still not met (Locke et al., 2018).

This study concluded that personalized cell therapy—despite its complexity—can be safely provided in a timely manner regardless of the coordination challenges between the treatment center and cell manufacturer. Axicabtagene ciloleucel can be administered safely following algorithms for the management of CRS and neurotoxicity. Most importantly, this study demonstrated an impressive benefit for participants with refractory NHL.

JULIET, a multicenter phase 2 trial of tisagenlecleucel conducted by Novartis Pharmaceuticals, included participants with relapsed or refractory DLBCL (Schuster, Bishop, et al., 2017). Tisagenlecleucel is transduced with a lentiviral vector and is made of a ScFv CD8 hinge, with a 4-1BB costimulatory and CD3-zeta intracellular domain that signals and initiates T-cell activation against CD19 found on B-cell malignancies (Havard & Stephens, 2018). The study enrolled 160 participants, and 106 received a CAR T-cell infusion, including 92 participants whose product was manufactured in the United States (Novartis Pharmaceuticals, 2018). Of the 160 participants enrolled, 11 did not receive the CAR T-cell infusion because of manufacturing errors. Thirty-eight other participants did not receive the infusion because of death, physician decision, or adverse events (Novartis Pharmaceuticals, 2018). The median age of participants was 56 years, with a range of 22–74 years. Of the 106 participants who received tisagenlecleucel, 68 were included in the analysis of outcomes submitted to the FDA for approval. Excluded from the analysis were those participants who did not receive bridging chemotherapy or who had measurable disease after completing the bridging chemotherapy (Novartis Pharmaceuticals, 2018). All participants had refractory or relapsed DLBCL and had received two or more lines of chemotherapy or had relapsed following autologous HSCT. Fifty-six percent had refractory disease. As in the ZUMA-1 study, the participants first received lymphodepleting chemotherapy; however, the chemotherapy doses and regimens varied. The chemotherapy regimen most commonly given was fludarabine at 25 mg/m^2 and cyclophosphamide at 250 mg/m^2 for three days. Additionally, 24% of participants received bendamustine at 90 mg/m^2 for two days, and 10% received no lymphodepleting chemotherapy (Novartis Pharmaceuticals, 2018). The median time from leukapheresis to cell infusion was 113 days (range 47–196 days) (Novartis Pharmaceuticals, 2018). The median dose of viable CAR T cells was 3.5×10^8, with a range of 1–5.2×10^8 cells. The majority of participants (73%) received tisagenlecleucel in the hospital. The lymphodepleting chemotherapy doses and drugs, manufacturing rate, and time to cell infusion varied dramatically between the ZUMA-1 and JULIET studies.

The Penn grading scale was used for grading CRS, which occurred in 74% of participants, with 23% experiencing a grade 3 or higher adverse event (Schuster, Bishop, et al., 2017). The median time to onset of CRS was three days (range 1–51 days), and the median time to resolution was eight days (range 1–36 days). Neurotoxicities occurred in 58% of the 106 participants, including 18% experiencing grade 3 or higher (Novartis Pharmaceuticals, 2018). Median time to onset of neurologic events was six days,

with a range of 1–359 days (Novartis Pharmaceuticals, 2018). Median duration of neurotoxicities was 14 days (Schuster, Bishop, et al., 2017). For 61% of participants, neurotoxicities resolved within three weeks, but encephalopathy lasting up to 50 days was observed (Novartis Pharmaceuticals, 2018). Neurotoxicity can occur concurrently with CRS, following CRS, or in the absence of CRS. The most common neurotoxicities observed were headache (21%), encephalopathy (16%), delirium (6%), anxiety (9%), sleep disorders (9%), dizziness (11%), tremors (7%), and peripheral neuropathies (8%) (Novartis Pharmaceuticals, 2018). Seizures, mutism, and aphasia were other observed toxicities (Novartis Pharmaceuticals, 2018). For CRS management, tocilizumab or corticosteroids were administered for 21% of participants (Novartis Pharmaceuticals, 2018). Eight percent received a single dose of tocilizumab; 13% received two doses of tocilizumab; and 13% received corticosteroids in addition to tocilizumab (Novartis Pharmaceuticals, 2018). Two patients received corticosteroids for CRS without tocilizumab, and two patients received corticosteroids for persistent neurotoxicities after resolution of CRS. Pharmacokinetics and cellular kinetics were measured and indicated that rapid CAR T-cell expansion occurred in a higher percentage of participants who received tocilizumab and steroids. Cytopenias that did not resolve by day 28 following infusion, including thrombocytopenia (40%) and neutropenia (25%), were also noted (Novartis Pharmaceuticals, 2018). Hypogammaglobulinemia-related B-cell aplasia may occur after tisagenlecleucel and was reported in 14% of participants with DLBCL.

Outcome measures were evaluable for 68 participants. The overall response rate was 50%, with 32% achieving complete remission and 18% achieving partial remission (Novartis Pharmaceuticals, 2018). Of the 22 participants who achieved complete remission, 9 achieved it within a month, 12 reached it by the third month, and an additional participant achieved complete at 6 months following CAR T-cell infusion (Novartis Pharmaceuticals, 2018).

CAR T-cell therapy is considered a living therapy because it continues to proliferate and actively target tumor cells long after the infusion, as evidenced by the participant achieving complete remission six months after cell infusion (Elahi et al., 2018). A therapy that remains active long after administration is an exciting new development in the treatment of cancer. The detailed evaluation of toxicity management in this study has formed the basis for algorithms used in clinical practice.

In the ELIANA study, 68 pediatric and young adult participants with relapsed or refractory B-cell ALL received a single infusion of tisagenlecleucel (Novartis Pharmaceuticals, 2018). A total of 88 participants with ALL were enrolled, and 68 received the CAR T-cell therapy, of which 63 were evaluable for outcomes. As a result of manufacturing failures, 9% did not receive therapy. The median age of participants was 12 years (range 3–23 years), with 35 male and 28 female participants. Six (10%) had primary refractory ALL, 30 (48%) underwent one prior HSCT, and six (10%) underwent two prior HSCTs (Novartis Pharmaceuticals, 2018). Lymphodepleting chemotherapy consisted of fludarabine at 30 mg/m² daily for four days and cyclophosphamide at 500 mg/m² daily for two days. Participants then received a single infusion of CAR T cells. Of the 22 participants with a white blood cell count less than 1,000/mm³, 20 received lymphodepleting chemotherapy (Novartis Pharmaceuticals, 2018). Bridging chemotherapy between leukapheresis and lymphodepleting chemotherapy was administered to 53% of participants (Novartis Pharmaceuticals, 2018).

Adverse reactions were observed in more than 20% of participants, and the symptoms were similar to those seen in adults with NHL. The most common adverse event was CRS, which occurred in 79% of participants; 49% of CRS was grade 3 or higher (Novartis Pharmaceuticals, 2018; O'Leary et al., 2019). The incidence of CRS was higher in this study compared to the JULIET study of adults with NHL. Risk factors for severe CRS in the pediatric relapsed or refractory ALL population included a large tumor burden (defined as more than 50% blasts in the marrow), uncontrolled or accelerating tumor burden following lymphodepleting chemotherapy, and active infections (Novartis Pharmaceuticals, 2018). Other adverse reactions included hypogammaglobulinemia (43%), unspecified infections (41%), pyrexia (40%), decreased appetite (37%), headache (37%), encephalopathy (36%), hypotension (31%), bleeding (31%), tachycardia (26%), nausea (26%), diarrhea (26%), vomiting (26%), viral infection (26%), hypoxia (24%), fatigue (25%), acute kidney injury (24%), edema (21%), cough (21%), and delirium (21%) (Novartis Pharmaceuticals, 2018). Neurotoxicities occurred in 72% of the participants, including 21% with grade 3 or higher (Novartis Pharmaceuticals, 2018). Median time to onset for neurotoxicities was six days after infusion, with a duration of six days, and resolution occurred within three weeks in 79% of the participants (Novartis Pharmaceuticals, 2018). Grade 3 or higher cytopenias that did not resolve by day 28 after infusion included neutropenia (40%) and thrombocytopenia (27%) (Novartis Pharmaceuticals, 2018). Prolonged neutropenia increases the risk of infection, and this risk is compounded by hypogammaglobulinemia.

Outcome measures included complete remission within three months of infusion and the number of participants achieving negative minimal residual disease as measured by less than 0.01% blasts in the blood or marrow on flow cytometry. Fifty-two participants (83%) achieved complete remission or complete remission with incomplete hematologic recovery, all of whom were minimal residual disease negative (Novartis Pharmaceuticals, 2018). With a median follow-up of 4.8 months, the median duration of complete remission or complete remission with incomplete hematologic recovery was not reached with a follow-up of 1.2–14.1 months (Novartis Pharmaceuticals, 2018).

U.S. Food and Drug Administration Approval

These pivotal trials led to the FDA approval of the first two CAR T-cell therapies. In August 2017, FDA approved tisagenlecleucel for children and young adults with relapsed or refractory B-cell ALL (O'Leary et al., 2019). In October 2017, axicabtagene ciloleucel was approved for the treatment of relapsed or refractory NHL, and in May 2018, tisagenlecleucel was approved for adults with refractory or relapsed B-cell NHL. Overall, CAR T-cell therapy can produce rapid and durable clinical responses in approximately 20%–80% of patients depending on disease (Graham, Hewitson, Pagliuca, & Benjamin, 2018; Kite Pharma, 2019b; Novartis Pharmaceuticals, 2018).

Tisagenlecleucel

FDA approved tisagenlecleucel in 2017 as the first gene therapy product for the treatment of patients up to 25 years of age with B-cell ALL that is refractory, a third complete remission or more, or relapsed disease. In May 2018, FDA approved the therapy for the indication of relapsed or refractory NHL, including DLBCL not otherwise specified, high-grade B-cell lymphoma, and DLBCL arising from follicular lymphoma, after two or more lines of systemic therapy. It is not approved for treatment of patients with primary central nervous system lymphoma (Novartis Pharmaceuticals, 2018).

Tisagenlecleucel was originally developed at the University of Pennsylvania and subsequently purchased by Novartis Pharmaceuticals (Havard & Stephens, 2018). For pediatric and young adult patients with relapsed or refractory ALL, a single dose of tisagenlecleucel may contain up to 2.5 × 10⁸ viable CAR T cells. For individuals with ALL, one or two doses may be administered depending on patient weight. For patients 50 kg or less, the dose range is 0.2–5 × 10⁶ viable CAR T cells/kg, and for patients greater than 50 kg, the dose range is 0.1–2.5 × 10⁸ viable CAR T cells and is not based on weight (Novartis Pharmaceuticals, 2018). For adults with relapsed or refractory DLBCL, a single dose of tisagenlecleucel may contain 0.6–6 × 10⁸ viable CAR T cells. The actual number of viable CAR T cells is recorded on the certificate of analysis provided by the manufacturer to the treatment center. CAR T cells are infused via IV without a filter at a rate of 10–20 ml per minute. Rate adjustments should be considered for smaller children. The volume of the infusion bag(s) ranges 10–50 ml.

Unsurprisingly, the costs of individualized CAR T-cell therapy is high, and the therapy is currently priced at $475,000 (Havard & Stephens, 2018). It is hoped that with additional clinical experience and advances in manufacturing processes, the cost of therapy will decrease.

Axicabtagene Ciloleucel

Axicabtagene ciloleucel was approved by FDA in October 2017 for the treatment of adult patients with relapsed or refractory large B-cell lymphoma, including DLBCL not otherwise specified, primary mediastinal large B-cell lymphoma, high-grade B-cell lymphoma, and DLBCL arising from follicular lymphoma, after two or more lines of systemic therapy (Kite Pharma, 2019b). Axicabtagene ciloleucel was originally developed at the National Cancer Institute before being acquired by Kite Pharma and subsequently purchased by Gilead Sciences (Havard & Stephens, 2018). The target dose is 2×10^6 viable CAR T cells/kg of body weight, with a maximum dose of 2×10^8 viable CAR T cells. Axicabtagene ciloleucel arrives at the treatment center without a certificate of analysis, so the specific number of viable CAR T cells is not known to the infusing center. The entire product has a volume of approximately 68 ml and is infused via IV without a filter either by gravity or by peristaltic pump within 30 minutes of thawing. Similar to tisagenlecleucel, this product is extremely expensive with a list price of $373,000 (Gallegos, 2018a).

Five Steps to Chimeric Antigen Receptor T-Cell Therapy

The five main steps to CAR T-cell therapy are leukapheresis, cell manufacturing, lymphodepleting chemotherapy, cell infusion, and follow-up.

Leukapheresis and Cell Manufacturing

CAR T-cell therapy requires a collection center and a manufacturing facility where the cells can be harvested, manufactured, and stored (Perica et al., 2018). Peripheral mononuclear cells are extracted from the patient by leukapheresis at a collection center. The process is similar to stem cell collection, usually taking approximately four hours, and patients generally tolerate the procedure well. Although the procedure can be performed though peripheral veins, an apheresis catheter or hemodialysis catheter usually is needed, as peripheral access may be challenging in this heavily treated population. Chapter 5 provides a more detailed discussion of apheresis. Multiple variables must be considered before scheduling a patient to start CAR T-cell therapy, including disease status, when the patient needs the next cycle of cytotoxic therapy, type of CAR T-cell product to be manufactured, clinical trial requirements for those enrolled in a research protocol, available manufacturing dates, anticipated manufacturing time, and insurance coverage. Aligning these multiple variables to set a date to begin the process is a significant challenge for the referring physician, physician to administer the therapy, nurse coordinator, and study coordinator. Systems, guidelines, or protocols that consider these multiple patient and institutional variables must be developed within institutions. Timing is a crucial factor for these patients with a challenging disease status.

Prior to cell collection, communication with the manufacturing site is critical to ensure the collected cells are processed correctly for the specified treatment plan. During the apheresis process, white blood cells are separated from whole blood by density using a continuous centrifuge. An anticoagulant is added during the process to prevent clumping. After collection, the white blood cells are sent to the manufacturer either fresh or cryopreserved. Cells collected for development for tisagenlecleucel are collected and frozen, and they can be stored for up to nine months at the treatment center. Cells collected for axicabtagene ciloleucel are shipped fresh and manufactured immediately (Perica et al., 2018).

Manufacturers of CAR T cells have contracts that establish both technical and quality standards and the expectations of collection centers and cell manufacturing. Manufacturers must consistently and reliably deliver a high-quality product. Tracking, manipulating, cryopreserving, storing, and verifying product identity are critical steps in CAR T-cell development and outlined in meticulous detail in the contracts between the manufacturer and treatment center (Perica et al., 2018). One of the Foundation for the Accreditation of Cellular Therapy (FACT) standards is ensuring a documented and traceable chain of custody of the cellular product. Maintaining the chain of custody for this genetically modified, individualized autologous cell product is of utmost importance (Perica et al., 2018).

Apheresis may occur weeks or months prior to the CAR T-cell infusion. Cells are collected for a specific CAR T-cell research protocol or commercial product and may not be used for any other clinical trial or commercial product (McConville et al., 2017). Manufacturing CAR T-cells begins with separating the T cells from the mononuclear white blood cells. Once the T cells are separated, a viral vector is used to introduce the genetically modified CAR, creating a CAR T cell. The CAR T cells are then expanded using a variety of cytokines. Prior to cryopreservation, the CAR T cells must pass quality control standards to ensure the safety and efficacy of the manufactured cells (Ghobadi, 2018). The typical manufacturing time for these therapies is 17 days for axicabtagene ciloleucel and 28 days for tisagenlecleucel. The manufacturing failure rate may be as low as 1% for axicabtagene ciloleucel and as high as 9% for tisagenlecleucel (Kite Pharma, 2019b; Novartis Pharmaceuticals, 2018). Manufacturing failures can be catastrophic for patients with advanced disease awaiting potentially curative CAR T-cell therapy. Minimizing the time from collection to cell manufacturing and infusion is of the upmost importance for patients who may have rapidly progressing disease.

Administration of Lymphodepleting Chemotherapy

Delivering lymphodepleting chemotherapy is an important component in the success of CAR T-cell therapy. According to Nair and Neelapu (2018), three principles support administration of lymphodepleting chemotherapy. The lymphodepleting chemotherapy improves the efficacy of CAR T-cell therapy by reducing the lymphocytes, thus creating space for the CAR T cells to proliferate. Second, lymphodepleting chemotherapy enhances the availability of homeostatic cytokines, such as IL-15, which promotes T-cell proliferation (Locke, Neelapu, Bartlett, Siddiqi, et al., 2017; Locke et al., 2018;). Finally, lymphodepleting chemotherapy decreases immunosuppressive cells, including regulatory T cells and myeloid suppressor cells, that might interfere with CAR T cell expansion and function, which helps to improve the antitumor efficiency of the CAR T cells (Kenderian, Porter, & Gill, 2017; Nair & Neelapu, 2018). One study demonstrated that for patients who received cyclophosphamide and fludarabine, expansion and persistence of CAR T cells was greater, and the rate of complete responses was higher, as compared to cyclophosphamide alone or cyclophosphamide and etoposide (Turtle et al., 2016).

Lymphodepleting chemotherapy is administered approximately one week prior to CAR T-cell infusion. CAR T cells may be delivered in the inpatient or outpatient setting depending on patient factors, research protocol or treatment plan, and type of chemotherapy to be administered (McConville et al., 2017). A typical lymphodepleting regimen includes cyclophosphamide and fludarabine for three days, similar to the regimens used in the pivotal trials (Kite Pharma, 2019b; Neelapu et al., 2017; Novartis Pharmaceuticals, 2018; Schuster, Bishop, et al., 2017).

Chimeric Antigen Receptor T-Cell Infusion

Chain of custody and verification of product are critical for this one-time, patient-specific treatment. The manufacturing site may be thousands of miles away from the treatment center, and the cells exchange hands many times through multiple departments. The journey these cells take is long and involves many steps, including collection, packaging for transport, shipping to the manufacturer, removal from shipping container, storage, genetic engineering, quality assessment, cryopreservation, packaging for transport to the treatment center, shipping, storage at the treatment center before infusion, thawing, and infusion. Given this complicated journey, maintaining the chain of custody and verification of the CAR T-cell product identity cannot be overemphasized.

Prior to thawing the product, patient identity is verified against the cassette containing the CAR T cells. This identification process usually involves a cell infusion technician and another healthcare professional—either a physician or nurse. Once identifiers have been confirmed, the thawing process may be initiated. Patient identification is verified against the labeling on the thawed product at the bedside. Prior to the cell infusion, the nurse must ensure that tocilizumab and emergency equipment (oxygen and suction) are available. Premedication with acetaminophen and diphenhydramine 30–60 minutes prior to the CAR T-cell infusion is recommended. Steroids should not be used as premedication. The dimethyl sulfoxide used during the cryopreservation of the CAR T cells may cause allergic reactions, including anaphylaxis. A critical step prior to thawing and infusing CAR T cells is an assessment to ensure the patient is free from an active uncontrolled infection,

which raises the risk of complications after infusion. CAR T cells are infused via IV using tubing without a filter. The IV tubing may be primed with normal saline. The nurse must ensure the entire contents of the bag are infused within 30 minutes of thawing. The cells may be infused by gravity or peristaltic pump and are administered quickly at a rate of 10–20 ml per minute. The volume of the infusion bag is 10–50 ml for tisagenlecleucel and approximately 70 ml for axicabtagene ciloleucel (Kite Pharma, 2019b; Novartis Pharmaceuticals, 2018). After the entire bag is infused, it should be rinsed with normal saline and infused to ensure the patient receives all remaining cells. If more than one bag of CAR T cells is to be infused, the first bag must be entirely infused prior to thawing of subsequent bags (Kite Pharma, 2019b; Novartis Pharmaceuticals, 2018).

Follow-Up and Monitoring

As with any new therapy, vigilant follow-up to assess for and identify side effects and late toxicities is essential. Following axicabtagene ciloleucel infusion, the manufacturer requires daily monitoring for seven days, and following tisagenlecleucel infusion, patients should be monitored two to three times a week for the first week. Following axicabtagene ciloleucel or tisagenlecleucel infusion, patients are to remain within close proximity (within two hours) of the treatment center for four weeks. Research protocols will specify follow-up requirements. Research protocols may also dictate if the CAR T-cell infusion must be administered in the hospital or can be administered in the outpatient setting. The type of CAR T-cell therapy and expected toxicities should also guide practitioners in determining if the cells are administered in the inpatient or outpatient setting. All follow-up and monitoring must occur at an authorized treatment center. Authorized treatment centers have met the commercial manufacturer's risk evaluation mitigation strategies (REMS) requirements. Laboratory monitoring includes C-reactive protein (CRP), ferritin, and complete blood count with differential. In addition to laboratory monitoring, assessments for neurotoxicity and CRS are critical.

Late effects of CAR T-cell therapy are unknown, as most patients have only been followed for a short period of time—less than two years. Concerns about late toxicities include B-cell aplasia, risk of secondary cancers, neurologic disorders, autoimmune disorders, reproductive toxicities, and late infectious complications (Lee et al., 2019; Zheng, Kros, & Li, 2018). As these patients move into post-treatment survivorship, quality-of-life issues and the true long-term benefits of CAR T-cell therapy and other immunotherapies can only be addressed through diligent long-term follow-up.

Toxicities and Side Effects of Chimeric Antigen Receptor T-Cell Therapy

Because CAR T-cell products are created using various methods, they have different side effect profiles and potential toxicities. These differences are the result of viral vectors used to genetically modify the T cell, costimulatory components, T-cell product composition, lymphodepleting chemotherapy regimens, tumor burden, and patient characteristics (Salter et al., 2018). It is imperative that nurses are aware of the differences between the CAR T-cell therapies because toxicities and side effects, as well as the timing of adverse events, are variable.

CRS and neurotoxicity are two serious and potentially life-threatening events often associated with CAR T-cell therapy. Because these toxicities can be severe, FDA requires that treatment centers administering commercially approved CAR T-cell therapy initiate and maintain a REMS program. The REMS program helps to mitigate the risks of the toxicities by imposing requirements for staff education and training prior to administering CAR T-cell therapy. Completing the REMS program is required before any treatment center can be authorized to perform CAR T-cell therapy. Each commercial manufacturer has a REMS program with specific criteria. All staff who administer, prescribe, or dispense CAR T cells must receive training and pass an assessment that emphasizes recognition and management of CRS and neurotoxicity. Additionally, all hospitals that administer CAR T cells must have two doses of tocilizumab available for each patient (Kite Pharma, 2019b; Novartis Pharmaceuticals, 2018). The commercial manufacturers provide the contracts for authorized treatment centers and ensure criteria are met.

In 2018, multiple experts from major academic centers and organizations in the field of oncology and hematology worked to develop consensus for grading criteria and definitions for these common adverse events. The consensus grading, published by American Society for Transplantation and Cellular Therapy (ASTCT), will hopefully provide clarity and facilitate comparisons across products (Lee et al., 2019).

Cytokine Release Syndrome

CRS is potentially life threatening and the most common reaction seen following CAR T-cell infusion. CRS is an uncontrolled inflammatory response caused by the proliferation and activation of CAR T cells (Neelapu et al., 2017). The activated T cells receive an exaggerated signal, stimulating them to release cytokines and chemokines (Graham et al., 2018). Cytokines that are secreted and elevated include tumor necrosis factor, granulocyte macrophage–colony-stimulating factor, IL-2, IL-6, IL-8, IL-10, IL-15, monocyte chemoattractant protein-1, tumor necrosis factor receptor p55, and macrophage inflammatory protein-1B (Davila et al., 2014; Hay et al., 2017; Kite Pharma, 2019b). These cytokines are responsible for the systemic inflammatory response seen after CAR T-cell therapy (Chavez & Locke, 2018; Davila et al., 2014; Lee et al., 2014). Currently, it is thought that high levels of IL-6 contribute to the organ toxicity seen in CRS (Graham et al., 2018). Release of these cytokines and chemokines activates macrophages and stimulates ongoing expansion of CAR T cells.

The incidence and severity of CRS may be higher in patients with a large tumor burden, which correlates with higher levels of T-cell activation. CRS symptoms appear to coincide with the time of maximal T-cell expansion (Lee et al., 2014, 2015). Other risk factors for severe CRS include comorbidities and onset of CRS within three days of cell infusion (Davila et al., 2014; Lee et al., 2015; Maude et al., 2014). CRS is mild for most patients, but vigilance is required, as CRS can quickly evolve to a serious and life-threatening reaction. Common signs and symptoms of CRS include fever, hypotension, tachycardia, and hypoxia. Fever is the hallmark sign. Other symptoms may include cardiac arrhythmias, including atrial fibrillation and ventricular tachycardia, as well as cardiac arrest and heart failure, although rare. Hepatic dysfunction (transaminitis), pleural effusions, renal insufficiency, coagulopathy, and hemophagocytic lymphohistiocytosis/macrophage activation syndrome may occur (Lee et al., 2019; Neelapu et al., 2017). Hypoxia and hypotension are the most common, and other manifestations usually occur concurrently (Lee et al., 2019). The onset of CRS typically occurs 24–48 hours after CAR T-cell infusion and may last up to seven days (Ogba et al., 2018). Serum ferritin and CRP are elevated and may aid in the diagnosis of CRS (Lee et al., 2015; Maude et al., 2014). If testing is available, cytokine levels, including elevated levels of IL-6, may also support a diagnosis of CRS (Graham et al., 2018; Maude et al., 2014). If CRS progresses, pulmonary edema and capillary leak syndrome may occur, requiring additional oxygenation and possible mechanical ventilation (Lee et al., 2019).

The grading used for CRS is developing as treatment centers gain more experience. For the pivotal studies described previously, each used a different grading scale for CRS, making comparison across studies and commercial products difficult. The different grading scales include the University of Pennsylvania scale, Lee scale, CTCAE, University of Texas MD Anderson Cancer Center scale, Memorial Sloan Kettering Cancer Center (MSKCC) scale, ASTCT consensus scale, and CARTOX Working Group scale (Brudno & Kochenderfer, 2018; Lee et al., 2014, 2019; Leick & Maus, 2018; Liu & Zhao, 2018). Table 16-1 shows a comparison of four grading systems used for CRS (Brudno & Kochenderfer, 2018). For pediatrics, the MD Anderson Cancer Center scale was modified with input from the Pediatric Acute Lung Injury and Sepsis Investigators Network and HSCT subgroup (Mahadeo et al., 2019). A notable difference in these scales is the grading of hypotension. In the Lee, MSKCC, and CARTOX scales, grade 2 is defined as hypotension responding to fluids or low-dose vasopressors and/or an oxygenation requirement of less than 40%; however, in the University of Pennsylvania scale, this constellation of symptoms is defined as grade 3. CTCAE was developed for CRS events caused by immunotherapies and for monoclonal antibody infusion reactions. The Lee scale redefined the CTCAE scoring as mild, moderate, severe, and life threatening to help guide treatment recommendations (Lee et al., 2014). The ASTCT consensus grading of CRS is the most recent published scale. It includes the following criteria (Lee et al., 2019):

- Fever of 38°C or higher for all grades
- Grade 1: no hypotension or hypoxia
- Grade 2: hypotension not requiring vasopressors and/or hypoxia requiring low-flow nasal cannula (< 6 L/minute) or blow-by (used in pediatrics)
- Grade 3: hypotension requiring one vasopressor with or without vasopressin and/or hypoxia requiring oxygen via high-flow nasal cannula (> 6 L/minute), nonrebreather mask, or Venturi mask
- Grade 4: hypotension requiring multiple vasopressors (except vasopressin) and/or hypoxia requiring positive

pressure, such as continuous positive airway pressure, bilevel positive airway pressure, intubation, or mechanical ventilation

In the ASTCT consensus grading for CRS, organ toxicity was removed with the recommendation that the CTCAE scale be used (Lee et al., 2019). Understanding the grading scales is important, as they form the basis of many treatment algorithms. It is also important for nurses to take into consideration how different toxicities are assessed in different clinical trials for CAR T-cell therapies, as well as knowing the different management strategies.

Grade 1–4 CRS occurred in up to 79% of pediatric and young adult patients with relapsed or refractory ALL and

Table 16-1. Comparison of Cytokine Release Syndrome Grading Systems[a]

CRS Grade	Consensus Group (Lee et al., 2014)	University of Pennsylvania (Porter et al., 2015)	Memorial Sloan Kettering Cancer Center (Park et al., 2018)	CARTOX Working Group (Neelapu, Tummala, Kebriaei, Wierda, Gutierrez, et al., 2018)
Grade 1	• Symptoms are not life threatening and require symptomatic treatment only, *e.g.*, fever, nausea, fatigue, headache, myalgias, malaise	• Mild reaction, treated with supportive care	• Mild symptoms requiring observation or symptomatic management only	• Temperature ≥ 38.0°C • SBP ≥ 90 mmHg • No oxygen required for SaO_2 > 90% • Grade 1 organ toxicities
Grade 2	• Symptoms require and respond to moderate intervention • Hypotension responsive to IV fluids or a low dose of a single vasopressor, not meeting criteria for grade 3 • Oxygen requirement < 40% FiO_2 • Grade 2 organ toxicity	• Hospitalization indicated – IV therapy – neutropenic fevers – parenteral nutrition • Grade 2 creatinine increase • Grade 3 LFT increase	• Moderate symptoms • Hypotension requiring any dose of vasopressors < 24 h, not meeting criteria for grade 3–4 • Hypoxia or dyspnea requiring supplemental oxygen, < 40%, up to 6 Liters by nasal cannula	• Hypotension with SBP < 90 mmHg, responding to IV fluids or vasopressors, at doses not meeting criteria for grade 3 • Hypoxia requiring supplemental oxygen, FiO_2 < 40% • Grade 2 organ toxicities
Grade 3	• Symptoms require and respond to aggressive intervention • Hypotension requiring multiple vasopressors or high dose vasopressors as defined: – norepinephrine ≥ 20 µg/min – dopamine ≥ 10 µg/kg/min – phenylephrine ≥ 200 µg/min – epinephrine ≥ 10 µg/min – vasopressin + norepinephrine ≥ 10 µg/min – other vasopressor dose equivalent to norepinephrine ≥ 20 µg/min • Oxygen requirement ≥ 40% FiO_2 • Grade 3 organ toxicity • Grade 4 transaminitis	• Hypotension requiring IV fluids or low-dose vasopressors, defined as not meeting criteria for grade 4 • Hypoxia requiring supplemental O_2, including CPAP/BiPAP • Coagulopathy requiring FFP or cryoprecipitate • Grade 3 creatinine increase • Grade 4 LFT increase	• Severe symptoms • Hypotension requiring any vasopressors ≥ 24 h, not meeting criteria for grade 4 • Hypoxia or dyspnea requiring supplemental oxygen ≥ 40%	• Hypotension requiring multiple or high dose vasopressors, as defined: – norepinephrine ≥ 20 µg/min – dopamine ≥ 10 µg/kg/min – phenylephrine ≥ 200 µg/min – epinephrine ≥ 10 µg/min – vasopressin + norepinephrine ≥ 10 µg/min – other vasopressor dose equivalent to norepinephrine ≥ 20 µg/min • Hypoxia requiring supplemental oxygen ≥ 40% • Grade 3 organ toxicities or Grade 4 transaminitis

(Continued on next page)

CRS Grade	Consensus Group (Lee et al., 2014)	University of Pennsylvania (Porter et al., 2015)	Memorial Sloan Kettering Cancer Center (Park et al., 2018)	CARTOX Working Group (Neelapu, Tummala, Kebriaei, Wierda, Gutierrez, et al., 2018)
Grade 4	• Life-threatening symptoms • Requirement for ventilator support • Grade 4 organ toxicity (excluding transaminitis)	• Hypotension requiring high dose vasopressors defined as: – norepinephrine ≥ 0.2 µg/kg/min – dopamine ≥ 10 µg/kg/min – phenylephrine ≥ 200 µg/min – epinephrine ≥ 0.1 µg/kg/min – other vasopressor dose equivalent to norepinephrine ≥ 0.2 µg/kg/min • Hypoxia requiring mechanical ventilation • Life-threatening toxicity	• Life threatening symptoms • Hypotension refractory to vasopressors with failure to reach target blood pressure despite use of vasopressors of the listed doses for ≥ 3 h – norepinephrine ≥ 20 µg/min – dopamine ≥ 10 µg/kg/min – phenylephrine ≥ 200 µg/min – epinephrine ≥ 10 µg/min – other vasopressor dose equivalent to norepinephrine ≥ 20 µg/min • Hypoxia or dyspnea requiring mechanical ventilation	• Hypotension that is life-threatening • Requirement for ventilator support • Grade 4 organ toxicity (excluding transaminitis)

[a] Unless otherwise indicated, the presence of any clinical criterion indicated by a bullet point results in classification as the listed Grade CRS.

Bi-PAP—bilevel positive airway pressure; CPAP—continuous positive airway pressure; CRS—cytokine release syndrome; FFP—fresh frozen plasma. FiO_2—fraction of inspired oxygen; LFT—liver function tests (transaminases); SaO_2—oxygen saturation of arterial blood; SBP—systolic blood pressure

Note. From "Recent Advances in CAR T-Cell Toxicity: Mechanisms, Manifestations and Management," by J.N. Brudno and J.N. Kochenderfer, 2018, Blood Reviews, 34, p. 49. Retrieved from https://doi.org/10.1016/j.blre.2018.11.002. Copyright 2018 by Elsevier. Reprinted with permission.

74%–94% of adult patients with relapsed or refractory DLBCL (Kite Pharma, 2019b; Novartis Pharmaceuticals, 2018). Grade 3–4 CRS occurred in 49% of patients with relapsed or refractory ALL, with an incidence of 13% following axicabtagene ciloleucel administration and 23% following tisagenlecleucel administration in adults with relapsed or refractory NHL (Kite Pharma, 2019b; Novartis Pharmaceuticals, 2018). Although direct comparison across these studies is difficult because of the use of multiple grading scales, the overall incidence of CRS is high. Staff and patient education regarding CRS and its signs and symptoms are key components of caring for recipients of CAR T-cell therapy. Patients should be encouraged to readily report hallmark signs of CRS, such as fever. For patients receiving CAR T-cell therapy in an outpatient setting, additional emphasis on reportable signs and symptoms is required.

The mainstay for managing mild CRS is supportive care. Fever is a common presentation and sign of CRS. An infectious disease workup should be initiated and include blood and urine cultures, chest x-ray, and initiation of antimicrobial therapy. Fevers should be aggressively managed with IV hydration, around-the-clock antipyretic, and cooling blankets and ice packs as needed. Astute and frequent monitoring of vital signs is essential. Orthostatic changes can be an indicator for intravascular volume changes. Maintaining blood perfusion to organs will min-

imize organ toxicity and can be evaluated by monitoring mean arterial blood pressure. Distinguishing signs and symptoms of CRS from sepsis or infection can be difficult. Therefore, the nurse should include both CRS and sepsis in the differential diagnosis, particularly if the patient is neutropenic. Arterial or venous blood gases may yield important clinical information on the acuity of a patient experiencing changes in respiratory rate and oxygen saturation at rest or with activity. Depending on institutional or research management guidelines, the administration of tocilizumab should be considered if a patient has ongoing fever or requires fluid boluses, vasoactive medications to maintain blood pressure, or additional oxygenation. Tocilizumab is an FDA-approved humanized anti-IL-6 monoclonal antibody that blocks binding and prevents signaling. The goal of treatment for a patient experiencing CRS is maintaining blood perfusion and oxygenation, as well as preventing organ damage. According to Lee et al. (2014), older adult patients or those with comorbidities may have less ability to withstand the stress of CRS and should be considered for earlier interventions. Patients with severe CRS may need an escalation of care; therefore, access to an intensive care unit (ICU) is essential. CRS can progress rapidly, and an ICU can provide vasopressors and ventilator support. A bedside or portable cardiac ultrasound to assess cardiac ejection fraction and obtain arterial blood gas assessments may be useful to determine fluid and oxygenation status to assist with decisions on whether to transfer a patient to the ICU.

CRP, a substance produced by the liver, is helpful as a nonspecific marker for inflammation. Trending CRP results may be used to identify the peak severity of CRS, and a declining CRP may signify resolution (Davila et al., 2014; Lee et al., 2014). One important caveat to interpreting CRP values is in the setting of corticosteroid or tocilizumab administration, which will decrease CRP values and may not truly reflect resolution of CRS (Davila et al., 2014). According to Lee et al. (2014), elevated ferritin was also noted in patients with CRS but did not predict CRS severity. CRP levels can also be elevated during infection, highlighting the nonspecific nature of CRP. In the pivotal studies, CRS occurred a median of two to three days following CAR T-cell infusion but as late as 51 days (Novartis Pharmaceuticals, 2018). Therefore, nurses must remain vigilant in assessing for CRS and infection given the frequent and persistent cytopenias observed 28 days or more after infusion.

Tocilizumab and corticosteroids are used to treat CRS. For patients weighing less than 30 kg, IV tocilizumab at 12 mg/kg is administered for one hour. For patients weighing more than 30 kg, IV tocilizumab at 8 mg/kg is administered every 6–8 hours. It is recommended that only three doses of tocilizumab be administered in a 24-hour period. However, if the clinical condition warrants, a fourth dose may be considered. Corticosteroids are recommended for severe CRS. Corticosteroids inhibit production of cytokines, including IL-2, IL-6, and IL-10, which are secreted by the activated CAR T cells. If CRS progresses to a more severe grade, despite administration of tocilizumab and corticosteroids, high doses of prednisolone, such as 1,000 mg IV for three days, may be recommended until symptoms resolve or CRS is downgraded to grade 1. After CRS symptoms resolve, a corticosteroids taper is initiated (Lee et al., 2014; Neelapu, Tummala, Kebriaei, Wierda, Locke, et al., 2018). Recommendations for corticosteroid dosing, length of administration, or tapering in CRS management vary. The use of tocilizumab and corticosteroids are often very effective in reducing the signs and symptoms of CRS, but nurses must remain vigilant because the symptoms may continue to worsen or reoccur. The goal of management is to prevent life-threatening toxicity while maximizing the antitumor efficacy of the CAR T cells. Initially, it was thought that corticosteroids may dampen the efficacy of CAR T-cell therapy because corticosteroids suppress T-cell function and induce T-cell apoptosis, but more recent experience indicates that the use of corticosteroids to manage toxicities is appropriate and does not appear to affect overall response rates (Davila et al., 2014; Locke et al., 2018; Locke, Neelapu, Bartlett, Lekakis, et al., 2017; Neelapu et al., 2017).

Patient education should include discussion of the signs and symptoms of CRS and what symptoms should be reported. As part of REMS requirements, a wallet card should be provided to all patients who received CAR T-cell therapy. The wallet card should specify the date of infusion, list physician name and contact information, and describe symptoms of CRS and neurotoxicity. Patients and families should be instructed to carry the card in their wallets so that it can be provided to the healthcare team if the patient presents to an emergency department.

Neurotoxicities

Neurotoxicity associated with CAR T-cell therapy has been called *chimeric antigen receptor T cell–related encephalopathy syndrome* (CRES); more recently it has been referred to as *immune effector cell–associated neurologic syndrome* (ICANS) (Lee et al., 2019; Neelapu, Tummala, Kebriaei, Wierda, Gutierrez, et al., 2018). ICANS encompasses other cellular immunotherapies and treatments, such as blinatumomab, which have similar neurologic side effects (Lee et al., 2019; Leick & Maus, 2018). The pathophysiology of ICANS is not fully understood. The neurologic changes may be a result of an inflammatory process in the brain secondary to the proliferation and expansion of CAR T cells. Passive diffusion of cytokines, such as IL-6, IL-8, interferon gamma–induced protein 10, and monocyte chemoattractant protein-1, into the brain or trafficking of T cells into the central nervous system have been hypothesized (Neelapu, Locke, & Go, 2018; Santomasso et al., 2018). Disruption of the blood–brain barrier causes neurologic changes as a result of passive diffusion of inflammatory cytokines. Higher numbers of CAR T cells have been found in the cerebrospinal fluid of patients who developed neurotoxicity and a higher peak of CAR T-cell expansion in the blood correlated with neurotoxicity (Lee et al., 2015; Neelapu et al., 2017; Santomasso et al., 2018). Early systemic inflammation triggering endothelial cell activation, blood–brain barrier disruption, or vascular dysfunction are additional hypotheses proposed to explain the pathophysiology of neurotoxicity (Gust et al., 2017; Ogba et al., 2018; Santomasso et al., 2018). In a review of 33 patients who developed neurotoxicity, Santomasso et al. (2018) found a strong correlation between the presence and severity of CRS and the development of neurotoxicity. The onset of neurotoxicity in relation to CRS was variable in these 33 patients. Neurotoxicity most often occurs after the start of CRS but may occur concurrently or after resolution. Of note, severe neurotoxicity can occur simultaneously with CRS or without CRS. Santomasso et al. (2018) found that neurotoxicity did not respond to tocilizumab in most patients. They also found that 73.9% of patients who had a baseline platelet count of less than $50,000/mm^3$ and a fever of greater than $38°C$ on day 3 after CAR T-cell infusion proceeded to develop severe neurotoxicity (Santomasso et al., 2018).

Manifestations of neurotoxicities include headache, confusion, tremors, aphasia, loss of consciousness, and seizures. Signs and symptoms may include diminished attention, language or word-finding problems, impaired handwriting, disorientation, agitation, and somnolence (Neelapu,

Tummala, Kebriaei, Wierda, Gutierrez, et al., 2018). More severe neurologic changes include somnolence, disorientation, impaired attention, global aphasia, twitching, decreased consciousness, encephalopathy, and seizures (Santomasso et al., 2018). Headache has been reported in up to 45% of patients, but as a nonspecific symptom, headaches may have many other causes (Kite Pharma, 2019b; Lee et al., 2019; Novartis Pharmaceuticals, 2018). Expressive aphasia is a specific symptom of ICANS and has been reported in 3%–18% of recipients, but the incidence was 34% in one clinical trial (Gust et al., 2017; Kite Pharma, 2019b; Novartis Pharmaceuticals, 2018). Expressive aphasia may appear as hesitant speech, inability to name objects, unintended words or phrases, or repetition of a word over and over. Expressive aphasia may progress over hours to days to global aphasia. The range of symptoms is variable; patients may be awake and unable to follow commands or may have a decreased level of consciousness, including obtundation or coma (Lee et al., 2019). Electroencephalograph (EEG) findings often indicate cortical irritation by epileptiform discharges or nonconvulsive electrographic seizures. Diffuse generalized slowing with or without triphasic waves at 1–2 hertz represents an encephalopathic state and is commonly observed (Neelapu, Tummala, Kebriaei, Wierda, Gutierrez, et al., 2018). If seizures occur, they often follow the onset of global aphasia (Lee et al., 2019).

Neurotoxicities can be severe, life threatening, and in rare cases, fatal. Cerebral edema and hemorrhage have occurred. Neurotoxicity is common, occurring in 72% of patients with ALL, 58% of patients with NHL treated with tisagenlecleucel, and up to 87% of patients with NHL treated with axicabtagene ciloleucel (Kite Pharma, 2019b; Novartis Pharmaceuticals, 2018). Following tisagenlecleucel administration, 21% of patients with ALL and 18% of patients with NHL developed grade 3–4 neurotoxicity, and less than 31% of patients receiving axicabtagene ciloleucel developed grade 3–4 neurotoxicity. According to the prescribing information for axicabtagene ciloleucel, median time to onset is four to six days from infusion, and duration of symptoms was six days for patients with ALL and up to 17 days for patients with DLBCL (Kite Pharma, 2019b).

Historically in clinical trials, neurotoxicities were graded according to CTCAE, and each symptom was scored individually. Using the CTCAE scale, each of the following signs and symptoms would be graded independently: level of consciousness, orientation, ability to perform activities of daily living, changes in speech, tremors, seizures, incontinence, and motor weakness (Neelapu, Tummala, Kebriaei, Wierda, Gutierrez, et al., 2018). To simplify assessment neurotoxicity of CAR T-cell therapy, MD Anderson Cancer Center developed the CARTOX-10 scale. CARTOX is a 10-point neurologic assessment tool that includes elements of the mini-mental status examination and focuses on concentration, speech, and writing. One point is assigned for each question, and a patient with a normal neurologic examination would score 10 points. A patient receives one point for answering each of the following correctly: year, month, city, hospital name, President, and where he or she lives, as well as naming three objects and writing a sentence. Additional parameters to consider when grading neurotoxicity include seizures, motor weakness, papilledema, cerebrospinal fluid opening pressure, elevated intracranial pressure, and cerebral edema assessed with imaging studies. The presence of seizures elevates neurotoxicity to a grade 3 or 4 in the ICANS grading scale (Neelapu, Tummala, Kebriaei, Wierda, Gutierrez, et al., 2018). To overcome overlapping terms, including delirium, aphasia, confusion, encephalopathy, and ability to perform activities of daily living, the ASTCT consensus group modified the CARTOX tool and named it the Immune Effector Cell–Associated Encephalopathy (ICE) screening tool (Lee et al., 2019). The 10-point ICE screening tool is similar to the CARTOX tool; however, it adds an assessment of receptive aphasia, replacing the element of naming the President with a command assessment, such as "show me two fingers." ICANS grading requires the 10-point ICE tool, as well as evaluation of other neurologic domains. The final ICANS grade is determined by the most severe event in the specific domain. Figure 16-2 summarizes the assessment tools for grading encephalopathy. Table 16-2 outlines the evaluation of other neurologic domains related to immune effector cell therapy. In a pediatric setting, depending on age, a child may not possess a level of cognitive development to complete the ICE assessment, so a different grading scale is used for pediatrics. The Cornell Assessment of Pediatric Delirium (CAPD) is recommended (Mahadeo et al., 2019). The CAPD assessment includes monitoring the child's eye contact, purposeful actions, awareness of surroundings, communication, and level of consciousness. The score from the CAPD is used with the ASTCT ICANS consensus to determine the grading for children (Lee et al., 2019).

The management of neurotoxicity is guided by severity and grading (Neelapu, Tummala, Kebriaei, Wierda, Gutierrez, et al., 2018). Manufacturers and individual institutions have established management guidelines, and additional guidelines have been based on research protocols. Grade 1–2 (mild) neurotoxicity is managed with supportive care and more frequent assessment, including neurologic assessent as frequently as every four hours depending on guidelines. A neurology consultation and further testing may be recommended including EEG or neuroimaging with magnetic resonance imaging or computed tomography (Neelapu, Tummala, Kebriaei, Wierda, Gutierrez, et al., 2018). With evidence of a severe change in neurologic status or grade 3–4 toxicity, in addition to administering corticosteroids, an immediate magnetic resonance imaging or computed tomography scan of the brain to rule out cerebral edema, hemorrhage, or other etiology may be required (Brudno & Kochenderfer, 2016; Kite Pharma, 2019b; Neelapu, Tummala, Kebriaei, Wierda, Gutierrez, et al., 2018; Novartis Pharmaceuticals,

2018). Repeated radiologic imaging may be necessary for a patient who continues to decompensate or shows no signs of improvement with treatment. A restless or delirious patient may not be able to cooperate with these imaging tests, and it can be challenging for nursing staff to help a patient comply. The additonal use of sedatives to help the patient comply is problematic, as it can further compromise the assessment of neurologic changes. If a patient experiences greater than grade 1 neurotoxicity concurrently with CRS, administration of tocilizumab is recommended (Kite Pharma, 2019b; Neelapu, Tummala, Kebriaei, Wierda, Gutierrez, et al., 2018). For grade 2 or higher neurotoxicty in the absence of CRS, administration of corticosteroids is recommended (Kite Pharma, 2019b; Neelapu, Tummala, Kebriaei, Wierda, Gutierrez, et al., 2018). However, specific research studies may have different criteria for management. The specific neurologic symptom and its severity and duration, coupled with the specific guidelines, may all be factors in consideration for treatment and urgency. On resolution of symptoms and a return to severity less than grade 2, corticosteroids should be tapered. Optimal duration and dosing of corticosteriods is unknown and may vary on a case-by-case basis depending on presentation. Patients need to be monitored closely for reoccurence of neurotoxicity after resolution of symptoms and discontinuation of corticosteroids (Neelapu, Tummala, Kebriaei, Wierda, Gutierrez, et al., 2018). Seizures may occur, and monitoring for nonclinical and clinical seizures by EEG activity is critical. Continuous EEG, with multiple lines secured to the head, can be difficult for the confused patient to tolerate. Seizure prophylaxis is considered a standard of care for CAR T-cell therapy at high risk for neurotoxicities such as axicabtagene ciloleucel. Levetiracetam is considered the first choice for seizure prophylaxis, as it has fewer side effects than other antiseizure medications and a lower risk of cardiac toxicity. Levetiracetam can also be administered in the setting of liver dysfunction, which may occur as a complication of CRS (Neelapu, Tummala, Kebriaei, Wierda, Gutierrez, et al., 2018). Nonconvulsive and convulsive epilepticus is managed with benzodiazepines and antiepileptic medications. The initiation of benzodiazepine is often helpful, resulting in rapid improvement in mental status and decreased seizure activity (Neelapu, Tummala, Kebriaei, Wierda, Gutierrez, et al., 2018).

A nursing neurology "bundle" is essential for the management of neurotoxicity. The neurology bundle needs to minimally include vigilant ongoing assessment and supportive care. Nurses should routinely administer a mini-mental status examination or thorough neurologic examination each shift and more frequently when a patient experiences a toxicity. Neurologic assessments should include cranial nerve evaluation; assessment for tremors, muscle weakness, cognitive changes, loss of attention, staring, twitching, and dozing off; and completion of the ICE screening instrument. Nurses play a key role in early identification of subtle decline or onset of cognitive or cerebellar symptoms. Assigning consistent nursing staff to a patient treated with CAR T-cell therapy can be helpful. Supportive care includes maintaining a safe environment and minimizing medications associated with drowsiness. Safety measures include preventing falls, keeping the head of bed elevated greater than 30°, calming a delirious patient, and more frequent neurologic assessments if ICE or neurologic score decreases. Involving a patient's family or caregiver is essential. A caregiver is in the best position to quickly note small personality or cognitive changes. Educating families on early changes is critical, especially if the patient is receiving care in the outpatient setting. Providing concrete examples of potential cognitive and neurologic changes is helpful. For example, experiencing hand tremors, brushing teeth without applying toothpaste, not initiating eating or drinking, having incontinence or missing the toilet when urinating, experiencing difficulty with word finding or verbalizing words, handwriting changes, and forgetting to perform routine habits, as well as changes in mental status (e.g., anxiety, anger, somnolence), are all

---

Figure 16-2. Encephalopathy Assessment Tools for Grading of Immune Effector Cell–Associated Neurotoxicity Syndrome

CARTOX-10
- Orientation: orientation to year, month, city, hospital, president/prime minister of country of residence: 5 points
- Naming: ability to name 3 objects (e.g., point to clock, pen, button): 3 points
- Writing: ability to write a standard sentence (e.g., Our national bird is the bald eagle): 1 point
- Attention: ability to count backwards from 100 by 10: 1 point

ICE
- Orientation: orientation to year, month, city, hospital: 4 points
- Naming: ability to name 3 objects (e.g., point to clock, pen, button): 3 points
- Following commands: ability of follow simple commands (e.g., "Show me 2 fingers" or "Close your eyes and stick out your tongue"): 1 point
- Writing: ability to write a standard sentence (e.g., Our national bird is the bald eagle): 1 point
- Attention: Count backwards from 100 by 10: 1 point

CARTOX-10 (left column) has been updated to the ICE tool (right column). ICE adds a command-following assessment in place of one of the CARTOX-10 orientation questions. The scoring remains the same.
Scoring: 10, no impairment;
7–9, grade 1 ICANS;
3–6, grade 2 ICANS;
0–2, grade 3 ICANS;
0 due to patient unarousable and unable to perform the ICE assessment, grade 4 ICANS.

Note. From "ASTCT Consensus Grading for Cytokine Release Syndrome and Neurologic Toxicity Associated With Immune Effector Cells," by D.W. Lee, B.D. Santomasso, F.L. Locke, A. Ghobadi, C.J. Turtle, J.N. Brudno, … S.S. Neelapu, 2018, *Biology of Blood and Marrow Transplantation, 25*, p. 634. Copyright 2018 by American Society for Blood and Marrow Transplantation. Retrieved from https://doi.org/10.1016/j.bbmt.2018.12.758. Licensed under CC BY-NC-ND 4.0 (https://creativecommons.org/licenses/by-nc-nd/4.0).

Table 16-2. American Society for Transplantation and Cellular Therapy Immune Effector Cell–Associated Neurotoxicity Syndrome Consensus Grading for Adults

Neurotoxicity Domain	Grade 1	Grade 2	Grade 3	Grade 4
ICE Score*	7–9	3–6	0–2	0 (patient is unarousable and unable to perform ICE)
Depressed level of consciousness†	Awakens spontaneously	Awakens to voice	Awakens only to tactile stimulus	Patient is unarousable or requires vigorous or repetitive tactile stimuli to arouse. Stupor or coma
Seizure‡	N/A	N/A	Any clinical seizure focal or generalized that resolves rapidly; or nonconvulsive seizures on EEG that resolve with intervention	Life threatening prolonged seizure (> 5min); or repetitive clinical or electrical seizures without return to baseline in between
Motor findings*	N/A	N/A	N/A	Deep focal motor weakness such as hemiparesis or paraparesis
Elevated ICP/Cerebral edema	N/A	N/A	Focal/local edema on neuroimaging§	Diffuse cerebral edema on neuroimaging; Decerebrate or decorticate posturing; or cranial nerve VI palsy; or Papilledema; or Cushing's triad

ICANS grade is determined by the most severe event (ICE score, level of consciousness, seizure, motor findings, raised ICP/cerebral edema) not attributable to any other cause; for example, a patient with an ICE score of 3 who has a generalized seizure is classified as grade 3 ICANS.

N/A indicates not applicable.

* A patient with an ICE score of 0 may be classified as grade 3 ICANS if awake with global aphasia, but a patient with an ICE score of 0 may be classified as grade 4 ICANS if unarousable.

† Depressed level of consciousness should be attributable to no other cause (e.g., no sedating medication).

‡ Tremors and myoclonus associated with immune effector cell therapies may be graded according to CTCAE v5.0, but they do not influence ICANS grading.

§ Intracranial hemorrhage with or without associated edema is not considered a neurotoxicity feature and is excluded from ICANS grading. It may be graded according to CTCAE v5.0.

CTCAE—Common Terminology Criteria for Adverse Events; EEG—electroencephalograph; ICANS—immune effector cell–associated neurotoxicity syndrome; ICE—immune effector cell–associated encephalopathy; ICP—intracranial pressure

Note. From "ASTCT Consensus Grading for Cytokine Release Syndrome and Neurologic Toxicity Associated With Immune Effector Cells," by D.W. Lee, B.D. Santomasso, F.L. Locke, A. Ghobadi, C.J. Turtle, J.N. Brudno, … S.S. Neelapu, 2018, *Biology of Blood and Marrow Transplantation, 25,* p. 634. Copyright 2018 by American Society for Blood and Marrow Transplantation. Retrieved from https://doi.org/10.1016/j.bbmt.2018.12.758. Licensed under CC BY-NC-ND 4.0 (https://creativecommons.org/licenses/by-nc-nd/4.0).

subtle signs that further assessment is warranted. Caregivers should be instructed to call about any subtle changes or concerns. It is not uncommon for patients to become irritated with repeated questions or requests from the nursing staff or caregiver, all of which may contribute to lack of compliance. Waking a sleeping patient for a neurologic assessment can be frustrating for the patient; however, it remains a critical nursing intervention to ascertain for changes or progression to a higher ICANS stage. Establishing other standard means to monitor attention and cognitive changes may be helpful for the nurse after frequent repetition of ICE screening questions. Mixing commands or using alternate questions may be helpful. The following are examples of commands that can be used to establish changes in cognition or strength:
• Stick your tongue out after you look at the ceiling.
• Touch your nose with your left hand.
• Draw a clock that shows 11:10.
• Write the word "man."
• Pretend to hold a pizza box with your left hand.

Requesting that a patient read several sentences or identify what objects are used for may also be useful in assessment.

Nurses should feel empowered to advocate for a neurologic consult and radiologic scans when a patient shows symptoms of neurotoxicity. Patients may wax and wane with their neurologic assessments. ICU care may be considered for patients with grade 3–4 toxicity, as more frequent neurologic assessment is required. Intubation may also be required in the event of airway compromise from status epilepticus or if a patient is unable to maintain the airway.

As the grading, assessment, and management of neurotoxicity evolves, clear and consistent communication among members of the healthcare team is paramount. It is essential that interprofessional and consulting team members, including neurology, critical care, and emergency department staff, are educated and aware of grading criteria to minimize gaps and provide patient safety and accurate diagnosis and management. Neurotoxicities start subtly, and astute recognition and communication of changes is critical. Each member of the team needs to understand a patient's grade of toxicity to be consistent and to ensure appropriate interventions and communication of the plan.

B-Cell Aplasia

B-cell aplasia, or acquired hypogammaglobulinemia, is an expected side effect of therapy targeting the CD19 antigen, which is located on healthy, mature B cells, as well as malignant cells of B-cell disorders. CAR T-cell therapy targets B-cell markers including CD19, CD20, and CD22; therefore, B-cell aplasia is an expected adverse event (June & Sadelain, 2018). B-cell aplasia is related to the depletion of all the cells of the B lineage that the therapy destroys. Persistent B-cell aplasia suggests ongoing CAR T-cell activity. However, in a two-year follow-up, ongoing responses were seen with recovered B cells, suggesting that with lymphoma, persistence of CAR T cells may not be required (Locke et al., 2018). Longer follow-up is necessary to fully appreciate B-cell aplasia and the impact of different CAR T-cell products (Maude & Barrett, 2016). However, hypogammaglobinemia is a consequence of B-cell aplasia that is associated with increased risk and frequency of infections, particularly sinopulmonary infections.

Hypogammaglobinemia was reported in 43% of patients with relapsed or refractory ALL and 14% of patients with DLBCL following tisagenlecleucel infusion (Novartis Pharmaceuticals, 2018). In a follow-up review of 12 patients in complete remission for six months after CAR T-cell infusion, those who did not receive prophylactic IV Ig were monitored for serum IgG levels, frequency of infection, and Ig recovery. Of these 12 patients, two patients received IV Ig for worsening sinopulmonary infections at 12 and 22 months after CAR T-cell therapy. Both had decreased IgG levels from baseline. Consideration should be given for routine monitoring of IgG levels, especially in patients with recurrent infections. As low IgG levels can be anticipated in the first year following CAR T-cell therapy, IgG level monitoring and replacement is expected (Schuster, Svoboda, et al., 2017).

Prolonged and Delayed Cytopenias

Generally, patients are referred back to their primary oncologist or hematologist 28 days after CAR T-cell therapy. In the ELIANA study of tisagenlecleucel in children and young adults with ALL, the incidence of grade 3 or higher cytopenias following infusion was 40% for neutropenia and 27% for thrombocytopenia (Novartis Pharmaceuticals, 2018). This study also reported that incidence of cytopenias lasting more than 56 days after CAR T-cell infusion was 17% for neutropenia and 12% for thrombocytopenia. In the JULIET study, prolonged cytopenia unresolved by day 28 with a grade 3 or higher toxicity following tisagenlecleucel infusion in the adult lymphoma group was reported at 40% for thrombocytopenia and 25% for neutropenia (Novartis Pharmaceuticals, 2018). Prolonged cytopenias unresolved by day 30 following axicabtagene

ciloleucel infusion occurred in 28% of patients, including thrombocytopenia (18%), neutropenia (15%), and anemia (3%) (Kite Pharma, 2019b). Infection prophylaxis guidelines and standards of care need to be developed and implemented. Patients receiving CAR T-cell therapy are at increased risk of infection. Fungal, bacterial, and viral infection prophylaxis and the duration of therapy vary among institutions (Mahmoudjafari et al., 2019). In a survey by the ASTCT Pharmacy Special Interest Group, bacterial prophylaxis with a fluoroquinolone, viral prophylaxis with acyclovir, fungal prophylaxis with fluconazole, and pneumocystis prophylaxis with trimethoprim-sulfamethoxazole were commonly used (Mahmoudjafari et al., 2019). Trimethoprim-sulfamethoxazole may result in bone marrow suppression, so an alternative medication, such as pentamidine, may be considered. However, no standards exist for duration or selection of high-risk groups, including disease or prior corticosteroid administration. The prescribing information for axicabtagene ciloleucel reports a 26% incidence of infections, and prescribing information for tisagenlecleucel reports the incidence at just over 41% in ALL and lymphoma patients (Kite Pharma, 2019b; Novartis Pharmaceuticals, 2018). The referring physician, patients, and caregivers need to be aware of the risk of prolonged or delayed cytopenias and be provided management guidelines. Frequent monitoring of blood counts and granulocyte–colony-stimulating factors, as well as transfusion support, may be necessary. Written education materials and patient and caregiver teaching should include strategies for infection prevention and bleeding precautions. As patients resume care with their primary hematologist or oncologist, data on long-term follow-up can be difficult. Patient self-reporting tools, including computer applications or surveys, may be useful.

Building an Immunotherapy Program: Teams and Infrastructure

Recent FDA approvals of CAR T-cell treatments has catapulted this relatively new therapy into the front lines of therapy for relapsed or refractory ALL and NHL. In addition to the cell manufacturers, other organizations provide standards and regulations overseeing CAR T-cell programs. FDA approves and regulates products and manages adverse event reporting with the individual manufacturers. FDA also mandates REMS training for sites administering commercially approved products. FACT works in conjunction with the manufacturers to provide collection, clinical, and processing standards. The Center for International Blood and Marrow Transplant Research functions as a data repository and bridges authorized treatment centers and FDA requirements (Perica et al., 2018). ASTCT used the Center for International Blood and Marrow Transplant Research database to establish consensus recommendations (Lee et al., 2019). ASTCT, American Society of Hematology, FACT, the International Society for Cellular Therapy, and other professional organizations are working to establish guidelines for toxicity management, but these are not yet fully utilized in practice (Lee et al., 2019). FACT, which has a long history of establishing standards and accreditation for blood and marrow transplant (BMT) programs, has released standards for immune effector cells, including CAR T-cell therapy (London, 2018). The first immune effector cell standards were released in 2017 (Maus & Nikiforow, 2017).

CAR T-cell therapy and future immunotherapy treatments will require highly specialized medical and nursing care. Many institutions have made the decision to administer and merge CAR T-cell therapy into the existing BMT units, recognizing the unique knowledge and skills of BMT nurses in managing and caring for acutely ill patients undergoing complex therapies. Managing the unique toxicities of CAR T-cell therapy and immunotherapy is expanding the knowledge and skills of BMT nursing, particularly related to the common toxicities of CRS and neurologic changes.

Coordination of Care

Whether therapy is provided in an inpatient or outpatient setting, with relapsed or refractory large disease burden or minimal disease, with a low or high performance status, or through clinical trials or as an approved treatment, CAR T-cell therapy is a complex process. Cell collection, cell manufacturing and processing, infusion, post-infusion care, and follow-up require collaboration from multiple disciplines and many departments. Establishing standards of care, educating staff, developing workflows, writing policies and procedures, and developing checks and balances are vital components to the safe administration of CAR T-cell therapy and patient care. Successful development of a CAR T-cell therapy program and optimal patient care require a coordinated care path and ongoing review of toxicities and outcomes. In their article discussing the CAR T-cell therapy program at MSKCC, Perica et al. (2018) described the eight essential steps to establishing a therapy program. These eight essential steps are patient intake; consultation; cell collection, ordering, shipping, and receiving; bridging chemotherapy; infusion; early postinfusion care; late postinfusion care; and regulation (Perica et al., 2018). Intake and developing a consultation service should include physicians, nurses, social workers, and research assistants experienced in CAR T-cell therapy. As options for clinical trials and standards of care grow, choices for the best pathway will become more complicated. For a successful collection process, apheresis centers, cell therapy technicians, administrative personnel, and nursing coordinators are essential components. All staff must be trained on the required regulations for cell collection, including washout periods for certain medications. The time to collect and manufacture cells and the time for insurance authorization varies, making the development of care paths challenging. The disease status of the patient becomes a critical factor in developing a timeline for CAR T-cell therapy and the need for bridging chemotherapy. Additional considerations include the time to manufacture cells and manufacturing failure rate. Safe cell infusion requires development and implementation of electronic orders, standards of care, and policies and procedures regarding product identification. As CAR T-cell therapy develops as a specialty, many centers are training nurse coordinators specifically for these therapies to follow the patients through the treatment process. Early or immediate postinfusion care prior to day 30 may require additional consults from other disciplines, including emergency department staff, pain service, psychiatry, neurology, and critical care. Providing education to these consulting services is essential. Patient management algorithms for CRS and neurotoxicities, policies, and orders should be developed and evaluated for outcomes. These algorithms and standards of care need to be easily accessible for all staff. Pharmacy staff must ensure two doses of tocilizumab are available for each patient during the follow-up period. Postinfusion care occurs in the outpatient setting and requires a dedicated staff to monitor and educate patients and caregivers. Housing, transportation, and expenses must also be taken into consideration. Postinfusion care occurs from day 30 onward and includes transitioning the patient back to the referring physician. Standards of practice, documentation, and follow-up procedures need to be developed. Clear communication for the referring physician to follow recommendations for long-term side effect recognition and management is important. Cytopenias, infections, relapse, and any other unexpected toxicities that may occur should be reported back to the treatment center. Financial, regulatory, and reporting requirements are the last elements in building a strong program. Insurance authorization and reimbursement protocols need to be developed. CAR T-cell therapy is expensive, and insurance coverage of this innovative and expensive treatment is still being developed. Data management systems to ensure the collection and reporting of information on toxicities, outcomes, and adverse events are essential. CRS and neurotoxicity reporting must be sent to either FDA or the manufacturer. Clinical, financial, internal system, regulatory, and administrative challenges are part of the complex process of providing this innovative treatment. However, as experience is gained and institutions and professional organizations continue working together to standardize management and reduce toxicities, the challenges of establishing these programs will be overcome. In the end, patients will have access to a potentially curative therapy delivered by teams that have established experience and expertise.

Cost and Insurance Coverage

The complex processes of developing CAR T cells, the patient-specific nature of CAR T-cell therapy, and the high risk of adverse events are coupled with a high financial cost. The wholesale price of a single infusion of tisagenlecleucel is $475,000, and axicabtagene ciloleucel is priced at $373,000. The total care costs for CAR T-cell therapy are estimated to be as high as $1.5 million per patient (Gallegos, 2018a). These costs include cell collection, processing, manufacturing, chemotherapy administration, hospitalization, infusion, side effect management, and follow-up (London, 2018). Private payers and the Centers for Medicare and Medicaid Services (CMS) have established reimbursement policies, International Classification of Disease codes, and diagnosis-related group codes for CAR T-cell therapy. CMS reimbursement rates are set at 6% above the wholesale costs. Manufacturers have requested CMS to apply a separate technology add-on payment for CAR T cells (Gallegos, 2018a). To provide additional payments for breakthrough technology, CMS approved CAR T-cell therapy through the new technology add-on payment program, which covers a maximum reimbursement of $186,500 in addition to a specific payment for a diagnosis-related group for the inpatient hospital stay. This amount does not come close to covering the costs of products or hospitalization. ASTCT has been working with payers and CMS to help establish and guide CAR T-cell therapy reimbursement policies (London, 2018). All aspects of therapy need to be considered in the cost for standardization for protocols to guide insurance coverage (Ogba et al., 2018). In May 2019, CMS hoped to complete a national coverage determination analysis on CAR T-cell therapy for Medicare patients with advanced cancer (Gallegos, 2018b). As CAR T-cell therapy expands to other types of cancers, many academic centers or early adopters have been risking financial loss as government payers determine reimbursement protocols (Ogba et al., 2018). To complicate the matter more, if the infusion is given in the outpatient setting and the patient experiences an adverse event and needs inpatient care within 72 hours, all payments become part of the inpatient stay, so the outpatient area loses revenue (Gallegos, 2018b). If the infusion occurs during the inpatient stay, Medicare reimburses one payment. Although outpatient reimbursement may appear to cover costs for treatment, it does not guarantee appropriate costs for the inpatient stay. This innovative therapy is laying the groundwork for how payers and insurance companies will reimburse for future cancer therapies, but it is also influencing hospitals to advocate for appropriate standard of care and reimbursement. It is an ever-changing dynamic process. Some hospitals have chosen not to provide this type of cellular therapy without the reimbursement of costs. Active research in biomedical and instrumentation is ongoing to build a cost-effective CAR T-cell product to improve affordability.

Summary

The future of immunotherapy as the fourth pillar of cancer therapy with a focus on cellular therapies and CAR T-cell treatment is exciting. From the initial research on CAR T cells to the currently approved treatments and current phase 3 clinical trials, CAR T-cell therapy is moving into clinical practice quickly. As more patients are treated and more CAR T-cell therapies become available, the future will shed light on which is the best treatment, when is the best time to provide the treatment, and which patients are the best candidates for that treatment. As professional organizations, payers, pharmaceutical companies, physicians, and hospitals work together for the same goal of providing the best outcomes possible for patients with cancer, the barriers will slowly be tackled—just as they were for BMT. The future promises to hold standardized algorithms for grading and toxicity management, insights into the best viral vectors, costimulatory domains, lymphodepleting chemotherapy regimens, and identification of the patients likely to experience the greatest benefit. The current success of CAR T-cell therapy is promising, and more work is needed to refine this therapy. These are exciting times for the oncology field.

References

Adaniya, S.P.S., Cohen, A.D., & Garfall, A.L. (2019). Chimeric antigen receptor T cell immunotherapy for multiple myeloma: A review of current data and potential clinical applications. *American Journal of Hematology, 94*(Suppl. 1), S28–S33. https://doi.org/10.1002/ajh.25428

Bayer, V., Amaya, B., Baniewicz, D., Callahan, C., Marsh, L., & McCoy, A.S. (2017). Cancer immunotherapy: An evidence-based overview and implications for practice. *Clinical Journal of Oncology Nursing, 21*(Suppl. 2), 13–21. https://doi.org/10.1188/17.cjon.s2.13-21

Brudno, J.N., & Kochenderfer, J.N. (2016). Toxicities of chimeric antigen receptor T cells: Recognition and management. *Blood, 127,* 3321–3330. https://doi.org/10.1182/blood-2016-04-703751

Brudno, J.N., & Kochenderfer, J.N. (2018). Recent advances in CAR T-cell toxicity: Mechanisms, manifestations and management. *Blood Reviews, 34,* 45–55. https://doi.org/10.1016/j.blre.2018.11.002

Chavez, J.C., & Locke, F.L. (2017). A possible cure for refractory DLBCL: CARs are headed in the right direction. *Molecular Therapy, 25,* 2241–2243. https://doi.org/10.1016/j.ymthe.2017.09.005

Chavez, J.C., & Locke, F.L. (2018). CAR T cell therapy for B-cell lymphomas. *Best Practice and Research Clinical Haematology, 31,* 135–146. https://doi.org/10.1016/j.beha.2018.04.001

Davila, M.L., Riviere, I., Wang, X., Bartido, S., Park, J., Curran, K., … Brentjens, R. (2014). Efficacy and toxicity management of 19-28z CAR T cell therapy in B cell acute lymphoblastic leukemia. *Science Translational Medicine, 6,* 224ra225. https://doi.org/10.1126/scitranslmed.3008226

Elahi, R., Khosh, E., Tahmasebi, S., & Esmaeilzadeh, A. (2018). Immune cell hacking: Challenges and clinical approaches to create smarter generations of chimeric antigen receptor T cells. *Frontiers in Immunology, 9,* 1717. https://doi.org/10.3389/fimmu.2018.01717

Gallegos, A. (2018a, April 27). Medicare sets outpatient CAR T-cell therapy rates. Retrieved from https://www.mdedge.com/hematology-oncology/article/164403/business-medicine/medicare-sets-outpatient-car-t-cell-therapy

Gallegos, A. (2018b, August 21). CMS finalizes CAR T-cell therapy inpatient payments. Retrieved from https://www.mdedge.com/jcomjournal/article/173086/practice-management/cms-finalizes-car-t-cell-therapy-inpatient-payments

Ghobadi, A. (2018). Chimeric antigen receptor T cell therapy for non-Hodgkin lymphoma. *Current Research in Translational Medicine, 66,* 43–49. https://doi.org/10.1016/j.retram.2018.03.005

Graham, C., Hewitson, R., Pagliuca, A., & Benjamin, R. (2018). Cancer immunotherapy with CAR-T cells—Behold the future. *Clinical Medicine, 18*, 324–328. https://doi.org/10.7861/clinmedicine.18-4-324

Gust, J., Hay, K.A., Hanafi, L.-A., Li, D., Myerson, D., Gonzalez-Cuyar, L.F., … Turtle, C.J. (2017). Endothelial activation and blood–brain barrier disruption in neurotoxicity after adoptive immunotherapy with CD19 CAR-T cells. *Cancer Discovery, 7*, 1404–1419. https://doi.org/10.1158/2159-8290.cd-17-0698

Havard, R., & Stephens, D.M. (2018). Anti-CD19 chimeric antigen receptor T cell therapies: Harnessing the power of the immune system to fight diffuse large B cell lymphoma. *Current Hematologic Malignancy Reports, 13*, 534–542. https://doi.org/10.1007/s11899-018-0482-6

Hay, K.A., Hanafi, L.-A., Li, D., Gust, J., Liles, W.C., Wurfel, M.M., … Turtle, C.J. (2017). Kinetics and biomarkers of severe cytokine release syndrome after CD19 chimeric antigen receptor–modified T-cell therapy. *Blood, 130*, 2295–2306. https://doi.org/10.1182/blood-2017-06-793141

Heyman, B., & Yang, Y. (2018). New developments in immunotherapy for lymphoma. *Cancer Biology and Medicine, 15*, 189–209. https://doi.org/10.20892/j.issn.2095-3941.2018.0037

June, C.H., & Sadelain, M. (2018). Chimeric antigen receptor therapy. *New England Journal of Medicine, 379*, 64–73. https://doi.org/10.1056/nejmra1706169

Kenderian, S.S., Porter, D.L., & Gill, S. (2017). Chimeric antigen receptor T cells and hematopoietic cell transplantation: How not to put the CART before the horse. *Biology of Blood and Marrow Transplantation, 23*, 235–246. https://doi.org/10.1016/j.bbmt.2016.09.002

Kite Pharma. (2019a). *Efficacy of axicabtagene ciloleucel compared to standard of care therapy in subjects with relapsed/refractory diffuse large B cell lymphoma* (ClinicalTrials.gov Identifier: NCT03391466). Retrieved from https://clinicaltrials.gov/ct2/show/record/NCT03391466

Kite Pharma. (2019b). *Yescarta™ (axicabtagene ciloleucel)* [Package insert]. Santa Monica, CA: Author.

Lee, D.W., Gardner, R., Porter, D.L., Louis, C.U., Ahmed, N., Jensen, M., … Mackall, C.L. (2014). Current concepts in the diagnosis and management of cytokine release syndrome. *Blood, 124*, 188–195. https://doi.org/10.1182/blood-2014-05-552729

Lee, D.W., Kochenderfer, J.N., Stetler-Stevenson, M., Cui, Y.K., Delbrook, C., Feldman, S.A., … Mackall, C.L. (2015). T cells expressing CD19 chimeric antigen receptors for acute lymphoblastic leukaemia in children and young adults: A phase 1 dose-escalation trial. *Lancet, 385*, 517–528. https://doi.org/10.1016/s0140-6736(14)61403-3

Lee, D.W., Santomasso, B.D., Locke, F.L., Ghobadi, A., Turtle, C.J., Brudno, J.N., … Neelapu, S.S. (2019). ASTCT consensus grading for cytokine release syndrome and neurologic toxicity associated with immune effector cells. *Biology of Blood and Marrow Transplantation, 25*, 625–638. https://doi.org/10.1016/j.bbmt.2018.12.758

Leick, M.B., & Maus, M.V. (2018). Toxicities associated with immunotherapies for hematologic malignancies. *Best Practice and Research Clinical Haematology, 31*, 158–165. https://doi.org/10.1016/j.beha.2018.03.004

Liu, D., & Zhao, J. (2018). Cytokine release syndrome: Grading, modeling, and new therapy. *Journal of Hematology and Oncology, 11*, 121. https://doi.org/10.1186/s13045-018-0653-x

Locke, F.L., Ghobadi, A., Jacobson, C.A., Miklos, D.B., Lekakis, L.J., Oluwole, O.O., … Neelapu, S.S. (2018). Long-term safety and activity of axicabtagene ciloleucel in refractory large B-cell lymphoma (ZUMA-1): A single-arm, multicentre, phase 1–2 trial. *Lancet Oncology, 20*, 31–42. https://doi.org/10.1016/S1470-2045(18)30864-7

Locke, F.L., Neelapu, S.S., Bartlett, N.L., Lekakis, L.J., Miklos, D.B., Jacobson, C.A., … Go, W.Y. (2017). Clinical and biologic covariates of outcomes in ZUMA-1: A pivotal trial of axicabtagene ciloleucel (axi-cel; KTE-C19) in patients with refractory aggressive non-Hodgkin lymphoma (r-NHL) [Abstract]. *Journal of Clinical Oncology, 35*(Suppl. 15), 7512. https://doi.org/10.1200/jco.2017.35.15_suppl.7512

Locke, F.L., Neelapu, S.S., Bartlett, N.L., Siddiqi, T., Chavez, J.C., Hosing, C.M., … Go, W.Y. (2017). Phase 1 results of ZUMA-1: A multicenter study of KTE-C19 anti-CD19 CAR T cell therapy in refractory aggressive lymphoma. *Molecular Therapy, 25*, 285–295. https://doi.org/10.1016/j.ymthe.2016.10.020

London, S. (2018, May 25). Logistics of CAR T-cell therapy in real-world practice. *ASCO Post.* Retrieved from https://www.ascopost.com/issues/may-25-2018/logistics-of-car-t-cell-therapy-in-real-world-practice

Mahadeo, K.M., Khazal, S.J., Abdel-Azim, H., Fitzgerald, J.C., Taraseviciute, A., Bollard, C.M., … Shpall, E.J. (2019). Management guidelines for paediatric patients receiving chimeric antigen receptor T cell therapy. *Nature Reviews Clinical Oncology, 16*, 45–63. https://doi.org/10.1038/s41571-018-0075-2

Mahmoudjafari, Z., Hawks, K.G., Hsieh, A.A., Plesca, D., Gatwood, K.S., & Culos, K.A. (2019). American Society for Blood and Marrow Transplantation Pharmacy Special Interest Group Survey on chimeric antigen receptor T cell therapy administrative, logistic, and toxicity management practices in the United States. *Biology of Blood and Marrow Transplantation, 25*, 26–33. https://doi.org/10.1016/j.bbmt.2018.09.024

Maude, S.L. (2017). CAR emissions: Cytokines tell the story. *Blood, 130*, 2238–2240. https://doi.org/10.1182/blood-2017-10-808592

Maude, S.L., & Barrett, D.M. (2016). Current status of chimeric antigen receptor therapy for haematological malignancies. *British Journal of Haematology, 172*, 11–22. https://doi.org/10.1111/bjh.13792

Maude, S.L., Frey, N., Shaw, P.A., Aplenc, R., Barrett, D.M., Bunin, N.J., … Grupp, S.A. (2014). Chimeric antigen receptor T cells for sustained remissions in leukemia. *New England Journal of Medicine, 371*, 1507–1517. https://doi.org/10.1056/nejmoa1407222

Maus, M.V., & Nikiforow, S. (2017). The why, what, and how of the new FACT standards for immune effector cells. *Journal for Immunotherapy of Cancer, 5*, 36. https://doi.org/10.1186/s40425-017-0239-0

McConville, H., Harvey, M., Callahan, C., Motley, L., Difilippo, H., & White, C. (2017). Car T-cell therapy effects: Review of procedures and patient education [Online exclusive]. *Clinical Journal of Oncology Nursing, 21*, E79–E86. https://doi.org/10.1188/17.cjon.e79-e86

McCune, J.S. (2018). Rapid advances in immunotherapy to treat cancer. *Clinical Pharmacology and Therapeutics, 103*, 540–544. https://doi.org/10.1002/cpt.985

Nair, R., & Neelapu, S.S. (2018). The promise of CAR T-cell therapy in aggressive B-cell lymphoma. *Best Practice & Research Clinical Haematology, 31*, 293–298. https://doi.org/10.1016/j.beha.2018.07.011

Neelapu, S.S., Locke, F.L., Bartlett, N.L., Lekakis, L.J., Miklos, D.B., Jacobson, C.A., … Go, W.Y. (2017). Axicabtagene ciloleucel CAR T-cell therapy in refractory large B-cell lymphoma. *New England Journal of Medicine, 377*, 2531–2544. https://doi.org/10.1056/NEJMoa1707447

Neelapu, S.S., Locke, F.L., & Go, W.Y. (2018). CAR T-cell therapy in large B-cell lymphoma. *New England Journal of Medicine, 378*, 1065. https://doi.org/10.1056/NEJMc1800913

Neelapu, S.S., Tummala, S., Kebriaei, P., Wierda, W., Gutierrez, C., Locke, F.L., … Shpall, E.J. (2018). Chimeric antigen receptor T-cell therapy—Assessment and management of toxicities. *Nature Reviews Clinical Oncology, 15*, 47–62. https://doi.org/10.1038/nrclinonc.2017.148

Neelapu, S.S., Tummala, S., Kebriaei, P., Wierda, W., Locke, F.L., Lin, Y., … Shpall, E.J. (2018). Toxicity management after chimeric antigen receptor T cell therapy: One size does not fit 'ALL.' *Nature Reviews Clinical Oncology, 15*, 218. https://doi.org/10.1038/nrclinonc.2018.20

Novartis Pharmaceuticals. (2018, May). *Kymriah™ (tisagenlecleucel)* [Package insert]. East Hanover, NJ: Author.

Novartis Pharmaceuticals. (2019a). *Tisagenlecleucel in adult patients with aggressive B-cell non-Hodgkin lymphoma* (ClinicalTrials.gov Identifier: NCT03570892). Retrieved from https://clinicaltrials.gov/ct2/show/NCT03570892

Novartis Pharmaceuticals. (2019b). *Tisagenlecleucel vs blinatumomab or inotuzumab for patients with relapsed/refractory B-cell precursor acute lymphoblastic leukemia* (ClinicalTrials.gov Identifier: NCT03628053). Retrieved from https://clinicaltrials.gov/ct2/show/NCT03628053

Novick, S. (2019). *Efficacy and safety study of bb2121 versus standard triplet regimens in subjects with relapsed and refractory multiple myeloma (RRMM)* (ClinicalTrials.gov Identifier: NCT03651128). Retrieved from https://clinicaltrials.gov/ct2/show/study/NCT03651128

Ogba, N., Arwood, N.M., Bartlett, N.L., Bloom, M., Brown, P., Brown, C., … Rosen, S.T. (2018). Chimeric antigen receptor T-cell therapy. *Journal of the National Comprehensive Cancer Network, 16*, 1092–1106. https://doi.org/10.6004/jnccn.2018.0073

O'Leary, M.C., Lu, X., Huang, Y., Lin, X., Mahmood, I., Przepiorka, D., … Pazdur, R. (2019). FDA approval summary: Tisagenlecleucel for treatment of patients with relapsed or refractory B-cell precursor acute lymphoblastic leukemia. *Clinical Cancer Research, 25*, 1142–1146. https://doi.org/10.1158/1078-0432.ccr-18-2035

Park, J.H., Rivière, I., Gonen, M., Wang, X., Sénéchal, B., Curran, K.J., … Sadelain, M. (2018). Long-term follow-up of CD19 CAR therapy in acute lymphoblastic leukemia. *New England Journal of Medicine, 378*, 449–459. https://doi.org/10.1056/NEJMoa1709919

Perica, K., Curran, K.J., Brentjens, R.J., & Giralt, S.A. (2018). Building a CAR garage: Preparing for the delivery of commercial CAR T cell products at Memorial Sloan Kettering Cancer Center. *Biology of Blood and Marrow Transplantation, 24*, 1135–1141. https://doi.org/10.1016/j.bbmt.2018.02.018

Porter, D.L., Hwang, W.-T., Frey, N.V., Lacey, S.F., Shaw, P.A., Loren, A.W., … June, C.H. (2015). Chimeric antigen receptor T cells persist and induce sustained remissions in relapsed refractory chronic lymphocytic leukemia. *Science Translational Medicine, 7*, 303ra139. https://doi.org/10.1126/scitranslmed.aac5415

Salter, A.I., Pont, M.J., & Riddell, S.R. (2018). Chimeric antigen receptor-modified T cells: CD19 and the road beyond. *Blood, 131*, 2621–2629. https://doi.org/10.1182/blood-2018-01-785840

Santomasso, B.D., Park, J.H., Salloum, D., Riviere, I., Flynn, J., Mead, E., … Brentjens, R.J. (2018). Clinical and biological correlates of neurotoxicity associated with CAR T-cell therapy in patients with B-cell acute lymphoblastic leukemia. *Cancer Discovery, 8*, 958–971. https://doi.org/10.1158/2159-8290.cd-17-1319

Schuster, S.J., Bishop, M.R., Tam, C.S., Waller, E.K., Borchmann, P., McGuirk, J.P., … Maziarz, T. (2017). Primary analysis of Juliet: A global,

pivotal, phase 2 trial of CTL019 in adult patients with relapsed or refractory diffuse large B-cell lymphoma [Abstract]. *Blood, 130*(Suppl. 1), 577. https://doi.org/10.1182/blood.V130.Suppl_1.577.577

Schuster, S.J., Svoboda, J., Chong, E.A., Nasta, S.D., Mato, A.R., Anak, Ö., … June, C.H. (2017). Chimeric antigen receptor T cells in refractory B-cell lymphomas. *New England Journal of Medicine, 377*, 2545–2554. https://doi.org/10.1056/nejmoa1708566

Turtle, C.J., Hanafi, L.-A., Berger, C., Hudecek, M., Pender, B., Robinson, E., … Maloney, D.G. (2016). Immunotherapy of non-Hodgkin's lymphoma with a defined ratio of CD8$^+$ and CD4$^+$ CD19-specific chimeric antigen receptor-modified T cells. *Science Translational Medicine, 8*, 355ra116. https://doi.org/10.1126/scitranslmed.aaf8621

Vormittag, P., Gunn, R., Ghorashian, S., & Veraitch, F.S. (2018). A guide to manufacturing CAR T cell therapies. *Current Opinion in Biotechnology, 53*, 164–181. https://doi.org/10.1016/j.copbio.2018.01.025

Whilding, L.M., & Maher, J. (2015). CAR T-cell immunotherapy: The path from the by-road to the freeway? *Molecular Oncology, 9*, 1994–2018. https://doi.org/10.1016/j.molonc.2015.10.012

Zhang, J., Medeiros, L.J., & Young, K.H. (2018). Cancer immunotherapy in diffuse large B-cell lymphoma. *Frontiers in Oncology, 8*, 351. https://doi.org/10.3389/fonc.2018.00351

Zheng, P.-P., Kros, J.M., & Li, J. (2018). Approved CAR T cell therapies: Ice bucket challenges on glaring safety risks and long-term impacts. *Drug Discovery Today, 23*, 1175–1182. https://doi.org/10.1016/j.drudis.2018.02.012

CHAPTER 17

Professional Practice

Kelli Thoele, PhD, RN, ACNS-BC, BMTCN®, OCN®

Introduction

Individuals with little or no formal education often performed nursing care prior to the foundation of modern nursing. Nursing practice was based on trial and error, observations of other caregivers, and information verbally passed down through generations (Egenes, 2018). In the early 19th century in Europe, nurses were often lower-class women who were unable to find other work or women who were trained in religious instruction and nursing care (Egenes, 2018). Florence Nightingale, widely considered the founder of modern nursing, established the first professional nursing school with a curriculum that addressed theory and clinical practice (Egenes, 2018).

To understand what it means to be a professional nurse, it is first necessary to understand the meaning of *profession*. A profession is defined as an "organized set of institutions, roles, and [people] whose business it is to apply or improve the procedures and techniques" (Toulmin, 1972, p. 142) of the discipline. In other words, a profession is a group of individuals with a specific set of knowledge that is formally taught. Members of a profession have autonomous practice and a responsibility to adhere to the role, behave ethically and legally, and improve the profession (Houle, 1980).

The American Nurses Association (ANA, 2010) defines nursing as "the protection, promotion, and optimization of health and abilities; prevention of illness and injury; alleviation of suffering through the diagnosis and treatment of human response; and advocacy in the care of individuals, families, communities, and populations" (p. 10). Although lay caregivers may provide support for the health of others, professional nurses have knowledge, expectations, credentialing, and accountability that are unique to the profession. Several characteristics differentiate individuals who perform a task (e.g., early nurses without formal education, family caregivers) from a profession (e.g., modern nursing). Figure 17-1 outlines the characteristics of a profession.

Professional Regulation

Several mechanisms of oversight, monitoring, and control regulate the nursing profession. Several resources are also available to provide a foundation for the nursing profession. ANA (2010, 2015a, 2015b) has developed the scope and standards of nursing practice, a code of nursing ethics, and a social policy statement. These publications provide a definition of nursing practice and the professional role, a framework for ethical analysis and decision making, and a description of nursing's value within and accountability to society. The International Council of Nurses (ICN, 2012, 2013) has also developed publications regarding the scope of nursing practice and a code of ethics for nurses. Specialty certification demonstrates competency in a particular nursing field.

Another form of oversight for nursing is through legal and government regulation (ANA, 2010). Each state in the United States has a nurse practice act that governs nursing within the state. Individual nurses are responsible for practicing according to the laws of the state nurse practice act and the rules and regulations established by the state board of nursing (Russell, 2012). Nurses also practice according to rules and regulations that are not limited to the nursing profession. For example, *United States Pharmacopeia* provides standards for the safe handling of hazardous drugs in multiple professions, including nurses, physicians, pharmacists, and veterinarians (Bonner, 2016).

Institutional policies and procedures also regulate nursing practice and should be based on the scope, standards, and ethics of the nursing profession. Institutional policies

---

Figure 17-1. Characteristics of a Profession

- Formal training or education
- Creation of a subculture
- Mastery of theoretical knowledge
- Self-enhancement of knowledge and skill
- Credentialing
- Ethical practice
- Clarification of the mission and functions of the profession
- Penalties for unethical and incompetent practice
- Use of practical knowledge
- Legal reinforcement of the rights and privileges of practitioners
- Autonomous practice
- Public awareness and acceptance
- Capacity to solve problems
- Relationships between the practitioners and those who use their services

Note. Based on information from Houle, 1980.

---

and procedures should align with applicable laws, rules, and regulations, as well as support evidence-based care that improves quality and safety (ANA, 2010). Finally, individual nurses regulate their own practice. Self-determination includes autonomy to choose actions, self-regulated control over practice based on personal values, and accountability for practice (ANA, 2010).

Hematopoietic Stem Cell Transplantation Nursing Specialty

In addition to general nursing practice, nurses who practice in hematopoietic stem cell transplantation (HSCT) must have knowledge about the unique needs of this patient population.

All nurses are accountable for meeting the standards of the profession (Brant & Wickham, 2013; Nelson & Guelcher, 2014; see Table 17-1). HSCT nurses, in addition to the general nursing profession, may also develop and demonstrate competency in knowledge specific to the care of transplant donors and recipients. As such, it is necessary to outline several aspects of professional practice, including education, self-care, advocacy, evidence-based practice (EBP), research, communication, leadership, interprofessional collaboration, and professional practice evaluation.

Education

Just as science and knowledge advance and evolve, a nurse's knowledge and competence also evolve through lifelong learning (ANA, 2015b; Brant & Wickham, 2013). Life-long learning may occur through formal education, informal discussions, self-reflection, academic publications, or new experiences. In addition to gaining new knowledge, nurses also contribute to the knowledge of others through mentoring, role modeling, or sharing educational findings (ANA, 2015b; Brant & Wickham, 2013).

Formal Education

One of the characteristics of a profession is formal training or education, and formal education for a nurse begins before licensure (Houle, 1980). In the United States, this education may include a diploma, associate degree, or baccalaureate degree. An individual is eligible to take the licensure examination with either degree, but evidence suggests that the baccalaureate degree better prepares nurses for practice. In a groundbreaking study, investigators found that hospitals with higher proportions of surgical nurses with a baccalaureate degree or higher had lower patient mortality and lower rates of failure to rescue (Aiken, Clarke, Cheung, Sloane, & Silber, 2003). Based on this study, as well as subsequent evidence demonstrating a link between nurse education level and patient outcomes, the baccalaureate degree is the recommended degree for entry into the nursing profession (Shalala et al., 2011).

Formal education may also include a postgraduate degree. Some nurses may choose to pursue postgraduate degrees in related fields, such as public health or business. Nurses who would like to learn more about nursing administration or nursing education may pursue a master's degree in nursing with a focus on leadership or education. To become an advanced practice registered nurse (APRN),

Table 17-1. Examples of Standards of Professional Performance

Performance Area	Standard
Education	"The oncology nurse acquires and expands a personal knowledge base that reflects the current evidence-based state of cancer care and oncology nursing and that incorporates enhanced competence and critical-thinking skills. The oncology nurse contributes to the professional development of licensed peers, assistive personnel, and inter-professional colleagues" (Brant & Wickham, 2013, p. 47).
Communication	"The oncology nurse interacts and communicates effectively with the interprofessional healthcare team and with the patient and family and uses a variety of strategies to foster mutual respect and shared decision making that enhance clinical outcomes and patient satisfaction in all practice settings" (Brant & Wickham, 2013, pp. 53–54).
Collaboration	"The oncology nurse partners with the patient and family, the interprofessional team, and community resources to optimize cancer care" (Brant & Wickham, 2013, p. 57).
Leadership	"The oncology nurse demonstrates leadership in the practice setting and in the nursing profession by actively acknowledging the dynamic nature of cancer care and the necessity to prepare for evolving technologies, modalities of treatment, and supportive care" (Brant & Wickham, 2013, p. 55).
Professional practice evaluation	"The oncology nurse consistently evaluates his or her own nursing practice in relation to national oncology nursing professional standards and guidelines, the state nurse practice act, relevant statewide relevant regulatory requirements, and job-specific performance expectations" (Brant & Wickham, 2013, p. 58).
Evidence-based practice and research	"The oncology nurse contributes to the scientific base of cancer nursing practice, education, management, quality improvement, and research through multiple avenues: identifying clinical dilemmas and problems appropriate for rigorous study, collecting data, critiquing existing research, and integrating relevant research into clinical practice to improve patient outcomes" (Brant & Wickham, 2013, p. 49).

master's degrees in nursing are available for clinical nurse specialists, nurse practitioners, nurse midwives, and registered nurse anesthetists. More than 250,000 APRNs practice in the United States, and the Consensus Model for APRN Regulation provides guidelines for regulation through education, licensure, accreditation, and certification (National Council of State Boards of Nursing [NCSBN], 2008). Doctoral degrees in nursing prepare nurses to lead research and generate new knowledge (PhD) or lead complex change (Doctor of Nursing Practice).

Credentialing

Credentialing, or a formal process to ensure professional standards are met, is another characteristic of a profession (Houle, 1980). Individual nurses are credentialed through licensure. Individuals who obtain a nursing degree must then pass a licensure examination to demonstrate competency for entry into the nursing profession (NCSBN, 2011). In the United States, licensure of nurses is through individual state boards of nursing. Nurses in participating states may have a multistate license through an enhanced Nurse Licensure Compact (NCSBN, n.d.). On the academic level, two organizations, the Accreditation Commission for Education in Nursing and the Commission on Collegiate Nursing Education, provide accreditation for nursing schools in the United States. This process ensures that nursing schools meet certain standards of nursing education.

Specialty certification demonstrates continued learning and development of expertise in a specific patient population (Brant & Wickham, 2013). The Oncology Nursing Certification Corporation (www.oncc.org) offers a certification to validate an individual's knowledge of caring for HSCT donors and recipients. Nurses are eligible to apply for the blood and marrow transplant certified nurse (BMTCN®) accreditation test if they meet specific requirements related to licensure, experience, HSCT nursing practice, and continuing education.

Lifelong Learning

Lifelong learning is necessary to maintain competency in the nursing profession. Academic journals are sources of new knowledge about HSCT and nursing care. Lifelong learning for HSCT nurses should include review of the literature, but nurses may not have access to journals or the necessary skills to critique the literature. One strategy to facilitate lifelong learning is a journal club—a group of individuals who gather to review and evaluate literature together. By reviewing journal articles together, nurses report increased enthusiasm about professional development, as well as improvements in skills and familiarity with research, personal and professional growth, learning, and implementation of research into practice (Häggman-Laitila, Mattila, & Melender, 2016). The Oncology Nursing Society (ONS) has developed a toolkit to facilitate journal clubs. This toolkit is publicly available and includes steps to create a journal club, a flyer to publicize meetings, tips to facilitate participation, participation guidelines, a glossary of research terminology, and resources to guide review and critique of selected articles (ONS, 2010).

Self-Care

The nursing profession is focused on the health and well-being of others; however, this focus should not be to the detriment of the individual nurse. The *Code of Ethics for Nurses* states "the nurse owes the same duties to self as to others" (ANA, 2015a, p. 19). Self-care is the ability of individuals, families, and communities to care for themselves in terms of hygiene, nutrition, environmental factors, social factors, and lifestyle in order to promote health and prevent and manage illness (World Health Organization, 1998, 2009). In addition to self-care, nurses must act with strong moral principles, maintain competence in the nursing profession, and continue to grow personally and professionally (ANA, 2015a). Self-care in nurses should not be viewed as a selfish activity but as a necessary component of well-being and a foundation for compassionate nursing practice (Mills, Wand, & Fraser, 2014). Despite believing that self-care is effective and important, nurses do not consistently practice self-care strategies (Mills, Wand, & Fraser, 2017).

Burnout and Moral Distress

Healthcare providers caring for patients in the HSCT setting report high levels of job satisfaction but report challenges with maintaining work–life balance, addressing ethical issues, and working in stressful environments (Denzen et al., 2013; Neumann et al., 2018). Nurses often experience burnout, compassion fatigue, and moral distress, and these issues may result in negative outcomes for patients, nurses, and healthcare organizations. An important part of self-care is preventing and managing stress associated with providing care for others.

In response to occupational stressors, some people develop burnout, emotional exhaustion, depersonalization, and decreased feelings of accomplishment (Maslach & Leiter, 2016). Approximately one-third of oncology and HSCT nurses report burnout, which is associated with decreased job satisfaction, stress, negative health outcomes in nurses, increased errors, and decreased patient safety (Cañadas-De la Fuente et al., 2018; Hall, Johnson, Watt, Tsipa, & O'Connor, 2016; Khamisa, Peltzer, & Oldenburg, 2013; Neumann et al., 2018). To prevent and manage burnout, nurses should get adequate nutrition, sleep, and exercise; participate in hobbies outside of work; develop skills to cope with stress; and have supportive relationships with colleagues and friends (Maslach & Leiter, 2016).

In addition to burnout, nurses may also experience moral distress, which results from the inability to pursue the morally correct action because of institutional constraints (Jameton, 1984). For example, nurses may feel moral distress when a patient refuses appropriate treatment, the ethical climate is negative, patients and families behave inappropriately toward the nurse, or when care is perceived as futile (Oh & Gastmans, 2015). More than one-third of nurses working in the HSCT setting report high levels of moral distress, which is associated with feelings of guilt and shame, withdrawal from patient care, distrust of others, higher intent to leave a job, and decreased professional quality of life (Austin, Saylor, & Finley, 2017; Neumann et al., 2018; Oh & Gastmans, 2015). The American Association of Critical-Care Nurses (n.d.) developed a framework to address moral distress known as the 4A's: ask, affirm, assess, and act. The nurse should ask about the nature of the problem, affirm a commitment to self-care and the obligation to act, assess sources of distress and the severity of distress, and act to address moral distress while remaining authentic to oneself.

Self-Reflection

To care for oneself, the nurse should reflect on self-care practices. For example, questions could include the following:

- Am I eating healthy food and drinking enough water?
- Do I exercise regularly?
- Am I getting adequate sleep?
- Do I set boundaries and avoid taking on too much responsibility?
- Do I express gratitude?
- Am I experiencing burnout at work?
- Do I feel moral distress when providing care?
- How often do I spend time with people who are important to me?
- Do I contribute to causes that align with my values?
- Do I have supportive relationships with friends, families, and colleagues?

Self-Care Practices

Once individuals reflect on self-care and identify opportunities for improvement, a wide variety of self-care activities can promote physical, psychological, emotional, and spiritual self-care. Nurses may perform some self-care activities during the workday, including being aware of one's needs, remaining hydrated, eating nutritious food, praying, and practicing mindfulness. Other practices, such as exercise, meditation, and journaling, require additional time. The number of self-care practices is limitless; a few practices are listed in Table 17-2.

As individuals in a caring profession, nurses may experience burnout and moral distress. Self-care is as necessary as providing care for others and includes caring for aspects of physical, emotional, mental, and spiritual life. Nurses should regularly reflect on their self-care needs and identify and implement practices to promote self-care.

Advocacy

Advocacy, or acting in support of oneself or another person, is a defining characteristic of the nursing profession. ANA (2015b) states that in addition to promoting health,

Table 17-2. Examples of Self-Care Activities

Activity	Potential Benefits
Nutrition	Decreased risk of chronic diseases (e.g., cancer, heart disease, diabetes mellitus, obesity) Overall health promotion
Exercise	Decreased risk of chronic disease Healthier bones and muscles Improved mood and mental health Longer life expectancy
Mindfulness	Weight loss Reduction in anxiety, stress, and burnout Improved mood, focus, and empathy
Adequate sleep	Fewer patient care errors Improved mood and energy, higher cognitive functioning Decreased risk of chronic disease
Journaling	Improved feeling of well-being
Forgiveness	Improved mental health, reduced depression and anxiety Increased levels of hope Higher social support and life satisfaction

Note. Based on information from Carrière et al., 2018; Centers for Disease Control and Prevention, 2018, 2019; Cirelli, 2019; Johnson et al., 2014; O'Connell et al., 2017; Smith, 2014; U.S. Department of Health and Human Services, 2017; VanderWeele, 2018; Wade et al., 2014.

preventing illness, and alleviating suffering, nursing involves "advocacy in the care of individuals, families, groups, communities, and populations" (p. 1). Nurses advocate for the health of communities by supporting social and environmental justice, access to equitable health care, policies to promote health, and community engagement. Nurses also advocate for the comfort, safety, well-being, humanity, dignity, and rights of others (ANA, 2015a, 2015b).

Advocating for Individuals

In addition to acting on behalf of patients, nurses should encourage patient self-advocacy. Cancer survivors report self-advocating regarding cancer treatment, symptom management, relationships with the care team, and support from friends and family (Hagan, Rosenzweig, Zorn, van Londen, & Donovan, 2017). To self-advocate, patients should have skills related to seeking information, communicating with others, solving problems, and negotiating (Hagan & Medberry, 2016). Nurses can help individuals seek information by directing them to several organizations that provide information to promote self-advocacy for donors and recipients, including the Blood and Marrow Transplant Information Network, National Bone Marrow Transplant Link, National Coalition for Cancer Survivorship, and National Marrow Donor Program. Nurses may also facilitate communication, problem-solving, and negotiation skills.

In situations in which the nurse advocates for another individual, the nurse must first understand the situation and patient. The nurse must engage in interpersonal dialogue regarding the experiences and wishes of the individual to understand the situation. This type of situation also requires maturity and skills to advocate for the patient. Both the nurse and patient should be empowered to make decisions (Vaartio, Leino-Kilpi, Salanterä, & Suominen, 2006). Advocating for an individual is an iterative process that includes analyzing, counseling, and responding to the patient's preferences about care and self-determination (Vaartio-Rajalin & Leino-Kilpi, 2011; see Figure 17-2).

Advocating for Populations

Health disparities are present in cancer care, and nurses are in the position to advocate for equitable health care. People who are poor, uninsured, or have limited access to health care have a greater burden of disease. In some types of cancer, race is associated with a higher incidence of cancer and higher rates of mortality (National Cancer Institute, n.d.). Disparities also exist in HSCT care. In a review of patients with multiple myeloma who were eligible for HSCT, African American patients had higher mortality rates and were less likely to undergo HSCT than Caucasian patients (Fiala & Wildes, 2017).

Nurses, through leadership in clinical care, healthcare delivery, policy, and research, can advocate for health equity and elimination of health disparities. The National Quality Forum (2017) has presented a roadmap for reducing health disparities with four necessary actions for stakeholders: identify disparities that exist and prioritize health equity, implement evidence-based interventions, invest in performance measures that assess health equity, and incentivize the achievement of health equity. Individuals from minority backgrounds are underrepresented in the nursing profession in the United States. Increasing diversity within the profession is another strategy to reduce health disparities (Phillips & Malone, 2014).

Another way to advocate for groups of individuals is through the development and implementation of local, state, and national policies. In a clinical setting, nurses can advocate for patients by ensuring that institutional policies are evidence based and patient centered. On a state or national level, nurses may advocate for policies to promote health, alleviate suffering, and prevent illness in populations. For example, the National Cancer Moonshot Initiative was a project to increase interprofessional collaboration, funding, and resources to prevent and treat cancer (National Cancer Advisory Board, 2016). To participate in this initiative, oncology nurses provided feedback and suggestions, and an oncology nurse participated in a panel of experts to ensure evidence-based approaches to initiatives (Mayer & Nasso, 2017; National Cancer Advisory Board, 2016). ONS (n.d.) supports policies that improve the quality of cancer care through meaningful quality measures and opportunities for emerging healthcare delivery models.

Advocating for the Nursing Profession

In addition to promoting self-advocacy and advocating for individuals and populations, nurses can also advocate for the nursing profession. For example, nurse leaders in a clinical setting can advocate for a healthy work environment, nurse participation in decision making, and resources to provide safe care (Tomajan, 2012). On a national level, nursing organizations have prioritized issues such as safe staffing, nursing workforce development, nurses practicing to the full scope of their license, and payment models that incorporate nurse work (ANA, n.d.; ONS, n.d.).

Communication

Communication is an essential part of health care, and it takes place via telephone, electronic systems, written word, and face-to-face interactions. In addition to verbal communication, nonverbal exchange of information may also occur through facial expressions, eye contact, gestures, distances between people, and tone of voice. Nurses must be able to effectively communicate and convey authenticity, caring, respect, and trust (ANA, 2015b). Communication also supports shared decision making between patients and healthcare providers (Brant & Wickham, 2013). By communicating effectively with patients, nurses can enhance patient outcomes, promote patient safety and adherence to self-care measures, and contribute to patient satisfaction (Brant & Wickham, 2013).

Communication With Patients and Families

Six core functions of patient–clinician communication contribute to outcomes in cancer care (see Figure

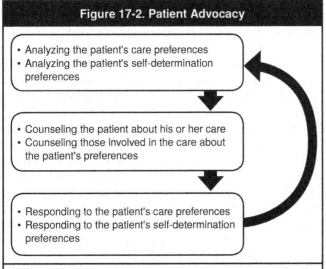

Figure 17-2. Patient Advocacy

- Analyzing the patient's care preferences
- Analyzing the patient's self-determination preferences

↓

- Counseling the patient about his or her care
- Counseling those involved in the care about the patient's preferences

↓

- Responding to the patient's care preferences
- Responding to the patient's self-determination preferences

Note. Based on information from Vaartio et al., 2009.

From "Nurses as Patient Advocates in Oncology Care: Activities Based on Literature," by H. Vaartio-Rajalin and H. Leino-Kilpi, 2011, *Clinical Journal of Oncology Nursing, 15*, p. 527. Copyright 2011 by Oncology Nursing Society. Reprinted with permission.

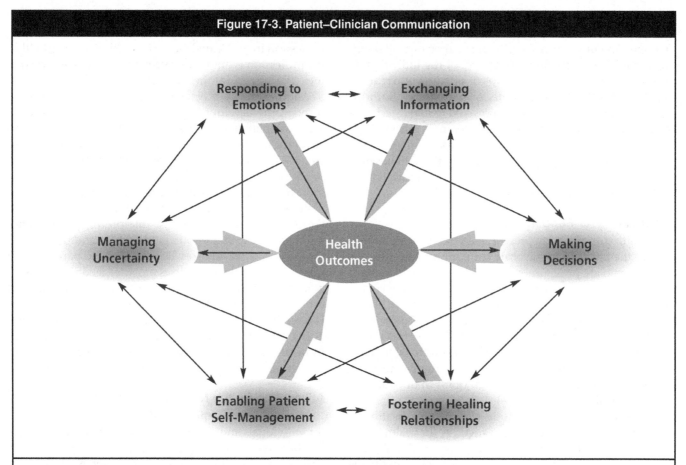

Figure 17-3. Patient–Clinician Communication

Note. From *Patient-Centered Communication in Cancer Care: Promoting Healing and Reducing Suffering* (NIH Publication No. 07-6225), by R.M. Epstein and R.L. Street Jr., 2007, p. 18. Retrieved from https://pubs.cancer.gov/ncipl/detail.aspx?prodid=T099.

17-3). When nurses and patients interact, it is necessary to foster healthy relationships in which patients perceive that nurses are committed to their best interests, accepting, competent, respectful, and empathetic. Information should be exchanged between the patient and nurse based on the needs of the patient, and decisions should be made based on that information. Optimal decision making includes ensuring that the perspectives of the patient and clinician are understood, differences in opinion are reconciled, and a mutual agreement is made regarding the best evidence-based course of action (Epstein & Street, 2007).

Nurses should recognize and respond to the dynamic emotional states of patients and intervene as appropriate. Interventions may include legitimation and validation of a patient's emotions, expression of empathy, or tangible help. Uncertainty is common in cancer care, and nurses can provide information and support to patients dealing with uncertainty. Finally, a function of patient-centered communication is to support and advocate for patient self-management (Epstein & Street, 2007).

Health literacy—the ability to understand health information needed to make decisions—is essential to patient–clinician communication and affects health outcomes including knowledge, use of preventive services, rates of hospitalization, healthcare costs, and health status (U.S. Department of Health and Human Services, n.d.). According to the most recent national data available in the United States, half of adults had intermediate health literacy, and 12% of respondents had proficient health literacy (Kutner, Greenberg, Jin, & Paulsen, 2006). The National Institutes of Health (n.d.) recommends communication based on cultural respect and presented in plain language to facilitate understanding by patients and other lay individuals.

When communicating with people from different cultures, it is important to understand the individual's health beliefs and cultural values. For example, discussing a potentially negative health outcome is avoided in some cultures, and eye contact may be viewed as offensive or appropriate in different cultures. Consideration of cultural beliefs may include asking a patient about personal beliefs and preferences and learning about a patient's culture through community organizations or interpreters (Brega et al., 2015). Language is a potential barrier to communication if the patient speaks a different language than the nurse or is unable to read. Trained medical interpreters and visual and written material are essential to facilitate communication in the presence of language barriers.

Plain language is a strategy to increase the clarity of verbal and written communication. The federal government has developed plain language guidelines to improve the clarity of communication from the government to the public, and these strategies are also used in health care. Components of plain language include writing for the intended audience, organizing the information to meet the needs of the audience, presenting information in simple terms, and using active voice (Plain Language Action and Information Network, 2011; U.S. Department of Health and Human Services, n.d.).

Communication With Healthcare Providers

Inadequate communication among healthcare providers can lead to diagnostic errors, medication errors, patient falls, wrong-site surgery, delays in treatment, medical malpractice lawsuits, increased healthcare costs, and death (Balogh, Miller, & Ball, 2015; Joint Commission, 2017; Ruoff, 2015). Nurses may use techniques to exchange information and effectively communicate in order to improve communication and prevent errors and delays in treatment.

One technique to improve communication is known as SBAR (situation, background, assessment, and recommendation). This structure helps frame information exchange regarding a situation that requires action by another individual. Using the SBAR technique, a nurse can briefly explain the situation and current problem, provide background information pertinent to the situation, discuss findings from the assessment of the situation, and recommend a course of action (Institute for Healthcare Improvement, 2017). SBAR has been used in multiple clinical settings and is associated with improvements in efficiency, perception of effective communication, culture of patient safety, and provider confidence in communication (Stewart, 2016).

Another technique to improve communication is known as I-PASS (illness severity, patient summary, action list, situation awareness and contingency planning, and synthesis by receiver). This method can be used when communicating during patient hand-off and includes information about the patient's severity of illness, a summary of the patient's current state and plan of care, a timeline and ownership of action items that still need to be completed, current and anticipated situation, and a summary by the receiver of information (Starmer et al., 2012). When studied in medical residents, the use of I-PASS was associated with a 23% decrease in medical errors and a 30% decrease in preventable adverse events (Starmer et al., 2014). I-PASS is also associated with improved communication in nurse handoff (Starmer et al., 2017). Figure 17-4 provides examples of communication using SBAR and I-PASS.

Interprofessional Collaboration

In addition to providing nursing care, nurses are part of an interprofessional team and collaborate with other

---

Figure 17-4. Examples of SBAR and I-PASS

SBAR
To communicate about a situation that requires action

Situation
Mr. Smith, a 24-year-old hematopoietic stem cell transplant recipient, is neutropenic and has a temperature of 38.4°C.

Background
- He has a history of germ cell tumor.
- He received an autologous stem cell transplant and is currently on day +7.
- His blood pressure is 92/64 mm Hg, pulse is 84 beats per minute (bpm), and respirations are 20 breaths per minute.
- His last blood cultures were 8 days ago, and he is allergic to cefepime.

Assessment
The patient is neutropenic and febrile.

Recommendation
I would like to obtain blood cultures and start antibiotics right away, and you need to assess the patient soon.

I-PASS
To hand-off patient care to another provider

Illness Severity
Mr. Smith is stable but currently febrile and hypotensive.

Patient Summary
- He is a 24-year-old male with a history of germ cell tumor.
- He received an autologous stem cell transplant and is on day +7.
- His blood pressure is 92/64 mm Hg, pulse is 84 bpm, and respirations are 20 breaths per minute.
- The physician was notified about the patient's fever and is on his way to assess the patient.

Action List
- I already sent blood cultures.
- The nursing assistant is going to check the patient's vital signs in 1 hour and will notify you of the results.
- The pharmacy technician is delivering antibiotics soon, and you will need to start the antibiotics within the next 15 minutes.

Situation Awareness and Contingency Planning
If the patient's blood pressure continues to drop, he may need to be transferred to the intensive care unit.

Synthesis by Receiver
The patient received an autologous transplant and has a neutropenic fever. Blood cultures have been sent, and I will monitor the patient's status and start antibiotics as soon as possible. I will notify the charge nurse that the patient may need to be transferred to the intensive care unit.

---

stakeholders and disciplines to promote quality care (ANA, 2015b). Interprofessional collaboration is a process of people from different professions working together (Reeves, Pelone, Harrison, Goldman, & Zwarenstein, 2017). Nurses collaborate with many different professions including medicine, pharmacy, social services, dietetics, and physical therapy. Members of each discipline have unique knowledge, and a team approach is necessary to manage the complexity of patient care and the healthcare system (Brant & Wickham, 2013).

Framework for Interprofessional Collaboration

The Interprofessional Education Collaborative (IPEC, 2016), a formation of six national associations of schools for health professions, developed a framework for interprofessional collaborative practice (see Figure 17-5). This framework provides interprofessional competencies to improve health and the patient experience while reducing costs (IPEC, 2016). The competencies within the framework can be applied in multiple professions and in a variety of educational and practice settings (IPEC, 2016).

When working with other professionals, there should be a climate of mutual trust and shared values. In addition to maintaining competence in the nursing scope of practice and demonstrating ethical conduct, nurses should respect the expertise of other professions and the diversity of patients and the healthcare team (IPEC, 2016). Each nurse should understand the skills, knowledge, and abilities of the nursing profession and communicate about the roles and responsibilities of the profession with patients and other team members. Interprofessional communication should be effective and respectful to facilitate collaboration. Finally, teamwork and shared accountability are a component of interprofessional collaboration (IPEC, 2016).

Interprofessional Education and Practice

Collaboration may begin before nursing licensure in an educational setting and continue in clinical practice. Interprofessional education is the interactive learning of members of multiple professions to improve collaboration and patient care (Reeves, Perrier, Goldman, Freeth, & Zwarenstein, 2013). The content of interprofessional education may be created based on the needs of the learners, or the content may be modified from an existing program, such as TeamSTEPPS or Crew Resource Management (Brashers, Phillips, Malpass, & Owen, 2015). Research on interprofessional education in practice has shown that education is associated with improved communication, teamwork, quality of care, and efficiency, as well as fewer adverse events (Brashers et al., 2015). For example, interprofessional education via a code blue simulation was associated with improved code team performance and improved patient survival to discharge (Knight et al., 2014).

In clinical practice, interventions to improve interprofessional collaboration include interprofessional activities, rounds, meetings, and checklists. These strategies may improve patient functional status, use of healthcare resources, and providers' adherence to recommended practices (Reeves et al., 2017). For example, exercise in HSCT recipients is an intervention that improves fatigue, lower extremity strength, and cardiopulmonary fitness (Persoon et al., 2013). To provide resources to support patient functional status, an interprofessional team worked together to design and construct a gym on an inpatient HSCT unit. Interprofessional collaboration facilitated the implementation of this project (Blackburn, Presson, Laufman, Tomczak, & Brassil, 2016).

Interprofessional collaboration is not a one-time project but part of an organization's culture. In an assessment of several healthcare organizations, six practices were found to support interprofessional collaboration. First, providers should make needs of patients and families the primary focus and align the work of professionals to provide care based on what is best for the patient. Second, leaders within the organization, including the chief medical officer and chief nurse executive, should work collaboratively and demonstrate commitment to interprofessional collaboration. Third, all professionals should understand the role and value of their professions and work at the top of their licenses. Fourth, communication should be continuous, effective, and respectful. Fifth, the structure of the organization should support interprofessional practice. Sixth, different disciplines should be trained together (Tomasik & Fleming, 2015).

Nurses have knowledge and skills that are unique to the nursing profession and collaborate with people from other professions to provide comprehensive care to patients. By

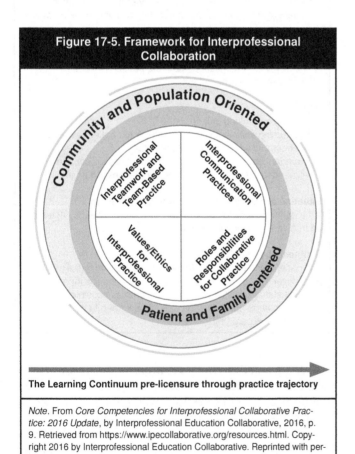

Figure 17-5. Framework for Interprofessional Collaboration

Community and Population Oriented

Interprofessional Teamwork and Team-Based Practice

Interprofessional Communication Practices

Values/Ethics for Interprofessional Practice

Roles and Responsibilities for Collaborative Practice

Patient and Family Centered

The Learning Continuum pre-licensure through practice trajectory

Note. From *Core Competencies for Interprofessional Collaborative Practice: 2016 Update,* by Interprofessional Education Collaborative, 2016, p. 9. Retrieved from https://www.ipecollaborative.org/resources.html. Copyright 2016 by Interprofessional Education Collaborative. Reprinted with permission.

collaborating with others through education and practice, nurses can improve communication, teamwork, and patient outcomes, as well as reduce healthcare costs. Interprofessional collaboration is essential to a positive organizational culture.

Leadership

Leadership, or influencing others toward a common goal, is an essential component of professional practice. One of the tenets of nursing practice is partnering with others to work toward a common goal of safe and quality health care (ANA, 2015b). As partners in the provision of health care, all nurses must work with and influence other people, whether working in direct patient care, education, research, a formal leadership role, a committee or board role, or public policy.

Because oncology nurses must provide safe, high-quality, and cost-effective care in an ever-changing environment, leadership is an expected role for all professional nurses (Brant & Wickham, 2013). Leadership may be in clinical practice or in the nursing profession. For example, nurses may develop and direct the nursing care plan, advocate for patients, mentor other nurses, develop patient and family education programs, and participate in committees or professional organization (Brant & Wickham, 2013). APRNs may show leadership skills by promoting interprofessional teamwork, sharing knowledge of research findings and EBP, serving as mentors or preceptors, or serving as liaisons to professional organizations or legislative bodies (Brant & Wickham, 2013).

The Future of Nursing: Leading Change, Advancing Health, a report published by the Institute of Medicine (now the Health and Medicine Division of the National Academies of Sciences, Engineering, and Medicine), presented recommendations for transforming the nursing profession. The report recommended that nurses should be prepared and enabled to lead change within the healthcare field (Shalala et al., 2011). This includes individual nurses taking responsibility for their personal and professional growth, nursing organizations providing opportunities for growth to their members, nursing educators teaching about leadership theories and practices, and healthcare decision makers including nurses in leadership positions (Shalala et al., 2011).

Leadership Styles

Several different leadership styles have been identified, including authoritarian, democratic, transactional, and transformational. Different leadership styles may be used in different situations. For example, a nurse leading patient care during an emergency will likely use a different leadership style than when leading an EBP improvement initiative with peers or developing the strategic plan of an organization.

Lewin, Lippitt, and White (1939) categorized leadership styles based on decision-making authority. In authoritarian leadership, the leader directs and controls activities and tells followers what to do, without obtaining input from the followers. This contrasts with the democratic leadership style, in which the leader shares decision making with the followers, and the laissez-faire leadership style, in which leaders allow followers to independently make decisions (Lewin et al., 1939).

More recent leadership styles include transactional leadership and transformational leadership (Byrne, 2015). Transactional leadership is a style in which the leader focuses on the completion of tasks and provides rewards for performance. Leaders who are transactional and notice deviations from the established rules and standards intervene and take corrective action (Bass, 1990; Burns, 1978). Transformational leadership is when "leaders broaden and elevate the interests of their employees, when they generate awareness and acceptance of the purposes and mission of the group, and when they stir their employees to look beyond their own self-interest for the good of the group" (Bass, 1990, p. 21). Transformational leaders may inspire employees, meet the emotional needs of employees, and intellectually stimulate employees in order to influence others (Bass, 1990).

Leadership style is related to individual and organizational outcomes. Nurses report higher job satisfaction when leaders have relationship-oriented leadership styles rather than task-oriented leadership styles (McCay, Lyles, & Larkey, 2017). Transformational leadership is directly associated with increased structural empowerment and indirectly associated with increased job satisfaction and decreased adverse patient outcomes (Boamah, Laschinger, Wong, & Clarke, 2018). In addition, transformational leadership by nurse executives is associated with increased commitment of nurses to the organization (Leach, 2005).

Transformational Leadership and Magnet® Certification

In the United States, the Magnet Recognition Program® recognizes healthcare organizations for nursing excellence and high-quality patient care (American Nurses Credentialing Center [ANCC], n.d.-a). The Magnet Model is a framework for nursing excellence and has five domains: structural empowerment; exemplary professional practice; new knowledge, innovations, and improvements; empirical outcomes; and transformational leadership (ANCC, n.d.-b).

To create an environment of nursing excellence and high-quality care, nurses should have attributes of transformational leaders. While transformational leadership is required to obtain Magnet status, it is also a key component of sustaining this designation (Hayden, Wolf, & Zedreck-Gonzalez, 2016). In a study of chief nursing officers (CNOs) at Magnet hospitals, transformational leadership was measured using a scale of the five practices of exemplary leadership (see Table 17-3), and the authors found that the top characteristics of Magnet CNOs were

Table 17-3. Practices of Exemplary Leadership

Practice	Characteristics
Model the way	Clarify your personal values, honor the values of others, and align your actions with shared values; be credible
Inspire a shared vision	Envision future possibilities and share with others; engage others in the vision by creating a sense of common purpose
Challenge the process	Try new ways of working and ways to improve, take chances, and learn from the experience
Enable others to act	Build trust and foster collaboration; increase the development of competence and self-determination in others
Encourage the heart	Provide clear expectations and encourage others; provide recognition that is personal and specific; support a spirit of community; recognize the contributions of others

Note. Based on information from Kouzes et al., 2015.

enabling others to act and modeling the way (i.e., demonstrating values and setting an example) (Clavelle, Drenkard, Tullai-McGuinness, & Fitzpatrick, 2012).

Leadership Framework

For oncology nurses working in all settings and roles, ONS has developed a framework for leadership development (see Figure 17-6). The skills described within the framework may guide self-assessment or leadership education and are divided into five domains: personal mastery vision, knowledge, interpersonal effectiveness, and systems thinking. The model includes three levels of competency to align with skills needed at an individual, group, or governance level of practice (ONS, 2012).

Within the first domain, personal mastery, the nurse must reflect on his or her beliefs and values. Although leaders must adapt in response to intrinsic or extrinsic factors, the nurse must remain authentic to his or her beliefs and values. Self-care is another aspect of personal mastery and includes physical, mental, spiritual, and emotional self-care. Lifelong learning is another competency associated with personal mastery (ONS, 2012).

Vision, the second leadership domain, is an idea of future goals. Nurses should look ahead, anticipate outcomes, and establish a direction for one's own practice. Nurse leaders may also identify a vision for a group of nurses, the nursing profession, or health care. Communication about a goal or vision and inspiring others to work toward the vision are also leadership competencies (ONS, 2012).

The third domain of leadership is knowledge. Nurses should pursue knowledge in order to answer questions, improve practice, and facilitate knowledge acquisition by others. This knowledge should be transferred to others and

applied to practice. Then, outcomes from application of this knowledge can be evaluated (ONS, 2012).

Within the fourth domain, interpersonal effectiveness, nurses build and maintain relationships with others and demonstrate empathy and a desire to help others. Verbal and nonverbal communication and emotional intelligence are necessary skills to develop interpersonal effectiveness. Nurses must also set boundaries and manage multiple demands by creating balance. On a group or governance level of leadership, nurses support interpersonal effectiveness by creating a supportive environment that fosters collaboration, empathy, accountability, and balance (ONS, 2012).

The fifth and final leadership domain is systems thinking. Nurses do not care for individual patients in isolation but care for multiple patients within a complex system. Navigation of the system is necessary to promote positive outcomes. Diversity is a component of systems thinking because, within the system, nurses work with and care for people with different viewpoints. In addition, nurses advocate for others and support ethical practice. Through interprofessional collaboration, the use of technology, and stewardship of resources, nurses can navigate change within a system to promote quality outcomes (ONS, 2012).

All nurses are leaders in some capacity, including leadership in clinical care, education, research, and public policy. Although different leadership styles may be used in different situations, relationship-based leadership and trans-

Figure 17-6. Nurse Leadership Competencies

Note. From *Oncology Nursing Society Leadership Competencies*, by Oncology Nursing Society, 2012, p. 8. Retrieved from https://www.ons.org/sites/default/files/leadershipcomps.pdf. Copyright 2012 by Oncology Nursing Society. Reprinted with permission.

formational leadership improve individual and organizational outcomes.

Professional Practice Evaluation

When providing clinical care, nurses assess patients, determine potential diagnoses, plan and implement interventions, and evaluate the results. Nurses may intervene again based on the evaluation. For example, if an HSCT recipient has pain related to mucositis, a nurse may administer pain medication, then reassess the pain. Without evaluating the outcome, the nurse will not know if the intervention was effective. Similarly, nurses must evaluate professional practice to determine if their nursing practice is safe, competent, and high quality (Brant & Wickham, 2013). Evaluating professional practice includes self-reflection, self-evaluation, and feedback from peers, colleagues, and supervisors (ANA, 2015b).

In addition, nurses should ensure that they are adhering to organizational policies, the state nurse practice act, regulatory requirements, and professional guidelines. By evaluating professional practice, nurses can identify areas of strength and potential growth and establish goals for professional growth (ANA, 2015b; Brant & Wickham, 2013). Professional practice evaluation may be an informal process or part of a formal performance management process. Table 17-4 provides sample questions for professional practice evaluation.

Evidence-Based Practice

EBP is the integration of research, clinical expertise, and patient preferences and values into clinical practice. The goal of EBP is providing high-quality, cost-efficient health care that results in optimal patient outcomes (Melnyk & Fineout-Overholt, 2015). EBP is different than quality improvement or research, but the three activities share characteristics (Newhouse, 2007). Nurses report that EBP is valuable for improving patient care but do not feel prepared to implement EBP or consistently use the best evidence in practice (Saunders & Vehviläinen-Julkunen, 2016; Underhill, Roper, Siefert, Boucher, & Berry, 2015).

EBP is a foundation of quality care and an expectation of professional performance for oncology nurses (ANA, 2010; Brant & Wickham, 2013). Oncology nurses report several challenges to the implementation of EBP, including resistance to change and lack of time and knowledge. However, support from individuals and the organization results in personal and professional transformation and empowerment to act (Fridman & Frederickson, 2014).

Steps of Evidence-Based Practice

Melnyk, Fineout-Overholt, Stillwell, and Williamson (2010) identified seven steps of the EBP process. These steps provide a framework for EBP and can be used in multiple

Table 17-4. Example Questions of a Professional Practice Evaluation

Professional Practice Topic	Questions for Self-Reflection
Education	Is my knowledge current? How do I seek opportunities to learn new knowledge and skills? How do I share knowledge with others through mentoring, role modeling, or formal presentations? Have I validated my knowledge through specialty certification?
Self-care	How do I focus on my own health and well-being? How do I prevent, identify, or manage burnout and moral distress?
Advocacy	How do I advocate for individual patients? How do I advocate for populations? How do I advocate for the nursing profession?
Communication	Is my communication patient centered? Do I consider health literacy when communicating with others? How do I use different communication strategies to promote effective communication?
Interprofessional collaboration	How do I support a culture of interprofessional collaboration? When I communicate with others, how do I foster mutual trust and shared values?
Leadership	How do I influence others toward a shared goal? How am I working to improve my proficiency within the five domains of leadership (personal mastery, vision, knowledge, interpersonal effectiveness, and systems thinking)?
Evidence-based practice	Do I ask questions about patient care and challenge current practice? How do I incorporate evidence (research, clinical expertise, and patient preferences/values) into my practice and evaluate outcomes?
Research	How do I integrate research findings into my practice? If I provide care for human participants in research, how do I ensure that their rights are protected?
Overall	Do I adhere to organizational policies, the state nurse practice act, regulatory requirements, and professional guidelines? Do I seek feedback from peers, colleagues, and my supervisor? What are my strengths and weaknesses? What are my goals for professional growth?

practice settings and for a variety of patient care outcomes. For example, the steps of EBP may be followed if nurses are trying to prevent hospital-acquired infections, prevent or treat mucositis, increase physical activity in HSCT recipients, reduce costs associated with unplanned readmissions, or improve patient and family coping.

Spirit of Inquiry

The first step of EBP is to create a culture and environment in which nurses can ask questions about patient care and challenge current practice (Melnyk et al., 2010). A spirit of inquiry may be supported by embedding EBP into the organizational mission and evaluation process, providing EBP mentors and resources, modeling EBP by leaders within the organization, and recognizing nurses who implement EBP (Melnyk & Fineout-Overholt, 2015). A spirit of inquiry is essential for the implementation and sustainability of EBP. To promote EBP sustainability, EBP projects must align with organizational goals, nurse champions should support and promote EBP, and leaders must support EBP and stakeholders (Chambers, 2015).

Formulating a Question

The next step of EBP is formulation of a clinical question. For questions seeking scientific evidence about interventions, prognosis, diagnosis, etiology, or experiences, the PICOT format may be used to ask the question (Fineout-Overholt & Stillwell, 2015). This format includes components about the patient population, intervention or issue, comparison intervention or issue, outcome of interest, and time to demonstrate the outcome (Fineout-Overholt & Stillwell, 2015; Stillwell, Fineout-Overholt, Melnyk, & Williamson, 2010a). All components of the PICOT format may not apply to each clinical question. Figure 17-7 provides sample PICOT questions.

Searching for Evidence

After formulating a clinical question, the next step is to search for evidence. Several databases are available to search for research and guidelines related to a topic of interest (see Table 17-5). Each database may contain millions of articles. To find relevant articles, it is necessary to use keywords and limit the search according to year published or the type of article. Using keywords from the PICOT question may help identify appropriate articles (Stillwell, Fineout-Overholt, Melnyk, & Williamson, 2010b). Librarians are an invaluable resource when searching for external evidence.

Appraising the Evidence

After finding evidence for practice, it is necessary to review each publication to determine the level of evidence, how well the study was conducted, and the usefulness for practice (Fineout-Overholt, Melnyk, Stillwell, & Williamson, 2010a). The level of evidence is based on the study design. For example, publications that synthesize research findings, such as systematic reviews or meta-analyses, are the highest level of evidence (Fineout-Overholt et al., 2010a). Experimental studies, such as controlled trials with or without randomization, are the next level of evidence. The lowest levels of evidence include nonexperimental studies, qualitative studies, and expert opinion (Fineout-Overholt et al., 2010a). To determine how well the study was conducted, it is necessary to determine if rigorous methods were used to increase the validity of the study and reduce bias (Fineout-Overholt, Melnyk, Stillwell, & Williamson, 2010b). Once relevant articles have been identified, information should be extracted from each article to synthesize the results (Fineout-Overholt et al., 2010b). Finally, appraisal of evidence includes reviewing the risks and benefits of the proposed intervention, importance of the outcome, feasibility in the practice setting, and values of your patient population (O'Mathúna & Fineout-Overholt, 2015).

Integrating External Evidence, Clinical Expertise, and Patient Values

The next step of EBP is to integrate the external evidence (research, reviews, and guidelines), clinical expertise, and patient values and preferences into a practice change (Melnyk et al., 2010). For example, opioids are an evidence-based intervention for the management of acute pain. A patient with a history of opioid addiction may prefer to avoid opioids. The nurse caring for the patient may instead suggest heat or cold application, music therapy, or repositioning to help the patient manage pain without opioids.

Evaluating Outcomes

After a practice change, the next step is to evaluate outcomes related to that change. This includes the expected outcomes, as well as any unintentional outcomes of the practice (Melnyk et al., 2010). If the EBP should improve patient outcomes, did those patient outcomes improve? What were the costs and cost savings associated with the practice change? Did this practice change result in unintended outcomes related to resources, nursing staff, or patient care?

Figure 17-7. Sample PICOT Questions

- In hematopoietic stem cell transplant (HSCT) recipients (patient population), how does exercise (intervention), compared to no exercise (comparison intervention), affect fatigue (outcome of interest) in the first month after the transplantation (time to demonstrate)?
- In HSCT recipients (P), do central line dressings containing chlorhexidine gluconate (I), compared to central line dressings without chlorhexidine gluconate (C), reduce central line–associated infections (O) when the patient is severely neutropenic (T)?
- Are nurses caring for HSCT donors and recipients (P), who participate in an evidence-based practice program (I), when compared to nurses who don't participate in an evidence-based practice program (C), more likely to implement evidence-based practice (O) within the next year (T)?
- Do pediatric HSCT recipients with acute leukemia (P) who have matched sibling donors (I), compared to mismatched related or matched unrelated donors (C), have less transplant-related mortality and acute or chronic graft-versus-host disease (O) in the first five years after transplantation (T)?
- How do adults (P) who are donating stem cells (I) perceive the meaning of stem cell donation (O) after donation (T)?

Table 17-5. Sources of External Evidence

Resource	Focus	Website
Cochrane Database of Systematic Reviews	Healthcare systematic reviews	www.cochrane.org
Cumulative Index to Nursing and Allied Health Literature	Nursing and allied health	www.cinahl.com
Embase	Biomedical literature	www.embase.com (login required)
Joanna Briggs Institute EBP Database	Evidence-based health care	https://joannabriggs .org/ebp
PubMed	Biomedical literature and life science journals	www.pubmed.gov

Disseminating the Outcomes

The final step of EBP is to disseminate the outcomes related to an evidence-based change. This may include dissemination within a healthcare organization, within a professional organization, at conferences, through podium and poster presentations, or through publication (Betz, Smith, & Melnyk, 2015). By sharing the results of collection and appraisal of evidence, implementation of a practice change, and identification of associated outcomes, other healthcare providers may be able to integrate evidence into other practice settings to improve outcomes.

Evidence-Based Practice Models

Although nurses report challenges implementing EBP, several theories, frameworks, and models are available to guide the translation of research into practice. These models may guide the EBP process, examine factors that influence implementation, or guide the evaluation of implementation (Nilsen, 2015). For clinical nurses, several models have been developed to guide the EBP process.

The Iowa Model of Evidence-Based Practice starts with identification of an issue or opportunity and guides users through the necessary steps to appraise and synthesize evidence, pilot a practice change, then implement and sustain the practice change before disseminating results (Buckwalter et al., 2017). Additional resources related to this model have been published to guide the adoption and implementation of EBP (Cullen et al., 2018). The Iowa model was designed for use by practitioners working in teams in a clinical setting, but this model has also been used in education and research (Titler, 2010).

The Johns Hopkins Nursing Evidence-Based Practice Model provides a 19-step process for the translation of evidence into practice. This process occurs in three phases: clinicians identify a practice question, appraise and synthesize evidence, and then translate evidence into practice. This

model was designed for use by practicing nurses, and several tools and guides are available for this process (Dang & Dearholt, 2018).

The Stetler Model of Research Utilization includes five phases: preparation by determining the purpose, influential factors, outcomes and resources; validation of the critiqued and synthesized relevant research; evaluation of the evidence and decision-making regarding a practice change; application of evidence into practice; and evaluation of the change and outcomes (Stetler, 2010). The most recent version of the Stetler model was intended for use by APRNs who lead EBP, but this model has been used by all levels of nurses in clinical settings, education, and research (Stetler, 2010).

Development of the Advancing Research and Clinical Practice Through Close Collaboration (ARCC®) Model was guided by control theory, cognitive behavioral theory, and input from nurses regarding barriers and facilitators to EBP (Dang et al., 2015). The ARCC model provides a process for the implementation of EBP and depends on mentors to work with clinicians to champion the value of EBP (Dang et al., 2015). The major steps of the EBP process in the ARCC model include assessment of organizational culture, identification of barriers and facilitators to EBP, development of mentors, implementation of EBP, and outcomes (Dang et al., 2015).

Research

Research is the systematic investigation of a topic and results in the generation of new knowledge (Protection of Human Subjects, 2009). The research process includes developing a research question; evaluating the current knowledge and literature regarding the topic; designing a study; accessing, collecting, and analyzing data; and disseminating the results (Lacey, 2015). As part of professional practice, nurses may be indirectly or directly involved in the research process by identifying clinical problems that could be addressed by research, appraising and sharing research findings, and integrating research into practice (ANA, 2015b). Additionally, nurses may conduct literature searches, participate in journal clubs or research committees, or seek input from researchers (Brant & Wickham, 2013). Nurses may conduct research, participate as a coinvestigator, coordinate research studies, or care for patients who are research participants.

Protection of Human Participants

To protect the rights of human participants in research, the National Commission for the Protection of Human Subjects of Biomedical and Behavioral Research (1979) published the Belmont Report. This report summarizes three ethical principles applicable to human research and provides guidelines for the protection of research participants. The first ethical principle is respect for people: individuals are autonomous agents and should be informed and voluntarily agree to research participation. Individuals with diminished autonomy, such as prisoners or people with mental disability, are entitled to protection from unethical treatment. The second ethical principle is beneficence: researchers should not harm patients and should aim to maximize the potential benefits of participating in a study while minimizing the potential risks. The third ethical principle is justice: the potential burden and benefits of the research should be distributed fairly (National Commission for the Protection of Human Subjects of Biomedical and Behavioral Research, 1979).

The Belmont Report provides three applications of the described ethical principles. First, research participants should provide informed consent. To satisfy this condition, investigators must inform the participant of the research procedures, potential risks and benefits, and alternatives to participating in research. The information should be presented in a way that is easily understood, and the participant should have adequate time to consider the information. Participation should be voluntary, and the individual should be allowed to stop participation at any time without repercussion. Second, the investigator should assess risks and benefits of participation in research and design the study to minimize risk while optimizing benefits. Review committees should ensure that risks to participants are justified. Third, the selection of participants should follow the principle of justice. For example, vulnerable participants including children, prisoners, and people with mental illness should not be the first population selected to participate in research, and vulnerable populations should have additional protections (National Commission for the Protection of Human Subjects of Biomedical and Behavioral Research, 1979). In the United States, institutional review boards assess all research proposals involving human participants and ensure that their rights and welfare are protected (U.S. Food and Drug Administration, 2019).

Nursing Roles in Research

Nursing research generates knowledge to provide a scientific foundation for clinical practice. The National Institute of Nursing Research (2016), part of the National Institutes of Health, supports and conducts research with the aim of promoting health and quality of life. Areas of scientific focus include symptom management, wellness, end-of-life and palliative care, and self-management. In addition to general nursing research priorities identified by the National Institute of Nursing Research, ONS has identified priorities for research to promote quality care and excellence in oncology nursing. To identify research priorities, oncology nurse leaders and content experts reviewed the literature and national priorities for research, surveyed oncology nurses, and used a consensus-building approach. Knobf et al. (2015) recognized eight priority areas for oncology nursing research and four themes of research (see Figure 17-8).

Nurses at all levels may be coinvestigators in research, and nurses with additional education may conduct

Figure 17-8. Oncology Nursing Society Research Priorities
Themes • Biomarkers • Bioinformatics • Comparative effectiveness research • Dissemination and implementation science **Research Priorities** • Aging • Family and caregivers • Improving healthcare systems • Palliative and end-of-life care • Risk reduction • Self-management • Survivorship and late effects of cancer treatment • Symptoms
Note. Based on information from Knobf et al., 2015.

research. Examples of nursing research are numerous in the literature. In the HSCT field, Dee, Toro, Lee, Sherwood, and Haile (2017) investigated falls in hospitalized autologous transplant recipients and found that fall risk increased 1.2 times for each day the patient experienced diarrhea. In addition, patients with a high score on the Morse Fall Scale, compared to patients with a low score on the scale, were 5.3 times more likely to fall (Dee et al., 2017). This study adds to scientific knowledge and is a source of evidence for nurse decision making.

Coordination of clinical trials is another role for nurses in the research process. Clinical trial nurses coordinate trials and manage patients who participate in trials (ONS, 2016). To provide effective, safe, and competent care, clinical trial nurses must advocate for patient safety and the integrity of the study protocol, adhere to the standards of nursing and the code of ethics, and have effective written and verbal communication skills (ONS, 2016; see Figure 17-9).

Nurses who provide care for research participants have several responsibilities. Nurses may support the informed consent process by ensuring that patients and family members understand the study, are informed about the risks and benefits of the study, have adequate time to review the information, and ask questions. Nurses should also advocate for ethical care for patients and provide education about the trial to patients and family members. As direct care providers, nurses may administer study medications, monitor patient responses to the intervention, collect biospecimens, and record data for the study (ONS, 2016; Parreco, Ness, Galassi, & O'Mara, 2012).

Clinical Trials and Hematopoietic Stem Cell Transplantation

The Foundation for the Accreditation of Cellular Therapy (FACT) and Joint Accreditation Committee of the International Society for Cellular Therapy and European Society for Blood and Marrow Transplantation

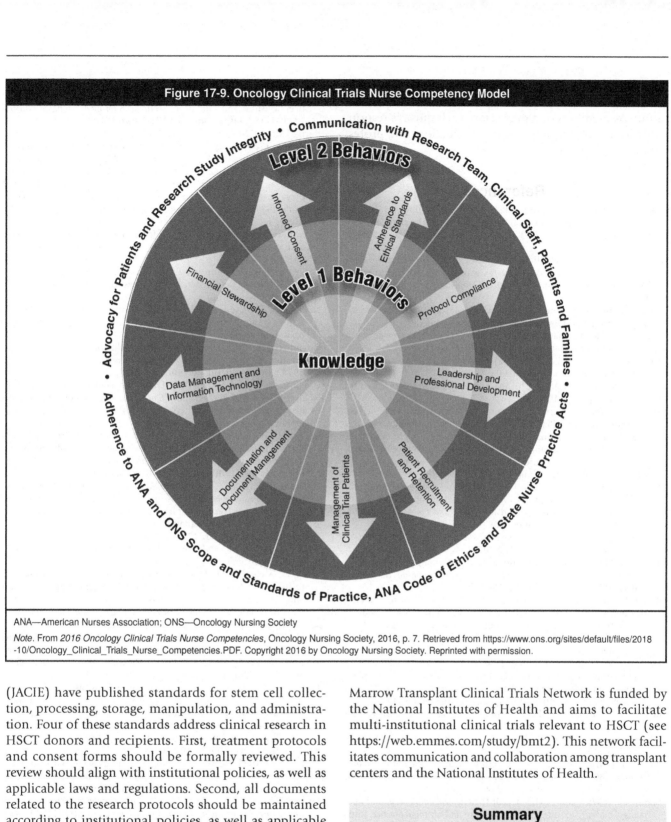

Figure 17-9. Oncology Clinical Trials Nurse Competency Model

ANA—American Nurses Association; ONS—Oncology Nursing Society

Note. From *2016 Oncology Clinical Trials Nurse Competencies*, Oncology Nursing Society, 2016, p. 7. Retrieved from https://www.ons.org/sites/default/files/2018 -10/Oncology_Clinical_Trials_Nurse_Competencies.PDF. Copyright 2016 by Oncology Nursing Society. Reprinted with permission.

(JACIE) have published standards for stem cell collection, processing, storage, manipulation, and administration. Four of these standards address clinical research in HSCT donors and recipients. First, treatment protocols and consent forms should be formally reviewed. This review should align with institutional policies, as well as applicable laws and regulations. Second, all documents related to the research protocols should be maintained according to institutional policies, as well as applicable laws and regulations. Third, informed consent should be obtained from participants or a legally authorized representative in a manner that minimizes undue influence or coercion. Fourth, a process should address potential conflicts of interest (FACT & JACIE, 2018). These standards support ethical treatment of HSCT donors and recipients who participate in clinical research.

Although clinical research may occur in one site, some trials are conducted at multiple sites. The Blood and Marrow Transplant Clinical Trials Network is funded by the National Institutes of Health and aims to facilitate multi-institutional clinical trials relevant to HSCT (see https://web.emmes.com/study/bmt2). This network facilitates communication and collaboration among transplant centers and the National Institutes of Health.

Summary

Nursing is a profession with a specific set of knowledge, autonomous practice, and a responsibility to improve the procedures and techniques of the discipline. The scope and standards of the profession are clearly defined (ANA, 2010; ICN, 2013); codes of ethics have been developed (ANA, 2015b; ICN, 2012); and the social contract between the nursing profession and society has been published (ANA, 2015a). Professional practice is multifaceted and includes concepts such as education, self-care, advocacy, EBP, research, communication, leadership, interprofessional collaboration, and professional practice evaluation. As members of a profession, each nurse is responsible for his or her own practice, evaluation, and professional development.

References

Aiken, L.H., Clarke, S.P., Cheung, R.B., Sloane, D.M., & Silber, J.H. (2003). Educational levels of hospital nurses and surgical patient mortality. *JAMA, 290*, 1617–1623. https://doi.org/10.1001/jama.290.12.1617

American Association of Critical-Care Nurses. (n.d.). *The 4A's to rise above moral distress.* Retrieved from https://www.trinity-health.org/documents/Ethics/1%20EthicsTopics/M/Moral%20Distress/Moral%20Distress%204A%27s.pdf

American Nurses Association. (n.d.). *Federal issues.* Retrieved from https://www.nursingworld.org/practice-policy/advocacy/federal

American Nurses Association. (2010). *Nursing's social policy statement: The essence of the profession.* Silver Spring, MD: Author.

American Nurses Association. (2015a). *Code of ethics for nurses with interpretive statements.* Silver Spring, MD: Author.

American Nurses Association. (2015b). *Scope and standards of practice* (3rd ed.). Silver Spring, MD: Author.

American Nurses Credentialing Center. (n.d.-a). ANCC Magnet Recognition Program®. Retrieved from https://www.nursingworld.org/organizational-programs/magnet

American Nurses Credentialing Center. (n.d.-b). Magnet model—Creating a Magnet culture. Retrieved from https://www.nursingworld.org/organizational-programs/magnet/magnet-model

Austin, C.L., Saylor, R., & Finley, P.J. (2017). Moral distress in physicians and nurses: Impact on professional quality of life and turnover. *Psychological Trauma: Theory, Research, Practice, and Policy, 9*, 399–406. https://doi.org/10.1037/tra0000201

Balogh, E.P., Miller, B.T., & Ball, J.R. (Eds.). (2015). *Improving diagnosis in health care.* https://doi.org/10.17226/21794

Bass, B.M. (1990). From transactional to transformational leadership: Learning to share the vision. *Organizational Dynamics, 18*, 19–31. https://doi.org/10.1016/0090-2616(90)90061-s

Betz, C.L., Smith, K.N., & Melnyk, B.M. (2015). Disseminating evidence through publications, presentations, health policy briefs, and the media. In B.M. Melnyk & E. Fineout-Overholt (Eds.), *Evidence-based practice in nursing and healthcare* (3rd ed., pp. 391–436). Philadelphia, PA: Wolters Kluwer.

Blackburn, R., Presson, K., Laufman, R., Tomczak, N., & Brassil, K.J. (2016). Establishing an inpatient gym for recipients of stem cell transplantation: A multidisciplinary collaborative. *Clinical Journal of Oncology Nursing, 20*, 66–71. https://doi.org/10.1188/16.cjon.66-71

Boamah, S.A., Laschinger, H.K.S., Wong, C., & Clarke, S. (2018). Effect of transformational leadership on job satisfaction and patient safety outcomes. *Nursing Outlook, 66*, 180–189. https://doi.org/10.1016/j.outlook.2017.10.004

Bonner, L. (2016). Safe handling of hazardous drugs: USP publishes new chapter <800>. *Pharmacy Today, 22*, 42. Retrieved from https://www.pharmacytoday.org/article/S1042-0991(16)00517-X/pdf

Brant, J.M., & Wickham, R. (Eds.). (2013). *Statement on the scope and standards of oncology nursing practice: Generalist and advanced practice.* Pittsburgh, PA: Oncology Nursing Society.

Brashers, B., Phillips, E., Malpass, J., & Owen, J. (2015). Appendix A review: Measuring the impact of interprofessional education (IPE) on collaborative practice and patient outcomes. In M. Cox, B.F. Brandt, J. Palaganas, S. Reeves, A.W. Wu, & B. Zierler (Eds.), *Measuring the impact of interprofessional education on collaborative practice and patient outcomes.* https://doi.org/10.17226/21726

Brega, A.G., Freedman, M.A.G., LeBlanc, W.G., Barnard, J., Mabachi, N.M., Cifuentes, M., ... West, D.R. (2015). Using the Health Literacy Universal Precautions Toolkit to improve the quality of patient materials. *Journal of Health Communication, 20*(Suppl. 2), 69–76. https://doi.org/10.1080/10810730.2015.1081997

Buckwalter, K.C., Cullen, L., Hanrahan, K., Kleiber, C., McCarthy, A.M., Rakel, B., ... Tucker, S. (2017). Iowa model of evidence-based practice: Revisions and validation. *Worldviews on Evidence-Based Nursing, 14*, 175–182. https://doi.org/10.1111/wvn.12223

Burns, J.M. (1978). *Leadership.* New York, NY: Harper and Row.

Byrne, Z.S. (2015). *Organizational psychology and behavior: An integrated approach to understanding the workplace.* Dubuque, IA: Kendall Hunt.

Cañadas-De la Fuente, G.A., Gómez-Urquiza, J.L., Ortega-Campos, E.M., Cañadas, G.R., Albendín-García, L., & De la Fuente-Solana, E.I. (2018). Prevalence of burnout syndrome in oncology nursing: A meta-analytic study. *Psycho-Oncology, 27*, 1–8. https://doi.org/10.1002/pon.4632

Carrière, K., Khoury, B., Günak, M.M., & Knäuper, B. (2018). Mindfulness-based interventions for weight loss: A systematic review and meta-analysis. *Obesity Reviews, 19*, 164–177. https://doi.org/10.1111/obr.12623

Centers for Disease Control and Prevention. (2018, August 8). Sleep and chronic disease. Retrieved from https://www.cdc.gov/sleep/about_sleep/chronic_disease.html

Centers for Disease Control and Prevention. (2019, July 2). Physical activity basics. Retrieved from https://www.cdc.gov/physicalactivity/basics/index.htm

Chambers, L.L. (2015). Factors for sustainability of evidence-based practice innovations: Part I. *Research and Theory for Nursing Practice, 29*, 89–93. https://doi.org/10.1891/1541-6577.29.2.89

Cirelli, C. (2019). Insufficient sleep: Definition, epidemiology, and adverse outcomes. In A.F. Eichler (Ed.). *UpToDate.* Retrieved October 1, 2019, from https://www.uptodate.com/contents/insufficient-sleep-definition-epidemiology-and-adverse-outcomes

Clavelle, J.T., Drenkard, K., Tullai-McGuinness, S., & Fitzpatrick, J.J. (2012). Transformational leadership practices of chief nursing officers in Magnet® organizations. *Journal of Nursing Administration, 42*, 195–201. https://doi.org/10.1097/nna.0b013e31824ccd7b

Cullen, L., Hanrahan, K., Farrington, M., DeBerg, J., Tucker, S., & Kleiber, C. (2018). *Evidence-based practice in action: Comprehensive strategies, tools, and tips from the University of Iowa Hospitals and Clinics.* Indianapolis, IN: Sigma Theta Tau International.

Dang, D., & Dearholt, S.L. (2018). *Johns Hopkins nursing evidence-based practice: Model and guidelines* (3rd ed.). Indianapolis, IN: Sigma Theta Tau International.

Dang, D., Melnyk, B.M., Fineout-Overholt, E., Ciliska, D., DiCenso, A., Cullen, L., ... Stevens, K.R. (2015). Models to guide implementation and sustainability of evidence-based practice. In B.M. Melnyk & E. Fineout-Overholt (Eds.), *Evidence-based practice in nursing and healthcare* (3rd ed., pp. 274–315). Philadelphia, PA: Wolters Kluwer.

Dee, V., Toro, J., Lee, S., Sherwood, P., & Haile, D. (2017). Autologous stem cell transplantation: The predictive value of the Morse Fall Scale in hospitalized patients. *Clinical Journal of Oncology Nursing, 21*, 599–603. https://doi.org/10.1188/17.cjon.599-603

Denzen, E.M., Majhail, N.S., Ferguson, S.S., Anasetti, C., Bracey, A., Burns, L., ... Murphy, E.A. (2013). Hematopoietic cell transplantation in 2020: Summary of year 2 recommendations of the National Marrow Donor Program's System Capacity Initiative. *Biology of Blood and Marrow Transplantation, 19*, 4–11. https://doi.org/10.1016/j.bbmt.2012.10.005

Egenes, K.J. (2018). History of nursing. In G. Roux & J.A. Halstead (Eds.), *Issues and trends in nursing: Practice, policy, and leadership* (2nd ed., pp. 3–30). Burlington, MA: Jones & Bartlett Learning.

Epstein, R.M., & Street, R.L., Jr. (2007). *Patient-centered communication in cancer care: Promoting healing and reducing suffering* (NIH Publication No. 07-6225). Retrieved from https://cancercontrol.cancer.gov/brp/docs/pcc_monograph.pdf

Fiala, M.A., & Wildes, T.M. (2017). Racial disparities in treatment use for multiple myeloma. *Cancer, 123*, 1590–1596. https://doi.org/10.1002/cncr.30526

Fineout-Overholt, E., Melnyk, B.M., Stillwell, S.B., & Williamson, K.M. (2010a). Evidence-based practice, step by step: Critical appraisal of the evidence: Part I. *American Journal of Nursing, 110*, 47–52. https://doi.org/10.1097/01.NAJ.0000383935.22721.9c

Fineout-Overholt, E., Melnyk, B.M., Stillwell, S.B., & Williamson, K.M. (2010b). Evidence-based practice, step by step: Critical appraisal of the evidence: Part II: Digging deeper—Examining the "keeper" studies. *American Journal of Nursing, 110,* 41–48. https://doi.org/10.1097/01.NAJ.0000388264.49427.f9

Fineout-Overholt, E., & Stillwell, S.B. (2015). Asking compelling, clinical questions. In B.M. Melnyk & E. Fineout-Overholt (Eds.), *Evidence-based practice in nursing and healthcare: A guide to best practice* (3rd ed., pp. 24–39). Philadelphia, PA: Wolters Kluwer.

Foundation for the Accreditation of Cellular Therapy & Joint Accreditation Committee–ISCT and EBMT. (2018, March). *FACT-JACIE international standards for hematopoietic cellular therapy: Product collection, processing, and administration* (7th ed.). Retrieved from https://www.ebmt.org/sites/default/files/2018-06/FACT-JACIE%207th%20Edition%20Standards.pdf

Fridman, M., & Frederickson, K. (2014). Oncology nurses and the experience of participation in an evidence-based practice project. *Oncology Nursing Forum, 41,* 382–388. https://doi.org/10.1188/14.onf.382-388

Hagan, T.L., & Medberry, E. (2016). Patient education vs. patient experiences of self-advocacy: Changing the discourse to support cancer survivors. *Journal of Cancer Education, 31,* 375–381. https://doi.org/10.1007/s13187-015-0828-x

Hagan, T.L., Rosenzweig, M.Q., Zorn, K.K., van Londen, G.J., & Donovan, H.S. (2017). Perspectives on self-advocacy: Comparing perceived uses, benefits, and drawbacks among survivors and providers. *Oncology Nursing Forum, 44,* 52–59. https://doi.org/10.1188/17.onf.52-59

Häggman-Laitila, A., Mattila, L.-R., & Melender, H.-L. (2016). A systematic review of journal clubs for nurses. *Worldviews on Evidence-Based Nursing, 13,* 163–171. https://doi.org/10.1111/wvn.12131

Hall, L.H., Johnson, J., Watt, I., Tsipa, A., & O'Connor, D.B. (2016). Healthcare staff wellbeing, burnout, and patient safety: A systematic review. *PLOS ONE, 11,* e0159015. https://doi.org/10.1371/journal.pone.0159015

Hayden, M.A., Wolf, G.A., & Zedreck-Gonzalez, J.F. (2016). Beyond Magnet® designation: Perspectives from nurse managers on factors of sustainability and high-performance programming. *Journal of Nursing Administration, 46,* 530–534. https://doi.org/10.1097/nna.0000000000000397

Houle, C.O. (1980). *Continuing learning in the professions.* San Francisco, CA: Jossey-Bass.

Institute for Healthcare Improvement. (2017). *SBAR: Situation-background-assessment-recommendation.* Retrieved from https://www.lsqin.org/wp-content/uploads/2017/08/SBARTechniqueforCommunication.pdf

International Council of Nurses. (2012). *The ICN code of ethics for nurses.* Retrieved from https://www.icn.ch/sites/default/files/inline-files/2012_ICN_Codeofethicsfornurses_%20eng.pdf

International Council of Nurses. (2013). *Scope of nursing practice* [Position statement]. Retrieved from https://www.icn.ch/sites/default/files/inline-files/B07_Scope_Nsg_Practice.pdf

Interprofessional Education Collaborative. (2016). *Core competencies for interprofessional collaborative practice: 2016 update.* Retrieved from https://hsc.unm.edu/ipe/resources/ipec-2016-core-competencies.pdf

Jameton, A. (1984). *Nursing practice: The ethical issues.* Englewood Cliffs, NJ: Prentice-Hall.

Johnson, A.L., Jung, L., Brown, K., Weaver, M.T., & Richards, K.C. (2014). Sleep deprivation and error in nurses who work the night shift. *Journal of Nursing Administration, 44,* 17–22. https://doi.org/10.1097/nna.0000000000000016

Joint Commission. (2017, September 12). *Sentinel event alert 58: Inadequate hand-off communication.* Retrieved from https://www.jointcommission.org/sentinel_event_alert_58_inadequate_handoff_communications

Khamisa, N., Peltzer, K., & Oldenburg, B. (2013). Burnout in relation to specific contributing factors and health outcomes among nurses: A systematic review. *International Journal of Environmental Research and Public Health, 10,* 2214–2240. https://doi.org/10.3390/ijerph10062214

Knight, L.J., Gabhart, J.M., Earnest, K.S., Leong, K.M., Anglemyer, A., & Franzon, D. (2014). Improving code team performance and survival outcomes: Implementation of pediatric resuscitation team training. *Critical Care Medicine, 42,* 243–251. https://doi.org/10.1097/ccm.0b013e3182a6439d

Knobf, M.T., Cooley, M.E., Duffy, S., Doorenbos, A., Eaton, L., Given, B., … Mallory, G. (2015). The 2014–2018 Oncology Nursing Society

research agenda. *Oncology Nursing Forum, 42,* 450–465. https://doi.org/10.1188/15.onf.450-465

Kouzes, J., Posner, B., & Bunting, M. (2015). *Extraordinary leadership in Australia and New Zealand: The five practices that create great workplaces.* Milton, Queensland, Australia: John Wiley and Sons Australia.

Kutner, M., Greenberg, E., Jin, Y., & Paulsen, C. (2006, September). *The health literacy of America's adults: Results from the 2003 National Assessment of Adult Literacy* (NCES 2006–483). Retrieved from https://nces.ed.gov/pubs2006/2006483.pdf

Lacey, A. (2015). The research process. In K. Gerrish & J. Lathlean (Eds.), *The research process in nursing* (7th ed., pp. 15–30). Hoboken, NJ: Wiley-Blackwell.

Leach, L.S. (2005). Nurse executive transformational leadership and organizational commitment. *Journal of Nursing Administration, 35,* 228–237. https://doi.org/10.1097/00005110-200505000-00006

Lewin, K., Lippitt, R., & White, R.K. (1939). Patterns of aggressive behavior in experimentally created "social climates". *Journal of Social Psychology, 10,* 269–299. https://doi.org/10.1080/00224545.1939.9713366

Maslach, C., & Leiter, M.P. (2016). Understanding the burnout experience: Recent research and its implications for psychiatry. *World Psychiatry, 15,* 103–111. https://doi.org/10.1002/wps.20311

Mayer, D.K., & Nasso, S.F. (2017). Cancer Moonshot: What it means for patients. *Clinical Journal of Oncology Nursing, 21,* 141–142. https://doi.org/10.1188/17.cjon.141-142

McCay, R., Lyles, A., & Larkey, L. (2018). Nurse leadership style, nurse satisfaction, and patient satisfaction: A systematic review. *Journal of Nursing Care Quality, 33,* 361–367. https://doi.org/10.1097/ncq.0000000000000317

Melnyk, B.M., & Fineout-Overholt, E. (2015). Making the case for evidence-based practice and cultivating a spirit of inquiry. In B.M. Melnyk & E. Fineout-Overholt (Eds.), *Evidence-based practice in nursing and healthcare* (3rd ed., pp. 3–23). Philadelphia, PA: Wolters Kluwer.

Melnyk, B.M., Fineout-Overholt, E., Stillwell, S., & Williamson, K. (2010). Evidence-based practice: Step by step: The seven steps of evidence-based practice. *American Journal of Nursing, 110,* 51–53. https://doi.org/10.1097/01.naj.0000366056.06605.d2

Mills, J., Wand, T., & Fraser, J.A. (2014). On self-compassion and self-care in nursing: Selfish or essential for compassionate care? *International Journal of Nursing Studies, 52,* 791–793. https://doi.org/10.1016/j.ijnurstu.2014.10.009

Mills, J., Wand, T., & Fraser, J.A. (2017). Self-care in palliative care nursing and medical professionals: A cross-sectional survey. *Journal of Palliative Medicine, 20,* 625–630. https://doi.org/10.1089/jpm.2016.0470

National Cancer Advisory Board. (2016, October 17). *Cancer moonshot blue ribbon panel report 2016.* Retrieved from https://www.cancer.gov/research/key-initiatives/moonshot-cancer-initiative/blue-ribbon-panel/blue-ribbon-panel-report-2016.pdf

National Cancer Institute. (n.d.). Examples of cancer health disparities. Retrieved from https://www.cancer.gov/about-nci/organization/crchd/about-health-disparities/examples

National Commission for the Protection of Human Subjects of Biomedical and Behavioral Research. (1979, April 18). *The Belmont Report: Ethical principles and guidelines for the protection of human subjects of research.* Retrieved from http://www.hhs.gov/ohrp/policy/belmont.html

National Council of State Boards of Nursing. (n.d.). Nurse Licensure Compact (NLC). Retrieved from https://www.ncsbn.org/enhanced-nlc-implementation.htm

National Council of State Boards of Nursing. (2008, July 7). *Consensus model for APRN regulation: Licensure, accreditation, certification and education.* Retrieved from https://www.ncsbn.org/Consensus_Model_for_APRN_Regulation_July_2008.pdf

National Council of State Boards of Nursing. (2011, October). *Understanding the NCLEX® examination through the core values of NCSBN.* Retrieved from https://www.ncsbn.org/NCLEX_Core_Values.pdf

National Institute of Nursing Research. (2016, September). *The NINR strategic plan: Advancing science, improving lives: A vision for nursing science.* Retrieved from https://www.ninr.nih.gov/sites/www.ninr.nih.gov/files/NINR_StratPlan2016_reduced.pdf

National Institutes of Health. (n.d.). Clear communication. Retrieved from https://www.nih.gov/institutes-nih/nih-office-director/office-communications-public-liaison/clear-communication

National Quality Forum. (2017, September 14). *A roadmap for promoting health equity and eliminating disparities: The four I's for health equity.* Retrieved from https://www.qualityforum.org/Publications/2017/09/A_Roadmap_for_Promoting_Health_Equity_and_Eliminating_Disparities__The_Four_I_s_for_Health_Equity.aspx

Nelson, M.B., & Guelcher, C. (2014). *Scope and standards of pediatric hematology/oncology nursing practice.* Chicago, IL: Association of Pediatric Hematology/Oncology Nurses.

Neumann, J.L., Mau, L.-W., Virani, S., Denzen, E.M., Boyle, D.A., Boyle, M.J., … Burns, L.J. (2018). Burnout, moral distress, work–life balance, and career satisfaction among hematopoietic cell transplantation professionals. *Biology of Blood and Marrow Transplantation, 24,* 849–860. https://doi.org/10.1016/j.bbmt.2017.11.015

Newhouse, R.P. (2007). Diffusing confusion among evidence-based practice, quality improvement, and research. *Journal of Nursing Administration, 37,* 432–435. https://doi.org/10.1097/01.nna.0000285156.58903.d3

Nilsen, P. (2015). Making sense of implementation theories, models and frameworks. *Implementation Science, 10,* 53. https://doi.org/10.1186/s13012-015-0242-0

O'Connell, B.H., O'Shea, D., & Gallagher, S. (2017). Examining psychosocial pathways underlying gratitude interventions: A randomized controlled trial. *Journal of Happiness Studies, 19,* 2421–2444. https://doi.org/10.1007/s10902-017-9931-5

Oh, Y., & Gastmans, C. (2015). Moral distress experienced by nurses: A quantitative literature review. *Nursing Ethics, 22,* 15–31. https://doi.org/10.1177/0969733013502803

O'Mathúna, D.P., & Fineout-Overholt, E. (2015). Critically appraising quantitative evidence for clinical decision making. In B.M. Melnyk & E. Fineout-Overholt (Eds.), *Evidence-based practice in nursing and healthcare* (3rd ed., pp. 87–138). Philadelphia, PA: Wolters Kluwer.

Oncology Nursing Society. (n.d.). Policy priorities. Retrieved from https://www.ons.org/make-difference/ons-center-advocacy-and-health-policy/policy-priorities

Oncology Nursing Society. (2010). *A how-to guide: Designing and creating a journal club for oncology nurses.* Retrieved from https://www.ons.org/sites/default/files/Journal%20Club%20Toolkit.pdf

Oncology Nursing Society. (2012). *Oncology Nursing Society leadership competencies.* Retrieved from https://www.ons.org/sites/default/files/leadershipcomps.pdf

Oncology Nursing Society. (2016). *2016 oncology clinical trials nurse competencies.* Retrieved from https://www.ons.org/sites/default/files/2018-10/Oncology_Clinical_Trials_Nurse_Competencies.PDF

Parreco, L.K., Ness, E., Galassi, A., & O'Mara, A.M. (2012, June 11). Care of clinical trial participants: What nurses need to know. *American Nurse Today, 7,* 3. Retrieved from https://www.americannursetoday.com/care-of-clinical-trial-participants-what-nurses-need-to-know

Persoon, S., Kersten, M.J., van der Weiden, K., Buffart, L.M., Nollet, F., Brug, J., & Chinapaw, M.J.M. (2013). Effects of exercise in patients treated with stem cell transplantation for a hematologic malignancy: A systematic review and meta-analysis. *Cancer Treatment Reviews, 39,* 682–690. https://doi.org/10.1016/j.ctrv.2013.01.001

Phillips, J.M., & Malone, B. (2014). Increasing racial/ethnic diversity in nursing to reduce health disparities and achieve health equity. *Public Health Reports, 129*(Suppl. 2), 45–50. https://doi.org/10.1177/00333549141291s209

Plain Language Action and Information Network. (2011, May). *Federal plain language guidelines.* Retrieved from https://www.plainlanguage.gov/media/FederalPLGuidelines.pdf

Protection of Human Subjects, 45 C.F.R. § 46. (2009). Retrieved from https://www.ecfr.gov/cgi-bin/text-idx?SID=d02a16ecf12e6149fadaac16045a464f&pitd=20190719&node=pt45.1.46&rgn=div5

Reeves, S., Pelone, F., Harrison, R., Goldman, J., & Zwarenstein, M. (2017). Interprofessional collaboration to improve professional practice and healthcare outcomes. *Cochrane Database of Systematic Reviews, 2017*(6). https://doi.org/10.1002/14651858.cd000072.pub3

Reeves, S., Perrier, L., Goldman, J., Freeth, D., & Zwarenstein, M. (2013). Interprofessional education: Effects on professional practice and healthcare outcomes. *Cochrane Database of Systematic Reviews, 2013*(3). https://doi.org/10.1002/14651858.cd002213.pub3

Ruoff, G. (Ed.). (2015). *Malpractice risks in communication failures: 2015 annual benchmarking report.* Boston, MA: CRICO Strategies.

Russell, K.A. (2012). Nurse practice acts guide and govern nursing practice. *Journal of Nursing Regulation, 3,* 36–42. https://doi.org/10.1016/s2155-8256(15)30197-6

Saunders, H., & Vehviläinen-Julkunen, K. (2016). The state of readiness for evidence-based practice among nurses: An integrative review. *International Journal of Nursing Studies, 56,* 128–140. https://doi.org/10.1016/j.ijnurstu.2015.10.018

Shalala, D.E., Bolton, L.B., Bleich, M.R., Brennan, T.A., Campbell, R.E., Devlin, L., … Vladeck, B.C. (2011). *The future of nursing: Leading change, advancing health.* https://doi.org/10.17226/12956

Smith, S.A. (2014). Mindfulness-based stress reduction: An intervention to enhance the effectiveness of nurses' coping with work-related stress. *International Journal of Nursing Knowledge, 25,* 119–130. https://doi.org/10.1111/2047-3095.12025

Starmer, A.J., Schnock, K.O., Lyons, A., Hehn, R.S., Graham, D.A., Keohane, C., & Landrigan, C.P. (2017). Effects of I-PASS Nursing Hand-off Bundle on communication quality and workflow. *BMJ Quality and Safety, 26,* 949–957. https://doi.org/10.1136/bmjqs-2016-006224

Starmer, A.J., Spector, N.D., Srivastava, R., Allen, A.D., Landrigan, C.P., & Sectish, T.C. (2012). I-PASS, a mnemonic to standardize verbal hand-offs. *Pediatrics, 129,* 201–204. https://doi.org/10.1542/peds.2011-2966

Starmer, A.J., Spector, N.D., Srivastava, R., West, D.C., Rosenbluth, G., Allen, A.D., … Landrigan, C.P. (2014). Changes in medical errors after implementation of a handoff program. *New England Journal of Medicine, 371,* 1803–1812. https://doi.org/10.1056/NEJMsa1405556

Stetler, C.B. (2010). Stetler model. In J. Rycroft-Malone & T. Bucknall (Eds.), *Models and frameworks for implementing evidence-based practice: Linking evidence to action* (pp. 51–82). Hoboken, NJ: Wiley-Blackwell.

Stewart, K.R. (2016, December). *SBAR, communication, and patient safety: An integrated literature review* [Honors thesis, University of Tennessee at Chattanooga]. Retrieved from https://scholar.utc.edu/cgi/viewcontent.cgi?referer=https://www.google.com/&httpsredir=1&article=1070&context=honors-theses

Stillwell, S.B., Fineout-Overholt, E., Melnyk, B.M., & Williamson, K.M. (2010a). Evidence-based practice, step by step: Asking the clinical question: A key step in evidence-based practice. *American Journal of Nursing, 110,* 58–61. https://doi.org/10.1097/01.naj.0000368959.11129.79

Stillwell, S.B., Fineout-Overholt, E., Melnyk, B.M., & Williamson, K.M. (2010b). Evidence-based practice, step by step: Searching for evidence: Strategies to help you conduct a successful search. *American Journal of Nursing, 110,* 41–47. https://doi.org/10.1097/01.naj.0000372071.24134.7e

Titler, M. (2010). Iowa Model of Evidence-Based Practice. In J. Rycroft-Malone & T. Bucknall (Eds.), *Models and frameworks for implementing evidence-based practice: Linking evidence to action* (pp. 137–146). Hoboken, NJ: Wiley-Blackwell.

Tomajan, K. (2012). Advocating for nurses and nursing. *Online Journal of Issues in Nursing, 17,* 4. Retrieved from http://ojin.nursingworld.org/MainMenuCategories/ANAMarketplace/ANAPeriodicals/OJIN/TableofContents/Vol-17-2012/No1-Jan-2012/Advocating-for-Nurses.html

Tomasik, J., & Fleming, C. (2015). *Lessons from the field: Promising interprofessional collaborative practices.* Retrieved from https://www.rwjf.org/en/library/research/2015/03/lessons-from-the-field.html

Toulmin, S.E. (1972). *Human understanding.* Princeton, NJ: Princeton University Press.

Underhill, M., Roper, K., Siefert, M.L., Boucher, J., & Berry, D. (2015). Evidence-based practice beliefs and implementation before and after an initiative to promote evidence-based nursing in an ambulatory oncology setting. *Worldviews on Evidence-Based Nursing, 12,* 70–78. https://doi.org/10.1111/wvn.12080

U.S. Department of Health and Human Services. (2015, June 23). *Quick guide to health literacy.* Retrieved from https://health.gov/communication/literacy/quickguide/Quickguide.pdf

U.S. Department of Health and Human Services. (2017). Importance of good nutrition. Retrieved from https://www.hhs.gov/fitness/eat-healthy/importance-of-good-nutrition/index.html

U.S. Food and Drug Administration. (2019, April 18). Information sheet: Institutional review boards frequently asked questions: Guidance for institutional review boards and clinical investigators. Retrieved from https://www.fda.gov/RegulatoryInformation/Guidances/ucm126420.htm#IRBMember

Vaartio, H., Leino-Kilpi, H., Salanterä, S., & Suominen, T. (2006). Nursing advocacy: How is it defined by patients and nurses, what does it involve and how is it experienced? *Scandinavian Journal of Caring Sciences, 20,* 282–292. https://doi.org/10.1111/j.1471-6712.2006.00406.x

Vaartio, H., Leino-Kilpi, H., Suominen, T., & Puukka, P. (2009). Nursing advocacy in procedural pain care. *Nursing Ethics, 16,* 340–362. https://doi.org/10.1177/0969733009097992

Vaartio-Rajalin, H., & Leino-Kilpi, H. (2011). Nurses as patient advocates in oncology care: Activities based on literature. *Clinical Journal of Oncology Nursing, 15,* 526–532. https://doi.org/10.1188/11.cjon.526-532

VanderWeele, T.J. (2018). Is forgiveness a public health issue? *American Journal of Public Health, 108,* 189–190. https://doi.org/10.2105/ajph.2017.304210

Wade, N.G., Hoyt, W.T., Kidwell, J.E.M., & Worthington, E.L., Jr. (2014). Efficacy of psychotherapeutic interventions to promote forgiveness: A meta-analysis. *Journal of Consulting and Clinical Psychology, 82,* 154–170. https://doi.org/10.1037/a0035268

World Health Organization. (1998). *The role of the pharmacist in self-care and self-medication.* Retrieved from http://apps.who.int/medicinedocs/pdf/whozip32e/whozip32e.pdf

World Health Organization. (2009). *Self-care in the context of primary health care.* Retrieved from http://apps.who.int/iris/bitstream/10665/206352/1/B4301.pdf

Index

The letter f after a page number indicates that relevant content appears in a figure; the letter t, in a table.

diarrhea with, 215–216
with GVHD, 165, 187t–188t
late, 316–321
neurologic, 289–290
oral, 204
pre-engraftment, 186
prevention of, 253
pulmonary, 249, 252–253
transmitted in blood products, 198
Bacteroides fragilis infection, 216
Baltimore Criteria, for diagnosing HSOS, 223, 225f
basiliximab, 158
basophils, 5, 186
B-cell aplasia, 364
BEAM conditioning regimen, 113, 213
BELINDA trial, 351
Belmont Report, 381–382
beneficence, principle of, 337–339, 337f
benefit-burden principle, 337f, 338
benzodiazepine, 362
"Berlin patient," 53
beta-thalassemia (β-thalassemia), 44
Be The Match program, 14, 17, 28–30, 29f, 101
biafungin, for pulmonary aspergillosis, 254
Billingham, Rupert E., 133
bioethical principles, 337, 337f
biologic agents
cardiotoxicity of, 267f
as conditioning regimen, 118
pulmonary toxicity of, 257
biomarkers
of kidney injury, 235
to predict GVHD, 141, 148
biosimilars, 91, 191
BK polyomavirus, 238–240
bladder irrigation, 240
Blood and Marrow Transplant Clinical Trials Network (BMT CTN), 27–28, 29f, 383
blood and marrow transplant certified nurse (BMTCN®), 73, 75, 371
B lymphocytes, 4t, 7, 186, 349
BMT data manager, 71
board-certified oncology pharmacists (BCOPs), 70
Board of Oncology Social Work Certification, 70
bone marrow
harvest of, 85–89
reconstitution of, 9
as stem cell source, 16
Bone Marrow and Cord Blood Donation and Transplantation, 29f

bone marrow microenvironment, 1–3
bone marrow stroma, 1
bone marrow transplantation (BMT), 13–14, 85
bone mineral density (BMD), loss of, 325
bortezomib
as conditioning regimen, 113
HBV reactivation from, 230
peripheral neuropathy from, 295
bottled water, safety of, 211
brain abscess, 289
breakthrough nausea and vomiting, 211. See also nausea/vomiting
bronchiolitis obliterans, 146–147, 164, 255, 258, 260, 261t, 328
bronchiolitis obliterans organizing pneumonia. See cryptogenic organizing pneumonia
bronchoalveolar lavage (BAL), for pulmonary diagnosis, 248
bronchodilators, 260
bronchoscopy, 248
Bu/Cy regimen, 112–113
Bu/Flu regimen, 112
BuMelTT conditioning regimen, 113
bupivacaine, for bone marrow harvest pain, 89
burnout, 371–372
busulfan
cardiotoxicity of, 267
as conditioning regimen, 112–113
hepatotoxicity of, 221
neurotoxicity of, 284, 285t
pulmonary toxicity of, 256
side effects of, 115t–116t

C

cadherins, 3
calcineurin inhibitor-induced pain syndrome, 292
calcineurin inhibitors, neurotoxicity of, 292
Canadian Cancer Trials Group (CCTG), 27t
Candida infection, 164, 186, 187t, 253, 268, 321
carboplatin
as conditioning regimen, 113
side effects of, 115t–116t
cardiac complications, 115t, 247, 261–266
from chemotherapy, 115t, 266–267, 267f
nursing management of, 271

from radiation therapy, 267–268
in survivorship, 324
cardiac function tests, 267
cardiac tamponade, 269–270
cardiomyopathy, 269
care continuum, in HSCT program, 64–67, 66f
care contracts, 340
caregiver support, 76–77, 329–330. See also patient/family education
carmustine
as conditioning regimen, 113
neurotoxicity of, 286
pulmonary toxicity of, 257
side effects of, 115t–116t
CAR T-cells
infusion of, 356
manufacture of, 350, 355
mechanism of action, 350–351, 352f
CAR T-cell therapy. See chimeric antigen receptor T-cell therapy
CARTOX grading scales, 357, 358t–359t, 361, 362f
carvedilol, 267
cataracts, 116t, 327
cathepsin G, 4
catheters
for apheresis, 96
care of, 96, 99
complications with, 96, 97t
for infusion, 120
occlusion of, 99
CBV conditioning regimen, 113
CD34 marker, 2, 99, 191
cell elimination, in gene therapy, 43
Cell Therapy Transplant Canada, 29f
cellular adhesion molecules (CAMs), 1, 3–4
Center for International Blood and Marrow Transplant Research (CIBMTR), 27–28, 29f, 31, 71, 168
Central Institutional Review Board (CIRB), 29f
central memory cells (TCMs), 6, 6t
cerebellar atrophy, 285
cerebrovascular disease, 290
certification, for nurse practitioners, 73
Certified Nurse Educator (CNE®) certification, 73
chaplaincy services, 70–71
checkpoint inhibitors, 349
chemokine antagonists, 4, 92–93
chemokines, 1, 4, 136
chemoreceptor trigger zone (CTZ), 212

chemotherapy agents
cardiotoxicity of, 266–267, 267f
as conditioning regimen, 111–113, 114t
diarrhea with, 214–215
kidney injury from, 236–237, 237f
nausea/vomiting with, 212
neurocognitive effects from, 326t
neurotoxicity of, 116t, 284–286, 285t, 295
nursing management of, 118
pulmonary toxicity of, 255–257, 256f, 262f
toxicities of, 113, 115t–116t
chemotherapy-induced nausea and vomiting (CINV), 211. See also nausea/vomiting
chest x-ray, for pulmonary diagnosis, 248, 265, 270
children
critical care for, 65
diarrhea in, 215
education issues for, 20
endocrine complications in, 323–324
ethical issues affecting, 340–341
HSOS in, 223–224
kidney injury in, 235, 237
long-term follow-up foe, 316
musculoskeletal effects in, 325
neurocognitive effects in, 325–327
oral complications in, 207t, 327
second HSCTs for, 304
stem cell collection from, 102
subsequent malignancies in, 306, 308–309
Children's Oncology Group (COG), 27t, 316
chimeric antigen receptor T cell-related encephalopathy syndrome (CRES), 360
chimeric antigen receptor (CAR) T-cell therapy, 44, 349. See also CAR T cells
building program for, 364–366
clinical trials on, 352–354
coordination of care in, 365
costs/insurance coverage of, 365–366
FDA approval of, 354–355
late effects of, 356
neurologic complications with, 283, 291–292, 292t
program development for, 63–64
steps of, 355–356

toxicities of, 119–120, 120t, 237, 286

donor evaluation, 19, 85, 86f

donor lymphocyte infusions (DLIs), 133, 174, 260, 303–304, 304f

donor registries, 14

donor-versus-HIV effect, 53

do-not-resuscitate (DNR) orders, 341–345, 342t

dopamine, 212

duloxetine, 295

dysgeusia, 209

E

early discharge models, of HSCT care, 65–66

early menopause, 323–324

echinocandins, for fungal infection, 321

echocardiogram, 270

ECOG-ACRIN Cancer Research Group, 27t

effector memory cells (TEMs), 6, 6t

efferent lymph vessels, 7

elastase, 4

electrolyte imbalances, 115t, 122–124

ELIANA study, 353–354, 364

encephalitis, 287–288

encephalopathy, 284, 290, 360–364, 362f

endocarditis, 268

endocrine complications, 323–324

endocytosis, 43

end-of-life, ethical issues in, 341–345, 342t, 343f–344f

endothelial cells, 2

engraftment phase, 9, 128–130, 190–191. See also delayed engraftment

engraftment syndrome, 129

entecavir, for hepatitis, 231

enteral nutrition, 210

Enterobacter infection, 204

Enterococcus infection, 186, 249

enterocolitis, 215

eosinophilic pulmonary syndrome (EPS), 258–259

eosinophils, 5, 186

epoetin alfa, for stem cell mobilization, 92

Epstein-Barr virus (EBV), 187t, 189, 250–251

erythema, 115t

erythematous maculopapular skin rash, 137–138, 139f

erythrocytes, 4t

Escherichia coli infection, 186, 187t, 204

etanercept, 158, 259

ethical issues

related to HSC donation/donors, 102–103, 341

related to patient/donor selection, 338t

ethical principles, 337, 337f

ethics, professional standards of, 337, 369

ethics consults, 345

etoposide

as conditioning regimen, 113

pulmonary toxicity of, 257

side effects of, 115t–116t

European League Against Rheumatism (EULAR), 52

European Organisation for Research and Treatment of Cancer (EORTC), 29f

European Society for Blood and Marrow Transplantation (EBMT), 29f, 32, 52

HSOS diagnostic criteria, 223, 225f

euthanasia, 342

evidence-based practice (EBT), 32, 379–381, 380f, 381t

Ewart sign, 270

experimental treatments, 338–340

expressive aphasia, 361

extracorporeal photopheresis (ECP), for chronic GVHD, 160, 164

extramedullary hematopoiesis, 1

exudative/elicited macrophages, 5

ex vivo expansion, of stem cell products, 105

F

FACT-JACIE International Standards for Hematopoietic Cellular Therapy, 67–68, 382–383

fear of cancer recurrence/progression (FCR), 305, 310. See also subsequent malignancies

feasibility analysis, for HSCT program, 63, 64f

Fenwal apheresis device, 98

fertility issues, 116t, 323–324

fever, 115t, 125, 127

fibrin degradation products (FDPs), 123

fibrin formation, 123

fibroblasts, 2

filgrastim

for HSC mobilization, 16, 90–92, 100

neutropenia decreased by, 191

financial analysis, for HSCT program, 63–64

fine-needle aspiration biopsy, for pulmonary diagnosis, 248–249

5-HT$_3$, and nausea/vomiting, 212–213

fluconazole, 127, 188, 254

fludarabine

as conditioning regimen, 112–113, 118

HBV reactivation from, 230–231

neurotoxicity of, 284–285

side effects of, 115t–116t

stem cell mobilization failure from, 93

subsequent cancer risk from, 308

fluid-attenuated inversion recovery (FLAIR) hyperintensity, 287

fluoroquinolone, for bacterial infections, 186

fluticasone, 260

follow-up care, 67–68, 308–310, 310f, 315–316, 317t–320t

food safety, 209–210, 210t, 211f

Food Safety for People With Cancer (FDA), 210

fosaprepitant, 213–214

foscarnet, 252, 287–288, 322

fractionated TBI, 113–114, 117

fragment antigen-binding (Fab) region, of antibodies, 7

Fresenius Kabi apheresis device, 98

fungal infections, 127, 186–189, 187t–188t

late, 321

neurological, 288–289

oral, 204

pulmonary, 249, 253–255

furosemide, for hyponatremia, 124

Fusarium infection, 188

Fusobacterium infection, 204

The Future of Nursing: Leading Change, Advancing Health, 377

G

gabapentin, 295

ganciclovir, 252, 287–288, 321

gastrointestinal effects

of acute GVHD, 138–140, 139f

of chronic GVHD, 143–144, 149t

nutritional management of, 166, 167t

gastrointestinal side effects, of conditioning regimens, 115t, 117

gene addition, 42

gene connection, 42

gene gun, 43

gene silencing, 42

gene therapy, 42–44

genetic basis, of HSCT, 8

genitourinary effects, of chronic GVHD, 150t

genitourinary side effects, of conditioning regimens, 115t

GI mucositis, 203. See also mucositis

Glucksberg staging/grading criteria, for acute GVHD, 140, 141t

graft engineering, 173

graft failure, 199

graft-versus-host disease (GVHD), 111, 133–134

acute *vs.* chronic, 133, 258f (See also acute GVHD; chronic GVHD)

cardiac effects of, 270–271

care coordination/monitoring for, 168–171, 169f–172f

infection with, 165–166

interprofessional care of, 166–168

neurologic effects of, 295

outcomes evaluation for, 171, 173t

prevention of, 133, 148–161, 151t

pulmonary effects of, 258–259

supportive/rehabilitative care, 164–165

graft-versus-leukemia effect, 111–112

graft-versus-tumor effect, 15, 174–175, 303, 350

gram-negative bacterial infections, 186, 187t–188t, 204, 252

gram-positive bacterial infections, 186, 187t–188t, 204, 252

granisetron, 213

granulocyte–colony-stimulating factor (G-CSF), 5, 16, 90–92

granulocyte macrophage–colony-stimulating factor (GM-CSF), 5, 16, 90–92

granulocyte-monocyte progenitor, 2, 4t

granulocyte recovery, 129–130

granulocytes, 4t, 5, 186

growth factors, 3, 16

side effects of, 91

grading of, 361, 362f–363f
management of, 361–362
in survivorship, 325–327
neurology bundle, for nursing management, 362–363
neuropathy, 147
neurotransmitters, affecting nausea/vomiting, 212
neutropenia, 185–186, 185t
after CAR T-cell therapy, 364
post-engraftment, 187t–188t, 191–192
pre-engraftment, 186–190, 187t
neutropenic enterocolitis, 215
neutrophil engraftment, 190–191
neutrophils, 5, 186
nivolumab, 349
NK-1 inhibitors, 212–213
non-Hodgkin lymphoma, 301, 302t, 349
nonmaleficence, principle of, 337–339, 337f
nonmalignant diseases, treated with HSCT, 44–53
nonmyeloablative regimens, 15, 18, 111–112, 118, 191, 308
nonvector method, of gene therapy, 43
NRG Oncology, 27t
nucleus tractus solitarius (NTS) neutrons, 212
nurse educators, 73
nurse leadership roles, in HSCT program, 72–74
Nurse Licensure Compact, 371
nurse navigators, 73–74
nurse practice acts, 369
nursing education, 370–371
nursing profession
advocating for, 373
defined, 369, 369f
standards of, 370, 370t
Nursing Professional Development Certification, 73
nursing research, 30–32, 33t–42t, 379–383, 381t, 382f–383f
nutritional support, enteral vs. parenteral, 210
nutrition management, 69, 209–211, 210t, 211f
with GVHD, 149t, 166, 167t
with oral mucositis, 208
nutrition plan, 69

O

OBERON trial, 351
obinutuzumab, HBV reactivation from, 230
obstructive lung disease, 146–147

occupational therapy, 71
octreotide, for chronic GVHD, 159–160
ocular complications, 145–146, 149t, 164, 327
ondansetron, 213
olanzapine, 214
older patients, 339, 341
OncoLink, 29f
oncology nurse navigators (ONNs), 73–74
Oncology Nursing Certification Corporation, 73, 75, 371
Oncology Nursing Society (ONS)
BMTSCT SIG, 31
chemotherapy guidelines, 118
clinical nurse specialist core competencies, 73
communities, 77
journal club toolkit, 371
leadership framework, 378–379, 378f
mucositis guidelines, 205–207
nurse practitioner core competencies, 73
Putting Evidence Into Practice (PEP) resources, 32
research priorities of, 382
Safe Handling of Hazardous Drugs, 118
Scope and Standards of Practice, 337
oncology social work, 70
oncolytic viral therapies, 349
open lung biopsy, 248–249
opioid therapy, 208
opportunistic infections. *See* infection
oral complications
of chronic GVHD, 146, 146f, 149t, 164
late, 327–328
oral cryotherapy, 205
oral hygiene, 205–207, 328
oral mucositis, 203
assessment of, 204, 205t
prevention/management of, 204–208, 206f, 207t
risk factors for, 204, 204f
oral pain, 146, 208
order for collection, 85, 87f–88f
organs, of immune system, 7–9
orientation program, for transplant nurses, 74, 74f
Osoba Nausea and Vomiting Module, 212
osteoblasts, 2
osteoclasts, 2, 5
osteoporosis/osteopenia, 325
ototoxicity, 116t
outcomes
patient expectations of, 340, 340t
reporting of, 79

outpatient care, for HSCT patients, 65–66, 66f
ovarian failure, 323–324

P

palifermin, for mucositis management, 207
parainfluenza, 127, 188t, 189, 249–250, 322
parenteral nutrition, 210
parotitis, 116t, 121
patient-centered outcomes research (PCOR) agenda, 28–30
Patient-Centered Outcomes Research Institute, 338
patient evaluation, before HSCT, 18–19, 19f
patient/family education, on HSCT, 19–20, 76–77, 118, 130
Patient Protection and Affordable Care Act (2010), 338
patient self-advocacy, 372–373, 373f
Patient Self-Determination Act (1990), 341
Patients for Affordable Drugs, 338
patient surrogates, 339
Pediatric Blood and Marrow Transplant Consortium (PBMTC), 29f
pediatric patients
critical care for, 65
diarrhea in, 215
education concerns for, 20
endocrine complications in, 323–324
ethical issues affecting, 340–341
HSOS in, 223–224
kidney injury in, 235, 237
long-term follow-up for, 316
musculoskeletal effects in, 325
neurocognitive effects in, 325–327
oral complications in, 207t, 327
second HSCTs for, 304
stem cell collection from, 102
subsequent malignancies in, 306, 308–309
pegylated filgrastim (pegfilgrastim), for stem cell mobilization, 92
pembrolizumab, 349
pentamidine, 255
pericardial effusion, 269–270
pericarditis, 268
periodontal infections, 208
peripheral blood stem cells (PBSCs), 16

advantages of, 85, 129, 137
collection of, 89
peripheral neuropathy, 116t, 147, 294–295, 295t
perirectal skin assessment, 216
personal autonomy, 337f, 342
Pesaro classification system, for thalassemia major, 46–47
phagocytosis, 5
Pharmacy SIG, 69
phototherapy, for chronic GVHD, 151f, 160
physical therapy, 71
Physician Data Query (PDQ*), 29f
physician teams, for HSCT program, 68, 69f
Physician Workforce Group, 68
PICOT clinical question format, 380, 380f
PIXY321, for stem cell mobilization, 92
plain language guidelines, 375
plasma cells, 7
platelet count, during engraftment phase, 128
platelet refractoriness, 193
plerixafor, 4, 92–96
pleural effusion, 263
pleurodesis, 263
pleuroparenchymal fibroelastosis (PPFE), 265
Pneumococcus infection, 165, 188t, 248
Pneumocystis jirovecii infection, 165, 187t–188t, 190, 255, 321
pneumonia, 127, 251–252, 257
pneumonitis, 116t, 257–258
polyclonal antibodies, for chronic GVHD, 151f, 158–159
polyenes, for fungal infection, 321
polymerase chain reaction (PCR), 287
pomalidomide, for chronic GVHD, 159
pooled platelets, 194
posaconazole, 127, 188, 254, 289
positron-emission tomography (PET) scans, for pulmonary diagnosis, 248
posterior reversible encephalopathy syndrome (PRES), 290–291
post-transplant acute limbic encephalitis (PALE), 287
post-transplant lymphoproliferative disorder (PTLD), 306
prednisone, 163t, 230
preparative regimens. *See* conditioning regimens
pRIFLE criteria, for pediatric kidney injury, 235

primary immunodeficiency diseases, treated with HSCT, 44–46

profession
 defined, 369, 369f
 standards of, 370, 370t

professional development, 74–75, 74f

professional practice evaluation, 379, 379t

pro forma, for HSCT program, 63–64

progenitor cells, types of, 2

program development, 63–64

program director, for HSCT program, 68

progressive multifocal leukoencephalopathy (PML), 287–288, 290

proinflammatory cytokines, 134

protozoal infections, 249

Pseudomonas infection, 186, 187t, 191, 204, 252, 268

psychological issues, related to HSC donation, 102–103

psychological/psychiatric services, in HSCT program, 70

pulmonary aspergillosis, 253–254

pulmonary complications, 247
 from bacterial infections, 249, 252–253
 from chemotherapy, 255–257, 256f, 262f
 of chronic GVHD, 146–147, 149t, 164, 247, 258–259
 diagnosis of, 248–249
 late, 328
 nursing management of, 265–266
 from radiation therapy, 257–258
 typical onset of, 248f
 from viral infections, 247, 249–251, 322

pulmonary embolism, 262–263

pulmonary fibrosis, 116t, 146, 257

pulmonary function tests (PFTs), 256, 265

pulmonary sinusoidal obstruction syndrome, 264

pure red cell aplasia, 196

Putting Evidence Into Practice (PEP) resources (ONS), 32

Q

quality management, of HSCT program, 77, 78f

quality plan/committee, for HSCT program, 77–79

quinolone, for bacterial infections, 186

R

radiation fibrosis, 258

radiation pneumonitis, 257–258

radiation therapy. *See also* total body irradiation
 cardiotoxicity of, 267–268
 neurotoxicity of, 286
 pulmonary toxicity of, 257–258

radioimmunotherapy, as conditioning regimen, 113

random donor platelets, 194

rapamycin, 155t

rasburicase, for TLS prevention, 122

rash, 137–138, 139f

recombinant human erythropoietin, for stem cell mobilization, 92

recombinant human stem cell factor, for stem cell mobilization, 92

recombinant urate, for TLS prevention, 122

reconstitution, of bone marrow, post-HSCT, 9

red blood cell (RBC) transfusions, 197–198

red marrow, 1

reduced-intensity conditioning, 111–112, 137, 196, 308

refractory nausea and vomiting, 211. *See also* nausea/vomiting

registries, for donors, 14

regulation
 of HSCT program, 78–79
 of nursing profession, 369–371

regulatory T cells (Treg cells), 6, 6t, 136

rehabilitation services, 71

relapse, 329
 after allogeneic transplantation, 303–304
 after autologous transplantation, 301–303, 302t
 nursing management of, 305–306

RELP analysis, 199

remestemcel-L, 174

REMS program, to mitigate toxicities, 357

renal disease/renal failure, 122, 231–237, 328–329. *See also* acute kidney injury

reproductive side effects, of conditioning regimens, 116t, 323–324

reprogramming, in gene therapy, 42–43

resident macrophages, 5

resource utilization, in HSCT programs, 75–76

respiratory syncytial virus (RSV), 127, 187t–188t, 189, 249–250, 322

retching, defined, 211. *See also* nausea/vomiting

rhinovirus, 249–250

RIFLE criteria, for kidney injury, 235, 236f

"right to try" laws, 338

rituximab, 155t, 158, 164, 349
 HBV reactivation from, 230–231
 pulmonary toxicity of, 257

rotavirus, 187t

Rule of Nines, 140, 142f

S

salivary gland dysfunction, 146, 208–209

sanctity of life, principle of, 337f

sargramostim
 neutropenia decreased by, 191
 for stem cell mobilization, 90–92

SBAR communication technique, 375, 375f

Scedosporium infection, 188

scientific review committees (SRCs), for clinical trials, 23–24

scleroderma, 51–52

Scleroderma: Cyclophosphamide or Transplantation trial, 30f

sclerodermatous skin effects, 143

scope and standards, of nursing practice, 369

screening, for subsequent malignancies, 308–310, 310f, 317t–320t. *See also* survivorship care

SDF-1α chemokine, 4

Seattle Criteria, for diagnosing HSOS, 223, 225f

secondary malignancies, 116t. *See also* subsequent malignancies

seizures, 116t, 284, 285t, 362

selectins, 3

self-care, for nurses, 371–372, 372t

sepsis, 125t, 126–128, 126f

serotonin, 212

Serratia infection, 204

serum sickness, 118, 159

severe acute respiratory syndrome (SARS), 249

severe combined immunodeficiency (SCID), 43–46

short-term HSCs (ST-HSCs), 2

sickle cell disease (SCD)
 as filgrastim side effect, 91–92

treated with HSCT, 48–49

signaling domains, 350

single-chain variable fragment (ScFv), 350

single-donor platelets, 194

sinusoidal obstruction syndrome (SOS), 111, 115t, 117, 264. *See also* hepatic sinusoidal obstruction syndrome; pulmonary sinusoidal obstruction syndrome

sirolimus
 dosage of, 152, 156
 drug interactions with, 156–157, 157t
 for GVHD, 151

skin
 involvement in acute GVHD, 137–138, 139f
 involvement in chronic GVHD, 143, 143f–145f, 149t

SNP analysis, 199

spermatogenesis, affected by HSCT, 323

spiritual care, 70–71

spleen, 8

sputum samples, for pulmonary diagnosis, 248

stakeholder team, development of, 64

Staphylococcus infection, 186, 187t, 204, 216, 249, 252, 268

STAT study, 52

stem cell collection, 98–99
 allogeneic, 99–101
 facilities for, 72
 future directions in, 105–106
 order form for, 85, 87f–88f
 side effects from, 99–101, 100t
 from unrelated donors, 101

stem cell factor, for stem cell mobilization, 92

stem cell manipulation, 105

stem cell mobilization, 16, 90
 algorithm for, 94f–95f
 by chemotherapy, 90
 failure of, 93–96
 future directions in, 96
 by growth factors, 90–92

stem cell processing, 105

Stem Cell Therapeutic Outcomes Database (SCTOD), 71

stem cell transduction, 43–44

Stetler Model of Research Utilization, 381

stomatitis, 115t. *See also* oral mucositis

STR analysis, 199

Streptococcus infection, 186, 187t–188t, 191, 199, 204, 252, 268, 316–321

stromal cells, 2, 4

subsequent malignancies, after HSCT, 306–310, 307t, 309t, 329